BONE AND SOFT TISSUE TUMORS

A Multidisciplinary Review with Case Presentations

BONE AND SOFT TISSUE TUMORS

A Multidisciplinary Review with Case Presentations

THERESE J. BOCKLAGE, MD
Professor of Pathology
University of New Mexico School of Medicine Health Sciences Center
Director, University of New Mexico Human Tissue Repository
Albuquerque, New Mexico, USA

ROBERT H. QUINN, MD
Department Chair and Professor
Residency Program Director
John J. Hinchey MD and Kathryn Hinchey Chair in Orthopaedics
Department of Orthopaedic Surgery
University of Texas Health Science Center at San Antonio
San Antonio, Texas, USA

BERNDT P. SCHMIT, MD
Assistant Clinical Professor of Radiology
University of Pittsburgh, UPMC East
Radiology Department
Monroeville, Pennsylvania, USA

CLAIRE F. VERSCHRAEGEN, MD
Irwin H. Krakoff Professor of Medicine
Director, Hematology Division
Director, Fletcher Allen Health Care Cancer Service Line
Co-Director, Vermont Cancer Center
Burlington, Vermont, USA

JP medical publishers

London • Philadelphia • Panama City • New Delhi

Published by JP Medical Ltd, 83 Victoria Street, London, SW1H 0HW, UK
Tel: +44 (0)20 3170 8910 Fax: +44 (0)20 3008 6180
Email: info@jpmedpub.com Web: www.jpmedpub.com

ISBN: 978-1-907816-22-2

British Library Cataloguing in Publication Data
A catalogue record for this book is available from the British Library

Library of Congress Cataloging in Publication Data
A catalog record for this book is available from the Library of Congress

JP Medical Ltd is a subsidiary of Jaypee Brothers Medical Publishers (P) Ltd, New Delhi, India.

Publisher:	Geoff Greenwood
Development Editors:	Gavin Smith, Katie Pattullo
Design:	Designers Collective Ltd

Typeset, printed and bound in India.

Preface

Patients with a bone or soft tissue tumor require a highly efficient, multidisciplinary team of physicians for optimal care. These tumors are rarely encountered in routine practice and often require diagnosis and treatment at specialized centers. However, patients frequently present to practices and institutions that are not specialized centers. Unfortunately, the information sources available to the frontline providers working in these centers are limited and rarely available in a concise, accessible format. We hope this textbook will meet the needs of these providers, and also serve as a valuable resource for specialty clinicians.

We wrote this book with two main objectives; firstly, we wanted to provide, in one volume, a practical guide to the diagnosis of bone and soft tissue tumors and the management of patients with these conditions; secondly, we wanted to optimize learning by presenting the information in two formats. The first format comprises the introduction to each chapter which presents reference information efficiently and informatively, allowing rapid review of a specific category of tumors. The second format comprises the remainder of each chapter, where the tumors are presented in more depth using case presentations that enhance learning thanks to their problem-based approach. The cases are not hypothetical and derive from our clinical experience. They illustrate that not every patient follows the textbook description in terms of presentation, diagnostic features and outcome.

This book grew out of a partnership of equals: an orthopaedic surgeon, an oncologist, a musculoskeletal radiologist, two radiation oncologists and a pathologist. We all found that the whole was, indeed, greater than the sum of the parts: that frank, respectful team discussion about each patient resulted in improved care. In light of this, our text is grounded in clinical reality, comprehensive and genuinely multidisciplinary; experts from participating disciplines have contributed to all chapters.

Having experienced for ourselves the increasing complexity of caring for patients in terms of new imaging modalities, surgical approaches, drugs, protocols and classification schemes, we understand the deluge of information a postgraduate medical trainee faces. We hope this book helps to alleviate this, while also engaging and educating the reader.

Therese J. Bocklage
Robert H. Quinn
Berndt P. Schmit
Claire F. Verschraegen
March 2014

Contents

Acknowledgements

We wish to thank the contributing authors listed below for providing content as follows:

Angela Meisner, MPH: SEER epidemiology in all chapters.

Ben Liem, MD: Radiation oncology in chapters 7, 8, 12, 13, 14, 17, 18, 21, 22, 26, 27.

Thomas Schroeder, MD: Radiation oncology in chapters 4, 5, 6, 9, 11, 15, 16, 19, 24, 25.

Sagus Sampath, MD: Radiation oncology in chapters 10, 20, 23.

Thomas Williams, MD: Molecular genetics of bone and soft tissue tumors in chapter 1.

David Meredith, MD: UNM epidemiology data and bone and soft tissue statistics.

Samuel Reynolds, MD: UNM epidemiology data bone and soft tissue statistics.

Jennifer Pincus, MD: UNM epidemiology data bone and soft tissue statistics.

Aaron Pritchard, MD: UNM epidemiology data bone and soft tissue statistics.

Myra Zucker, PA: Gross pathology photographs.

We are deeply grateful to Teresa Quintana, our impeccably organized, efficient and dedicated administrative assistant who cheerfully and expertly performed multiple tasks for this project, and to Michael Grady, a specialist in optimizing images for publication who carefully improved the quality of every image in the text.

We thank Charles Key for his expertise and guidance with the SEER epidemiology portions and we appreciate the many hours of work Julia Kreger performed in sourcing radiology images and reviewing patient charts.

We thank Gavin Smith of JP Medical Publishers for his discerning editing and responsive, cordial communication.

TB, RQ, BS, CV

Dedications

To our families who patiently supported us:
My parents, Jeanne and Bill, and my sisters, Cam and Paula (Therese Bocklage)
Stephanie, Taryn, Hunter and Devin (Robert Quinn)
Julie, my wonderful wife; Lukas, Karina and Carsten, my precious children (Berndt Schmit)
Ram Murthy, my husband, and my children, Victor and Adeline for tolerating my long stay at the computer (Claire Verschraegen)
My beautiful daughter, Brooke, and my husband, Ben (Angela Meisner)
My wife, Ann and my daughter, Sophia (Ben Liem)
Piper, Electra, & Remington; and especially Sabrina (Thomas Schroeder)

To our trainees whose enthusiasm inspired us.

To our patients who continue to teach us.

WORLD HEALTH ORGANIZATION (WHO) 2013 CLASSIFICATION OF BONE TUMORS				
	Benign	**Intermediate (locally aggressive)**	**Intermediate (rarely metastasizing)**	**Malignant**
Chondrogenic tumors	1. Osteochondroma 2. Enchondrdoma 3. Periosteal chondroma 4. Osteochondromyxoma 5. Subungual exostosis 6. Bizarre parosteal osteochondromatous proliferation (BPOP) 7. Synovial chondromatosis	1. Chondromyxoid fibroma (CMF) 2. Atypical cartilaginous tumor/chondrosarcoma grade I	Chondroblastoma	1. Chondrosarcoma grade II, grade III 2. Dedifferentiated chondrosarcoma 3. Mesenchymal chondrosarcoma 4. Clear cell chondrosarcoma
Osteogenic tumors	1. Osteoma 2. Osteiod osteoma	1. Osteoblastoma	None	1. Low-grade central osteosarcoma 2. Conventional osteosarcoma including fibroblastic, chondroblastic, and osteoblastic types 3. Telangiectatic osteosarcoma 4. Small cell osteosarcoma 5. Secondary osteosarcoma 6. Parosteal osteosarcoma 7. Periosteal osteosarcoma 8. High-grade surface osteosarcoma
Fibrogenic tumors	None	1. Desmoplastic fibroma of bone	None	1. Fibrosarcoma of bone
Fibrohistiocytic tumors	1. Benign fibrous histiocytoma/non-ossifying fibroma	None	None	None
Hematopoietic neoplasms	None	None	None	1. Plasma cell myeloma 2. Solitary plasmacytoma of bone 3. Primary non-Hodgkin lymphoma of bone
Osteoclastic giant cell rich tumors	1. Giant cell lesion of the small bones	Giant cell tumor of bone	Giant cell tumor of bone	1. Malignancy in giant cell tumor of bone
Notochordal tumors	1. Benign notochordal tumor	None	None	1. Chordoma
Vascular tumors	1. Hemangioma	1. Epithelioid hemangioma	1. Epithelioid hemangioma	1. Epithelioid hemangioendothelioma (EHE) 2. Angiosarcoma
Myogenic tumors	1. Leiomyoma	None	None	1. Leiomyosarcoma
Lipogenic tumors	1. Lipoma	None	None	1. Liposarcoma
Tumors of undefined neoplastic nature	1. Simple bone cyst 2. Fibrous dysplasia 3. Osteofibrous dysplasia 4. Chondromesenchymal hamartoma 5. Rosai-Dorfman disease	1. Aneurysmal bone cyst 2. Langerhans cell histiocytosis, monostotic and polyostotic 3. Erdheim-Chester disease	None	None
Miscellaneous tumors	None	None	None	1. Ewing sarcoma 2. Adamantinoma 3. Undifferentiated high-grade pleomorphic sarcoma of bone
Rarely, other sarcomas of soft tissue, in addition to those listed in the WHO 2013 Classification of Bone Tumors, have been described as originating in bone (in scattered case reports).				

WORLD HEALTH ORGANIZATION (WHO) 2013 CLASSIFICATION OF SOFT TISSUE TUMORS				
	Benign	**Intermediate (locally aggressive)**	**Intermediate (rarely metastasizing)**	**Malignant**
Adipocytic tumors	1. Lipoma 2. Lipomatosis 3. Lipomatosis of nerve 4. Lipoblastoma/lipoblastomatosis 5. Angiolipoma 6. Myolipoma 7. Chondroid lipoma 8. Extra-renal angiomyolipoma 9. Extra-adrenal myelolipoma 10. Spindle cell/pleomorphic lipoma 11. Hibernoma	1. Atypical lipomatous tumor/well differentiated liposarcoma	None	1. Dedifferentiated liposarcoma 2. Myxoid liposarcoma 3. Pleomorphic liposarcoma 4. Liposarcoma, NOS
Fibroblastic/ myofibroblastic tumors	1. Nodular fasciitis 2. Proliferative fasciitis 3. Proliferative myositis 4. Ischemic fasciitis 5. Myositis ossificans 6. Fibro-osseous pseudotumor of digits 7. Elastofibroma 8. Fibrous hamartoma of infancy 9. Fibromatosis colli 10. Juvenile hyaline fibromatosis 11. Inclusion body fibromatosis 12. Fibroma of tendon sheath 13. Desmoplastic fibroblastoma 14. Mammary-type myofibroblastoma 15. Calcifying aponeurotic fibroma 16. Angiomyofibroblastoma 17. Cellular angiofibroma 18. Nuchal-type fibroma 19. Gardner fibroma 20. Calcifying fibrous tumor	1. Palmar/plantar fibromatosis 2. Desmoid-type fibromatosis 3. Lipofibromatosis 4. Giant cell fibroblastoma	1. Dermatofibrosarcoma protuberans (DFSP) including fibrosarcomatous and pigmented versions 2. Solitary fibrous tumor (SFT) 3. Inflammatory myofibroblastic tumor (IMFT) 4. Myxoinflammatory fibroblastic sarcoma (MIFS) including atypical variant 5. Infantile fibrosarcoma	1. Adult fibrosarcoma 2. Myxofibrosarcoma 3. Low-grade fibromyxoid sarcoma (LGFMS) 4. Sclerosing epithelioid fibrosarcoma (SEFS) 5. Malignant solitary fibrous tumor (malignant SFT)
So-called fibrohistiocytic tumors	1. Tenosynovial giant cell tumor comprising localized type and diffuse type (the latter also commonly called pigmented villonodular synovitis) 2. Deep benign fibrous histiocytoma	None	1. Plexiform fibrohistiocytic tumor 2. Giant cell tumor of soft tissues	1. Malignant variant of diffuse type of tenosynovial giant cell tumor
Smooth muscle tumors	1. Deep leiomyoma	None	None	2. Leiomyosarcoma (excluding skin)
Pericytic/ perivascular tumors	1. Glomus tumor and benign variants 2. Myopericytoma including myofibroma 3. Angioleiomyoma	1. Glomangiomatosis 2. Myofibromatosis	None	1. Malignant glomus tumor 2. Malignant myopericytoma
Skeletal muscle tumors	1. Rhabdomyoma including adult type, fetal type, genital type	None	None	1. Embryonal rhabdomyosarcoma (E-RMS) including anaplastic and botryoid cases 2. Alveolar rhabdomyosarcoma (A-RMS) including solid and anaplastic cases 3. Pleomorphic rhabdomyosarcoma (pleomorphic RMS) 4. Spindle cell/Sclerosing rhabdomyosarcoma (spindle cell/sclerosing RMS)

	Benign	Intermediate (locally aggressive)	Intermediate (rarely metastasizing)	Malignant
Vascular tumors	1. Hemangioma including synovial, venous, ateriovenous hemangioma/malformation 2. Intramuscular hemangioma 3. Epithelioid hemangioma 4. Angiomatosis 5. Lymphangioma	1. Kaposiform hemangioendothelioma (kaposiform HE)	1. Retiform hemangioendothelioma (retiform HE) 2. Papillary intralymphatic angioendothelioma 3. Composite hemangioendothelioma (composite HE) 4. Pseudomyogenic (epithelioid-sarcoma like) hemangioendothelioma (pseudomyogenic HE) 5. Kaposi sarcoma	1. Epithelioid hemangioendothelioma (EHE) 2. Angiosarcoma
Chondro-osseous tumors	1. Soft tissue chondroma	None	None	1. Extraskeletal mesenchymal chondrosarcoma 2. Extraskeletal osteosarcoma
Gastrointestinal stromal tumors	1. Benign gastrointestinal stromal tumor (benign GIST)	None	1. Gastrointestinal stromal tumor, uncertain malignant potential (GIST-UMP)	1. Gastrointestinal stromal tumor, malignant (GIST-Mal)
Nerve sheath tumors	1. Schwannoma (including variants) 2. Melanotic schwannoma 3. Neurofibroma (including variants such as plexiform neurofibroma) 4. Perineurioma 5. Granular cell tumor 6. Dermal nerve sheath myxoma 7. Solitary circumscribed neuroma 8. Ectopic meningioma 9. Nasal glial heterotopia 10. Benign Triton tumor 11. Hybrid nerve sheath tumors	None	None	1. Malignant peripheral nerve sheath tumor (MPNST) 2. Epithelioid malignant peripheral nerve sheath tumor (epithelioid MPNST) 3. Malignant Triton tumor 4. Malignant granular cell tumor 5. Ectomesenchymoma 6. Malignant perineurioma
Tumors of uncertain differentiation	1. Acral fibromyxoma 2. Intramuscular myxoma (including cellular variant) 3. Juxta-articular myxoma 4. Deep ('aggressive') angiomyxoma 5. Pleomorphic hyalinizing angiectatic tumor (PHAT) [may have borderline behavior] 6. Ectopic hamartomatous thymoma	1. Hemosiderotic fibrolipomatous tumor	1. Atypical fibroxanthoma (AFX) 2. Angiomatoid fibrous histiocytoma (AFH) 3. Ossifying fibromyxoid tumor (OFMT) 4. Mixed tumor, NOS 5. Myoepithelioma 6. Phosphaturic mesenchymal tumor 7. Perivascular epithelioid cell tumor (PEComa)	1. Synovial sarcoma (spindle cell, biphasic and NOS) 2. Epithelioid sarcoma 3. Alveolar soft part sarcoma (ASPS) 4. Clear cell sarcoma of soft tissue 5. Extraskeletal myxoid chondrosarcoma (ESMCS) 6. Extraskeletal Ewing sarcoma 7. Desmoplastic small round cell tumor (DSRCT) 8. Extra-renal rhabdoid tumor 9. Perivascular epithelioid cell tumor, malignant (malignant PEComa) 10. Intimal sarcoma 11. Ossifying fibromyxoid tumor, malignant (malignant OFMT-M) 12. Myoepithelial carcinoma 13. Phosphaturic mesenchymal tumor, malignant
Undifferentiated/ unclassified sarcomas	None	None	None	1. Undifferentiated spindle cell sarcoma 2. Undifferentiated pleomorphic sarcoma 3. Undifferentiated round cell sarcoma 4. Undifferentiated epithelioid sarcoma 5. Undifferentiated sarcoma, NOS

Chapter 1 Pathology overview of musculoskeletal tumors and principles of diagnosis

RATIONALE

Individuals learn the practice of medicine not only through lectures and laboratory sessions but also through daily experiential learning guided by senior practitioners. This form of apprenticeship learning defines this text, which combines succinct overviews of the tumors followed by actual patient cases.

Problem-based learning

The current term for such case-based learning is problem-based learning (PBL). This book parallels the PBL curriculum popular in many medical schools.

Problem-based learning not only recognizes but also capitalizes on the concept that human beings are storytellers and story listeners by nature. Consequently, students naturally absorb key medical elements of a personal story and may find learning passive sets of data both more difficult and less engaging. One complements the other, and this book presents both. The text is arranged in the flow in which patients are treated. The histories are trimmed to key facets.

Evidence-based data

Where feasible, the information provided in this text is evidence based. However, extensively verified facts are few in rare entities, and the realm of bone and soft tissue tumors is replete with such rarities. Thus, the approach to treating a patient with a rare tumor is one that is comparative, sometimes requiring a trial and error approach. However, with careful documentation of these patients' care along with data aggregation, even rare tumors become better characterized, advancing the field of musculoskeletal oncology.

Team approach

Close collaboration that bridges medical disciplines yields optimal care of a patient with a mesenchymal tumor. This is facilitated by regular review of patient cases in the setting of a working tumor board, including a surgical oncologist, medical oncologist, radiation oncologist, radiologist and pathologist. Students should always be welcome.

The treatment of a complex patient also relies on contributions from nurses, social workers, nutritionists, counselors, psychiatrists, laboratorians, pathologists' assistants, physical and occupational therapists and others, and this book acknowledges the dedicated attention of these medical professionals.

The value of exploring a disease course in a single patient

In many books on bone and soft tissue pathology, tumors often appear clear and easily identifiable as the images shown are the result of the cumulative experience of the author, who has distilled his or her knowledge to present 'perfect' examples of the tumor(s) in question.

The reality is that tumors do not always present so unambiguously. Each real case presented in this text outlines the patient's history, laboratory findings, disease progress, and outcomes. They are the actual findings in one patient, intended to illustrate in practical terms the real (and often not so clear-cut) presentation, diagnosis, treatment and outcome in an individual with a specific bone or soft tissue lesion.

PATHOLOGY TRIAGE OF BONE AND SOFT TISSUE TUMORS

Gross specimens

The role of the anatomic pathologist is to ensure the proper handling, processing, and diagnosis of the patient's specimen beginning with a fine needle aspiration biopsy, a needle core biopsy or incisional biopsy and commonly ending with a large, complex resection. Although occasionally undervalued, careful gross examination of soft tissue and bone tumors is critical to ensure subsequent accurate diagnosis, to assign the correct tumor grade and to record response to therapy.

Gross assessment of necrosis

Depending on the specific sarcoma type, the amount of pre-treatment necrosis influences grade and prognosis. Percent necrosis is estimated by careful gross review of complete cross sections of tumor. **Figure 1.1** is an example of a mixed viable and necrotic tumor.

Value of gross photos

Digital cameras have made photographing gross specimens more convenient. Moreover, some pathology software programs enable integration of photographs into the final report. Gross photos illustrate to the medical team features such as margin status and chemotherapy response. **Figures 1.2** through **1.6** compare the gross appearances of multiple tumors.

Tissue banking for research

Collecting fresh tumor (and paired normal tissue, when possible) for biobanking for future research investigations is worthwhile. A small amount (1 cm^3, for example) can be frozen and stored for years. At hospitals without sufficient freezer capacity, new solutions are available to store tissue at room temperature while adequately preserving RNA. This banking effort is essential for improving the diagnostic categorization of mesenchymal tumors, identifying biomarkers, and developing targeted therapy. Formalin-fixed, paraffin embedded blocks are also capable of being mined for more limited nucleic acid and protein information.

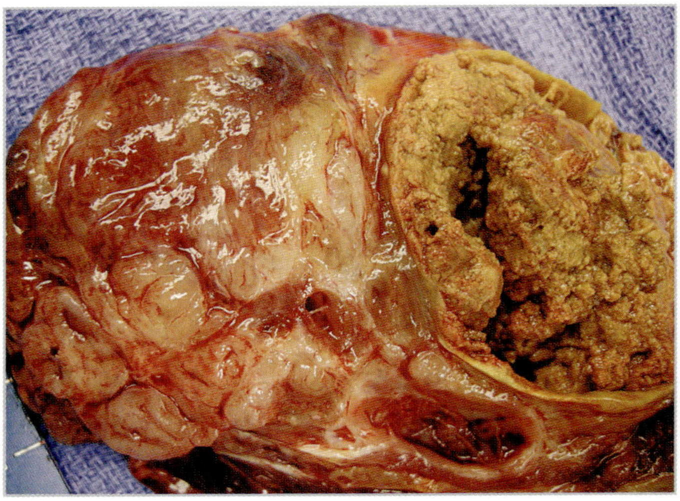

Figure 1.1 Extraskeletal myxoid chondrosarcoma, gross cut section. This tumor starkly contrasts viable myxoid gelatinous tumor (left) with an area of abrupt necrotic cavitated yellow friable tumor (right). The necrotic, partly cystic area may represent infarction after prior biopsy.

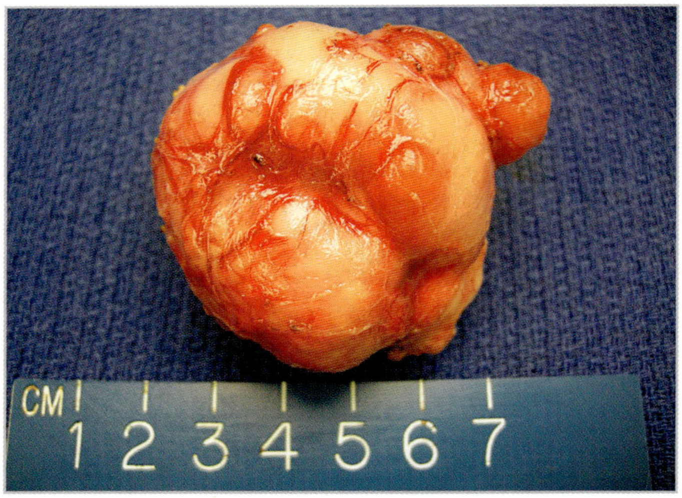

Figure 1.2 Lipoblastoma, external surface of tumor, gross photo. The external surface of many tumors exhibits a thin translucent membranous covering.

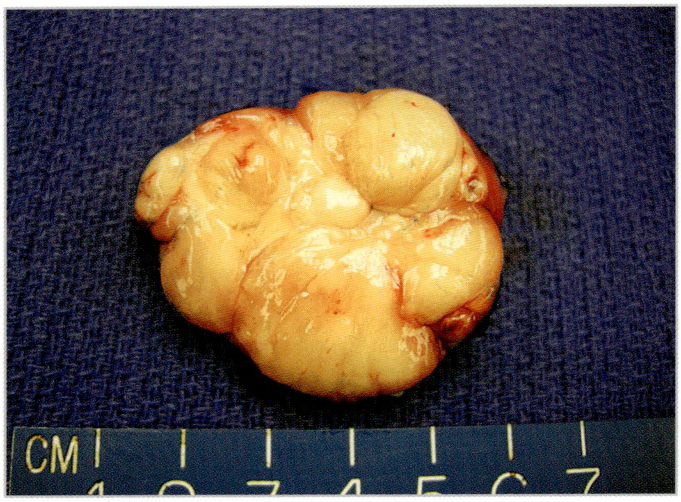

Figure 1.3 Lipoblastoma, cut surface, gross photo. On cross sections, a adipocytic tumor may resemble mature adipose tissue with a pale yellow soft, glistening cut surface. Subtle additional clues to the diagnosis may also be present. Lipoblastoma is typically lobulated on microscopic review, and the lobulation can be appreciable also grossly, as in this example.

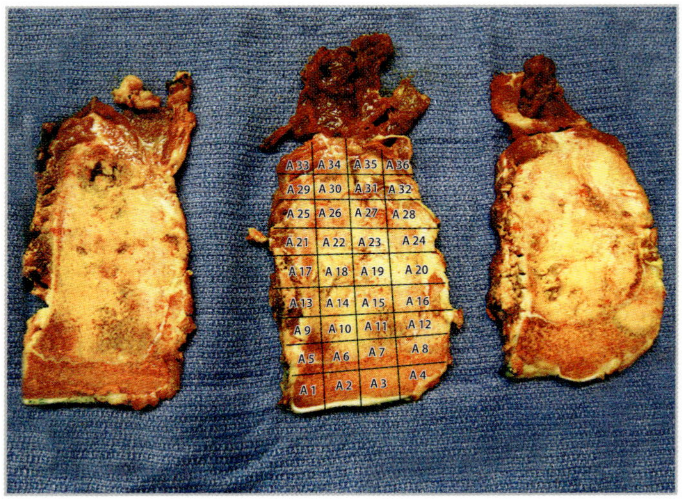

Figure 1.4 Osteosarcoma, gridding post chemotherapy. A band saw cuts thin sections of fresh tumor amenable to careful gridding to assess percent necrosis after neoadjuvant chemotherapy.

Ancillary studies to confirm the diagnosis

In addition to harvesting fresh tumor for banking, it may be advisable to conduct cytogenetic analysis, and this will require sending a small sterile sample to the cytogenetic laboratory for karyotyping. In some cases, it is also helpful to prepare touch preps of tumor on unfixed slides for potential fluorescent in situ hybridization (FISH) analysis. These slides can be stored at room temperature.

Very few tumors are subjected to electron microscopy (EM), and therefore tumor aliquots for EM are seldom prepared.

When feasible with bone tumors, it is advisable to submit a portion of tumor without decalcification in order to optimize antigenicity for potential IHC staining (molecular genetic analysis may also be compromised after decalcification). To avoid this harsh pretreatment, a small sample dissected free of bone and cartilage fragments is submitted to the histology department. With heavily calcified or ossified lesions, it may not be possible to obtain a tumor sample that does not require decalcification.

DIAGNOSING A LESION IN SOFT TISSUE OR BONE

John S. J. Brooks, American bone and soft tissue pathologist, suggests asking four questions when dealing with a possible mesenchymal tumor (Brooks, 2010 – questions are paraphrased):

1. Is the mass an actual neoplasm?

Some non-neoplastic lesions can mimic a neoplasm, and the most common of these are myofibroblastic proliferations such as nodular fasciitis and proliferative fasciitis. Other entities that may raise concern for a neoplasm comprise reactive entities such as a maturing

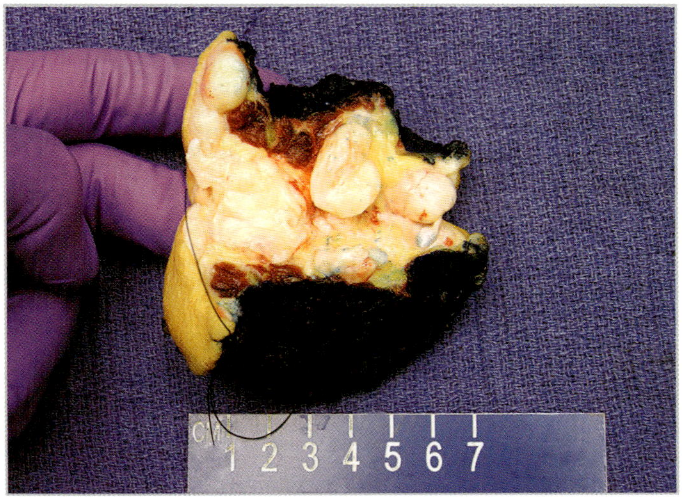

Figure 1.5 Epithelioid hemangioendothelioma, gross photo of cut section. Epithelioid hemangioendothelioma does not reveal its vascular nature on gross inspection. This is true of many intermediate and high grade blood vessel tumors. Notice the multiple discrete nodules, which can be seen in benign and malignant tumors.

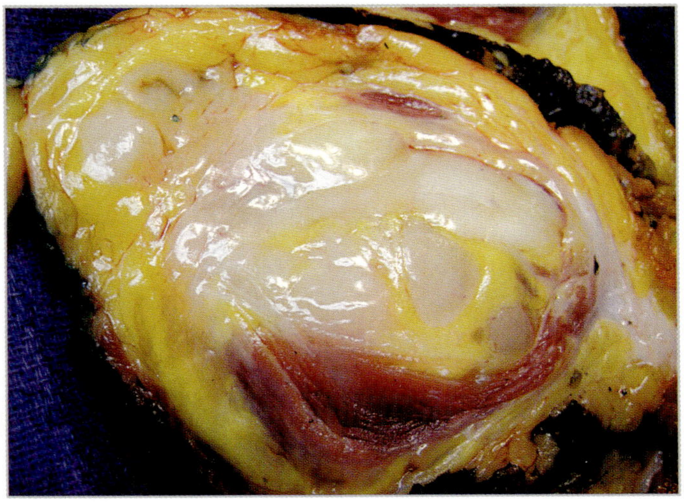

Figure 1.6 Malignant peripheral nerve sheath tumor, gross photo of cut section. This large, deep seated sarcoma demonstrates aggressive features with multiple, subfascial, coalescing, infiltrating tumor nodules.

fracture callus. To correctly answer whether the lesion is neoplastic, one must have a working knowledge of the histology of non-neoplastic mimics of mesenchymal neoplasms. In histologically ambiguous situations, one must rely upon the contributions of colleagues: clinicians and radiologists who can be counted upon for critical patient history and imaging information.

2. If it is a neoplasm, is it malignant?

Once a lesion is determined to be neoplastic, the next step is to ascertain whether it is benign or malignant. A pathologist begins with general histologic rules of malignancy and benignancy (see below).

3. If this is a malignant neoplasm, is it a sarcoma or could it represent a metastatic carcinoma, melanoma or lymphoma?

For example, not all fascicular spindle cell tumors are mesenchymal. If the lesion is deemed malignant, the origin of the tumor is the next question: primary mesenchymal versus metastatic non-mesenchymal tumor? For example, a spindle cell tumor of the head and neck in an older man is more likely sarcomatoid carcinoma (such as spindle cell squamous carcinoma) or melanoma than sarcoma. Clinical history of melanoma should never be summarily dismissed as irrelevant.

4. Is the diagnosis thoroughly defensible?

In other words, have the other entities in the differential been completely excluded? Painstaking effort should be exerted to be confidently conclusive especially in cases where treatment is dictated by and differs by diagnosis.

This final question is a critical query that is faced by many pathologists who may have limited experience with bone and soft tissue pathology due to the rarity of some of these lesions. If a pathologist cannot be completely confident of the specific diagnosis, the most prudent option is to consult with an acknowledged bone or soft tissue expert pathologist. This has two desirable consequences: optimal diagnosis for the patient and convergence of data pertaining to unusual tumors.

Rules of histology

Benign features of mesenchymal tumors

Table 1.1 lists some of the histologic features that are associated most commonly with benign behavior in mesenchymal tumors. Of course, there are exceptions to this list of features because some malignant tumors may look deceptively benign, while some benign tumors may appear high grade malignant.

Malignant features of mesenchymal tumors

Table 1.2 lists the histologic features of mesenchymal tumors that are commonly associated with malignant (aggressive local or metastatic) behavior. Just as for the benign histologic features listed in **Table 1.1**, the general histologic features of malignancy in **Table 1.2** are not 100% sensitive and specific. Both tables merely provide starting guidelines.

Immunohistochemistry does not supersede histology

The development of consistent, reliable immunohistochemistry (IHC) to detect cell antigens was revolutionary in surgical pathology and dramatically advanced pathology diagnostics. However, IHC cannot replace careful review of the standard histologic characteristics of a tumor. This is because nearly all antigens tested by IHC are not specific, and because quite a few tumors, typically those that are less differentiated, aberrantly express antigens that can obscure the diagnosis. In all instances, the IHC reactivity pattern should be examined in the context of the general overall histologic appearance of the tumor, clinical history and radiologic findings.

Today, thousands of antibodies are available for use in formalin fixed, paraffin embedded tissues. Judicious rather than opulent use of these antibodies is both less costly and less confusing. **Table 1.3** provides a broad overall delineation of the more common antibodies useful in bone and soft tissue tumors showing reactivity in the analogous normal tissue, benign lesions, and malignant tumors. **Table 1.4** lists tumors that have relatively more specific antibody signatures.

Table 1.1 Histologic features commonly associated with benign behavior in mesenchymal tumors

Feature	Example of low magnification	Example of high magnification
Hypocellularity	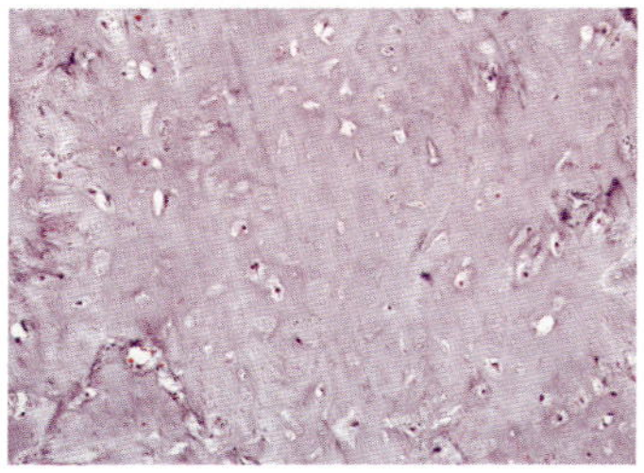	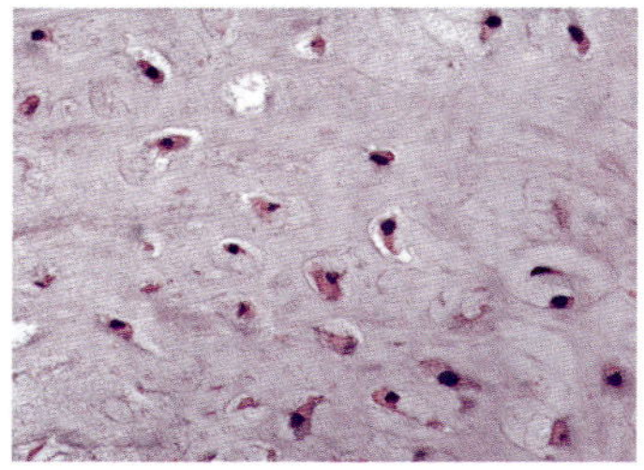
Pushing rather than invasive border	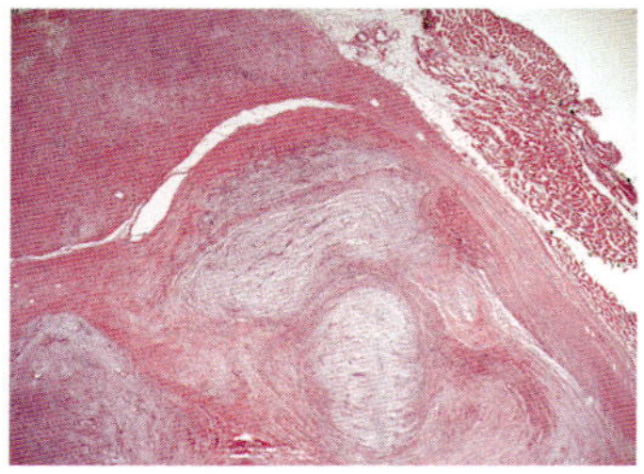	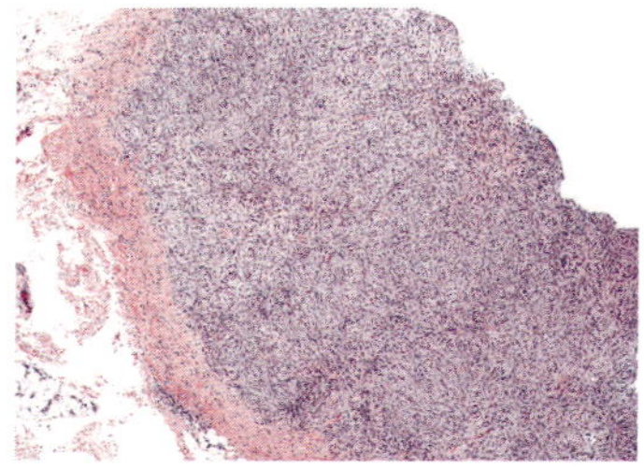
No necrosis	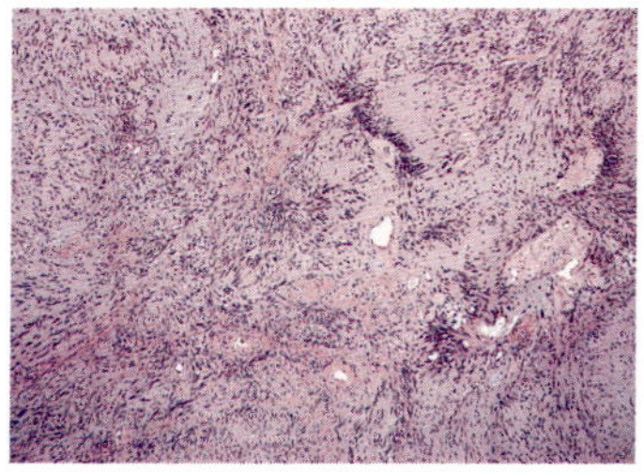	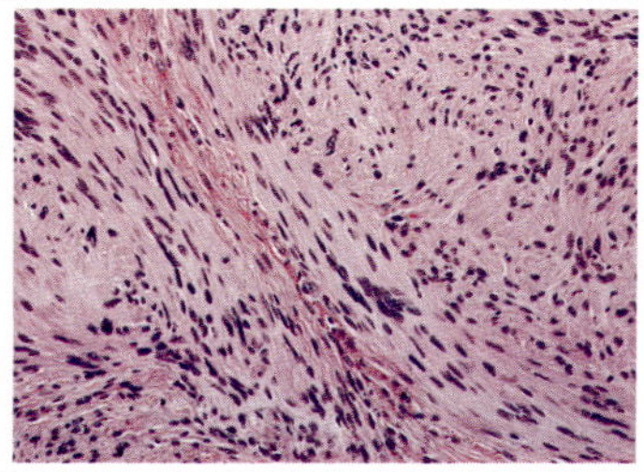
Few if any mitotic figures and no abnormal mitotic figures	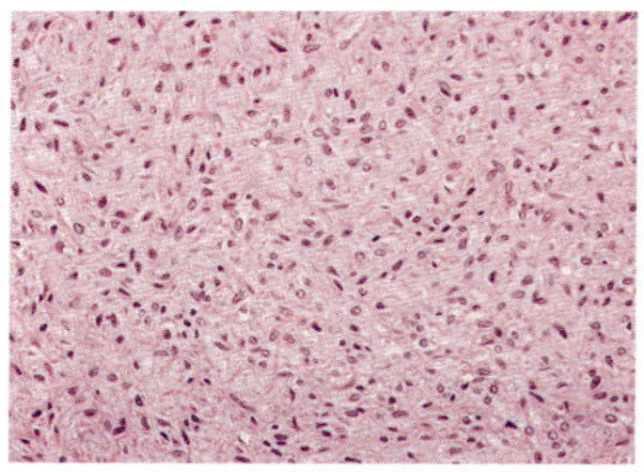	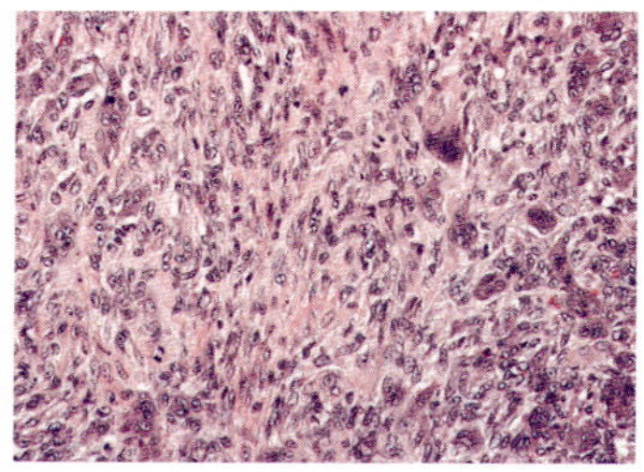
Pale uniform nuclei with fine chromatin	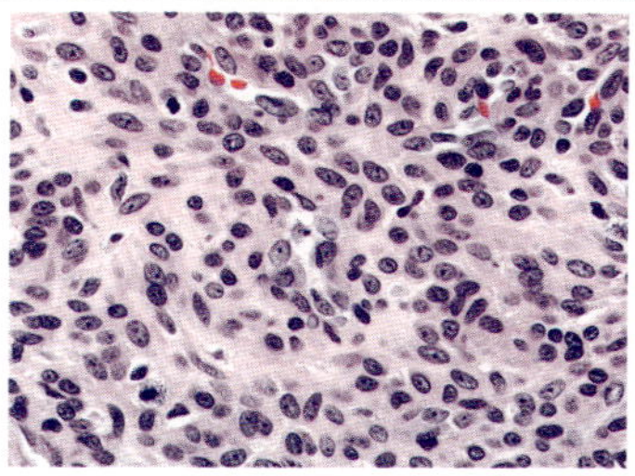	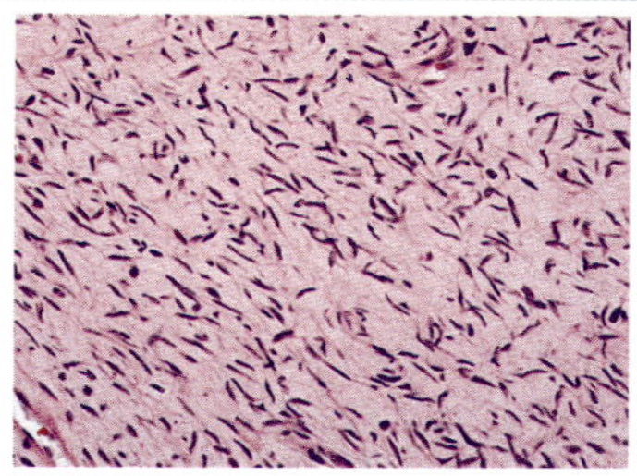

Figure 1.7 shows a prominently positive keratin IHC stain in high grade sarcoma. This aberrant epithelial keratin expression illustrates a misleading result, which is especially dangerous if examined in isolation of clinical and radiologic findings, histomorphology and other IHC results. **Table 1.5** lists common cell and architectural features found in bone and soft tissue tumors.

Additional figures of characteristic immunohistochemical staining patterns demonstrate that the intracellular location of reactivity can be critical in the diagnostic value of the antibody (**Figs 1.8** through **1.10**).

MOLECULAR GENETICS

Like other neoplasms, benign and malignant mesenchymal tumor cells may contain acquired genetic lesions that result in the activation of oncogenes and/or the inactivation of tumor suppressor genes. Soft tissue and bone tumors are characterized by the acquisition of a series of mutations as they develop. These mutations generally occur in the regulatory or coding regions of genes that are transcribed into mRNAs that are translated into proteins. The result is either an abnormally

Table 1.2 Histologic features commonly associated with malignant behavior in mesenchymal tumors

Feature	Example of low magnification	Example of high magnification
Hypercellularity	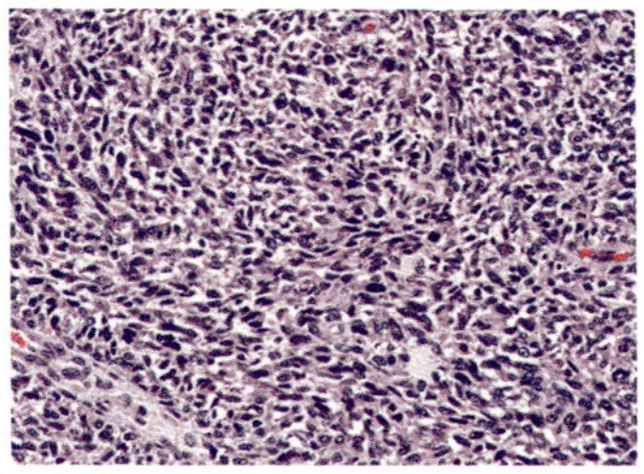	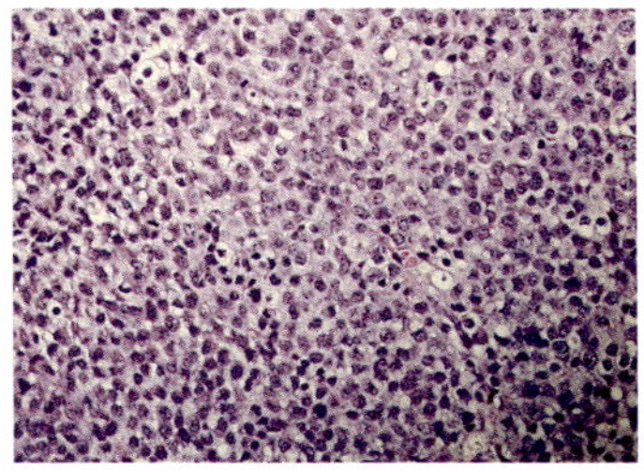
Invasive or permeative border	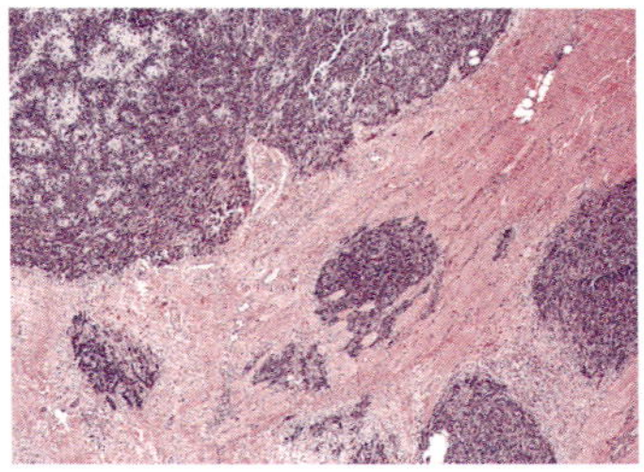	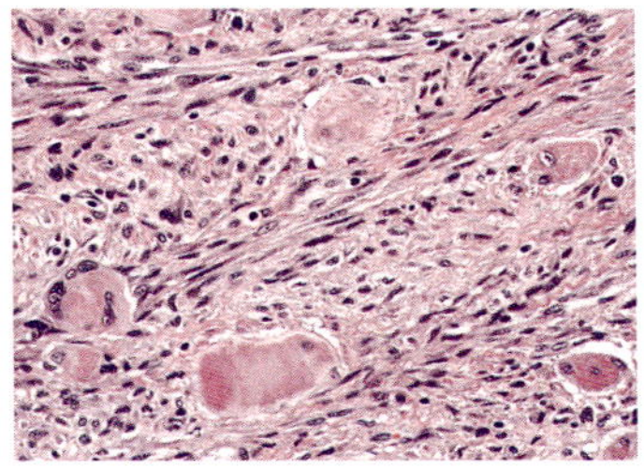
Necrosis	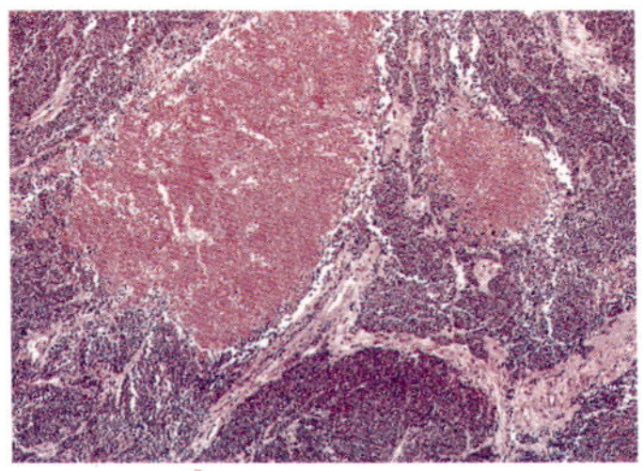	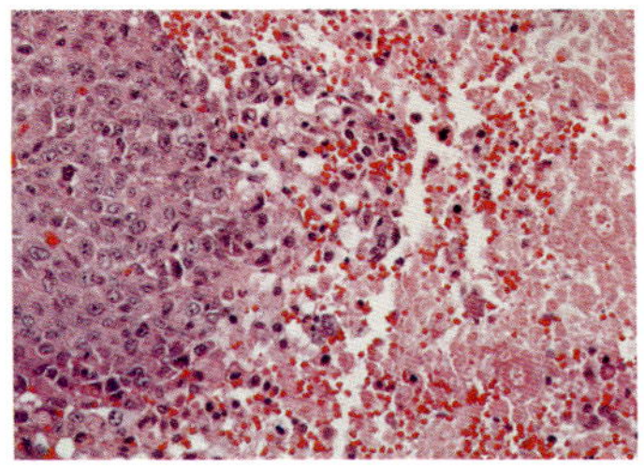
Nuclear pleomorphism	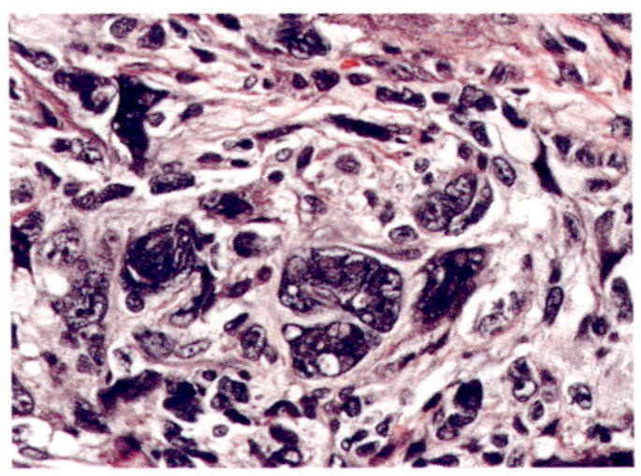	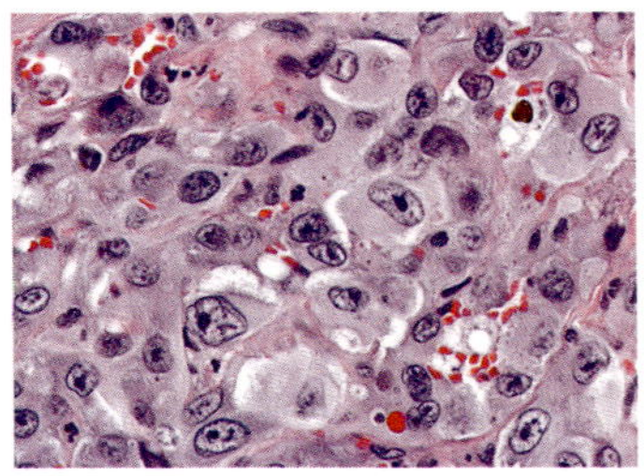
Primitive blastic (small blue round cell) look	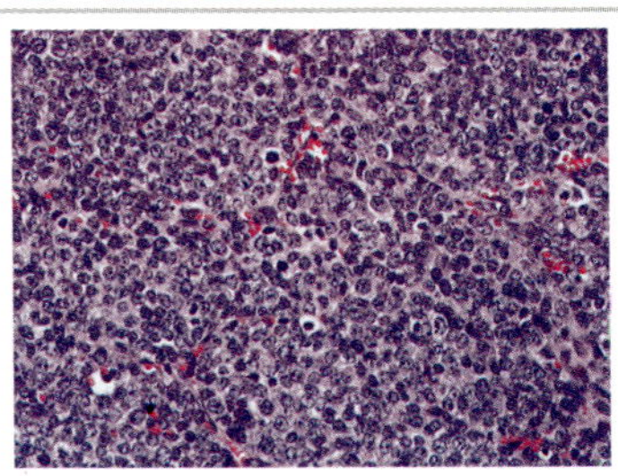	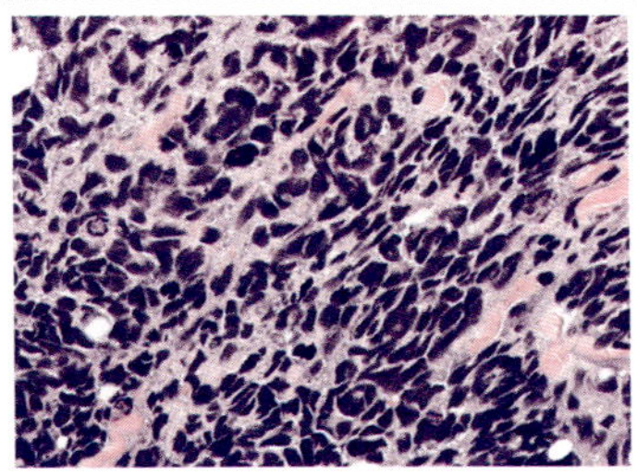
Nuclear hyperchromasia	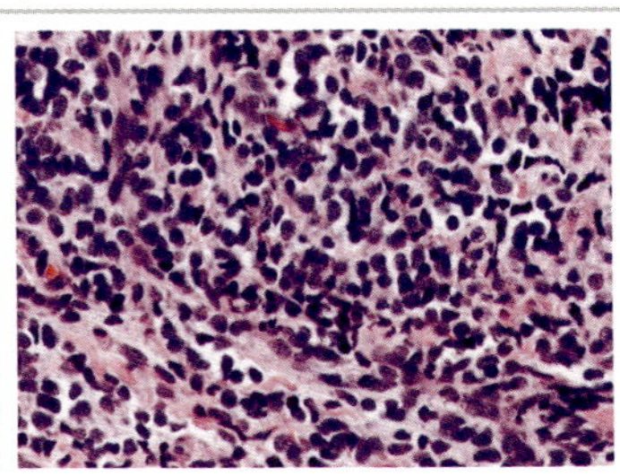	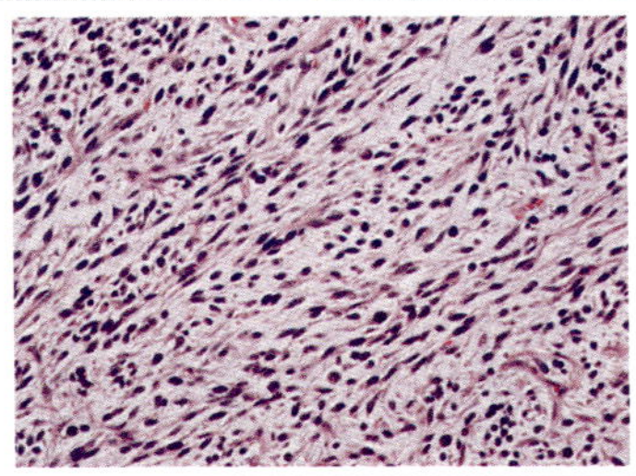

Table 1.2 Continued from page 5

Feature	Example at low magnification	Example at high magnification
Coarse and often irregularly distributed chromatin	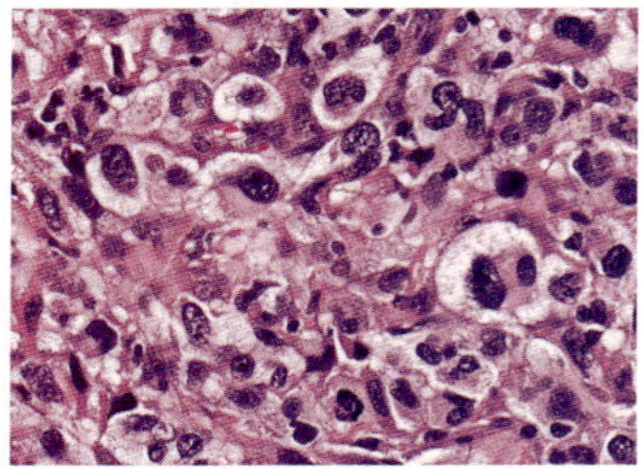	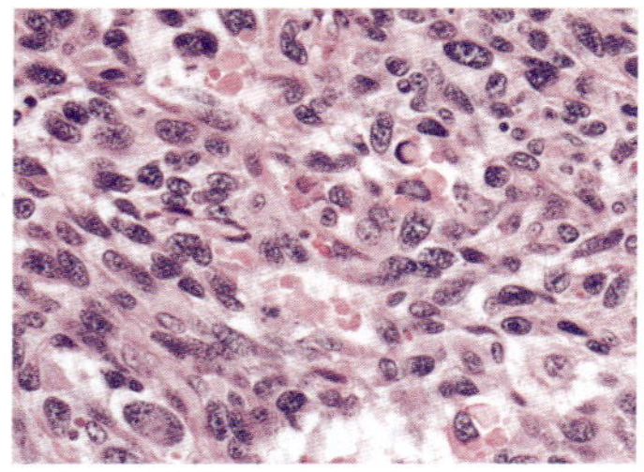
High mitotic rate	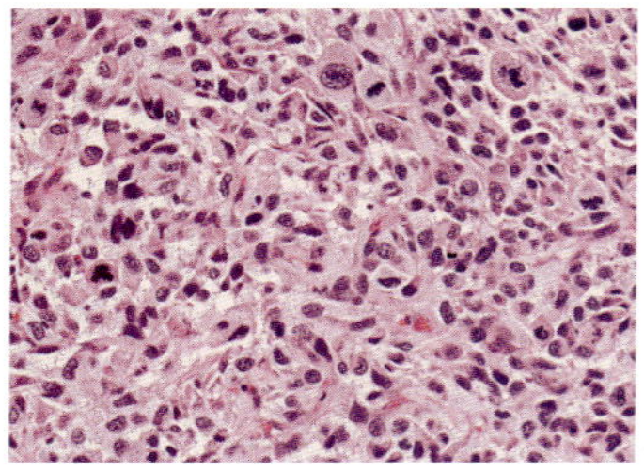	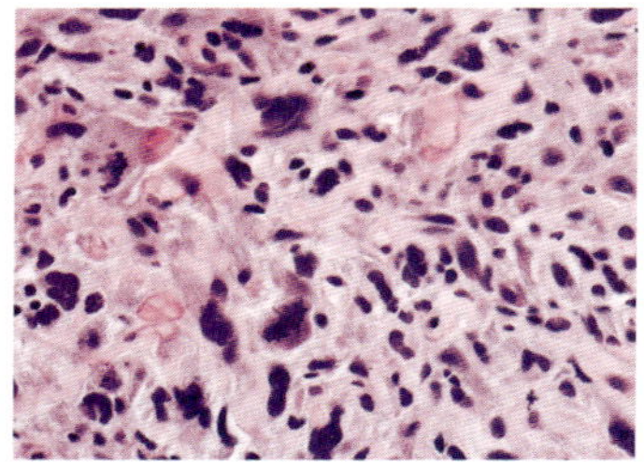
Atypical mitotic figures	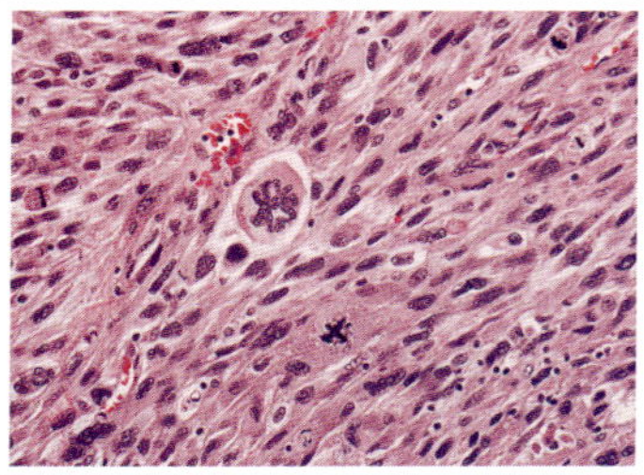	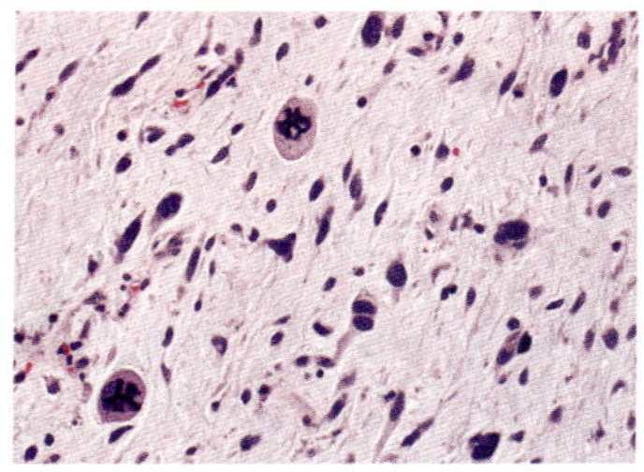

high or low concentration of the protein or a protein with aberrant or reduced function. Mutations may also cause the production of abnormal regulatory RNAs. Mutations that may be found in these lesions range from large scale chromosomal rearrangements, detectable by cytogenetic assays to single nucleotide 'point mutations' that must be identified by sensitive molecular diagnostic techniques.

Classic cytogenetic, FISH cytogenetic, and molecular diagnostic tests have several basic features in common. A cell or tissue sample from the patient is obtained. Target cellular DNA or RNA is either made readily accessible for DNA hybridization within the cells via enzymatic treatment, or the DNA or RNA is completely isolated and purified from the cells and re-suspended in water. The target DNA is then made single stranded by heating, disrupting the hydrogen bonds that join the complementary Gs and Cs and As and Ts (guanine, cytosine, adenine and thymine respectively). This makes the target DNA accessible to hybridization with a DNA probe specific for a chromosomal region, for a gene, or for a gene region. DNA probes may be synthetic or cloned DNA of known sequence and may range in size from 12 nucleotides to several hundred thousand nucleotides.

When cells are studied with cytogenetic techniques, a karyotype is prepared in which the autosomal pairs of metaphase chromosomes and sex chromosomes are arranged in order from largest to smallest for identification and inspection. Benign and malignant mesenchymal lesions may have normal appearing karyotypes, karyotypes with specific isolated translocations involving the rearrangement of two genes, or bizarre karyotypes with massive chromosomal duplications and deletions and the presence of multiple unidentifiable 'marker' chromosomes. Chromosomal abnormalities in mesenchymal lesions may result in the duplication, amplification, or deletion of chromosomes or chromosome regions and the genes contained therein. Alternatively, translocations occurring at specific breakpoints between two chromosomes may alter the regulation of expression of a critical gene or join portions of two genes together resulting in the production of a chimeric mRNA and an encoded protein with an oncogenic function.

Cytogenetic assays allow the study of chromosomes and chromosome regions within cells. A sample from the tumor can be collected under sterile conditions, placed in tissue culture fluid and sent to the laboratory for analysis. Freezing the sample or placing it in fixative makes cytogenetic studies for which the cells must be cultured impossible. In the laboratory, the tumor cells may be cultured for several days before arresting dividing cells in metaphase when the chromatin is condensed, making the chromosomes relatively easy to analyze.

A wide range of molecular genetic technology and clinical techniques have been developed to assist in the detection of acquired mutations in tumor cells. **Table 1.6** describes the major clinical genetic assays and techniques used in assessment of bone and soft tissue tumor lesions.

Table 1.7 lists the genetic findings in bone tumors. **Table 1.8** lists the genetic findings in soft tissue tumors. These do not capture all genetic abnormalities, as new findings are continuously being reported.

Table 1.3 Common antibodies useful in mesenchymal tumor diagnosis

Antibody or antibody set	Distribution in normal tissue	Some benign tumors reactive for this antibody	Some malignant tumors reactive for this antibody	Other antibodies uncommonly expressed
Desmin, SMA, MSA, caldesmon, smooth muscle myosin heavy chain	Smooth muscle	Leiomyoma	Leiomyosarcoma	Pankeratin S-100 protein
Myogenin, desmin, MyoD, α-sarcomeric actin, CD56	Skeletal muscle	Rhabdomyoma	Rhabdomyosarcoma	Smooth muscle actin S-100 protein (rare)
SMA, MSA; desmin less frequently	Myofibroblasts	Myofibroma	Myofibrosarcoma	Pankeratin (fairly common)
S-100 protein (less frequent in high grade tumors) CDK4 and MDM2 in low grade tumors and dedifferentiated LPS	Adipose tissue	Lipoma (S-100 protein only)	Liposarcoma	Dedifferentiated LPS may form muscle that will be SMA and/or desmin reactive
S-100 protein, HMB45, Melan-A, MiTF	Melanocytes	Nevi	Melanoma and clear cell sarcoma	Some melanomas are negative for all melanocytic markers Clear cell sarcoma may express only one marker
S-100 protein	Chondrocytes	Enchondroma, synovial chondromatosis	Chondrosarcoma	No others in common use
S-100 protein	Peripheral schwann cells	Schwannoma, neurofibroma	Malignant peripheral nerve sheath tumor (MPNST) (50% of cases, usually focal but epithelioid variant is usually diffusely positive for S-100 protein)	GFAP +/-. Keratins may be positive, especially in MPNST. Desmin and myogenin in Malignant Triton Tumor
EMA, Claudin, GLUT1	Perineurial cells	Perineurioma	MPNST with perineurial differentiation	CD34 in sclerosing perineurioma
Neurofilaments, GFAP, NSE, CD56	Axonal cells	Neurofibroma	MPNST with axonal differentiation	CD56 also stains other tumors S-100 and CD34 are also positive in neurofibroma
CD34, CD31, FLI-1, ERG (C terminus directed)	Endothelial cells	Hemangioma	Angiosarcoma	D2-40 is expressed in normal lymphatics and some angiosarcomas CD34 is also expressed in nonvascular tumors such as DFSP, GIST and SFT Keratins may be expressed especially in epithelioid vascular tumors
CD99 (membranous reactivity only), Fli-1	No known normal cell counterpart	No known benign tumor	Ewing sarcoma family of tumors	Pankeratin, S-100 protein

Antibodies in bold font are the main antibodies used for the particular tumor. SMA: smooth muscle actin, MSA: muscle specific actin (HHF-35 actin), MiTF: Microphthalmia-associated transcription factor, EMA: epithelial membrane antigen, GFAP: glial fibrillary acidic protein, NSE: neuron specific enolase, FLI-1: Friend leukemia virus integration 1, GLUT1: Glucose transporter 1, HMB45: Melanosome clone HMB45, CD56: NCAM, neural cell adhesion molecule, Melan-A: Melanocyte A antibody (A103), CDK4: cyclin-dependent kinase 4, MDM2: Mdm2 [murine double minute] p53 binding protein homolog (mouse), DFSP: Dermatofibrosarcoma protuberans, GIST: Gastrointestinal stroma tumor, SFT: Solitary fibrous tumor

Table 1.4 Some tumors with relatively specific antigen reactivity patterns

Tumor	Antibody reactivity pattern	Additional confirmatory studies
Alveolar soft part sarcoma	TFE3 (nuclear) positive +/- : desmin, S-100 protein, SMA	FISH for translocation
Atypical lipomatous tumor (ALT)/ Well differentiated liposarcoma	CDK4 and/or MDM2 (both nuclear) positive p16: nuclear +/- cytoplasmic positive (must be diffusely positive to be diagnostically useful)	FISH for CDK4/MDM2 amplification
Chordoma	Brachyury, keratins positive +/-: S-100 protein	Imaging may be very helpful
Clear cell sarcoma	S-100, HMB45, Melan-A one or more positive	FISH for translocation
Dermatofibrosarcoma protuberans	CD34 diffusely positive except in areas of fibrosarcomatous transformation	FISH for translocation
Desmoid type fibromatosis	Aberrant nuclear β-catenin expression (70-80%)	Mutation analysis not commonly performed
Desmoplastic small round cell tumor	Odd tetrad reactivity: WT1, NSE, keratin/EMA, dot-like desmin	FISH for translocation
Epithelioid sarcoma	INI-1 loss of expression, EGFR expression, keratins, CD34 (50%)	PCR

Table 1.4 Continued from page 7

Tumor	Antibody reactivity pattern	Additional confirmatory studies
Gastrointestinal stroma tumor	c-kit (95%), DOG-1 (95%), CD34 (60%), +/-: smooth muscle actin	PCR for c-kit, PDGFRa mutations
Leiomyosarcoma	Actin and desmin both positive in most cases, caldesmon also commonly positive (~70%) and most specific for smooth muscle differentiation	No specific genetic findings
Low grade fibromyxoid sarcoma	MUC4 positive	FISH for translocation
Rhabdomyosarcoma	Myogenin, desmin positive Rarely smooth muscle actin	FISH for translocations in alveolar RMS almost always required by protocol
Synovial sarcoma	EMA, keratins, TLE1 (90%) +/-: S-100 protein, calponin	FISH for translocation almost always required

Positive = typically positive (85% or more), +/- = 10-20% positive, Rarely positive = 3-5% positive. TFE3 = Transcription factor binding to IGHM enhancer 3, WT1= Wilms tumor 1, INI-1 = Integrase interacter 1 = SMARCB1, DOG-1 = Discovered on GIST-1, MUC4 = Mucin 4, TLE1 = Transducin-like enhancer of split 1, c-kit = CD117, mast/stem cell growth factor receptor (homolog of a feline sarcoma viral oncogene: v-kit)

Table 1.5 Cell shapes, architectural patterns and stromal components in mesenchymal tumors

Feature	Low magnification example	High magnification example
Spindle cells	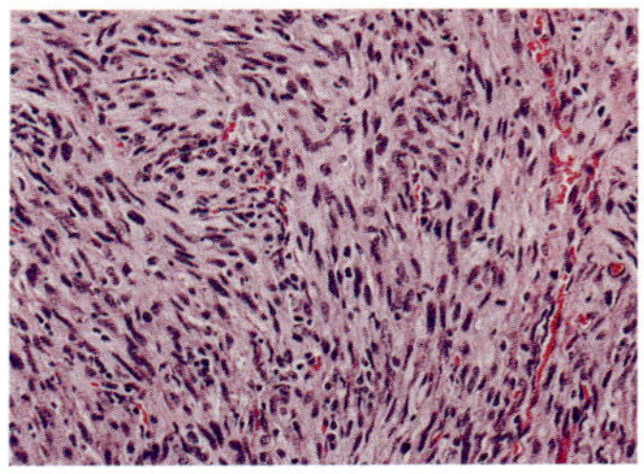	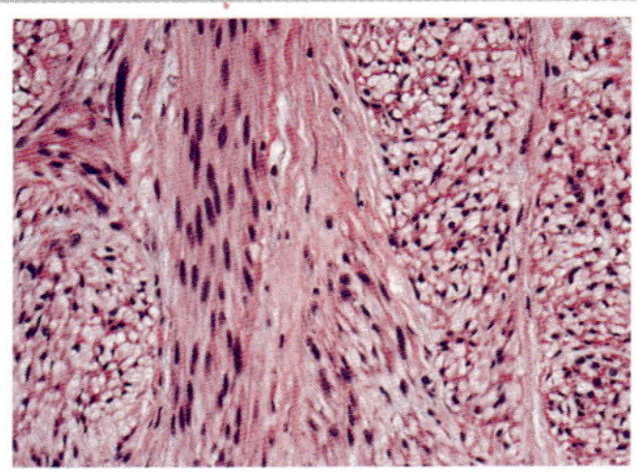
Stellate cells	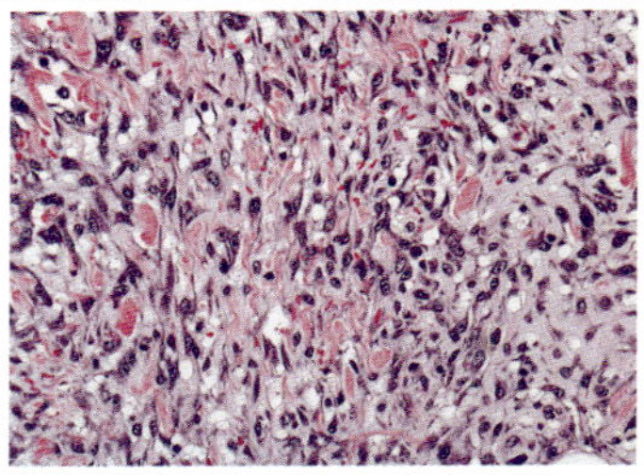	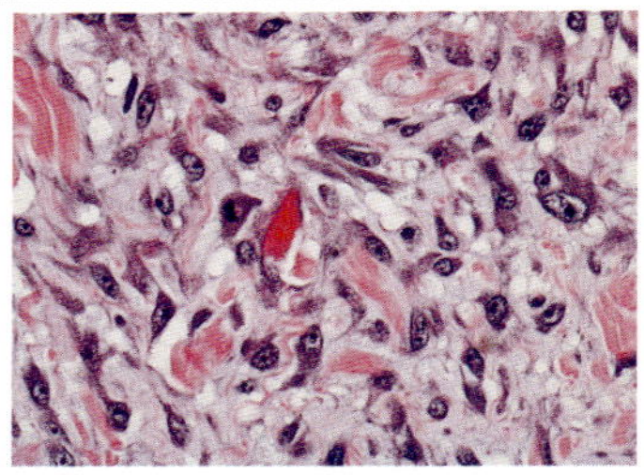
Epithelioid cells	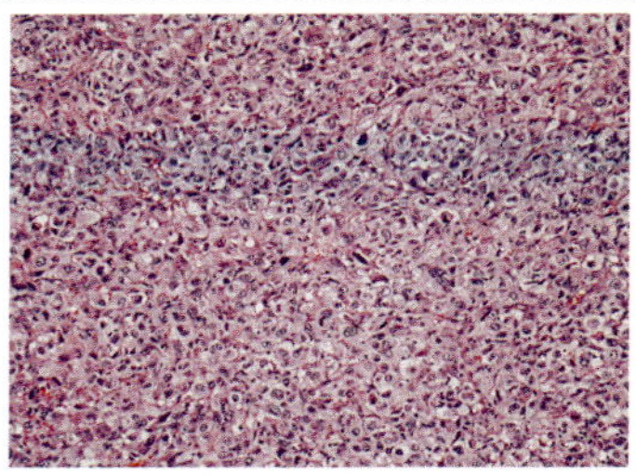	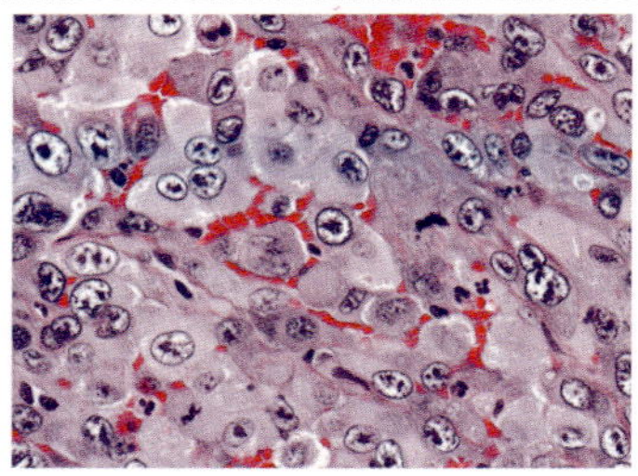
Small round blue cells	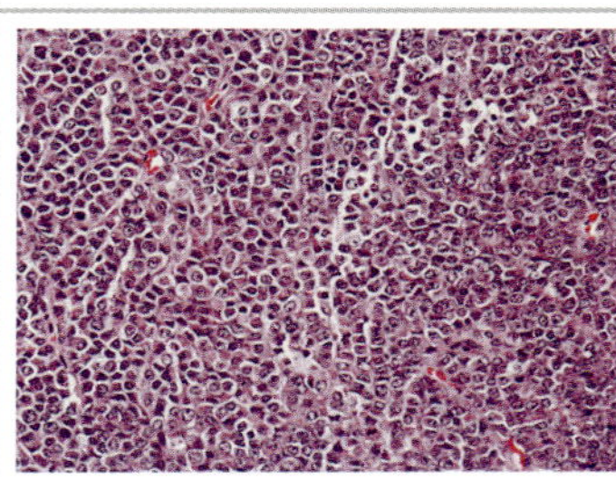	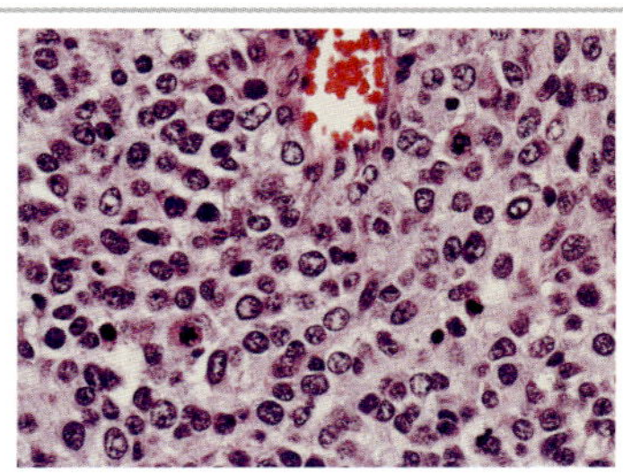

Table 1.5: Continued from page 8

Feature	Low magnification example	High magnification example
Tumor giant cells	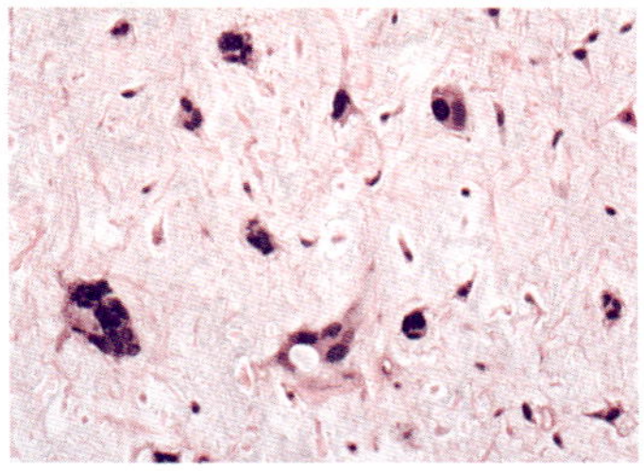	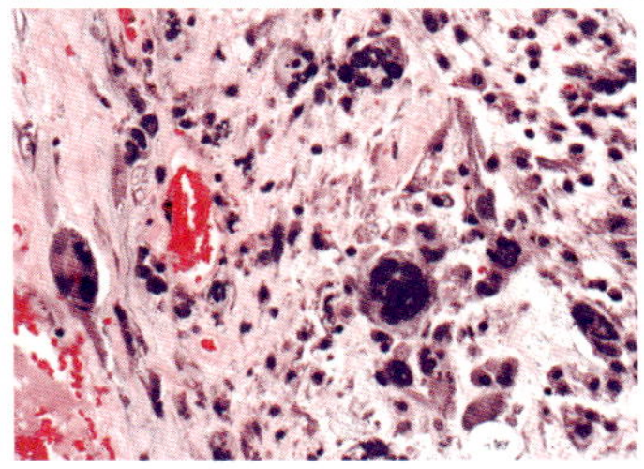
Osteoclastic giant cells	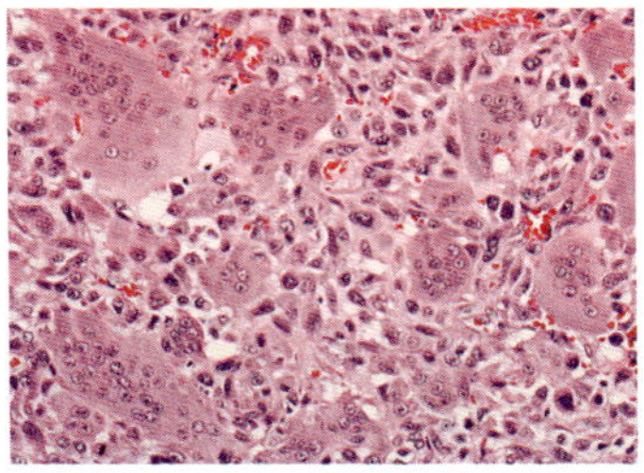	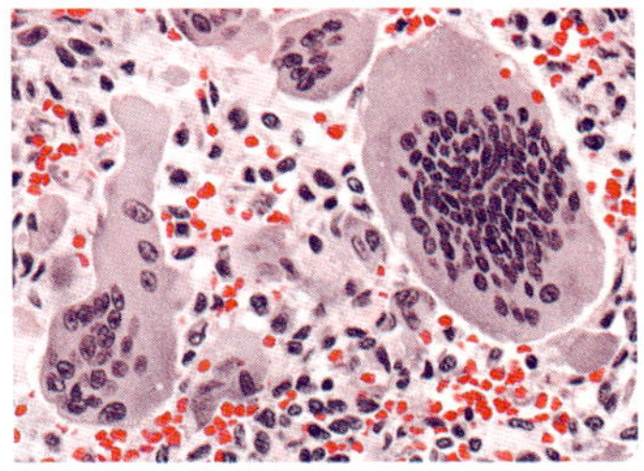
Pleomorphic tumor cells	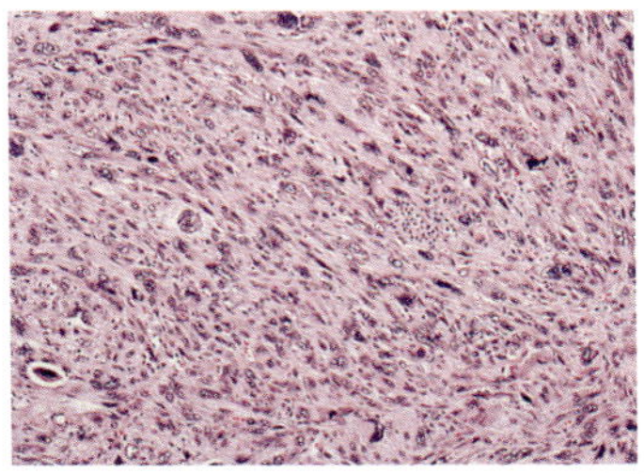	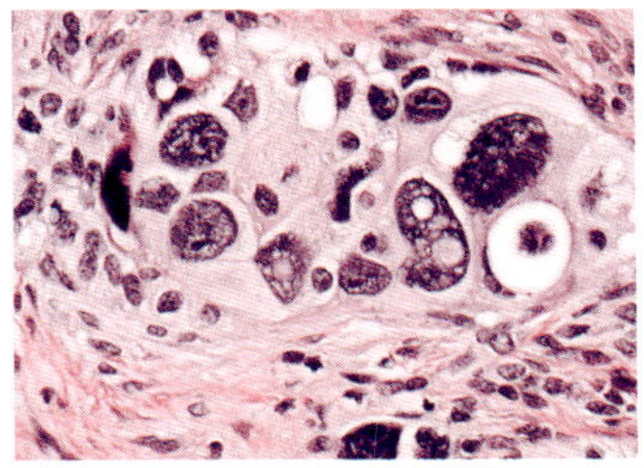
Myxoid matrix	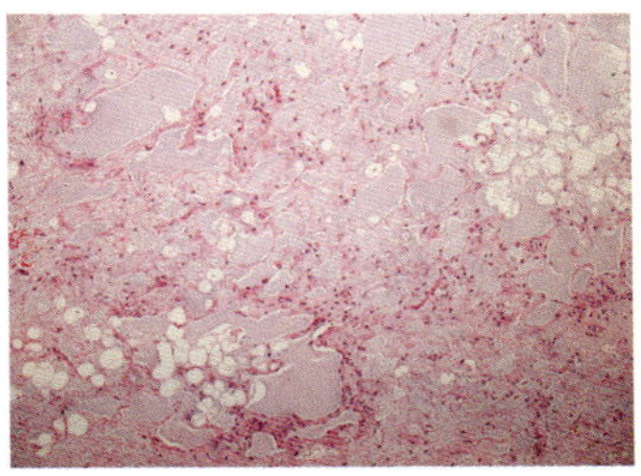	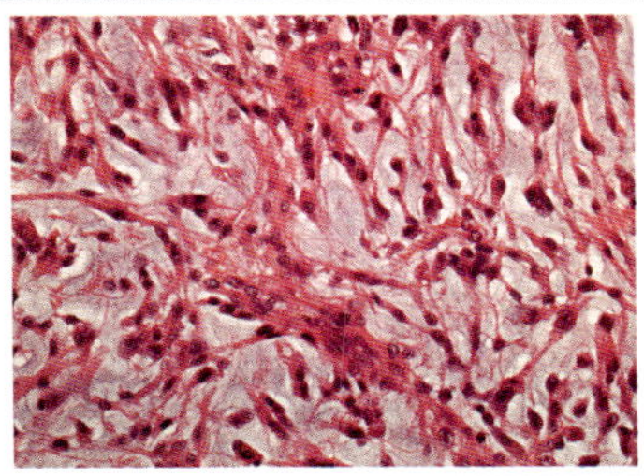
Fibrous matrix	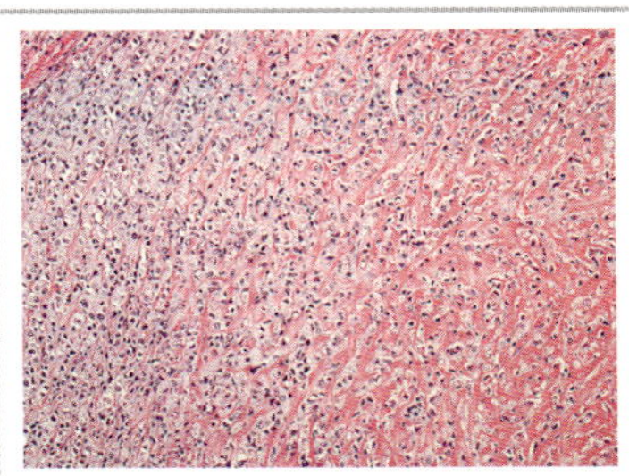	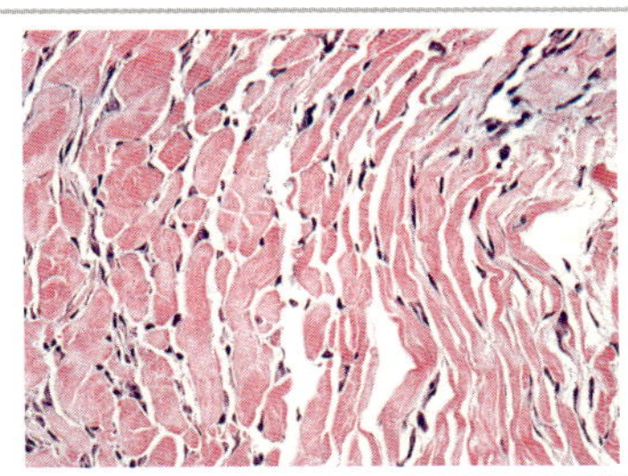
Osteoid	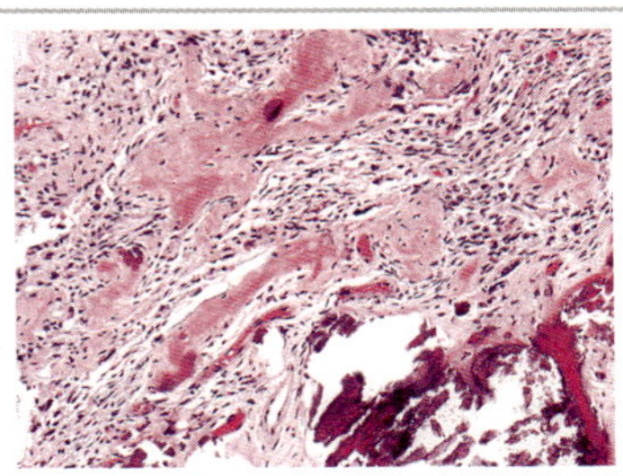	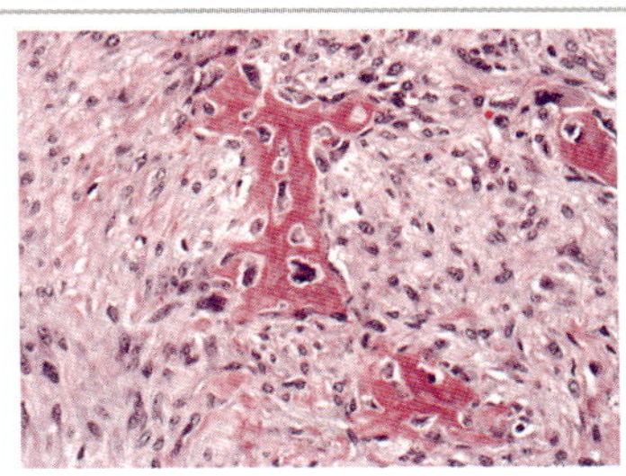

Table 1.5: Continued from page 9

Feature	Low magnification example	High magnification example
Bone (mineralized osteoid)	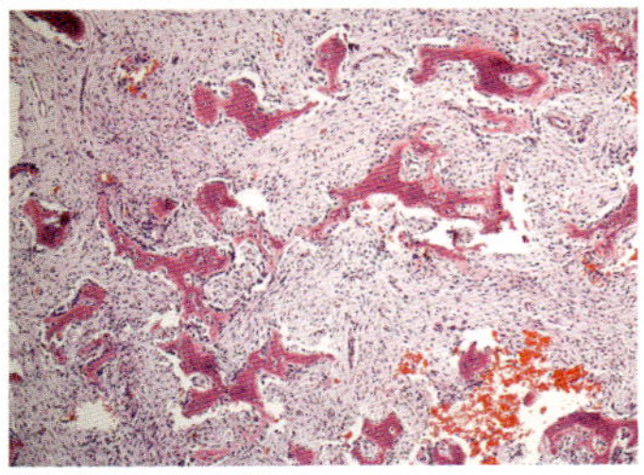	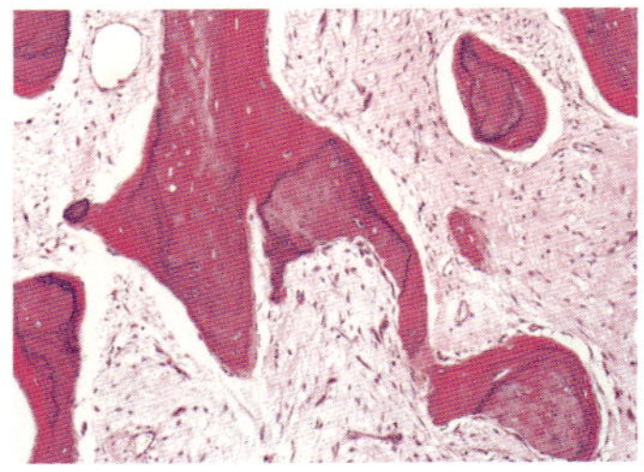
Cartilage	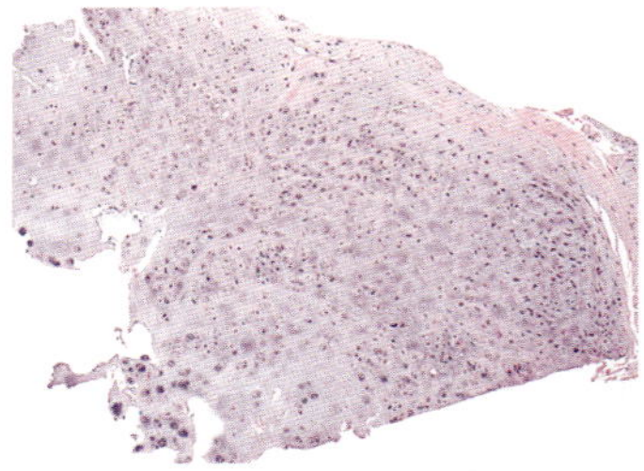	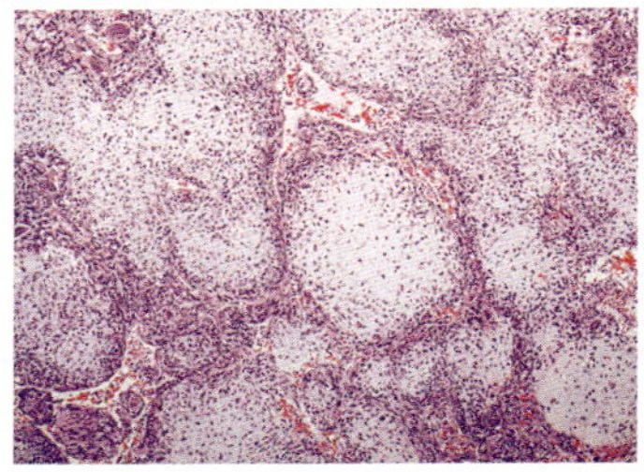
Calcifications	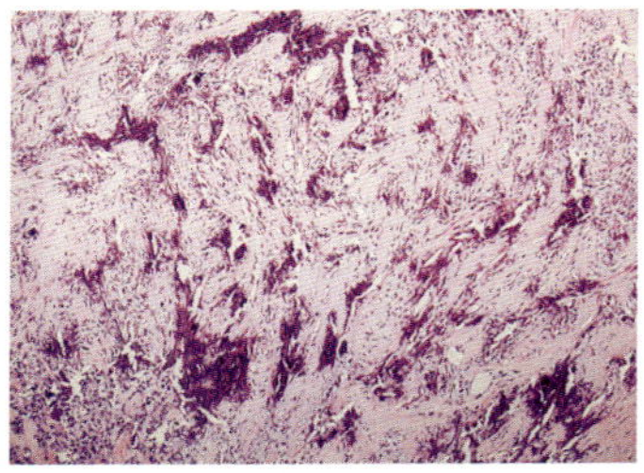	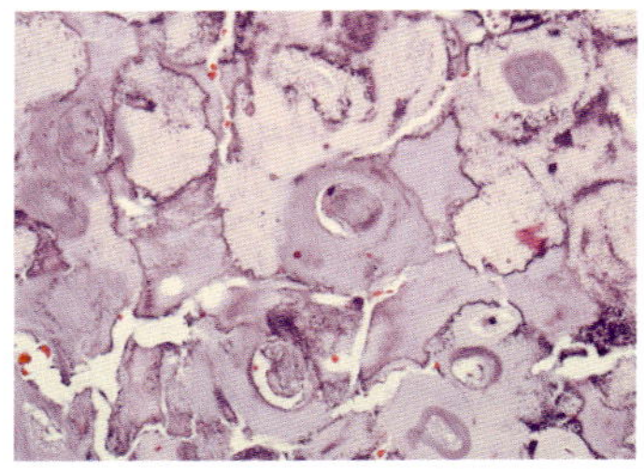
Sheets of cells	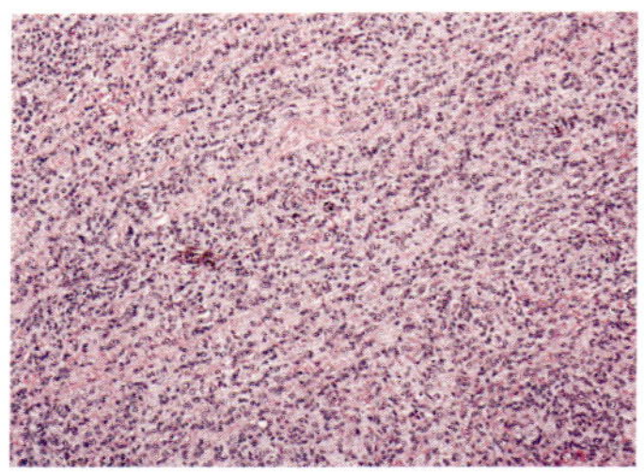	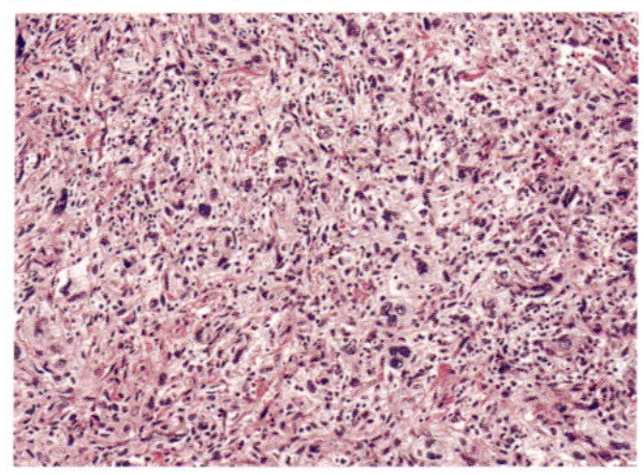
Fascicles of cells	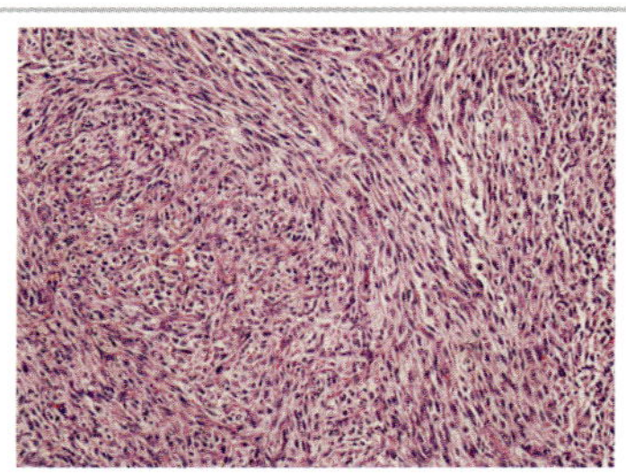	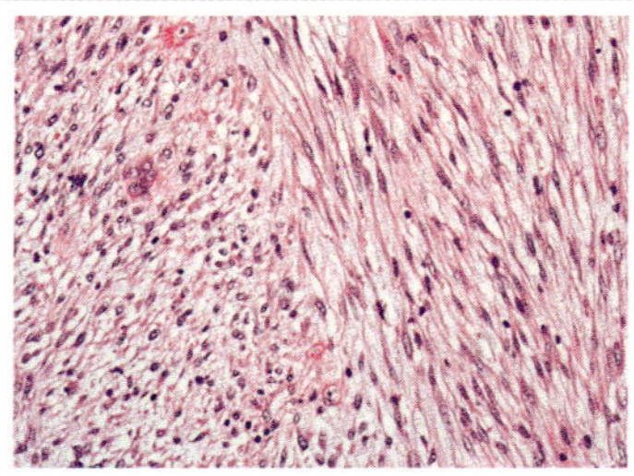
Storiforming mats of cells	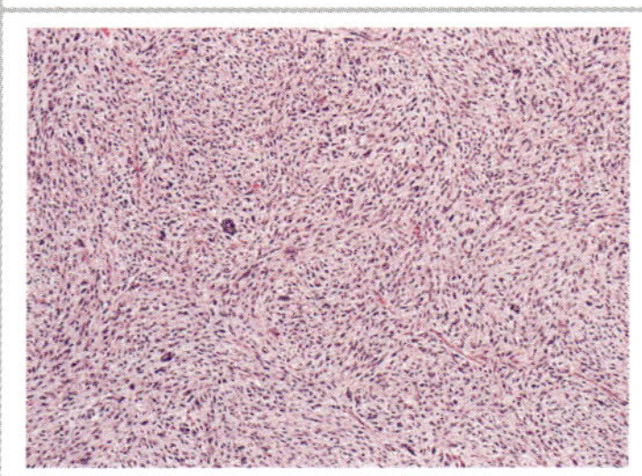	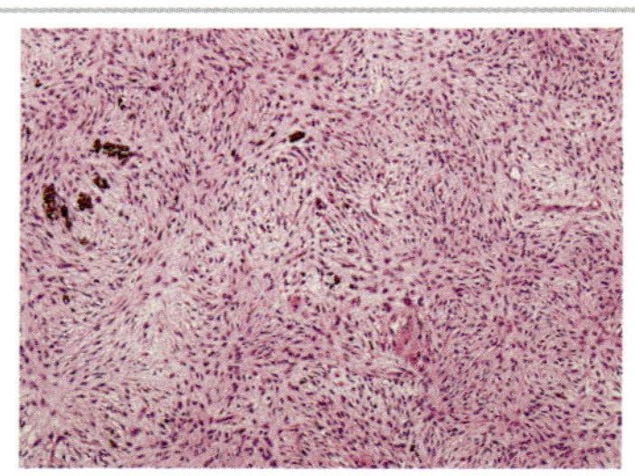

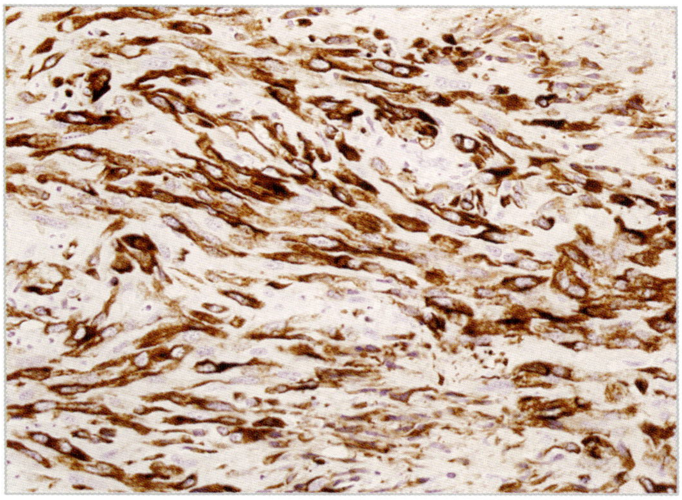

Figure 1.7 Malignant peripheral nerve sheath tumor, pankeratin IHC stain. Sarcomas may strongly and diffusely express epithelial markers such as keratins and EMA. Such reactivity is usually focal but when strong and diffuse can be a confusing finding.

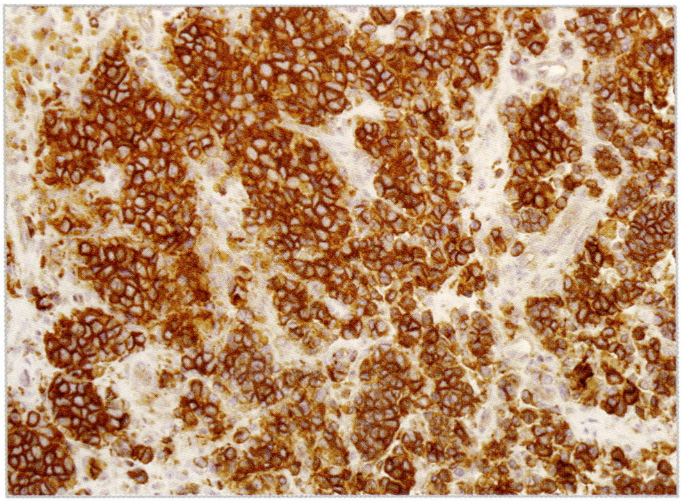

Figure 1.8 Ewing sarcoma, high magnification, CD99 IHC stain. Characteristically, the Ewing sarcoma family of tumors expresses CD99 in a relatively specific membranous pattern of reactivity (brown chromogen).

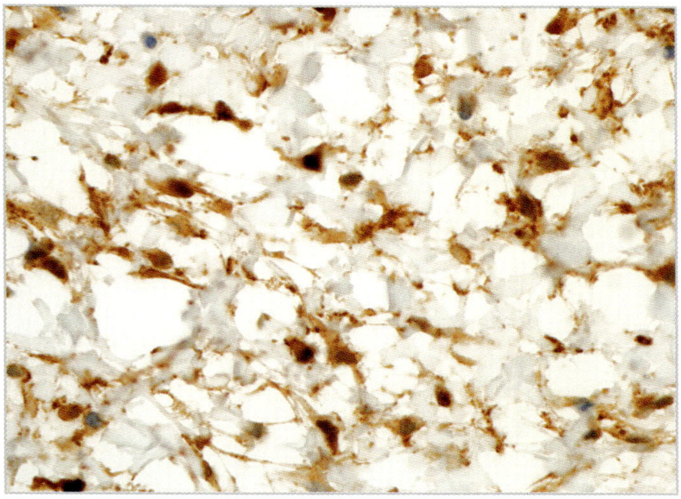

Figure 1.9 Desmoid-type fibromatosis, high magnification, β-catenin IHC stain, brown chromogen. Approximately 80% of soft tissue desmoid tumors aberrantly express nuclear β-catenin. Nuclear reactivity is a relatively specific feature and helps differentiate the tumor from reactive scar tissue. It may be focal and associated with cytoplasmic and membranous reactivity also present in this example.

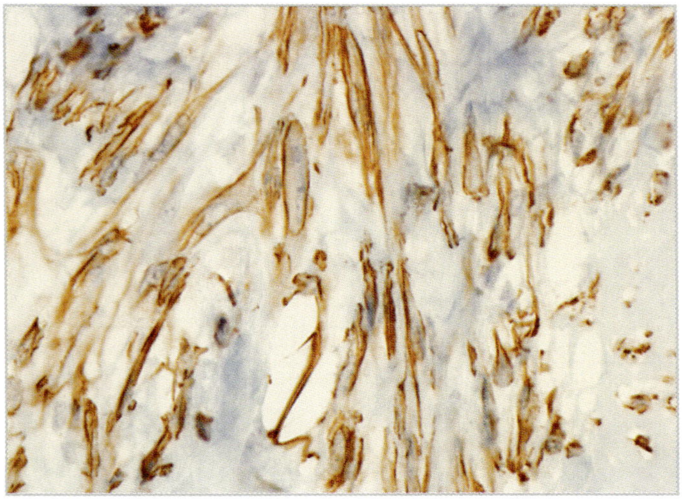

Figure 1.10 Low grade myofibrosarcoma, high magnification, smooth muscle actin (SMA) IHC stain, brown chromogen. Myofibroblasts often demonstrate a parallel subplasmalemmal pattern of SMA expression ('tram track' reactivity). In contrast, smooth muscle cells exhibit diffuse cytoplasmic reactivity for SMA. This is an example of the diagnostic clues provided by the cellular location of antigen expression.

CAUTIONARY TALES

Benign lesions that look malignant

Some benign mesenchymal lesions, by virtue of hypercellularity, high mitotic activity and/or nuclear variability, readily appear malignant. **Table 1.9** lists some of these tumors.

Malignant lesions that look benign

By contrast, a few sarcomas may look deceptively benign with minimal cytologic atypia, sparse to absent mitotic activity and no necrosis. **Table 1.10** lists these tumors.

Malignant tumors that look like sarcomas

Sarcoma mimickers encompass non-mesenchymal tumors, and these may be encountered with consternating frequency, especially in the head and neck. **Table 1.11** lists these malignant mimics of sarcoma.

Manifold appearance of some bone and soft tissue tumors

A single specific bone or soft tissue tumor may present diverse histologic appearances. This increases the complexity of the diagnosis of bone and

Table 1.6 Genetic assays used in the clinical assessment of bone and soft tissue tumors

Method	Description	Sample	Utility	Limit of resolution	Sensitivity
Traditional cytogenetics	Chromosomes examined in metaphase	Fresh cells or tissue, not fixed or frozen	Detection of large scale chromosomal duplication, deletions, translocations	5-10 megabases	One molecule of DNA (one chromosome)
Fluorescent in situ hybridization cytogenetics	Examination of specific chromosome regions with fluorescent DNA probes	Fresh or fixed cells or tissue	Detection of finer scale chromosomal duplication, deletions, translocations	100,000 nucleotides	One molecule of DNA (one chromosomal region)
Reverse transcriptase PCR	Polymerase chain reaction amplification of nucleic acids	Fresh cells or tissues	Detection and quantitation of chimeric mRNAs	Several hundred nucleotide target	A few molecules of target mRNA
High resolution melting assays	PCR with controlled melting to detect sequence variation	Fresh or fixed cells and tissue	Detect point mutations in DNA	Single nucleotide mutations	Few percent cells containing mutation in mixture of benign cells
DNA sequencing	Multiple methods for determining DNA sequence of a genomic region	Fresh or fixed cells and tissue	Determine DNA sequence of a region of the genome or the entire genome	Single nucleotide variation	Can begin with one, a few, or many cells

Table 1.7 Representative genetic findings in bone tumors or lesions

Tumor	Behavior	Genetic finding	Utility
Aneurysmal bone cyst	Benign to intermediate	USP6 (17p13) gene translocations: t(16;17) = *CDH11-USP6* t(1;17) = *THRAP3-USP6* t(3;17) = *CNBP-USP6* t(9;17) = *OMD-USP6* t(17;17) = *COL1A1-USP6*	Dx but not commonly needed
Chondroblastoma	Intermediate (rarely malignant)	Heterogeneous rearrangements	Not helpful
Chondromyxoid fibroma	Benign	6q12-15,6p23-25, 6q23-27 rearrangements Rare other translocations	Dx but not commonly needed
Chordoma	Malignant	T (brachyury homolog) and *EGFR* copy number gains	Dx but not commonly used
Clear cell chondrosarcoma	Malignant	May have extra copies of 20 or 9p loss or rearrangement Retinoblastoma pathway commonly altered.	Not helpful
Enchondroma	Benign	Normal karyotype usually	Not helpful
Conventional chondrosarcoma, low grade	Intermediate	More complex karyotype than most enchondromas	May be helpful
Conventional chondrosarcoma, high grade	Malignant	Complex aneuploidy	Not helpful
Ewing sarcoma family of tumors	Malignant	t(11;22)(q24;q12) = *EWSR1-FLI1* t(21;22)(q22;q12) = *EWSR1-ERG* t(7;22)(p22;q12) = *EWSR1-ETV1* t(17;22)(q21;q12) = *EWSR1-ETV4* t(2;22)(q33;q12) = *EWSR1-FEV* t(16;21)(p11;q22) = *FUS-ERG* t(2;16) = *FUS-FEV* inv (22) = *EWSR1-ZSG* t(2;22)(q31;q12) = *EWSR1-SP3* t(20;22)(q13;q12) = *EWSR1- NFATC2* t(4;22)(q31;q12) = *EWSR1- SMARCA5*	Dx (90% are *EWSR1-FLI1*) A few of the rare translocations have only been described in soft tissue cases
Fibrous dysplasia	Benign	*GNAS1* gene mutations	Dx but not commonly needed
Giant cell tumor of bone	Intermediate	Telomeric associations Secondary findings	Dx but not commonly needed
Mesenchymal chondrosarcoma	Malignant	*t(8;8)(q21;q13) = HEY1-NCOA2*	Dx
Osteosarcoma, low grade	Intermediate to malignant	Normal karyotype	Not helpful
Osteosarcoma, high grade	Malignant	Complex aneuploidy	Not helpful

Dx = diagnosis. Benign = does not recur (or only rarely), Intermediate = locally aggressive or recurrent or rarely metastasizes (<5%), Malignant = commonly metastasizes and often locally aggressive and recurrent.

Table 1.8 Representative genetic findings in soft tissue tumors

Tumor	Behavior	Genetic finding	Utility
Deep (aggressive) angiomyxoma	Intermediate	12q15 rearrangements = *HMGA2*	Dx but not commonly needed
Alveolar soft part sarcoma	Malignant	t(X;17)(p11;q25) = *ASPSCR1(ASPL)-TFE3*	Dx
Angiomatoid fibrous histiocytoma	Intermediate	t(12;16)(q13;p11) = *FUS/TLS-ATF1* t(12;22)(q13;q12) = *EWSR1-ATF1* t(2;22)(q33;q12) = *EWSR1-CREB1*	Dx
Angiosarcoma	Malignant	Complex aneuploidy	Not useful
Clear cell sarcoma	Malignant	t(12;22)(q13;q12) = *EWSR1-ATF1* t(2;22)(q33;q12) = *EWSR1-CREB1*	Dx
Dermatofibrosarcoma protuberans	Intermediate	Ring chromosome composed of 17q21 and 22q10-q31 sequences t(17;22)(q22;q13) = *COL1A-PDGFβ*	Dx but not commonly needed
Desmoid-type fibromatosis	Benign to intermediate	CTNNB1 mutations Trisomy 8, 20 5q21-22 loss or mutations = *APC*	Dx but not commonly needed
Desmoplastic fibroblastoma		t(2;11)(q31;q12) = ? t(11;17)(q12;p11.2) = ?	Dx but not commonly needed
Desmoplastic small round cell tumor	Malignant	t(11;22)(p13;q12) = *EWSR1-WT1* t(21;22)(q22;q12) = *EWSR1-ERG*	Dx
Epithelioid hemangioendothelioma (EHE)	Intermediate to malignant	t(1;3)(p36;q25) = *WWTR1-CAMTA1*	Dx
Epithelioid sarcoma	Malignant	Complex changes by CGH 22q11 abnormalities = *INI1* (*SMARCB1*)	Not useful
Extraskeletal myxoid chondrosarcoma	Malignant	t(9;22)(q22;q12) = *EWSR1-NR4A3* t(9;17)(q22;q11) = *TAF2N-NR4A3* t(9;15)(q22;q21) = *TCF12-NR4A3* t(9;22)(q22;q15) = *TFG-NR4A3*	Dx
Fibroma of tendon sheath	Benign	t(2;11)(q31-32;q12) = ?	Dx but not commonly needed
GIST	Malignant	c-kit gene mutation (majority) PDGFRa gene mutation (minority)	Dx but not commonly needed
Hibernoma	Benign	11q13-21 rearrangements	Dx but not commonly needed
Inflammatory myofibroblastic tumor (IMFT)	Intermediate	*ALK1* gene fusions (2p23 translocations): t(1;2)(q25;q23) = *TPM3-ALk* t(2;19)(q23;q13) = *TPM4-ALK* t(2;17)(q23;q23) = *CLTC-ALK* t(2;2)(p23;q13) = *RANBP2-ALK*	Dx but not commonly needed
Leiomyosarcoma	Malignant	Complex aneuploidy	Not useful
Lipoblastoma	Benign to intermediate	8q11-13 rearrangements = *PLAG1*	Dx but not commonly needed
Lipoma, conventional	Benign	12q15 rearrangements = *HMGA2* 6p21 rearrangements = *HMGA1*	Dx but not needed
Liposarcoma **> Myxoid/round cell LPS**	Malignant	Myxoid/RC LPS: t(12;16)(q13;p11) = *FUS-DDIT3* t(12;22)(q13;q12) = *EWSR1-DDIT3*	Dx but not commonly needed
Low grade fibromyxoid sarcoma	Malignant	t(7;16)(q34;p11) = FUS-CREB3L2 t(11;16)(p11;p11) = FUS-CREB3L1	Dx
Malignant peripheral nerve sheath tumor (MPNST)	Malignant	Complex aneuploidy 22q11.2 abnormalities = *INI1* (*SMARCB1*) in some epithelioid MPNST	Not useful
Myoepithelial carcinoma of soft tissue	Malignant	t(1;22)(q23;q12) = *EWSR1-PBX1* t(19;22)(q13;q12) = *EWSR1-ZNF444* t(6;22)(p21;q12) = *EWSR1-POU5F1* 16p11.2 rearrangement = *FUS-?*	Dx
Myxofibrosarcoma	Malignant	Complex aneuploidy	Not useful
Myxoinflammatory fibroblastic sarcoma	Malignant	t(1;10)(p22;q24) = *FGF8* and *NPM3*	Dx
Neurofibroma	Benign	Monoallelic or biallelic loss of 17q11.2 = *NF1* (neurofibromin)	Not useful
Pericytoma	Benign	t(7;12)(p22;q13) = *ACTB-GLI1*	Dx but not commonly needed
Perineurioma	Benign	10q22-24 deletions rearrangements not *ALK1* (sclerosing perineurioma) 22q11.2 alterations in some cases of both types	Dx but not commonly needed
Rhabdoid tumor of ST	Malignant	Del 22q11.22 = del *SMARCB1*	Dx

Table 1.8: Continued from page 13

Tumor	Behavior	Genetic finding	Utility
Rhabdomyosarcoma	Malignant	A-RMS: t(2;13)(q35;q14) = *PAX3-FOX01A* t(1;13)(q36;q14) = *PAX7- FOXO1A* t(2;X)(p35;q13) = *PAX3-MLLT7* t(2;2)(q35;q23) = *PAX3-NCOAI* E-RMS, adult sclerosing/spindle RMS, pleomorphic RMS: complex aneuploidy	Dx (for A-RMS)
Schwannoma	Benign	22q12 loss = *NF2* (Merlin, Schwannomin)	Not useful
Sclerosing epithelioid fibrosarcoma	Malignant	t(7;16)(q34;p11) = *FUS-CREB3L2* t(11;16)(p11;p11) = *FUS-CREB3L1*	Dx
Soft tissue angiofibroma	Benign	t(5;8)(p15;q13) = *AHRR-NCOA2*	Dx
Solitary fibrous tumor	Intermediate	NAB2-STAT6 fusion (both genes on 12q13) 12q13-15 rearrangements	May be useful in Dx
Spindle cell lipoma/pleomorphic lipoma	Benign	16q13-qter rearrangements monosomy 13 partial del(13q)	Dx but not commonly needed
Synovial sarcoma	Malignant	t(X;18)(p11;q11) = *SS18-SSX1* t(X;18)(p11;q11) = *SS18-SSX2* t(X;18)(p11;q13) = *SS18-SSX4* t(X; 20)(p11;q13) = *SS18L1- SSX1*	Dx
Tenosynovial giant cell tumor, diffuse or localized	Benign to intermediate	t(1;2)(p13;q37) = *CSF1-COL6A3* Trisomy 5,7	Dx but not commonly needed

Dx = diagnosis, Benign = a tumor that will not recur (or only rarely) and does not metastasize, Intermediate = a tumor that can be locally aggressive and/or recur and/or has a low risk (</= 5%) of metastasis, Malignant = a tumor that has a high risk for metastasis and may be locally aggressive also. This list of genetic abnormalities is necessarily incomplete because new discoveries are ongoing.

Table 1.9 Some benign mesenchymal lesions that appear histologically malignant

Tumor	Example at low magnification	Example at high magnification
Nodular fasciitis	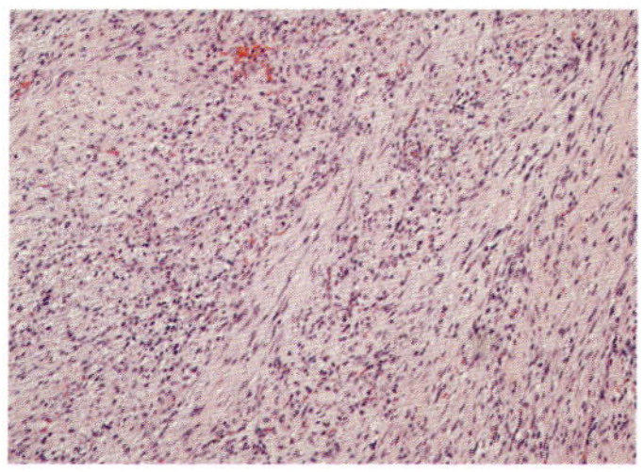	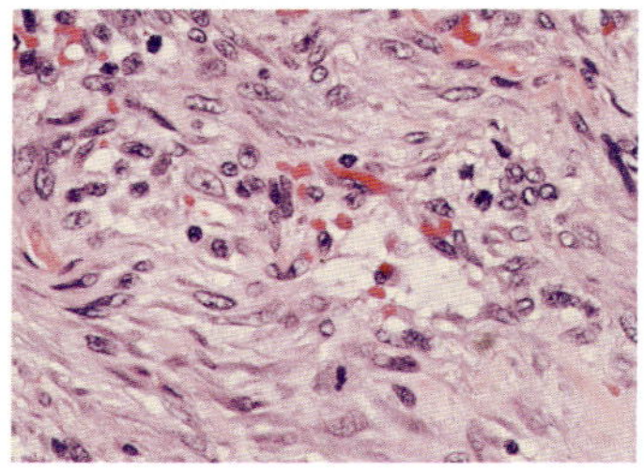
Myositis ossificans	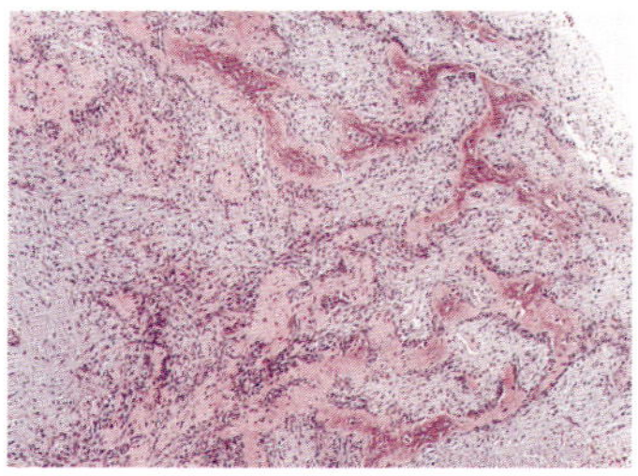	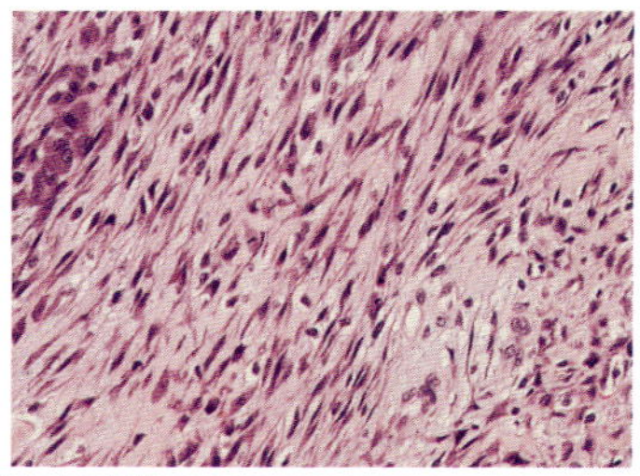
Neurofibroma	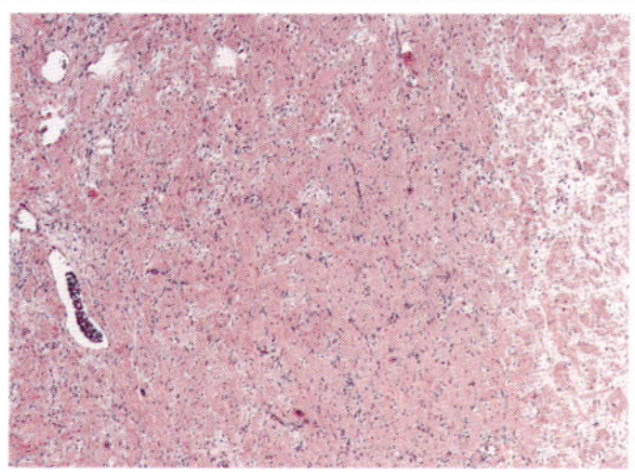	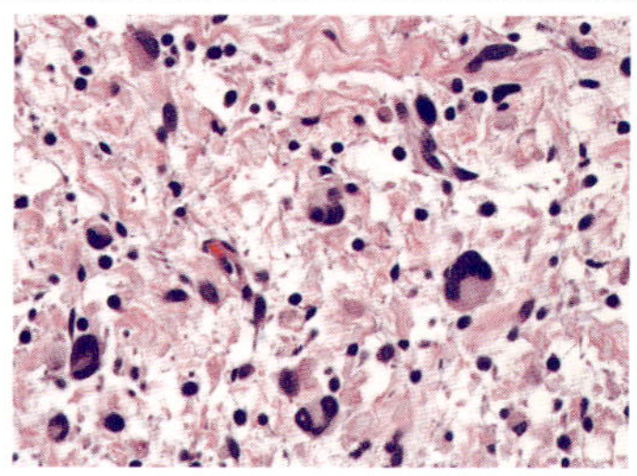

Table 1.9: Continued from page 14

Tumor	Example at low magnification	Example at high magnification
Pleomorphic hyalinizing angiectatic tumor (PHAT)	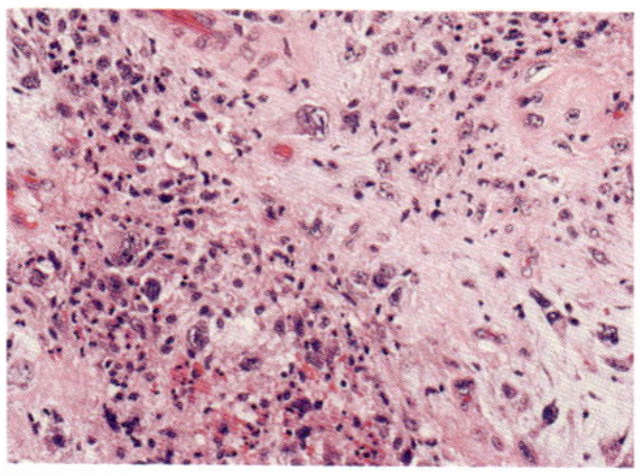	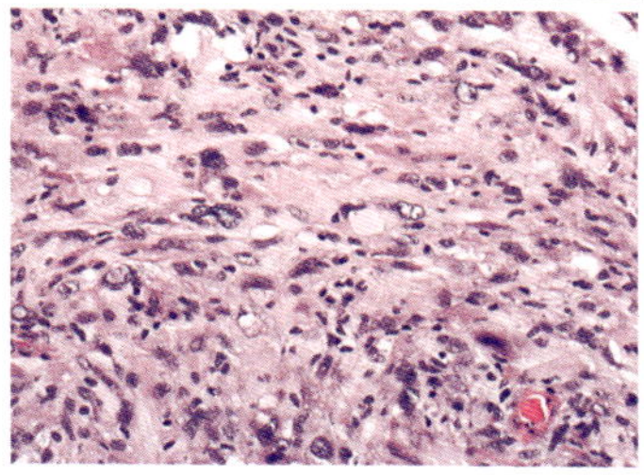
Cellular schwannoma	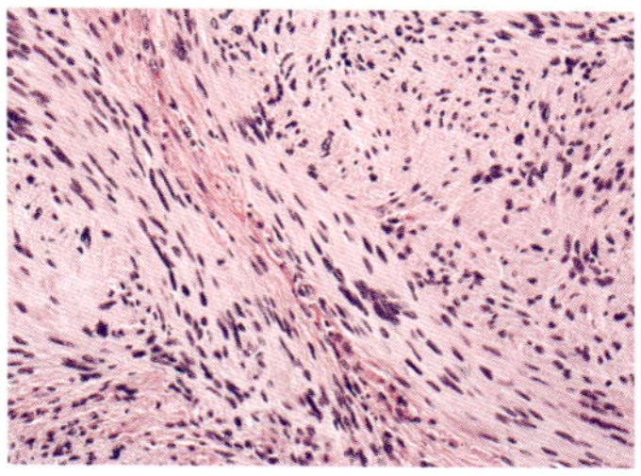	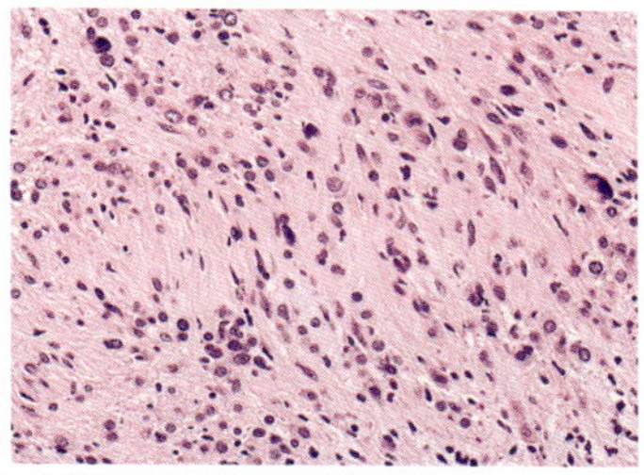
Unstable fracture	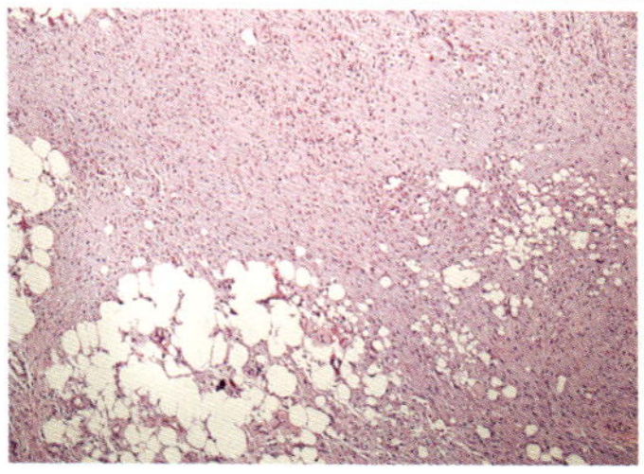	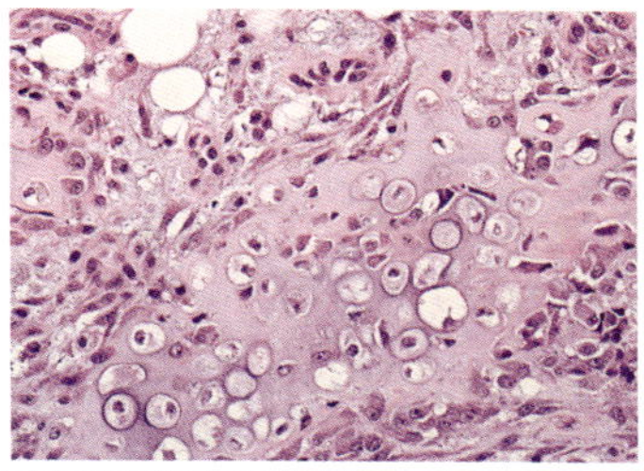

Table 1.10 Some malignant mesenchymal tumors that appear histologically benign

Tumor	Example at low magnification	Example at high magnification
Clear cell sarcoma, sclerosing type	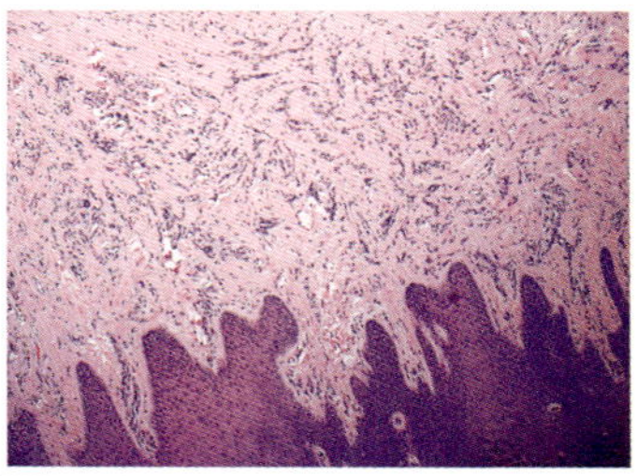	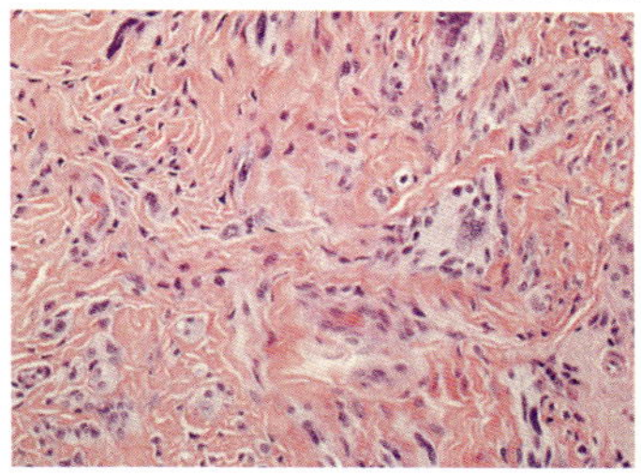
Epithelioid sarcoma	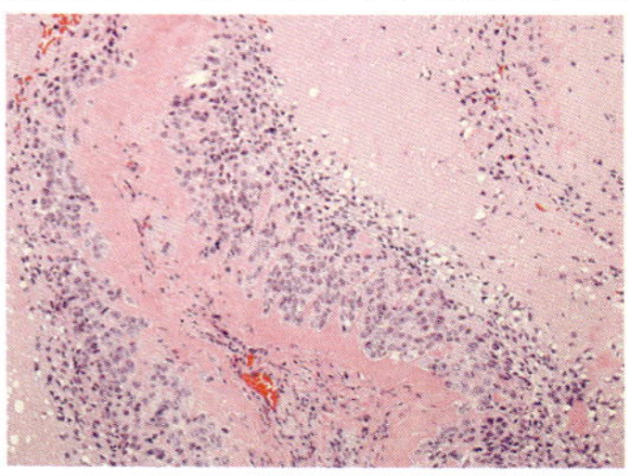	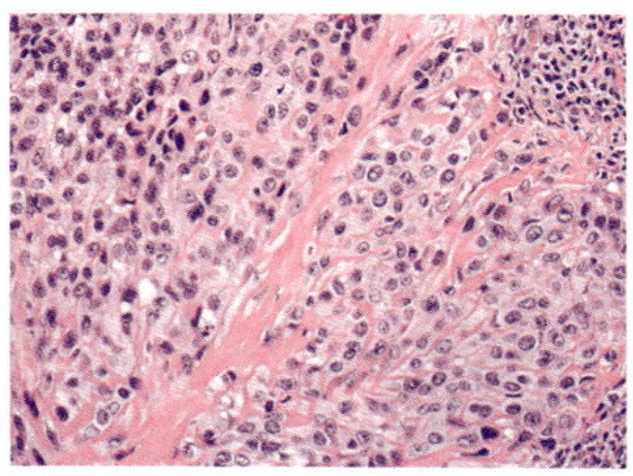

Table 1.10: Continued from page 15

Tumor	Example at low magnification	Example at high magnification
Low grade myofibroblastic sarcoma	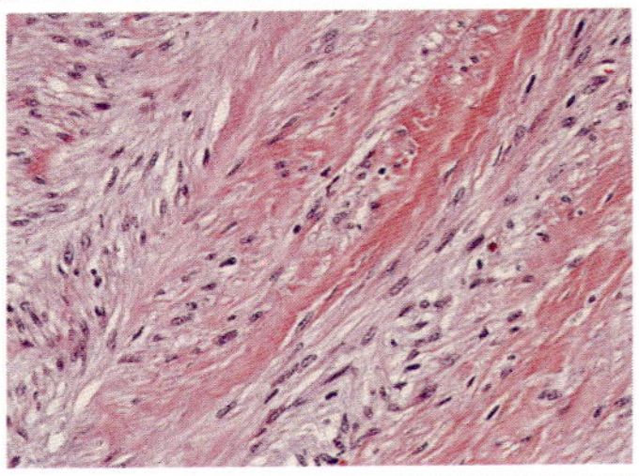	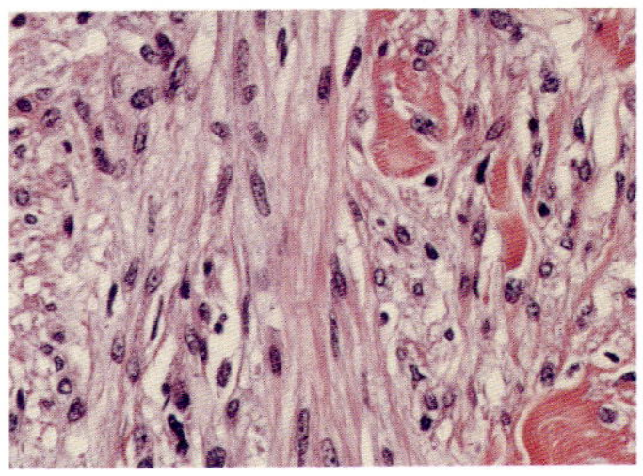
Low grade fibromyxoid sarcoma	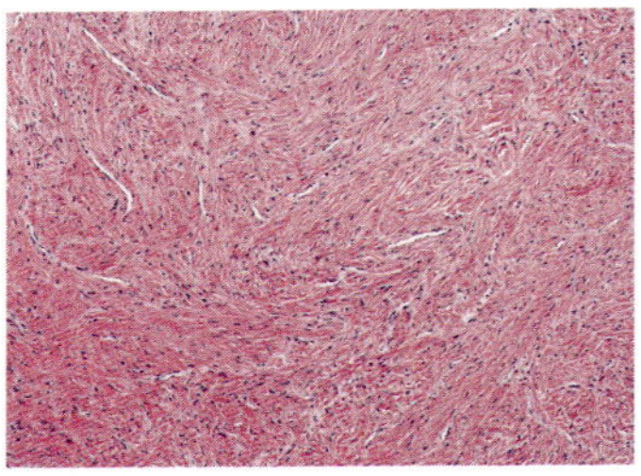	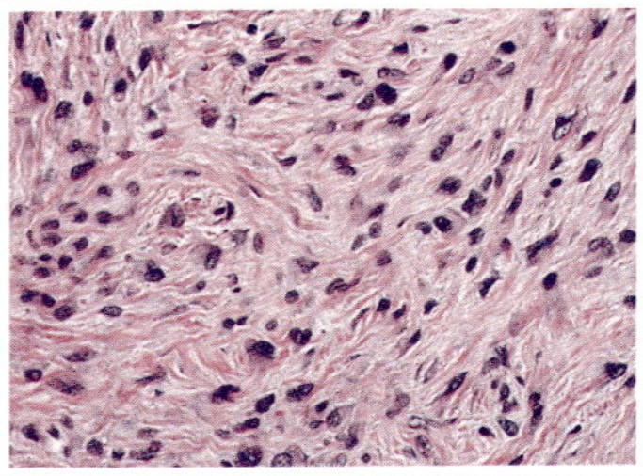
Parosteal osteosarcoma	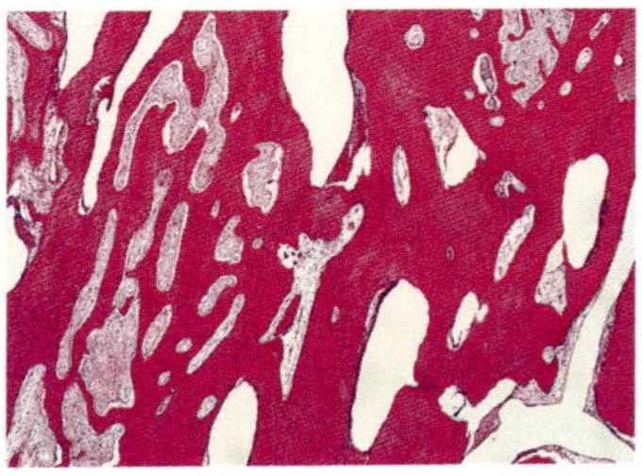	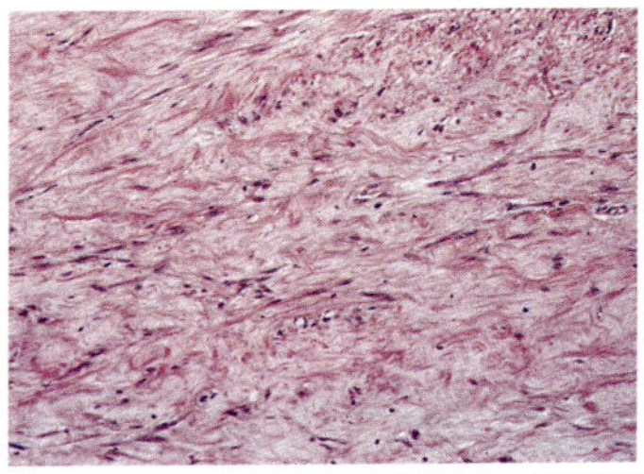

Table 1.11 Nonmesenchymal tumors that may histologically mimic sarcoma

Tumor	Histopathology	Helpful clinical scenario	Useful IHC or molecular tests
Sarcomatoid carcinoma mimicking a spindle cell sarcoma	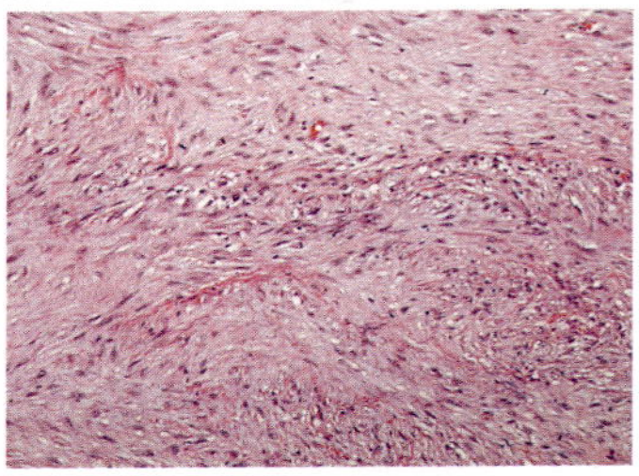	Head and neck tumor in older patient	Keratins and p63 are positive in sarcomatoid squamous carcinoma
Sarcomatoid breast carcinoma mimicking angiosarcoma	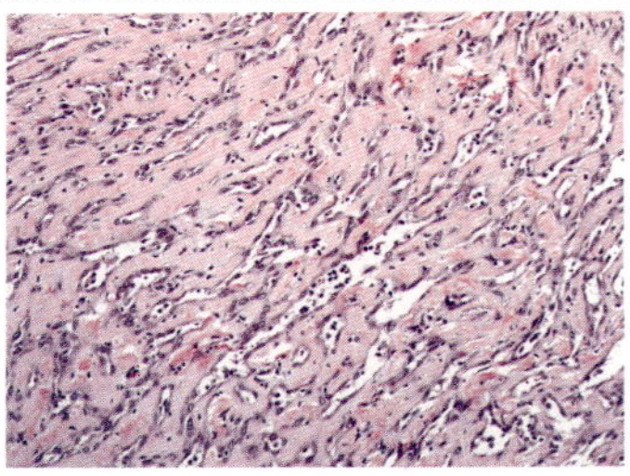	Breast location or history of breast carcinoma	Keratins, MOC31, ER, PR (unlikely to be reactive, however). Lack of reactivity for endothelial markers such as CD34, CD31, ERG (C terminus directed)
Melanoma which can mimic a small round blue cell sarcoma, a sarcoma with epithelioid cells, a spindle cell sarcoma or pleomorphic sarcoma	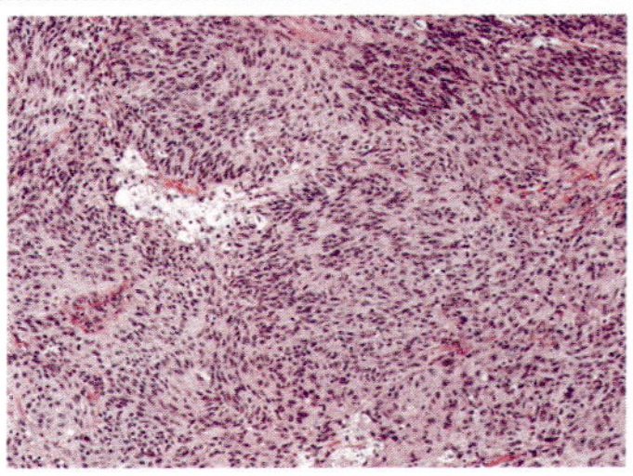	History of melanoma, even if remote	Melanocytic markers including S-100 protein, HMB45, Melan-A, MiTF, BRAF mutation analysis, c-kit mutation analysis

Table 1.11: Continued from page 16

Tumor	Histopathology	Helpful clinical scenario	Useful IHC or molecular tests
Follicular dendritic cell sarcoma mimicking a spindle cell sarcoma	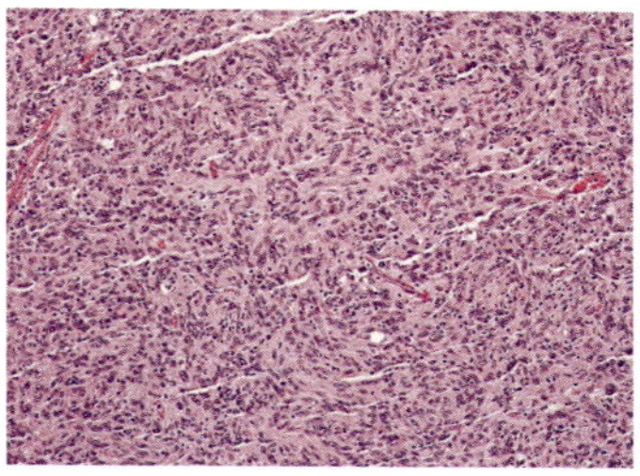	May arise in a lymph node or in soft tissue	Clusterin, fascin, CD21, CD23, CD35
True histiocytic sarcoma mimicking a spindle cell or polygonal cell sarcoma	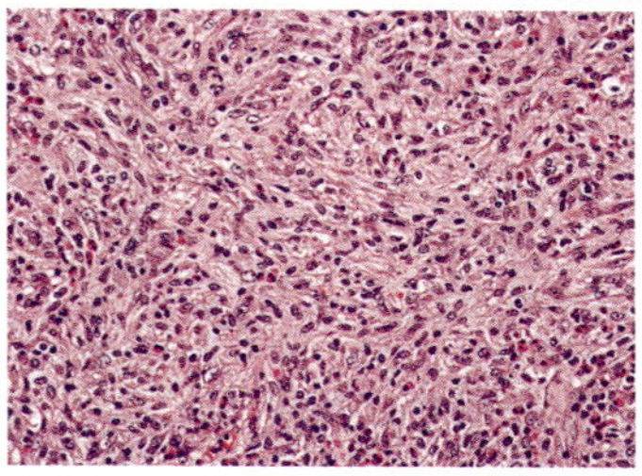	This can easily present as a soft tissue neoplasm, but it is very rare	CD163, CD68, lysozyme positive in tumor cells

soft tissue tumors which otherwise might seem straightforward from the relatively few number of actual entities (WHO 2013 lists 112 soft tissue tumors and 51 bone tumors). **Table 1.12** lists some of the mesenchymal tumors that can exhibit a diverse range of histologic appearances.

Some genetic findings are not tumor specific

Mesenchymal tumors, including sarcomas, may be normal diploid in chromosome complement. Finding a normal karyotype can be helpful when a tumor with a known specific translocation is in the diagnostic differential. However, it is important to establish the level of confidence in a diploid karyotype, as it may represent overgrowth of normal cells and thus an artifact of the assay.

Approximately half of sarcomas exhibit a complex aneuploid karyotype without distinguishing, consistently recurrent abnormalities. Another, approximately 50% of sarcomas demonstrate a specific finding, typically a balanced translocation, on genetic analysis. This can be immensely helpful diagnostically and may prove increasingly useful in targeted therapy development. Some translocation specific sarcoma, as this group is termed, also may show secondary genetic abnormalities, and some of these may affect prognosis.

Finally, a few tumors that are discordant histologically and in behavior contain identical translocations (this has been termed 'tumor infidelity for fusion transcripts')(Romeo et al. 2010). One paired example is angiomatoid fibrous histiocytoma and clear cell sarcoma which share two translocations: t(12;22) = *EWS-ATF1* and t(2;22) = *EWS-CREB1*. These two tumors look different microscopically, show a different antibody staining profile, and one is usually benign, while the other is malignant. Thus, clinical, radiologic, histologic, antigenic, and even genetic findings must be evaluated in context and in toto to guarantee a conclusive, accurate diagnosis.

Cytogenetic analysis may be unsuccessful

Despite rapidly triaging fresh tumor in a sterile fashion and submitting it quickly to the cytogenetics laboratory for processing, up to 50% of mesenchymal tumors do not subsequently grow in culture, and therefore karyotyping fails. Fortunately, for some specific tumors, an alternate path may be taken to uncover the genetic profile of the tumor. Formalin-fixed, paraffin embedded blocks or touch preps may be used for FISH examination for translocations and other aberrations such as gene amplification. The polymerase chain reaction (PCR) can reveal specific mutational changes. Direct sequencing can provide voluminous information but also can be 'directed' to specific genetic sites. The costs of these tests vary, the availability may be limited, and for FISH and PCR, a specific pre-test probability drives the choice of probes: these are not 'fishing expeditions'. Despite its expense and test complexity, genetic evaluation is becoming increasing important not just diagnostically, but it can also predict behavior and response to therapy.

Still in many cases, it is not yet essential for patient care.

Mesenchymal sarcomas are not always specifically diagnosable

Even an expert soft tissue or bone pathologist will be unable to classify ~5-10% of cases in terms of rendering a specific tumor diagnosis. This impairs prognostication and therapy selection. An example of an unclassifiable tumor is provided in **Figure 1.11**. With continuing refinement of the molecular classification of mesenchymal tumors, the percentage of unclassifiable lesions should fall.

Consulting a bone or soft tissue pathologist in difficult cases is advantageous, as these individuals not only have personal depth of experience but can also access the most advanced diagnostic techniques. Most importantly, the patient's treatment may be optimized as a consequence of subspecialist pathologist review; at a minimum, the patient will be counseled regarding the likely disease course.

OVERVIEW OF EPIDEMIOLOGY OF SARCOMAS

Compared with lung, prostate, breast, and colorectal carcinoma, sarcomas afflict only a few. Bone sarcomas are 5-6 fold less common

Table 1.12 Some mesenchymal tumors that have a diverse array of histologic appearances

Tumor	Possible histologic appearances	Example 1	Example 2
Myxofibrosarcoma	Low grade myxoid hypocellular tumor ranging to high grade sarcomatous areas with sheets of pleomorphic tumor cells, epithelioid areas, osteoclastic giant cell rich areas	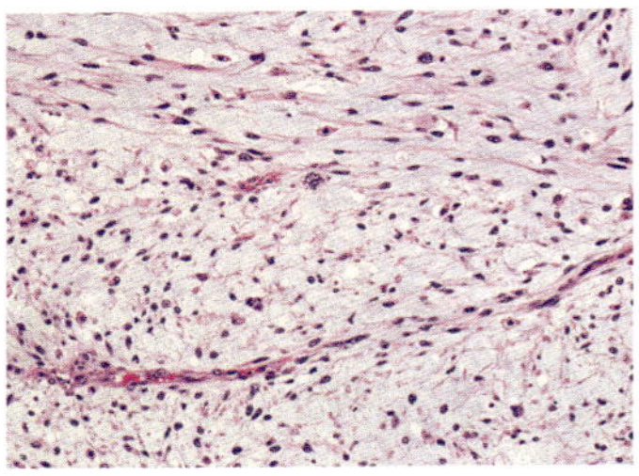	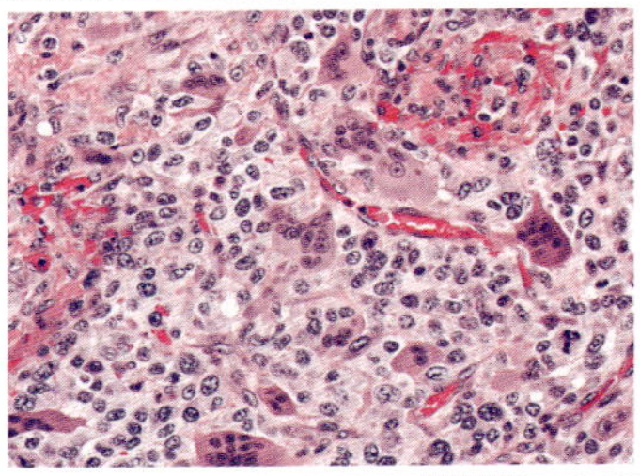
Dedifferentiated liposarcoma	May have well-differentiated areas, metaplastic malignant cartilage, bone, muscle, obscuring inflammation	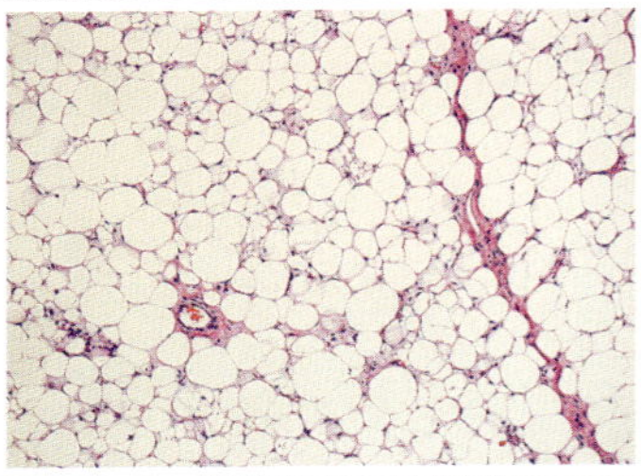	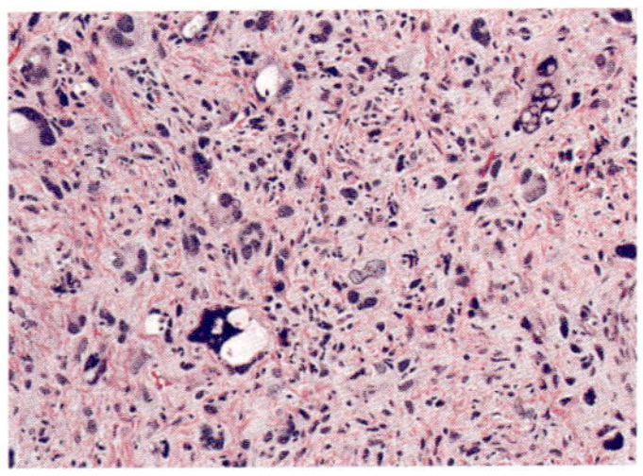
Synovial sarcoma	Fascicles of crowded plump spindle cells that overlap to hypocellular collagenized calcified areas to areas with true epithelial gland formation to focal myxoid areas	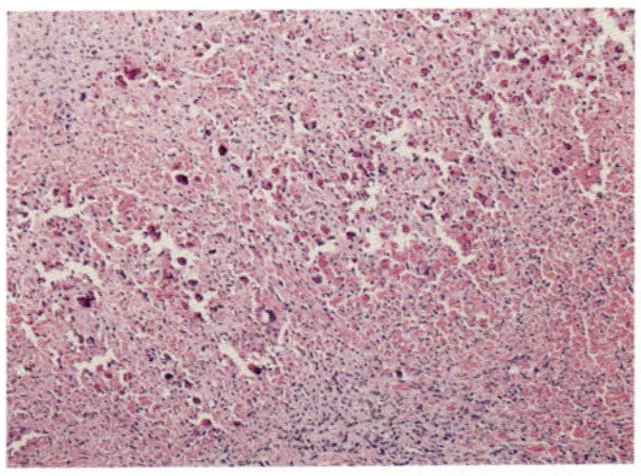	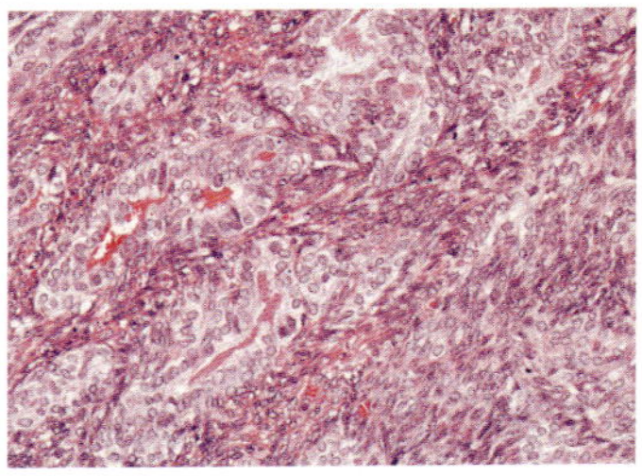
Malignant PEComa	High grade perivascular epithelioid tumor cells to fascicles of lower grade spindle cells	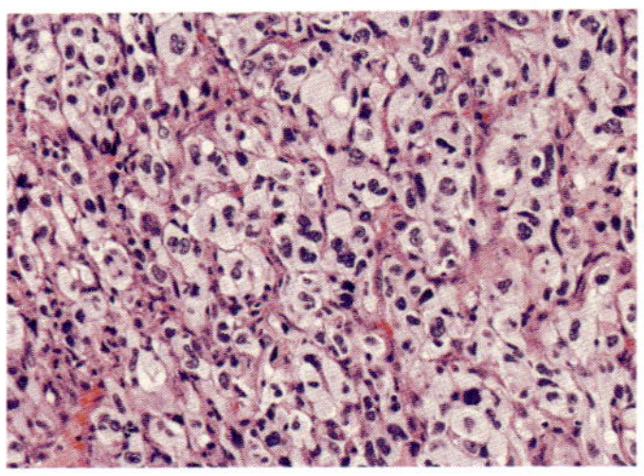	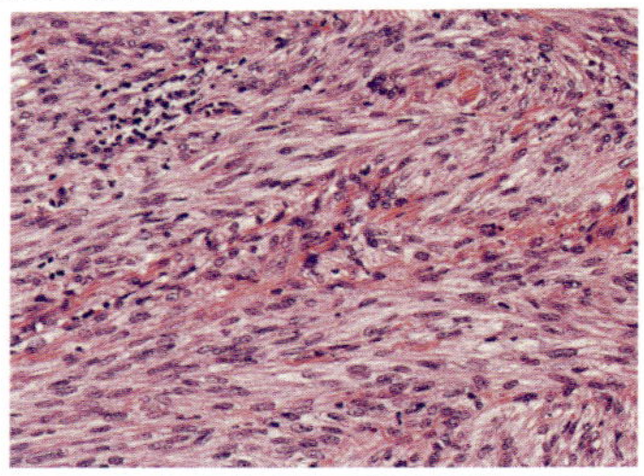
Leiomyosarcoma	Fascicles of spindled eosinophilic cells with scattered markedly atypical cells to myxoid tumors to epithelioid tumors, to heavily inflamed tumors to tumors with many osteoclastic giant cells	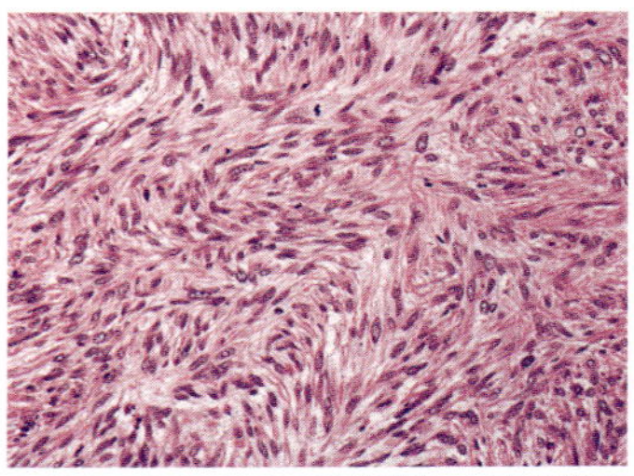	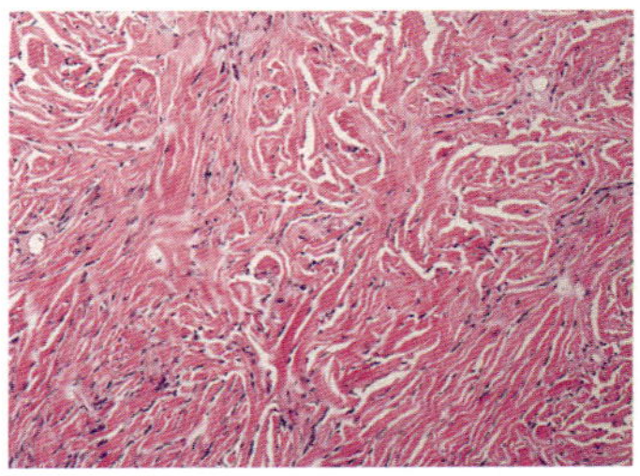
Malignant peripheral nerve sheath MPNST	Fascicles and herringbones of overlapping spindled tumor cells (mimicking classic spindle cell SS) to epithelioid tumors, to low grade hypocellular myxoid tumors to tumors with glands or skeletal muscle differentiation	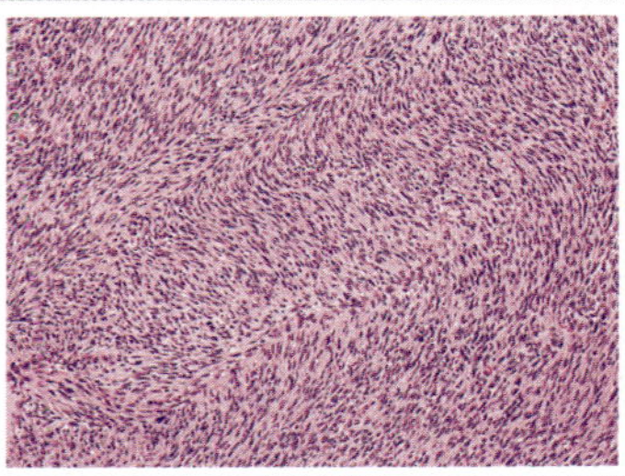	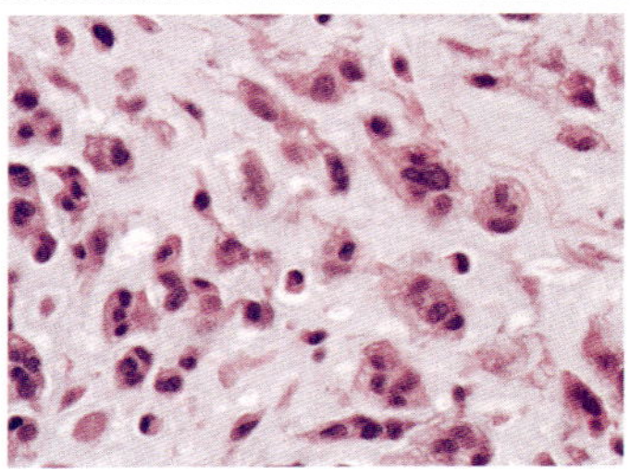

All of the tumors in this table can exhibit multiple histologic appearances, not just the two patterns shown.

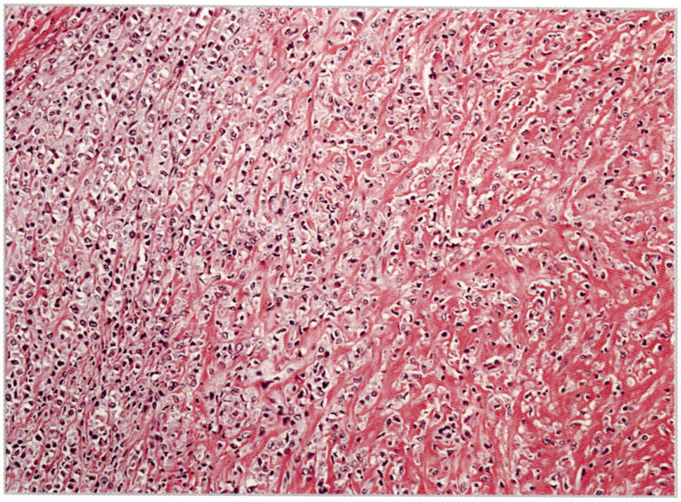

Figure 1.11 Sarcoma with epithelioid features unable to further classify, medium magnification. This is an example of a tumor that could not be specifically subclassified. It was reviewed by an expert sarcoma pathologist who employed IHC and FISH to attempt to better define it. The consultant concluded that it was difficult to predict its behavior but would likely at least locally recur. The patient, a woman in her 20s, rapidly developed multiple bone metastases and died of disease within 8 months of presentation despite complete resection and intensive chemotherapy. This case indicates there is still work to be done in mesenchymal tumor classification and prognostication.

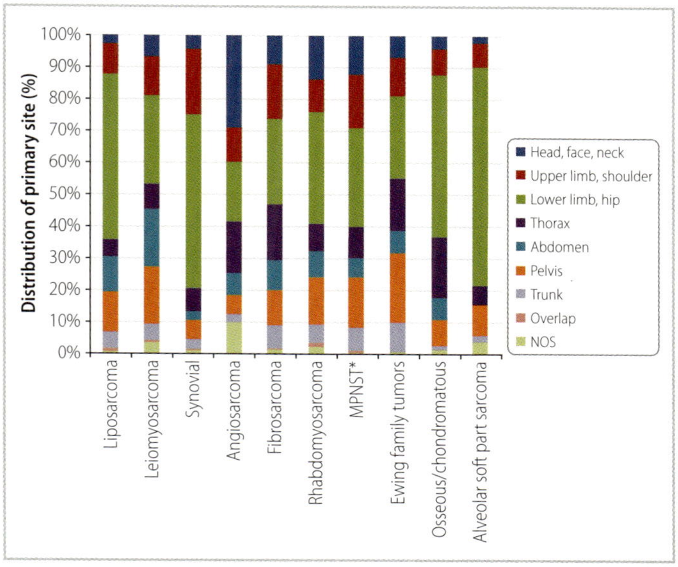

Figure 1.12 Distribution of primary site by soft tissue tumor type for adults aged 20 years and older in 13 SEER registries diagnosed between 1994 and 2008.

than soft tissue sarcomas. A recent review of cases occurring in the Rhone-Alpes region of 6 million inhabitants noted age standardized incidence rates of soft tissue, visceral and bone sarcomas of 3.6, 2.0, and 0.6 per 100,000/year with GIST (18%), unclassified sarcoma (16%), liposarcoma (15%), and leiomyosarcoma (11%) as the most common diagnoses (Ducimetiere et al. 2011). Surveillance Epidemiology and End Results (SEER) U.S. data not subject to central pathology review recorded leiomyosarcoma (many in the uterus), 'malignant fibrous histiocytoma', liposarcoma, and dermatofibrosarcoma protuberans as the most common soft tissue and visceral sarcomas (n = 26,758 cases, years 1978-2001) (Toro et al. 2006). For soft tissue sarcomas, international age adjusted incidence rates range from 1.8-5/year (Wibmer et al. 2010). There is some controversy over whether the incidence is increasing, with some studies reporting, and others refuting, such a trend. Median overall survival of metastatic sarcoma improved by 50% over 1987-2006 according to a French Sarcoma Group study (Italiano et al. 2011).

Figure 1.12 depicts in a histogram format the distribution of major soft tissue sarcomas by primary site according to SEER cases abstracted at 13 SEER sites from 1994-2008. **Figure 1.13** illustrates the same sarcomas according to stage at presentation. Consistent with expectations, most liposarcomas present as localized lesions, while alveolar soft part sarcoma more commonly is high stage at presentation. There are no clear gender differences in the distribution of the major sarcomas (**Fig. 1.14**). Median age and age ranges are provided in **Table 1.13** (again, SEER data for adults over 20 years from 1994-2008, 11 major sarcoma types). Five year relative survival rates are lowest overall for rhabdomyosarcoma and highest overall for liposarcoma (**Fig. 1.15**). In general, younger adults survive longer than older adults though the differences may be minor for some types. Tumors categorized as fibrosarcoma would likely benefit from central pathology review as diagnostic criteria and technological advances may permit reclassification of most tumors in this category.

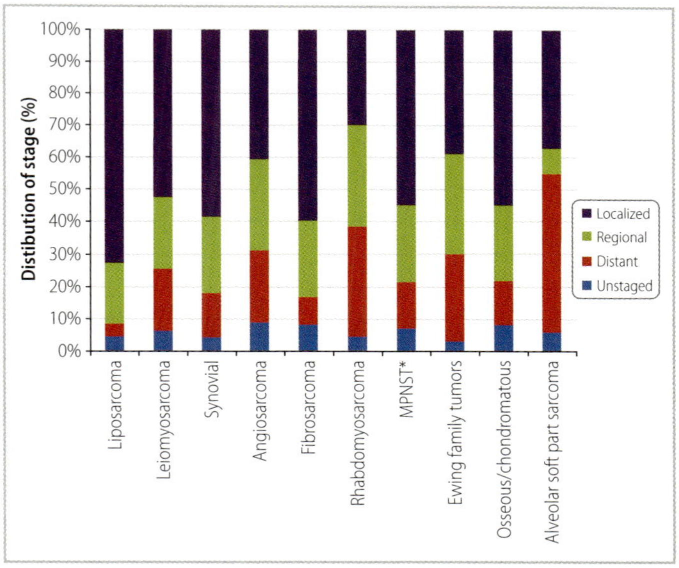

Figure 1.13 Distribution of stage by soft tissue tumor type for adults patients aged 20 years and older in 13 SEER registries diagnosed between 1994 and 2008.

The Surveillance, Epidemiology and End Results (SEER) Program is the data source for the epidemiology sections of this book. SEER was established by the National Cancer Institute in 1973, and it is the primary source for comprehensive, population-based cancer statistics in the US. Currently, the entire program covers 28% of the US population.

The data presented in this book are from cases diagnosed between 1994 and 2008 within 13 SEER Program registries (statewide

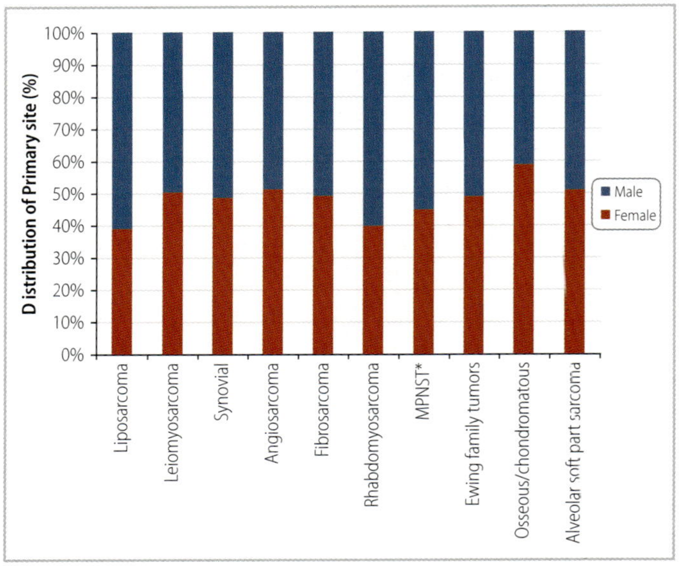

Figure 1.14 Distribution of sex by soft tissue tumor type for adults patients ages 20 years and older in 13 SEER registries diagnosed between 1994 and 2008.

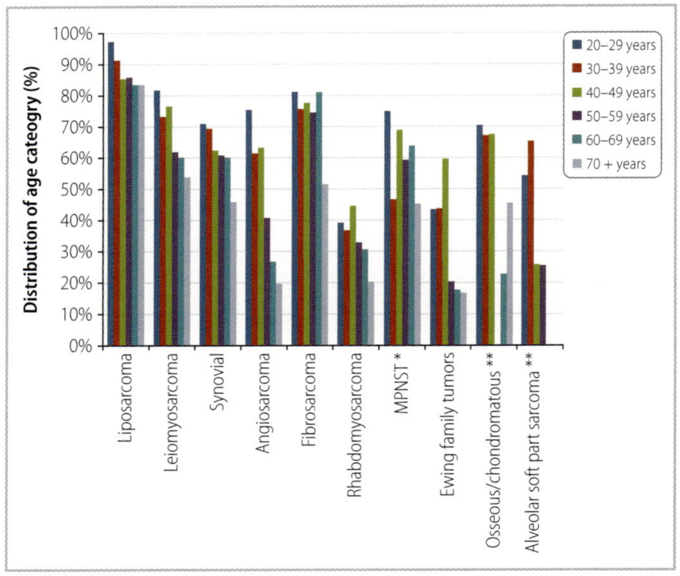

Figure 1.15 Five year relative survival rate of soft tissue tumor types by age category for cases diagnosed in 13 SEER registries diagnosed between 1994 and 2008. [*MPNST = malignant peripheral nerve sheath tumor. ** Relative survival could not be calculated for osseous/chondromatous tumors (50-59 years) and alveolar soft part sarcoma tumors (60-69 years and 70+ years)]

Table 1.13 Characterization of age by soft tissue tumor type for cases diagnosed in 13 SEER registries diagnosed between 1994 and 2008

Tumor type	Total number of cases	Percent pediatric cases**	Median age (years)	Age range (years)
Liposarcoma	2733	1.5%	58.0	1-100
Leiomyosarcoma	2122	1.0%	62.0	0-102
Synovial	794	19.1%	35.0	2-94
Rhabdomyosarcoma	624	60.4%	14.0	0-96
Angiosarcoma	523	2.1%	68.0	0-10
Ewing family tumors	367	40.3%	23.0	0-88
Fibrosarcoma	331	8.2%	52.0	0-97
MPNST *	270	11.5%	46.5	0-93
Osseous/chondromatous	79	7.6%	62.0	10-87
Alveolar soft part sarcoma	71	28.2%	24.0	9-56

* MPNST = Malignant peripheral nerve sheath tumors
** Pediatric cases are ages 0 – 19 years

registries: Connecticut, Hawaii, Iowa, New Mexico, Utah; metropolitan areas: Atlanta, Detroit, Los Angeles, San Francisco-Oakland, San Jose-Monterey, Seattle-Puget Sound; rural areas of Georgia; Alaska Native populations residing in Alaska). The analyses were restricted to malignant tumors and the histology codes are from the International Classification of Diseases for Oncology - Third Edition (ICDO-3). The ICDO-3 coding system was used for the site of the tumor at diagnosis as well. Codes C40.0-C41.9 were used for tumors of the bone (bones, joints and articular cartilage), and C49.0-C49.9 for tumors of the soft tissue (connective, subcutaneous and other soft tissues).

All SEER incidence rates in the upcoming chapters are per million and are age-adjusted to the 2000 US standard population. SEER obtains the population estimates to calculate these rates from the US Census Bureau, and the mortality data are provided by the National Center for Health Statistics.

FUTURE OF MUSCULOSKELETAL PATHOLOGY

The next 10 years should yield major advances in cellular pathobiology that will directly impact the care of patients with bone and soft tissue tumors. Because the human genome has been entirely sequenced, and the 'omes' (proteome, metabolome, epigenome and others) are steadily being explored, increasing numbers of specific, cell pathway-based aberrations will be uncovered in mesenchymal tumors. Molecular genetic approaches, bioinformatics analyses and mathematical tumor modeling will be required to make and understand these discoveries. Eventually, best practice may entail successively biopsying a patient's sarcoma over time to progressively assess tumor evolution and tumor response to therapy.

In 25 years, with enhanced radiologic and serologic tumor detection, many patients will present with smaller lesions amenable to refined surgical excision. Most sarcomas may then be contained, if not cured, by a combination of surgery and targeted, flexible therapy that shifts as the tumor shifts genetically and molecularly.

ADVICE TO MEDICAL STUDENTS AND PATHOLOGY RESIDENTS

Medical students interested in pathology as a career should discuss the field with a pathologist. Shadowing a pathologist would best reveal the vital role this physician plays in patient care. Pathology needs dedicated, inquisitive creative individuals.

Pathology residents particularly fascinated by bone and soft tissue pathology would do well to take an active stance in learning this field by studying as many individual cases as possible including case presentations presented on national pathology websites and actively participating in case sign outs and tumor boards. Few fellowships exist in bone and soft tissue pathology. However, anatomic pathology is edging ever more into the submicroscopic realm, and a combination of a strong traditional surgical pathology background with expertise in genetic molecular analysis of tumors is an optimal preparation for addressing these tumors in one's professional career.

The practice of pathology is not an independent one. The anatomic pathologist depends on the clinical members of the patient care team including the radiologist, medical oncologist, surgeon, and radiation-oncologist. In return, the musculoskeletal pathologist, by typing the tumor, fundamentally determines the patient's therapy. Close collaboration with clinical colleagues impels improved diagnosis and opens opportunities for advancing the field. This collegiality catalyzes the pathologist and champions the patient.

REFERENCES

Barretina J, Taylor BS, Banerji S, et al. Subtype specific genome alterations define new targets for soft-tissue sarcoma therapy. Nat Genetics 2010;42:715–723.

Bridge JA. Advances and limitations of cytogenetic, molecular cytogenetic and molecular diagnostic testing in mesenchymal neoplasms. J Orthop Science 2008;13:273–282.

Brooks, SJ. Disorders of soft tissue. In: Mills, SE. Sternberg's Diagnostic Surgical Pathology, 5th ed. Baltimore: Wolters Kluwer/Lippincott Williams and Wilkins: 2010.

Ducimetiere F, Lurkin A, Ranchere-Vince D, et al. Incidence of sarcoma histotypes and molecular subtypes in a prospective epidemiological study with central pathology review and molecular testing. PLOS One 2011;6:e20294. 1–14.

Fisher C. Soft tissue sarcomas with non-EWS translocations: molecular genetic features and pathologic and clinical correlations. Virch Arch 2010;456:153–166.

Gibault L, Perot G, Chibon F, et al. New insights in sarcoma oncogenesis: a comprehensive analysis of a large series of 160 soft tissue sarcomas with complex genomics. J Pathol 2011;223:64–71.

Guillou L, Aurias A. Soft tissue sarcomas with complex genomic profiles. Virch Arch 2010;456:201–217.

Italiano A, Mathoulin-Pelissier S, Le Cesne A, et al. Trends in survival for patients with metastatic soft tissue sarcoma. Cancer 2011;117:1049–1054.

Jin Y, Moller E, Nord KH, et al. Fusion of the AHRR and NCOA2 genes through a recurrent translocation t(5;8)(p15;q13) in soft tissue angiofibroma results in upregulation of aryl hydrocarbon receptor target genes. Genes Chromosomes Cancer 2012;51:510–520.

Ordonez JL, Osuna D, Garcia-Dominguez DJ, et al. The clinical relevance of molecular genetics in soft tissue sarcomas. Adv Anat Pathol 2010;17:162–181.

Romeo S, Duim RA, Bridge JA, et al. Heterogeneous and complex rearrangements of chromosome arm 6q in chondromyxoid fibroma: delineation of breakpoints and analysis of candidate genes. Am J Pathol 2010;177:1365–76.

Sjogren H, Orndal C, Tingby O, et al. Cytogenetic and spectral karyotype analysis of benign and malignant cartilage tumors. Int J Oncol 2004;24:1385–91.

Toro JR, Travis LB, Wu HJ, et al. Incidence patterns of soft tissue sarcomas, regardless of primary site, in the Surveillance, Epidemiology and End Results program, 1978-2001: an analysis of 26,758 cases. Int J Cancer 2006;119:2922–2930.

Toro JR, Travis LB, Wu HJ, et al. Incidence patterns of soft tissue sarcomas, regardless of primary site, in the Surveillance, Epidemiology, and End Results program, 1978-2001: an analysis of 26,758 cases. Int J Cancer 2006;119:2922–2930.

Verweij J, Baker LH. Future treatment of soft tissue sarcomas will be driven by histological subtype and molecular alterations. Eur J Cancer 2010;46:863-868.

Wang L, Motoi T, Khanin R, et al. Identification of a novel, recurrent HEY1-NCOA2 fusion in mesenchymal chondrosarcoma based on a genome-wide screen of exon-level expression data. Genes Chromosomes Cancer 2012;51:127–139.

Wibmer C, Leithner A, Zielonke N, et al. Increasing incidence rates of soft tissue sarcomas? A population-based epidemiologic study and literature review. Ann Oncol 2010;21(5):1106–11.

Yasuda T, Nishio J, Sumegi J, et al. Aberrations of 6q13 mapped to the COL12A1 locus in chondromyxoid fibroma. Mod Pathol 2009;22:1499–506.

FURTHER READING

Fletcher CDM, Bridge JA, Hogendoorn P, Mertens F (eds). World Health Organization Classification of Tumours of Soft Tissue and Bone, 4th Ed. Lyon: IARC Press, 2013.

Chapter 2 Radiology overview of soft tissue and bone tumors

RADIOLOGY

Sarcoma imaging is a challenging and at times daunting task for the radiologist. There are a myriad of differing tumors that occur throughout the musculoskeletal system and the imaging appearances of the benign and malignant tumors have extensive overlap. The radiologist plays a crucial role in the multidisciplinary care of a patient with sarcoma. In this section, we will discuss the imaging modalities, imaging strategies and the various tasks of the radiologist in caring for sarcoma patients.

The radiologist fulfills multiple roles in the care of sarcoma patients. At some institutions, the diagnostic or interventional radiologist may acquire the tissue for diagnosis by performing imaging guided percutaneous needle biopsy of a lesion. This should always be done after conferring with the sarcoma surgeon to assure that an appropriate biopsy route is used. There is a potential for tumor seeding of the needle tract and many surgeons will actually excise the needle tract to assure local tumor control. An error in biopsy route could potentially prevent limb salvage surgery resulting instead in unnecessary amputation. Also, the physician performing the biopsy should carefully consider the target area within a tumor. The non-enhancing portion of a tumor could represent matrix or necrotic material and may not yield diagnostic tissue for the pathologist. Some tumors have large feeding or draining vessels, these should be avoided to minimize potential hemorrhage risk. Depending on the vessels and surgical setting, interventional radiologist at some institutions will provide preoperative embolization of tumors to mitigate surgical blood loss.

Diagnostically, the radiologist has a difficult and often humbling task in sarcoma imaging. The referral environment of a given case affects the radiologist's role. In the United States, a primary care provider ordering, say an MR exam of a new palpable mass may be a physician assistant, nurse practitioner or a physician. Each may work in relative isolation or may have ready access to specialist consultation. The radiologist must be responsive to these differing practice situations to be optimally helpful to the patient. Our recommendations to 'follow up' or 'correlate clinically' may be pointless without detailed instructions. As a radiologist, we need to specify the imaging modality to be used and time frame for follow up. Also, we must specify what exactly is to be clinically correlated. Typically, masses that are painful or enlarging are much more ominous for malignancy, and we should be explicit about these symptoms and history being important for correct interpretation of the imaging study. Best is for the radiologist to contact the referring provider to discuss the findings and specific next steps. Of course, if the referring provider is a sarcoma specialist, then such detailed instructions are likely superfluous.

As for diagnostic interpretation, the radiologist should provide basic information such as tumor size, location and effect on adjacent structures. Generally speaking the larger a tumor, the greater the risk of malignancy and the greater the risk a given malignancy has already metastasized. The radiologist should be precise in their description of location within a given bone; diaphysis, metaphysis or epiphysis as well as intramedullary, eccentric or cortical. Measuring the lesion's distance from an easily identifiable landmark, such as a joint line, can aid others in locating the lesion at time of surgery or biopsy or when correlating findings with other imaging modalities. Likewise, the location of a soft tissue tumor in a given compartment and its proximity or invasion of vital structures such as nerve and vessels is crucial for treatment planning. Surgical planning may change depending on the tumor's effect on adjacent structures such as the presence of neural foraminal encroachment or bowel involvement.

The tumor's effect on adjacent structures may reveal its chronicity and aggressiveness. A tumor may show pressure-like 'erosion' of bone where the surface of the cortex remains smooth and intact with minimal or no thinning of the cortex. This absence of invasion suggesting the lesion is long standing and likely benign. A non-aggressive lesion may appear to 'push' or displace adjacent muscle and vessels as opposed to invading or encasing them. Aggressive tumors usually show frank invasion and actual destruction of adjacent soft tissues. However, early in a tumor's course, invasion may occur focally and the radiologist must analyze the entire tumor's margin carefully.

Radiologists often interpret non-enhancing portions of the tumor as necrotic tissue. This is generally true for other tumors, say in the liver or brain, but with sarcomas, the non-enhancing tissue may represent viable hypovascular tissue such as matrix or fibrous tissue. Additionally, sarcomas may have non-enhancing portions due to cystic or gelatinous areas without necrosis, or they may have spontaneous hemorrhage with accumulated blood degradation products. The distinction from necrosis is important because tumors with more necrotic areas tend to be higher grade with more aggressive behavior and poorer prognosis. Unfortunately, correct identification of sarcoma necrosis is difficult with any imaging modality. Dynamic enhancement MR imaging may prove to be useful to distinguish sarcoma necrosis and may be an important field for future research. Furthermore, on follow up imaging, radiologists tend to interpret the development of non-enhancing portions of a tumor as indicative of positive response to radiation or chemotherapy. This conclusion may not be true for sarcoma and the care team must be guarded in their optimism about new areas without enhancement.

A central diagnostic task for the radiologist is the assessment of a tumor's aggressiveness. In general, a homogeneous soft tissue mass without enhancement, destructive features or adjacent reactive changes is less worrisome for malignancy and the radiologist can report the tumor as 'non-aggressive'. Since the imaging appearance cannot render a definitive histologic diagnosis, the radiologist should refrain from reporting such a non-aggressive tumor as 'benign'. Even a non-aggressive appearing tumor could represent an indolent malignancy. Regardless of this fundamental uncertainty, the radiologist's non-aggressive label can reassure the patient and referring doctors that a conservative approach may be reasonable. Conservative management may simply involve monitoring the tumor size over time with physical exam or imaging studies. The interval for surveillance is based on judgment and experience. There are patient factors relevant to this decision. If the patient is a competent individual and an excellent historian, then one might be confident with a long surveillance interval of say, 1 year. On the other hand, many patients in reality are not sure when their mass developed. Often there are associated symptoms such as pain; however the etiology of the pain is uncertain because there may be an adjacent arthritic joint or recent injury compounding the clinical setting. This common confusing clinical situation may undermine confidence in conservative management pushing the care team to pursue immediate tissue diagnosis or at least a shorter interval for imaging surveillance. The radiologist must avoid allowing imaging intervals less than 3 months as tumors usually won't have changed significantly. Rendering an interpretation that a tumor is stable during a 1 or 2 month interval may be falsely reassuring to the patient and referring team.

Occasionally, we encounter a case that proves to be a cyst on imaging. The radiologist must exercise discipline in diagnosing a cyst which should have no enhancement, no nodularity, minimal if any septation and must show fluid characteristics on the imaging study. Each imaging modality has a distinct strategy for correctly identifying fluid and a fastidious approach is necessary to avoid errantly diagnosing a featureless solid tumor as a cyst. Cysts of the musculoskeletal system are relatively rare and can be seen from remote prior injury with resulting seroma. An adventitial bursa can form de novo from repetitive mechanical irritation of a site. Usually, a referral for possible cyst will actually reveal a lymph node or solid mass that requires further workup or, at least follow up to establish stability. The radiologist must avoid the pitfall of a fluid collection that is actually a cyst dissecting from elsewhere such as a Baker's cyst of the knee extending into the calf, or a paralabral or parameniscal cyst extending away from the joint. As always the radiologist must be wary of an unusual bowel hernia or vascular lesion such as an aneurysm accounting for the clinically suspected 'cyst'.

Finding a tumor with aggressive features such as heterogeneity, hemorrhage, enhancement, invasion or destruction of adjacent tissues, the radiologist can report a worrisome or aggressive tumor and recommend referral to a sarcoma surgeon. However, even an aggressive appearing lesion may be benign as abscess and hematoma can look similar to a sarcoma. If the clinical setting strongly supports the diagnosis of hematoma or abscess, then appropriate conservative management can be initiated. At our institution we recommend follow up to document complete resolution. Depending on the specific case, adequate follow up may simply entail physical exam alone or may require imaging if the lesion is deep seated. The underlying concern is a sarcoma can have hemorrhage and/or hematoma which may obscure the underlying true pathology. Furthermore, the hematoma could conceivably become secondarily infected and develop an abscess. It is important to perform the follow up imaging after complete clinical resolution has occurred or else the imaging study will simply show a resolving process and an underlying occult neoplasm will not yet be excludable without another follow up imaging exam.

When faced with the numerous tumors that have non-specific and overlapping appearances, the radiologist may become inured to their diagnostic task. But we must not surrender our efforts to find the subtle or unique features that may enable a more specific diagnosis. Patient age and tumor location alone can often generate a useful differential diagnosis for bone tumors. Occasionally, we can discern a specific tumor matrix such as cartilage, fibrous or bone tissue that can narrow the differential diagnosis significantly. Soft tissue tumors are generally more difficult to diagnose specifically. However, there may be identifiable tissues such as fat, calcification or hemorrhage that can help narrow the diagnosis. Likewise, there may be an association with a nerve or vessel that can aid in diagnosis.

In the follow up phase of sarcoma patient care, the radiologist must image the location of tumor origin for recurrence and search for distant metastasis. Generally, the lung is the most common site for sarcoma metastasis, with marrow and liver being less common and regional adenopathy being an unusual site of metastasis. The typical imaging surveillance interval is 6 months. However, if there is greater clinical concern due to high tumor grade or tumor involvement of surgical margins, a 3-month interval is sometimes employed. Generally, the chest is imaged with contrast enhanced CT to assess for lung metastasis. The bone or soft tissue compartment of origin is imaged with contrast enhanced MRI. The radiologist must assure that the entire bone or soft tissue compartment is included in the exam. Recurrences usually occur at the original tumor site, but can occur anywhere within the surgical bed or compartment. To facilitate adequate imaging coverage and interpretation, we have surface imaging markers placed on any palpable lesion, as well as, at the proximal and distal ends of the surgical scar. Ideally, the MR exams should be performed with the identical imaging sequences, slice thickness and field of view to minimize inter-exam variation and foster accuracy in assessing the stability of a lesion or evolution of post-operative change. PET imaging is rarely utilized for sarcoma imaging due to the variable and unreliable uptake by these tumors and their metastasis. Overall, patient care is best optimized by a thoughtful and dedicated radiologist who can work well with the sarcoma team of care givers.

FUTURE DIRECTIONS OF SARCOMA IMAGING

The future of sarcoma imaging will likely gain in specificity as more sophisticated imaging technology develops. Molecular imaging based on tissue specific or even tumor specific markers may improve diagnostic accuracy and increase the sensitivity and specificity of surveillance imaging.

Dynamic enhanced imaging techniques may better characterize tumor vascularity. This is currently employed with breast MR imaging where a graph showing the speed of contrast wash in and wash out from a tumor has proven to be useful to distinguish benign from malignant breast lesion. A similar graph of dynamic MR enhancement may help distinguish benign from malignant soft tissue tumor, and may allow imaging assessment of tumor grade. Furthermore, changes in a tumor's dynamic enhancement may indicate response to radiation or chemotherapy in the neoadjuvant treatment setting.

Another avenue of future sarcoma imaging research may lie in the mathematical modeling and study of the imaging data set. Cross sectional imaging provides three dimensional imaging data of a tumor which could provide the basis for applying mathematical interrogation techniques of a tumor for specific objective features. Vittorio Cristini has performed mathematical modeling of the surface of brain tumors showing correlation with tumor grade and invasiveness (Bearer 2009). In the setting of sarcoma, there are two potential surfaces of interest. The outer surface of a sarcoma interfaces with normal host tissue and its features may correlate with invasive potential. Additionally, sarcomas often are quite heterogeneous internally and hence, have other tissue interfaces that may be of interest, such as between enhancing and non-enhancing areas. Such an internal interface may represent a boundary between matrix producing portions and cellular portions of the tumor.

A different avenue for mathematical modeling would be to study the voxel to voxel (VTV) heterogeneity of a tumor. MR imaging is capable of demonstrating tissue based on different molecular features (i.e. T1 or T2 relaxation, enhancement, diffusion, etc.). For instance, the study of a tumor's T2 relaxation heterogeneity may prove to correlate with differences in intercellular water or may indicate differences in cellular density. Presumably, high grade tumors would show greater VTV heterogeneity, say on T2 images, and this may correlate with the presence of multiple cell lines. Or, there may be high VTV on post contrast images which might correlate with high levels of neo-angiogenesis and greater metastatic potential.

INFORMATION FOR MEDICAL STUDENTS AND RESIDENTS

Sarcoma imaging is a subspecialty of musculoskeletal diagnostic radiology. Those interested in the field would typically complete a diagnostic radiology residency and then a fellowship in musculoskeletal imaging. As sarcomas are relatively rare, it can take considerable time to acquire relevant experience and large referral centers would offer an educational advantage to an interested student.

RADIOGRAPHS

It may seem surprising that in the age of cross sectional imaging the simple plain radiograph remains the imaging cornerstone of diagnosis in bone tumors. The radiograph is easy and inexpensive to acquire yet usually shows fundamental features such as location, matrix and aggressiveness. The radiograph in fact is often the best overall depiction of a tumor's aggressiveness by showing its zone of transition, periosteal reaction and bone destruction.

As described above, an indolent lesion may cause thinning of the overlying cortex presumably from pressure of the slow growing lesion against the cortex resulting in bone remodeling. A more aggressive lesion would have destroyed the cortex and created frayed lesion margins. Pressure erosion can create a gently scalloped appearance to the thinned cortex. **Figure 2.1** shows an enchondroma of the finger with scalloped thinning of the cortex but no breakthrough and no fraying of bone.

Aggressive lesions cause bone destruction which appears as cortical erosion or trabecular loss. Generally, any loss of cortex is worrisome and may indicate a destructive or aggressive process. However, cortical erosion is not specific and can be seen with infection, rheumatologic disease, metabolic disease such as hyperparathyroidism and neoplastic process. Active cortical erosion will have indistinct margins that look frayed or will appear as if the bone is melting. **Figure 2.2** shows active erosive destruction of the plantar calcaneus in a patient with Reiter's (Reactive) arthropathy. Note how the bone appears to be melting away resulting in an indistinct and fuzzy margin. **Figure 2.3** shows a patient with psoriatic arthropathy who has both active and healed appearing erosions of the interphalangeal joints. All of the erosions show loss of bone, however, the active erosions has the indistinct edges while the healed erosions show white cortical bone margin.

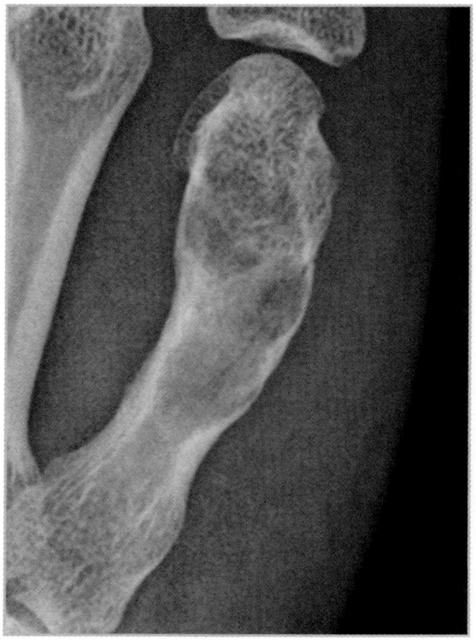

Figure 2.1 Enchondroma. Anteroposterior radiograph of the hand showing a lucent mildly expansile lesion of the 5th metacarpal. There is a non-displaced pathologic fracture. There is no identifiable matrix. Note the endosteal scalloping and smooth cortical thinning. This is a typical appearance of an enchondroma in the hand, these typically do not have calcified matrix.

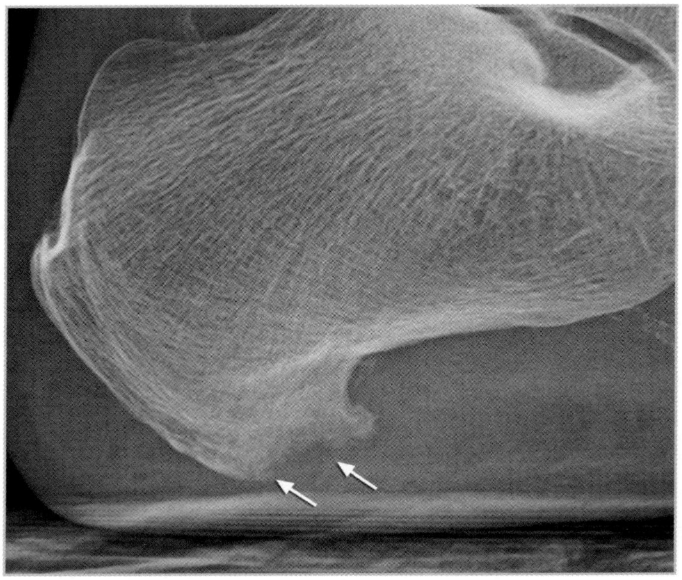

Figure 2.2 Reiter's disease erosion. Lateral radiograph of the heel in a 64 year old man with Reiter's (reactive) arthropathy. There is active erosion of bone along the plantar aspect of the calcaneus, arrows. Note how active erosion appears to melt the bone away.

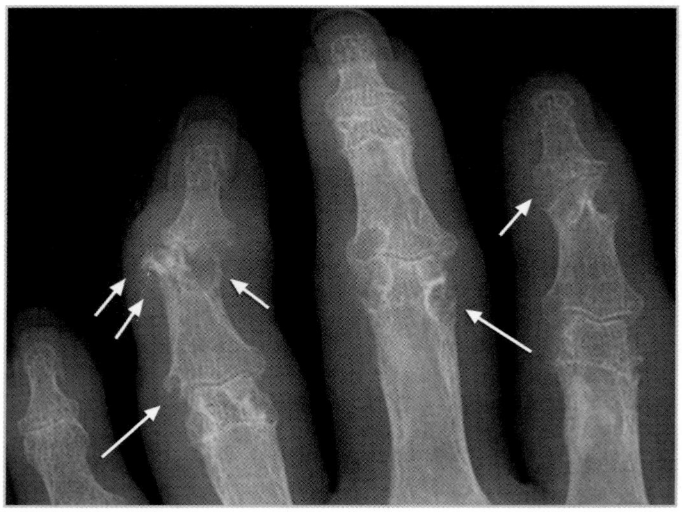

Figure 2.3 Psoriatic arthropathy. Close up of an anteroposterior view of the fingers in a 75 year old woman. There are active erosions shown by the small arrows. The active erosions show indistinct margins. The large arrows indicate healed or quiescent erosions which have corticated, smooth margins.

Cortical erosion can involve the outer surface or the endosteal surface of the cortex. Bone destruction can involve a broad area, as seen in a large osteosarcoma or may be focal as seen with a portion of an enchondroma that has dedifferentiated into a chondrosarcoma, see **Figure 2.4**. Loss of trabeculae can be a subtle finding only visible as decreased density, loss of trabecular crispness or an area with homogeneous, featureless appearance. **Figure 2.5** shows an osteosarcoma causing trabecular destruction and loss of density along the lateral femoral metaphysis. Frank bone destruction can result in a permeative pattern as seen in **Figure 2.6**. This highly aggressive bone destruction gives the appearance that the bone is melting away. **Figure 2.7** shows numerous lytic defects of the skull which has been termed; 'moth-eaten' pattern or the 'pepper pot' pattern of bone destruction classically seen in multiple myeloma.

The zone of transition is a geometric concept that describes the shortest distance between a point that is entirely in normal bone and a point that is entirely inside the lesion. A wide zone of transition indicates invasive margins of an aggressive lesion. **Figure 2.8** shows a metastasis with permeative destruction of the femoral diaphysis and a wide zone of transition. On the other hand, a narrow zone of transition indicates an indolent lesion with normal, healthy bone abutting the surface of the lesion. The extreme example of a narrow zone of transition is a sclerotic boarder indicating there has been prolong period of lesion stability allowing normal bone to form a corticated boarder successfully containing the lesion. **Figure 2.9** shows a non-ossifying fibroma with a sclerotic margin of uniform thickness. There is also a pathologic fracture of the medial cortex.

Periosteal reaction is a sign of bone inflammation and healing. Initially, periosteal reaction is lucent and with time ossifies and becomes dense, eventually remodeling into a thickened cortex. Laminated periosteal reaction (**Fig. 2.10**) may form if there is a rapid or stuttering course of disease causing layers of healing, alternating

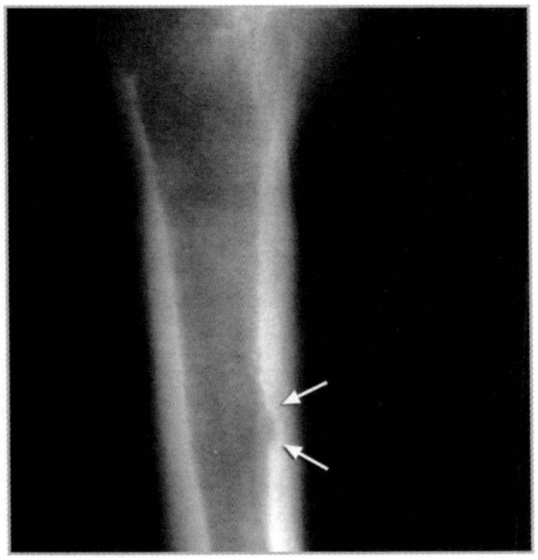

Figure 2.4 Grade 3 chondrosarcoma. Close up of an anteroposterior radiograph of the proximal femur. The arrows indicate a focus of endosteal erosion. The chondrosarcoma was very large involving the entire proximal femur yet only this small focus of tumor was destroying cortex.

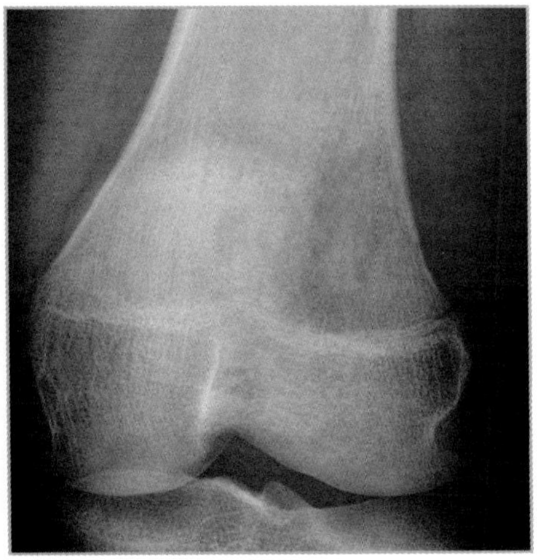

Figure 2.5 Osteosarcoma. Anteroposterior radiograph of the distal femur shows subtle loss of bone density in the lateral aspect of the metaphysis indicating a lesion destroying trabeculae. The cortex appears intact and no soft tissue mass is yet evident.

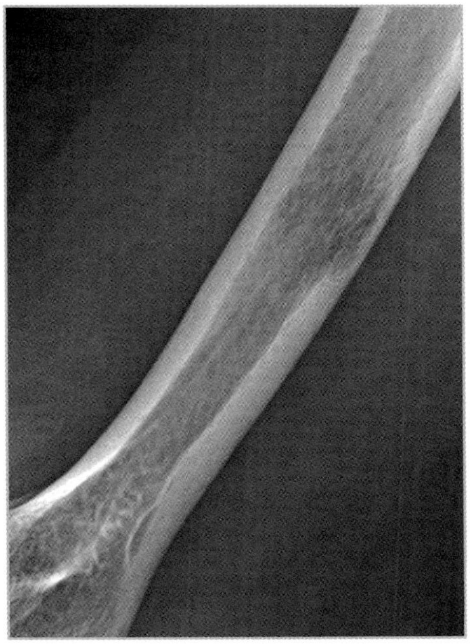

Figure 2.6 Metastasis. Anteroposterior radiograph of the humerus in a patient with small cell cancer of unknown primary. There is permeative destruction of bone with frayed erosion of the endosteal surface. This is a highly aggressive lesion and pathologic fracture is likely imminent. The lesion margins are indistinct and it is difficult to discern where the lesion ends and normal bone resumes. This indicates a wide zone of transition, another hallmark of an aggressive lesion.

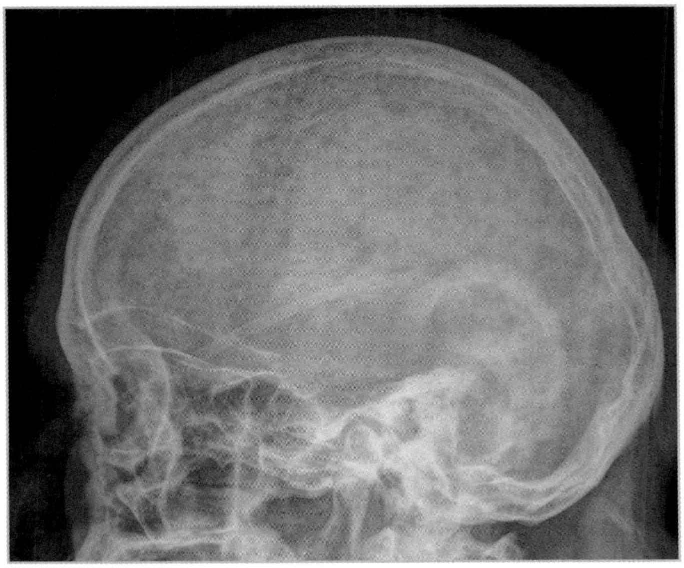

Figure 2.7 Multiple myeloma. Lateral radiograph of the skull shows numerous lytic lesions. This has been termed 'moth-eaten' or 'pepper pot' appearance indicating aggressive bone destruction. Although this is classic appearance for multiple myeloma, conceivably metastatic disease could look similar.

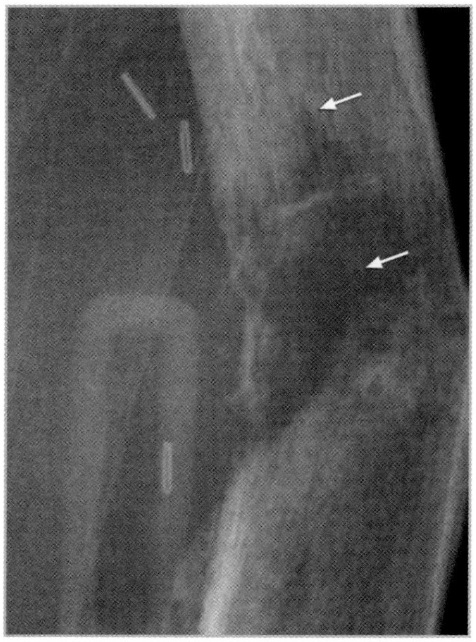

Figure 2.8 Metastasis. Anteroposterior radiograph of the femur shows a metastasis with permeative destruction with a pathologic fracture. There is a wide zone of transition which spans between the arrows.

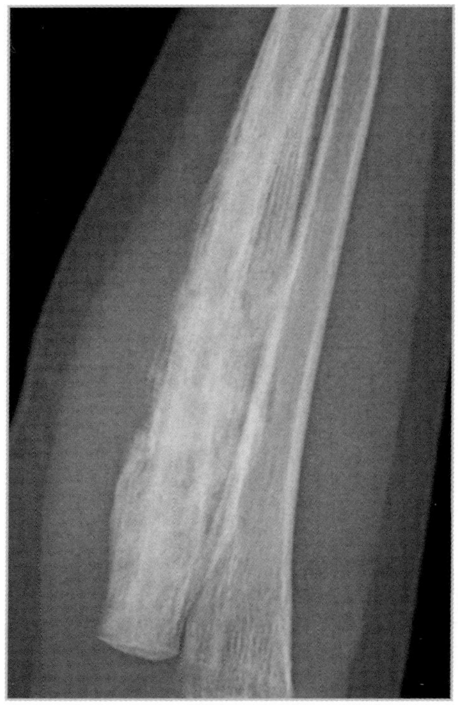

Figure 2.10 Ewing sarcoma. Lateral radiograph of the forearm in a 3 year old boy. There is laminated periosteal reaction along several areas of the radial diaphysis. The laminated periosteal reaction probably results from a stuttering disease course with alternating layers of healing. Although this is malignant periosteal reaction, it is not as aggressive as the sunburst or hair-on-end pattern of periosteal reaction.

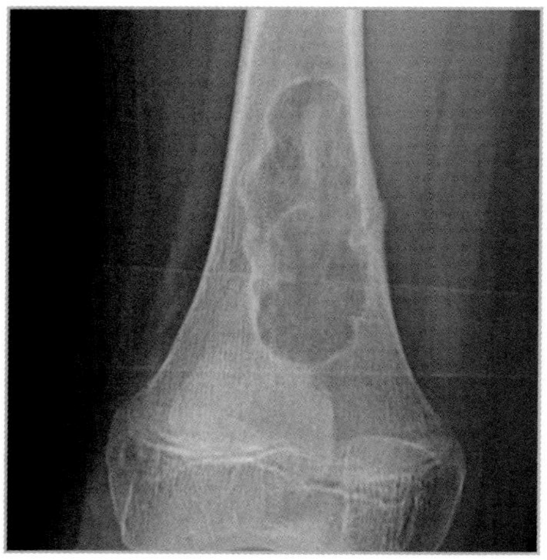

Figure 2.9 Non-ossifying fibroma. Anteroposterior radiograph of the distal femur shows a lucent lesion with uniform thickness undulating sclerotic margins. There is a medial pathologic fracture. The sclerotic margin indicates a non-aggressive lesion with a stable margin.

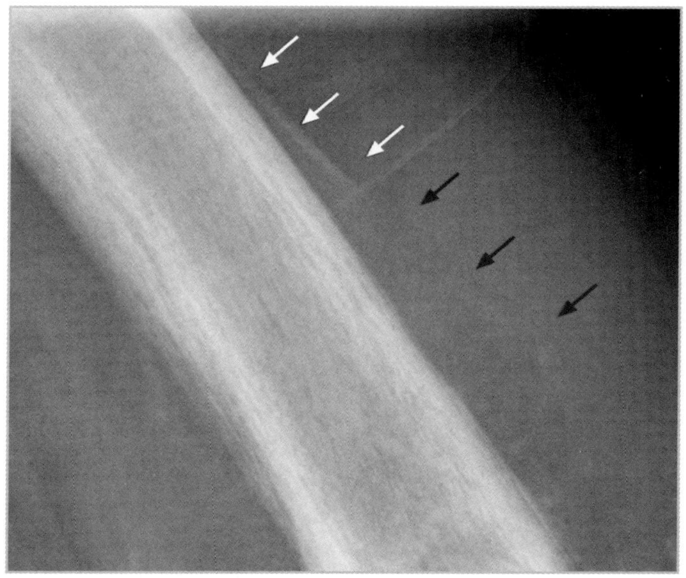

Figure 2.11 Osteosarcoma. Lateral radiograph of the distal femur shows a Codman triangle, white arrows, of preserved periosteal reaction. The black arrows indicate where the tumor has destroyed the periosteal reaction. The Codman triangle indicates a highly aggressive lesion.

with overlying layers of new periosteal reaction. In general, continuous smooth periosteal reaction is seen with benign processes such as infection and fracture healing. Discontinuous periosteal reaction is worrisome for underlying neoplasm where the tumor has destroyed both the bone cortex and its overlying periosteum and then spread into the soft tissues. The discontinuous periosteal reaction can result in the Codman triangle sign **Figure 2.11**. The triangle represents the remaining periosteal reaction that is not destroyed by the tumor. Highly aggressive periosteal reaction will have a sunburst or 'hair on end' appearance due to tumor streaming through the periosteal reaction resulting in thin columns of mineralized tissue that are oriented perpendicular to the bone surface. **Figure 2.12** and **2.13** are radiographs of osteosarcomas and a Ewing sarcoma, respectively, showing highly aggressive periosteal reaction with the hair-on-end or starburst appearance. There are three types of bone tumor matrix including fibrous, cartilaginous and osteoid. A radiograph can usually demonstrate the matrix type. **Figure 2.14** shows the ground glass appearance of fibrous matrix as seen in an 11 year old boy with fibrous dysplasia. Note the homogeneous, featureless appearance of fibrous matrix. A cystic lesion can have a similar featureless appearance due to the absence of trabeculae. **Figure 2.15** shows the arc and ring pattern of calcification seen in an enchondroma of the proximal humerus in a young adult. The arcs represent a partially calcified ring or a partially visualized ring. Note the rings tend to be 2-4 mm in diameter. **Figure 2.16a** is another case of an enchondroma with arc and ring calcification pattern involving the distal femur. **Figures 2.16b** and **2.16c** are

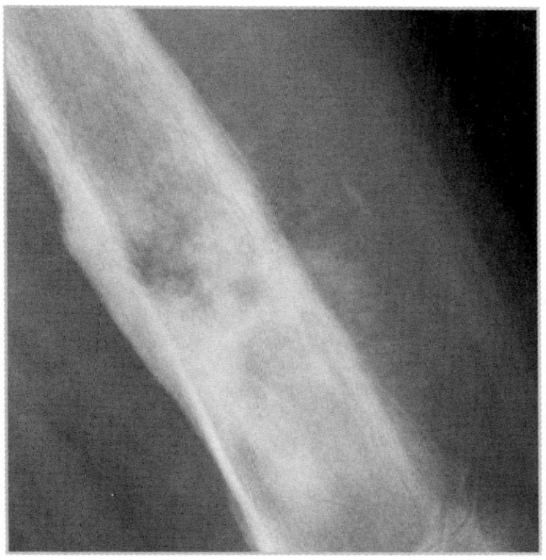

Figure 2.12 Osteosarcoma. Lateral radiograph of the distal femur shows the sunburst or hair-on-end pattern of periosteal reaction. This is indicates a highly aggressive lesion with soft tissue extension of tumor. There are areas of calcified osteoid projecting within the marrow of the distal metaphysis.

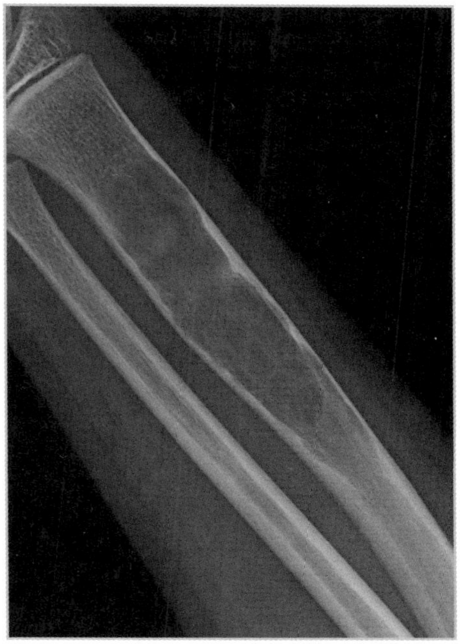

Figure 2.14 Fibrous dysplasia. Anteroposterior radiograph of the distal radius in an 11 year old boy shows a mildly expansile lucent lesion with endosteal smooth scalloping. The lesion has ground glass density matrix indicating fibrous tissue.

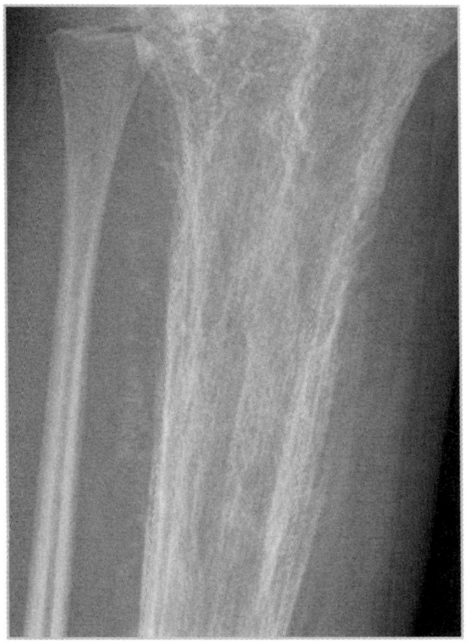

Figure 2.13 Ewing sarcoma. Anteroposterior radiograph of the proximal tibia in a 7 year old girl shows the sunburst or hair-on-end pattern of highly aggressive periosteal reaction. There is laminated periosteal reaction along the medial aspect of the tibial diaphysis. The cortex is destroyed along the proximal lateral aspect of the tibial metaphysis.

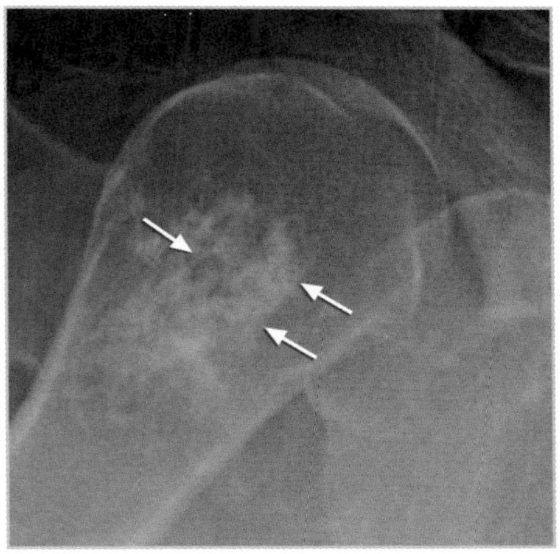

Figure 2.15 Enchondroma. Anteroposterior radiograph of the proximal humerus shows calcified arc and ring matrix pattern, arrows, characteristic of a cartilage lesion. Note the individual rings are approximately 2-4 mm in diameter.

the accompanying MR images. Note the spherical lobules of cartilage tissue which again are about 2-4 mm in size. Some have described these as popcorn in appearance. The MR appearance is quite variable in signal as some lobules are calcified resulting in low signal on all MR sequences. **Figure 2.17** shows osteoid matrix from a healing fracture that is 2 months status post open reduction and internal fixation (ORIF). Note the fluffy yet homogeneously calcified appearance of this new bone. **Figure 2.18** shows the osteoid formation from calcifying heterotopic ossification 23 days after ORIF. **Figure 2.19a** and **2.19b** are radiographs from an osteosarcoma in the proximal tibia of a 13 year old boy. Note the extensive periosteal reaction and the abundant calcifying osteoid. The diagnosis of osteosarcoma is straight forward when there is a clearly destructive malignancy producing osteoid.

ULTRASOUND

Although ultrasound plays a dominant role in clinical areas such as obstetrics, it has only a limited role in the imaging of soft tissue tumors of the musculoskeletal system. Ultrasound can definitively diagnose fluid and hence can be used to correctly identify a cyst. However, in our experience, a cyst is rarely the cause of a patient's soft tissue mass. Many of the palpable lesions felt by patients are tumors of the skin and likely are lipomas or prominent lobules of subcutaneous adipose tissue. Ultrasound is not specific for diagnosing fat tissue and no imaging modality can definitively exclude malignant histology. At our institution we find ultrasound is of little value in the initial workup of soft tissue tumor, except when hernia or aneurysm is suspected.

COMPUTED TOMOGRAPHY

CT scanning is a fast and robust imaging modality that uses a rotating beam of radiation to create two dimensional image 'slices' of a patient. Helical (spiral) scanning entails continuous movement of the patient through the scanner with simultaneous continuous rotation of the radiation beam around the patient. This allows for faster scanning and better reconstruction of images into other planes (coronal and

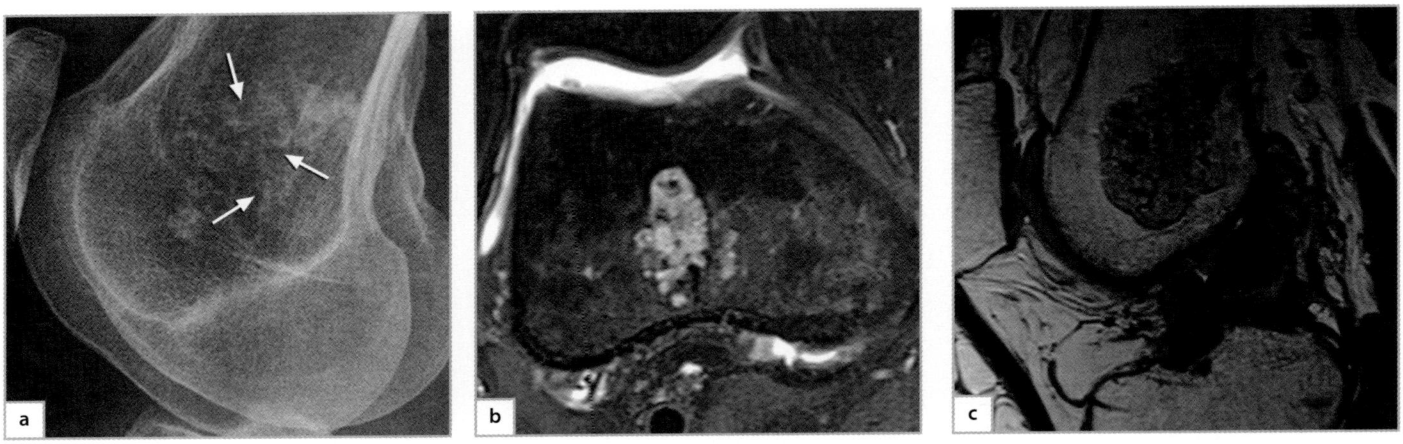

Figure 2.16 Enchondroma. **2.16a** is a lateral radiograph of the distal femur shows calcified arc and ring matrix pattern, arrows, indicating a cartilage lesion. MR Figures are presented of the same lesion including; **2.16b** axial proton density fat saturated and **2.16c** sagittal proton density Figures. Cartilage matrix has a lobulated appearance some have described as emulating popcorn. The signal of cartilage lesions is highly variable depending on the extent of calcification. Uncalcified cartilage will appear T1 isointense and high signal on T2 and STIR Figures similar to the appearance of water on MRI. The calcified portions will be low signal on all sequences and may show blooming on T2 Figures, especially T2* gradient echo Figures. Note again the individual lobules are about 2-4 mm is size correlating with the size of the arcs and rings as seen by radiographs.

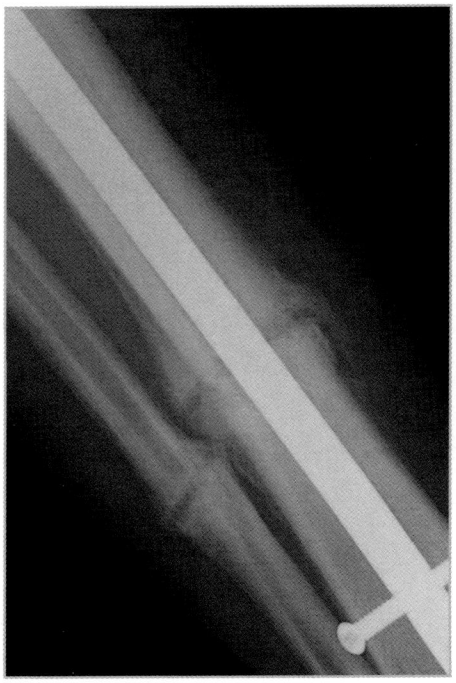

Figure 2.17 Healing fracture. Anteroposterior radiograph of the leg after open reduction and internal fixation (ORIF) of the tibial fracture 2 months prior shows healing osteoid bridging the fractures. Calcifying osteoid has a homogeneous, cloud like appearance.

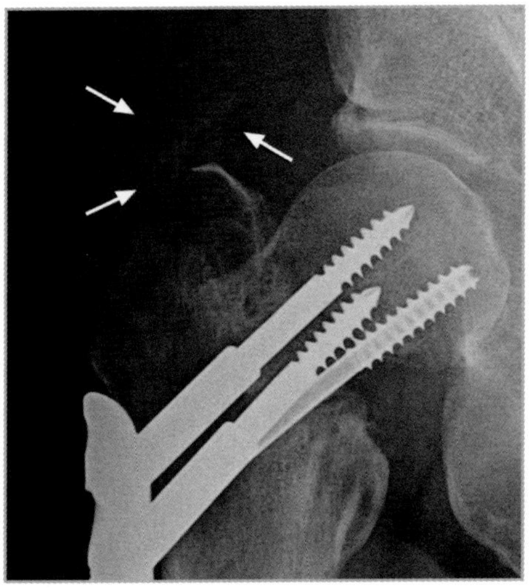

Figure 2.18 Heterotopic ossification. Anteroposterior radiograph of the hip in a patient with ORIF 23 days prior. There is calcifying osteoid developing in the soft tissues adjacent to the fracture and surgery, arrows. Note the cloud like appearance of this mildly calcified, immature osteoid. With time, the osteoid will ossify developing internal trabeculae of cancellous bone and a corticated surface.

sagittal). Also, modern scanners have multiple detectors (16 slice, 64 slice, etc.) which enable both thinner slices and greater speed of coverage. A standard CT scanning technique (1-3 mm slice thickness) with reformations in the sagittal and coronal planes is a sufficient exam protocol for most cases. CT contrast contains iodine and is rapidly excreted into the urine. Because iodine contrast agents are potentially nephrotoxic, renal insufficiency is a relative contraindication. There is an occasional patient who is allergic to iodine contrast, rarely is the reaction severe or fatal. Patients with prior reaction must be premedicated with steroid and anti-histamine. At our institution, IV contrast is not usually given for CT scan of an extremity tumor because we typically already have an MRI with contrast to assess vascularity and tumor enhancement. Occasionally, high resolution CT scanning is needed (sub 1 mm slices) to assess a lesion, for example, a small suspected enchondroma in the finger, and the radiologist may protocol especially thin slices with higher beam strength (higher mA setting) to decrease imaging noise.

CT can play an important role in the initial diagnosis of a bone tumor in certain situations. If radiography is equivocal regarding cortical erosion or breakthrough, CT can provide definitive visualization of cortical integrity and the fine detail that allows determination if an erosion is active or healing. Additionally, CT can offer improved visualization of matrix type when radiographs do not definitively demonstrate the presence or the type of matrix.

CT plays a central role in the systemic surveillance of the patient for metastatic disease, especially for disease spread to the lung. CT is also valuable for surveillance of retroperitoneal tumors. However, typically, MR is used to image the extremities for follow up, and occasionally,

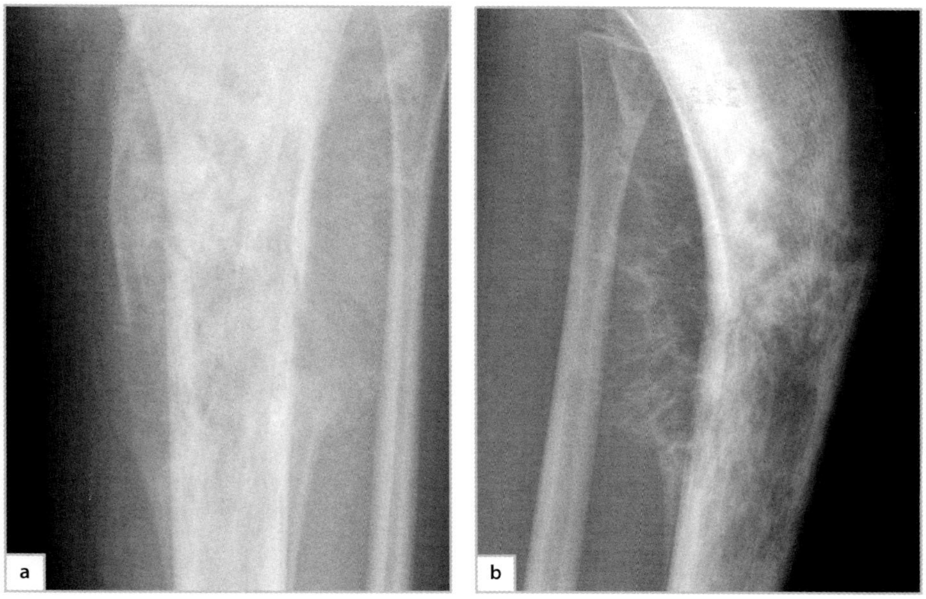

Figure 2.19 Osteosarcoma. 2.19a is an anteroposterior and 2.19b is a lateral radiograph of the proximal tibia in a 13 year old boy. There is soft tissue mass with areas of calcifying osteoid indicating an osteosarcoma. There is a Codman triangle of periosteal reaction along the distal aspect of the tumor as seen on the AP view. There is a pathologic fracture of the tibia. There are areas of densely calcified osteoid projecting within the proximal tibial marrow space best seen on the lateral view.

CT may be employed if there is extensive metallic hardware causing limiting artifact on MR. Any heavy density material, such as metal or barium will attenuate the CT scan beam and may cause spray artifact affecting the slices that go through the dense material. Hence, extensive metallic hardware may render an area uninterpretable on both CT and MR imaging.

MAGNETIC RESONANCE IMAGING

MR imaging is the dominant imaging modality for soft tissue tumors and sarcoma evaluation and follow up. The soft tissue contrast and multiplanar imaging capability make MR an invaluable imaging tool. Medical MRI is based on the imaging of protons whose appearance depends on their molecular environment. Thus MR can identify fat, water and edematous tissue. To a lesser extent, MRI can identify hemorrhage, protein and mineral (calcium). Air and metal will be devoid of signal and actually disturbs the magnetic environment often ruining visualization in the immediate surrounding environment. With the injection of intravenous gadolinium contrast, tissues brighten as demonstrated on T1 weighted images which indicate high vascularity, pooling of blood or leakage of the contrast from the intravascular environment into the interstitial tissue space. The main MR contrast agents use chelated gadolinium which is excreted by the kidneys, but is not nephrotoxic. Allergies to gadolinium contrast are rare. There is a relative contraindication against gadolinium contrast agents in patient with renal insufficiency due to the rare association of nephrogenic systemic fibrosis.

There are a number of technical considerations that effect sarcoma MR imaging. In the US, most scanners are 1.5 tesla field strength and serve well for sarcoma imaging. For the obese or claustrophobic patient, a so called 'open' MR scanner may need to be utilized. These scanners have a more open architecture to accommodate patients but have lower field strength resulting in generally lesser imaging quality. The radiologist can attempt to design sequences to mitigate this loss of image quality, never the less; the exam will typically take longer and have lesser image quality on a low field scanner.

The proper imaging coil must be chosen to provide adequate coverage of the tumor and its compartment. Generally, the smallest coil to cover the region of clinical interest should be used to optimize signal. Some coils give poor image homogeneity in tissues close to the coil. This can compromise visualization of the skin and superficial structures when using some surface or flex coils. The radiologist must be familiar with their imaging equipment to best optimize studies of sarcoma patients.

The radiologist should carefully design the imaging sequences to obtain maximum tissue information and anatomy in the least possible time. Patient motion related image degradation is a constant problem and the radiologist must design imaging protocols that are time efficient. Each MR sequence typically take 2-5 minutes to perform and requires the patient hold absolutely still for the entire imaging sequence. Any movement during the sequence results in motion blurring of all slices in that sequence. There is no way to repeat a single MR image slice (as on can do with CT scanning). If there is motion, the entire sequence must be redone. Unfortunately, many patients believe they can hold still, perhaps imagining reading a book while sitting on the couch. However, for many patients, lying flat on their back in a noisy scanner, results in back pain, restless legs and pressure points. The technologist plays a crucial role in achieving patient comfort before the exam by thoughtfully placing pillows, towels and sponges to position the patient comfortably and hopefully minimize motion.

For the initial tumor MR imaging study, T1, T2, fluid sensitive, and matching pre and post contrast T1 weighted fat saturated sequences should be performed. Although not specific, tissue enhancement has significant implications. The absence of enhancement is the cornerstone of fluid diagnosis with MR imaging. Without intravenous contrast, the definitive diagnosis of cyst cannot me made with MRI.

NOTE ON MRI TERMINOLOGY

For the sake of brevity, we will omit stating 'weighted' when describing a T1 weighted or T2 weighted sequence. The weighting of an image is an important concept for those wanting to design or understand chemical and physics basis of MR sequences.

In general, enhancing tissue indicates a solid lesion with viable tissue. Whereas, a non-enhancing portion of a tumor may represent hypovascular or avascular tissue such as fibrous tissue, matrix, fluid or necrosis. In the follow up setting, new areas of non-enhancement may indicate ongoing matrix formation or may indicate new necrosis from successful therapy. It is important for pre and post contrast images to be created with identical sequences parameters (same slice, field of view, matrix, TR (repetition time), TE (echo time), shim, bandwidth etc.) so that subtle enhancement can be correctly identified. Ideally, all three imaging planes are obtained on the exam; however, often two imaging planes are sufficient for interpretation.

A fluid sensitive sequence refers to an image where adipose tissues appear low signal (dark or black) and water or edematous tissues appear high signal (bright or white). The radiologist can employ different fluid sensitive sequences including; T2 fat saturated or short T1 inversion recovery (STIR) sequences. STIR has the advantage of providing uniform decrease in fat signal when field homogeneity is compromised. Hence, STIR sequence should generally be used for large fields of view and when there is metallic hardware or a foreign body that limits homogeneity. The STIR sequences requires slightly more time and will have slightly less image quality than a comparable T2 fat saturated sequence but the clinical robustness of STIR sequences is invaluable.

Generally, we use a 10% gap between slices. Only if there is a small tumor do we utilize intercalated slices with no interslice gap. Since soft tissue tumors tend to be large, thin slice imaging is not emphasized. Instead coverage is paramount so the exam does not miss a skip lesion or area of tumor spread.

Ideally, the initial MR exam would include T1, T2, STIR and enhancement information on a tumor. The radiologist has then performed an 'imaging biopsy' of the lesion (**Table 2.2**). This full palate of MR sequences can tell the radiologist about the nature of tissue in the tumor. The T2 sequence can be sacrificed on follow up studies when the purpose of imaging shifts to recurrence detection and not tumor diagnosis. Of note, T2 fast spin echo sequences tend to show fat as moderately high signal whereas conventional spin echo T2 sequence will show fat as moderately low signal. In most practices, fast spin echo sequences have virtually replaced conventional spin echo due to the substantially shortened sequence time.

There is extensive overlap in sarcoma appearance on MRI. The majorities of sarcomas have heterogeneous isointense or low signal on T1 with heterogeneous high signal on T2 and STIR sequences. Most sarcomas enhance intensely and heterogeneously. The utility of MR lies in its exquisite ability to show location, spread and adjacent structure involvement. The MR exam can have some tissue specificity, like a biopsy, and can identify fat tissue, viable tissue, water, edema and hemorrhage. There are some imaging appearances of tumors on MR that can be helpful in diagnosis but these are discussed in each tumor subsection but the radiologist is cautioned that specificity is often modest.

Table 2.1 Typical MR protocol for imaging an extremity tumor

	Plane	Weighting	Coverage	Slice
1	Coronal	T1	Joint to joint	5-8 mm
2	Coronal	STIR, T2 fat sat	Joint to joint	5-8 mm
3	Axial	T1 fat sat	Tumor	5-15 mm
4	Axial - optional	T2	Tumor	5-15 mm
5	Axial	STIR, T2 fat sat	Tumor	5-15 mm
6	Axial post	T1 fat sat	Tumor	5-15 mm
7	Sagittal post	T1 fat sat	Joint to joint	5-8 mm

Table 2.2 Imaging biopsy: signal characteristics of various tissues

T1	T2	STIR	Enhances	Tissue type
+	I/–	–	V	Fat
–	–	–	–/V	Fibrous
–	+	+	–	Water, edema
+	+	V	–	Proteinaceous fluid
I	I/+	V/+	+/V	Tumor tissue
–	B	–	–	Hemosiderin, Ca++

+ High signal (White); – Low signal (Black); V Variable; I Isointense signal (grey, similar to normal muscle); B Blooms – a low signal area on T1 becomes larger on T2. This effect is most pronounced on T2* gradient echo sequences.

REFERENCES

Bearer EL, Lowengrub JS, Frieboes HB, et al. Multiparameter computational modeling of tumor invasion. Cancer Res 2009;69(10):4493–501.

Chapter 3 Surgery of musculoskeletal tumors

SURGERY

Overview

Surgery plays a crucial role in the treatment of many of the musculoskeletal neoplasms. The goals of surgery are to balance the risks and consequences of local recurrence with the desire to preserve function and minimize complications. Surgery should be performed in coordination with the other crucial treatment modalities. The purpose of this section is to provide a broad overview of surgical management. Specific surgical techniques, including those of biopsy, are beyond the scope of this text.

Staging

Two staging systems are commonly employed when planning treatment of musculoskeletal neoplasms. The Musculoskeletal Tumor Society (MSTS) system stages both benign and malignant neoplasms of bone and soft tissue. The American Joint Committee on Cancer (AJCC) system stages malignant neoplasms and has a separate system for tumors of bone and soft tissue.

In the MSTS system (**Table 3.1**), benign tumors are assigned a stage of 1 (latent tumors), 2 (active tumors), or 3 (aggressive tumors). Malignant tumors are assigned a stage of I (low grade malignant) or II (high grade malignant). Malignant tumors are further subdivided based on whether they are contained within the anatomic compartment of origin (A), or have extended beyond it (B). Malignant tumors are assigned a stage of III if metastases are present.

With the AJCC system (**Table 3.2a-c**), assessment is made concerning the histologic grade of the tumor (G), qualities of the primary tumor (T), and the presence of lymphatic spread (N) or metastasis beyond regional lymph nodes (M).

Biopsy

Although often mistakenly considered as a minor procedure, the biopsy is an integral part of surgical management. Improper placement, orientation, or technique of a biopsy can contaminate vital structures necessitating amputation where a limb salvage procedure could be performed, or unnecessarily adding to the complexity of a limb salvage procedure.

A carefully planned biopsy should provide adequate diagnostic tissue without compromising the definitive procedure while minimizing complications of the biopsy itself. Options for procurement of diagnostic tissue include fine needle aspiration, core-needle biopsy, and open incisional or excisional biopsy.

Surgical margins

Some tumors are surrounded by a thin and well defined fibrous capsule (in soft tissue) or sclerotic margin (in bone) which completely contains the tumor. These characteristics are generally true of inactive benign tumors. High grade malignant tumors generally have no capsule at all and may send finger-like extensions into surrounding normal tissue. Intermediate grade benign and malignant tumors may have an incomplete pseudocapsule. Between the tumor (including its capsule or pseudocapsule) and normal tissue exists a real, or virtual,

Table 3.1: MSTS staging system

MSTS stage	Description	Examples: Bone tumor	Examples: Soft tissue tumor
1	Latent benign tumor	Nonossifying fibroma, unicameral bone cyst, enchondroma	Lipoma, fibroma, schwannoma
2	Active benign tumor	Chondroblastoma, osteoblastoma, aneurysmal bone cyst	Myxoma, hemangioma, pigmented villonodular synovitis
3	Aggressive benign tumor	Giant cell tumor	Fibromatosis
IA	Low grade malignant tumor contained within its compartment of origin	Parosteal osteosarcoma	Low grade soft tissue sarcoma
IB	Low grade malignant tumor extending beyond its compartment of origin		
IIA	High grade malignant tumor contained within its compartment of origin	Conventional osteosarcoma	Intermediate or high grade soft tissue sarcoma
IIB	High grade malignant tumor extending beyond its compartment of origin		
IIIA	Low or high grade malignant tumor, with metastasis, primary tumor contained within its compartment of origin	Any	Any
IIIB	Low or high grade malignant tumor, with metastasis, primary tumor extending beyond its compartment of origin		

Table 3.2a AJCC staging system descriptors

AJCC descriptor	Bone tumor	Soft tissue tumor (see Table 4.4)
G1	Well differentiated – low grade	Well differentiated
G2	Moderately differentiated – low grade	Moderately differentiated
G3	Poorly differentiated – high grade	Poorly differentiated
G4	Undifferentiated – high grade	Poorly differentiated or undifferentiated
T1	Primary tumor 8 cm or less in greatest dimension	N/A
T1a	N/A	Primary tumor 5 cm or less in greatest dimension, superficial
T1b		Primary tumor 5 cm or less in greatest dimension, deep
T2	Primary tumor > 8 cm in greatest dimension	N/A
T2a	N/A	Primary tumor > 5 cm in greatest dimension, superficial
T2b		Primary tumor > 5 cm in greatest dimension, deep
T3	Discontinuous tumors in the primary bone site	N/A
N0	No regional lymph node metastasis	
N1	Regional lymph node metastasis	
M0	No distant metastasis	
M1	N/A	Distant metastasis
M1a	Metastasis to lung	N/A
M1b	Metastasis to other distant sites	N/A

Table 3.2b AJCC staging system for bone tumors

AJCC stage	Primary tumor	Regional metastasis	Distant metastasis	Tumor grade
IA	T1	N0	M0	G1,2 low grade, GX
IB	T2,T3	N0	M0	G1,2 low grade, GX
IIA	T1	N0	M0	G3,4 high grade
IIB	T2	N0	M0	G3,4 high grade
III	T3	N0	M0	Any G
IVA	Any T	N0	M1a	Any G
IVB	Any T	N1	Any M	Any G
	Any T	Any N	M1b	Any G

Table 3.2c AJCC staging system for soft tissue tumors

AJCC stage	Primary tumor	Regional metastasis	Distant metastasis	Tumor grade
IA	T1a, T1b	N0	M0	G1, GX
IB	T2a, T2b	N0	M0	G1, GX
IIA	T1a, 1b	N0	M0	G2, G3
IIB	T2a, T2b	N0	M0	G2
III	T2a, T2b	N0	M0	G3
	Any T2b	N1	M0	Any G
IV	Any T	Any N	M1	Any G

space termed the 'reactive zone'. This area may contain satellites of tumor cells, reactive inflammatory tissue, or both. Although some tumors may, in fact, have neither it is difficult to know what cells are present in this reactive zone by imaging studies, independent of what one knows is generally true from the clinical behavior and pathologic examination of each tumor type. The 'width' of the reactive zone is quite variable.

Any surgical decision must consider the consequences of leaving real or potential tumor behind. Many tumors will rarely recur even if a small amount of gross tumor is left behind (enchondroma, lipoma, and myxoma) whereas high grade malignant tumors may recur even when an amputation is performed through a presumably normal level of tissue. In general, low recurrence rates can be acceptable in the treatment of benign tumors where the additional morbidity and functional deficits outweigh the consequences of tumor recurrence. Conversely, recurrence rates should be minimized in the treatment of high grade malignancies where tumor recurrence may contribute to mortality and increasingly morbid resection procedures. All of this must be further tempered by the likelihood of cure; the surgeon provides little benefit to patients by subjecting them to complex debilitating procedures if the likelihood of cure is remote.

An intralesional procedure is one performed within the capsule or pseudocapsule of the tumor. Curettage of a bone tumor or piecemeal excision of a soft-tissue tumor would be examples of an intralesional tumor excision. By definition, gross or microscopic tumor is left behind.

Marginal excision of a tumor occurs when the plane of dissection is through the reactive zone of the tumor. Examples would include the 'shelling out' of a lipoma or excision of an osteochondroma by cleaving the stalk. With a marginal margin, there is a risk that microscopic tumor is left behind in the reactive zone.

An 'extended' intralesional or marginal procedure is performed when all gross tumor is removed from the capsule or pseudocapsule (if intralesional) or reactive zone (if marginal) and then an effort is made to extend the plane of dissection further. This may be accomplished mechanically (e. g. the use of a burr in the treatment of a bone tumor), physically (by freezing the surrounding tissue with liquid nitrogen, cautery, or with the exothermic production of heat with polymethylmethacrylate), or chemically (e. g. phenol or alcohol). Margin extension in this manner decreases the risk of microscopic tumor being left behind in the reactive zone.

A wide resection occurs when the plane of dissection is through normal tissue. It is important to note that this represents a qualitative, not quantitative, description. As long as the dissection occurs through normal tissue, beyond the reactive zone, a wide margin is claimed. If the plane of dissection truly occurs through normal tissue, the risk of leaving microscopic tumor behind should theoretically be zero. The term 'contaminated wide margin' is often used to describe a procedure which ultimately resulted in a wide surgical margin, however, exposure of the tumor occurred at some point during the procedure.

A radical resection is performed by removing the entire anatomic compartment in which the tumor originated. Although rarely performed today, this procedure was used historically for the treatment of many sarcomas which were at one time believed to contain 'skip lesions' in a high percentage. A skip lesion is a nodule of isolated tumor within the same compartment as the primary tumor but separated by an interval of normal tissue beyond the reactive zone.

Table 3.3 associates the generally preferred procedure associated with the MSTS classification system. **Figures 3.1a** and **3.1b** show specific types of resection associated with a representative bone and soft tissue tumor.

Once the decision is made as to the type of surgical margin desired, the risks and benefits of limb salvage surgery versus amputation must be weighed. Although amputation will rarely be considered for treatment of benign tumors, it may play a role in the scenario of multiply recurrent tumors associated with increasing disability as a result of the multiple recurrences, multiple surgeries, or associated complications. Modern reconstruction techniques (utilizing internal prosthetic components of increasingly sophisticated design, allograft tissue, or a combination of both) has made limb salvage surgery popular and, in many cases, the treatment of choice. No long-term differences in outcome have been demonstrated between amputation and limb salvage procedures in the treatment of primary malignancy. Nevertheless, amputation always has a role and should be considered based on the patient's lifestyle preferences and the predicted functionality of the proposed limb salvage procedure. If significant disability will exist after the limb salvage, particularly if major nerves and or vessels must be resected along with the tumor, amputation may offer a more optimal functional result.

Best practice in surgical oncology of bone and soft tissue tumors

Musculoskeletal oncology is a complex discipline and is best practiced by those with adequate training, generally in the form of a specialized fellowship following an orthopaedic or general surgery residency.

Because this represents a truly multi-disciplinary field, close collaboration should occur with colleagues in medical oncology (including pediatric oncology), radiation oncology, pathology, radiology, and plastic/reconstructive surgery. Practice will typically take place in a sophisticated tertiary care center where technology is readily available along with the appropriate clinical expertise to support complex surgical procedures in compromised patients.

Future of musculoskeletal oncology surgery

The future looks bright for our patients, from a multidisciplinary perspective. From the surgical standpoint, expect improved technology to assist with surgical precision (e.g. computerized surgical navigation).

Table 3.3: Surgical margins as a function of MSTS stage

MSTS stage	Procedure	Examples	
		Bone tumor	Soft tissue tumor
1	Intralesional	Curettage	Piecemeal excision
2	Marginal	Complete curettage of intraosseous tumor, resection of osteochondroma	Shelling out of entire tumor
3	Aggressive benign tumor	Extended curettage, possible wide resection in expendable bones	Marginal resection with adjuvant, possible wide resection
IA	Wide resection	Wide bone resection	Wide soft tissue resection
IB			
IIA			
IIB			
IIIA	Wide resection with metastatectomy if resectable	Wide bone resection with metastatectomy if resectable	Wide soft tissue resection with metastatectomy if resectable

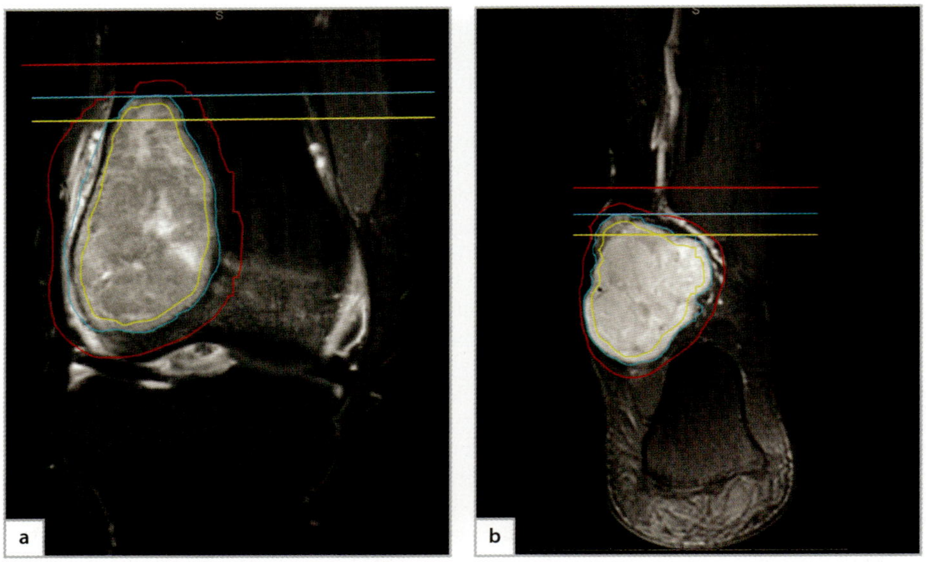

Figure 3.1: Shown are MRI images of a bone tumor (**3.1a**) and a soft tissue tumor (**3.1b**). Yellow lines represent the plane of dissection for an intralesional resection or amputation. Blue lines represent the plane of dissection for a marginal resection or amputation. Red lines represent the plane of dissection for a marginal resection or amputation.

Improvements in the technology of implants and external prosthetic devices will improve the functionality, durability, and longevity of devices for both limb salvage procedures and amputations.

Advice for medical students

Medical students interested in surgical oncology need to first explore the differences between general surgery and orthopaedic surgery. Although there is much overlap in practice, the concentrations tend to be very different. While orthopaedic oncologists will concentrate their cancer practice in sarcoma and metastatic disease, the general surgical oncologist will typically focus heavily on the management of carcinomas.

Advice for residents

Residents in general or orthopaedic surgery should spend time on the surgical oncology service. Particularly in orthopaedics, the specialty can be markedly different from other subspecialties. Most orthopaedic oncologists will spend 60-70% of their practice managing soft tissue tumors. Cases tend to be long, complex, and often involve types of surgical technique more closely related to general surgery than orthopaedic surgery. Additionally, patients are generally more compromised and complications more common than with most other areas of orthopaedics.

REFERENCES

Enneking WF. A system of staging musculoskeletal neoplasms. Clin Orthop Relat Res 1986;204:9–24.

Mankin, JH, Mankin CJ, Simon M. The hazards of biopsy, revisited. J Bone Joint Surg 1996;78-A:656–663.

Ogilvie CM, Torbert JT, Finstein JL, et al. Clinical utility of percutaneous biopsies of musculoskeletal tumors. Clin Orthop Relat Res 2006;450:95–100.

Simon MA. Biopsy of musculoskeletal tumors. J Bone Joint Surg 1982;64:1253–1257.

Virkus WW, Marshall D, Enneking WF, et al. The effect of contaminated surgical margins revisited. Clin Orthop Relat Res 2002;397:89–94.

Wolf RE, Enneking WF. The staging and surgery of musculoskeletal neoplasms. Orthop Clin North Am 1996;27(3):473–481.

Chapter 4 Medical and radiation oncology of musculoskeletal tumors: principles of diagnosis and treatment

MEDICAL ONCOLOGY

Introduction

Medical oncologists participate in the multidisciplinary approach to adult (and sometimes teenager) patients with malignant sarcomas and pediatric oncologists treat these tumors in children. Thus benign or low malignant potential musculoskeletal neoplasms are usually not treated by medical or pediatric oncologists, except for rare exceptions such as fibromatosis. Soft tissue sarcomas are rare malignancies in adults (Jemal, et al. 2009). There are over 50 different types of sarcomas, some more sensitive to chemotherapy than others. Traditionally, the activity of a new drug in soft tissue sarcomas was determined by studying it in all subtypes. Bone sarcomas (Ewing and osteosarcomas in particular) have been better studied as single entities. However, as data accumulates for the sensitivity of certain subtypes to particular chemotherapies, efforts are made to define histology-driven treatment approach. New therapies are also being identified based on the unique molecular signatures of the various sarcomas (**Table 4.1**). For patients with advanced sarcomas, the goals of care are to prolong life while maintaining or improving quality of life. In this scenario, stabilization of disease can be a meaningful endpoint.

Standard chemotherapy drugs

Doxorubicin either alone or in combination with other agents is the standard of care for most unresectable or metastatic sarcomas. Response rates for single agent doxorubicin range from 9% to 27% (Judson, et al. 2001, Schoenfeld, et al. 1982). There is a dose-response curve for doxorubicin, with higher response rates in patients receiving doses over 60 mg/m^2 (Borden, et al. 1987, Patel, et al. 1998). **Table 4.2** shows the main side effects of chemotherapy agents used for sarcoma. The addition of either ifosfamide, dacarbazine or both to doxorubicin increases response rate, with no improvement in overall survival (Antman, et al. 1993, Borden, et al. 1987, Edmonson, et al. 1993). Filgrastim should then be administered to promote timely recovery of the neutrophil count.

Ifosfamide is an alkylating agent with similar single agent activity as doxorubicin (Antman, et al. 1989, Bramwell, et al. 1993) and a dose-response curve (Buesa, et al. 1998, Patel, et al. 1997). Because of the potential toxicity, ifosfamide is usually administered in the inpatient setting. Ifosfamide appears to be particularly active in synovial sarcoma (Rosen, et al. 1994, Sleijfer, et al.). This drug is not indicated in elderly patients and in those with pre-existing renal impairment.

Dacarbazine also has activity as a single agent and patients with leiomyosarcoma (LMS) appears to be more sensitive to this agent (Buesa, et al. 1991, Gottlieb, et al. 1976, Zucali, et al. 2008).

Pegylated liposomal doxorubicin (PLD) is a formulation of doxorubicin which increases area under the curve and tumor penetration of the drug. PLD activity might be similar to the one of doxorubicin (Judson, et al. 2001, Toma, et al. 2000) but strong evidence is lacking.

Gemcitabine is a nucleoside analogue. Tumor responses to single agent gemcitabine are low (under 10% in the first line and refractory settings) (Maki, et al. 2007, Svancarova, et al. 2002, Von Burton, et al. 2006). Data from the pancreatic cancer setting suggest that patients who receive gemcitabine at a fixed dose rate of 10 mg/m^2/min have improved survival over those who receive gemcitabine as a standard 30 minute infusion (Tempero, et al. 2003). Fixed dosing of gemcitabine is currently used in combination with docetaxel,(Hensley, et al. 2002) a microtubule inhibitor of the taxane family (Hensley, et al. 2002), (van Hoesel, et al. 1994, Verweij, et al. 1995). Objective response rates vary from 25 to 50% (Hensley, et al. 2008, Leu, et al. 2004, Maki, et al. 2007). Vinorelbine a vinca alkaloid combined to fixed dose gemcitabine also has activity, with an overall response rate of 25% (Dileo, et al. 2007). Vinorelbine might offer an alternative for patients who do not tolerate docetaxel.

Similarly to docetaxel, paclitaxel has shown clinical benefit in patients with angiosarcoma or Kaposi sarcoma (Cianfrocca, et al. , Penel, et al. 2008). Dramatic responses to various doses of paclitaxel have been observed in these patients (Casper, et al. 1998). Unfortunately, median time to progression remains short at 4 months with an overall survival of 8 months. The combination of docetaxel, gemcitabine and bevacizumab induced responses in all 4 patients with angiosarcoma with two confirmed complete pathological responses and a long term survival of 75% (Verschraegen, et al. 2012). In combination with radiotherapy, taxanes and doxorubicin have induced long term remissions in this disease (Penel, et al. 2011).

Experimental chemotherapy treatments for sarcomas

Pal ifosfamide-tris (ZIO-201; Ziopharm Inc.) and 2-nitroimidazole phosphoramidite conjugate (TH-302; Threshold Pharmaceuticals, Inc.) are active metabolites of ifosfamide with activity against sarcoma cell lines (Kolb EA 2006) with theoretically less toxic effects. The combination of pal ifosfamide and doxorubicin is tolerated as an outpatient regimen and has activity in sarcoma (Chawla et al. 2008, Verschraegen et al. 2010). The combination of TH-302 and doxorubicin is equally well tolerated (Ganjoo, et al. 2011). To confirm these preliminary results, randomized phase III trials are being performed. Ifosfamide might soon be replaced by such less toxic analogues.

Trabectedin (ET-743; Johnson and Johnson) is a marine derived alkaloid that binds DNA through the minor groove. It is approved in Europe for patients with sarcoma who have failed prior anthracycline

Table 4.1 Fusion transcripts in soft tissue sarcoma

Diagnosis	Chromosomal abnormality	Genes involved	Potential targeted therapy	References
Alveolar rhabdomyosarcoma	t(2;13)(q35;q14) t(1;13)(p36;q14)	PAX3-FKHR PAX7-FKHR		
Alveolar soft part sarcoma	t(X;17)(p11.2;q25)	TFE3-ASPL	Sunitinib Cediranib	Stacchiotti, 2011 Kummar, 2013
Angiomatoid fibrous histiocytoma	t(12;16)(q13;p11)	FUS-ATF1		
Clear cell sarcoma	t(12;22)(q13;q12)	EWS-ATF1	Tivantinib	Wagner, 2012
Congenital fibrosarcoma/congenital mesoblastic nephroma	t(12;15)(p13;q25)	ETV6-NTRK3		
Dermatofibrosarcoma protuberans	t(17;22)(q22;q13)	PDFGB-COL1A1	Imatinib	Rutkowski, 2010
Desmoplastic small round cell tumor	t(11;22)(p13;q12)	EWS-WT1		
Endometrial stromal sarcoma	t(7;17)(p15;q21)	JAZF1-JJAZ1		
Ewing's sarcoma/peripheral primitive neuroectodermal tumor	t(11;22)(q24;q12) t(21;22)(q22;q12) t(7;22)(p22;q12) t(17;22)(q12;q12) t(2;22)(q33;q12) t(16;21)(p11;q22)	EWS-FLI1 EWS-ERG EWS-ETV1 EWS-FEV EWS-E1AF FUS-ERG	YK-4-279	Erkizan, 2009
Low grade fibromyxoid sarcoma	t(7;16)((q33;p11)	FUS-CREB3I2		
Inflammatory myofibroblastic tumor	t(1;2)(q22;p23) t(2;19)(p23;p13) t(2;17)(p23;q23)	TPM3-ALK TPM4-ALK CLTC-ALK	Crizotinib	Butrynski, 2010
Myxoid chondrosarcoma	t(9;22)(q22;q12) t(9;15)(q22;q21) t(9;17)q22;q11)	EWS-CHN TFC12-CHN TAF2N-CHN		
Myxoid liposarcoma	t(12;16)(q13;p11) t(12;22)(q13;q12)	TLS-CHOP EWS-CHOP		
Synovial sarcoma	t(X;18)(p11;q11)	SSX1-SYT SSX2-SYT SSX4-SYT		

Table 4.2 Main side effects of chemotherapy agents

	Doxorubicin[1]	PLD[2]	Ifosfamide[3]	Dacarbazine	Gemcitabine	Paclitaxel	Docetaxel	Vinorelbine
Myelosuppression	+++	+	+++	+++	++	+++	+++	++
Nausea/vomiting	++	++	++	+++	+	++	++	+
Neurotoxicity			++			+++	+	++
Cardiotoxic	+++ cumulative							
Nephrotoxic			++					
Alopecia	+++		+++	+++		+++	+++	
Bladder toxic			+++ use Mesna					
Skin Toxicity		+++					+	
Infusion reactions		++				+++	+	

[1] A minority of patients may develop cardiotoxicity with anthracyclines (Schein, et al. 1975). Infusional rather than bolus administration, or the use of dexrazoxane, a chelating agent that interferes with iron-mediated free radical generation may decrease the risk of cardiomyopathy (Seifert, et al. 1994).

[2]PLD, pegylated liposomal doxorubicin. Causes palmar plantar erythrodysesthesia (hand-foot syndrome).

[3] Ifosfamide should be administered with a good hydration. The renal toxicity is tubular acidosis (Cohen, et al. 1975).

therapy. The response to single agent therapy in the first line setting (5 to 17%) parallels that of doxorubicin and ifosfamide (Garcia-Carbonero, et al. 2004, Le Cesne, et al. 2005, Yovine, et al. 2004). Phase I studies of the combination of trabectedin with other drugs such as doxorubicin, paclitaxel and platinum compounds have been conducted and show tolerability and potential activity in sarcomas (Blay, et al. 2008).

Eribulin mesylate is a non-taxane inhibitor of microtubule growth. It is a synthetic analog of halichondrin B, a marine sponge product and is currently FDA approved for refractory metastatic breast cancer (Schoffski, et al. 2011). Preclinical activity has been seen in sarcoma. This drug is now being tested for patients with refractory disease to doxorubicin regimens.

Targeted therapies

m-TOR pathway

Mutations in the cytoplasmic tuberous sclerosis complex (TSC)1 and TSC2 proteins, which prevent interaction and inhibition of mTOR activity, are seen various tumors, including perivascular epithelioid cell tumors (PEComas) (Martignoni, et al. 2010). PTEN can also be altered in sarcomas (Gibault, et al. 2011).

Ridaforolimus (AP23573; Ariad Pharmaceuticals and Merck & Company) is an mTOR inhibitor which stabilizes about 28% of patients with advanced refractory bone and soft tissue sarcomas (Chawla, et al. 2012). The Sarcoma mUlti-Center Clinical Evaluation of the Efficacy of riDaforolimus (SUCCEED) study tested maintenance with oral ridaforolimus versus a placebo. Temsirolimus, another mTOR inhibitor has been studied with at best stabilization of disease (Movva, et al. 2011).

IGF1R pathway

The insulin like growth factor 1 receptor (IGF1R) pathway is a commonly activated pathway in many sarcomas (Maki 2010). Insulin growth factor 1 and 2 (IGFs) bind to IGF1R activating the receptor and stimulate intracellular signaling primarily through the RAS–RAF–MAPK and the PI3-K/AKT-mTOR pathways (Rikhof, et al. 2009). Overexpression of IGF2 by immunohistochemistry has been seen in patients with solitary fibrous tumors, chondrosarcomas, undifferentiated pleomorphic sarcomas, Ewing's sarcomas, tenosynovial giant cell tumors, gastrointestinal stromal tumors, malignant peripheral nerve sheath tumors, myxoid liposarcomas and synovial sarcomas (Steigen, et al. 2009). Figitumumab is a fully human IgG2 monoclonal antibody targeting the insulin-like growth-factor-1 receptor (IGF-1R). In a phase 1 trial, figitumumab had antitumor activity in patients with refractory Ewing's sarcoma (Olmos, et al. 2010). Cixutumumab is another IGFR monoclonal antibody which was tested in patients with refractory Ewing sarcoma with some antitumor activity (Malempati, et al. 2012).

Antiangiogenic agents

Studies have shown a correlation between expression of tumor vascular endothelial growth factor (VEGF) and grade, stage, disease free and overall survival in soft tissue sarcomas (STS) (Hoffmann, et al. 2009, Kilvaer, et al. 2010). Sorafenib, sunitinib, imatinib, dasatinib, and pazopanib have all demonstrated activity in the phase II setting of advanced metastatic or recurrent STS (**Table 4.3**) (Cassier, et al. 2007). When clinical responses are seen it is commonly in patients with soft part alveolar sarcoma, LMS, and angiosarcoma, but the usual best clinical response is stable disease.

Bevacizumab, a monoclonal antibody to circulating VEGF, has been combined with various chemotherapy agents in the management of metastatic sarcoma. When combined with doxorubicin the response rate, however, was lower than that of the historical response rate to single agent doxorubicin and 35% of patients had a grade 2 or worse decline in left ventricular ejection fraction, making this combination intolerable (D'Adamo, et al. 2005). In combination with gemcitabine and docetaxel, response rate is around 30% (Verschraegen, et al. 2012)

Best practices in medical oncology of bone and soft tissue tumors

Musculoskeletal oncology is a complex discipline and is best practiced by those with adequate training through a specialized fellowship in medical oncology following a general internal medicine residency. However, post fellowship mentoring in a center specialized in sarcoma treatment is essential.

The multi-disciplinary nature of sarcoma management brings together medical oncology (including pediatric oncology), radiation oncology, pathology, radiology, and plastic/reconstructive surgery. Practice will typically take place in a sophisticated tertiary care center where technology is readily available along with the appropriate clinical expertise to support complex chemotherapy administration in tight collaboration with pathologists and radiologists for diagnosis, and surgeons and radiation oncologists for treatment.

Advice for medical students and residents

Residents and students will not have the opportunity to see many of the patients with sarcoma who require chemotherapy administration. Any interested student or resident should seek a special elective in a hospital that has a multi-disciplinary sarcoma team to familiarize themselves with these rare tumors.

Table 4.3 Tyrosine kinase therapy in soft tissue sarcoma

Study	Agent	N	PFS rate at 3 months	Best response (N)	Progression-free survival (months)	Overall survival (months)
(Maki, et al. 2009)	Sorafenib 400 mg bid	147	53% (entire population)	Angiosarcoma (5) LMS (1)	3.2	14.3
(Sleijfer, et al. 2009)	Pazopanib 800 mg daily	142	26% (adipocytic) 44% (LMS) 49% (synovial) 39% (other)	LMS (1) Synovial (5) Other (3)	2.6 (adipocytic) 3.0 (LMS) 5.4 (synovial) 3 (other)	6.6 (adipocytic) 11.8 (LMS) 10.3 (synovial) 10.0 (other)
(George, et al. 2009)	Sunitinib 37.5 mg daily	53	NA	DSRCT(1)	1.8	NA
(Chugh, et al. 2009)	Imatinib 300 mg bid	190	NA	Angiosarcoma Fibrosarcoma LMS Liposarcoma MFH Osteosarcoma MPNST Synovial	2.8 (angiosarcoma) 1.9 (fibrosarcoma) 2.8 (LMS) 3.7(liposarcoma) 1.9 (MFH) 1.9 (MPNST) 1.9(synovial) 2.5 (rhabdomyosarcoma)	NA

LMS: leiomyosarcoma, MPNST: malignant peripheral nerve sheath tumor, MFH: malignant fibrous histiocytoma, DSRCT: desmoplastic round cell tumor, bid: twice per day, NA: not available

RADIATION ONCOLOGY

Overview

The appropriate approach to the patient with sarcoma is clearly multidisciplinary. It requires expertise in pathology, radiology, surgery, medical oncology, and radiation oncology. Radiation oncology plays an important role in the treatment of sarcomas. The main role for radiation therapy is as adjuvant treatment to surgery to improve local control of disease. Radiation therapy also is an important part of palliative treatment for patients with incurable disease as well as the treatment of patients with disease not amenable to surgery. As the pathological description of sarcomas has evolved, so has the treatment with radiation therapy. Today diagnosis and treatment is clearly more challenging for all practitioners, and radiation oncology has not been excluded.

In the chapters that follow, specific cases will be explored. In general, the comments regarding radiation therapy are largely restricted to indications and sequencing. Specifics details regarding dose, fractionation, target, technique, and modality are not discussed as that was felt to be outside the purpose of this book. This case exploration will hopefully yield understanding of the complex world of musculoskeletal neoplasms and the importance of the multidisciplinary approach.

Grade

Traditionally radiation therapy largely reduced treatment of sarcoma to two main groups: intermediate-high grade and low grade sarcoma. Nearly all experts will recommend radiation therapy as part of limb-sparing treatment for high grade sarcomas. This is based to a large degree on the randomized study conducted by Steven Rosenberg in the late 1970's, which demonstrate no difference in local control and overall survival between amputation and wide local excision with adjuvant radiation therapy (Rosenberg et al, 1982). Radiation for low grade sarcomas is a more debatable proposition. A randomized study conducted by James Yang did demonstrate a reduction in local recurrence in low grade sarcoma, but showed no survival benefit. Consequently, if a local recurrence is unlikely to affect mobility or function, some will advocate for observation followed by re-excision and potential radiation if the tumor recurs. The preferred grading system due to reproducibility and ease of use is the French FNCLCC (Fédération Nationale des Centres de Lutte Contre le Cancer) system shown below (Guillou et al, 1997) (**Table 4.4**). This is currently the recommended system by the AJCC. Today, grade plays a critical role in selection of appropriate treatment, but anatomic location, histology, genetic abnormalities, patient age, and sequencing of treatment modalities can significantly complicate therapy decisions.

Sequencing of radiation

One important consideration in treatment of sarcomas is the sequencing of surgery and radiation therapy. Many or even most radiation oncologists will advocate for the neo-adjuvant application of radiation as it allows for a lower dose and a smaller treatment volume. The randomized study performed by Brian O'Sullivan demonstrated no difference in local control rates when radiation therapy was applied prior to surgery compared with after surgery (O'Sullivan et al, 2002). There was increased wound complications following upfront radiation, but a follow-up paper showed a trend towards decreased late toxicity, especially fibrosis (Davis et al, 2005).

Future of musculoskeletal radiation oncology

The future for radiation of musculoskeletal neoplasms will likely be in two arenas: an evolution of indications for radiation therapy and improvement in techniques.

A preview of the evolution of indications can be seen in small series and case reports that have identified excellent responses correlated with specific genetic abnormalities within the neoplasm. Some of these will be described in the chapters that follow. An example is myxoid liposarcoma. This malignancy is associated with a translocation of chromosomes 12 and 16, t(12;16)(q13;p11), case reports and small series have demonstrated marked responses to radiation and chemotherapy. As techniques for genetic sequencing improve in both cost and speed, these techniques will be increasingly utilized and correlated with outcomes. This will clarify indications for both radiation therapy and chemotherapy.

The future for radiation oncology with regard to technology will like rely on better utilization of imaging. Imaging, both anatomical and functional, continues to improve. These improvements have already impacted the target for radiation. As imaging improves, these improvements will be utilized in radiation treatment planning. This will result in improved definition of the target and allow for greater sparing of normal tissue. Currently, a preview of this can be seen in the development of a consensus paper on targets for intensity modulated radiation therapy (IMRT) for extremity sarcoma (Wang et al, 2011).

Advice for medical students

Radiation oncology is very different from most medical or surgical practices. The aspiring medical student should first explore general radiation oncology. The best way to explore the application of radiation in sarcoma is through research. Opportunities for research in sarcoma will largely be available only at high volume academic centers.

Advice for residents

The specifics of indications, techniques, sequencing, doses, and definition of targets for radiation in sarcoma can be very confusing to the physician in training. As an example, there is a smattering of special indications for radiation therapy in both benign and malignant musculoskeletal neoplasms, some are debatable and some are not. These include: keloids, heterotopic ossifications, myxoid liposarcomas, desmoids tumors, chondrosarcoma of the clivus, and others. Many of these are discussed in the chapters that follow. Techniques can also be confusing as different high volume centers will utilize different techniques. These include intraoperative radiation (IORT), interstitial brachytherapy, and particle beam technology. Utilization of these techniques is dependent on local availability and expertise. Residents interested in sarcoma should pursue a residency or fellowship position at a high volume academic center and pursue research.

Table 4.4 FNCLCC grading system (add tumor differentiation, mitotic count, and tumor necrosis scores)

Final grade	Total score
1	2-3
2	4-5
3	6-8

Tumor differentiation	Score
Resembles mature normal mesenchymal tissue	1
Sarcomas of definite histologic type	2
Undifferentiated and unknown tumor type, synovial and embryonal sarcomas	3

Mitotic count	Score
0-9 mitoses per 10 hpfs	1
10-19 mitoses per 10 hpfs	2
20+ mitoses per 10 hpfs	3

Tumor necrosis	Score
No necrosis	0
Less than or equal to 50%	1
Greater than 50%	2

Histologic type	Score
Well-differentiated liposarcoma	1
Myxoid liposarcoma	2
Round-cell liposarcoma	3
Pleomorphic liposarcoma	3
Dedifferentiated liposarcoma	3
Well-differentiated fibrosarcoma	1
Conventional fibrosarcoma	2
Poorly differentiated fibrosarcoma	3
Well-differentiated malignant schwannoma (malignant neurofibroma)	1
Conventional malignant schwannoma	2
Poorly differentiated malignant schwannoma	3
Epithelioid malignant schwannoma	3
Malignant triton tumor	3
Well-differentiated malignant hemangiopericytoma	2
Conventional malignant hemangiopericytoma	3
Myxoid MFH	2
Typical storiform/pleomorphic MFH	2
Giant-cell and inflammatory MFH	3
Well-differentiated leiomyosarcoma	1
Conventional leiomyosarcoma	2
Poorly differentiated/pleomorphic/ epithelioid leiomyosarcoma	3
Biphasic/monophasic synovial sarcoma	3
Embryonal/alveolar/pleomorphic rhabdomyosarcoma	3
Well-differentiated chondrosarcoma	1
Myxoid chondrosarcoma	2
Mesenchymal chondrosarcoma	3
Conventional angiosarcoma	2
Poorly differentiated/epithelioid angiosarcoma	3
Extraskeletal osteosarcoma	3
Ewing's sarcoma/PNET	3
Alveolar soft tissue sarcoma	3
Epithelioid sarcoma	3
Malignant rhabdoid tumor	3
Clear-cell sarcoma	3
Undifferentiated sarcoma	3

MFH: malignant fibrous histiocytoma; PNET: primitive neurectodermal tumour

REFERENCES

Antman K, Crowley J, Balcerzak SP, et al. An intergroup phase II randomizes study of doxorubicin and dacarbazine with or without ifosfamide and mesna in advanced soft tissue and bone sarcomas. J Clin Oncol 1993;11:1276–85.

Antman KH, Ryan L, Elias A, et al. response to ifosfamide and mesna: 124 previously treated patients with metastatic or unresectable sarcoma. J Clin Oncol 1989;7:126–31.

Bileo P, Morgan JA, Zahrieh D, et al. Gemcitabine and vinorelbine combination chemotherapy for patients with advanced soft tissue sarcomas: results of a phase II trial. Cancer 2007:109:1863–9.

Blay JV, von Mehren M, Samuels BL, et al. Phase I combination study of trabectedin and doxorubicin in patients with soft-tissue sarcoma. Clin Cancer Res 2008;14:6656–62.

Borden EC, Amato DA, Rosenbaum C, et al. Randomized comparison of three adriamycin regimens for metastatic soft tissue sarcomas. J Clin Oncol 1987;5:840–50.

Bramwell VH, Mouridsen HT, Santoro A, et al. Cyclophosphamide versus ifosfamide: a randomized phase II trial in adult soft-tissue sarcomas. The European Organization for Research and Treatment of Cancer [EORTC], Soft Tissue and Bone Sarcoma Group. Cancer Chemother Pharmacol 1993;31 Suppl 2:S180–4.

Buesa JM, Lopez-Pousa A, Martin J, et al. Phase II rial of first-line high-dose ifosfamide in advanced soft tissue sarcomas of the adult: a study of the Spanish Group for Research on Sarcomas (GEIS). Ann Oncol 1998;9:871–6.

Buesa JM, Mouridsen HT, van Oosterom AT, et al. High-dose DTIC in advanced soft-tissue sarcomas in the adult. A phase II study of the EORTC Soft Tissue and Bone Sarcoma Group. Ann Oncol 1991;2:307–9.

Butrynski JE, D'Adamo DR, Hornick JL, et al. Crizotinib in ALK-rearranged inflammatory myofibroblastic tumor. N Engl J Med 2010;363:1727-1733.

Casper ES, Waltzman RJ, Schwartz GK, et al. Phase II trial of paclitaxel in patient with soft-tissue sarcoma. Cancer Invest 1998;16:442–6.

Cassier PA, Dufresne A, Fayette J, et al. Emerging drugs for the treatment of soft tissue sarcomas. Expert Opin Emerg Drugs 2007;12:139–53.

Chawla SP, Staddon AP, Baker LH, et al. Phase II study of the mammalian target for rapamycin inhibitor ridaforolimus in patients with advanced bone and soft tissue sarcomas. J Clin Oncol 2012;30:78–84.

Chugh R, Wathen KJ, Maki RG, et al. Phase II multicenter trial of imatinib in 10 histologic subtypes of sarcoma using a bayesian hierarchical statistical model. J Clin Oncol 2009;27:3148–53.

Cianfrocca M, Lee S, Von Roenn J, et al. Randomized trial of paclitaxel versus pegylated liposomal doxorubicin for advanced human immunodeficiency virus-associated Kaposi sarcoma: evidence of symptom palliation from chemotherapy. Cancer 116:3969–77.

Cohen MH, Creaven PJ, Tajada F, et al. Phase I clinical trial of isophosphamide (MSC-109724). Cancer Chemother Rep 1975;59:751–5.

D'Adamo DR, Anderson SR, Albritton K, et al. Phase II study of doxorubicin and bevacizumab for patients with metastatic soft-tissue sarcomas. J Clin Oncol 2005;23:7135–42.
Davis AM, O'Sullivan B, Turcotte R, et al. Late radiation morbidity following randomization to preoperative versus postoperative radiotherapy in extremity soft tissue sarcoma. Radiother Oncol 2005 Apr;75(1):48–53.
Dileo P, Morgan JA, Zahrieh D, et al. Gemcitabine and vinorelbine combination chemotherapy for patients with advanced soft tissue sarcomas: results of a phase II trial. Cancer 2007;109:1863–9.
Edmonson JH, Ryan LM, Blum RH, et al. Randomized comparison of doxorubicin alone versus ifosfamide plus doxorubicin or mitomycin, doxorubicin, and cisplatin against advanced soft tissue sarcomas. J Clin Oncol 1993;11:1269–75.
Erkizan HV, Kong Y, Merchant M, et al. A small molecule blocking oncogenic protein EWS-FLI1 interaction with RNA helicase A inhibits growth of Ewing's sarcoma. Nat Med 2009;15(7):750-6.
Ganjoo, KN, Cranmer LD, Butrynski JE, et al. A Phase I study of the safety and pharmacokinetics of the hypoxia-activated prodrug TH-302 in combination with doxorubicin in patients with advanced soft tissue sarcoma. Oncology 2011;80:50–6.
Garcia-Carbonero R, Supko JG, Manola J, et al. Phase II and pharmacokinetic study of ecteinascidin 743 in patients with progressive sarcomas of soft tissues refractory to chemotherapy. J Clin Oncol 2004;22:1480–90.
George S, Merriam P, Maki RG, et al. Multicenter phase II trial of sunitinib in the treatment of nongastrointestinal stromal tumor sarcomas. J Clin Oncol 2009;27:3154–60.
Gibault L, Perot G, Chibon F, et al. New insights in sarcoma oncogenesis: a comprehensive analysis of a large series of 160 soft tissue sarcomas with complex genomics. J Pathol 2011;223:64–71.
Gottlieb JA, Benjamin RS, Baker LH, et al. Role of DTIC (NSC-45388) in the chemotherapy of sarcomas. Cancer Treat Rep 1976;60:199–203.
Guillou L, Coindre JM, Bonichon F, et al. Comparative study of the National Cancer Institute and French Federation of Cancer Centers Sarcoma Group grading systems in a population of 410 adult patients with soft tissue sarcoma. J Clin Oncol 1997;15(1):350–62.
Hensley ML, Blessing JA, Mannel R, et al. Fixed-dose rate gemcitabine plus docetaxel as first-line therapy for metastatic uterine leiomyosarcoma: a Gynecologic Oncology group phase II trial. Gynecol Oncol 2008;109:329–34.
Hensley ML, Maki R, Venjatraman E, et al. Gemcitabine and docetaxel in patients with unresectable leiomyosarcoma: results of a phase II trial. J Clin Oncol 2002;20:2824–31.
Hoffmann AC, Danenberg KD, Taubert H, et al. A three-gene signature for outcome in soft tissue sarcoma. Clin Cancer Res 2009;15:5191–8.
Jemal A, Siegel R, Ward E, et al. Cancer statistics, 2009. CA Cancer J Clin 2009;59:225–49.
Judson I, Radford JA, Harris M, et al. Randomized phase II trial of pegylated liposomal doxorubicin (DOXIL/CAELYX) vesus doxorubicin in the treatment of advanced or metastatic soft tissue sarcoma: a study by the EORTC Soft Tissue and Bone Sarcoma Group. Eur J Cancer 2001;37:870–7.
Kilvaer TK, Valkov A, Sorbye S, et al. Profiling of VEFGs and VEFGRs as prognostic factors in soft tissue sarcoma: VEGFR-3 is an independent predictor of poor prognosis. PLoS One 2010;5:e15368.
Kummar S, Allen D, Monks A, et al. Cediranib for metastatic alveolar soft part sarcoma. J Clin Oncol 2013:20;31(18):2296-302.
Le Cesne A, Play JY, Judson I, et al. Phase II study of ET-743 in advanced soft tissue sarcomas: a European Organization for the Research and Treatment of Cancer (EORTC) soft tissue and bone sarcoma group trial. J Clin Oncol 2005;23:576–84.
Leu KM, Ostruszka Li, Shewach D, et al. Laboratory and clinical evidence of synergistic cytotoxicity of sequential treatment with gemcitabine followed by docetaxel in the treatment of sarcoma. J Clin Oncol 2004;22:1706–12.
Maki RG, D'Adamo DR, Kehan ML, et al. Phase II study of sorafenib in patients with metastatic or recurrent sarcomas. J Clin Oncol 2009;27:3133–40.
Maki RG, Wathen JK, Patel SR, et al. Randomized phase II study of gemcitabine and docetaxel compared with gemcitabine alone in patients with metastatic soft tissue sarcomas: results of sarcoma alliance for research through collaboration study 002 [corrected]. J Clin Oncol 2007;25:2755–63.
Maki RG. Small is beautiful: insulin-like growth factors and their role in growth, development, and cancer. J Clin Oncol 2010;28:4985–95.
Malempati S, Weigel B, Ingle AM, et al. Phase I/II trial and pharmacokinetic study of cixutumumab in pediatric patients with refractory solid tumors and Ewing sarcoma: a report from the Children's Oncology Group. J Clin Oncol 2012;30:256–62.
Martignoni G, Pea M, Reghelllin D, et al. Molecular pathology of lymphangioleiomyomatosis and other perivascular epithelioid cell tumors. Arch Pathol Lab Med 2010;134:33–40.
Movva S, Bocklage T, Schmit B, et al. Phase I study of irinotecan and temsirolimus in patients with refractory sarcomas. J Clin Oncol 2011;29S:A10027.
O'Sullivan B, Davis AM, Turcotte R, et al. Preoperative versus postoperative radiotherapy in soft-tissue sarcoma of the limbs: a randomized trial. Lancet 2002;359(9325):2235–41.
Olmos D, Postel-Vinay S, Molife LR, et al. Safety, pharmacokinetics, and preliminary activity of the anti-IGF-1R antibody figitumumab (CP-751,871) in patients with sarcoma and Ewing's sarcoma: a phase 1 expansion cohort study. Lancet Oncol 2010;11:129–35.
Patel SR, Vadhan-Raj S, Burgess MA, et al. Results of two consecutive trials of dose-intensive chemotherapy with doxorubicin and ifosfamide in patients with sarcomas. Am J Clin Oncol 1998;21:317–21.
Patel SR, Vadhan-Raj S, Papadopolous N, et al. High-dose ifosfamide in bone and soft tissue sarcomas: results of phase II and pilot studies—dose-response and schedule dependence. J Clin Oncol 1997;15:2378–84.
Penel N, Bui BN, Bay JO, et al. Phase II trials of weekly paclitaxel for unresectable angiosarcoma: the ANGIOTAX Study. J Clin Oncol 2008;26:5269–74.
Penel N, Marreaud S, Robin YM, et al. Angiosarcoma: state of the art and perspectives. Crit Rev Oncol Hematol 2011;80:257–63.
Rikhof B, de Jong S, Suurmeijer AJ, et al. The insulin-like growth factor system and sarcoma. J Pathol 2009;217:469–82.
Rosen G, Forscher C, Lowenbraun S, et al. Synovial sarcoma. Uniform response of metastases to high dose ifosfamide. Cancer 1994;73:2506–11.
Rosenberg SA, Tepper J, Glatstein E, et al. The treatment of soft-tissue sarcomas of the extremities: prospective randomized evaluations of (1) limb-sparing surgery plus radiation therapy compared with amputation and (2) the role of adjuvant chemotherapy. Ann Surg 1982;196(3):305–15.
Rutkowski P, Van Glabbeke M, Rankin CJ, et al. Imatinib mesylate in advanced dermatofibrosarcoma protuberans: pooled analysis of two phase II clinical trials. J Clin Oncol 2010;28(10):1772-9.
Schein PS, Winokur SH. Immunosuppressive and cytotoxic chemotherapy: long-term complications. Ann Intern Med 1975;82:84–95.
Schoenfeld DA, Rosenbaum C, Horton J, et al. A comparison of Adriamycin versus vincristine and adriamycin, and cyclophosphamide versus vincristine, actinomycin-D, and cyclophosphamide for advanced sarcoma. Cancer 1982;50:2757–62.
Schoffski P, Ray-Coquard IL, Cioffi A, et al. Activity of eribulin mesylate in patients with soft-tissue sarcoma: a phase 2 studyin four independent histological subtypes. Lancet Oncol 2011;12:1045–52.
Seifert CF, Nesser ME, Thompson DR. Dexrazoxane in the prevention of doxorubicin-induced cardiotoxicity. Ann Pharmacother 1994;28:1063–72.
Sleijfer S, Ouali M, van Glabbeke M, et al. Prognostic and predictive factors for outcome to first-line ifosfamide-containing chemotherapy for adult patients with advanced soft tissue sarcomas: an exploratory, retrospective analysis on large series from the European Organization for Research and Treatment of Cancer-Soft Tissue and Bone Sarcoma Group (EORTC-STBSG). Eur J Cancer 46:72–83.
Sleijfer S, Ray-Coquard I, Papai Z, et al. Pazopanib, a multikinase angiogenesis inhibitor, in patients with relapsed or refractory advanced soft tissue sarcoma: a phase II study from the European organization for research and treatment of cancer-soft tissue and bone sarcoma group (EORTC study 62043). J Clin Oncol 2009;27:3126–32.
Stacchiotti S, Negri T, Zaffaroni N, et al. Sunitinib in advanced alveolar soft part sarcoma: evidence of a direct antitumor effect. Ann Oncol 2011;22(7):1682-90.
Steigen SE, Schaeffer DF, West RB, et al. Expression of insulin-like growth factor 2 in mesenchymal neoplasms. Mod Pathol 2009;22:914–21.
Svancarova L, Blay JY, Judson IR, et al. Gemcitabine in advanced adult soft-tissue sarcomas. A phase II study of the EORTC Soft Tissue and Boone Sarcoma Group. Eur J Cancer 2002;38:556–9.
Tempero M, Plunkett W, Ruiz Van Haperen V, et al. Randomized phase II comparison of dose-intense gemcitabine: thirty-minute infusion and fixed dose rate infusion in patients with pancreatic adenocarcinoma. J Clin Oncol 2003;21:3402–8.

Toma S, Tucci A, Villani G, et al. Liposomal doxorubicin (Caelyx) in advanced pretreated soft tissue sarcomas: a phase II study of the Italian Sarcoma Group (ISG). Anticancer Res 2000;20:485–91.

van Hoesel QG, Verweij J, Catimel G, et al. Phase II study with docetaxel (Taxotere) in advanced soft tissue sarcomas of the adult. EORTC Soft Tissue and Bone Sarcoma Group. Ann Oncol 1994;5:539–42.

Vermeij J, Catimel G, Sulkes A, et al. Phase II studies of docetaxel in the treatment of various solid tumours. EORTC Early Clinical Trials Group and the EORTC Soft Tissue and Bone Sarcoma Group. Eur J Cancer 1995;31A Suppl 4:S21–4.

Verschraegen CF, Arias-Pulido H, Lee SJ, et al. Phase IB study of the combination of docetaxel, gemcitabine, and bevacizumab in patients with advanced or recurrent soft tissue sarcoma: the Axtell regimen. Ann Oncol 2012;23:785–.90.

Von Burton G, Rankin C, Zalupski MM, et al. Phase II trial of gemcitabine as first line chemotherapy in patients with metastatic or unresectable soft tissue sarcoma. Am J Clin Oncol 2006;29:59–61.

Wagner AJ, Goldberg JM, Dubois SG, et al. Tivantinib (ARQ 197), a selective inhibitor of MET, in patients with microphthalmia transcription factor-associated tumors: results of a multicenter phase 2 trial. Cancer 2012;118(23):5894-902.

Wang D, Bosch W, Roberge D, et al. RTOG sarcoma radiation oncologists reach consensus on gross tumor volume and clinical target volume on computed tomographic images for preoperative radiotherapy of primary soft tissue sarcoma of extremity in Radiation therapy Oncology Group Studies. Int J Radiat Oncol Biol Phys 2011;81(4):e525–8.

Yang JC, Chang AE, Baker AR, et al. Randomized prospective study of the benefit of adjuvant radiation therapy in the treatment of soft tissue sarcomas of the extremity. J Clin Oncol 1998;16(1):197–203.

Yovine A, Riofrio M, Blay JY, et al. Phase II study of ecteinascidin-743 in advanced pretreated soft tissue sarcoma patients. J Clin Oncol 2004;22:890–9.

Zucali PA, Bertuzzi A, Parra HJ, et al. The 'old drug' dacarbazine as a second/third line chemotherapy in advanced soft tissue sarcomas. Invest New Drugs 2008;26:175–81.

Chapter 5 Adipocytic tumors

OVERVIEW

The most common soft tissue tumor that is resected is the lipoma. Despite its ubiquity, it is a true monoclonal neoplasm composed of mature adipocytes with characteristic, sometimes surprisingly complex genetic changes.

Besides the abundant lipoma, adipocytic tumors range from other benign types to aggressive liposarcomas. Not only is the lipoma the most common benign adult soft tissue tumor**,** liposarcoma is the most common adult sarcoma (for example, liposarcoma comprises 25% of all soft tissue sarcomas in a European database: www.conticabase.org)(Coindre et al. 2010).

In describing adipocytic tumors we will follow a plan used for all the ensuing chapters: 1) classify adipocytic tumors according to the World Health Organization (WHO) classification of 2013; 2) review the demographics of adipocytic tumors; 3) summarize the pathologic and molecular genetic features of these tumors; 4) list soft tissue tumors composed partly of fat that are excluded from the adipocytic tumor family, although adipocytes may form a considerable portion of the tumor, and finally; 5) discuss the radiology, surgery, and oncology of adipocytic tumors.

CLASSIFICATION

The 2013 WHO classification of adipocytic tumors is provided in **Table 5.1** below according to behavior.

As is the case with other bone and soft tissue tumors, enthusiastic pathologists occasionally report new variants of adipocytic tumors. However, the adipocytic tumors officially recognized by the World Health Organization are listed in **Table 5.1**. These are tumors that occur more often than in a boutique case report or two, feature reproducible histologic features, and behave in a predictable fashion, perhaps not within a single patient but across groups of patients.

Figure 5.1 indicates the total number of liposarcomas diagnosed in 13 Surveillance, Epidemiology and End Results (SEER) registries from 1994-2008 according to major type. Notably, although liposarcoma is the most common adult sarcoma, less than 4000 were diagnosed over these 14 years (about 270 per year; culled from 15% of the US population). Also, note that the third most common 'type' diagnosed by US pathologists (private and academic) was not otherwise specified (NOS); in other words, 18% were not specifically subtyped. Pathologists specializing in sarcoma diagnosis have a much lower rate of NOS cases, in part due to expertise accrued by the large

Table 5.1 WHO classification of adipocytic tumors of soft tissue (2013)

Tumor	Behavior	Additional comments
Lipoma • Lipoma • Fibrolipoma • Intramuscular or intermuscular lipoma • Others such as osteolipoma or chondrolipoma	Benign	Abundant tumor in adults; rare in children
Lipomatosis	Benign	Many lipomas; may be associated with liver disease or certain ethnicities
Lipomatosis of nerve	Benign	Rare, predominantly affects median or ulnar nerve
Lipoblastoma/lipoblastomatosis	Benign	Almost exclusive to pediatric age group
Angiolipoma	Benign	Often occurs as multiple subcutaneous nodules < 3 cm
Myolipoma	Benign	Rare tumor composed of smooth muscle and fat
Chondroid lipoma	Benign	Benign fat tumor that contains lipoblasts as well as mature fat cells
Extra-renal angiomyolipoma	Benign	Not discussed in this text as it is an intra-abdominal tumor
Extra-adrenal myelolipoma	Benign	Not discussed in this text as it is an intra-abdominal tumor
Spindle cell/pleomorphic lipoma	Benign	These two tumors share the exact same genetic findings and occur in the same body sites
Atypical lipomatous tumor/well differentiated liposarcoma • Lipoma like • Sclerosing • Inflammatory • Spindle cell	Intermediate	ALT is the term for this tumor when it occurs in extremities and head and neck. Well diff liposarcoma is the term used when it occurs in the retroperitoneum or mediastinum. Spindle cell liposarcoma is currently classified as a type of atypical lipomatous tumor/well differentiated liposarcoma. However, it has different IHC and genetic findings and may represent a unique type of LPS, albeit one that behaves as an ALT/well differentiated liposarcoma
Dedifferentiated liposarcoma	Malignant	May occur de novo or may arise in an ALT or well diff liposarcoma
Myxoid liposarcoma	Malignant	High grade variant is called round cell liposarcoma
Pleomorphic liposarcoma	Malignant	Contains markedly atypical lipoblasts
Liposarcoma, not otherwise specified	Malignant	Features do not allow specific subtyping

Benign: does not recur or recurs non-aggressively and does not metastasize. Intermediate: can recur aggressively and/or may rarely (<5%) metastasize. Malignant: can recur and commonly metastasizes.

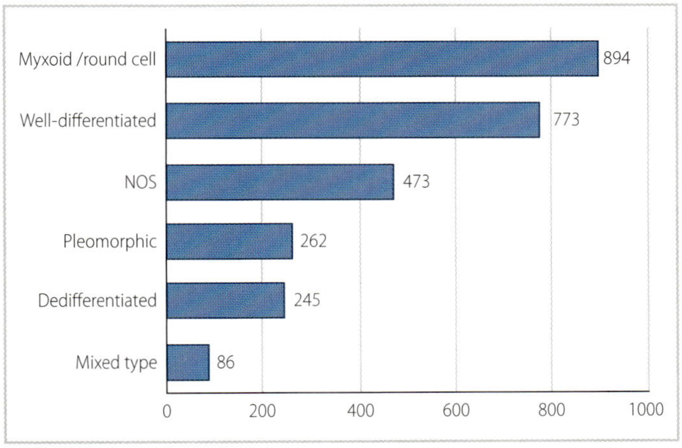

Figure 5.1 Frequency of liposarcoma subtypes in 13 SEER registries between 1994 and 2008 (SEER US National Cancer Institute Multicenter Epidemiology Project).

number of specimens they review and because of access to ancillary diagnostic tests.

Several adipocytic tumors include subvariants distinguished by distinct histologic features. However, the subvariants share genetic abnormalities (Hameed et al. 2007). For example, the well-differentiated liposarcoma has three variants: 1) lipoma-like; 2) sclerosing; and 3) inflammatory. The lipoma-like is the most common and histologically looks similar to a lipoma, the sclerosing type has large areas of fibrosis, and the inflammatory type may have so many inflammatory cells that they obscure the neoplastic adipocytes. All three types behave similarly and contain giant marker and supernumerary ring chromosomes that comprise many duplications of the 13-15 bands of the long arm of chromosome 12 (12q13-15).

Spindle cell liposarcoma has been classified as a type of well-differentiated liposarcoma. However, genetically it is dissimilar and may behave differently as well. In fact, it may be closely related to the benign spindle cell/pleomorphic lipoma, a tumor it resembles histologically (Mentzel et al, 2010).

DEMOGRAPHICS

In line with many other soft tissue sarcomas, malignant adipocytic tumors usually occur in an older age group. However, even benign fat tumors such as lipoma are uncommon in children. Most tumors of fat afflict adults. Lipoblastoma is the exception, and it is virtually always restricted to infancy and childhood. **Figure 5.2** depicts the age range of liposarcoma types from 1994-2008 in the US (SEER). Note that there is a large age range per type but that the average age of the myxoid/round cell and mixed types is younger. The 'mixed' type of liposarcoma recorded in SEER records may include a substantial number of myxoid/round cell liposarcomas which can exhibit histologic heterogeneity and thus be misclassified as 'mixed'. Thus, classification slippage may explain the younger age of 'mixed' liposarcomas in the SEER data.

Liposarcomas occur slightly more commonly in men (see **Table 5.2**), and men more frequently develop hibernomas and spindle cell lipomas/pleomorphic lipomas (Kempson et al. 2001).

PATHOGENESIS

As with many other soft tissue tumors, the exact etiology of adipocytic tumors is not established. Do obese patients develop more adipocytic tumors? Partly, because lipomas but not the other types of adipocytic tumors seem to be more common in overweight individuals. Genetic perturbances play a large role, because specific chromosomal abnormalities occur for many of the tumor types (refer to **Table 5.3** describing the genetics of specific adipocytic tumors).

What is known about the cause of most adipocytic tumors implicates abnormalities of genes on the long arm of Chromosome 12 position q13-15. This region contains 164 genes of which a few are amplified and over expressed (*MDM2*, *CDK4*, and *HMGA2*; important players in well-differentiated/dedifferentiated liposarcoma) and a few display structural changes (*HMGA2* and *DDIT3*, important players in lipoma and myxoid/round cell liposarcoma, respectively). In general, the abnormalities match a specific type of adipocytic tumor. Interestingly, a few of the genes involved in fat tumor generation, such as *HMGA2* and *DYRK2*, also contribute to the formation of a considerable number of non-adipocytic tumors such as chondromas and deep angiomyxoma among others (Italiano A et al. 2008). See **Table 5.2** for the genetic findings in adipocytic tumors, as is understood currently, of course.

Although abnormalities of the 12q13-15 region are crucial to the pathogenesis of many lipomatous tumors, several adipocytic tumors lack 12q13-15 alterations. These comprise: 1) angiolipoma, 2) spindle cell/pleomorphic lipoma, 3) lipoblastoma, 4) hibernoma, 5) chondroid lipoma, and 6) spindle cell liposarcoma.

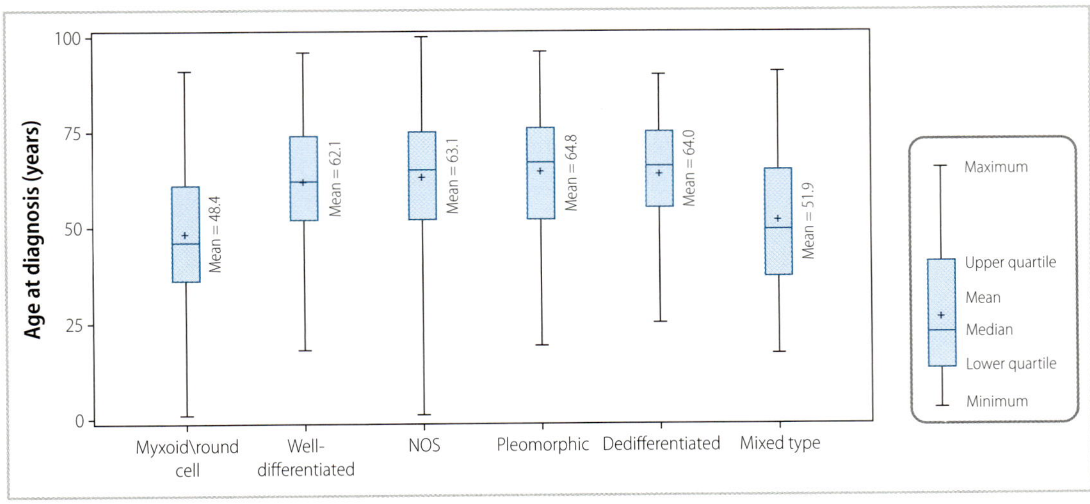

Figure 5.2 Age distribution of liposarcoma subtypes among cases in 13 SEER registries during 1994-2008 (N=2,733).

Table 5.2 Average annual incidence rates of liposarcoma tumors in 13 SEER registries between 1994 and 2008.

	Age-adjusted incidence rate per million (standard error)		
Liposarcoma subtype	**Overall**	**Male**	**Female**
Myxoid/round cell	1.6 (0.1)	2.0 (0.1)	1.2 (0.1)
Well differentiated	1.4 (0.1)	1.9 (0.1)	1.0 (0.1)
NOS	0.9 (0.0)	1.1 (0.1)	0.7 (0.0)
Dedifferentiated	0.4 (0.0)	0.7 (0.1)	0.3 (0.0)
Pleomorphic	0.5 (0.0)	0.7 (0.1)	0.4 (0.0)
Mixed type	0.2 (0.0)	0.2 (0.0)	0.1 (0.0)

SEER data were evaluated from 13 registries during a 15 year period (1994-2008). This section will focus on 6 malignant liposarcoma subtypes (with the ICDO-3 code presented parenthetically): well-differentiated (8851/3), myxoid/round cell (8852/3 and 8853/3), pleomorphic (8854/3), mixed type (8855/3), de-differentiated (8858/3), and not otherwise specified (NOS) (8850/3). All tumors presented here arise in the connective, subcutaneous and other soft tissues. Of these cases, the overall age-adjusted incidence rate for liposarcoma is 4.9 per million. Males have statistically higher incidence rates of every liposarcoma subtype compared to females (**Table 5.2**). The number of cases reported in 13 SEER registries is shown in **Figure 5.3**.

Table 5.3 Genetics of adipocytic tumors

Tumor	Chromosomal abnormality	Genes involved	Percentage of tumors with abnormality
Lipoma	Mostly translocations or insertions at 12q13-15 (most often t(3;12)), 6p21-23, and loss of 13q; these occur in separate tumors or less commonly together	*HMGA2* and LPP as well as others The key finding is structural rearrangements not amplification of *HMGA2* (there are rare exceptions)	55-75%, higher % in older patients 67% have 12q13-15 aberrations 33% have 6p21-23 or loss of 13q etc.
Angiolipoma	Normal karyotype	Aberrant *HMGA2* gene expression	100% have normal karyotype
Hibernoma	Rearrangements and losses at 11q13-21	Loss of *MEN1* and/or *AIP* (11q13) with losses of other genes at this site and abnormal high expression of other genes including *UCP1*	Majority
Spindle cell lipoma/ pleomorphic lipoma	Monosomy or partial loss of 13 and/or 16 (most commonly 16q13-qter and 13q12 and 13q14-q22)	RB1 gene deletion (13q14)	>90%
Chondroid lipoma	t(11;16)(q13;p12-13)	C11orf95 (11q13) – *MKL2* (16p13.3) gene fusion	Unknown
Lipoblastoma	Rearrangements of 8q11-13 +/- gain of chromosome 8	*PLAG1* (8q12.1) rearranged. Partners include HAS2 (8q24.13) and *COL1A2* (7q21.3)	>95%
Atypical lipomatous tumor/well-differentiated liposarcoma	Supernumerary ring and giant marker chromosomes (comprise amplification of 12q13-q15)	*MDM2, HDM2* or *HDMX* (p53 binding protein gene), *CDK4, SAS, HMGA2*	100%
Dediffentiated liposarcoma	Supernumerary ring and giant marker chromosomes (comprises amplification of 12q13-q15 +/- others)	*MDM2, HDM2* or *HDMX* (p53 binding protein gene), *CDK4, SAS, HMGA2*	100%
Myxoid/round cell liposarcoma	t(12;16)(q13;p11)	*CHOP-FUS* gene translocation (*CHOP* is also called *DDIT3* (12q13)-*FUS* (16p11). Other mutations also present especially in round cell liposarcoma	95%
	t(12;22)(q13;q12)	*EWSR1* (22q12)-*DDIT3* (12q13) Other mutations also present	5%
Pleomorphic liposarcoma	Aneuploid Amplification of MDM2 gene at 12q13-15*.	Additional numerous abnormalities as seen in other high grade sarcomas. *MDM2**	33%*. 100% have additional numerous abnormalities as seen non-specifically in high grade sarcomas

Table 5.3: Continued from page 44

Tumor	Chromosomal abnormality	Genes involved	Percentage of tumors with abnormality
The rare pleomorphic epithelioid liposarcoma may actually be a type of myxoid/round cell liposarcoma	t(12;16)(q13;p11)	*DDIT3-FUS*	Too few cases to know at this point
Spindle cell liposarcoma	Monosomy 7	Not applicable	Too few cases to know at this point (n=2 to date)
Some information in this table may be preliminary and based on only a few reports. Therefore, caution is warranted. New findings are regularly being reported, and therefore this list may be incomplete.			

Why are there only four types of liposarcoma and not 15, for example? A recent elegant study partially addresses this question by comparing normal adipocytes arrested at various stages of differentiation with the liposarcoma types. By analyzing gene expression profiles, the authors found that liposarcomas that look more mature microscopically actually express genes in common with the mature fat cell. In contrast, the less histologically mature liposarcomas, such as dedifferentiated liposarcoma and pleomorphic liposarcoma, share gene expression profiles with immature, early developing fat cells (Days 7 and 10 of a 21 day maturation period). Moreover, the dedifferentiated and pleomorphic liposarcomas retain expression of genes that are associated with mesenchymal stem cells; these genes are turned off in the more mature tumors (well-differentiated liposarcoma, and myxoid/round cell liposarcoma) (Matushansky et al. 2008).

So, it appears that there may be particularly vulnerable times (four times) in the maturation of fat cells when they can undergo mutations that lead to specific types of liposarcoma (four types). Perhaps further gene expression work will show that many high grade pleomorphic sarcomas, not otherwise specified (sarcomas with no histological observable lines of differentiation) are in actuality a fifth type of liposarcoma, one that is molecularly related to Day 1 or Day 2 cells of the 21 day fat cell maturation cycle.

Interestingly, two recent reviews of dedifferentiated liposarcoma support a notion that historically was heretical: pleomorphic liposarcoma can compose the dedifferentiated component in dedifferentiated liposarcoma (Marino-Enriquez et al. 2010, Boland et al. 2010). The contenders of this proposal suggest that in such a case, the tumor should no longer be diagnosed as mixed liposarcoma (e.g. a combination of dedifferentiated liposarcoma and pleomorphic liposarcoma) but as dedifferentiated liposarcoma in which pleomorphic liposarcoma forms the dedifferentiated component. At the protein level, it seems that the pleomorphic liposarcoma portion of these dedifferentiated liposarcomas displays reactivity for MDM2 and CDK4 consistent with dedifferentiation from a well-differentiated component (de novo pleomorphic liposarcoma not associated with well-differentiated liposarcoma does not usually over-express MDM2 and CDK4). From these observations, it seems reasonable to assume that the category of 'mixed liposarcoma' will decline in future reported cases of liposarcoma.

Why don't lipomas transform to liposarcomas? After all, for many carcinomas such as squamous carcinoma, there is a premalignant stage known as dysplasia. Why isn't a lipoma the premalignant stage of liposarcoma? The answer seems to reside, as usual, in the genes. Almost all lipomas exhibit structural rearrangements of the HMGA2 gene (usually in the form of various translocations or inversions). Liposarcomas, on the other hand, show amplification as well as structural rearrangements of the HMGA2 gene and neighboring genes, MDM2, CDK4 and less frequently SAS/TSPAN31. These genetic differences are distinct and lead to lipoma on the benign end and well-differentiated and dedifferentiated liposarcoma on the malignant end of the scale. Of course, remember that myxoid/round cell liposarcoma, spindle cell liposarcoma, and spindle cell/pleomorphic lipoma do not contain aberrations of the 12q13-15 region but rather abnormalities of other genes (see **Table 5.3** for details).

Of course, biology, including the human variety, is not 100% predictable: rarely, a lipoma may show the same genetic changes as a well-differentiated liposarcoma, and yet it looks and behaves like a lipoma (Italiano et al. 2007). However, the few tumors so described do not produce the proteins MDM2 and CDK4, as is seen in the majority of well-differentiated/dedifferentiated liposarcoma, a profound difference. Some groups advocate that histologically classic lipomas that feature the genetics of well-differentiated liposarcoma/dedifferentiated liposarcoma should be treated as the latter (Billing et al. 2008). Time will tell whether histology trumps genetics in terms of how best to classify and treat these tumors.

Both lipomas and liposarcomas often have additional abnormalities of other genes that also undoubtedly play a role in the divergence of the tumors. For example, dedifferentiated liposarcoma may also show amplification of the *JUN* gene in the 1p32 band and the *ASK1* gene in the 6q23 band in addition to amplification of specific genes at 12q14-15 (Coindre et al. 2010).

PATHOLOGY

The importance of being a lipoblast

A fat tumor with lipoblasts is not always malignant! A fat tumor without lipoblasts is not always benign!

A lipoblast was once considered the most reliable means of confirming the malignant nature of a fat tumor. Unfortunately, lipoblasts are not exclusively found in liposarcomas. In fact, it is now recognized that there are quite a few tumors that may contain lipoblasts but which are not malignant, such as spindle cell lipoma/plemorphic lipoma and lipoblastoma. Furthermore, some tumors contain cells that simulate lipoblasts (myxofibrosarcoma, most notoriously), some primitive cells that actually are lipoblasts cannot be recognized as such because they don't meet the classic cytologic criteria (true for the round cells of myxoid liposarcoma), and some well-differentiated liposarcomas don't seem to have any lipoblasts despite careful review of many sections of the tumor.

If lipoblasts are found (such as in **Figs 5.3** and **5.4**), these cells suggest a differential rather than conclusively confirm one. Lipoblasts come in several forms from histologically bland to starkly atypical (the latter are termed 'pleomorphic lipoblasts' meaning marked nuclear atypia is present as well as the requisite cytoplasmic fat vacuole(s) indenting the nucleus). While minimally atypical lipoblasts can be seen in both benign and malignant tumors, pleomorphic lipoblasts remain good indicators of a liposarcoma. Importantly, clinical and radiologic findings and newer pathology laboratory tests such as immunohistochemistry and cytogenetics enable pathologists to accurately classify adipocytic tumors without undue reliance on lipoblasts.

Histologic grading of adipocytic tumors

Benign adipocytic tumors are not graded.

According to the various grading systems, well-differentiated liposarcomas are Grade 1, myxoid liposarcomas are Grade 1 or 2, round cell liposarcomas are Grade 2 or 3, and dedifferentiated liposarcomas and pleomorphic liposarcomas are Grade 3. Please refer to the introductory chapters for more details regarding the National Cancer Institute, TNM Classification of Malignant Tumors and French Federation of Cancers grading systems.

Grading has importance, as it contributes to predicting behavior and outcome.

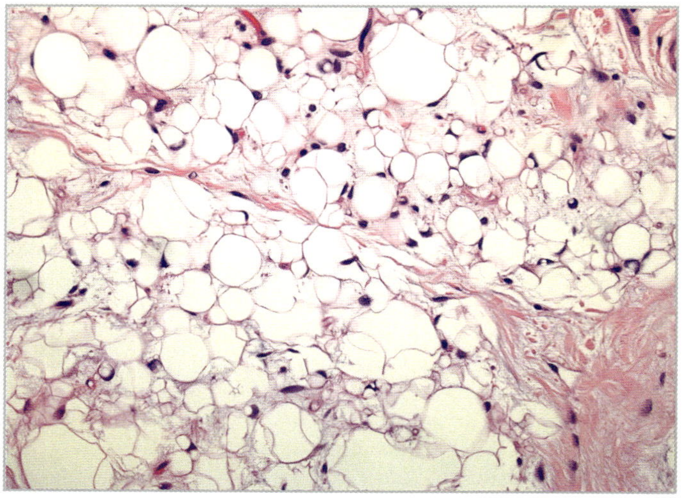

Figure 5.3 Univacuolar (including signet ring type) lipoblasts in a myxoid liposarcoma. This type of lipoblast with only nuclear atypia can be found in both malignant tumors and in benign tumors (examples of the latter include spindle cell/pleomorphic lipoma and lipoblastoma).

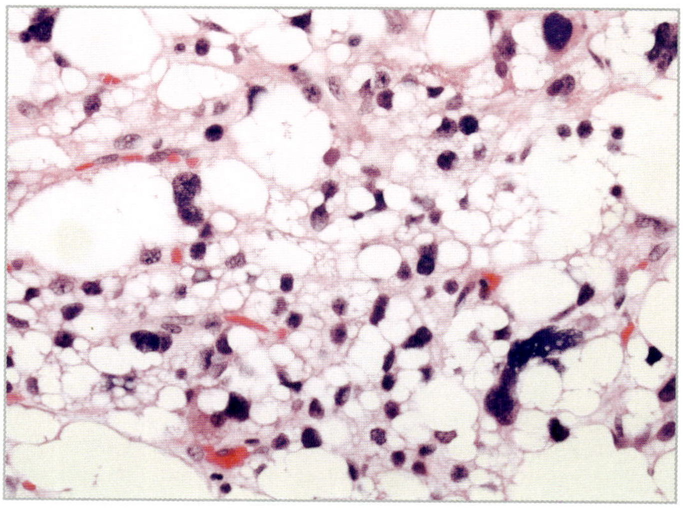

Figure 5.4 'Pleomorphic' lipoblasts in a pleomorphic liposarcoma. This marked degree of nuclear atypia is almost never seen in a benign lesion.

Behavior of adipocytic tumors

Behavior is related to the specific type of adipocytic tumor. Importantly, tumor size and location, both of which pertain to resectability, each play a role in outcome. Once a specific diagnosis such as myxoid liposarcoma is rendered, histologic grade also affects prognosis, the major reason why pathologists bother, although stage exerts a stronger effect in predicting outcome. A recently developed nomogram to predict outcome following surgery of liposarcomas includes the following independent predictors of five year and 12 year disease specific survival: age, presentation status (biopsy, no treatment or prior excision), histologic type, primary site, tumor size, and excision margin status (n= 801 patients treated at Memorial Sloan Kettering Medical Center from 1982-2005)(Moore Dalal et al. 2006). Interestingly, behavior does not seem to directly correlate with molecular findings, although this may change as more is discovered at the genetic level.

Of the benign tumors, intramuscular lipoma and lipoblastomatosis can recur locally because they may be difficult to entirely remove with conservative excision, and because some have the potential to regrow.

Among the malignant adipocytic tumors, pleomorphic liposarcoma is the most aggressive with a 30-50% metastasis rate and death due to tumor of 30-50% (Miettinen 2010). However, as noted from SEER data, pleomorphic liposarcoma shows a better survival than dedifferentiated liposarcoma. This is because of the inclusion of retroperitoneal tumors. Dedifferentiated liposarcoma invariably recurs locally even if the time interval is up to 20 years, and distant metastases occur in 15-20%. However, as with pleomorphic liposarcoma, smaller size and location in the extremities or superficial tissue improves survival and reduces the metastatic rate (Henricks 1997). Somewhat controversial is whether the histologic grade of the dedifferentiated component influences behavior, e.g. low grade dedifferentiated areas may portend a better behavior than high grade dedifferentiated regions. Interestingly, dedifferentiated liposarcomas one might expect to behave worse; those with smooth muscle or skeletal muscle malignant components (these comprise about 5% of dedifferentiated liposarcoma cases), do not behave any differently than dedifferentiated liposarcoma without muscle type sarcomatous areas (Binh et al. 2007).

High grade myxoid liposarcomas exhibit a much higher metastasis and mortality rate than lower grade myxoid liposarcomas. Grading of myxoid liposarcomas comprises evaluation of percentage of round cells (the higher grade area of myxoid/round cell liposarcoma) and presence of necrosis. Overexpression of p53 protein has also been reported to be a poor prognostic indicator in myxoid liposarcomas. Multifocal myxoid liposarcomas, even of low grade, also behave poorly, and some experts believe this represents soft tissue metastases rather than multiple metachronous primaries (Miettinen 2010). **Table 5.4** lists the ten year relative survival of liposarcoma patients diagnosed in the US from 1994-2008 (SEER data; 13 registries).

Figure 5.5 graphically depicts the most common body site locations of liposarcomas (SEER data from 13 registries 1994-2008). **Table 5.5** provides an abbreviated pathology description of adult adipocytic tumors grouped by behavior. **Table 5.6** lists the pediatric adipocytic tumors.

The last pathology table regarding adipocytic tumors actually describes tumors that can contain fat but are NOT classified as adipocytic tumors (**Table 5.7**). Why is that? Some of these neoplasms contain fat that is acting as a reactive space filler subsequent to skeletal muscle atrophy (such as with angiomatosis). Others are formed

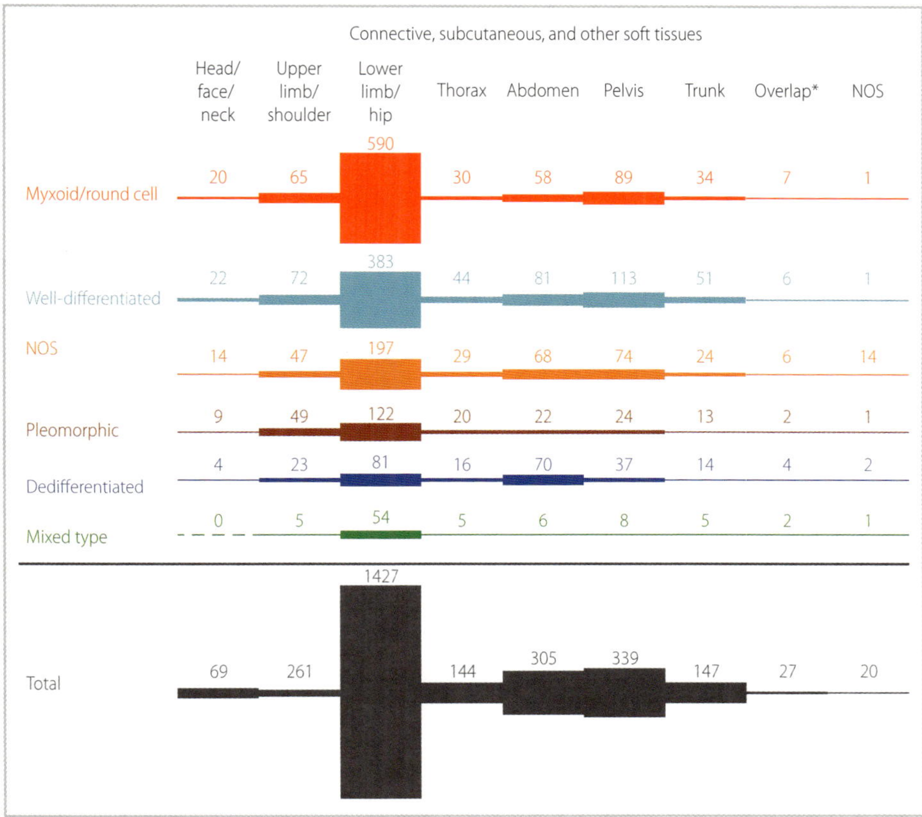

Figure 5.5 Liposarcoma tumors by site for cases In 13 SEER registries diagnosed between 1994 and 2008.

Table 5.4 Ten-year relative survival rate by liposarcoma subtype between 1994 and 2008, percent survival

Liposarcoma subtype	Relative survival (SE)
Myxoid	83.7% (2.4%)
Round cell	53.8% (7.0%)
Well-differentiated	98.7% (1.5%)
NOS	81.6% (3.3%)
Mixed type	76.9% (8.3%)
Pleomorphic	60.8% (5.5%)
Dedifferentiated	61.8% (6.2%)

Patients diagnosed with well-differentiated liposarcoma had the best prognosis compared to the other subtypes (10-year relative survival=98.7%). Furthermore, 53.8% of round cell liposarcoma patients survive their cancer at least 10 years from diagnosis after adjusting for normal life expectancy. (SE= Standard Error)

of cells that differentiate into several distinctive types with adipocytic cells forming only one contributor (such as fibrous hamartoma of infancy). Others in the list may only uncommonly contain fat (such as solitary fibrous tumor). However, on a case by case basis, these tumors may contain substantial amounts of fat, therefore, it is prudent to know about them and not to mistake them for actual WHO classified adipocytic tumors.

Special stains used to diagnose adipocytic tumors

S-100 Protein

Positive in most tumors with fat cells: most adipocytic tumor cells express S-100 protein that is commonly both nuclear and cytoplasmic. The function of this protein is not known, and it is also produced by other mesenchymal and non-mesenchymal cells such as chondrocytes, melanocytes, Schwann cells, neuronal cells, some myoepithelial cells, and some inflammatory cells, among others. So, it is not exclusively expressed in fat cells. However, one would expect some positivity in a tumor of fat, although where it might be more helpful, such as in dedifferentiated liposarcoma, it is seldom strongly and diffusely reactive. This is because S-100 reacts most strongly with mature adipocytes with progressively weaker staining of immature adipocytes and lipoblasts, and malignant counterparts of these last two cells compose the bulk of higher grade tumors.

CD34

Positive in spindle cell lipoma/pleomorphic lipoma and spindle cell liposarcoma. Expression of this protein is also not specific. It is expressed in spindle cell lipoma/pleomorphic lipoma and to a lesser extent in spindle cell liposarcoma (the degree of extent, unfortunately, may be in the eye of the beholder, so percent reactivity does not really help distinguish the two lesions). CD34 reactivity occurs in the neoplastic spindle and pleomorphic cells and NOT in the neoplastic fat cells.

CDK4 and MDM2

Positive in well-differentiated lps and dedifferentiated liposarcoma. These are proteins whose genes are often altered in well-differentiated liposarcoma and dedifferentiated liposarcoma. These are very useful in the diagnosis of well-differentiated liposarcoma and dedifferentiated liposarcoma, especially when trying to determine if the former is not just a lipoma and the latter is not another type of sarcoma. For well-differentiated liposarcoma, CDK4 and/or MDM2 are usually expressed in scattered adipocyte nuclei (around one positive nucleus per high power microscopic field). MDM2 is more commonly expressed than

Table 5.5 Adult adipocytic tumors grouped by behavior

Tumor	Incidence	Age and sex distribution	Body site	Histopathology description including immunohistochemistry (IHC)	
				Medium magnification	High magnification
Benign: does not recur or does not do so aggressively and does not metastasize					
Lipoma	Very common	Adults, most commonly 40-60 years M = F	Anywhere but trunk most common	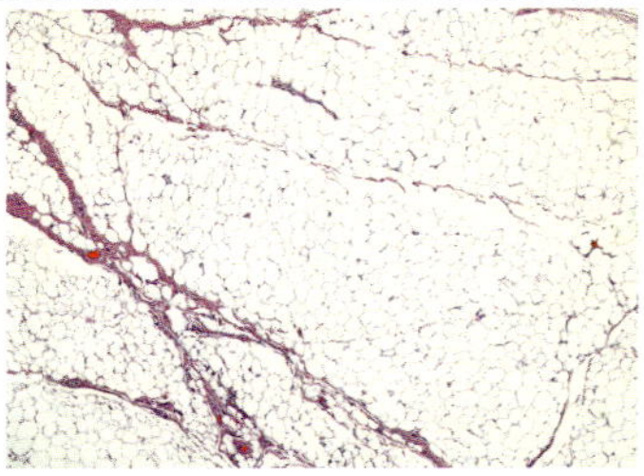	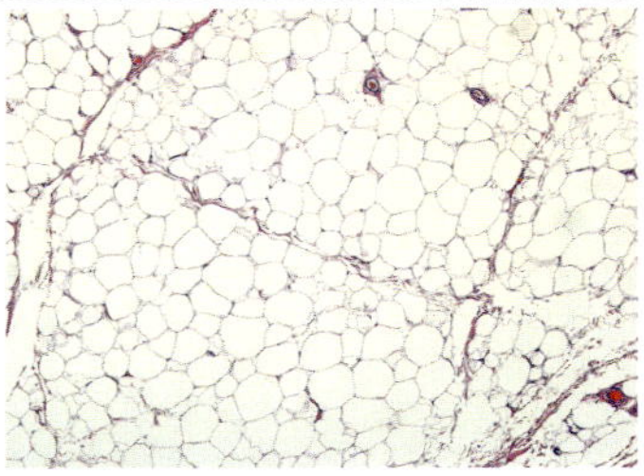
Looks like adult fat; all variants have mature fat cells with minimal size variation except in areas of fat necrosis.. Variants include fibrolipoma, myolipoma, osteolipoma, and myxolipoma (with added fibrous tissue, smooth muscle, bone and myxoid matrix, respectively). IHC: the mature fat cells are S-100 protein positive. Negative for MDM2 and CDK4. p16 may be positive but is usually only diffuse in areas of fat necrosis.					
Angiolipoma	Common	Adolescents and Young Adults in 20's M=F	Forearm typical Often multiple	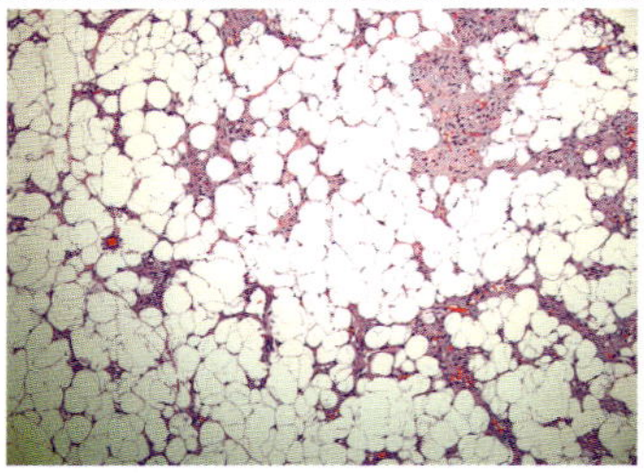	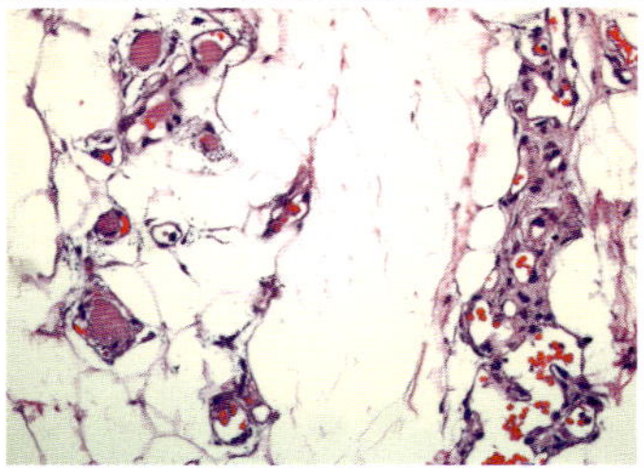
Mature fat cells with clusters of small vessels. IHC: fat cells are S-100 positive. Vessels commonly thrombosed. Tumors with many vessels can mimic histologically a vascular tumor (fat cells obscured).					
Hibernoma	Rare	Younger adults in 30's and 40's M slightly > F	Limbs, Trunk, Head and Neck	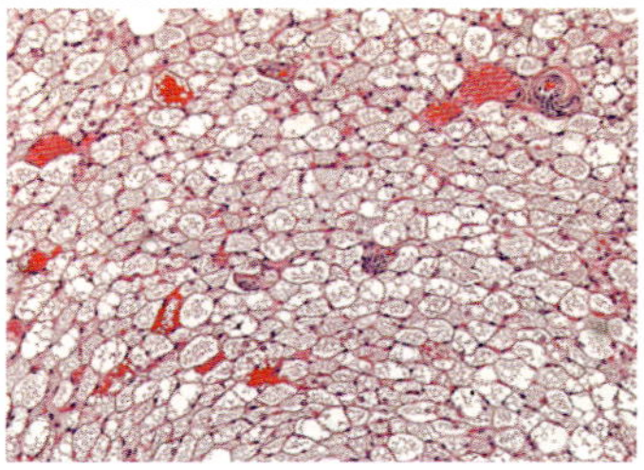	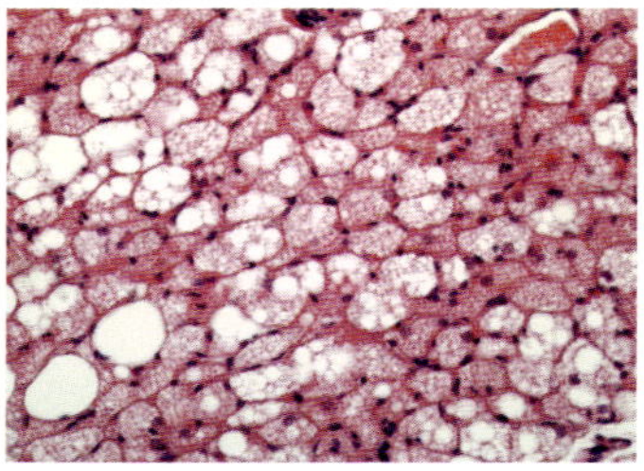
Looks like brown fat but can also contain mature adipocytes. Six variants occur including lipoma-like, myxoid, and spindle. IHC: S-100 protein positive. Negative for CDK4 and MDM2.					
Spindle cell lipoma/ pleomorphic lipoma	Common	Middle aged to older adults M >> F	Shoulder and Neck Rarely elsewhere	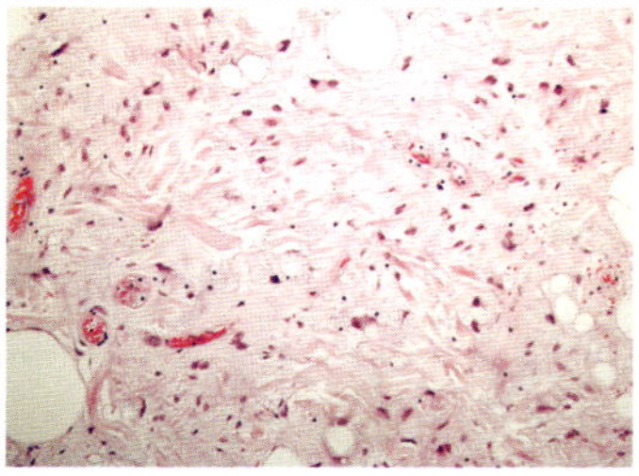	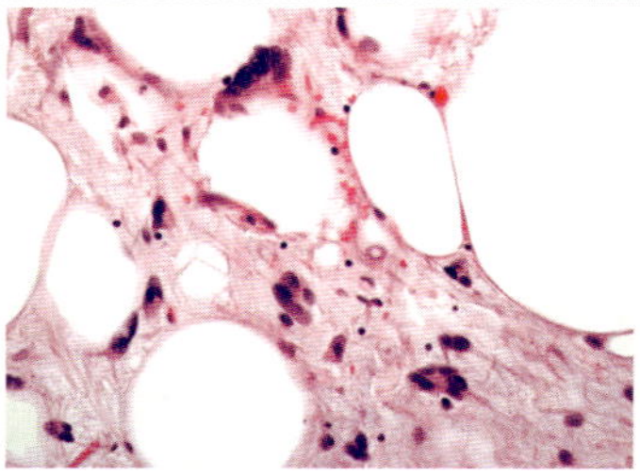
Mature adipocytes with mild size variation and spindle cells +/- pleomorphic cells including 'floret cells'. Lipoblasts may be present. Some minor variants. IHC: fat cells are S-100 protein positive. Spindle and pleomorphic cells are CD34 positive and usually negative for S-100 protein.					
Chondroid lipoma	Rare	Young adults F >> M	Limbs, back	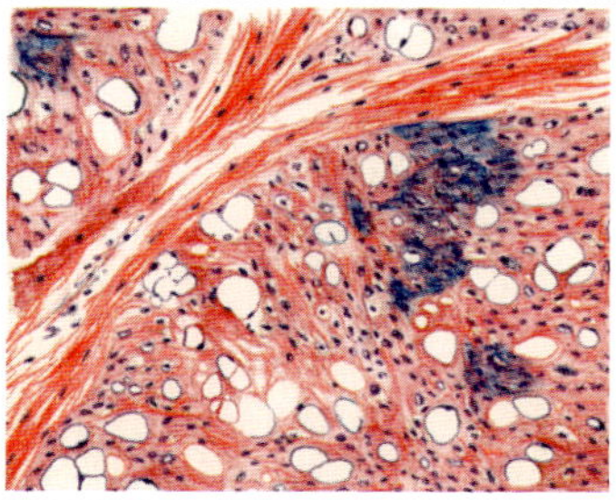	
Mature fat cells mixed with cells that have multiple vacuolations (like hibernoma cells) and cells with relatively high nuclear to cytoplasmic ratios. Cells sit in lacunae or in a myxoid to vaguely chondroid matrix. True cartilage is absent.					

Table 5.5: Continued from page 48

<table>
<tr><th rowspan="2">Tumor</th><th rowspan="2">Incidence</th><th rowspan="2">Age and sex distribution</th><th rowspan="2">Body site</th><th colspan="2">Histopathology description including IHC</th></tr>
<tr><th>Medium magnification</th><th>High magnification</th></tr>
<tr><td>Intramuscular lipoma (Intermuscular lipoma, a related lesion, occurs between but not in muscles.)</td><td>Common</td><td>Adults
M = F</td><td>Limbs</td><td>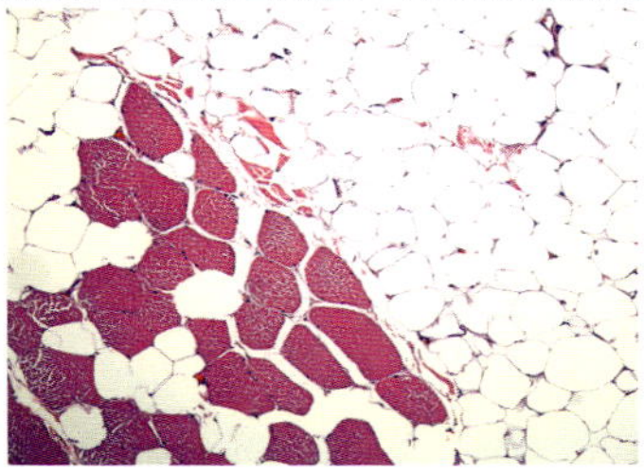</td><td>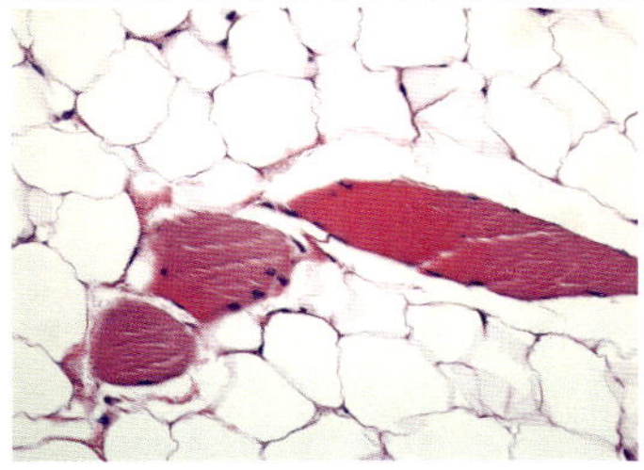</td></tr>
<tr><td colspan="6">Looks like mature fat with nearly evenly sized fat cells. However, the 'mature fat' infiltrates skeletal muscle at tumor margin and even within the tumor. This is benign but can locally recur (~20% of those with infiltrative borders) but aggressive surgery is NOT required or recommended. IHC: Negative for MDM2 and CDK4.</td></tr>
<tr><td colspan="6">Intermediate: can recur aggressively/may rarely (<5%) metastasize</td></tr>
<tr><td>Atypical lipomatous tumor (ALT)</td><td>Common</td><td>Middle aged to older adults
M = F</td><td>Limbs: deep (sub-fascial) most commonly but superficial also</td><td>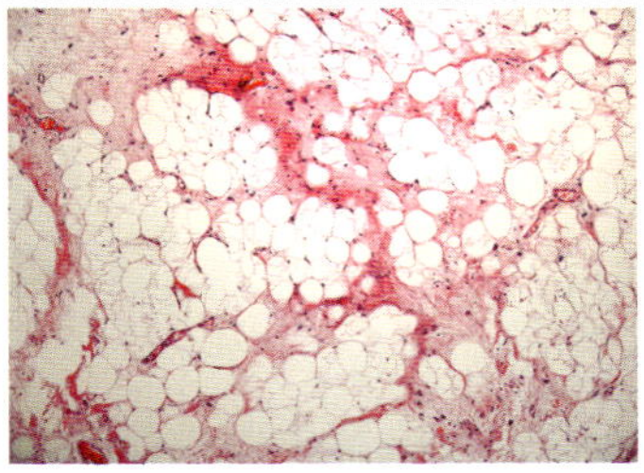</td><td>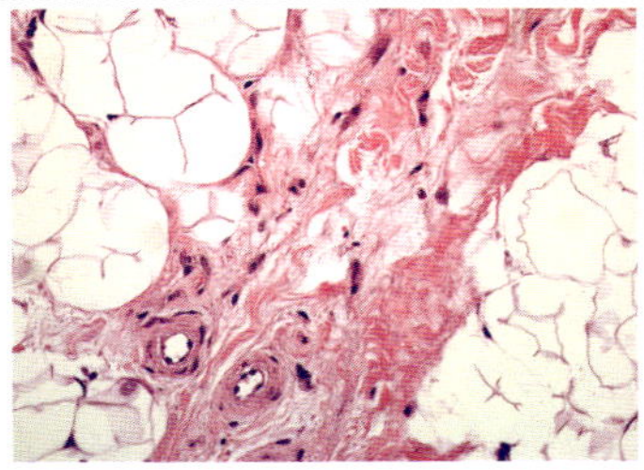</td></tr>
<tr><td colspan="6">'Lipoma-like' variant looks deceptively like a lipoma but it has greater range in fat cell size, enlarged fat cell nuclei, and scattered atypical stromal cells mostly in fibrous bands, Lipoblasts are absent to rare. By definition it is superficial or intramuscular rather than retroperitoneal or mediastinal. Three variants.
IHC: Nearly all tumors are positive for CDK4 or MDM2, most are positive for both. However, FISH may need to be done to confirm amplification of rare IHC negative tumors.</td></tr>
<tr><td colspan="6">Malignant: can recur aggressively and commonly metastasizes</td></tr>
<tr><td>Well-differentiated liposarcoma</td><td>Common</td><td>Middle aged to older adults
M = F</td><td>Retroperitoneum and mediastinum</td><td>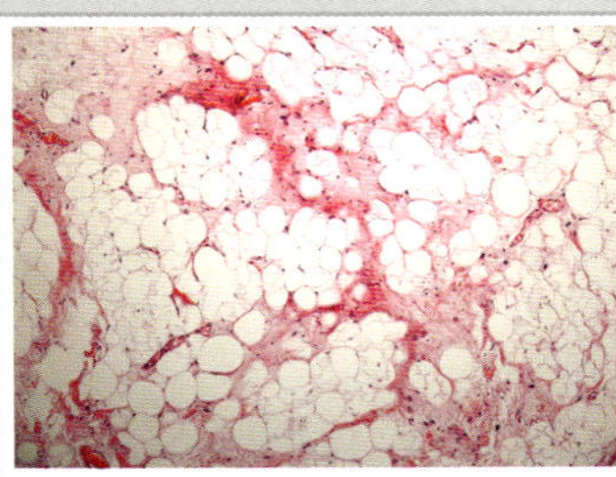</td><td>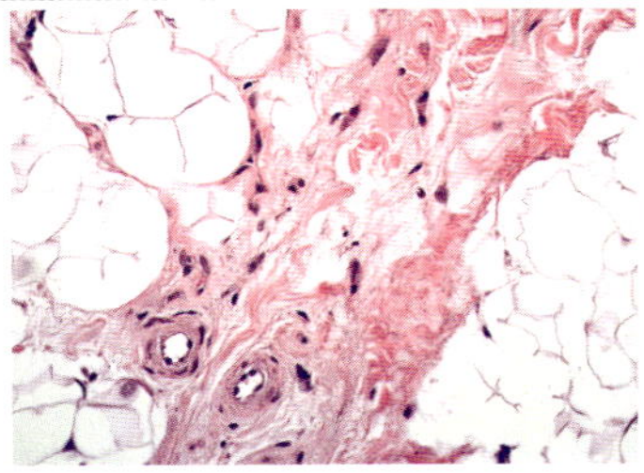</td></tr>
<tr><td colspan="6">Looks exactly like an ALT. Same three variants as with ALT above: 1) lipoma-like, 2) sclerosing, and 3) inflammatory. IHC as for atypical lipomatous tumor.</td></tr>
<tr><td>Myxoid liposarcoma</td><td>Common</td><td>Young adults (30's, 40's, up to 50's)
M = F</td><td>Limbs, often the thigh</td><td>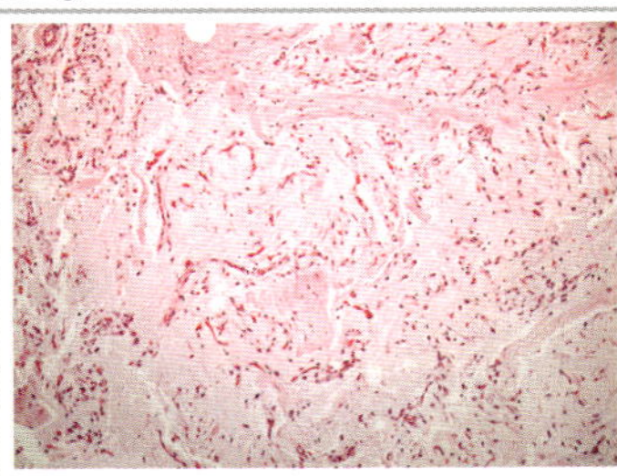</td><td>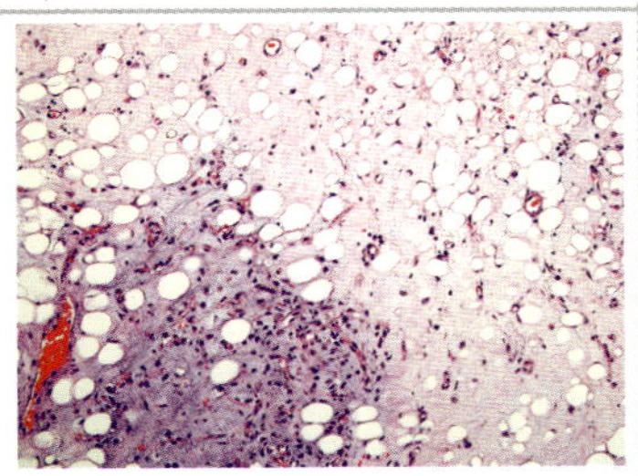</td></tr>
<tr><td colspan="6">Heterogeneous with myxoid areas, cysts, more cellular areas and 'chicken wire' vessels. Cells comprise unevenly sized adipocytes, bona fide lipoblasts some of which may look like signet ring cells, and spindle cells.
IHC: S-100 protein positive. Negative for CDK4 and MDM2.</td></tr>
</table>

Table 5.5: Continued from page 49

Tumor	Incidence	Age and sex distribution	Body site	Histopathology description including IHC	
				Medium magnification	High magnification
Round cell liposarcoma	Uncommon	Young adults (30's, 40's, up to 50's) M = F	Same as above	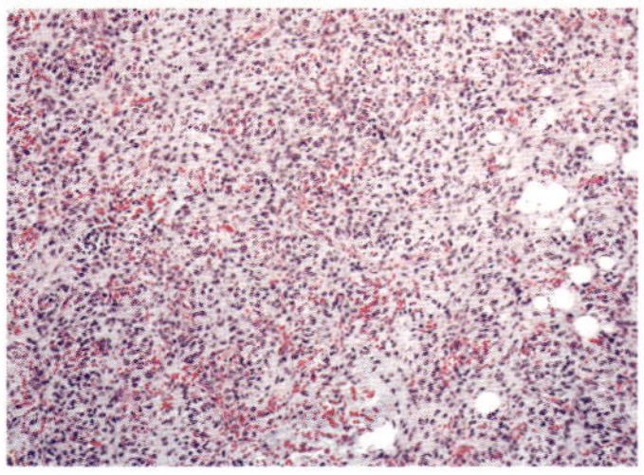	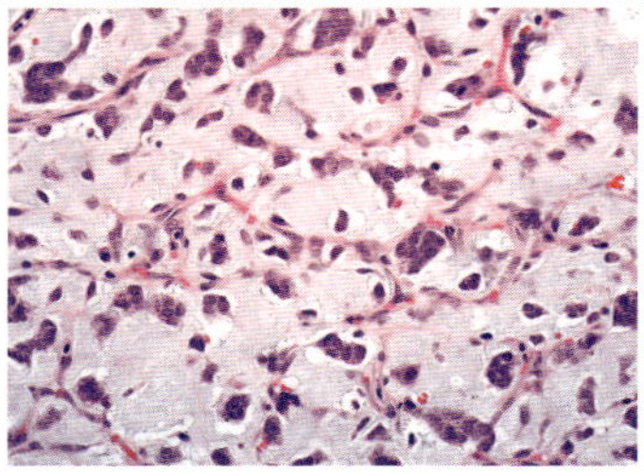
A more malevolent version of myxoid liposarcoma with at least some part of the tumor containing primitive lipoblasts ('round cells') that don't contain fat vacuoles. Some or most of the tumor can be morphologically identical to myxoid liposarcoma. IHC: As for myxoid liposarcoma. CD34 can highlight characteristic chicken wire vascular pattern in difficult cases.					
Dedifferentiated liposarcoma	Common	Middle aged to older adults M = F	Retroperitoneum most commonly then spermatic cord, limbs, trunk and head and neck	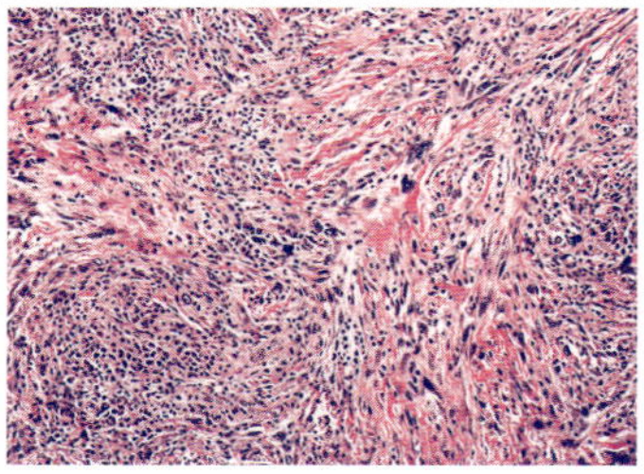	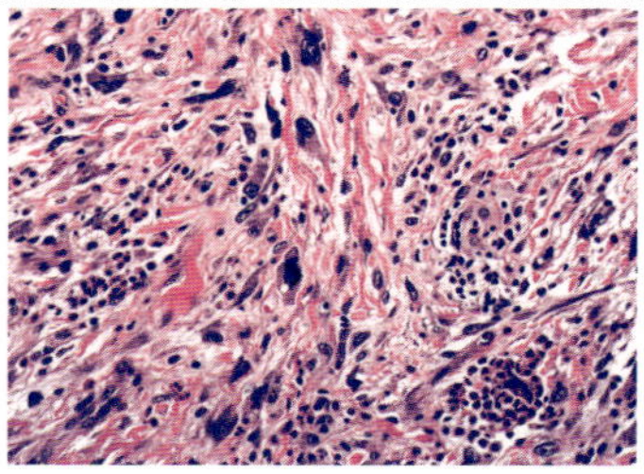
Combination of well-differentiated liposarcoma and some other sarcoma such as chondrosarcoma, osteosarcoma, sarcoma high grade NOS., etc. Can include low grade sarcoma, also Rare cases may resemble myxoid LPS even including 'chicken wire' vessels. In these cases, IHC and genetics are very helpful. Differentiated liposarcoma can occur de novo or also as a recurrence of well-differentiated liposarcoma (in which case metastasis becomes a risk). IHC: Fat cells positive for S-100 protein. Most cases are positive for CDK4 and MDM2.					
Pleomorphic liposarcoma	Rare	Middle aged to older adults M = F	Limbs most commonly then retroperitoneum and trunk	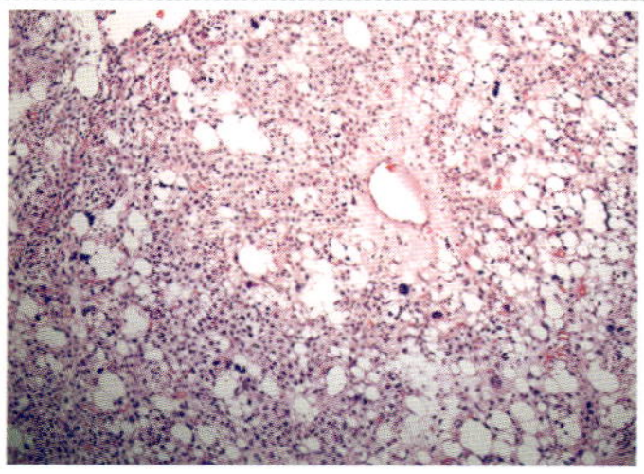	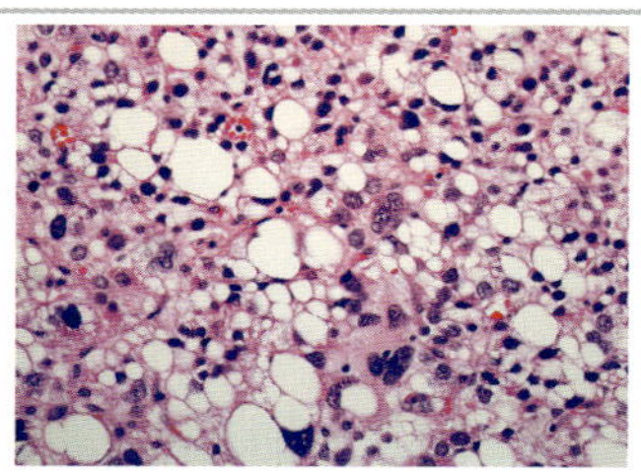
Pleomorphic lipoblasts are usually easy to spot, even at low magnification. There is no low grade liposarcoma or another type of sarcoma. Rare variant: 'epithelioid liposarcoma'; it features round epithelial-looking cells but should have a few pleomorphic lipoblasts that may require careful hunting to find. IHC: Some of the lipoblasts may be S-100 protein positive (but often pleomorphic lipoblasts are negative). CDK4 or MDM2 may be positive; usually negative. Epithelioid variant may be also positive for keratins AE1/AE3, melan-A and smooth muscle actin.					
Spindle cell liposarcoma	Rare	Adults, mostly middle aged to older M > F	Limbs, both superficial and deep and inguinal region	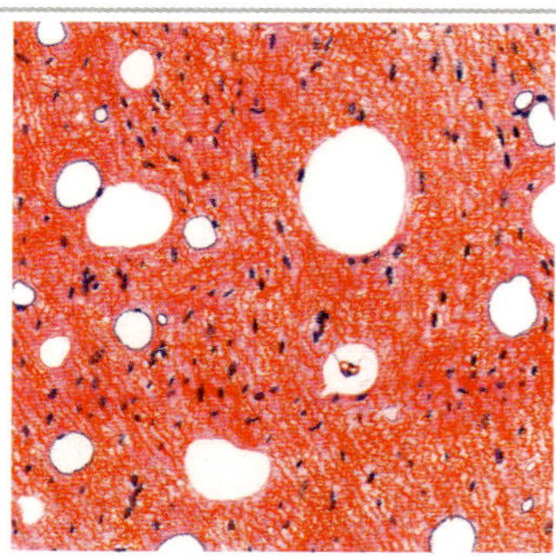	
Streaming uniform spindle cells with wiry collagen fibers and intermixed lipoblasts and mature fat cells. IHC: Spindle cells are CD34 positive. Fat cells are S-100 protein positive. Usually negative for CDK4 and MDM2.					

Table 5.5: Continued from page 50

Tumor	Incidence	Age and sex distribution	Body site	Histopathology description including IHC: Medium magnification	Histopathology description including IHC: High magnification
Mixed type liposarcoma	Rare	Adults, mostly middle aged to older M > F	Limbs, deep	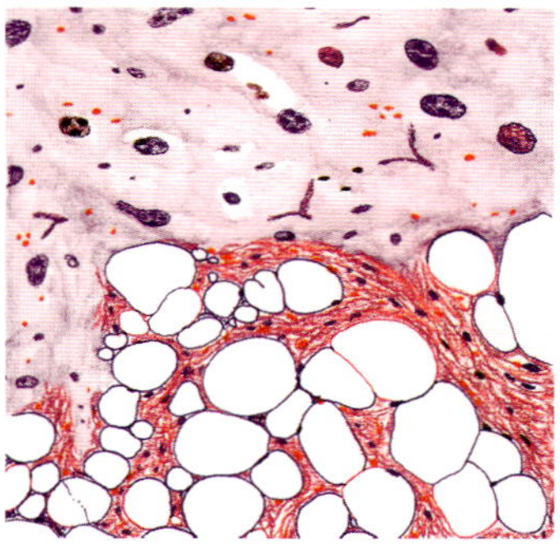	
Contains two or more distinct types of liposarcoma such as well-differentiated liposarcoma and myxoid liposarcoma. Differential includes pure myxoid liposarcoma with lots of mature looking lipoblasts and pure well-differentiated liposarcoma with myxoid stroma. Remember: dedifferentiated liposarcoma is not considered a mixed type liposarcoma even though it commonly has a well-differentiated liposarcoma component. IHC: Should be positive for CDK4 and MDM2 in well-differentiated liposarcoma regions.					
Incidence note: 'Common to very common' indicates that a medium sized practice will treat at least several to dozens of patients with the lesion annually, 'Uncommon to rare' indicates the same practice size will treat one to two patients with the lesion every five years, 'Rare to very rare' indicates the same sized practice will see zero to one patient with the lesion every 20 years. M: male, F: female.					

Table 5.6 Pediatric adipocytic tumors grouped by behavior

Tumor	Incidence	Age and sex distribution	Body site	Medium magnification (photo or text description)	Histopathology including IHC
Benign: does not recur or recurs non-aggressively and does not metastasize					
Lipoblastoma (lipoblastomatosis when growth is diffuse)	Common	Infants and young children (most under 3 years) M > F	Limbs most common; trunk, head and neck, mediastinal less common	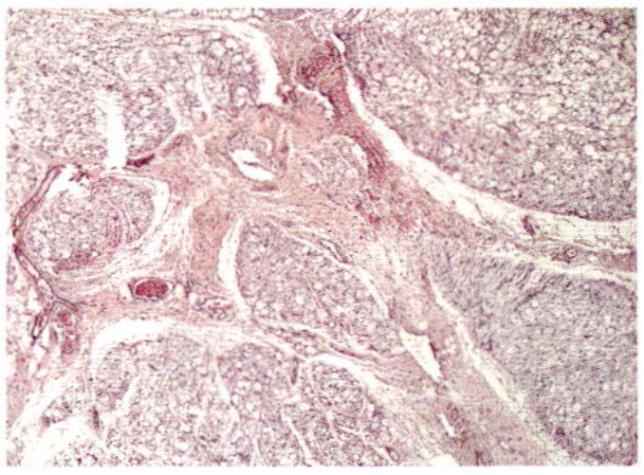	Looks like a myxoid liposarcoma but is more lobulated (this is not always appreciable; fortunately, the two can be distinguished by cytogenetics) and age of patient. The lesion can mature as patient ages and develops a large mature adipocyte component
Lipomatosis of nerve	Very rare	Children to young adults. M = F	Hand/arm, rarely elsewhere	Mature adipose tissue and fibrous tissue infiltrate the nerve separating nerve bundles. Concentric perineurial fibrosis and 'onion bulb' nerve twig sepations. No atypia, necrosis, or mitotic activity	This may be a hamartoma in that it involves mature fat and hypocellular fibrous tissue infiltrating a large peripheral nerve (most commonly the median and ulnar). May be associated with macrodactyly (33%)
Incidence note: 'Common to very common' indicates that a medium sized practice will treat at least several to dozens of patients with the lesion annually, 'Uncommon to rare' indicates the same practice size will treat one to two patients with the lesion every five years, 'Rare to very rare' indicates the same sized practice will see zero to one patient with the lesion every 20 years.					

Table 5.7 Non-adipocytic tumors that contain fat. These are tumors that can contain fat but are not considered tumors of fat (usually the fat is minor component or, at most, one of several components of the tumor, or only occurs occasionally in the tumor).

Tumor	Incidence	Age and sex distribution	Body site (in order of occurrence)	Cell types	Histopathology including IHC
Benign: does not recur or recurs non-aggressively and does not metastasize					
Fibrous hamartoma of infancy	Rare	Young children up to 3 years M > F	Arm, shoulder (especially axillary folds), lower limbs, trunk. Not hands/feet	Mature adipocytes and primitive mesenchymal cells	Tripartate pattern of: 1) mature adipocytes, 2) hypocellular fibrocollagenous tissue, and 3) streaming spindle cells
Renal angiomyolipoma	Rare	Children to middle aged adults. Children more likely to have tuberous sclerosis. F >> M	Kidney, liver retroperitoneum	Perivascular epithelioid cells, spindle myoid cells, mature adipocytes usually present. Cases with atypia and mitoses may possibly behave malignantly	Tripartate pattern of: vessels, fat, and smooth muscle in varying proportions. Rare malignant version

Table 5.7: Continued from page 51

Tumor	Incidence	Age and sex distribution	Body site (in order of occurrence)	Cell types	Histopathology including IHC
Angioleiomyoma	Uncommon	Middle-aged to older adults, less commonly all other ages M > F	Superficial limbs including hands and feet, head and neck	Endothelial cells, smooth muscle cells, may rarely have mature adipocytes	Three types depending on prominence of vessels 1) solid, 2) venous, 3) cavernous; rarely will have some intermixed fat
Leiomyoma of deep soft tissue	Very rare	Adults	Limbs, scrotum,	Smooth muscle cells some contain intermixed mature adipocytes	Bland smooth muscle fascicles with foci of degeneration, fat can be present. Very rare. Any mitotic activity or atypia makes it at least of uncertain malignant potential. IHC: Cells are positive for markers of smooth muscle including desmin, smooth muscle actin, caldesmon.
Mammary-type myofibroblastoma	Rare	Adults M > F	Breast, trunk, groin, vaginal wall	Mature adipocytes and myofibroblasts	Swirling bland spindle cells with a few intermixed fat cell clusters. No atypia. Spindle cells are positive for CD34 and desmin
Angiomyofibroblastoma	Rare	Adults F > M	Genital region	Endothelial cells, myofibroblasts and sometimes mature adipocytes	10% have prominent mature fat, otherwise delicate vessels in edematous background with roundish myofibroblasts, the latter often aggregating around vessels. IHC: Myofibroblasts are positive for hormone receptors and may be positive for CD34, desmin, and smooth muscle actin. Rare malignant version
Intermediate: can recur aggressively/may rarely (<5%) metastasize					
Lipofibromatosis	Rare	Infants to 2 years old M > F	Hands (fingers), feet, less commonly elsewhere	Mature adipocytes, lipoblast-like adipocytes, oval to spindle fibroblasts	Clusters of adipocytes surrounded by variably cellular fibrous bands. May infiltrate muscle but usually superficial. IHC: fat cells and sometimes fibroblasts are S-100 positive; CD34 and BCL2 may also be positive. NEGATIVE: keratins and desmin
Intramuscular hemangioma	Common	Children to young adults (most younger than 20 years) F = M	Limbs	Blood vessel components and mature adipocytes	Looks a lot like angiomatosis (except the increased mural capillaries in vessels) but is limited to one tissue plane or muscle. Can contain mature fat
Angiomatosis	Uncommon	Children to young adults. F > M	Limbs, most commonly leg including foot, then trunk	Blood vessel components and mature adipocytes	Variably sized vessels in fat crossing contiguous tissue planes or involving multiple muscles. May see increased capillaries in vein walls
Mixedtumor/ myoepith-elioma/ parachordoma	Rare	Adults, young to middle aged, children uncommonly M > F	Limbs, usually superficial, head and neck	Myoepithelium and divergent differentiation to include mature adipocytes	Myoepithelium with epithelium (called mixed tumor) or purely myoepithelial (called myoepithelioma) in myxoid or chondroid matrix; fat is sometimes present. IHC: keratins, p63, commonly also S-100 protein, GFAP, smooth muscle actin, calponin. Rare malignant version
Extravisceral solitary fibrous tumor	Rare	Adults, but extrathoracic in all tumors occur all ages M = F	Superficial (40%) and deep limbs, head and neck	Myofibroblasts and a few tumors have mature adipocytes	'Patternless pattern' of alternating hypo-and hypercellular areas with blunt spindle cells, collagenization, rarely, prominent fat is present. IHC: Cells are positive for CD34, sometimes bcl-2 Mitotic rate >4/10hpf, pleomorphism, necrosis associated with malignant behavior; rare bland versions can metastasize

Table 5.7: Continued from page 52

Tumor	Incidence	Age and sex distribution	Body site (in order of occurrence)	Cell types	Histopathology including IHC
Hemosiderotic fibrohistiocytic lipomatous lesion	Very rare	Middle aged adults, few children F > M	Ankles/Feet, rarely hand or elsewhere	Mature adipocytes, spindle cells that are CD34 positive, histiocytes and mast cells	Looks like traumatized fat: clusters of mature fat cells partitioned by strands of fibrous tissue containing spindle cells, histiocytes, mast cells and coarse hemosiderin deposits. Fresh hemorrhage and multinucleated osteoclast like giant cells may also be present. No atypia
Ectopic hamartomatous thymoma (branchial anlage mixed tumor)	Very rare	Young to middle aged adults. M >> F	Superficial or deep supraclavicular and peristernal	Epithelial cells commonly including squamous cells, spindle cells many of which may be epithelial in keratin expression, and mature adipocytes	Tripartate pattern: 1) spindle cells, 2) epithelial cells, 3) fat cells in varying proportions. Despite the name, thymic elements are absent IHC: epithelial cells positive for keratins and sometimes EMA Spindle cells can be keratin positive and also positive for myoepithelial markers such as calponin and smooth muscle actin Both cell types can be positive for CD34, CEA and calretinin
Cellular angiofibroma	Rare	Adults F = M	Genital region	Endothelial cells, spindle cells probably specialized genital myofibroblasts and sometimes mature adipocytes	Fat in small, peripheral clusters in up to 50%; otherwise small and medium vessels, at least some with fibrinoid change, set in spindle cell stroma. Stroma is fibrous and/or edematous. Spindle cells are short and plump. IHC: May stain for hormone receptors, CD34, desmin or smooth muscle actin (similar to angiomyofibroblastoma, with which it previously had been confused)

Incidence note: 'Common to very common' indicates that a medium sized practice will treat at least several to dozens of patients with the lesion annually, 'Uncommon to rare' indicates the same practice size will treat one to two patients with the lesion every five years, 'Rare to very rare' indicates the same sized practice will see zero to one patient with the lesion every 20 years. M: Male. F: Female.

CDK4. Perhaps reflective of its higher grade, in most cases of dedifferentiated liposarcoma, many tumor fat cells are positive (30% or more) for one or both markers. These markers, however, are not specific for liposarcoma, as a few pleomorphic sarcomas may be strongly positive for one or the other. Dual reactivity is more specific, as ~90% of well-differentiated/dedifferentiated. liposarcoma show expression of both proteins by IHC, while only ~4% of other sarcomas are reactive for both MDM2 and CDK4 (Bui et al. 2005).

FISH for CDK4 and MDM2 gene abnormalities

In situ-hybridization examining amplification of the CDK4 gene and the MDM2 gene does appear to be more sensitive and specific in the diagnosis of well-differentiated and dedifferentiated-liposarcoma but only modestly so. In particular cases, however, it can be very helpful, such as confirming a diagnosis of dedifferentiated liposarcoma versus pleomorphic sarcoma, not otherwise specified (Coindre et al. 2010). Currently, just a few labs perform these FISH tests for CDK4 and MDM2.

p16

Reported to be positive in atypical lipomatous tumor/well-differentiated liposarcomas and dedifferentiated liposarcoma. This protein, a cell cycle regulator, may be over-expressed in atypical lipomatous tumors/well-differentiated liposarcomas (about 80% of cases) and when combined with MDM2 reactivity, it may be specific for this tumor (the single hibernoma and lipoblastoma in the paper cited were admittedly p16 positive but MDM2 negative) (He et al. 2009). A cautionary note: overexpression of p16 is a common occurrence in sarcomas, however, and is not specific for well-differentiated/differentiated liposarcoma. It may also be positive in the other liposarcoma variants but is touted as particularly discriminating in the setting of determining whether a fatty tumor is a lipoma or a well-differentiated liposarcoma/atypical lipomatous tumor. Positive staining can be both nuclear and/or cytoplasmic. A rare lipoma may show p16 expression diffusely or strong expression in areas of fat necrosis, but in these cases tumor cells are negative for MDM2 or CDK4. Most tumors of fat with diffuse strong p16 expression are atypical lipomatous tumors/well-differentiated liposarcomas.

RADIOLOGY

The imaging evaluation of a fatty tumor is a common clinical request but remains a complicated task fraught with perils for the radiologist. The difficulty lies in distinguishing the commonly occurring fat tumor, a lipoma, from the other fatty lesions including the various liposarcomas. The sprectrum of fat tumors includes simple lipomas, intra- and inter-muscular lipomas, pleomorphic lipoma and the subtypes of liposarcomas (well-differentiated or atypical lipomas, myxoid, round cell, pleomorphic, spindle cell and dedifferentiated liposarcomas). Compounding diagnostic efforts, benign lipomas can develop complications such as infarction, bruising and inflammation. Some patients will become unconsciously obsessed with their 'lump' and palpate them to the point of causing tissue irritation. This can result in edema seen on MRI, confounding accurate assessment.

Fatty lesions comprise a spectrum of tumors with a highly variable imaging features and significant overlap in their appearance. Imaging is limited in specificity and does best at diagnosing tumors at the extremes of biology. A completely bland, absolutely featureless tumor that has fat signal on MR or fat density on CT is undoubtedly a lipoma. If the clinical setting and practice environment are clearly reassuring, follow up may not be needed. At the other extreme, a fat tumor with complex appearance, enhancing tissue and invasive features is easy to correctly diagnoses as a liposarcoma. An important caveat is that often the highly malignant fat tumors have no discernible fat tissue on imaging and the radiologist can only give a generic diagnosis of a sarcoma. The real difficulty for radiologist is the overlapping appearance of those tumors that lie in the middle of the biologic spectrum; these are the tumors that show only moderately complexity and have minimally enhancement such as the atypical lipoma, well differentiated liposarcoma, pleomorphic lipoma. Furthermore, although most liposarcomas are simple to diagnose on imaging with frankly aggressive and invasive appearance, there are the occasional liposarcomas that can lie in the middle of this imaging spectrum having only modest heterogeneity and enhancement. The radiologist is faced with the classic conundrum of sensitivity versus specificity. We never want to miss the diagnosis of a liposarcoma which requires us to recommend follow up or biopsy of fat lesions that have this intermediate imaging appearance.

As with other sarcomas, the imager must define the mass – specifically, its location, size and proximity to important structures. The secondary role is an attempt to judge the risk of malignancy for the lesion. Unfortunately, even the bland appearing fatty tumor could harbor the atypia of low grade liposarcoma and warrant a pathologic diagnosis of malignancy. Thus, the imager should refrain from declaring any fatty tumor 'benign'. In the best of circumstances, a completely bland fatty tumor may be diagnosed as a 'simple fat tumor without worrisome features'. The need to follow up such a bland fat tumor is ultimately best decided by the referring physician who can accurately assess the patient's history, symptoms and the overall clinical setting. One feared complication of fatty tumors is dedifferentiation of an atypical or well-differentiated liposarcoma. This is fortunately rare, but the patient should be educated about the risk (Dei Tos 2000). The imager can help the clinical care team by offering the reassurance that no aggressive or malignant feature is found, thus emboldening the patient and his/her care team in embarking on a conservative management plan. If the clinical or imaging situation is unclear, than imaging follow up can be performed in 3-6 months to assess the lesion stability . Lesions that have worrisome or aggressive features should be referred to an orthopedic oncologist for biopsy or excisional evaluation.

There are many factors the radiologist should assess in a fatty tumor. The location of the fatty tumor has intrinsic bearing on the risk for malignancy. The superficial fatty tumors, entirely within the subcutaneous tissues, harbor the least overall malignant risk (Pang AK, et al 2000). The intramuscular or deep fatty tumors are at increased risk, while the retroperitoneal fatty tumors have the highest rate for malignancy.

MRI without and with contrast is the most useful single exam for imaging evaluation. CT is helpful for retroperitoneal tumor imaging and can be useful in the setting of an MR incompatible patient. The general imaging appearance of a simple fat tumor should show homogeneous fat on all imaging modalities without molestation of adjacent structures. The tumor should show uniform fat density by CT. Fat typically has CT Hounsfield density units of -40 to -80. MRI should show uniform high signal on T1 weighted images and low signal after fat saturation. Fluid sensitive sequences such as short T1 inversion recovery (STIR) and T2 fat saturated sequences should show no edema within or adjacent to the tumor. There should be no enhancement. The sensitivity for subtle enhancement can be optimized with matching pre- and post- contrast T1 fat saturated sequences.

A reassuring morphologic feature of a subcutaneous fat 'tumor' is one that has no capsule and thus blends imperceptibly with the adjacent subcutaneous fatty tissue. Indeed, such fat 'tumors' are only identifiable on imaging because the markers placed on the skin indicate where the patient feels the 'lump'. These clinically palpable 'masses' may simply represent a focally prominent locule of normal subcutaneous fat. Ultrasound typically shows an echogenic lesion but renders little specificity in the workup of fatty tumor. This modality is not recommended for soft tissue tumor evaluation unless there is a clinical question of possible aneurysm, hernia, or cyst.

The aggressive or malignant features of liposarcomas include increased vascularity, heterogeneous CT density or heterogeneous MR signal, edema, invasion, nodularity and septation. In general, malignant fat tumors look complex. Most liposarcomas will show a mixture of three tissue components. There may be some residual normal appearing fat. There is also abnormal fat tissue showing septation, edema and enhancement. Finally, there is the frankly cellular portion of the tumor which appears heterogeneous, may have visible invasion, , will show complex enhancement and may have areas of necrosis. The most aggressive liposarcomas show little or no discernible fat (Einarsdottir et al. 1999) and the radiologist can only diagnose a nonspecific 'sarcoma'.

Although imaging specificity can be limited, there are some characteristic features that can guide the radiologic differential.
In general, a lipoma should be a bland appearing fat tumor with simple thin capsule. A small series showed that all tumors which were completely composed of fat by imaging were in fact lipomas (Kransdorf et al. 2002). This means the appearance of the tumor tissue identically matched adjacent subcutaneous tissue on all imaging tests. Unfortunately, their study also showed, up to 9% of the proven lipomas can have less than 75% fat. This contradictory appearance emphasizes the difficulty in diagnosing a specific subtype of fat tumor based on imaging. Indeed, in our experience, the completely featureless, bland fat tumor is rare and most fat tumors have a few septations or mild heterogeneity.

Intramuscular lipomas are classically comprised of bland appearing fat. They usually have well defined margins, although less commonly, they can have infiltrative margins with intermingled muscle fibers. Unfortunately, this appearance overlaps with appearance of malignant sarcomas. Intramuscular lipomas may have septa which should be thin measuring less than 2 mm, without nodularity or significant enhancement (Matsumoto, et all. 1999). Intermuscular lipomas can have a dumbbell morphology as they insinuate between muscles (Nishida, et al. 2007).

The spindle cell lipoma is also known as a pleomorphic lipoma and is benign. They have a variable appearance with heterogeneous tissue and typically appear to be only 25–75% fat. They are predominately seen in the subcutaneous tissues of middle aged men. In a small series, 44% were located on the posterior neck (Bancroft et al. 2003). Spindle cell lipomas otherwise tend to occur on the shoulders and back (Usta et al. 2004). The non-adipose tissue components typically show intense enhancement. Thus the imaging appearance can be similar to a liposarcoma, however the location and demographic features are mildly suggestive of this benign diagnosis.

The entity of atypical lipoma is somewhat confusing because of terminology. It is also known as atypical lipomatous tumor or well differentiated liposarcoma depending of location of the tumor. These three related tumors can recur locally but have no metastatic potential (Dei Tos 2000). The WHO has indicated that the term 'atypical lipoma' should be used only for subcutaneous extremity lesions and the term 'well differentiated liposarcoma' should be used for all remaining sites. Atypical lipoma and well-differentiated liposarcomas have similar radiological appearance and commonly have thick, enhancing septa with patchy non-adipose components. These septal findings match well with the thick fibrous bands traversing such tumors as seen on pathology (Oghuri et al. 2003). Unfortunately, even thin septa can occur in both benign and malignant adipose tumors lending no specificity to diagnosis (Hosono et al. 1997, Kransdorf et al. 2002). Enhancement of a fatty tumor can help distinguish an atypical lipomatous tumor from a lipoma (Panzarella et al. 2005). Well differentiated liposarcoma usually have more than 75% fat while other liposarcomas usually have less that 25% fat (Kransdorf et al. 2002).

The higher grade liposarcomas are generally similar in appearance showing heterogeneous tissues with minimal adipose elements (<25%), irregular boarders and heterogeneous enhancement. The myxoid liposarcoma subtype is interesting for its tendency for extra-pulmonary metastasis, in particular to the spine, soft tissues, retroperitoneum, and peritoneal surface. Bone spread is not as common (Hanna et al. 2008). However, bone metastasis can be difficult to detect by bone scan or PET and MRI may be more sensitive for both bone and soft tissue metastasis. (Schwab et al. 2007, Sheah et al. 2008). Spindle cell liposarcoma tends to recur locally and may dedifferentiate (Dei Tos , 2000).

Lipoblastoma is a rare benign fat tumor typically occurring in infancy or early childhood. These are usually asymptomatic. Lipoblastomas are usually well circumscribed tumors; however, a diffuse form can occur called lipoblastomatosis. The MR imaging features include various degrees of non-enhancing cystic changes; mild to moderate internal fibrous septae intermixed with a few small enhancing soft tissue nodules, (Chen CW, et al. 2010).

As always, the imaging workup of a suspected sarcoma includes staging the patient, this is typically accomplished by anatomic imaging of the chest, abdomen and pelvis with CT scans with IV and oral contrast.

Key points in the radiology of adipocytic tumors

Imaging strategy

1. MRI is the technique of choice.
2. Ultrasound is limited.

Nonaggressive fat tumor

1. Uniform fat tumor without molestation of adjacent structures.
2. There should be no: septa, nodularity, vascularity, edema or enhancement.

Worrisome features

1. Deep or retroperitoneal location.
2. Firm, painful or enlarging.
3. Edema, infiltration, enhancement, thick septa, nodularity, non-fatty tissue.

SURGERY

Tumors for which MRI demonstrates a homogenous fatty signal, consistent with lipoma can be observed or, if enlarging and/or symptomatic, can be excised marginally with a low risk of local recurrence. When MRI demonstrates focal or diffuse heterogeneity, a formal biopsy should be performed with the most heterogenous area being the target for biopsy tissue. This is important, as homogeneous regions may fail to reveal a dedifferentiated or high grade component on biopsy.

With biopsy proven pleomorphic lipoma/spindle cell lipoma or circumscribed lipoblastoma, marginal excision will generally suffice.

With biopsy proven diffuse lipoblastoma or atypical lipomatous tumor/well-differentiated liposarcoma of the extremity, treatment should be individualized. Marginal excision will result in a measurable risk of local recurrence, and the possible risk (albeit low) of the tumor recurring as a higher grade neoplasm. Nevertheless, local recurrence (in the absence of dedifferentiation) may take years to become clinically evident and the added morbidity of wide resection, particularly with a large tumor in an elderly patient, may not be warranted.

All higher grade liposarcomas should be treated with wide resection, usually with the addition of adjuvant radiation therapy.

All tumors marginally excised, because of MRI appearance or biopsy, should be removed through an oncologically safe approach as the final pathology may reveal areas of higher grade tumor.

MEDICAL ONCOLOGY

Despite extensive reporting on the treatment of soft tissue sarcomas, as with all the other sarcoma subtypes, there are little data regarding specific treatments for liposarcoma. Moreover, all liposarcomas are not the same and, in fact, exhibit varied responses to multidisciplinary treatments.

Chemotherapy results in liposarcomas compared with other sarcomas

Two studies have examined large scale chemotherapy data for soft tissue sarcomas, and in both, liposarcomas stand out as having a better prognosis than most other soft tissue tumor subtypes.

The first study is a meta-analysis done by the European Organization for Research and Treatment of Cancers (EORTC) (Van Glabbeke et al 1999). Patients treated in seven randomized studies that were anthracyclin-based (doxorubicin or epirubicin) were pooled for the analysis. The overall survival was 51 weeks, and the overall response rate was 26%. By univariate analysis, patients with liposarcoma had a significantly better survival time (76 weeks), but when multivariate analysis was performed, liposarcoma dropped out when tumor grade was included. In all, there were 13% grade 1 soft tissue sarcomas, but for liposarcoma, these figures were grade 1, 39%, grade 2, 34%, and grade 3, 28%, respectively. By univariate analysis, the higher response rate seen in patients with liposarcoma (36%) was of borderline significance, however, in the multivariate analysis, absence of liver lesions ($P < 0.0001$), young age ($P < 0.0024$), high histopathologic grade ($P < 0.0051$), and liposarcoma ($P < 0.065$) were the only independent favorable prognostic factors of response.

The second study examined response and survival after first line chemotherapy treatment for advanced STS. Most regimens were anthracyclin based, with 299 patients treated with single agent versus 189 treated with a combination. Ninety-five patients did not receive an anthracyclin as the first treatment. A 33% overall response rate was seen with 22% having disease stabilization. The overall survival was 12 months. Interestingly, this study also demonstrated that patients treated with combination chemotherapy experienced longer survival than those treated with a single agent. A non-significant trend for improved survival was found for sarcoma patients who had locally advanced disease (15 months) compared with those who had either localized metastatic disease (13 months) or disseminated metastases (9 months) ($P < 0.06$). Patients with liposarcoma had a favorable survival (18 months, $P < .001$), but their response rate was not significantly better than as seen with other sarcomas (Karavasilis et al 2008). On multivariate analysis for overall survival, liposarcoma was found to be an independent favorable prognostic factor, with a relative risk of 0.70 (95% CI: 0.50–0.98, $P < 0.03$). In contrast with the EORTC cohort discussed above, this study found an improved survival for patients with liposarcoma, but liposarcoma was not particularly chemosensitive. However, in this study, grading of the tumor was not described.

In general, liposarcoma appears to be a chemosensitive tumor with a relatively good prognosis for extended survival. The distribution of tumor grades in this histologic subtype explains the favorable survival, but the high response rate is remarkable. In fact, if the patients with grade 1 liposarcoma were dropped from that model, the response rate may have been higher.

Oncology treatment according to histologic type of adipocytic tumor

As has been noted in the pathology portion of this chapter, well-differentiated liposarcoma and dedifferentiated liposarcoma occur predominantly in the retroperitoneum and can be multifocal, whereas myxoid, round-cell, and pure pleomorphic liposarcomas primarily occur in the extremities (Skubitz et al 2007). Certainly, options are more constrained when dealing with a retroperitoneal rather than distal extremity liposarcoma.

The 5-year survival and disease-free survival of patients with high grade extremity liposarcomas treated with ifosfamide were 92% (84%–100%) and 81% (70%–92%) compared with 65% (51%–79%) and 63% (50%–76%) for patients who did not receive chemotherapy (log-rank P value < 0.0003). Independent prognostic factors for improved survival were: 1) smaller size, 2) myxoid/round cell histologic subtype, and 3) treatment with ifosfamide. In patients with large, high-grade, primary extremity liposarcoma, doxorubicin was not associated with improved survival but ifosfamide was. Therefore, treatment with ifosfamide should be considered in patients with high-grade primary extremity liposarcoma (Eilber et al 2004).

While one study suggests the value of ifosfamide in liposarcoma treatment, in another study, the opposite findings were observed. In 88 patients with liposarcoma, the response rates to chemotherapy of the different histological subtypes were significantly better in patients with myxoid liposarcoma compared to de- and well-differentiated tumors, 48% versus 11%; this finding is in accord with the first study results in that this subtype is more responsive. However, all patients with myxoid liposarcoma who responded to chemotherapy were treated with a doxorubicin-based therapy. None of the patients treated with single agent ifosfamide responded (Jones et al 2005). This study included low and high grades sarcomas of any anatomical site which may account for the different findings. No significant difference in overall survival from first-line chemotherapy was observed between the subgroups. The median progression-free survival was 4 months for myxoid, 16 months for round cell liposarcoma, 11 months for well-differentiated, 2 months for dedifferentiated and 8 months for pleomorphic sarcoma. Median survival from diagnosis was 60 months. Myxoid liposarcoma patients had a statistically significant longer overall survival compared to patients with well-differentiated tumors (119 months versus 59 months, $P = 0.006$). This finding is not surprising, understanding that myxoid liposarcoma may be graded from '1+' to '3', while well-differentiated liposarcoma is always grade '1'.

Well-differentiated liposarcoma, a low grade tumor unlikely to metastasize, is usually treated solely by surgical resection (Lahat et al 2008). However these tumors may be huge, and the biopsy done to confirm the radiological findings may miss areas of dedifferentiation. The main treatment is surgical, and an attempt should be made to obtain negative margins while sparing as many organs as possible. Overall and local recurrences are 50% and 45%, and only 5% recur as high grade metastatic disease. Median time to recurrence is about 55 months, with a 5 year recurrence-free survival of 40% and a 5 year survival rate of 90%.

The treatment of dedifferentiated liposarcoma, a high grade tumor, must be multidisciplinary. There is no standard of care regarding the sequence of treatments. Surgeons again should attempt to remove all tumor while sparing normal organs when feasible. Chemotherapy can be given in neoadjuvant fashion or postoperatively. Radiotherapy is best delivered intraoperatively to minimize exposure to the viscera. Despite this combined multimodality approach, the prognosis of dedifferentiated liposarcoma is poor. Overall and local recurrence are 80% and 70%. Median time to recurrence is about 13 months, with a 5 year recurrence-free survival of 8% and a 5 year survival rate of 35% (Lahat et al 2008).

Myxoid liposarcoma is also classified as a low or intermediate-grade tumor depending on grade. Myxoid liposarcomas contain tumor cells that represent various stages of adipocyte differentiation in a myxoid matrix (Guadagnolo et al 2008). When they are mixed with round cell (with a round-cell component >5%), they are more aggressive with a lower survival rate (about 50% at 5 years with more risk for metastatic dissemination) (Guadagnolo et al 2008, Fiore et al 2007). Cytogenetically, almost all myxoid liposarcomas have a specific reciprocal translocation of chromosomes 12 and 16, t(12;16)(q13;p11), resulting in oncogenic hybrid proteins, DDIT3-FUS or DDIT3-WSR1 fusion proteins. Although the presence of this molecular genetic abnormality has not been shown to have prognostic significance, it does provide a method for confirmation of the diagnosis of myxoid liposarcoma. No therapy has been directed against the fusion protein to date. Myxoid liposarcomas also overexpress many ribosomal protein genes (Skubitz et al 2005). The overall survival rate at 5 years is about 80% and the local control rate, 97% (Fiore et al 2007). Distant metastases occur in 15% of patients at 5 years, but more patients will become metastatic with time, and patients should be followed for at least 10 years. The pattern of metastases is different than with most sarcomas. About half of the patients will develop retroperitoneal metastases, 20% in other extrapulmonary soft tissues, 20% in the lung, 15% in bone, and 5% in the liver. Staging and surveillance imaging should include the abdomen and pelvis, as well as the thorax, for patients with localized myxoid liposarcoma. Most patients are treated with a combination of surgery and radiotherapy.

Myxoid liposarcoma is particularly radiosensitive with impressive tumor regression and local control rates. But when the tumor is greater than 10 cm or when the tumor contains a round cell (higher grade) component, chemotherapy is recommended, and about 30% of patients are thus candidates for chemotherapy. Whether chemotherapy affects survival or the development of metastases is debatable. A significant objective response rate for doxorubicin- and dacarbazine-based chemotherapy has been observed (Patel et al 1994). This is pertinent for this malignancy, because patients tend to present with large, bulky tumors, and chemotherapy offers a means to reduce the primary tumor size and facilitate local therapy. Another effective chemotherapy is trabectedin. Fifty-one patients with advanced pretreated myxoid liposarcoma received trabectedin (24-h continuous infusion or as a 3-h infusion, every 21 days, at 1.1–1.5 mg/m^2) in a compassionate-use program. The median number of courses was 10 (range, 1–23). After a median follow-up of 14 months, two patients had a complete response and 24 patients had a partial response; the overall response was 51% (95% CI, 36–65). Five patients had early progressive disease. Median progression-free survival was 14.0 months, and progression-free survival at 6 months was 88% (Grosso et al 2007).

Pleomorphic liposarcoma is a high-grade tumor (Gebhard et al 2002) affecting the limbs in 70-80% of cases. Two series have been published, one from Memorial Sloan Kettering Cancer Center (Dalal et al, 2006), a tertiary referral center, and one from Italy (Fiore et al 2007). About 25% to 50% of patients will recur with distant metastases, mainly in the lungs and the pleura. The 5-year overall survival is about 50-80% (Dalal et al 2006, Fiore et al 2007). Poor prognostic factors include age over 60 years, truncal tumor location, deep location, tumor size greater than 5 cm, vascular invasion, and incomplete tumor excision. Progressive development of a painless soft tissue mass is the most common presenting symptom. The results of the Italian series were better, perhaps because their cohort reflected primary referrals. There is no specifically recommended chemotherapy regimen for this type of liposarcoma.

New therapies

Trabedectin is approved in Europe for the treatment of soft tissue sarcomas, and in particular, myxoid liposarcoma are known to be responsive to trabectedin (Grosso et al 2007, Yovine et al 2004). Of 41 refractory patients treated in a phase I combination study of trabectedin (0.9 to 1.3 mg/ m^2) plus doxorubicin (60mg/m^2) every 3 weeks, five patients had a response, including 3 patients with liposarcoma, and 37% had a 6 months progression-free interval. The maximum tolerated dose of trabedectin was 1.1 mg/ m^2 with the use of prophylactic granulocyte colony-stimulating factor (Blay et al 2008).

Expression of peroxisome proliferator-activated receptor (PPAR) is high in adipocytes. This receptor regulates adipogenesis, lipid metabolism and glucose homeostasis. PPAR - activation induces differentiation of preadipocytes to adipocytes and is associated with cell cycle arrest (Altiok et al 1997). PPAR ligands are also able to induce cell cycle arrest and terminal differentiation in liposarcoma cells, but in some other models, may have tumor promoting effects (Tontonoz et al 1997). Various PPAR ligands have antitumor effects on almost every kind of tumor cell. The first clinical trial of troglitazone demonstrated induction of differentiation in liposarcomas (Demetri et al 1999). Three patients with intermediate to high-grade liposarcomas were treated with troglitazone. Biopsies of tumors from each of these patients while on troglitazone demonstrated histologic evidence of extensive lipid accumulation by tumor cells (an indicator of maturation) and substantial increases in NMR-detectable tumor triglycerides compared with pretreatment biopsies. In addition, expression of several mRNA transcripts characteristic of differentiation in the adipocyte lineage was induced. There was also a marked reduction in immunohistochemical expression of Ki-67, a marker of cell proliferation. However, when rosiglitazone was tested in liposarcoma patients, it was inactive (Debrock et al 2003). Nine assessable patients with a liposarcoma received rosiglitazone 4 mg twice a day. The mean time to progression was 6 months (2-16+ months). There were no significant change in histologic appearance of the liposarcomas after treatment. The level of gene expression (peroxisome proliferator-activated receptor γ (PPAR γ), adipsin and fatty acid binding protein) changed significantly in two patients, but this did not result in a clinical response.

The murine double minute (MDM) 2 locus is amplified in liposarcomas such as well-differentiated, dedifferentiated, and a proportion of pleomorphic liposarcomas (see molecular genetics table in the pathology section of this chapter). Nutlin 3A is a MDM2-antagonist which induces apoptosis in osteosarcoma cell lines with amplified MDM2. Nutlins are cis-imidazoline analogs which inhibit the interaction between MDM2 and p53, and were discovered by screening a chemical library (Vassilev et al 2004). Nutlin-1, Nutlin-2 and Nutlin-3 were all identified in the same screen, however Nutlin-3 is the compound most commonly used in anti-cancer studies. Several liposarcoma cell lines, with or without MDM2 amplification, were treated with Nutlin 3A. Downstream p53 dependent transcription and apoptosis was observed in the cells with amplified MDM2 in vitro. There has been no clinical trials with this class of agents (Muller et al 2007).

Cancer/testis antigens (CTAGs) are a group of immunogenic proteins that are expressed selectively in some cancers but not in normal tissue except testis and ovary. Compared with normal tissues, CTAG-1, CTAG-2, and another CTAG known as PRAME have been found to be overexpressed in liposarcoma, suggesting that immunotherapy, including the use of tumor vaccines, may be useful in selected liposarcomas (Ayyoub et al, 2004).

RADIATION

Adipocyte tumors represent a heterogeneous group of tumors from the clinical perspective. The use of radiation therapy of these tumors is largely restricted to higher grade malignant tumors or in lower grade malignant tumors with tight or positive margins in an area where further surgery is likely to be morbid. The justification of this use of radiation therapy is not specific to adipocyte tumor, but based in a long history of using radiation in malignant soft-tissue sarcomas.

For low grade and benign tumors (pleomorphic lipoma/spindle cell lipoma, lipoblastoma, and atypical lipomatous tumor), adjuvant radiation therapy is generally not utilized. A possible exception to that list is the well-differentiated liposarcoma. Radiation therapy should be considered in cases of tight/positive margin where further surgery is not warranted as local recurrence rates can be high, and the tumor can harbor dedifferentiated components. This approach is justified as a randomized trial showed low grade tumors had decreased local recurrence when adjuvant radiation therapy was employed. This study included a small number of low-grade liposarcomas (Yang et al. 1998).

For the higher grade tumors (Dediffentiated Liposarcoma and Pleomorphic Liposarcoma), radiation therapy should be included in all patients with localized disease. When possible, neo-adjuvant radiation therapy is favored over adjuvant radiation as functional outcomes have been found to be superior in a randomized study (Davis et al. 2005).

Interestingly, the use of radiation therapy in myxoid liposarcomas (probably including pleomorphic epitheloid liposarcoma), specifically tumors with the FUS-DDIT3 or WSR1-DDIT3 translocations, shows excellent response rates. In one study, the pathological response rate of 'pure' myxoid liposarcomas was 100% to neo-adjuvant radiation therapy (de Vreeze et al. 2008). A larger retrospective study performed at the MD Anderson Cancer Center showed that the use of radiation therapy in myxoid liposarcoma resulted in local control rates of 97% with 10 year overall survival rates of 79% (Guadagnolo et al. 2008). Considering that soft-tissue sarcomas have been labeled by some as radio-resistant, the response of myxoid liposarcomas is quite significant. Consequently, all patients with myxoid liposarcomas should be considered for upfront radiation therapy as excellent response rates are the norm.

CASES

Case 5.1 Intramuscular lipoma

Clinical history and presentation

The patient is a 44 year old woman who presents with an chest mass of three months' duration. The mass was noted spontaneously. It is asymptomatic. Physical examination reveals a vague rubbery mass in the chest wall measuring approximately 10 cm maximally. It is non-tender.

Surgical findings and comments

Operative findings reveal an intramuscular fatty mass generally separable from the surrounding muscle except where individual muscle fibers enter into, or exit from, the tumor. MRI is often diagnostic for these tumors, and excision can generally be performed without a formal biopsy. Occasionally, muscle fibers traversing through the tumor can generate an appearance of heterogeneity on MRI. If the MRI appearance is not consistent with a lipoma, then biopsy should be performed. Treatment is marginal excision. Recurrence is rare.

SURGICAL GRAY AREA

Because these tumors are slow growing and minimally symptomatic, it is not unusual for patients to report that the mass was recently noted when, in fact, it is likely to have been present for a long period of time prior to recognition.

Radiology findings

MRI imaging of the patient's tumor, **Case fig. 5-1a** axial T1, **Case fig. 5.1b** axial STIR, **Case fig. 5.1c** axial T1 fat saturation, and **Case fig. 5.1d** axial T1 fat saturation post-contrast, reveals a 3.4 × 9.2 × 4.1cm mass in the anterior margin of the pectoralis muscle. The mass shows homogeneous T1 high signal and STIR low signal identical to adjacent subcutaneous fat. There is a single dominant septation measuring up to 1.9mm but no nodularity, edema or enhancement.

To include additional imaging findings of intramuscular lipoma, a second case is presented with MR images **Case fig. 5.1e** coronal T1, **Case fig. 5.1f** coronal STIR, and **Case fig. 5.1g** axial STIR. This 55 year old man has a 5.1 × 3.5 × 3.7 cm mass in the left abdominal wall musculature. The mass is T1 high signal and STIR low signal and matches the signal of adjacent fat tissue in the mesentery and skin. The mass has irregular margins but no nodularity, septations or edema.

Pathology findings

Gross features

Case fig. 5.1h is a representative slice of the tumor. The tumor comprises yellow, soft fatty tissue with interspersed red skeletal muscle not only present at the tumor edges but also within the tumor. The specimen is received unoriented, and the tumor grossly involves tissue edges suggesting margins will most likely be positive on microscopic review.

Microscopic features

Low magnification: **Case fig. 5.1i** depicts a typical low power view of the lesion. The tumor looks like normal fat but unlike normal fat, it infiltrates around and through skeletal muscle. Margins are involved.

High magnification: **Case fig. 5.1j** of the tumor comprises mature fat cells growing around muscle fibers. The tumor cells vary only mildly in size and shape. Multiple sections reveal that the tumor lacks marked lobularity, fibrous bands, atypical stromal cells and lipoblasts (these are all features of atypical lipomatous tumor/well-differentiated liposarcoma, lipoma-like variant).

Special studies: A portion of the tumor is sent for cytogenetics but, unfortunately, the cells do not successfully grow in culture (inability to obtain karyotype occurs in about 60% of adipocytic tumors). Immunohistochemistry: There is no expression of MDM2 and CDK4.

Pathologic differential or, why isn't it one of the following?

Atrophic skeletal muscle with partial fat replacement: Unlike intramuscular lipoma, this process doesn't form a discrete mass.

Atypical lipomatous tumor (ALT)/Well-differentiated liposarcoma: ALT shows more pronounced lobularity with transecting fibrous bands (septae). These bands often contain atypical stromal cells (absent in intramuscular lipoma). ALT cells exhibit a much greater range in size with fivefold or greater differences. Some cases will contain lipoblasts (not seen in lipomas). ALT/well-diff liposarcoma is positive in scattered cells for CDK4 and MDM2 by either immunohistochemistry or amplification of the genes (in most cases; only rare lipomas are positive by immunohistochemistry and usually not for both markers). ALT may be positive for p16 (lipomas are negative, according to two recent reports). Infiltration around and between skeletal muscle cells characteristic of intramuscular lipoma would be unusual for ALT/well-differentiated liposarcoma.

Case fig. 5.1k illustrates cases of intramuscular lipoma diagnosed at the University of New Mexico Health Sciences Center from the period 2000-2010 with location, age, and gender information.

Oncology approach

Medical oncology

This is a benign tumor with no role for chemotherapy.

Radiation oncology

Reports of this intramuscular lipoma site a recurrence rate as high as 40% (Bjerregaard et al. 1989). However, recurrence is typically managed with wider excision, as there is no known role for adjuvant radiation therapy.

Patient outcome

The patient is doing well with no signs of recurrent tumor three years after marginal surgical excision.

Case table 5.1a Summary pathology findings of Case 5.1

Diagnosis	Intramuscular lipoma
Size	5.0 cm
Location	Deep (intramuscular)
Margin status	Positive
Histologic grade	Not graded: benign
Pathologic stage (TNM classification)	Not graded: benign

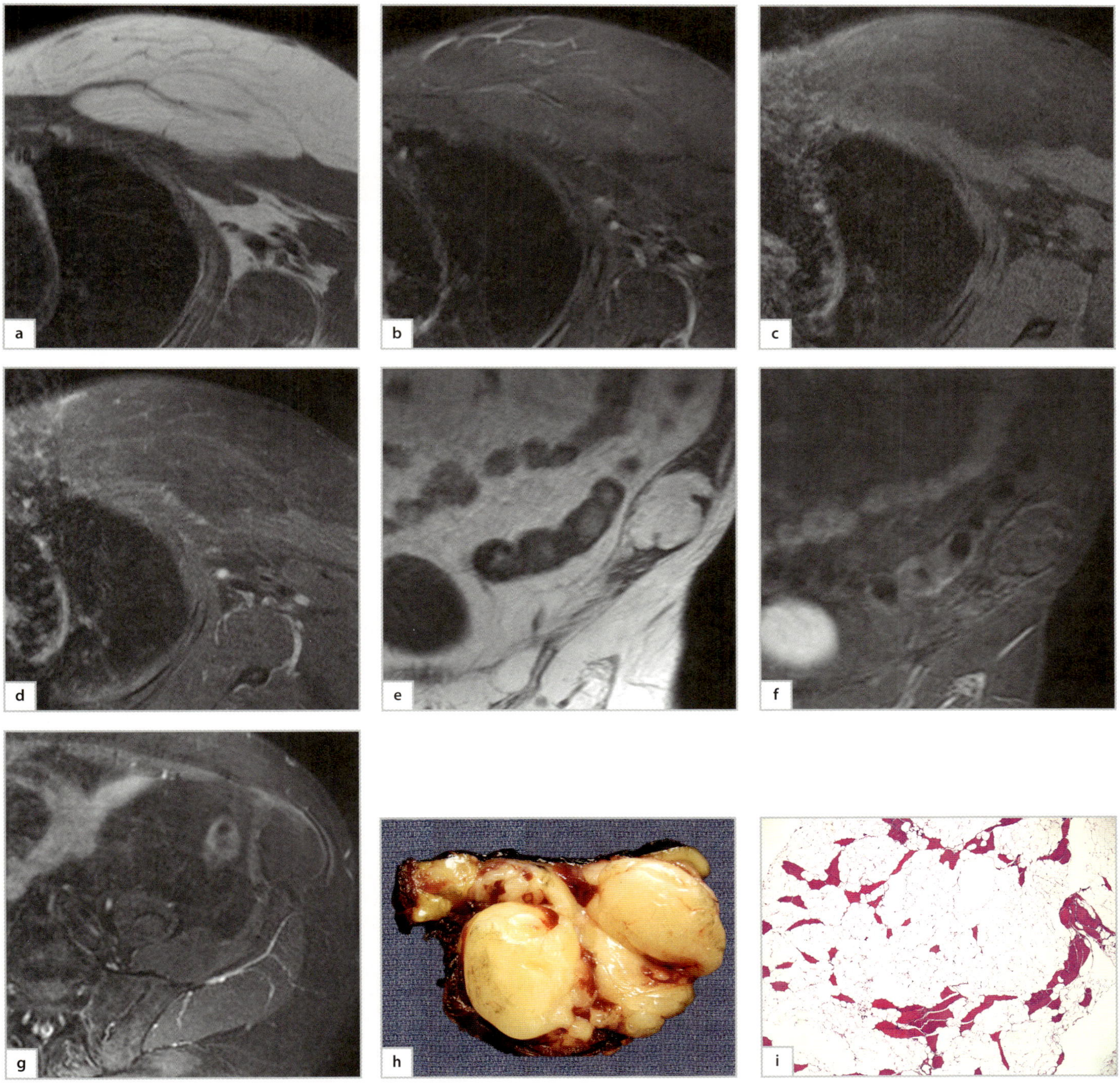

Cases figure 5.1 Intramuscular lipoma imaging. **5.1a:** Axial T1, **5.1b**: Axial STIR, **5.1c**: Axial T1 fat saturation, **5.1d**: Axial T1 fat saturation post-contrast. Nine centimeter mass in the anterior margin of the pectoralis muscle with homogeneous T1 high signal and STIR low signal, identical to adjacent subcutaneous fat. Second comparison case of Intramuscular lipoma imaging: **5.1e**: Coronal T1, **5.1f**: Coronal STIR, **5.1g**: Axial STIR. Mass in the left abdominal wall musculature. The mass is T1 high signal and STIR low signal and matches the signal of adjacent fat tissue in the mesentery and skin. The mass has irregular margins. **5.1h**: Gross section of intramuscular lipoma. Lobulated pale grossly fatty tissue grows around skeletal muscle bundles. The lesion grossly extends to blacked inked surgical margins. **5.1i**: Low magnification view of intramuscular lipoma. What looks like normal fat but is actually neoplastic fat is infiltrating through and pushing apart skeletal muscle fibers.

Case figure 5.1: Continued from page 59

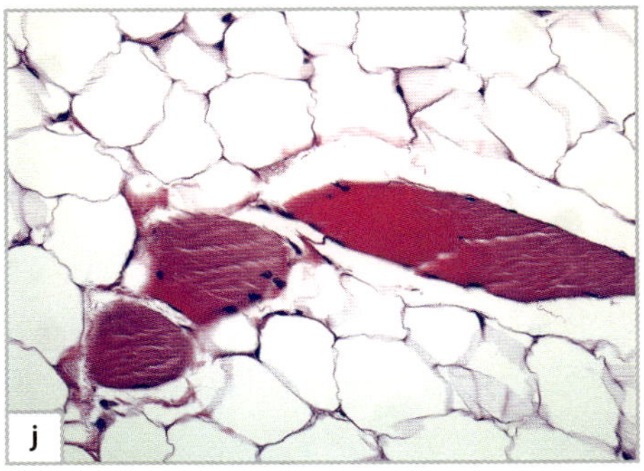

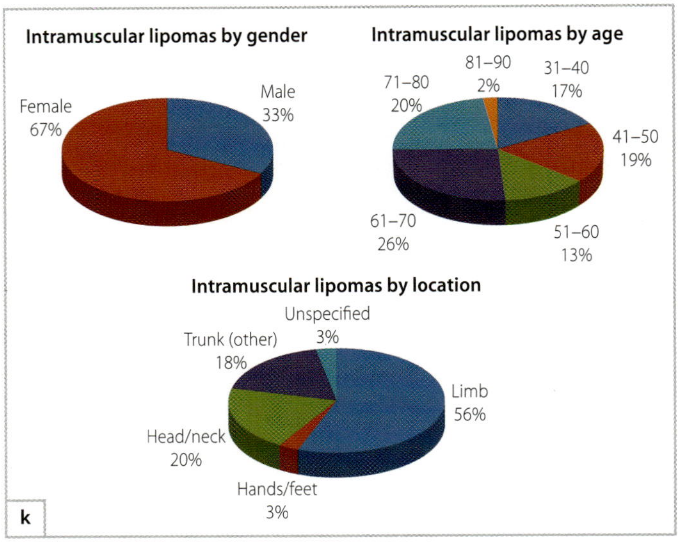

5.1j: High magnification view of intramuscular lipoma: The tumor cells still look like normal adult adipocytes. However, they insinuate themselves between skeletal muscle fibers. There are no lipoblasts, no atypical stromal cells, and no marked variation in adipocyte size and shape. **5.1k:** Cases of intramuscular lipoma resected at the University of New Mexico Health Sciences Center (UNMHSC) 2000-2010. Notice the broad age distribution and skewing towards more females for the UNM HSC cases; in the literature, men are considered to be slightly more commonly affected.

Case 5.2 Pleomorphic lipoma

Clinical history and presentation

The patient is a 56 year old man who presents with a dorsal thorax mass of several years' duration. The mass has recently increased slightly in size. It is asymptomatic.

Physical examination reveals a large rubbery mass deeply situated in the soft tissue of the posterior thorax adjacent to the spine. It is approximately 12 cm in maximum dimension. It has a rubbery consistency on palpation. It is non-tender.

SURGICAL KEY POINT

Because the imaging of spindle cell lipoma/pleomorphic lipoma will usually not allow differentiation from a well-differentiated liposarcoma, a biopsy will generally be indicated prior to excision.

Surgical findings and comments

At surgery, the mass is noted to be a well-defined neoplasm, relatively easily separable from surrounding muscle. The gross appearance is most consistent with a fatty neoplasm, however it is firmer and more edematous than a simple lipoma.

SURGICAL KEY POINT

Spindle cell lipoma/pleomorphic lipoma rarely recur after simple marginal excision, and metastases have not been reported.

Radiology findings

Case figs 5.2a through **5.2e** comprise MR images showing a fairly well-circumscribed back mass measuring 5.6 × 11.4 × 10.4 cm. The mass is heterogeneously T1 high signal and shows T2 and STIR high signal without enhancement. The mass has multiple septations with an overall lobulated morphology. The tumor causes mass effect on the paraspinal muscles without infiltration evident. This particular tumor shows approximately 75% fat composition. The extensive areas of high signal on STIR sequences indicate edema or cellularity; both findings are worrisome for a potential aggressive fat tumor. If the tumor showed enhancement, then liposarcoma would be strongly suspected. Despite the typical appearance and location for a spindle cell/pleomorphic lipoma, the mass has excessive heterogeneity and tissue diagnosis is needed. Although this tumor proved to be benign, its imaging appearance could overlap with one of the lower grade liposarcomas and underscores the difficulty in interpreting imaging studies of fat tumors.

Pathology findings

Gross features

The tumor consists of yellow lobulated tissue covered by a thin gray, semi-translucent membrane. Sectioning reveals a slightly firm, glistening, septated cut surface. The tumor is slightly firmer than a typical lipoma.

Microscopic features

Low magnification: At low power, the tumor consists of a mix of adipose cells of various sizes which are embedded in pink fibrous tissue

(**Case fig. 5.2f**). There are no areas of necrosis. The tumor does not infiltrate scant adjacent normal adipose tissue. The percentage of fat to fibrous areas is about 30:70.

High magnification: Higher magnification reveals adipocytes that vary markedly in size (**Case fig. 5.2g**). In the fibrous tissue, short, thick, 'ropy' collagen fibers are interspersed along with scattered monomorphic spindle cells. Multinucleated cells, many featuring a peripheral ring of nuclei ('floret' cells), are scattered throughout the tumor (**Case fig. 5.2h**). Mitoses are absent. Pleomorphic lipoblasts (lipoblasts with marked nuclear hyperchromasia) are absent. Numerous mast cells are also present dispersed as single cells throughout the tumor.

Special studies: Spindle cells in the lesion are strongly and diffusely positive for CD34 protein (**Case fig. 5.2i**), and only a rare cell (less than one per 10 high power fields) is positive for CDK4. There is no reactivity for MDM2 (all tested by immunohistochemistry using appropriate positive and negative controls). CD34 reactivity is characteristic of this tumor but not specific. Cytogenetics is attempted and is unsuccessful.

Case table 5.2a Summary pathology findings of Case 5.2

Diagnosis	Pleomorphic lipoma
Size	12.0 cm
Location	Deep
Margin status	Positive
Histologic grade	Not graded: benign
Pathologic stage (TNM classification)	Not graded: benign

Oncology approach

This is a benign tumor with no indication for chemotherapy or radiation treatment.

Patient outcome

Because this is a benign tumor with little propensity for local recurrence (5% or less), the patient is watched instead of undergoing re-excision. He has not developed recurrence thus far at 2.5 years after initial surgery.

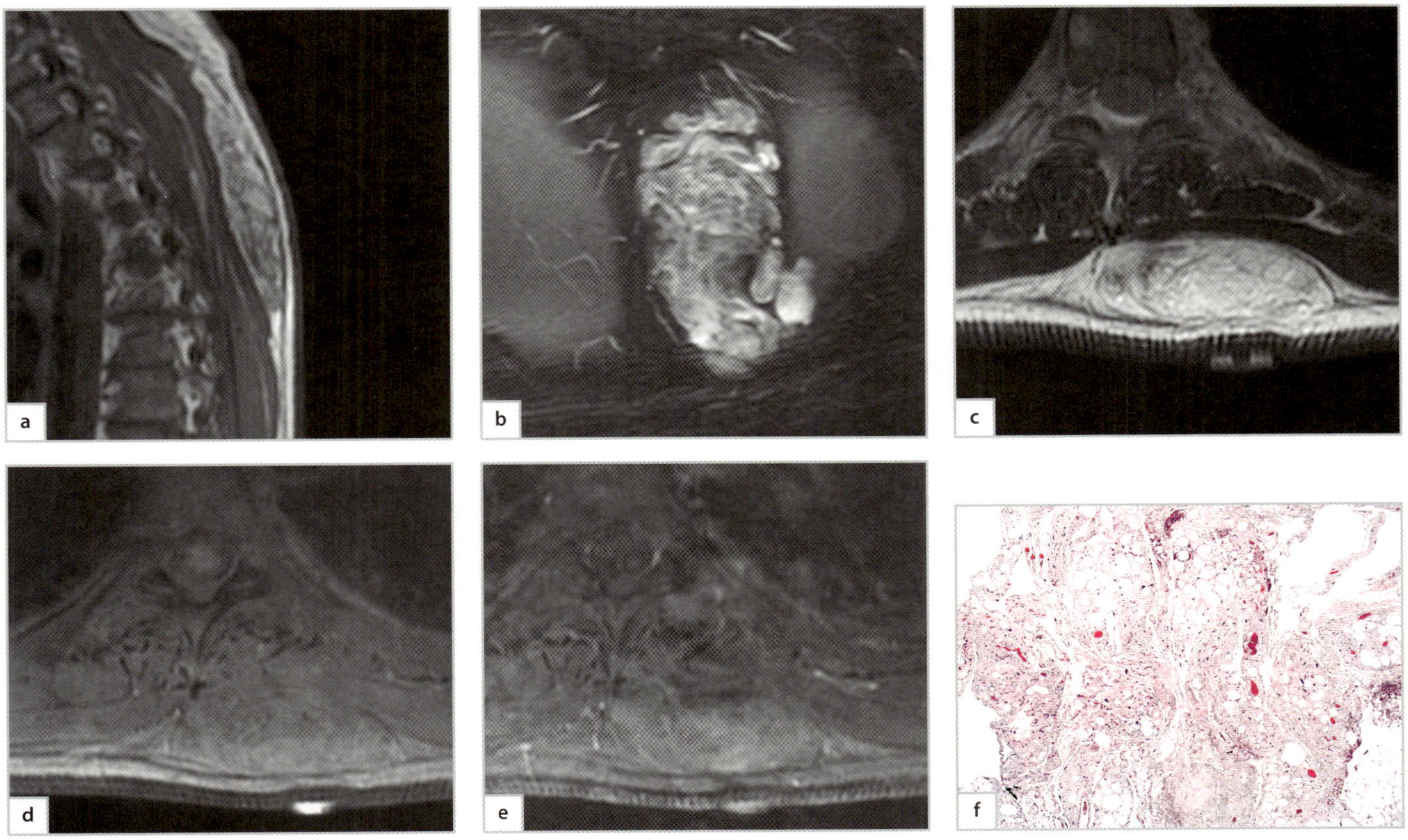

Case figure 5.2 Spindle cell/pleomorphic lipoma imaging. **5.2a**: Sagittal T1, **5.2b**: Coronal STIR, **5.2c**: Axial T2, **5.2d**: Axial T1 fat saturated, **5.2e**: Axial T1 fat saturated post-contrast. There is a subcutaneous, fairly well circumscribed mass measuring 5.6 × 11.4 × 10.4cm on the back. The mass is heterogeneously T1 high signal and shows T2 and STIR high signal without enhancement. The mass is multiseptated with an overall lobulated morphology. The tumor causes mass effect on the paraspinal muscles without evident infiltration. **5.2f**: Pleomorphic lipoma at low magnification. Notice the mixture of adipocytes and fibrous tissue. The fat cells vary markedly in size (like atypical lipomatous tumor/well-differentiated liposarcoma).

Case figure 5.2: Continued from page 61

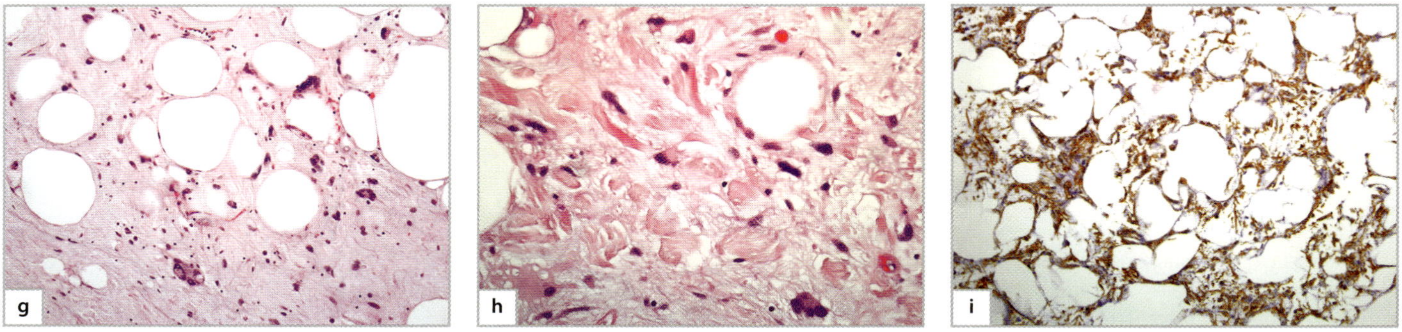

5.2g: Slightly higher magnification of pleomorphic lipoma. The fibrous areas contain short stumpy collagen fibers ('ropy collagen', and scattered cells with pink cytoplasm and irregular big nuclei. The nuclei of these cells is fine and not coarse or hyperchromatic (the latter two features would be concerning for malignant cells). **5.2h**: Pleomorphic lipoma high magnification. At higher magnification, a fibrous area reveals a multinucleated tumor cell with a flower petal arrangement of nuclei ('floret cell') in addition to more of the 'ropy' collagen fibers. **5.2i**: Pleomorphic lipoma with extensive expression of CD34 antigen. Typically, the spindle and pleomorphic cells of plemorphic and spindle cell lipomas strongly and diffusely express CD34.

Case 5.3 Atypical lipomatous tumor/well differentiated liposarcoma

Clinical history and presentation

The patient is a 77 year old woman who presents with a large calf mass which has been present for over 10 years.

Physical examination reveals a soft-tissue mass involving most of the calf. The limits between the mass and surrounding normal structures are not clearly delineated on palpation. It has a soft, rubbery consistency on palpation. It is non-tender.

SURGICAL KEY POINT

The typical low grade heterogeneity that will generally be seen with these tumors on pre-operative MRI will usually warrant a biopsy prior to definitive resection.

Surgical findings and comments

At surgery, the tumor is a multi-lobulated but encapsulated mass that separates easily from the surrounding soft tissues.

SURGICAL KEY POINT

Wide surgical resection is generally recommended as the treatment of choice. Atypical lipomatous tumors of the extremity can recur after marginal excision and can occasionally (5%) recur as a dedifferentiated neoplasm with a significant risk of metastasis. Atypical lipomatous tumors themselves do not metastasize.

SURGICAL GRAY AREA

Because of the relatively low risk of recurrence and low risk of dedifferentiation, wide resection in all cases may be overly aggressive, particularly in the elderly. Marginal resection with close, and prolonged, follow-up may be appropriate in many clinical situations.

Radiology findings

The radiology images (**Case figs 5.3a** through **5.3d**), show an infiltrative complex fat tumor involving much of the calf. The tumor shows areas of STIR high signal indicating edema or cellularity. The margins are ill-defined with infiltration or invasion evident. This fat tumor has clear aggressive features. One can imagine obtaining clean surgical margins would likely be difficult to achieve given the infiltrative nature of the tumor. A high grade liposarcoma could well have had this degree of heterogeneity, enhancement and invasive appearance.

Pathology findings

Gross features

The specimen comprises a 27 cm mass that on sectioning reveals a lobulated, firm tan tumor with focal acute hemorrhage. There is no normal tissue. Margins are inked.

Microscopic features

Low magnification: The view at low power (10x objective; **Case fig. 5.3e**) reveals abundant fat interspersed irregularly by strands of fibrous tissue. In a few areas, the fibrous strands become a little thicker and entrap fat cells. There is no necrosis or hypercellularity.

High magnification: At higher magnification, the tumor cells resemble mature adipocytes except they are markedly variable in size (**Case fig. 5.3f**). A rare lipoblast (fat cell with a nucleus indented by one or more cytoplasmic fat vacuoles) is identified (**Case fig. 5.3g**). Atypical polygonal cells with dark, angulated or multiple nuclei are dispersed in some of the collagen bands (**Case fig. 5.3h**). These cells do not contain lipid and are termed 'atypical stromal cells'. Blood vessels in the tumor also disclose a few of these atypical cells in their walls (**Case fig. 5.3i**).

Special studies: One to four neoplastic fat cells per high power microscopic field are positive for CDK4 and MDM2, enough to be considered a positive result (**Case figs 5.3j** and **5.3k**). A portion of the specimen sent for cytogenetics reveals the typical genetics of atypical lipomatous tumor/well-differentiated liposarcoma: supernumerary ring and giant marker chromosomes both of which consist of many copies of 12q13-15.

Pathologic differential or, why isn't it one of the following?

Deep lipoma: The main lesion in the differential is a large deep lipoma. Most lipomas don't reach the size of 28 cm, but it can happen. The histologic features that are *inconsistent* with lipoma are 1) marked range in adipocyte size, 2) strands of a collagen and blood vessels that contain scattered atypical stromal cells, and 3) rare lipoblasts. Adipocyte variability in size could occur in an area of fat necrosis in a lipoma, but such an area would also be associated with inflammation including foamy macrophages and even necrotic adipocytes which would be clues to the diagnosis of lipoma with trauma and not ALT/well-differentiated liposarcoma.

ALT and well-differentiated liposarcoma are the same entity: The only difference between them is location. Crucially, location = behavior = determines name. Extremity and non-cavity trunk tumors are ALT, while mediastinal and retroperitoneal examples are called well-differentiated liposarcoma. The former do not metastasize and only recur in a small percentage of cases. Dedifferentiation in extremity and non-cavity trunk tumors is rare but at that point, metastasis can occur. Mediastinal and retroperitoneal tumors de-differentiate more commonly, thereby acquiring metastatic capability. However, these tumors also can kill the patient through surgically uncontrollable local spread (due to growth around vital organs). This patient exemplifies the importance of location in behavior. She lived with this slowly growing ALT for a decade: plenty of time for it to have dedifferentiated and metastasized. Thankfully, dedifferentiation is unusual in extremity and non-cavity trunk sites.

Case table 5.3a Summary pathology findings of Case 5.3

Diagnosis	Atypical lipomatous tumor
Size	27.0 cm
Location	Deep extremity
Margin status	Positive
Histologic grade	Low grade = 1 of 3 by TNM, NCI, and FNCLCC systems
Pathologic stage (TNM classification)	T2b/n0/m0 (staging workup is negative) = stage ib

Case fig. 5.3l illustrates the spectrum of benign and malignant adipocytic tumors diagnosed on surgical resections from 2000-2010. Ninety three percent of the surgically excised tumors are benign (the great majority comprising standard lipoma).

Oncology approach

Medical oncology and radiation oncology

This is a low grade tumor that has a median time of recurrence of about 55 months and only a 5% risk for de-differentiation in residual tumor. Generally, atypical lipomatous tumor is treated by surgery only with an attempt, if possible, at achieving wide margins.

Patient outcome

Because the patient is elderly with significant co-morbidities, she and her care team decide to follow her carefully rather than re-excise the lesion. At three years, she is without local recurrence, and there is no evidence of metastatic disease.

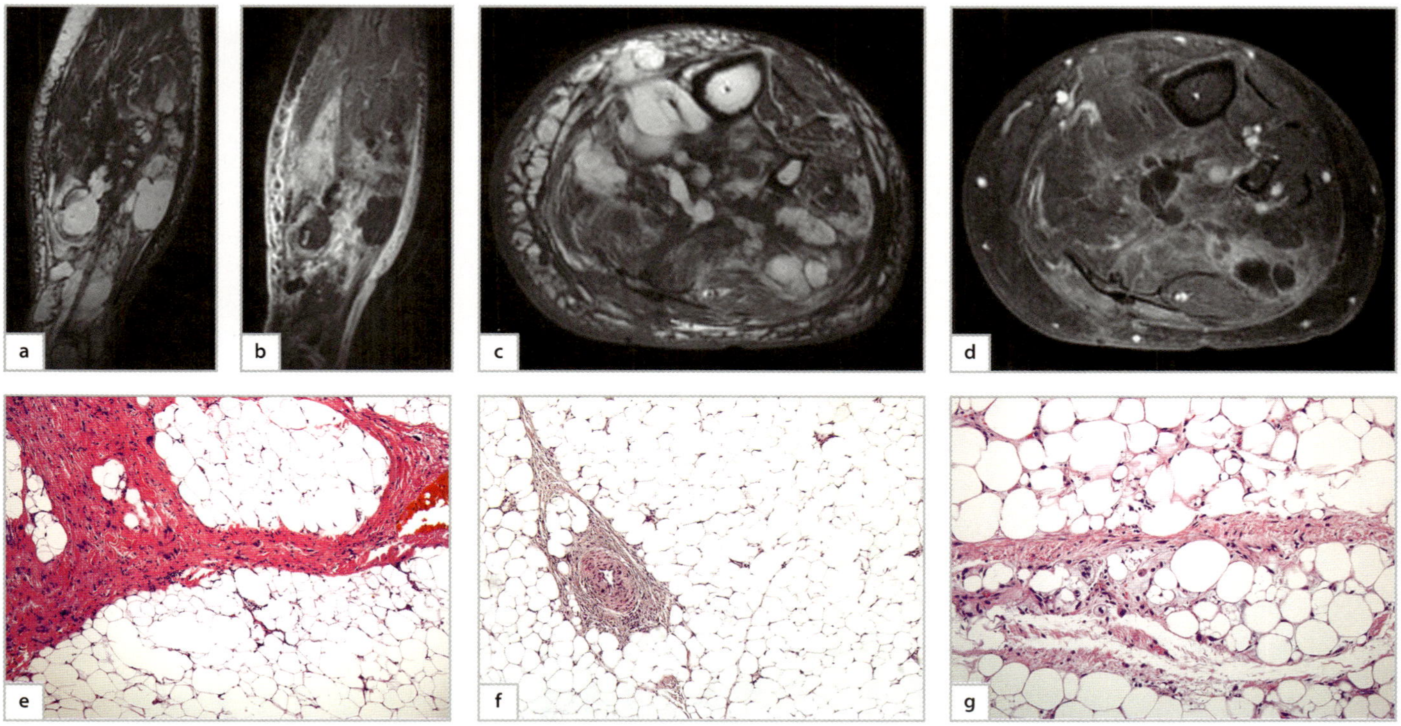

Case figure 5.3 Atypical lipomatous tumor/well differentiated liposarcoma imaging. 5.3a: Coronal T1, **5.3b**: Coronal STIR, **5.3c**: Axial T1, **5.3d**: Axial T1 fat saturated post-contrast. There is a heterogeneous complex mass involving most of the calf. The mass measures 27.1 × 7.3 × 11.5cm and has T1 high signal areas indicating fat tissue. There are heterogeneous areas of STIR high signal and patchy areas of moderate enhancement. The margins are ill defined with possible areas of infiltration.

Case figure 5.3: Continued from page 63

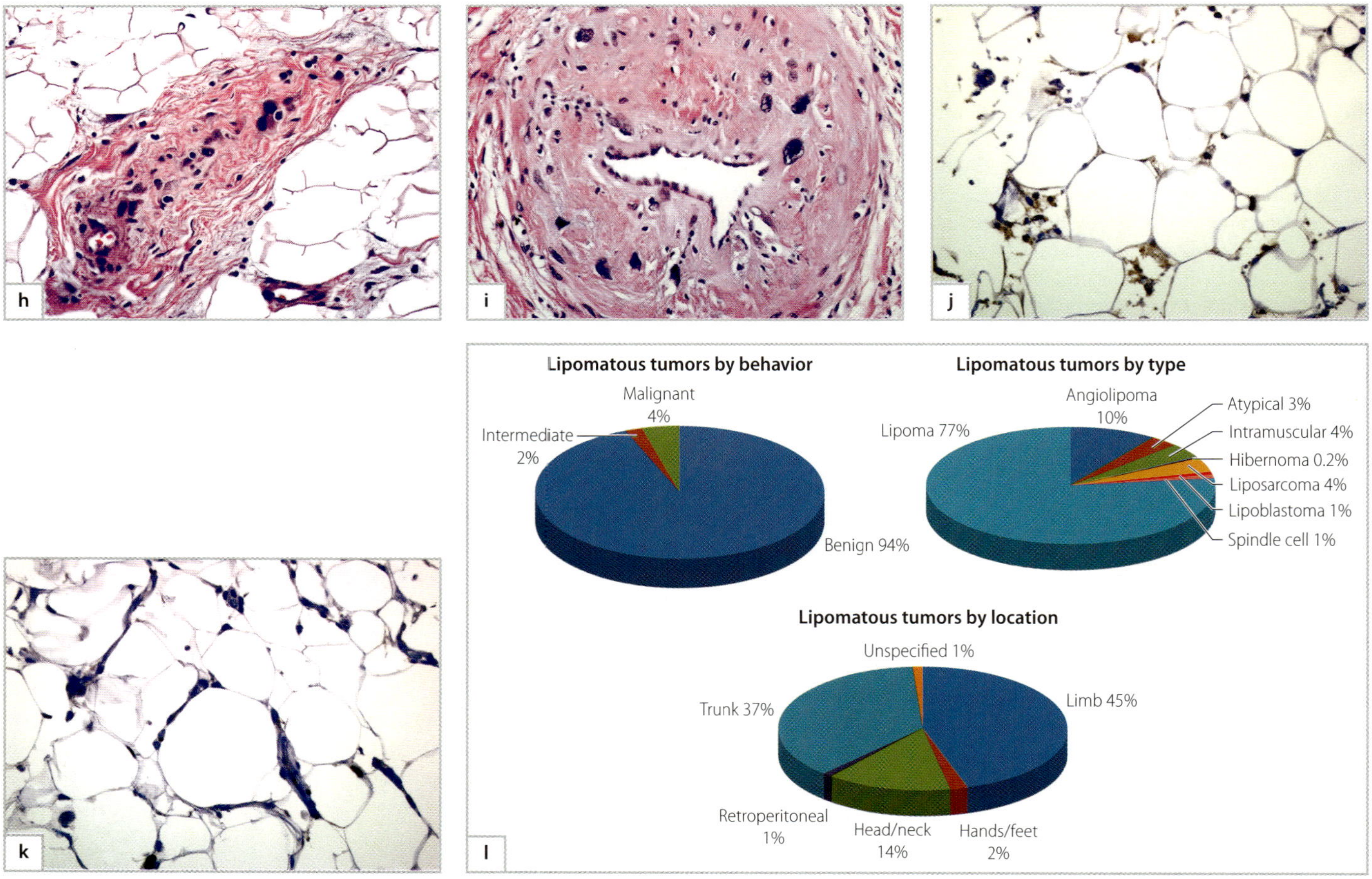

5.3e: Low magnification of atypical lipomatous tumor. The tumor at low power comprises mature looking fat divided haphazardly into lobules by bands of fibrous tissue. The long branching bands of fibrosis would be unusual for a lipoma, and the adipocytes vary in size markedly throughout the section, another feature unlike a lipoma (except if were mechanically traumatized with subsequent fat cell regeneration). **5.3f**: Medium magnification of atypical lipomatous tumor. Notice the fat cells differ in size. There is up to five-fold variation in adipocyte size. **5.3g**: Higher magnification of atypical lipomatous tumor. After responsibly scouring many tumor sections, the pathology resident finds one field containing lipoblasts. **5.3h**: Atypical lipomatous tumor, high magnification of fibrous band. These bands often contain atypical stromal cells as are seen here: the nuclei are variable in shape, hyperchromatic, and some cells contain multiple nuclei. **5.3i**: Atypical lipomatous tumor, high magnification. A blood vessel in the tumor contains atypical stromal cells in its wall. While fairly located in vessels of ALTs, most atypical stromal cells reside in the fibrous bands separating lobules of tumor. **5.3j**: CDK4 reactivity in atypical lipomatous tumor. Scattered cells exhibit nuclear positivity consistent with overexpression of the CDK4 protein. **5.3k**: MDM2 reactivity in ALT. Similar nuclear reactivity pattern as for CDK4 consistent with the diagnosis of ALT. **5.3l**: Distribution of benign and malignant adipocytic tumors resected at UNM HSC 2000-2010. As would be expected, the excised benign tumors far outnumber the excised malignant tumors (~10:1 ratio; n = 1040).

Case 5.4 Pleomorphic liposarcoma

Clinical history and presentation

The patient is a 56 year old man who presents with a right arm mass first noted four months ago. It has grown slowly, but progressively, since first noted. He relates mild tenderness associated with the mass.

Physical examination reveals a large, firm mass over the anterior aspect of the proximal arm. It is deeply situated and adherent to surrounding structures. It is minimally tender.

Surgical findings and comments

An incisional biopsy is performed based on the MRI findings. Subsequent to pathology evaluation, the tumor is resected with an attempt to obtain wide negative margins.

SURGICAL KEY POINT

These tumors will typically not appear fatty on MRI, therefore a biopsy will be required prior to resection. Wide resection is the treatment of choice for this tumor. With a margin < 1cm, radiation therapy should be considered.

Radiology findings

The radiology images (**Case figs 5.4a** through **5.4d**), show an aggressive, heterogeneous mass of the anterior arm. There are T1 high signal and STIR low signal areas indicating fat tissue (as opposed to T1 high signal hemorrhage or proteinaceous material). The presence of adipose tissue narrows the differential to one of the fat tumors. The heterogeneity, extensive edema and enhancement indicate this is an aggressive tumor and a liposarcoma is the leading diagnosis.

Pathology findings

Gross features

1. The incisional biopsy consists of fragments of firm tan tissue.
2. The final resection specimen comprises a 20 cm tumor that grossly appears circumscribed with a discrete interface with scant adjacent normal tissue. Serial sectioning reveals a slightly firm, tan tumor with areas of softening consistent with necrosis. Surgical margins are negative but close in multiple areas (approximately 1 mm in areas).
3. Three months after resection, the patient is noted to have new masses in the lungs consistent with metastatic disease. A wedge resection of the mass from the right lower lobe is consistent with metastatic pleomorphic liposarcoma.

Microscopic features

Low magnification: At low magnification (**Case fig. 5.4e**), the tumor is hypercellular with a sheet-like growth and large areas of necrosis. Some tumor cells appear vacuolated; these comprise about 30-50% of total tumor cells.

High magnification: Even at medium magnification it is easy to appreciate that adipocytes vary markedly in size (**Case fig. 5.4f**). High magnification reveals many cells containing crisply delineated clear cytoplasmic vacuoles. Some tumor cells are univacuolated, while others are multivacuolated. Most of these vacuolated cells contain hyperchromatic nuclei with coarse, grainy chromatin. These pleomorphic nuclei are sharply indented or deformed by the clear cytoplasmic vacuoles consistent with pleomorphic lipoblasts (**Case fig. 5.4g**). Mitoses are numerous, and atypical mitoses are scattered throughout the tumor. A few chronic inflammatory cells are present, mostly clustering around regions of necrosis. In addition to the clearly identifiable lipoblasts, up to half of the tumor cells are not vacuolated with pale eosinophilic cytoplasm and pleomorphic nuclei (**Case fig. 5.4h**).

Special studies: Tumor cells are negative for markers of dedifferentiated liposarcoma (MDM2 and CDK4) by immunohistochemistry. Cytogenetic analysis is not performed.

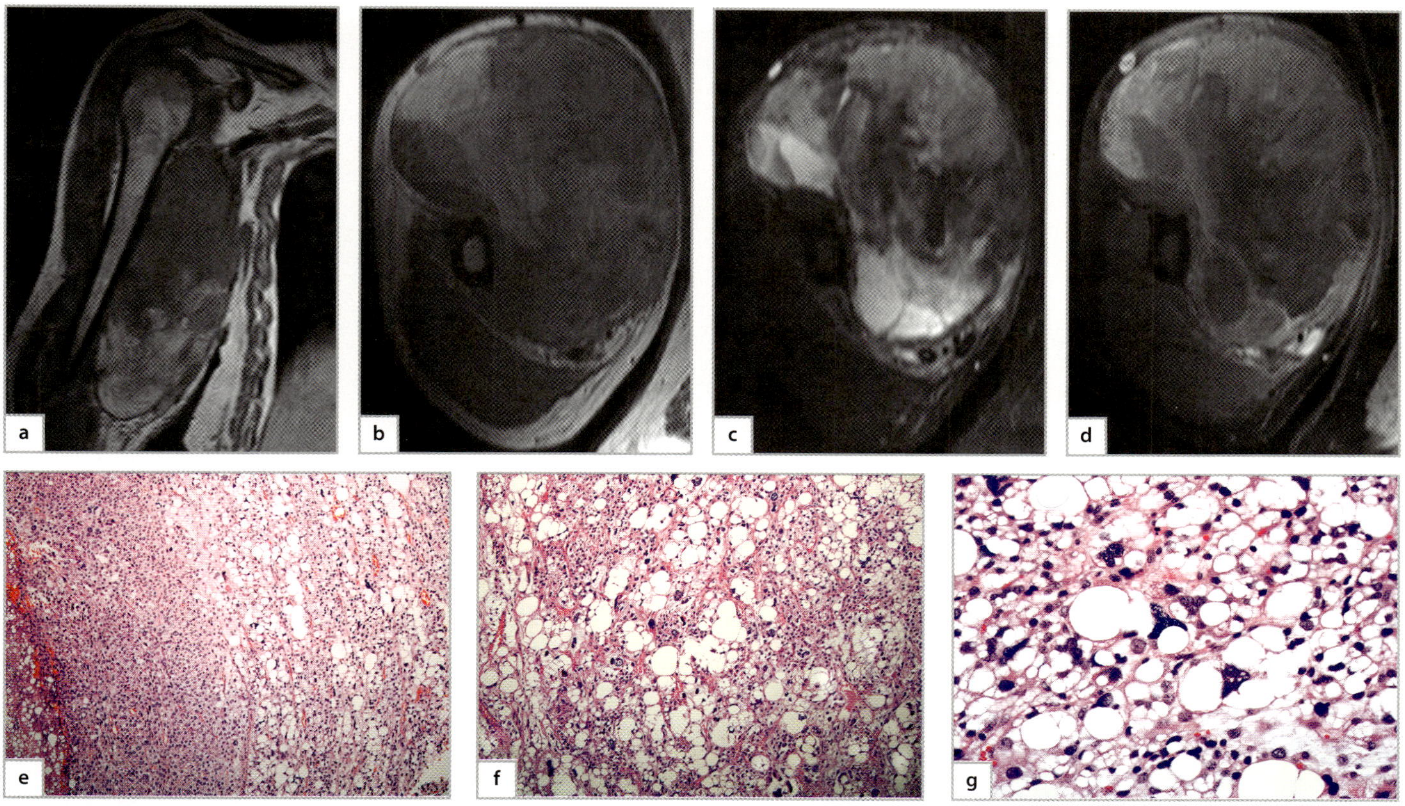

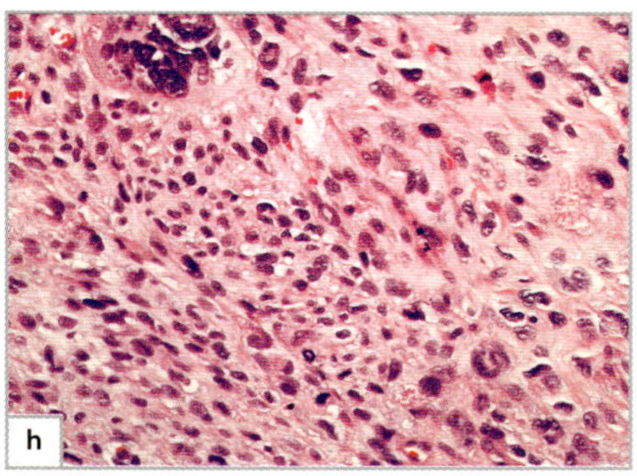

Case figure 5.4 Pleomorphic liposarcoma imaging 5.4a: Coronal T1, **5.4b**: Axial T1, **5.4c**: Axial STIR, **5.4d**: axial T1 fat saturated post-contrast. MR images reveal a heterogeneous mass measuring 16.6 × 11.4 × 10.4cm in the anterior arm. The mass has only a small percentage of fat tissue evident. There is extensive edema signal on STIR sequences and the mass shows significant heterogeneous enhancement. **5.4e**: Pleomorphic liposarcoma, low magnification. The tumor is cellular with a mixture of vacuolated cells and eosinophilic tumor cells. Even at this power, the cells clearly vary markedly in size. The very dark shapes comprise hyperchromatic tumor nuclei. **5.4f**: Pleomorphic liposarcoma, medium magnification. Marked variation (five-fold or more) in lipoblast size is easily appreciated. **5.4g**: Pleomorphic liposarcoma, high magnification. Many lipoblasts are present, some with angulated indented nuclei. The clear cytoplasmic vacuoles contained lipid which dissolves during histology processing leaving empty spaces. The nuclei are variably hyperchromatic with coarse chromatin. A few nuclei are smudgy consistent with apoptosis or necrosis. **5.4h**: Pleomorphic liposarcoma, high magnification. Notice that these tumor cells are not vacuolated. These are undoubtedly still primitive neoplastic adipocytes but are not identifiable as lipoblasts, as they do not contain fat vacuoles that sharply indent the nucleus. A few inflammatory cells are also present.

Pathologic differential or, why isn't it one of the following?

Dedifferentiated liposarcoma: The classic histologic definition of dedifferentiated liposarcoma is that it must contain a combination of well-differentiated liposarcoma and one or more malignant mesenchymal elements such as high grade pleomorphic sarcoma, NOS, osteosarcoma, chondrosarcoma, fibrosarcoma, leiomyosarcoma, etc. The dogma dictated that pleomorphic liposarcoma could not count as the other mesenchymal element. There is, however, some movement among experts to consider pleomorphic liposarcoma a valid dedifferentiated component of dedifferentiated liposarcoma. This is not a totally trivial matter, because of the difference in behavior between pleomorphic liposarcoma (worse) and dedifferentiated liposarcoma (slightly better). Sampling error could result in calling a dedifferentiated liposarcoma a pleomorphic liposarcoma, if only the latter area was biopsied. The potential for sampling error is another reason why discriminating pathologists prefer pear-sized rather than pea-sized initial incisional biopsies, although multiple needle core biopsies taken from different areas of a large tumor can also reduce sampling error.

Pleomorphic high grade undifferentiated sarcoma with pseudolipoblasts (PUS with pseudolipoblasts): The degree of cytologic atypia present in this tumor would be compatible with PUS. However, the incontrovertable, diagnostic lipoblasts so prominently noticeable in this patient's tumor excludes PUS. Pseudolipoblasts have clear cytoplasm, but they do not sharply indent the nucleus and do not generally have clearly marginated vacuoles. Unfortunately, fat stains (such Sudan Black and Oil Red O) would not help distinguish a pseudo-lipoblast from a true lipoblast, as lipid is destroyed in standard formalin/alcohol histology processing of tissues. Lipid staining only works on frozen sections or smears, preparations which are usually not made for soft tissue tumors.

Pleomorphic/spindle cell lipoma: Floret cells in pleomorphic lipoma don't usually exhibit the degree of nuclear hyperchromasia and granularity of chromatin as seen in at least some lipoblasts in pleomorphic liposarcoma. Ropy collagen fibers are also a characteristic feature of pleomorphic lipoma not present in pleomorphic liposarcoma. Pleomorphic lipoma also is CD34 strongly positive in the non-fat cell portion of the tumor; CD34 can be positive in pleomorphic liposarcoma but would be unusual. Pleomorphic lipoma usually contains mature fat cells (adult fat cells) and often will feature areas consistent with spindle cell lipoma. Cytogenetically, pleomorphic/spindle cell lipoma shows aberrations of 16q, 13q, or 6p without supernumerary ring chromosomes. In contrast, pleomorphic liposarcoma is characterized by a highly aneuploid karyotype with multiple non-specific alterations.

Oncology approach

Medical oncology

Prior to initiating radiation therapy, the patient developed a clinical recurrence as well as multiple bilateral metastases to the lung. He was started on chemotherapy (gemcitabine, taxotere, avastin). He appeared to be responding well, but prior to receiving his third cycle; he developed a right-sided pneumothorax. This was treated with a video-assisted thoracoscopic surgery (VATS) resection of a pleural tumor. The patient is subsequently on and off chemotherapy. He does have an excellent partial response to the initial gemcitabine, taxotere, and avastin.

Radiation oncology

In this patient, radiation therapy will not help overall survival. However, it may be helpful for palliation if any of his tumor causes pain or dysfunction. He does not experience pain or significant dysfunction.

Patient outcome

The patient succumbs to metastatic tumor in the lungs at 1.5 years after his tumor is excised.

Case table 5.4a Summary pathology findings of Case 5.4

Diagnosis	Pleomorphic liposarcoma
Size	20 cm
Location	Deep extremity
Margin status	Negative but some are close (1.0 mm from tumor)
Histologic grade	High grade = 3 of 3 by tnm, nci, and FNCLCC systems
Pathologic stage at presentation (TNM classification)	T2b/n0/m0 + high grade (staging workup is initially negative) = stage III

Case 5.5 Dedifferentiated liposarcoma

Clinical history and presentation

The patient is a 67 year old woman who presents with a one-year history of a progressively enlarging posterior thigh mass. Pressure from the mass makes sitting uncomfortable, but she otherwise has no symptoms.

Physical examination reveals a large firm mass deep in the posterior thigh. It is attached to surrounding deep structures. It is non-tender.

Surgical findings and comments

A needle core biopsy is performed with findings most consistent with low grade liposarcoma. Wide resection is then performed.

Radiology findings

The radiology images (**Case figs 5.5a** through **5.5d**), show a heterogeneous mass in the medial compartment. The tumor shows

SURGICAL KEY POINT

These tumors (or at least the dedifferentiated portion) will typically not appear fatty on MRI, therefore a biopsy will be required prior to resection Wide resection is the treatment of choice for this tumor. With a margin < 1 cm, radiation therapy should be considered.

SURGICAL GRAY AREA

Needle biopsies can often underestimate the grade of the neoplasm. When performed, the target should be the most heterogeneous area of the tumor as seen on imaging. Results of needle biopsies must be interpreted with caution.

intense enhancement and frankly invasive margins. There is no T1 high signal tissue to indicate fat tissue. This is clearly an aggressive tumor, and although the appearance is non-specific due to the absence of discernible fat tissue, the radiologist can at least diagnose a sarcoma.

One additional case, **Case 5.5f** through **5.5j**, shows a heterogeneous enhancing mass with a few areas of margin invasion. The mass in only moderately high signal on T2 and STIR sequences possibly due to high cellularity or calcification. The adjacent edema indicates inflammation or invasion of adjacent tissues. The lack of central enhancement could be from necrosis or matrix production. Again, no fat tissue is identifiable, and the radiologist can only diagnose a generic sarcoma.

Pathology findings

Gross features

Main resection: The tumor is received as a single large mass with attached fat and muscle. It measures 10 × 6 × 5 cm. Serial sections reveal one area that glistens and shines with a yellow soft consistency consistent with fat differentiation. Another separate area of the tumor is slightly firmer and white with a 'fish flesh' consistency. There are no identifiable areas of necrosis.

Microscopic features

Low magnification. Needle core biopsy: Unfortunately, the needle core biopsy only samples a lower grade area of the tumor leading to a diagnosis of low grade liposarcoma. Cytogenetics is not performed, as the tissue is too scant to spare for karyotyping.

Main resection

Low magnification: The resection specimen reveals areas consistent with well-differentiated liposarcoma comprising mildly varying adipocytes (**Case fig. 5.5k**). However, there are also areas of hypercellular tumor that don't contain identifiable fat cells.

High magnification. Main resection: The well-differentiated component consists of mature appearing sheets of adipocytes traversed by bands of sclerotic tissue. A few areas feature a myxoid matrix and increasing cellularity. One large region of tumor is hypercellular with markedly pleomorphic tumor cells that show irregularly shaped, hyperchromatic nuclei. In this area, there are no lipoblasts (**Case fig. 5.5l**). Other dedifferentiated areas are not so pleomorphic and resemble a non-specific low grade spindle cell sarcoma (**Case fig. 5.5m**). The outer layers of tumor transition discretely from well-differentiated liposarcoma-like to progressively higher grade sarcoma, not otherwise specified (**Case fig. 5.5n**). Dedifferentiated liposarcomas often feature sharp transitions from one grade to another but gradual changes also occur, even in the same tumor.

Special studies: Consistent with the diagnosis of dedifferentiated liposarcoma, the tumor is positive for CDK4, MDM2, and p16 (reactivity

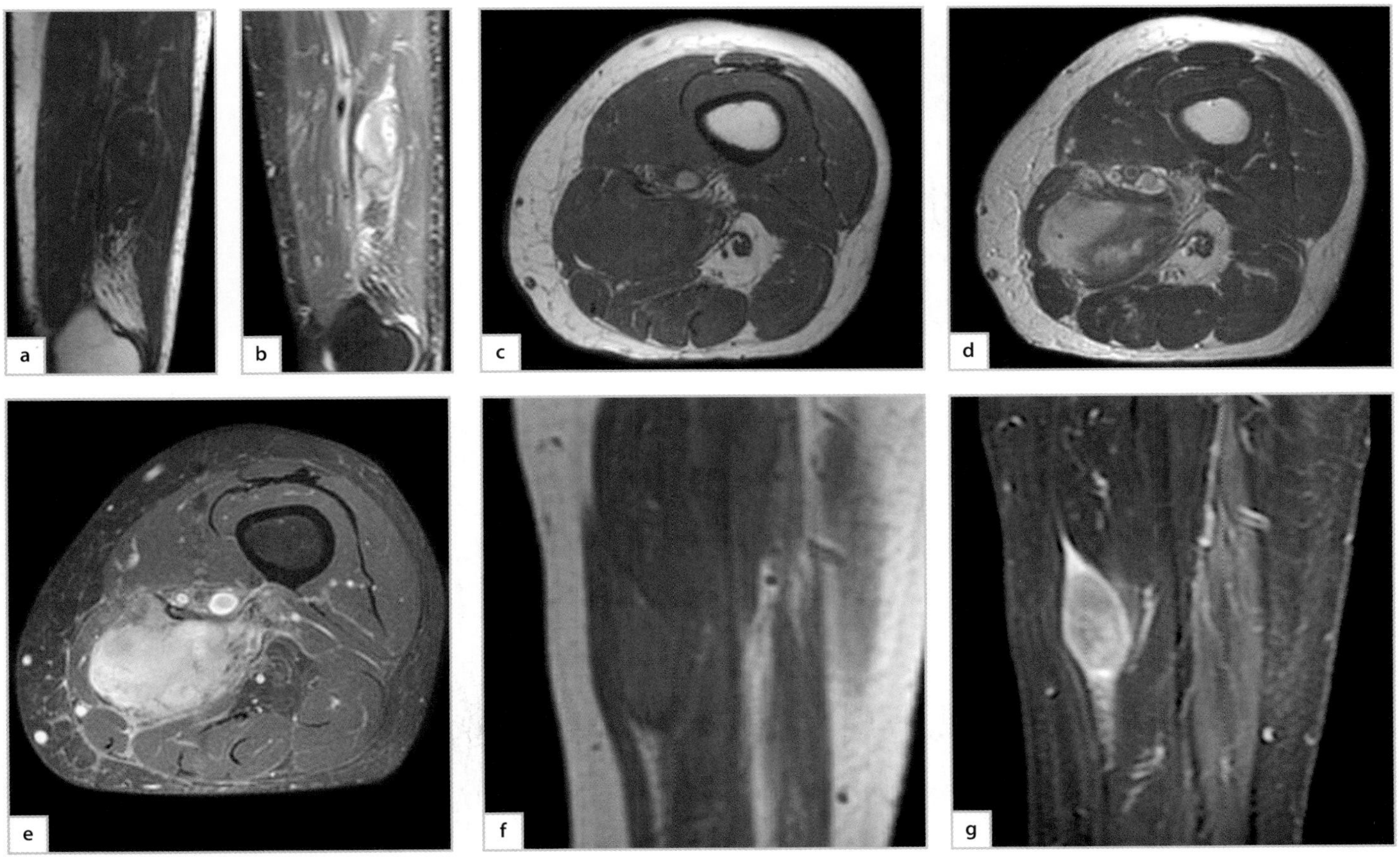

Case figure 5.5 Dedifferentiated liposarcoma imaging: MR images **5.5a**: Sagittal T1, **5.5b**: Sagittal STIR, **5.5c**: Axial T1, **5.5d**: Axial T2, **5.5e**: Axial T1 fat saturated post-contrast. There is a 9.9 × 3.6 × 6.4 cm T1 isointense, T2 and STIR high signal mass in the adductor magnus compartment of the thigh. The mass is heterogeneous and has intense diffuse enhancement. There is frank infiltration and invasion of the surrounding tissues. Anteriorly, the tumor contacts the superficial femoral artery and vein. The sciatic nerve is lateral to the mass and there is tumor surrounding the nerve inferiorly (images not included). Additional case of dedifferentiated liposarcoma with MR images including: **5.5f**: Coronal T1, **5.5g**: Coronal STIR.

Case figure 5.5: Continued from page 67

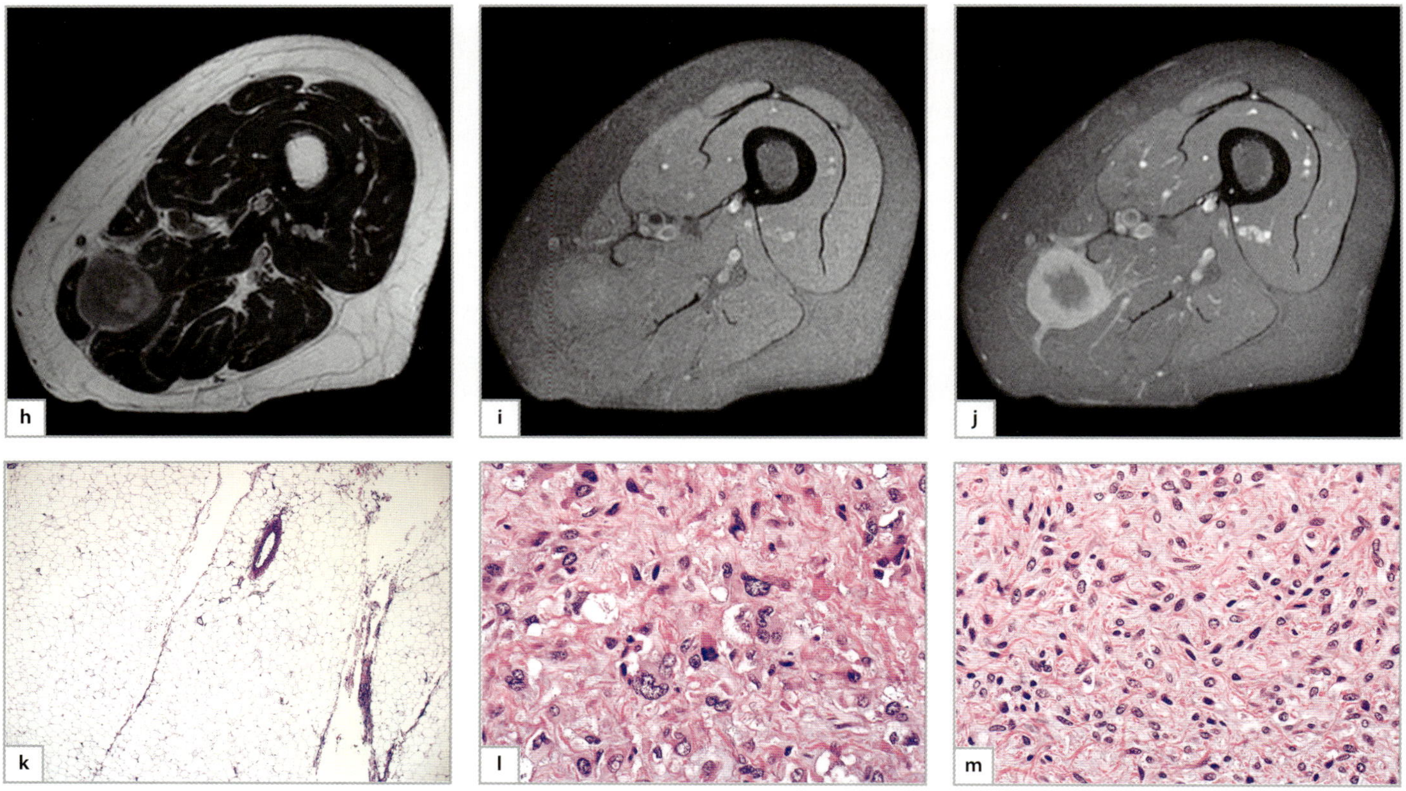

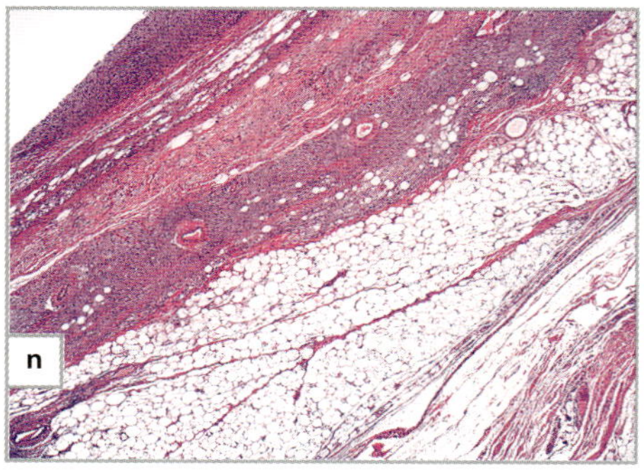

5.5h: Axial T2, **5.5i**: Axial T1 fat saturation and **5.5j**: Axial T1 fat saturated post-contrast. There is a 4.6 × 2.8 × 2.5 cm mass in the medial compartment of this 63 year old woman. The mass is T1 isointense with heterogeneous T2 and STIR intermediate signal. The mass shows intense rim enhancement. There is adjacent edema and enhancing tissue extending into the soft tissues. **5.5k**: Low grade area of dedifferentiated liposarcoma. This portion of the tumor is histologically consistent with well-differentiated liposarcoma. Notice the great variety of adipocyte size and myxoid background. **5.5l**: Medium power magnification of a dedifferentiated part of the tumor. Marked hypercellularity and cellular pleomorphism consistent with high grade sarcoma, not otherwise specified. As would be expected for most dedifferentiated liposarcoma, lipoblasts are absent. **5.5m**: High power view of dedifferentiated area of tumor. Another region of dedifferentiation exhibits much less cytologic atypia comparable in grade to a low grade spindle cell sarcoma. Not uncommonly, dedifferentiated areas will range in degree of atypia, but most tumors will contain some high grade dedifferentiated sarcoma. **5.5n**: Stratigraphy (variation) in this patient's dedifferentiated liposarcoma. At lower magnification, you can appreciate the discrete layer of low grade liposarcoma over which lie bands of increasingly cellular tumor. The most cellular region is at the top and would qualify as high grade dedifferentiated liposarcoma.

for all three markers is widespread in the dedifferentiated regions and spotty in the well differentiated areas).

Pathologic differential or, why isn't it one of the following?

Mixed type liposarcoma: This rare type of liposarcoma comprises mixtures of the other types including pleomorphic liposarcoma, myxoid liposarcoma, and ALT/well-differentiated liposarcoma. This patient's various findings are best explained by de novo dedifferentiation rather than mixed type liposarcoma, as there is a well-differentiated component and an obvious high grade sarcomatous component that

Case table 5.5a Summary pathology findings of Case 5.5

Diagnosis	Dedifferentiated liposarcoma
Size	10 cm
Location	Deep extremity
Margin status	Widely negative (all 1.0 cm or greater from tumor)
Histologic grade	High grade = 3 of 3 by TNM Classification of Malignant Tumours, National Cancer Institute, and FNCLCC systems
Pathologic stage at presentation (TNM classification)	T2b/n0/m0 + high grade (staging workup is initially negative) = stage iii

does not contain lipoblasts. Furthermore, the reactivity for CDK4 and MDM2 throughout all areas of tumor is consistent with de novo dedifferentiated liposarcoma, as pleomorphic liposarcoma areas should be negative for these markers in most cases, and myxoid liposarcoma areas would also be negative.

Oncology approach

Medical oncology

After being counseled about the risk of distant metastasis and the morbidity associated with chemotherapy, the patient elects to postpone chemotherapy until if and when she develops recurrent or distant tumor.

Radiation oncology

Adjuvant radiation therapy is recommended for this patient. This recommendation is based on the results of two randomized studies that showed a statistically significant benefit in local control with adjuvant radiation therapy (Mundt et al. 1995, Yang et al. 1998). Prior to the wide local excision, neoadjuvant radiation therapy may have been a good option, but the patient does not elect to have it.

Patient outcome

Despite a 40% risk for local recurrence and 15-20% risk of distant metastases, the patient remains free of disease at 3.5 years. She will need to be followed carefully over the long term, as overall disease free survival drops substantially by 10-20 years.

Case 5.6 Myxoid/round cell liposarcoma

Clinical history and presentation

The patient is a 31 year old man with schizophrenia whose caretaker noted a mass on the patient's mid lateral trunk two months ago. Physical examination reveals a firm mass deeply situated in the lattisimus dorsi muscle. It is adherent to underlying deep structures. It is non-tender.

Surgical findings and comments

Incisional biopsy is performed. After the pathologist renders the diagnosis, wide resection of the tumor is carried out. As the surgical approach is straight-forward, wide margins are achieved.

SURGICAL KEY POINT

These tumors will typically not appear fatty on MRI, therefore a biopsy will be required prior to resection. Wide resection is the treatment of choice for this tumor. With a margin < 1 cm, radiation therapy should be considered.

Radiology findings

The radiology images (**Case figs 5.6a** through **5.6d**), show a non-specific heterogeneous enhancing mass of the latissimus dorsi muscle. The small area of T1 high signal tissue is also high signal on STIR sequences indicating this may be hemorrhage. Alternatively, this tissue might represent fat tissue that is edematous or cellular. Given the absence of definitive fat tissue, the radiologist can only render a generic diagnosis of an aggressive tumor such as a sarcoma.

Pathology findings

Gross features

1. At biopsy, the specimen comprises multiple fragments of white to tan soft tissue.
2. Upon definitive resection, the tumor appears circumscribed and measures 12 × 7 × 7 cm. Serial sectioning reveals shiny white, almost sticky surfaces and firmer, 'fish-flesh' like areas (**Case fig. 5.6e**). Necrosis is not grossly appreciable. There is only scant adherent normal skeletal muscle and fascia.

Microscopic features

Low magnification: Main resection: At low magnification, this patient's tumor is vaguely lobulated with areas of clear cells intermixed with more densely cellular regions. The tumor focally invades fascia. There is no necrosis at low power. Multiple patterns of low to high cellularity with corresponding amounts of myxoid matrix are appreciable (**Case fig. 5.6f**).

High magnification: Main resection: Higher magnification reveals a blue-gray background matrix and a mesh-like network of small vessels about the size of capillaries. This vascular pattern is called 'chicken-wire' like or, more formally, a 'plexiform capillary network' (**Case fig. 5.6g**). It is characteristic of myxoid liposarcoma and lipoblastoma/lipoblastomatosis. Small pools of acellular myxoid matrix are interspersed among the more uniformly cellular areas (**Case fig. 5.6h**). Other areas resemble well-differentiated liposarcoma with many signet ring lipoblasts and a few stellate shaped lipoblasts (**Case fig. 5.6i**). Cellularity transitions from fairly dispersed cells with prominent matrix to gradually increasing numbers of cells (**Case fig. 5.6j**). On highest magnification, the very cellular areas comprise compact clusters of uniform, small round cells without vacuoles, with indistinct cell borders and round nuclei with mild hyperchromaticity ('round cells' of myxoid liposarcoma). The round cell component in this patient's tumor also exhibits a rare morphology of tight balls of round cells floating in mucin (**Case fig. 5.6k**). Mitoses are rare, and individual cell necrosis is absent. Geographic necrosis is likewise absent. Importantly, the percentage of round cell areas in this lavishly sampled tumor is about 25% of total tumor volume. (It is important to note if a round cell component is present, as such tumors metastasize with a greater frequency than myxoid liposarcoma and have a poorer long-term survival. Just how much the risk is increased when the round cell element is less than 25% is not precisely known. In any case, it is critical to carefully and extensively submit numerous sections of a myxoid liposarcoma to include all areas of tumor that grossly appear dissimilar; the round cell component may, for example, be firmer and paler grossly, and such areas should be sampled thoroughly.)

Special studies: Main resection: Antibody to S-100 protein stains many of the vacuolated fat cells; only a few of the non-vacuolated round cells

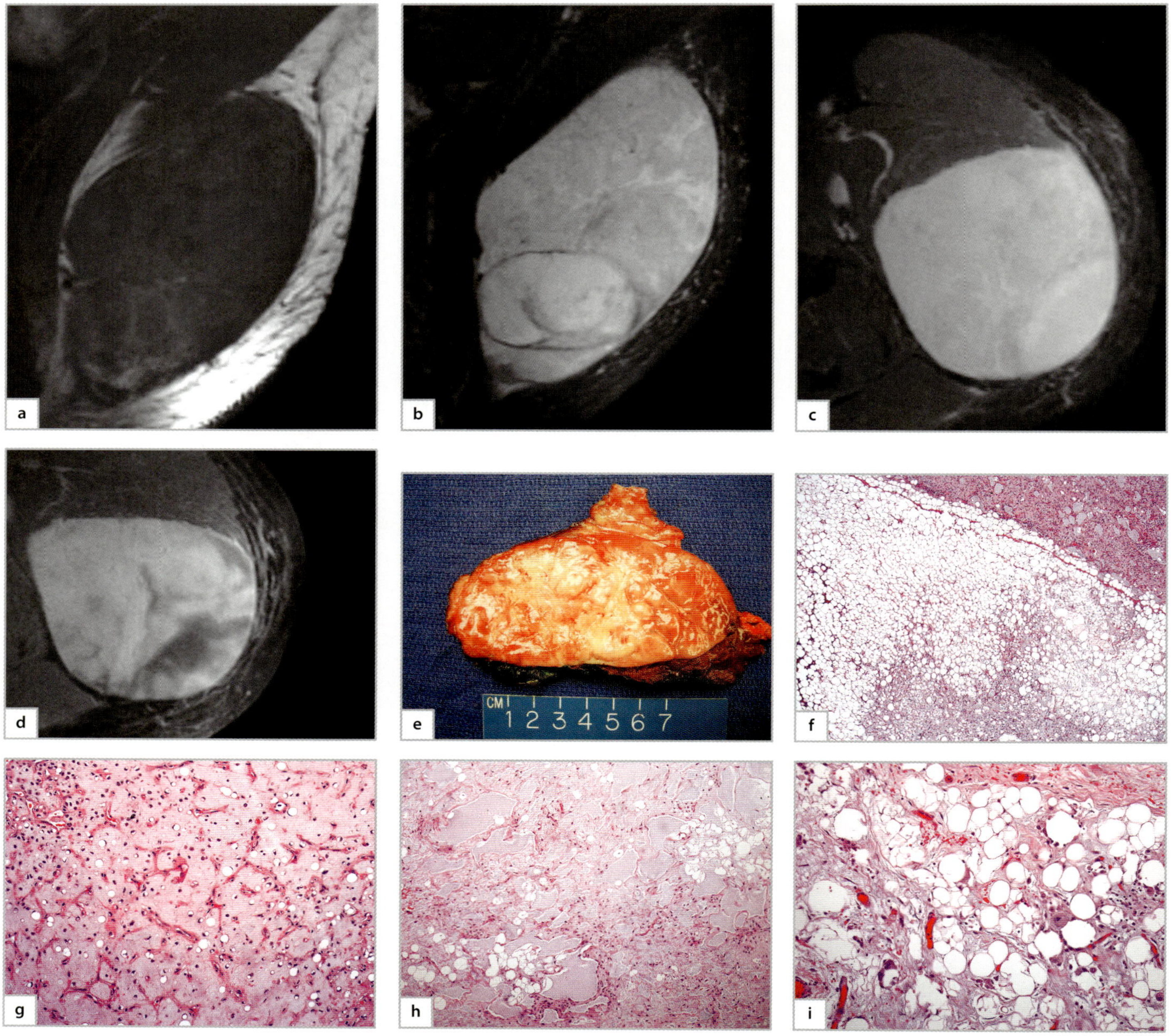

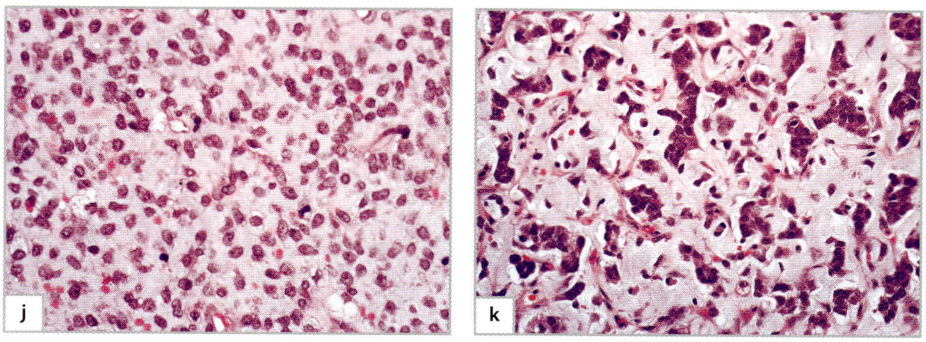

Case figure 5.6 Myxoid liposarcoma imaging: MR images **5.6a**: Coronal T1, **5.6b**: Coronal STIR, **5.6c**: Axial STIR and **5.6d**: Axial T1 fat saturated post-contrast. There is a 12.6 × 7.8 × 6.3 cm mass in the latissimus dorsi muscle. The tumor is almost entirely T1 isointense with STIR high signal and intense heterogeneous enhancement. There is a small area of striated T1 high signal tissue seen in the inferior aspect of the mass (Figure 5-6a) which corresponding high signal on STIR sequences that could represent hemorrhage. **5.6e**: Gross cut section of myxoid liposarcoma. Notice the glistening, mucoid appearance of the tumor surface. Other cross sections contain scattered denser, white nodules of slightly firmer consistency. **5.6f**: Low power of myxoid liposarcoma. Myxoid liposarcoma commonly exhibits multiple patterns in one tumor; here, one area looks like well-differentiated liposarcoma, another (upper right corner) is myxoid with pools of mucin, and the center also appears myxoid but with a prominent plexiform capillary network. **5.6g**: Myxoid liposarcoma, medium magnification. In this field, the plexiform or chicken wire capillary network and myxoid matrix stand out. A few obvious fat cells are also present, but most of the tumor cells do not have vacuoles. The cellularity is increased but is not to the point of labeling the region as a round cell component.

Case figure 5.6: Continued from page 70

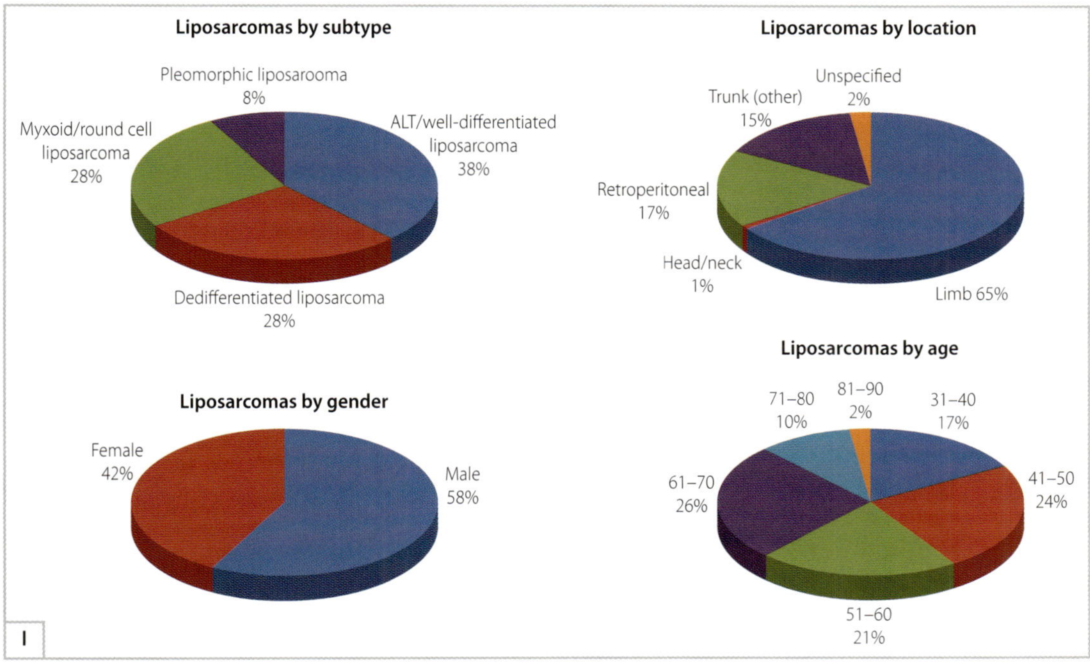

5.6h: Microscopic heterogeneity of myxoid liposarcoma. Yet another pattern of the tumor features mucin pools and clusters of more mature lipoblasts. Closely packed mucin pools outlined by plexiform capillaries can resemble fluid in lung alveoli thus meriting the description, 'pulmonary edema' pattern. Such a pattern seems specific to myxoid liposarcoma (but it can also occur in the mixed liposarcoma type when that type contains a component of myxoid liposarcoma). **5.6i**: Myxoid liposarcoma with signet ring lipoblasts. Note the signet ring and other types of lipoblasts supported by the plexiform capillary network. A bit of myxoid matrix intercolates between the neoplastic fat cells. A field like this would be very difficult to distinguish from well differentiated liposarcoma/ALT except that the chicken wire vasculature would not be seen in well-differentiated liposarcoma/ALT. **5.6j**: Transitional area bridging myxoid liposarcoma and round cell liposarcoma. Hypercellular areas of confluent growth of the round cells with no intervening stroma quality as the higher grade, round cell component. This area, while showing increased density of cells, does not yet grow as a solid sheet of back to back round cells. **5.6k**: Round cell Component of myxoid liposarcoma. This particular tumor illustrates a rare variant of the round cell component: tight clusters of the round cells floating in mucin. Note that these cells are only slightly atypical with small nucleoli and a high N/C ratio. **5.6l**: Resected liposarcomas at University of New Mexico Health Sciences Center from 2000-2010. Notice the broad adult age range, but a majority of patients are over forty years old. Extremities are the favored primary site.

are reactive. CD34 is negative as are CDK4 and MDM2 (all evaluated for expression by immunohistochemistry using appropriately reactive positive and negative controls).

Cytogenetics is performed and, after several days cosseted in ideal culture conditions, metaphase spreads of about 20 tumor cells disclose a distinctive and characteristic t(12;16)(q13;p11).

Pathologic differential or, why isn't it one of the following?

Before discussing specific entities in the differential, it is worth noting that myxoid liposarcoma can display a number of peculiar histologic appearances. In fact, a clue to the diagnosis of myxoid liposarcoma is the presence of an array of patterns, although the triad of 1) chicken wire vessels, 2) at least focal signet ring lipoblasts, and 3) myxoid background are usually the main defining features. In especially cellular, round cell areas of a myxoid/round cell liposarcoma, the plexiform capillary network may be obscured. If necessary, a CD34 antibody stain can highlight these vessels and confirm the presence of the chicken wire pattern. In table format below is a list of the microscopic features that are seen in myxoid liposarcoma (**Case table 5.6a**). This is a quixotic tumor histologically, and undoubtedly the list below is incomplete, but it should describe the majority of myxoid liposarcoma you will encounter in your practice.

Case fig. 5.6l details the number, types, age range, and location of liposarcomas resected at the University of New Mexico Health Sciences Center from 2000-2010. Unlike the SEER data, at the University of New Mexico Health Sciences Center, there were more atypical lipomatous tumors/well differentiated liposarcomas and dedifferentiated liposarcomas removed than myxoid liposarcomas. The number of dedifferentiated liposarcomas is high due to inclusion of retroperitoneal tumors, a site which rarely harbors myxoid liposarcoma (and then only as a metastasis).

Oncology approach

Medical oncology

This patient has a tumor greater than 10 cm. The National Comprehensive Cancer Network (NCCN) guidelines suggest considering neoadjuvant chemotherapy or radiotherapy for tumors greater than 10 cm. The patient's tumor is of the myxoid with round cell type, which is most sensitive to chemotherapy. A recommendation for participation in a clinical trial or standard of care with doxorubicin based chemotherapy was offered. However the patient declined the medical oncology consultation and never received chemotherapy.

Radiation oncology

Since his original resection, the patient has had multiple local recurrences. At the time of the first recurrence, radiation therapy was indicated. This is echoed in recent studies which have demonstrated that myxoid liposarcomas have an excellent response to radiation. With neoadjuvant radiation, a recent Swedish study showed a 76% partial response rate with four complete responses (small tumors) in 33 tumors. The study also demonstrated a change in the histology with more areas demonstrating mature lipomatous composition after radiation. Nearly all of the tumors had the FUS-DDIT3 (TLS/FUS-CHOP) translocation (Engstrom et al. 2007). A retrospective review from the MD Anderson Cancer Center demonstrated a 97% five year local control rate with wide-local excision and radiation therapy in 127 patients. The predominant area of failure was not locally, but in

Case table 5.6a Range of histologic findings in myxoid/round cell liposarcoma

Myxoid/round cell liposarcoma histologic feature	Frequency
Plexiform capillary network ('chicken wire' or 'crow's feet' capillaries)	Always (but may be obscured in the rare, pure round cell liposarcoma due to its high cellularity; CD34 antibody staining is helpful to ident fy the network)
Lipoblasts	Nearly always, most commonly in the form of signet ring type lipoblasts (single vacuole deforming the nucleus)
Myxoid matrix	Nearly always (may be obscured in the rare, pure round cell liposarcoma due to its high cellularity)
Sheets of mature-appearing fat cells (looks like well-differentiated liposarcoma/ALT but cells are smaller than in well diff liposarcoma/ALT)	Common
Many microcysts forming a 'pulmonary edema' look	Uncommon
Microvacuolated lipoblasts looking like brown fat of hibernoma	Uncommon
Hypercellular transitional zones with increased numbers of spindle tumor cells without back to back round cells	Uncommon and indicative of high grade myxoid liposarcoma if composing more than 25% of tumor
Clumping or stranding of the round cells	Rare
Dense collagen replacing some of the myxoid matrix	Rare
Metaplastic cartilage	Rare

Patterns described in individual unique case reports are not listed.

Case table 5.6b Summary pathology findings of Case 5.6

Diagnosis	Myxoid liposarcoma with a round cell component (25% of total tumor volume)
Size	12.6 cm
Location	Deep lateral trunk
Margin status	Negative but close (some margins are 1.0 mm from tumor)
Histologic grade	High grade = 3 of 3 by TNM, 2 by NCI (<15% necrosis), and 3 by fnclcc systems
Pathologic stage at presentation (TNM classification)	T2b/n0/m0 + high grade (staging workup is initially negative) = stage iii

the retroperitoneum (Guadagnolo et al. 2008). Probably the strongest argument in favor of adjuvant therapy is the randomized study by Yang, et al. This demonstrated a statistically significant decrease in local recurrence after radiation therapy for low grade sarcoma. This appeared to be particularly true in patients with <1 cm margins (Yang et al. 1998).

This patient was treated using adjuvant external beam radiation. Six MV photons were used to deliver a dose of 66 Gy in 33 fractions of 2 Gy. Initial field covered the lesion plus a wide margin due to the multiply recurrent nature of the tumor. The margins were 2 cm radially and 5 cm superior-inferiorly. Fields were reduced after the initial 50 Gy to the same lateral margins and a 3.5cm superior-inferior margin. Margins selection was based on a careful retrospective studies (Mundt et al. 1995).

Patient outcome

Eight months after resection, the patient develops a local recurrence that is treated by limited excision and radiation. Two more recurrences follow at 11 months and 15 months. The patient is currently alive with disease at 19 months post initial tumor resection.

Case 5.7 Lipoblastoma

Clinical history and presentation

The patient is a two year old girl who presents with a two month history of a suprascapular mass first noted by her parents. It has remained stable and appears not to cause her symptoms.

Physical examination reveals a rubbery deep mass over the scapula approximately 6 cm in diameter. It is mobile and non-tender.

Surgical findings and comments

The tumor is marginally excised.

SURGICAL KEY POINT

Marginal excision is generally curative in the circumscribed type. Recurrence is more common in the diffuse type, where wide resection may be warranted.

Radiology findings

The radiology images (**Case figures 5.7a** and **5.7b**), show a non-specific appearing mass with little vascularity. The exam reveals no fluid collection. The homogeneous mild echogenicity is suggestive of fat tissue but unfortunately, ultrasound is not specific for diagnosing fat tissue. The ultrasound confirms the presence of a tumor but offers little diagnostic direction other than the exclusion of a cyst. Hence, tissue diagnosis or MR imaging is needed for further evaluation.

Our second case of lipoblastoma, **Case fig. 5.7c** through **5.7f**, shows a tumor with fat signal in the medial thigh musculature. This is not a featureless or bland tumor as it has minimal striated edema and enhancing areas. It is reassuring that there is no nodularity or invasive margins seen. A heterogeneous fat lesion at this young age is likely a lipoblastoma, a liposarcoma could have identical appearance but would be quite unusual at this age.

Pathology findings

Gross features

The tumor is received as an ovoid portion of tissue covered by a thin membrane-like capsule measuring 5.6 × 4.4 × 2.2 cm (**Case fig. 5.7g**). The external surfaces are inked, and cut sectioning reveals pale yellow surfaces (**Case fig. 5.7h**). Lipoblastoma/lipoblastomatosis are generally relatively small; less than 5 cm in maximum dimensions; this tumor is a bit large but not exceptionally so.

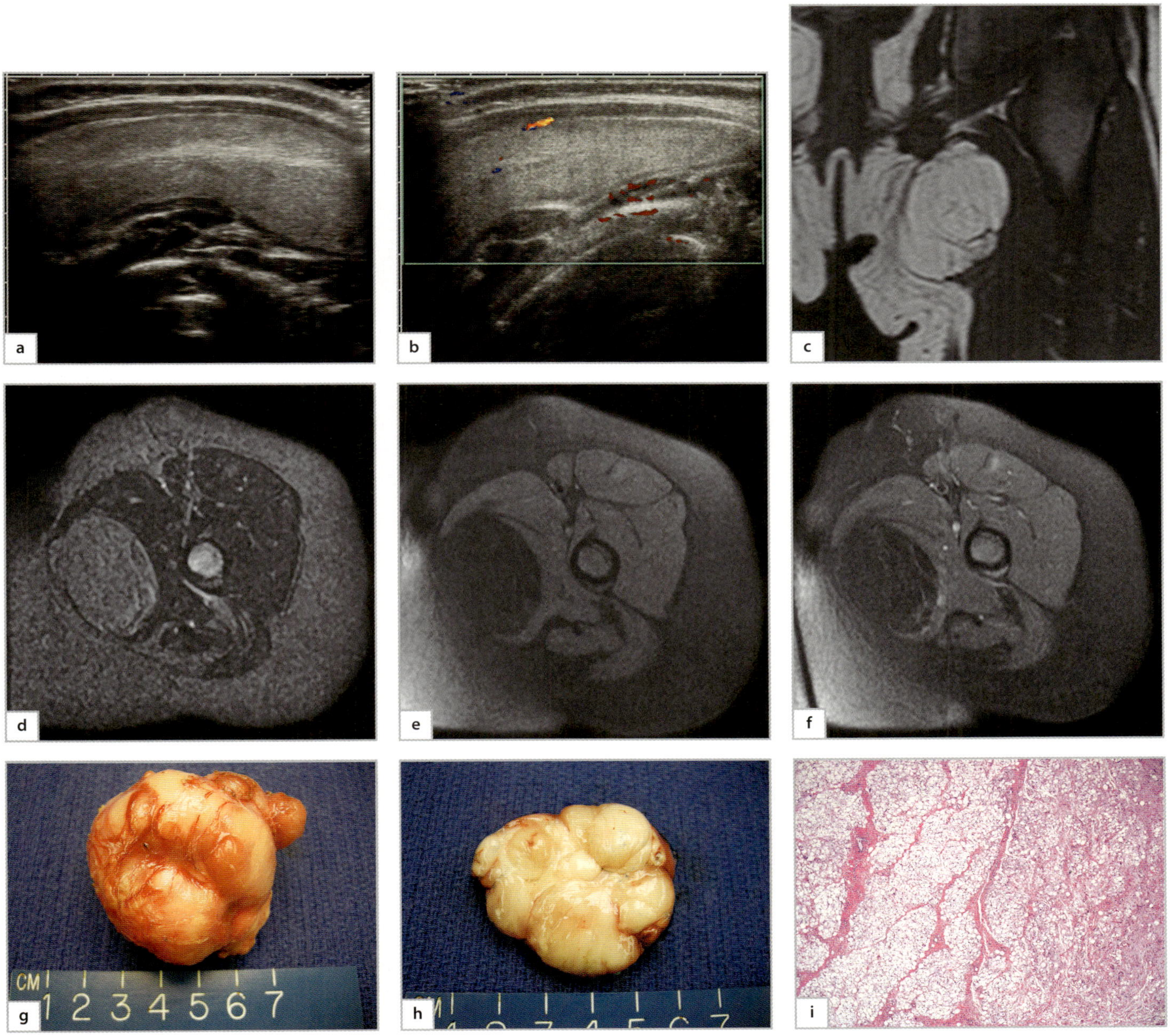

Case figure 5.7 Lipoblastoma imaging: 5.7a: Gray scale ultrasound, **5.7b**: Color Doppler (ultrasound) images of this 26 month old girl with a mass overlying the scapula. The mass is homogeneous and moderately echogenic with minimal Doppler signal. No fluid collection is seen. LIpoblastoma additional case imaging: MR images. **5.7c**: Coronal T1, **5.7d**: Axial STIR, **5.7e**: Axial T1 fat saturation, **5.7f**: Axial T1 fat saturation post-contrast. This lipoblastoma in a 14 month old girl is a 3.5 × 2.4 × 3.1cm forms a mass in the adductor magnus muscle showing T1 high signal and STIR low signal matching other fat tissue. There are several fine septations without nodularity or edema. There is minimal striated enhancement along the lateral aspect of the mass. **5.7g**: External surface of resected lipoblastoma. This patient's tumor is solitary and not diffusely infiltrative as in lipoblastomatosis. **5.7h**: Cut surface of resected lipoblastoma. Even grossly, the tumor is multi-lobulated. **5.7i**: Low magnification of lipoblastoma. In this image, obvious fat differentiation is on the left with a myxoid appearing area on the right. Fibrous septae separate groups of tumor cells into lobules.

Microscopic features

Low magnification: The tumor comprises lobules of obvious adipose tissue with scattered hypocellular myxoid areas (**Case fig. 5.7i**). Intermediate magnification reveals a network of capillaries exactly like that seen in myxoid liposarcoma (the 'chicken wire' arborizing capillary pattern) (**Case fig. 5.7j**).

High magnification: Some of the fat cells look like mature adipocytes, while others are consistent with signet ring lipoblasts (**Case fig. 5.7k**). Spindle cells are also present that focally aggregate but are uniform and bland appearing with slender nuclei, fine chromatin, and inconspicuous nucleoli. Mitoses and apoptotic bodies are not identified.

Case figure 5.7: Continued from page 73

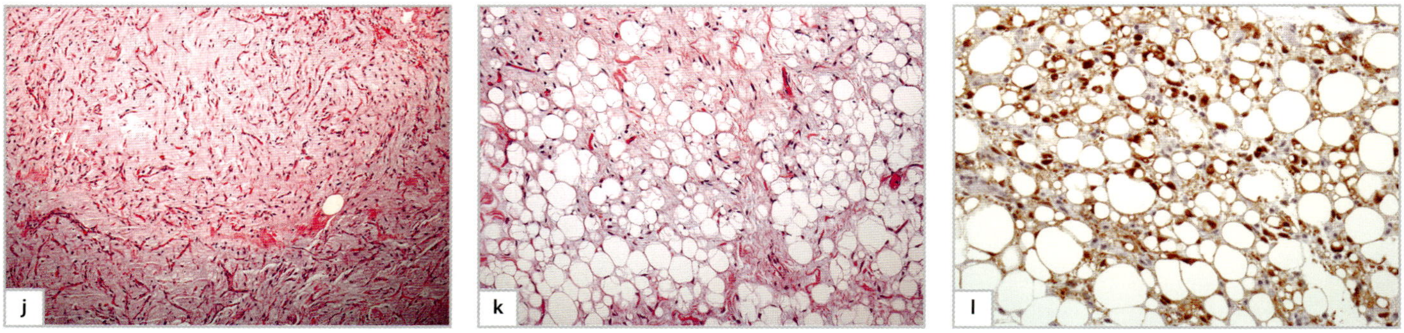

5.7j: Lipoblastoma at medium magnification. Myxoid region with plexiform capillary network ('chicken wire' capillaries). **5.7k**: Lipoblastoma with lipoblasts. This area of the tumor is more obviously adipocytic comprising variously sized adipocytes. The myxoid matrix and a few spindle cells are also present as well as the arborizing capillaries. **5.7l**: Lipoblastoma with strongly positive S-100 protein expression. Although unnecessary in this tumor because of the obvious diagnostic features, an S-100 antibody stains most of the adipocytes both in a membranous and nuclear pattern (a brown color is a positive reaction). Some cells are negative including a few small spindle cells.

Special studies: Many of the vacuolated cells are reactive for S-100 protein (more than 50%; **Case fig. 5.7l**), while only a few spindle cells (about 5%) are positive (performed using immunohistochemistry with appropriate controls).

Oncology approach

Medical oncology

As lipoblastomas are benign with no risk of metastasis, chemotherapy is not administered.

Radiation oncology

There is no known indication for radiation therapy of lipoblastomas, as they rarely recur. This patient does not receive radiation therapy.

If the patient had a liposarcoma, then adjuvant radiation therapy would be indicated due to the high local recurrence risk. At this young an age, the radiation would cause significant long term morbidity of her right shoulder. Lipoblastoma has upregulation of the PLAG1 gene (located on chromosome 8) (Hibbard et al. 2000). This abnormality can be detected and may be helpful in cases where it is difficult to distinguish a lipoblastoma from a liposarcoma.

Case table 5.7a Summary pathology findings of Case 5.7

Diagnosis	Lipoblastoma
Size	5.6 cm
Location	Deep shoulder
Margin Status	Positive
Histologic Grade	Not graded: Benign
Pathologic Stage at Presentation (TNM Classification)	Not graded: Benign

Patient outcome

The patient is doing well with no sequelae at 6 years post marginal excision.

Case 5.8 Angiolipoma

Clinical history and presentation

A 33 year old man is referred from his family doctor because of multiple superficial 'lumps'. He states he has had them for years but can't remember if they all appeared at the same time or sequentially. They have stayed the same size for many years. Two of them, however, are occasionally painful. The patient doesn't recall any other family members having similar tumors. Physical examination reveals five compressible subcutaneous masses ranging in size from approximately 2 to 4 cm maximally. Two are located in the right forearm, one in the left upper arm, one on the abdomen, and one in the right proximal thigh. Several are mildly tender to palpation. They are not associated with overlying skin changes.

Surgical findings and comments

All five lesions are marginally excised.

Radiology findings

Because of the superficial location and small size of the lesions and clinical impression that they most likely represent lipomas or angiolipomas, radiologic studies are not performed.

Pathology findings

Gross features

All five tumors are received intact and are covered by a thin translucent membrane through which yellow fatty appearing tissue is visible.

On cut sections, the tumors are predominantly yellow, shiny, and compressible consistent with adult fat, with streaks of fibrous tissue and a few pinpoint foci of red areas.

Microscopic features

Low magnification: The tumors comprise predominantly mature fat that is interspersed by aggregates of small blood vessels (**Case fig. 5.8a**). The proportion of fat to vessels varies from field to field, but in these five tumors, the fat forms the large majority of the tumor.

High magnification: The fat cells are without atypia and are consistent with mature adipocytes. The blood vessels are uniformly small consistent with venules and capillaries without atypia (**Case fig. 5.8b**). A small proportion of the vessels are occluded by fibrin thrombi and a few exhibit hyalinized walls consistent with prior damage (**Case fig. 5.8c**).

Variable features or types that can occur in these tumors (not seen in this case)

Vessel rich angiolipoma: may mimic a vascular tumor (see differential).

Fibrotic angiolipoma: Long-standing angiolipomas may exhibit fibrotic bands or fibrosis in the vascular areas.

Special studies: Because of the classic histologic findings and clinical presentation of this patient, tissue that was set aside for possible cytogenetics analysis is instead processed for routine histology, as it is not needed for diagnostic or prognostic information. However, if cytogenetics had been performed, it would have revealed a normal male karyotype.

Case table 5.8a Summary pathology findings of Case 5.8

Diagnosis	Angiolipoma (multiple)
Size	Up to 4 cm
Location	Subcutaneous trunk and extremities
Margin status	Positive
Histologic grade	Not graded: benign
Pathologic stage at presentation (TNM classification)	Not graded: benign

Pathologic differential or, why isn't it one of the following?

Lipoma: Lipomas certainly can occur as multiple lesions and are most often subcutaneous. However, the vascularity of lipomas is minimal in comparison with the clusters and bands of vessels seen in angiolipoma. Clinically, lipomas are not generally painful or tender.

Kaposi's sarcoma: Angiolipomas with prominent vasculature may mimic a vascular tumor such as Kaposi's sarcoma (KS). By the time it has reached the nodular stage, KS comprises a prominent cellular component of fascicles and whorls of spindled cells with only slit like lumina. This would be distinctly more cellular and spindled with less obvious vessel formation than in the vascular component of angiolipoma. Eosinophilic hyaline globules are often apparent, while conversely, vascular thrombi would not be found (angiolipomas often have thrombi and do not feature the extracellular or intracellular hyaline globules). Finally, Kaposi's sarcoma is reactive for antibody to human herpes simplex virus-8 (HHSV-8), which is absent in angiolipomas.

Oncology approach

Oncology and radiation oncology

Angiolipomas are benign with no significant morbidity or risk for local recurrence. Therefore, there is no role for oncology in treating these lesions. Interestingly (despite the normal diploid karyotype of angiolipoma), about 5% of patients with angiolipomas report a family history of such tumors. However, the patients with an angiolipoma family history have tumors that do not behave differently from the much more common sporadic cases.

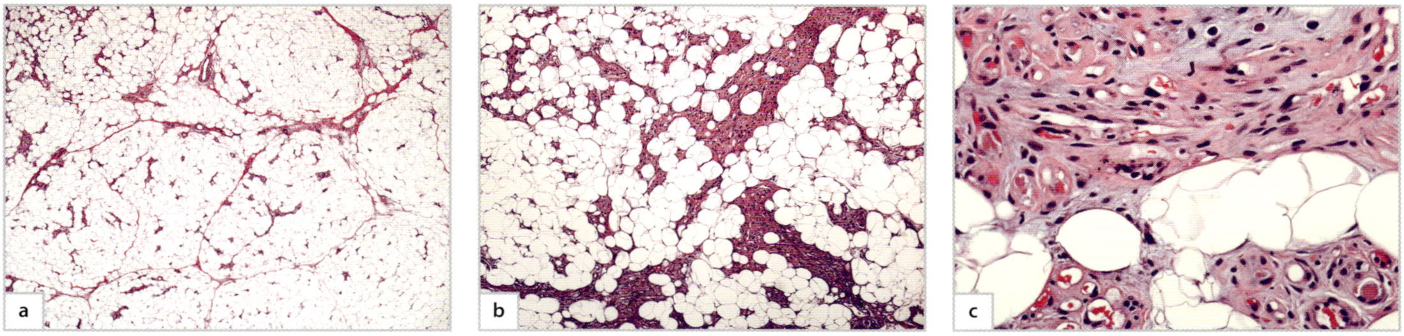

Case figure 5.8 Angiolipoma. **5.8a**: Medium magnification. A representative image reveals mature fat divided by thin fibrous bands into lobules. Interspersed blood vessels are embedded directly in fat or in strands of collagen. **5.8b**: Higher magnification. Another area shows increased blood vessels mixed with pink fibrous tissues traversing among the mature fat cells. **5.8c**: High magnification. Clustered together are capillary and venule sized vessels without atypia. At least two vessels contain fibrin thrombi comprising homogeneous pink intraluminal material. Some vessels also exhibit thickened pink walls (hyalinization) consistent with microdamage (secondary to prior episodes of thrombosis).

REFERENCES

Altiok S, Xu M, Spiegelman BM. PPAR γ induces cell cycle withdrawal: inhibition of E2F/DP DNA-binding activity via down-regulation of PP2A. Genes Dev 1997;11(15):1987–98.

Ayyoub M, Taub RN, Keohan ML, et al. The frequent expression of cancer/testis antigens provides opportunities for immunotherapeutic targeting of sarcoma. Cancer Immun 2004;4:7.

Bancroft LW, Kransdorf MJ, Peterson JJ, et al. Imaging characteristics of spindle cell lipoma. AJR 2003;181:1251–54.

Billing V, Mertens F, Domanski HA, et al. Deep-seated ordinary and atypical lipomas: histopathology, cytogenetics and clinical features and outcome in 215 tumours of the extremity and trunk wall. J Bone Joint Surg Br 2008;90(7):929–33.

Binh MB, Guillou L, Hostein I, et al. Dedifferentiated liposarcomas with divergent myosarcomatous differentiation developed in the internal trunk: a study of 27 cases and comparison to conventional dedifferentiated liposarcomas and leiomyosarcomas. Am J Surg Pathol 2007;31:1557–66.

Blay JR, von Mehren M, Samuels BL, et al. Phase I combination study of trabectedin and doxorubicin in patients with soft-tissue sarcoma. Clinical Cancer Research 2008;14(2):6656–62.

Boland JM, Weiss SW, Oliveira AM, et al. Liposarcomas with mixed well-differentiated and pleomorphic features: a clinicopathologic study of 12 cases. Am J Surg Pathol 2010;34:837–43.

Bui NBM, Sastre-Garau X, Guillou L, et al. MDM2 and CDK4 immunostainings are useful adjuncts in diagnosing well-differentiated and dedifferentiated liposarcoma subtypes. A comparative analysis of 559 soft tissue neoplasms with genetic data. Am J Surg Pathol 2005;29:1340–47.

Chen CW, Chang WC, Lee HS, et al. MRI features of lipoblastoma: differentiating from other palpable lipomatous tumor in pediatric patients. Clin Imaging 2010;34(6):453–7.

Coindre J-M, Pédeutour F, Aurias A. Well-differentiated and dedifferentiated liposarcomas. Virchows Arch 2010;456:167–79.

Dalal KM, Kattan MW, Antonescu CR, et al. Subtype specific prognostic nomogram for patients with primary liposarcoma of the retroperitoneum, extremity, or trunk. Ann Surg 2006;244(3):381–91.

Davis A, O'Sullivan B, Turcotte R, et al. Late radiation morbidity following randomization to preoperative versus postoperative radiotherapy in extremity soft tissue sarcoma. Radiother Oncol 2005;75:48–53.

de Vreeze RS, de Jong D, Haas RL, et al. Effectiveness of radiotherapy in myxoid sarcomas is associated with a dense vascular pattern. Int J Radiat Oncol Biol Phys 2008;72(5):1480–7.

Debrock G, Vanhentenrijk V, Sciot R, et al. A phase II trial with rosiglitazone in liposarcoma patients. British J Cancer 2003;89(8):1409–12.

Dei Tos AP, Doglioni C, Piccinin S, et al. Coordinated Expression and Amplification of the MDM2, CDK4, and HMGI-C Genes in Atypical Lipomatous Tumours. J Pathol 2000;190:531–6.

Dei Tos AP. Liposarcoma: New entities and evolving concepts. Ann Diagn Pathol 2000;4(4):252–66.

Demetri GD, Fletcher CD, Mueller E, et al. Induction of solid tumor differentiation by the peroxisome proliferator-activated receptor-gammma ligand troglitazone in patients with liposarcoma. Prox Natl Acad Sci USA 1999;96(7):3951–6.

Eilber FC, Eilber FR, Eckardt J, et al. The impact of chemotherapy of the survival of patients with high-grade primary extremity liposarcoma. Ann Surg 2004;240(4):686-95; discussion 695–7.

Einarsdottir H, Soderlund V, Larson D, et al. MR Imaging of lipoma and liposarcoma. Acta Radiol 1999;40(1):64–8.

Fiore M, Grosso F, Lo Vullo S, et al. Myxoid/round cell and Pleomorphic liposarcomas: prognostic factors and survival in a series of patients treated at a single institution. Cancer 2007;109(12):2522–31.

Fletcher CDM, Unni KK, Mertens F. World Health Organization Classification of Tumours Pathology and genetics of Tumours of Soft Tissue and Bone. IARC Press: Lyons, 2002.

Gebhard S, Coindre JM, Michels JJ, et al. Pleomorphic liposarcoma: Clincopathologic, immunohistochemical, and follow-up analysis of 63 cases: a study from the French Federation of Cancer Centers Sarcoma Group. Am J Surg Pathol 2002;26(5):601–16.

Grosso F, Jones RL, Demetri GD, et al. Efficacy of trabectedin (ecteinascidin-743) in advanced pretreated myxoid liposarcomas: a retrospective study. Lancet Oncol 2007;8(7):595–602.

Guadagnolo B, Zagars G, Ballo M, et al. Excellent Local Control Rates and Distinctive Patterns of Failure in Myxoid Liposarcoma Treated with Conservative Surgery and Radiotherapy. Int J Radiat Oncol Biol Phys 2008;70(3):760–5.

Hameed M. Pathology and Genetics of Adipocytic Tumors. Cytogenet Genome Res 2007;118:138–47.

Hanna SA, Qureshi YA, Bayliss, L, et al. Late widespread skeletal metastases from myxoid liposarcoma detected by MRI only. World J Surg Oncol 2008;18(6):62.

He M, Aisner S, Benevenia J, et al. p16 Immunohistochemistry as an alternative marker to distinguish atypical lipomatous tumor from deep-seated lipoma. Appl Immunohistochem Mol Morphol 2009;17:51–6.

Henricks W, Chu YC, Goldblum JR, et al. Dedifferentiated liposarcoma. A clinicopathologic analysis of 155 cases with a proposal for an expanded definition of dedifferentiation. Am J Surg Pathol 1997;21:271–81.

Hosono M, Kobayashi H, Fugimoto R, et al. Septum-like structures in lipoma and liposarcoma: MR imaging and pathologic correlation. Skeletal Radiol 1997;26(3):150–4.

Italiano A, Cardot N, Dupré F, et al. Gains and Complex rearrangements of the 12q13-15 chromosomal region in ordinary lipomas: The missing link between lipomas and liposarcoma? Int J Cancer 2007;121:308–15.

Jones RL, Fischer C, Al-Muderis, et al. Differential sensitivity of liposarcoma subtypes to chemotherapy. Eur J Cancer 2005;41(18):2853–60.

Karavasilis V, Seddon BM, Ashley S, et al. Significant clinical benefit of fist line palliative chemotherapy in advanced soft tissue sarcoma: retrospective analysis and identification of prognostic factors in 488 patients. Cancer 2008;112(7):1585–91.

Kempson RL, Fletcher CDM, Evans HL, et al. Atlas of Tumor Pathology Tumors of the Soft Tissues. Armed Forces Institute of Pathology: Washington, D.C., 2001.

Kransdorf MJ, Bancroft LW, Peterson JJ, et al. Imaging of fatty tumors: distinction of lipoma and well-differentiated liposarcoma. Radiology 2002;224(1):99–104.

Lahat G, Anaya DA, Wang X, et al. Resectable well-differentiated versus dedifferentiated liposarcomas: two different diseases possibly requiring different treatment approaches. Ann Surg Oncol 2008;15(6):1585–93.

Marino-Enriquez A, Fletcher CDM, Dal Cin P, et al. Dedifferentiated liposarcoma with 'homologous' lipoblastic (pleomorphic liposarcoma-like) differentiation: clinicopathologicand molecular analysis of a series suggesting revised diagnostic criteria. Am J Surg Pathol 2010;34:1122–31.

Matsumoto K, Hukuda S, Ishizawa M, et al. MRI findings in intramuscular lipomas. Skeletal Radiol 1999;28(3):145–52.

Matushansky I, Hernando E, Socci ND, et al. A Developmental Model of Sarcomagenesis Defines a Differentiation-Based Classification for Liposarcomas. Am J Pathol 2008;172:1069–80.

Mentzel T, Palmedo G, Kuhnen C. Well-differentiated spindle cell liposarcoma ('atypical spindle cell lipomatous tumor') does not belong to the spectrum of atypical lipomatous tumor but has a close relationship to spindle cell lipoma: clinicopathologic, immunohistochemical, and molecular analysis of six cases. Mod Pathol 2010;23:729–36.

Moore D, Antonescu CR, Singer S. Diagnosis and Management of Lipomatous Tumors. J Surg Oncol 2008;97:298–313.

Moore Dalal K, Kattan MW, Antonescu CR, et al. Subtype specific prognostic nomogram for patients with primary liposarcoma of the retroperitoneum, extremity or trunk. Ann Surg 2006;244:381–91.

Muller CR, Paulsen EB, Noordhuis P, et al. Potential for treatment of liposarcomas with the MDM2 antagonist Nutlin-3A. Int J Cancer 2007;121(1):199–205.

Nishida J, Morita T, Ogose A, et al. Imaging characteristics of deep-seated lipomatous tumors: Intramuscular lipoma, intermuscular lipoma, and lipoma-like liposarcoma. J Orthop Sci 2007;12(6):533–41.

Ohguri T, Aoki T, Hisaoka M, et al. Differential diagnosis of benign peripheral lipoma from well-differentiated liposarcoma on MR Imaging: is comparison of margins and internal characteristics useful? AJR Am J Roentgenol 2003;180(6):1689–94.

Pang AK, Hughes T. Magnetic resonance imaging of lipoma and liposarcoma: potential of short tau inversion recovery as a technique of fat suppression. Australas Radiol 2000;44(4):412–6.

Panzarella MJ, Nagvi AH, Cohen HE, et al. Predictive value of gadolinium enhancement in differentiating ALT/WD liposarcomas from benign fatty tumors. Skeletal Radiol 2005;34(5):272–8.

Patel SR, Burgess MA, Plager C, et al. Myxoid liposarcoma. Experience with chemotherapy. Cancer 1994;74(4):1265–9.

Schwab JH, Boland PJ, Antonescu C, et al. Spinal metastases form Myxoid Liposarcoma warrant screening with Magnetic resonance imaging. Cancer 2007;110(8):1815–22.
Sheah K, Ouellette HA, Torriani M, et al. Metastatic myxoid liposarcomas: imaging and histopathologic findings. Skeletal Radiol 2008;37(3):251–8.
Skubitz KM, Cheng EY, Clohisy DR, et al. Differential gene expression in liposarcoma, lipoma, and adipose tissue. Cancer Invest 2005;23(2):105–18.
Skubitz KM, D'Adamo DR. Sarcoma. Mayo Clin Proc 2007;82(11):1409–32.
Surveillance, Epidemiology, and End Results (SEER) Program (www.seer.cancer.gov) SEER*Stat Database: Incidence - SEER 13 Regs Research Data, Nov 2009 Sub (1992-2007) <Katrina/Rita Population Adjustment> - Linked To County Attributes - Total U.S., 1969-2007 Counties, National Cancer Institute, DCCPS, Surveillance Research Program, Cancer Statistics Branch, released April 2010, based on the November 2009 submission.
Tontonoz P, Singer S, Forman BM, et al. Terminal differentiation of human liposarcoma cells induced by ligands for peroxisome preliferator-activated receptor γ and the retinoid X receptor. Proc Natl Acad Sci USA 1997;94(1):237–41.
Usta U, Turkman E, Mizrak B, et al. Spindle cell lipoma in an intramuscular lipoma. Pathol Int 2004;54(9):734–49.
Van Glabbeke M, van Ooosterom AT, Oosterhuis JW, et al. Prognostic factors for the outcome of chemotherapy in advanced soft tissue sarcoma: an analysis of 2,185 patients treated with anthracycline-containing first-line regiments – a European Organization for Research and Treatment of Cancer Soft Tissue and Bone Sarcoma Group Study. J Clin Oncol 1999;17(1):150–7.
Vassilev LT, Vu BT, Graves B, et al. In vivo activation of the p53 pathway by small-molecule antagonists of MDM2. Science 2004;303(5659):844–8.
Yang JC, Chang AE, Baker AR, et al. Randomized prospective study of the benefit of adjuvant radiation therapy in the treatment of soft tissue sarcomas of the extremity. J Clin Oncol 1998;16(1):197–203.
Yovine A, Riofrio M, Blay JR, et al. Phase II study of ecteinasciindin-743 in advanced pretreated soft tissue sarcoma patients. J Clin Oncol 2004;22(5):890–9.

Chapter 6 Fibroblastic/myofibroblastic tumors of soft tissues

OVERVIEW

Tumors of fibroblastic and myofibroblastic differentiation are grouped together, because the two cell types are closely related and often jointly form a tumor. Even within one specific tumor type, the percentage of cells with myofibroblastic or fibroblastic features varies from specimen to specimen leading to plasticity in differentiation of these cells down to the level of a specific patient's tumor.

Myofibroblasts are fibroblasts that are able to contract because of myofilaments. They most commonly arise from fibroblasts but also may develop from smooth muscle cells, possibly pericytes and circulating bone marrow cells, and even epithelial cells, (the last origin is described as 'the epithelial to mesenchymal transition' or EMT, a phenomenon that may play a key role in carcinoma progression)(Fisher 2004). Although many tumors consist of neoplastic myofibroblasts and others may contain reactive myofibroblasts, this cell is normally inconspicuous in the human body and limited to the periphery of seminiferous tubules and perhaps a few other sites. However, myofibroblasts are indispensable in normal life, as they form the principal mesenchymal cell in the early stages of wound healing and tissue inflammation. In fact, some tumors of myofibroblasts/fibroblasts histologically mimic 'normal' wound healing to a remarkable degree (fibromatoses and inflammatory myofibroblastic tumors, for example). Actually, some tumors in this category may represent a skewed wound healing response or a 'transient neoplasia' rather than a persistent monoclonal neoplasm (such as the different types of fasciitis and myositis ossificans) (Erickson-Johnson et al. 2011).

It is most likely that this already large group of soft tissue tumors will continue to expand as lesions of uncertain differentiation become recognized as fibroblastic/myofibroblastic. Although seemingly a dull matter for non-pathologists, accurate classification of soft tissue tumors can lead the way to optimizing therapy and improving outcomes. To introduce a common American metaphor, apples and oranges are both fruit but differ in many ways. Similarly, combining mesenchymal tumors of various types, behaviors, and grades and then subjecting them to the same chemotherapy is like 'mixing apples and oranges'. For most mesenchymal tumors, the current therapies generally don't distinguish the apples from the oranges... or from the mangosteens. Therapeutic approaches can only become more fine-tuned if the responses of various tumors are specifically monitored according to tumor type (and eventually, according to the molecular signature of the tumor with understanding of modulating effects of epigenetic, immunologic and environmental factors).

CLASSIFICATION

The World Health Organization (WHO) classification of fibroblastic/myofibroblastic tumors (as of 2013) (see **Table 6.1**) consists of 32 tumors/tumorous lesions.

Table 6.1 WHO classification of fibroblastic/myofibroblastic tumors and tumorous conditions of soft tissue (2013)

Tumor	Behavior	Additional comments
Fasciitis - Nodular fasciitis - Proliferative fasciitis and myositis. - Myositis ossificans and fibro-osseous pseudotumor of the digits. - Ischemic fasciitis	Benign	Some lesions may spontaneously regress Myositis ossificans and ischemic fasciitis may uncommonly recur There is a less than 2% recurrence rate for the other types of fasciitis after simple excision
Elastofibroma	Benign	Site restricted almost exclusively to the posterior upper back. May be a tumorous lesion rather than a true neoplasm Genetic predisposition has been reported
Fibrous hamartoma of infancy	Benign	Simple excision is usually curative
Myofibroma/myofibromatosis	Benign*	Some cases may spontaneously regress. Myofibromatosis is the diffuse form. *The viscera (lungs most commonly) may also be involved; death may rarely occur from local invasive growth. Some cases show autosomal dominant inheritance
Fibromatosis colli	Benign	Rare and site restricted (distal third of sternocleidomastoid muscle) probably resulting from intra-uterine malpositioning or delivery complications
Juvenile hyaline fibromatosis	Benign*	Extremely rare condition with development of multiple soft tissue and bone nodules. *May cause death in some cases. Appears to be an autosomal recessive disease
Inclusion body fibromatosis	Benign	Site restricted in almost all cases to fingers and toes Commonly multifocal. Regression is common
Fibroma of tendon sheath	Benign to intermediate	Site restricted in most cases to the hand. Can recur in up to 25% of cases
Desmoplastic fibroblastoma	Benign	May reach a large size. Some cases have same translocation (t(2;11)) as noted in fibroma of tendon sheath

Table 6.1: Continued from page 78

Tumor	Behavior	Additional comments
Mammary-type myofibroblastoma	Benign	This tumor may be more closely related to smooth muscle than myofibroblasts. It shares the same genetic abnormalities with spindle cell lipoma and cellular angiofibroma and shows loss of Rb1 protein by IHC like these other tumors. Site restricted in most cases to inguinal region
Calcifying aponeurotic fibroma	Intermediate	Site restricted in most cases to the hands and feet. Tends to recur, often after a long period of time
Angiomyofibroblastoma	Benign*	Site restricted to vulva/vagina/perineum in females and testis/scrotum in males. *Rare malignant variant has been described
Cellular angiofibroma	Benign*	Site restricted almost exclusively to vulva and inguinal/scrotal regions. *Recently, malignant transformation has been described
Nuchal-type fibroma	Benign to intermediate	Some cases can recur locally. More common in males and 40% of patients have diabetes mellitus
Gardner fibroma	Benign to intermediate	Can look identical to nuchal-type fibroma. Occurs in the setting of Gardner syndrome. Recurrences may look like extra-abdominal fibromatosis
Calcifying fibrous tumor	Benign to intermediate	Can occur in body cavities and can reach a large size
Giant cell angiofibroma	Benign	A distinctive histologic variant of solitary fibrous tumor that usually occurs in the orbital region. Only rarely recurs
Palmar/plantar (Superficial) fibromatosis	Benign to intermediate	Site restrictied to three locations: hand, feet, penis. Patients with alcoholic liver disease, diabetes mellitus types 1 and 2, epilepsy (secondary to drug regimen) at increased risk. Genetic predisposition plays a role in some patients
Desmoid-type fibromatosis	Intermediate, locally aggressive	Mesenteric lesions may be sporadic or associated with Gardner syndrome or with familial desmoid syndrome
Lipofibromatosis	Intermediate, locally aggressive	Site restricted in most cases to hands and feet. High rate of local, non-destructive recurrence
Giant cell fibroblastoma	Intermediate, locally aggressive	This is a distinctive histologic variant of DFSP that usually occurs in children
Dermatofibrosarcoma protuberans (DFSP) – Fibrosarcomatous DFSP – Pigmented DFSP (Bednar tumor)	Intermediate, rarely metastasizing	Relatively common superficial myofibroblastic tumor with multiple variants
Solitary fibrous tumor (SFT)	Intermediate to malignant	Most do not metastasize but long term follow up is indicated. Wide distribution in body
Inflammatory myofibroblastic tumor (IMT)	Intermediate to malignant	Wide distribution in body; most are in lung, mesentery, and omentum
Low grade myofibroblastic sarcoma	Malignant	Site restricted in most cases to head and neck region especially tongue and oral cavity
Myxoinflammatory fibroblastic sarcoma (MIFS)	Malignant	Site restricted in most cases to hands and wrists or feet and ankles
Infantile fibrosarcoma	Intermediate to malignant	Only rarely metastasizes. Shows same translocation, t(12;15) and similar morphology as congenital mesoblastic nephroma
Adult fibrosarcoma	Malignant	A diagnosis now rarely rendered as most tumors with this histopathology are other types such as synovial sarcoma
Myxofibrosarcoma	Malignant	Previously termed myxoid malignant fibrous histiocytoma (myxoid MFH). Now recognized to differentiate along fibroblastic lines
Low grade fibromyxoid sarcoma (LGFMS)	Malignant	Metastases may occur many years after initial presentation
Sclerosing epithelioid fibrosarcoma (SEFS)	Malignant	Shares some of the genetic findings with low grade fibromyxoid sarcoma and most likely represents a more aggressive version of LGFMS

Benign: does not recur or does not recur aggressively and does not metastasize. Intermediate: can recur aggressively and/or can rarely metastasize. Malignant: can recur and commonly metastasizes.

DEMOGRAPHICS

As with other categories of soft tissue tumors, myofibroblastic/fibroblastic lesions affect a broad age range and both sexes. Some specific types are restricted to children (such as fibrous hamartoma of infancy, infantile fibrosarcoma, and fibromatosis colli) and others to adults (such as myxofibrosarcoma and elastofibroma). Others have a greater incidence in the pediatric age group but are also reported in adults (such as inclusion body (digital) fibromatosis, Gardner fibroma, and inflammatory myofibroblastic tumor). Likewise, a few predominantly adult tumors may uncommonly occur in children such as fibroma of tendon sheath and solitary fibrous tumor.

Only one tumor shows a predilection for a particular racial group: superficial fibromatoses. These are more common in Caucasians especially those of northern European ancestry.

A few tumors in this category exhibit marked selectivity for one sex. These include one specific body site for deep fibromatoses (abdominal wall musculature in young adult women) superficial fibromatoses particularly the palmar variant (much more common in white men), nuchal-type fibroma (also much more common in men) and angiomyofibroblastoma (much more common in women).

The incidence of the various fibroblastic/myofibroblastic tumors is not known precisely. This is because some tumors are rare, some have only been recently described, and some may be difficult to diagnose. SEER (Surveillance, Epidemiology and End Results) Registries in the US have tracked the incidence of the following three malignant myofibroblastic/fibroblastic tumors: myxofibrosarcoma, fibrosarcoma, not otherwise specified, and myofibrosarcoma. **Table 6.2** reveals the incidence of these three designations with five year relative survival. It is important to note that the fibrosarcoma category may encompass other lesions than adult fibrosarcoma such as synovial sarcoma, high grade dermatofibrosarcoma protuberans, and malignant peripheral nerve sheath tumor, three sarcomas that mimic histologically adult fibrosarcoma and that may only be distinguished from it by techniques not available to all SEER submitting pathologists. It is anticipated that future adult fibrosarcomas captured in the SEER data will comprise vanishingly few cases.

PATHOGENESIS/ETIOLOGY

Genetic abnormalities play a well-established role in the development of some of the myofibroblastic/fibroblastic tumors (see **Table 6.3** for the genetic abnormalities reported in these tumors). For example, deep fibromatoses (of which some mesenteric lesions occur in the

Table 6.2 Tumor grade and five year relative survival of myxofibrosarcoma, fibrosarcoma, not otherwise specified (presumed adult fibrosarcoma but most likely consisting of multiple sarcoma types; see text) and myofibrosarcoma from1994 through 2008 in 17 SEER registries

Grade	Histologic type		
	Myxofibro-sarcoma	**Fibrosarcoma, NOS**	**Myofibro-sarcoma**
Well-differentiated	142 (17.8%)	75 (14.5%)	2 (9.5%)
Moderately differentiated	322 (40.4%)	157 (30.3%)	8 (38.1%)
Poorly differentiated	96 (12.1%)	79 (15.2%)	3 (14.3%)
Undifferentiated; anaplastic	159 (20.0%)	88 (17.0%)	4 (19.1%)
Unknown	78 (9.8%)	120 (23.1%)	4 (19.1%)
Overall 5 year relative survival (standard error)	89.4% (2.0%)	73.6% (2.6%)	89.0% (8.4%)

The corresponding morphology codes of the International Classification of Diseases for Oncology and The Systematize Nomenclature of Medicine are in parenthesis): fibrosarcoma, NOS (8810/3), myxofibrosarcoma (8811/3), and myofibrosarcoma (8825/3). The average annual age-adjusted incidence rates are 0.1 per 100,000 for fibrosarcoma, NOS, 0.1 per 100,000 for myxofibrosarcoma, and 0.0 per 100,000 for myofibrosarcoma. All rates are age-adjusted to the 2000 U.S. standard population. Fibrosarcoma, NOS and myofibrosarcoma rates are similar when comparing males and females. The rates for myxofibrosarcoma are 0.1 per 100,000 for both males and females; however, the rates are *statistically* lower in females than males.

Table 6.3 Genetics of fibroblastic/myofibroblastic tumors of soft tissue

Tumor	Chromosomal abnormality	Genes involved	Percentage of tumors with abnormality
Fasciitis lesions	Nodular fasciitis may show rearrangements at 17p13 including t(17;22)(p13;q12.3-13)	Nodular fasciitis: *USP6* (17p13) rearrangements including t(17;22) = *MYH9-USP6* fusion *MYH9* (22q12.3-13)	Majority of nodular fasciitis cases (90%+) show 17p13 rearrangements including translocation to 22q12.3-13 in 65% of cases Unknown if these alterations are seen in the other types of fasciitis
Myositis ossificans and fibroosseous pseudotumor of digits	None = normal karyotype	None	0%: All lesions have a normal karyotype
Elastofibroma	Possible abnormalities of 1p, 13q, 19, 22, Xq12-22. No consistent abnormalities	Possible deletions of *CASR* (3q21), *GSTP1* (11q13), *BRCA2* (13q2) and gains on *APC* (5q21) and *PAH* (12q23) May be familial in some cases	Unknown No consistent abnormalities
Fibrous hamartoma of infancy	Various balanced translocations including t(2;3)(q31;q21) (less than 5 cases published)	Unknown	Unknown (less than 5 cases with genetic findings published)
Myofibroma/ Myofibromatosis	Little known. One report of interstitial deletion of 6q12q15.	Unknown	Unknown
Fibromatosis colli	None	None	None: considered a reactive condition post-birth or intra-uterine trauma
Juvenile hyaline fibromatosis	No detectable abnormalities on karyotype	Germline mutations of capillary morphogenetic protein 2 gene (4q21); autosomal recessive and very rare condition	100% have germline mutation
Inclusion body fibromatosis	Unknown	Unknown	Unknown
Fibroma of tendon sheath	t(2;11)(q31-32;q12) in one case report	Unknown	Unknown
Desmoplastic fibroblastoma	t(2;11)(q31;q12) in several cases and one t(11;17)(q12;p11.2)	Unknown	Unknown
Mammary-type myofibroblastoma	Partial monosomy of 13q and/or 16q	Loss of *Rb1* and *FKHR* (13q14)	Majority possibly up to 100%
Calcifying aponeurotic fibroma	Unknown	Unknown	Unknown
Angiomyofibroblastoma	Unknown	Unknown	Unknown

Table 6.3: Continued from page 80

Tumor	Chromosomal abnormality	Genes involved	Percentage of tumors with abnormality
Cellular angiofibroma	Partial monosomy of 13q and/or 16q (same change as in mammary type myofibroblastoma	Loss of *Rb1* (monoallelic deletion)	Majority up to 100%
Nuchal type fibroma	Unknown	Unknown	Unknown
Gardner fibroma	Loss of heterozygosity or mutations at 5q	APC gene LOH or mutation	Unknown. Most patients have Gardner syndrome, familial adenomatous polyposis (FAP) and/or *APC* mutations This diagnosis should prompt a work-up for associated findings
Calcifying fibrous tumor	Unknown	Unknown	Unknown
Giant cell angiofibroma	Possible 6q13 abnormalities One case of t(12;17)(q15;q23)	Unknown	Unknown No consistent abnormalities
Superficial fibromatosis	Unknown	Negative for mutations of the β-catenin and *APC* genes	Unknown
Desmoid-type fibromatosis	Trisomy 8, trisomy 20 and loss of Y	Sporadic deep fibromatosis shows mutations of *CTNNB1* (β catenin gene). Cases associated with *FAP* have inactivating germline mutations of *APC* (5q21)	Majority of cases show mutations or LOH of *CTNNB1* or *APC* gene
Lipofibromatosis	t(4;9;6) in one case report	Unknown	Unknown
Giant cell fibroblastoma	t(17;22)(q21.3;q13)	Fusion of *COL1A1* (17q21) with *PDGFB* (22q13)	~100% have balanced or unbalanced t(17;22)
Dermatofibrosarcoma protuberans (DFSP)	t(17;22)(q22;q13) Ring chromosomes comprising amplified portions of 17 and 22 One case of t(5;8) Secondary changes of trisomy 8, trisomy 5	t(17;22) = Fusion of *COL1A1* (17q21) with *PDGFB* (22q13)	~100% have unbalanced translocations also with additional gains of the two genes. Balanced translocations as found in giant cell fibroblastoma are absent
Solitary fibrous tumor (SFT) and hemangiopericytoma (HPC)	Diploid or near diploid karyotype in most cases. Trisomy 21, 4q13 and 12q rearrangements in some cases including t(12;19)(q13;q13)	Consistent finding of intrachromosomal gene fusion at 12q13 of *NAB2-STAT6*. Overexpression of some other genes: *IGF2*, *DDR1*, *ERBB2* and *FGFR1* (last three are tyrosine receptor kinases)	*NAB2-STAT6* gene fusion can only be detected by sequencing or *PCR*. This fusion is present in nearly all cases (close to 100%). Overexpression of *IGF2* gene may be revealed as a consistent finding and is a target gene of *EGR* which is abnormally upregulated by the *NAB2-STAT6* fusion protein
Inflammatory myofibroblastic tumor (IMFT)	Translocations of ALK (anaplastic lymphoma kinase) gene with other partners: t(2;1)(p23;p13), t(2;19)(p23;p13), t(2;17)(p23;q23), t(2;2)(p23;q35), t(2;4)(p23;q21), t(2;11)(p23;p15) and t(2;2)(p23;q13)	*ALK-TPM3* (1p13) *ALK-TPM4* (19p13) *ALK-CLTC* (17q23) *ALK-ATIC* (2q35) *ALK-SEC31L1* (4q21) *ALK-CARS* (11p15) *ALK-RANBP2* (2q13)	Most IMFT occurring in children show translocations of ALK gene. Translocation positive cases may have a better prognosis. Most adult IMFT are translocation negative. Type of translocation affects pattern of *ALK* protein expression in tissue sections (eg. nuclear, cytoplasmic, or membranous reactivity)
Low grade myofibroblastic sarcoma (LGMFS)	Alterations of 12p11 and 12q13-q22 in some cases	Unknown	Unknown
Myxoinflammatory fibroblastic sarcoma (MIFS)	t(1;10)(p22;q24) or der10(1;10)	Unknown	Unknown: reported in a few cases of MIFS and possible related tumor, hemosiderotic fibrolipomatous tumor
Infantile fibrosarcoma	t(12;15)(p13;q25) Trisomies of 8, 11, 17, 20	Translocation of ETV6 and NTRK3 genes	~100% (same translocation is also present in several other non-sarcoma tumors)
Adult fibrosarcoma	Unknown	Unknown	Unknown
Myxofibrosarcoma	Complex aneuploid karyotpe: may have 7q gains and 12q gains more frequently than gains and losses at other sites; ring chromosomes also may be present	Some cases have MET gene product overexpression (7q31.2)	Majority of low grade cases and all high grade cases have a complex aneuploid karyotype
Low grade fibromyxoid sarcoma (LGFMS)	t(7;16)(q33;p11) smay have ring forms also containing these genes t(11;16)(p11;p11) t(11;22)(p11;q12) in two cases	*FUS-CREB3L2* translocation (*FUS* is at 16p11) *FUS-CREB3L1* rarely *EWSR1-CREB3L1 rarely*	Most cases have *FUS-CREB3L2* translocation or ring forms. Few cases have *FUS-CREB3L1* translocation. Rare cases have *EWSR1-CREB3L1* translocation
Sclerosing epithelioid fibrosarcoma (SEFS)	Same translocations as in LGFMS. Also rearrangements of 10p11, 17q11, and 1p31 described in single case reports	Same genetic abnormalities as for LGFMS except *EWSR1-CREB3L1* not reported as of 2013	Most cases may have same genetic abnormalities as in low grade fibromyxoid sarcoma

LOH: loss of heterozygosity. See References for papers pertaining to this table. This static list should not be considered complete as new discoveries are continuous.

setting of Gardner syndrome [familial adenomatous polyposis]) are associated with mutations of the FAP gene on chromosome 5q or with mutations of the β-catenin gene, but they also may contain trisomies of chromosome 8 and/or 20 as well as retinoblastoma and p53 gene alterations. Sporadic examples of deep fibromatoses are associated with mutations of the β-catenin gene and or the APC gene, while familial desmoids are due to germline mutations in the APC gene (which manifest as Gardner syndrome or hereditary desmoid disease) (Lips et al. 2009).

Interestingly, some deep fibromatoses appear to be associated with prior tissue injury such as prior abdominal surgery or with recent pregnancy (in particular for the latter, the anterior abdominal wall desmoids). Other tumors in this category that may occur as a result of tissue injury include ischemic fasciitis, nodular fasciitis (NF), cranial fasciitis, myositis ossificans (MO), fibrous pseudotumor of the digits, and fibromatosis colli. Although usually considered an aberrant myofibroblastic/fibroblastic tissue response rather than a true monoclonal neoplasm, cases of NF have been reported featuring abnormal monoclonal karyotypes. Recently, a group from the Mayo Clinic reported rearrangements of the USP6 gene (17p13) in 92% of NF cases and a novel fusion gene: MYH9-USP6 in 65% of tested cases (Erickson-Johnson et al. 2011).

Several tumors are linked with abnormal metabolic conditions: superficial fibromatosis (associated with alcoholism, diabetes) and nuchal-type fibroma (Type 1 diabetes). Like deep fibromatosis, superficial fibromatosis may also arise in the setting of trauma. Thus, the pathogenesis of a single tumor may be multifactorial. Genetics alone or environment alone seldom accounts for tumor development; multifactoriality may be the rule and not the exception for most neoplasms including myofibroblastic/fibroblastic tumors.

Patient age inexplicably constrains some of these tumors. Why some tumors are exclusive to childhood and others are not is not known. Congenital fibrosarcoma and fibrous hamartoma of infancy simply do not affect adults, yet inclusion body fibromatosis (previously termed infantile digital fibromatosis) can occur in adults, though rarely. There are slight genetic differences in giant cell fibroblastoma and dermatofibrosarcoma protubernas which may help account for the former occurring mostly in children and the latter mostly in adults, although the two tumors are very closely related. A considerable number of myofibroblastic/fibroblastic tumors also affect young adults preferentially or older adults preferentially. Myxofibrosarcoma generally afflicts individuals 50 years and older, and one can speculate that the pro-carcinogenic conditions of advanced age (such as reduced ability to repair DNA mutations, accumulation of toxic exposures and impaired ability to clear harmful cellular substances) increases the risk for this relatively common sarcoma. However, the particulars leading to the specific development of myxofibrosarcoma have not been determined.

An example of a genetically well-characterized myofiberoblastic/fibroblastic tumor is dermatofibrosarcoma protuberans (DFSP). The tumor exhibits a consistent translocation involving the Collagen 1A1 gene (*COL1A1*) and the Platelet Derived Growth Factor β gene (*PDGFB*) resulting in a chimeric growth factor (t(17;22)(q22;q13))(O'Brien et al. 1998). A small percentage of DFSPs may harbor areas that look like a pleomorphic high grade undifferentiated sarcoma; it has been suggested that these tumor have a more aggressive behavior with a higher rate than 15% of metastasis (Miettinen 2010).

A final peculiar feature notable in myofibroblastic/fibroblastic tumors is the favoritism exhibited by some tumors for specific body sites. For example, inclusion body fibromatosis, calcifying aponeurotic fibroma, myxoinflammatory fibroblastic sarcoma, and most superficial fibromatoses occur in the hands and feet, while elastofibroma almost always affects the deep soft tissues of the upper posterior back. Alternatively, the inguinal area, scrotum, vulva and/or perineum are the most common locations for mammary type myofibroblastoma, angiomyofibroblastoma, cellular angiofibroma, and deep (aggressive angiomyxoma), among others. It is possible that the lower genital tract contains a specific type of myofibroblast/fibroblast. Certainly, some of the tumors at this site express hormone receptors akin to the normal fibrocytes of the region. There are no unique features yet reported for fibroblasts or fibrocytes in the hands and feet. However, the hands and feet may be prone to particular tumors for other milieu-specific reasons.

PATHOLOGY

Tables 6.4 and **6.5** describe the main pathologic features of myofibroblastic/fibroblastic tumors. Neoplastic and reactive myofibroblasts are usually distinguished from fibroblasts by immunohistochemistry (IHC): myofibroblasts usually are reactive for antibodies to smooth muscle actin while fibroblasts are non-reactive. However, myofibroblasts may show a range of reactivity to myoid markers. This can include cells that are both desmin and actin positive (but this dual positivity is much more common in smooth muscle cells), cells that are just desmin positive or cells negative for both actin and desmin. In the last instance, electron microscopy is required (at least currently) to distinguish myofibroblasts lacking actin and desmin reactivity (by conventional IHC) from fibroblasts. In practical terms, electron microscopy is seldom employed.

In contrast to neoplastic smooth muscle cells, neoplastic myofibroblasts are less eosinophilic (on standard hematoxylin and eosin staining), do not consistently feature blunt-ended, cigar shaped or train-car shaped nuclei, and often are not arranged in the long, sweeping fascicles characteristic of many smooth muscle tumors (this is variable, however). In some tumors, myofibroblasts are stellate or polygonal in shape in additional to spindled with tapered nuclei, and the cytoplasm can be a pale lavender (amphophilic) color. A few smooth muscle tumors and uncommon myofibroblastic tumors may comprise cells that are epithelioid in appearance, so this cell shape does not permit distinction between the two. While both smooth muscle cells and myofibroblasts usually express smooth muscle actin, the pattern of expression is often more diffusely cytoplasmic in smooth muscle cells and by contrast is more accentuated at the cell borders ('tram-track' or subplasmalemmal pattern) in myofibroblasts (this is also variable and can be difficult to appreciate). Also by IHC, smooth muscle cells more commonly express h-caldesmon than myofibroblasts.

Ultimately, to accurately render a diagnosis of a specific myofibroblastic/fibroblastic tumor, the pathologist must adhere to the published histologic criteria for the tumor, and where necessary, use IHC and genetic tests to support the diagnosis. Of course, clinical findings including body site location and patient age can and should significantly influence the diagnosis.

Table 6.6 lists tumors that were not considered myofibroblastic/fibroblastic in the 2013 WHO classification of soft tissue tumors. Based on some histologic features and IHC expression profiles, an argument can be made to assign them to the myofibroblastic/fibroblastic tumor group. Recognition of the line of differentiation of a neoplasm is the first step to better characterizing the tumor ultimately resulting in more effective treatment.

Table 6.4 Exclusively or predominantly pediatric fibroblastic/myofibroblastic tumors of soft tissue grouped by behavior

Tumor	Incidence	Age and sex distribution	Body site (in order of occurrence)	Histopathology description including IHC: Medium magnification	Histopathology description including IHC: High magnification
Benign: does not recur and does not metastasize					
Fibrous hamartoma of infancy	Rare	Up to 2 years usually. M > F by 2:1	Axillary soft tissue, chest wall, arm, shoulder, thigh, groin. Rarely hands/feet	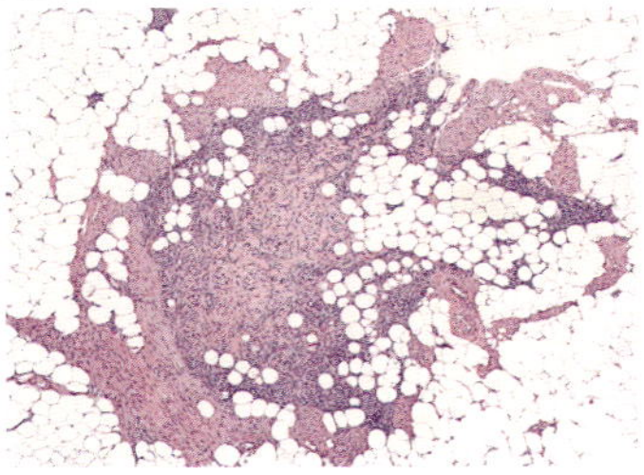	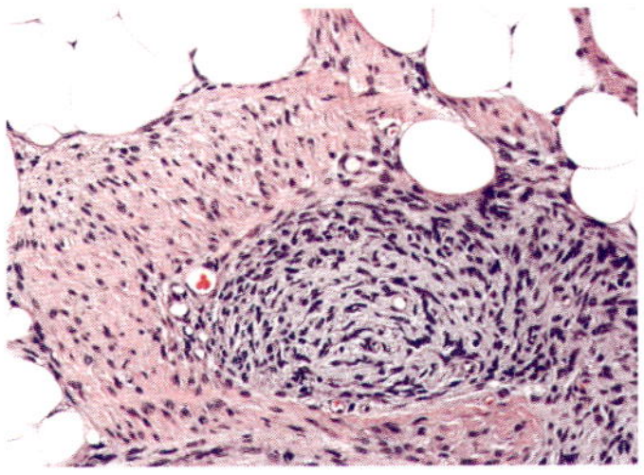
Triad of components: 1) mature fat, 2) myxoid islands of disordered cellular but bland spindle fibroblasts, 3) fibrous trabeculae of bland fibroblasts or myofibroblasts (latter are actin positive usually desmin negative). A few cases may be fibrotic only or composed of Component 2 only.					
Inclusion body fibromatosis (formerly termed infantile digital fibromatosis)	Rare	First year M = F (Rarely, adults may be affected.)	Dorsal, superficial aspect of fingers and toes #2-5 (rarely thumb or great toe). Can be multiple. Rarely occurs elsewhere	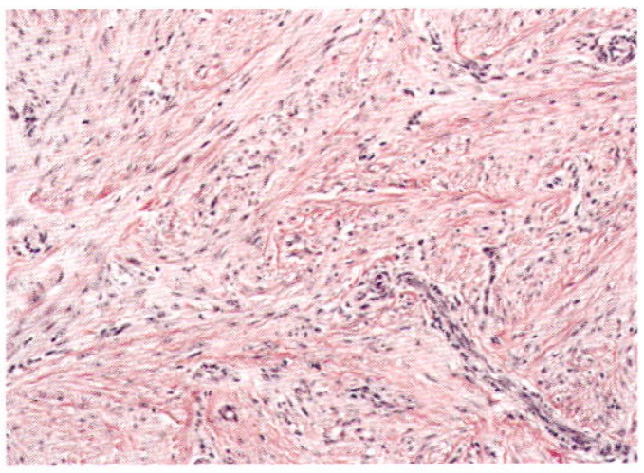	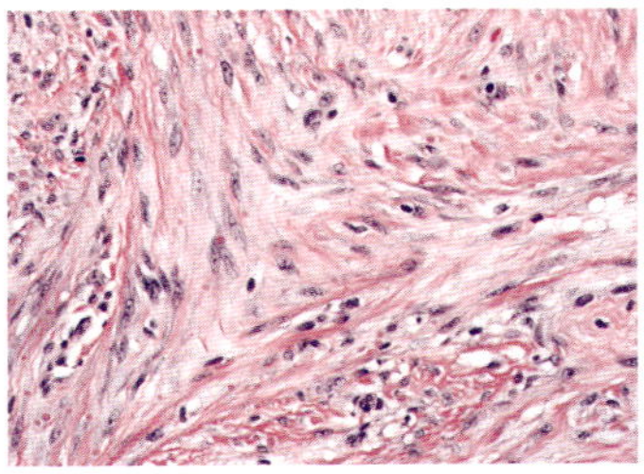
Streaming fascicles and sheets of uniform elongate spindle cells. Non-encapsulated. Background is sometim fibrotic. Characteristic trichrome stain-positive eosinophilic globular intracytoplasmic inclusions that are also commonly positive for actins.					
Fibromatosis colli	Common	Birth up to six months. M = F	Sternocleidomastoid muscle, usually lower third	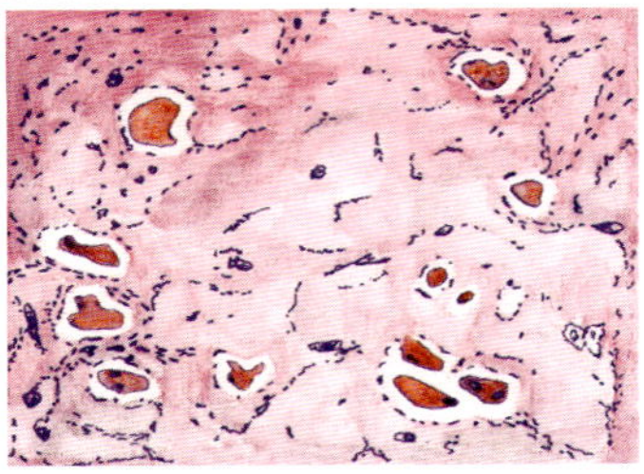	
Scar-like reactive process presumed secondary to birth trauma. Early stage is cellular with spindle myofibroblasts (actin positive) infiltrating and separating skeletal muscle fibers. Later stage is more fibrotic and less cellular.					
Juvenile hyaline fibromatosis	Very rare	Infancy and childhood	Multiple nodules in skin, around joints, and in bones; rarely in viscera also	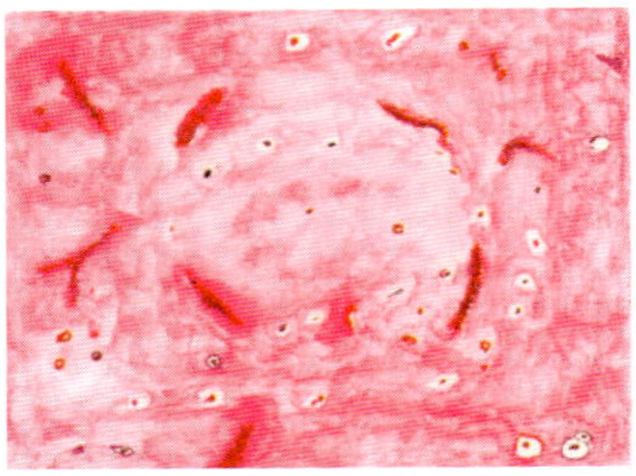	
Waxy eosinophilic nodules of very low to low cellularity. Matrix is PAS positive, diastase resistant. Lesional cells are fibroblasts with vacuolated cytoplasm. Capillaries are prominent.					
Calcifying aponeurotic fibroma	Rare	Usually children (median 12 years); rarely young adults M > F by 2:1	Superficial nodule in palms, soles, ankles, wrists, proximal extremities, trunk (>50% in hands)	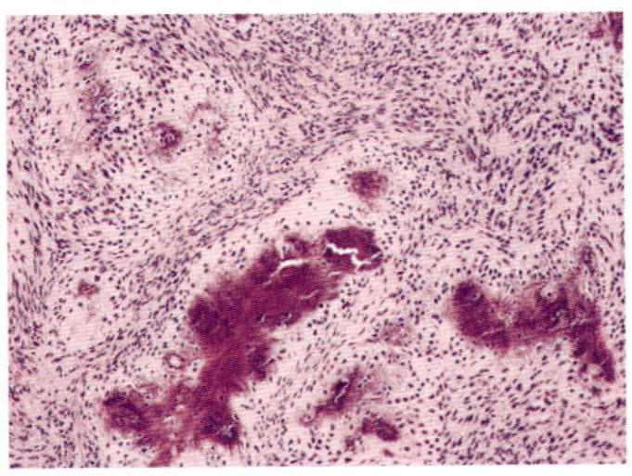	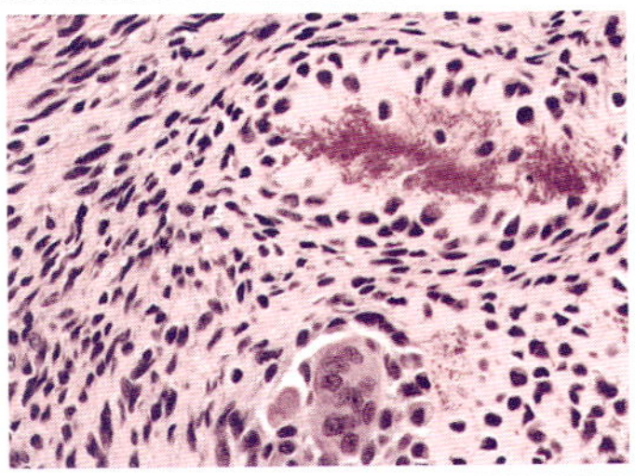
Two components: 1) well-defined nodules with central calcification and rim of epithelioid fibroblasts +/- osteoclasts, sometimes with chondroid in center also, 2) intervening spindle cell fibroblastic fascicular stroma. Younger patients have more of Component 2 and older patients more of Component 1. Variably positive for actins and S-100 protein.					

Table 6.4: Continued from page 83

Tumor	Incidence	Age and sex distribution	Body site (in order of occurrence)	Histopathology description including IHC Medium magnification	High magnification
Calcifying fibrous tumor	Rare	Children to young adults. (Rarely older adults.)	Subcutaneous and deep soft tissues of extremities, trunk, neck but also visceral sites (can be multiple) M = F	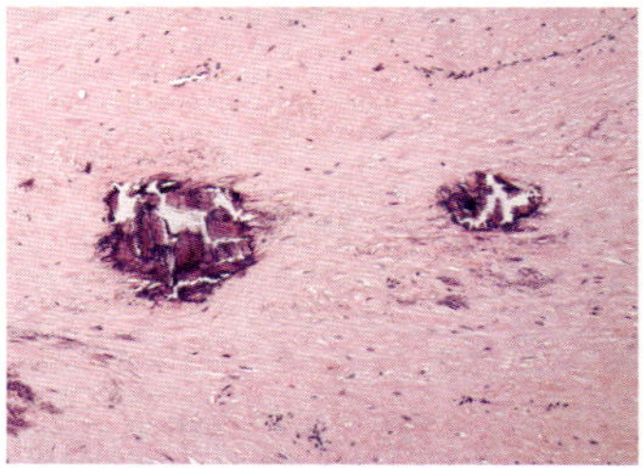	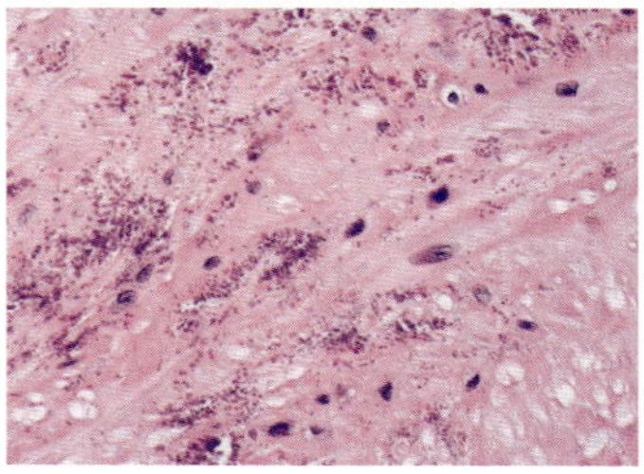
Fibrotic and hyalinized hypocellular scar-like tissue with scattered lymphocyte aggregates and psammomatous and/or dystrophic calcifications. The few lesional spindle cells may be CD34, desmin, and actin positive.					
Intermediate: can recur and/or rarely (<5%) metastasizes					
Lipofibromatosis (infantile fibromatosis of non-desmoid type)	Very rare	Young children usually 2 and under. M > F by 2:1	Usually superficial in hands, feet; less commonly thigh, trunk, head	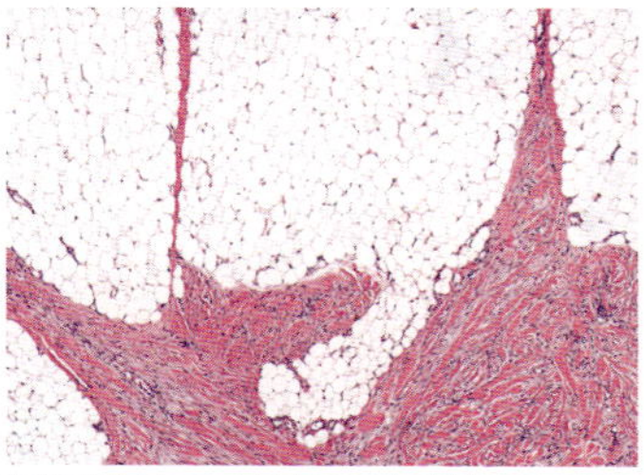	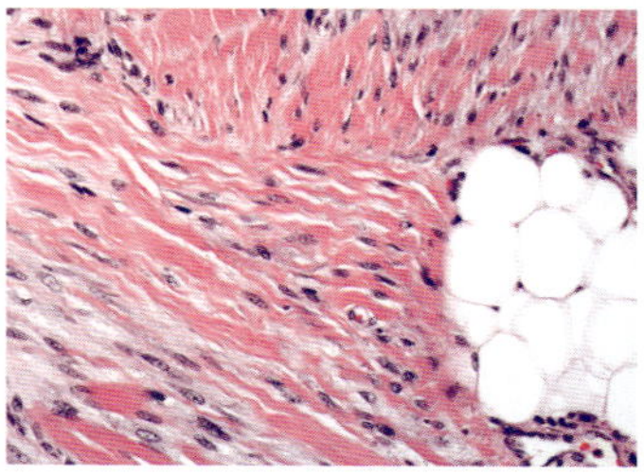
Biphasic: looks like fibrous hamartoma of infancy with 1) fat and 2) spindle cell trabeculations but no primitive myxoid spindle cell nodules. Spindle cells may be CD34 and actin positive.					
Giant cell fibroblastoma	Rare	Children and rarely in adults M > F	Usually superficial in trunk, groin, axilla; rare elsewhere		
Protruberant dermal and subcutaneous myxoid or fibrous hypocellular spindle cell tumor with scattered multinucleated tumor giant cells which sometimes line ectatic, non-vascular spaces. Minimal atypia, no necrosis and low mitotic rate. IHC: CD34 positive only. A few cases have areas of adult type DFSP.					
Gardner fibroma	Rare	Children to 10 years old (rarely up to young adult) M = F	Superficial or deep trunk, most commonly para-spinous area	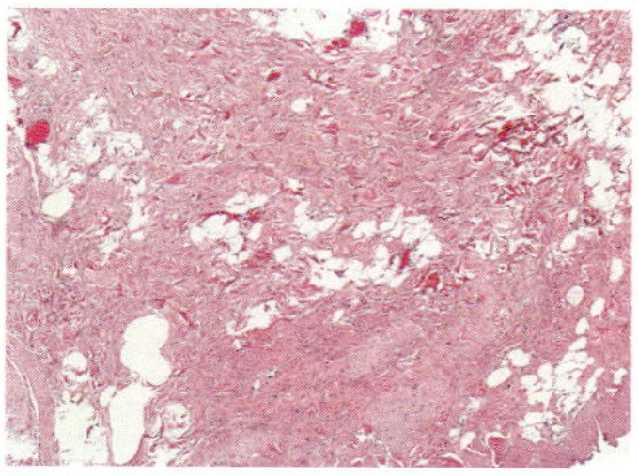	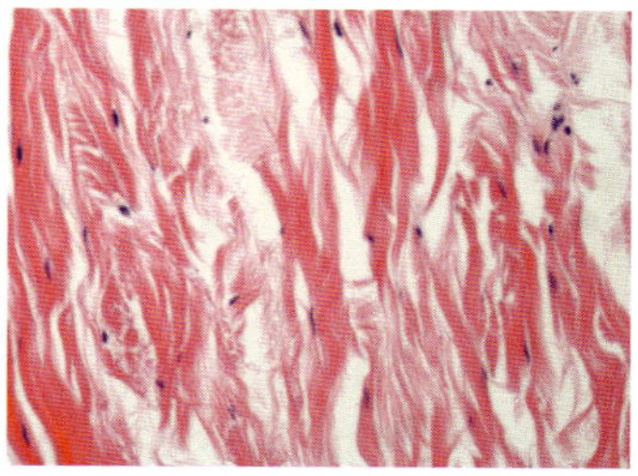
Hypocellular densely fibrotic tumor with thick and thin collagen bands that gap apart with scant small fibroblasts. Plaque-like growth entraps surrounding tissues like fat, nerves, and skeletal muscle. Majority show nuclear reactivity for β-catenin (similar to desmoid tumors).					
Myofibroma/ myofibromatosis	Rare	Most cases are birth to 2 years. Can occur later up to elderly. M > F	Usually superficial tissues of head and neck (and also oral cavity) but can occur in trunk, lower and upper extremities, bone (cranium most commonly) and viscera. Can be multicentric but solitary form more common	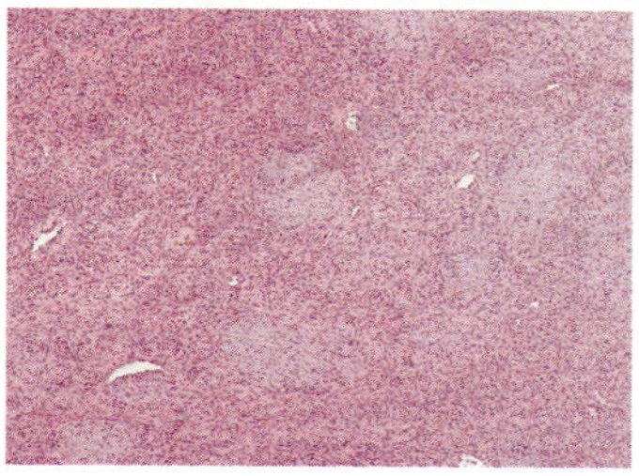	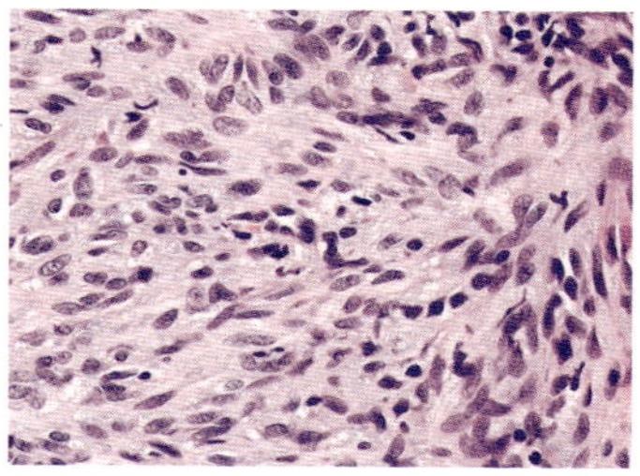
Usually biphasic growth of 1) nodules of mature elongate myofibroblasts distributed in pink matrix, 2) cellular, more primitive fibroblastic areas in between the less cellular pale pink myofibroblastic nodules. Component 2 can have ectatic, 'antler-horn' vessels (hemangiopericytomatous vascular pattern). Calcifications, necrosis, fibrosis, and intravascular growth common. Tumor cells are positive for smooth muscle actin (in myoid nodules) and CD34 in primitive fibroblastic areas (latter may also express HHF-34 actin).					

Table 6.4: Continued from page 84

Tumor	Incidence	Age and sex distribution	Body site (in order of occurrence)	Histopathology description including IHC: Medium magnification	High magnification
Inflammatory myofibroblastic tumor (IMT) (inflammatory fibrosarcoma)	Rare	Children to young adults (median is 9 years). Rarely older adults. F > M	Lung, mesentery, omentum, other organs, less commonly soft tissues (mostly head and neck) and bone	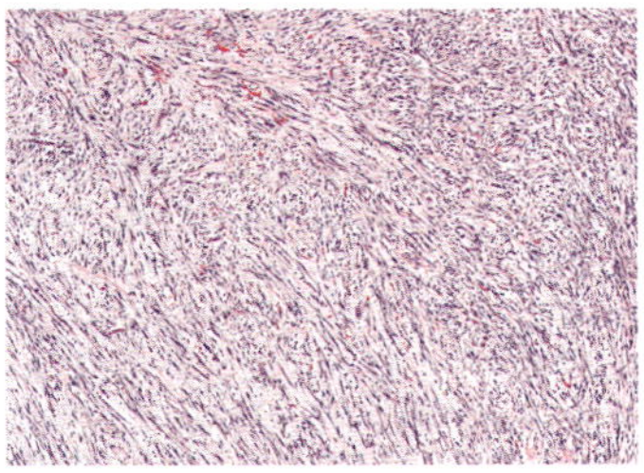	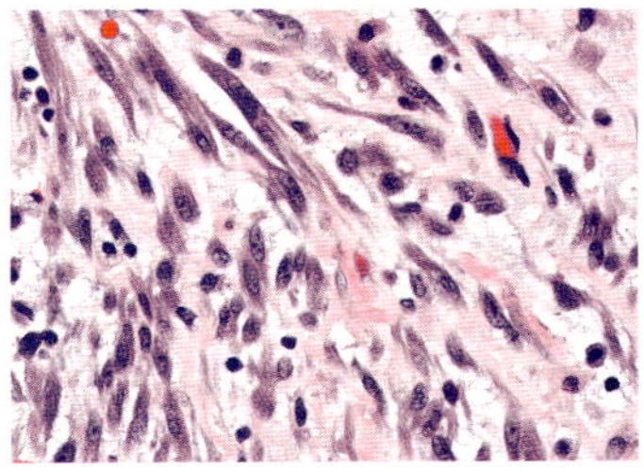
Three main patterns that can mimic other tumors or processes: A) granulation tissue or NF like, B) cellular spindle fascicular like, C) mature scar or desmoid like with lower cellularity and plate like collagen. Every pattern contains inflammatory cells, most commonly lymphocytes, plasma cells, and eosinophils. Marked nuclear atypia is rare, but ganglion like and Reed-Sternberg like cells may be seen. 50% of cases are positive for ALK-1 with variable positivity for actins, desmin, and AE1/AE3 or CAM5.2 keratins.					
Infantile fibrosarcoma (congenital fibrosarcoma)	Rare	Almost all patients are infants to 2 years. M > F by 3:2	Superficial and deep soft tissues of extremities, usually distal, trunk, head and neck. Rarely mesentery	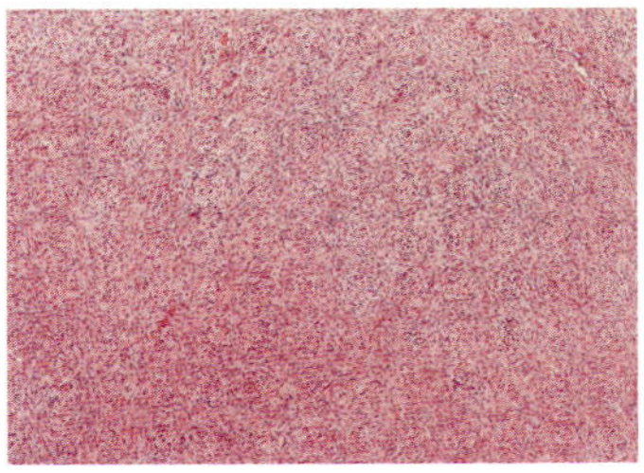	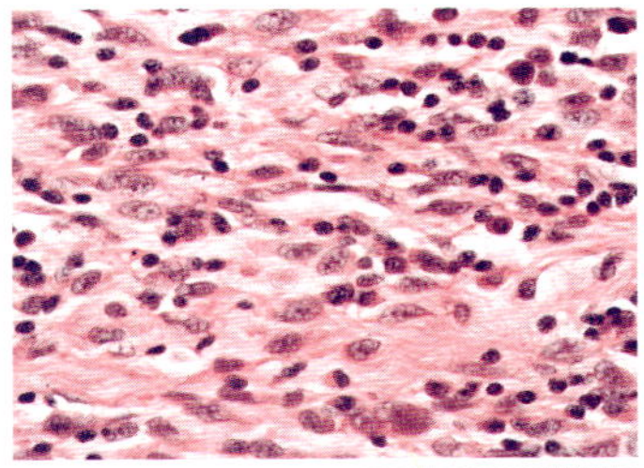
Cellular infiltrative tumor of spindle to oval fibroblasts (rarely round cells entirely) arranged in sheets, cords, herringbone pattern or in hemangiopericytomatous pattern. High mitotic rate, necrosis, hemorrhage, entrapment of normal tissues are common. Extramedullary hematopoieses, sparse chronic inflammatory cells, and calcifications may occur. Rare tumors have marked nuclear pleomorphism (may be more aggressive). Tumor cells are variably positive for actins. Genetic studies are required as some cases are atypical histologically.					
Incidence note: 'Common to very common' indicates that a medium sized practice will treat at least several to dozens of patients with the lesion annually, 'Uncommon to rare' indicates the same practice size will treat one to two patients with the lesion every five years, 'rare to very Rare' indicates the same sized practice will see zero to one patient with the lesion every 20 years. Note: Cutaneous and sino-nasal tumors classified as fibroblastic/myofibroblastic are not presented in this table.					

Table 6.5 Predominantly or exclusively adult fibroblastic/myofibroblastic tumors of soft tissue grouped by behavior

Tumor	Incidence	Age and sex distribution	Body site (in order of occurrence)	Histopathology (including IHC): Medium magnification	High magnification
Benign: does not recur or recurs non-aggressively and does not metastasize					
Fasciitis lesions – **Nodular fasciitis (NF)** – **Proliferative fasciitis and proliferative myositis (PFPM)** – **Ischemic fasciitis (IF) (atypical decubital fibroplasia)** – **Cranial fasciitis (CF)**	NF: common All others: rare	NF: most commonly young adults but all ages affected. CF: Infancy PFPM and IF: middle aged to older adults most commonly	NF: mostly subcutis of upper extremity, trunk and head and neck. PFPM: upper extremity, lower extremity and trunk. IF: Usually subcutis over bony prominences CF: outer table of skull and adjacent soft tissues	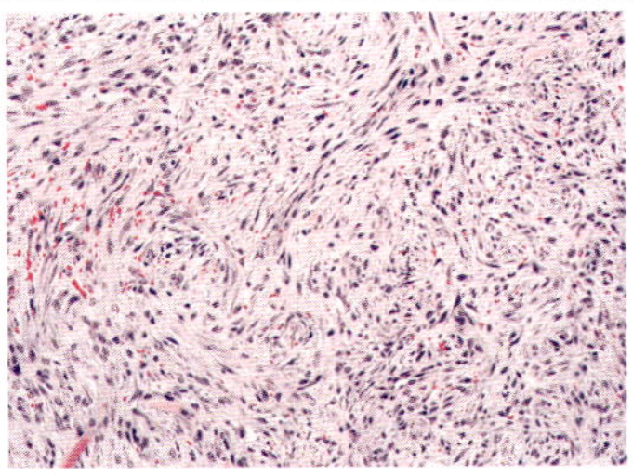 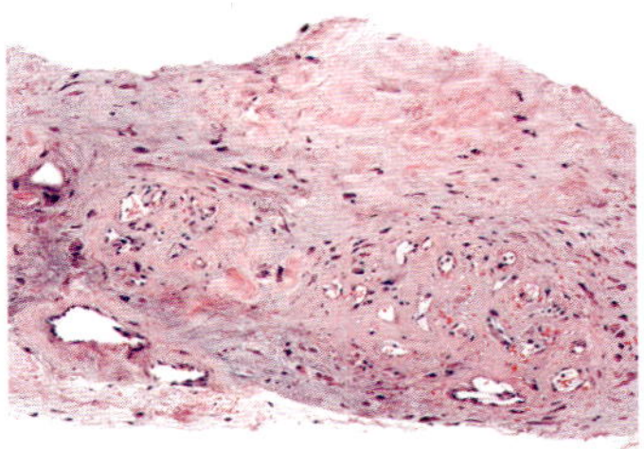	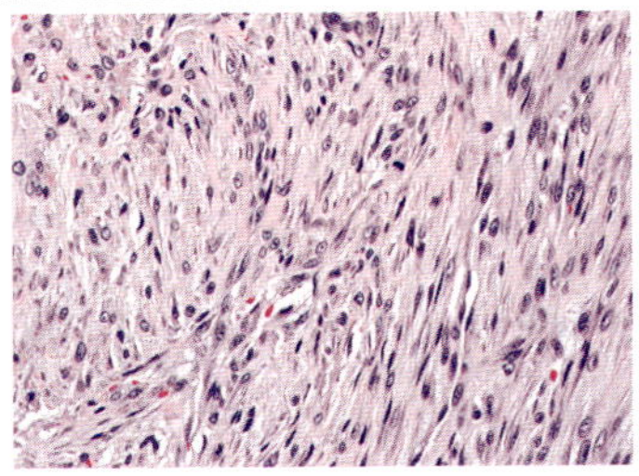 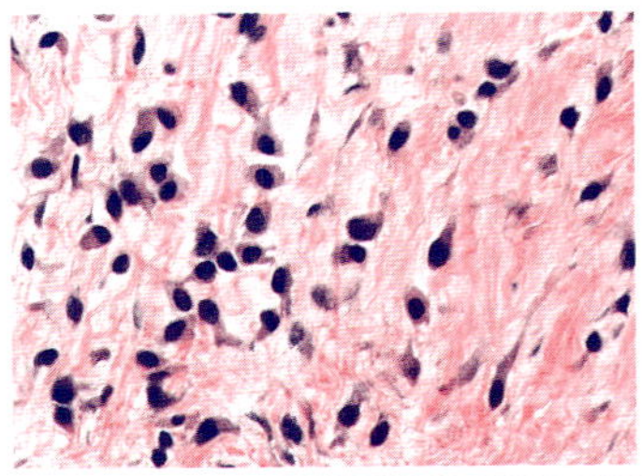
NF and CF: teased apart or cell culture appearance of plump to spindle fibroblasts and myofibroblasts, commonly has mitoses (none atypical) acute hemorrhage, and sprinkles of chronic inflammatory cells. May mature over time with fibrosis and cystic degeneration. May have osseous metaplasia. *Proliferative fasciitis*: as above but with ganglion cell-like myofibroblasts/fibroblasts also present. Proliferative myositis occurs in skeletal muscle. *Ischemic Fasciitis*: Reactive changes to tissue necrosis including spindle and ganglion-cell like fibroblasts, atypical fibroblasts (but with non-alarming smudgy chromatin) mixed with zones of fibrinoid necrosis, myxoid change, fibrosis, palisades of vessel proliferation around necrotic areas, and fibrinoid change of muscular vessels.					

Table 6.5: Continued from page 85

Tumor	Incidence	Age and sex distribution	Body site (in order of occurrence)	Histopathology (including IHC) Medium magnification	High magnification
Myositis ossificans (MO) and Fibroosseous pseudotumor of digits (FPD)	Rare	Broad age range but young adults most common. M > F for MO F > M for fibroosseous pseudotumor of digits	MO: muscle of extremities, trunk and head and neck [Same process can also occur in tendons, subcutis, and fascia] FPD: subcutis of fingers, less commonly toes	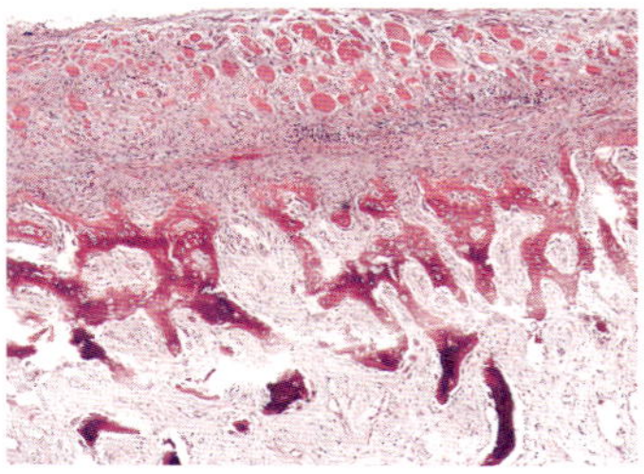	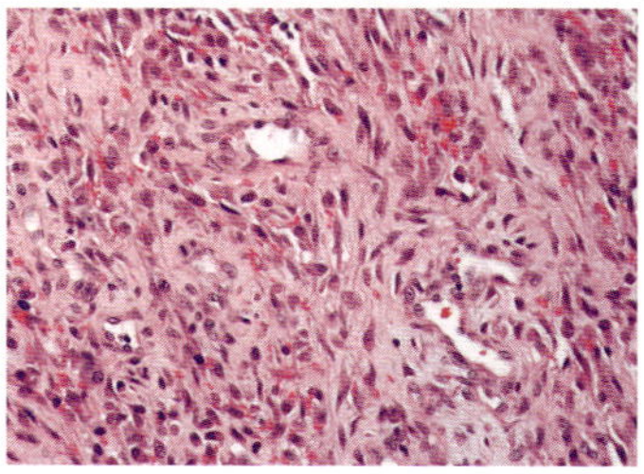
MO: Classically exhibits a zonal growth of cellular, NF center with peripheral woven bone formation and fibrous pseudocapsule. However, zonation may not always be present. Cartilage also can form. With time, the lesion may regress, fibrose, or may convert to lamellar bone. FPD: Like MO but disorganized with bone found throughout the mass. Both lesions can be cellular and mitotically active but there are no atypical mitoses and no convincing nuclear atypia. Woven bone component is rimmed by osteoblasts.					
Elastofibroma	Rare	Most patients are > 50 years. F >> M	Deep subscapular soft tissue. Rarely elsewhere	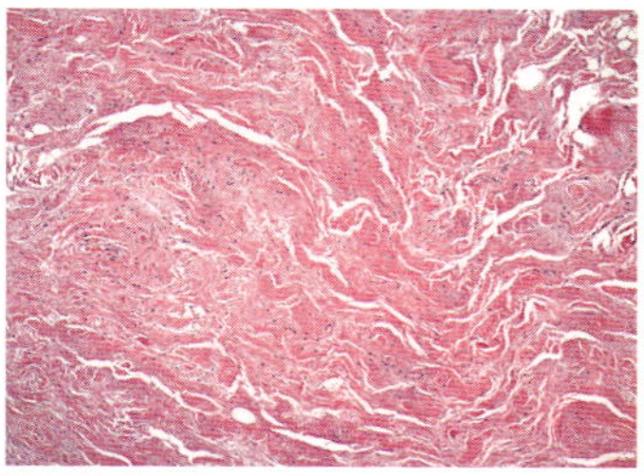	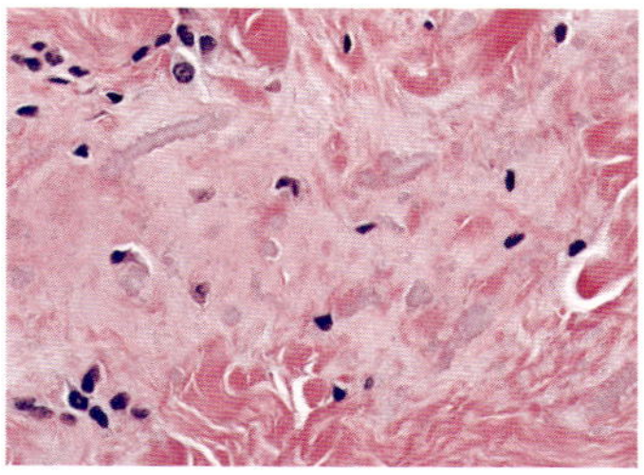
Hypocellular collagenous tumor with entrapped fat and prominent coarse beaded or fragmented elastic fibers simulating fungal hyphae or amyloid on H&E stain. Elastin stain highlights the fibers. Fibers are positive for collagen II and other tumor cells are positive for CD34.					
Fibroma of tendon sheath	Uncommon	Usually 30s-40s but any age is possible. M > F	Fingers, palm, wrist, less commonly knee, foot; rarely elsewhere	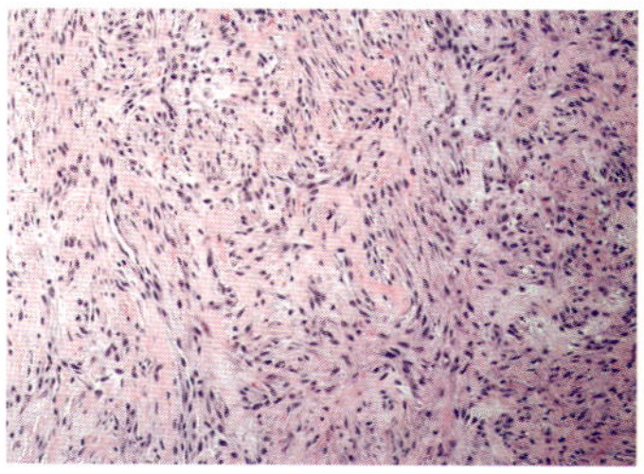	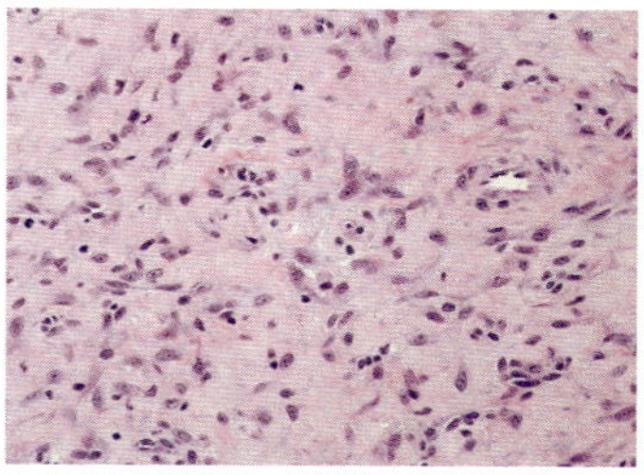
Circumscribed nodules of dense collagen with scattered spindle fibroblasts/myofibroblasts and slit-like vessels. May have hypercellular and myxoid areas and osseous metaplasia. Cells can be SMA positive; usually CD34 negative.					
Desmoplastic fibroblastoma (collagenous fibroma)	Uncommon	Usually 40s-60s; rare in children. M >> F	Arm, trunk, legs, neck, head. Usually in subcutis but may involve skeletal muscle	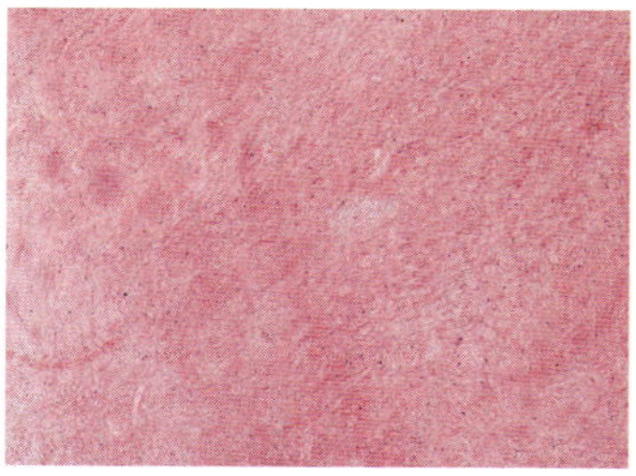	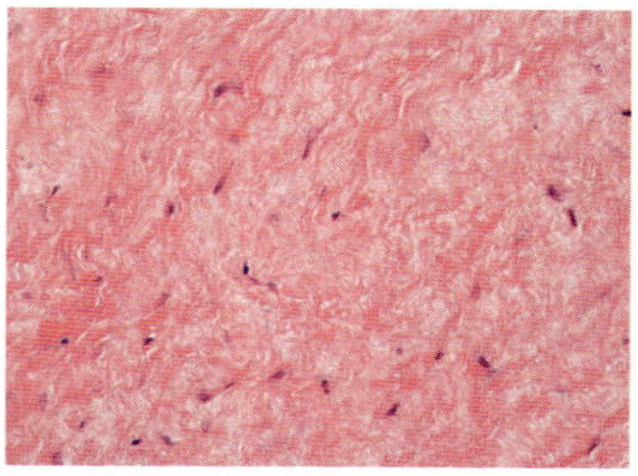
Hypocellular collagenous tumor with scattered uniform spindle or stellate fibro/myofibroblasts. May have myxoid change. Often positive for actin, may be keratin positive; negative for CD34.					
Mammary-type myofibroblastoma	Rare	Adults 40s-60s. M > F	Subcutis of groin, trunk, buttock, back. Rarely may occur in deep tissues	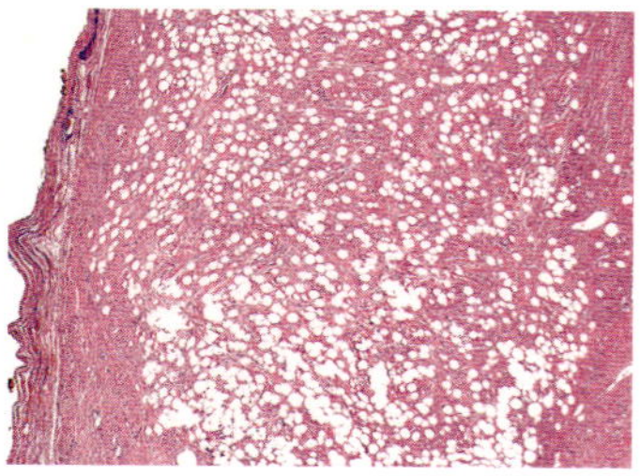	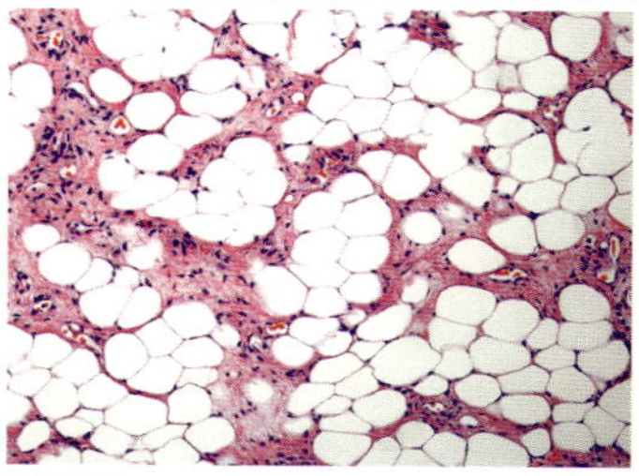
Fascicles of spindle cells with interspersed small foci of adipose tissue and prominent streaming coarse bands of collagen. Stromal mast cells present. Vessels may be hyalinized with lymphocyte aggregates. Usually desmin and CD34 positive. May be actin positive.					

Table 6.5: Continued from page 86

Tumor	Incidence	Age and sex distribution	Body site (in order of occurrence)	Histopathology (including IHC)	
				Medium magnification	High magnification
Angiomyofibroblastoma and Angiomyofibroblastoma-like tumors of male genital tract	Rare	Adults 20s-50s. F >> M	Perineal tissues, vagina. Scrotum or paratesticular in males	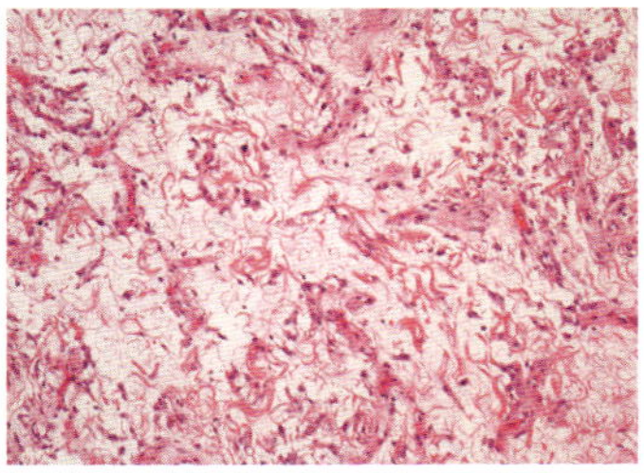	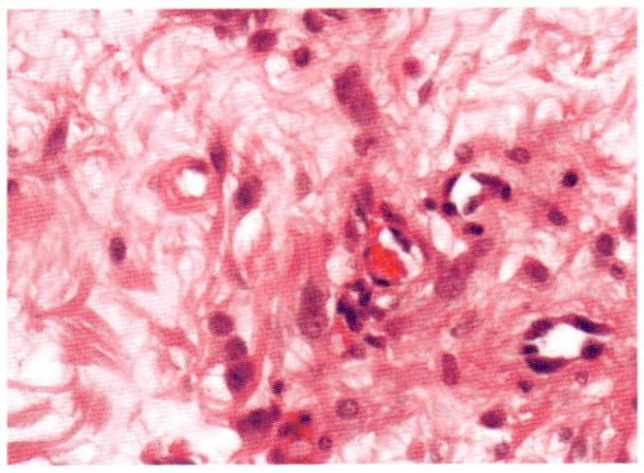
Myxoid matrix with embedded prominent network of small vessels. Round (epithelioid or plasmacytoid) or spindle tumor cells concentrate around the vessels. May be more fibrotic in older patients. 10% have fat. Tumor cells are positive for desmin (may be absent in older patients) and in females express ER and PR. Some may be CD34 positive. Rare malignant variant occurs with marked nuclear atypia, abnormal mitotic figures, and necrosis.					
Cellular angiofibroma	Rare	Adults 40s-60s. F > M	Perineal region, scrotum and para-testicular region in males	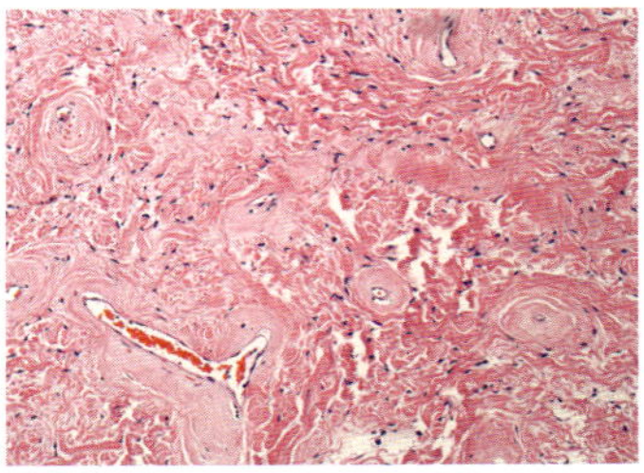	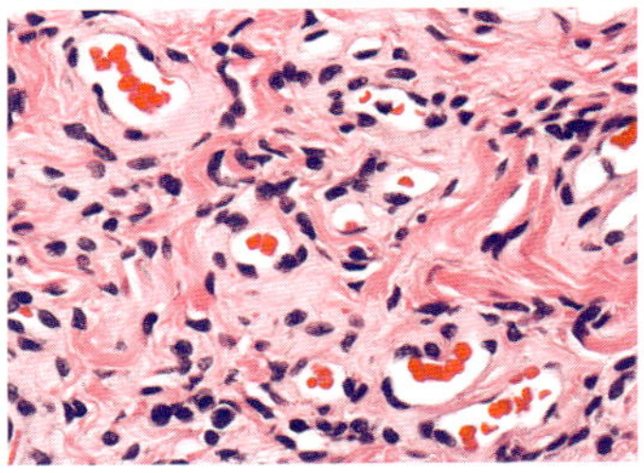
May be closely related to angiomyofibroblastoma. Differs by containing larger, hyalinized blood vessels with intervening moderately cellular stroma of spindle fibro/myo-fibroblasts. Stroma tends to be fibrotic unlike most angiomyofibroblastomas. Fat and mast cells may be present. Tumor cells are variably positive for desmin, CD34 and actin and PR/ER (the latter in females only).					
Nuchal type fibroma	Uncommon	Adults 20s-50s. M > F Forty percent of patients have diabetes mellitus	Neck, upper back, face, extremities. Dermis and subcutis; rarely extends to skeletal muscle	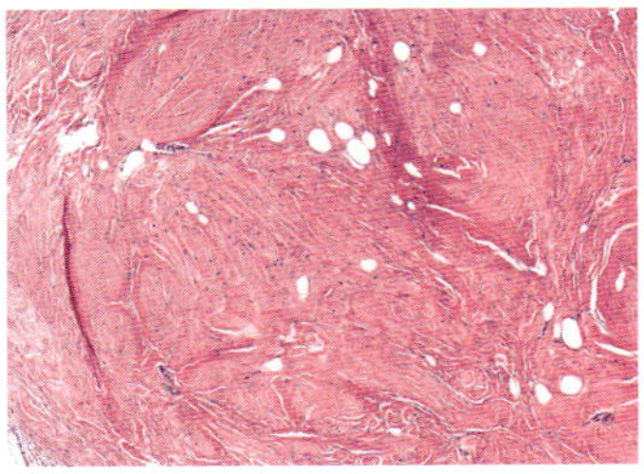	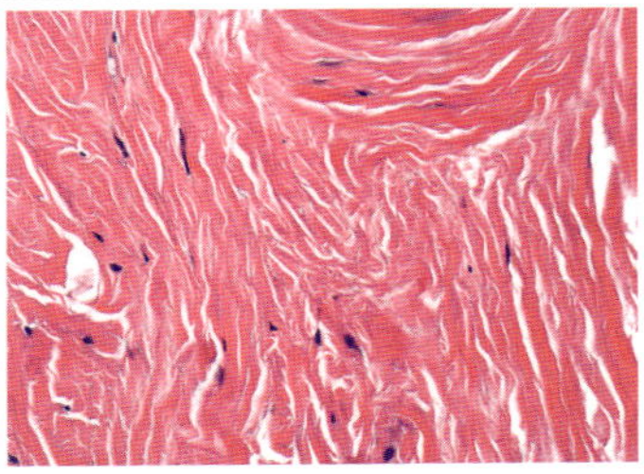
Thick bundles of collagen intersecting irregularly with few interspersed spindle fibroblasts. Entrapped fat, skin adnexae, and foci of reactive nerve twigs common. Tumor cells are negative for nuclear β-catenin.					
Intermediate: can recur, locally aggressive and/or rarely (<5%) metastasizes					
Dermatofibrosarcoma protuberans (DFSP)	Common	Most patients are young adults (20s to 40s). M > F	Trunk, proximal upper extremity, proximal lower extremity. Dermis extending into subcutis and epidermis	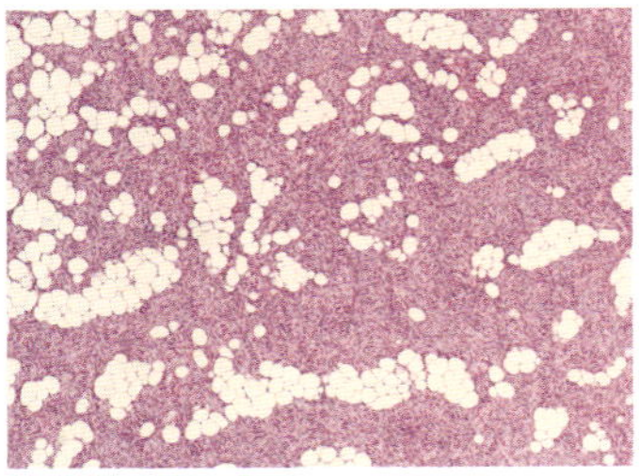	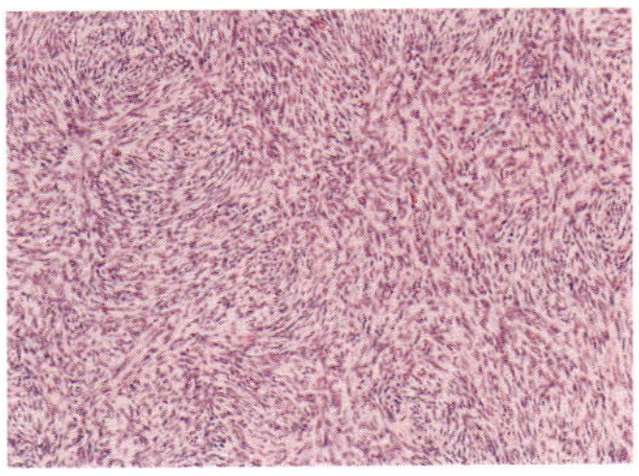
Storiform growth pattern comprising uniform ovoid to spindle cells with characteristic 'honeycomb' infiltration of subcutaneous fat (layers of tumor cells with interspersed fat cells). Unusual findings include: giant cell fibroblastoma areas (the pure pattern of giant cell fibroblastoma is almost exclusive to children), myoid nodules emanating from blood vessels, myxoid change, granular cell change, and a component of melanin-containing cells (Bednar variant). Rare transformation to higher grade occurs mostly in the form of adult type fibrosarcoma. IHC: CD34 strongly positive (may be less positive in fibrosarcomatous transformed areas), apolipoprotein D (APO D) and low affinity nerve growth factor receptor, p75.					

Table 6.5: Continued from page 87

Tumor	Incidence	Age and sex distribution	Body site (in order of occurrence)	Histopathology (including IHC) Medium magnification	High magnification
Giant cell angiofibroma (histologic variant of solitary fibrous tumor)	Rare	Adults, most commonly 40s-50s M > F in orbital tumors; F > M in extra-orbital tumors.	Orbital soft tissues and eyelids; rarely head and neck and trunk, perineal region in subcutaneous tissues	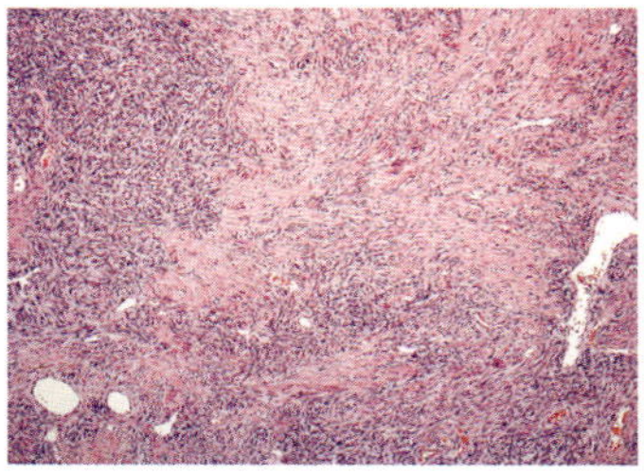	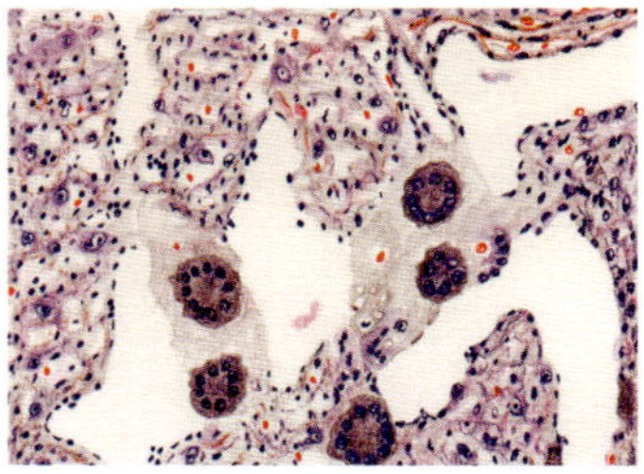
'Patternless pattern' of solitary fibrous tumor with the addition of pseudovascular spaces lined in part by multinucleate tumor cells. Sometimes the spaces are absent. Tumor cells are almost always CD34 and often bcl-2 positive like conventional solitary fibrous tumor.					
Superficial fibromatosis (palmar fibromatosis: Dupuytren disease, plantar fibromatosis: Ledderhose disease)	Common	Adults for palmar lesions, adults and children for plantar lesions M > F Trauma, alcohol use, and Northern European ancestry common	Palm and fingers in tendons and fascia. Plantar aponeurosis in lesions of feet May affect more than one site simultaneously	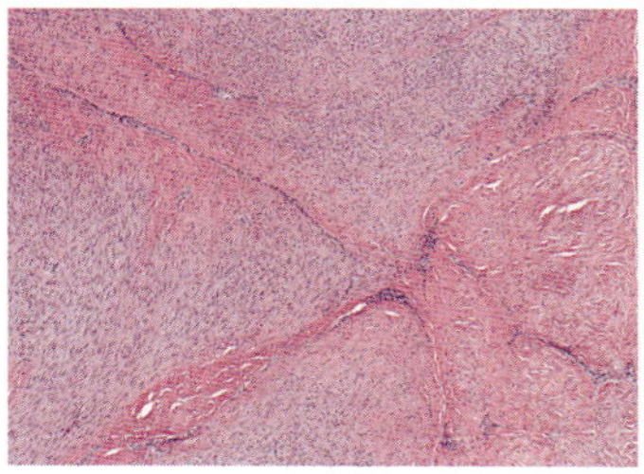	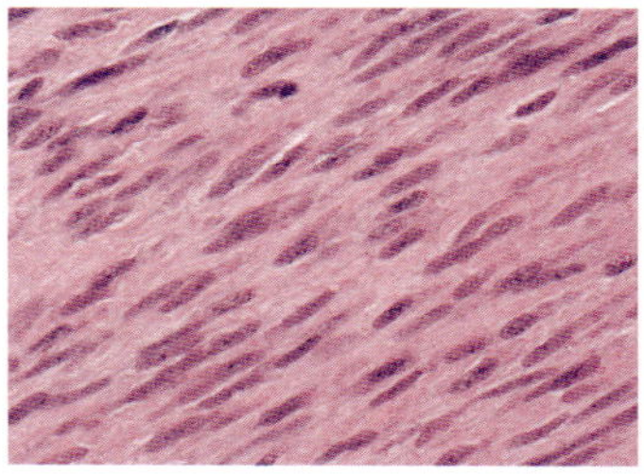
Temporal progression from cellular nodules composed of plump short spindle fibroblasts to fibrotic nodules of lower cellularity. The fibroblasts have pale vesicular nuclei. Mitoses may be present but are not atypical. There is no pleomorphism. Osteoclast-like giant cells may be seen, especially in plantar fibromatosis. Some cases have nuclear β-catenin expression. Some cells may express smooth muscle actin.					
Desmoid-type fibromatosis (deep fibromatosis, aggressive fibromatosis, desmoid tumor, extra-abdominal fibromatosis)	Common	Broad age range from children through middle-aged adults. M = F except for anterior abdominal wall tumors Some cases are familial	Shoulder, chest and back, thigh, head and neck: all deep. Others occur in abdominal wall (mostly young adult females)	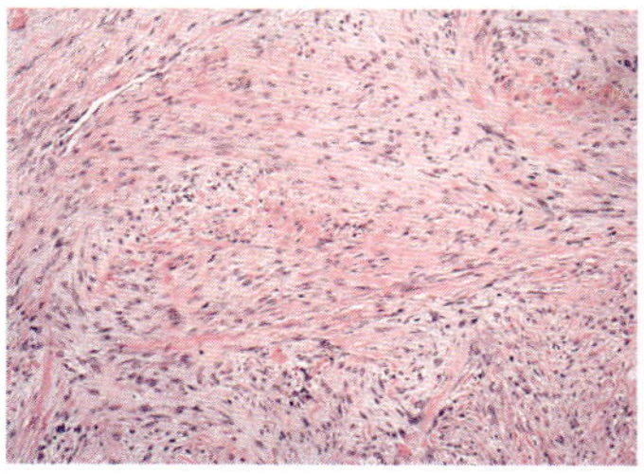	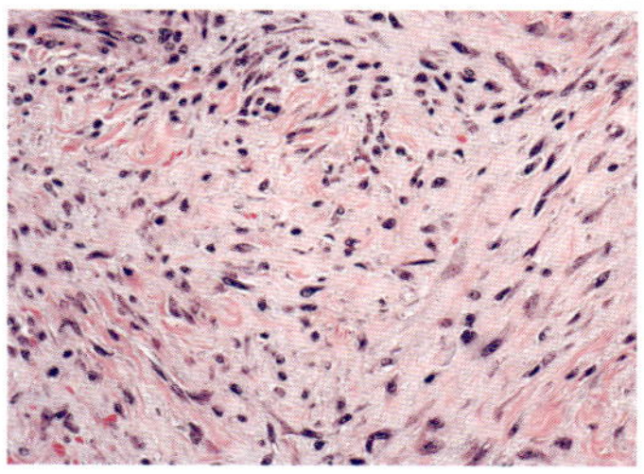
Long sweeping fascicles of slightly spindled fibroblasts and myofibroblasts generally with indistinct cell borders. Nuclei are vesicular and mitoses are not atypical. Mast cells, thin-walled, slightly curving vessels and small clusters of lymphocytes are typical. Some tumors may be myxoid or have keloidal like collagen deposition. A few cells may be actin positive. Eighty percent of cases show nuclear β-catenin by IHC. Usually permeative growth but no pleomorphism and no necrosis.					
Solitary fibrous tumor (SFT)	Rare			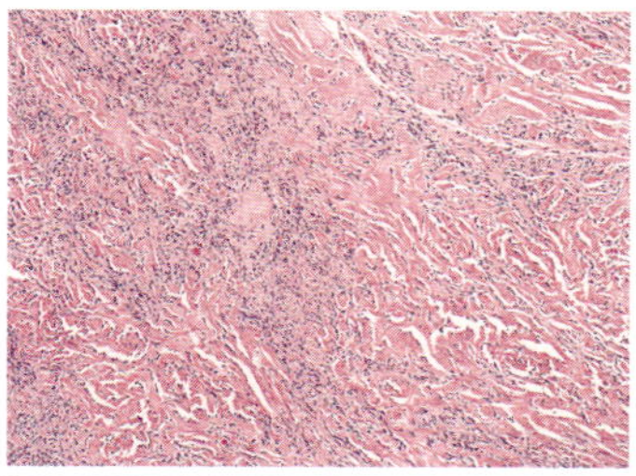	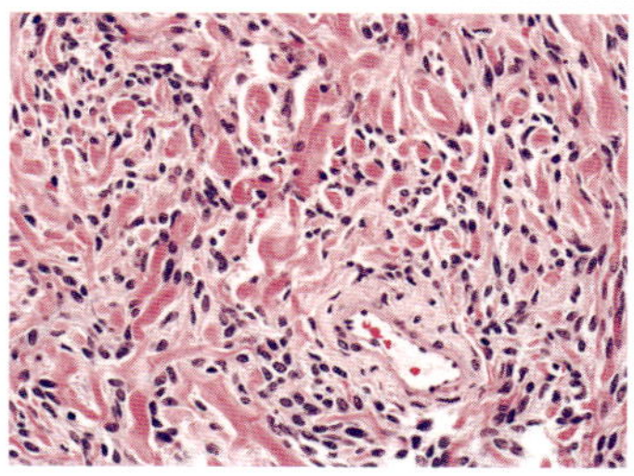
Characterized by haphazard intersecting dense hypocellular fibrous areas with myxoid and cellular regions = 'patternless pattern'. Tumor cells are plump spindle cells to elongate spindle cells. Degenerative atypia and multinucleate cells may be present. Staghorn shaped vessels may be prominent and others may show hyalinized walls. Mitoses usually <4/10hpf. HPC type tumors are uniformly cellular with plump spindle cells and staghorn vessels. Most are benign but may have unpredictable behavior: those with pleomorphism, increased mitoses, necrosis and infiltrative margins more likely to carry risk for metastasis.					

Table 6.5: Continued from page 88

Tumor	Incidence	Age and sex distribution	Body site (in order of occurrence)	Histopathology (including IHC) Medium magnification	 High magnification
Malignant: can recur and commonly metastasizes					
Low grade myofibroblastic sarcoma (myofibrosarcoma)	Rare	Adults > children. Males slightly more than females	Extremities, head and neck (especially tongue and oral cavirty) rarely elsewhere	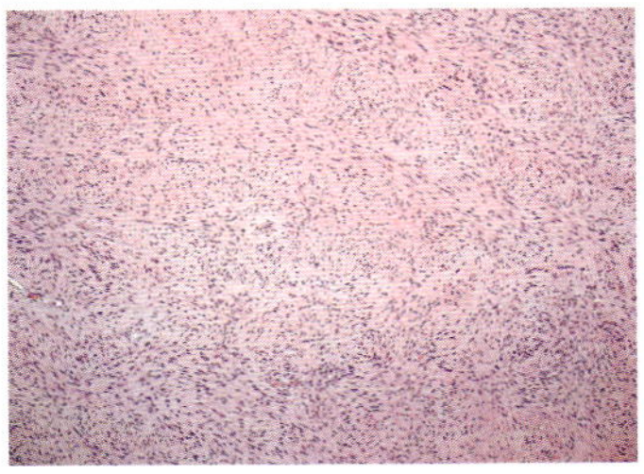	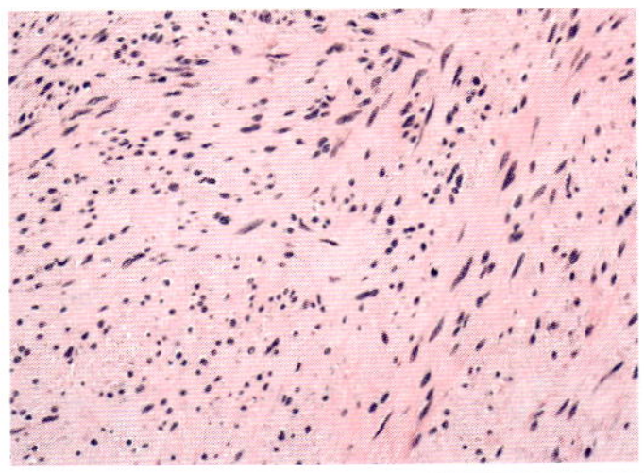
Fascicular and storiforming infiltrative tumor composed of spindle or fusiform cells with elongate to wavy nuclei or plumper rounded nuclei with small nucleoli. A few cases may be more collagenized. Moderate nuclear atypia is present at least focally (more irregularly shaped nuclei, hyperchromatic). Tumors may be well vascularized with numerous capillaries. Inflammation is inconspicuous. Many mitoses and necrosis are associated with more aggressive behavior. Tumor cells may be combinations of actin and desmin reactive but are caldesmon negative.					
Myxoinflammatory fibroblastic sarcoma (MIFS) (inflammatory myxohyaline tumor of distal extremities with virocyte or Reed-Sternberg-like cells, acral myxoinflammatory fibroblastic sarcoma, inflammatory myxoid tumor of the soft parts with bizarre giant cells)	Rare	Adults >> children. M = F	Hands/wrists, feet/ankles; rarely elbow or knee	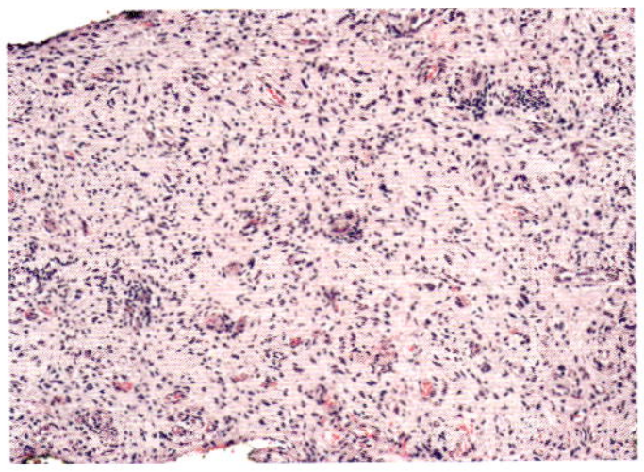	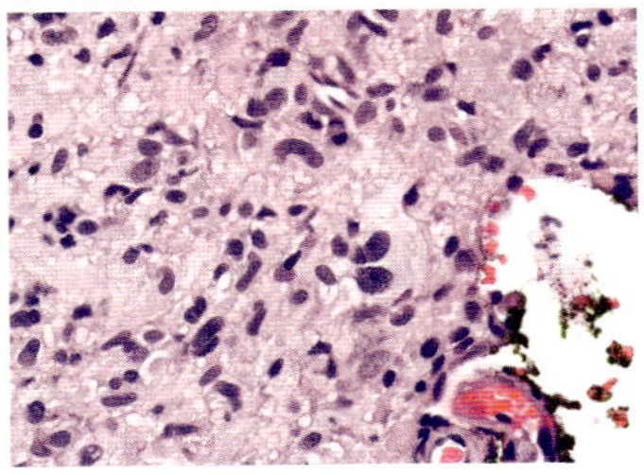
Predominantly subcutaneous but infiltrative multinodular tumor that can invade dermis and tendons but not skeletal muscle or bone. Heterogeneous with myxoid and fibrotic areas containing intense acute and chronic inflammation, bizarre giant cells mimicking Reed-Sternberg or virally infected cells or lipoblasts, and mononuclear epithelioid fibroblasts. Hemosiderin and multinucleated reactive giant cells may be present. Mitoses are rare (less than 1/10hpf). Tumor cells are vimentin positive with some focal keratin, CD68 or CD34 reactivity. Muscle markers and S-100 are negative.					
Adult fibrosarcoma	Very rare	Adults >> children. M = F	Extremities, trunk, head and neck	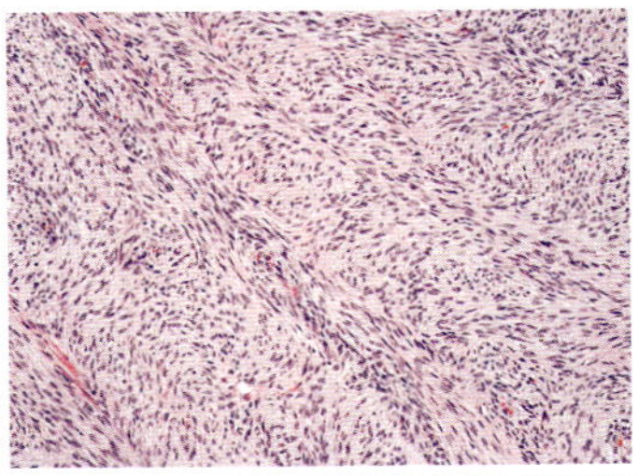	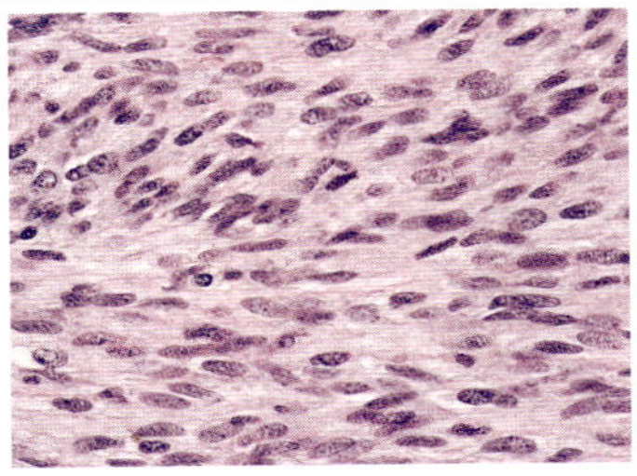
This is a diagnosis of exclusion as many tumors such as synovial sarcoma, malignant peripheral nerve sheath tumor, and high grade sarcoma arising in dermatofibrosarcoma protuberans look like adult FS. Classically, the tumor is deep, grows in long sweeping fascicles forming 'herringbone' like formations, and the cells are spindled with elongate, hyperchromatic nuclei. Collagen may be present and may be keloidal. Myxoid change may be present. Extreme pleomorphism is absent. Mitotic rate varies. Tumor cells may be very focally reactive for actin.					
Myxofibrosarcoma	Common	Older adults (50s upward) >>> young adults and children (20 and under). M slightly > F	Extremities including proximal, lower > upper; rarely in head and neck or hands/feet	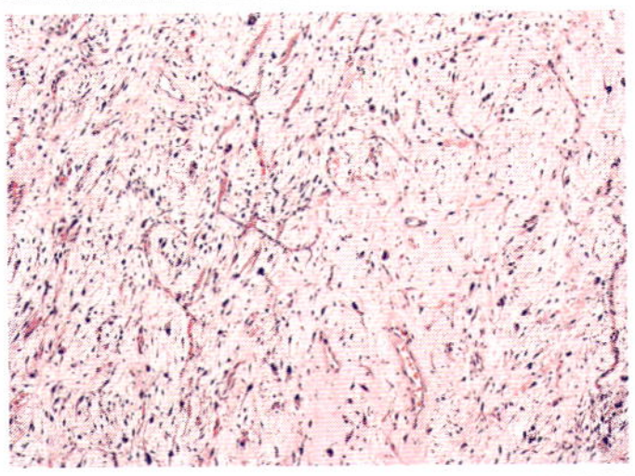	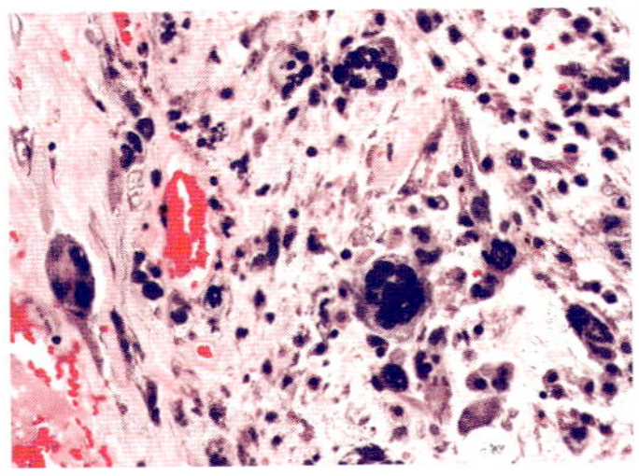
Infiltrative, often multinodular tumor with variable cellular and pronounced myxoid regions composed of stellate to spindle cells floating in hyaluronic acid matrix. Grade 1 tumors are hypocellular with scattered definitely atypical cells, Grade 2 tumors are more cellular, and Grade 3 tumors are highly cellular with marked nuclear pleomorphism and less abundant myxoid matrix. Higher grade tumors often contain regions of low grade tumor. Some tumor cells mimic lipoblasts but do not show the nuclear indentation of true lipoblasts. 'Curvilinear' (long slowly arching) vessels are characteristic, often with increased perivascular cellularity. Some tumors are reactive for CD34, and some cells may be positive for actins (desmin is negative).					

Table 6.5: Continued from page 89

Tumor	Incidence	Age and sex distribution	Body site (in order of occurrence)	Histopathology (including IHC) Medium magnification	High magnification
Low grade fibromyxoid sarcoma	Rare	Young to middle-aged adults; children. M slightly > F	Young to middle-aged adults; children. M slightly > F	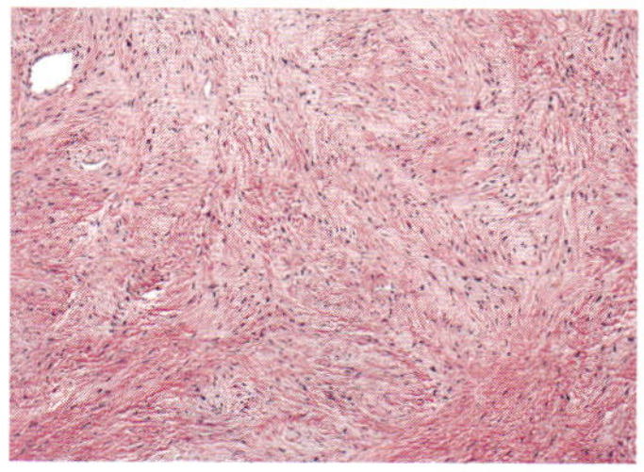	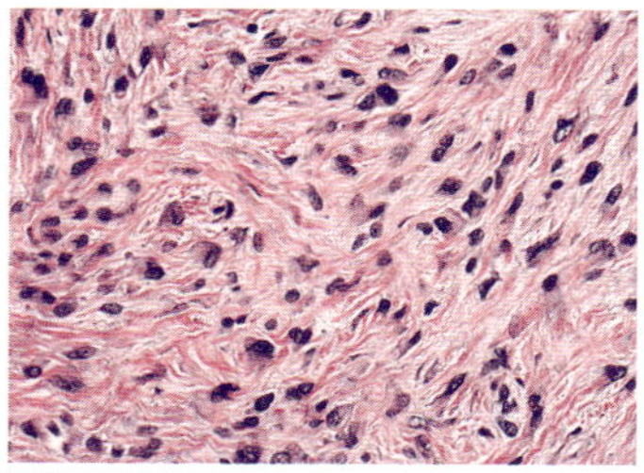
Infiltrative tumor comprising whorls and fascicles of spindled cells with ovoid or blunt ended nuclei. Fibrous areas resemble fibromatosis in cellularity. Myxoid regions usually are whirling with prominent arching vessels described as waterfalls or arcades. There is usually an abrupt transition between fibrous and myxoid areas. Some tumors have rounded collagen nodules surrounded by round cells ('giant rosettes'). Up to 20% of tumors at presentation may contain higher grade, more cellular regions. Mitoses are uncommon except in high grade areas. Recurrences may be all high grade. Tumor cells may be positive for EMA, claudin-1, rarely actin and S-100 protein. MUC4 is sensitive and specific for this tumor (also SEFS) in the setting of fibroblastic tumors. The round cells bordering the giant rosettes are often S-100 positive (also NSE and Leu-7).					
Sclerosing epithelioid fibrosarcoma (SEFS)	Rare	Adults (average age ~45 years). F slightly > M	Lower limbs, shoulder, trunk, neck; rarely in viscera and bone. Deep location	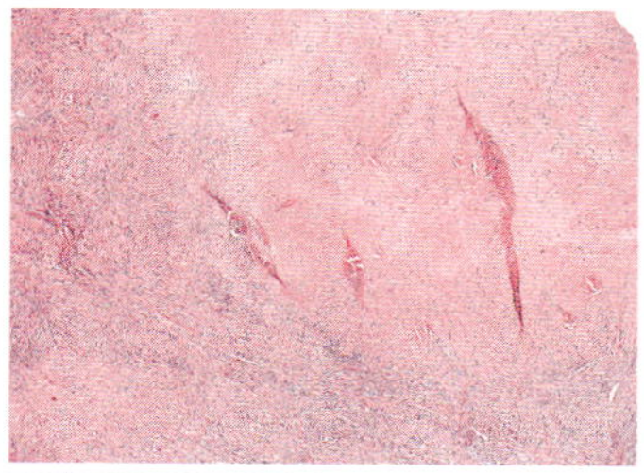	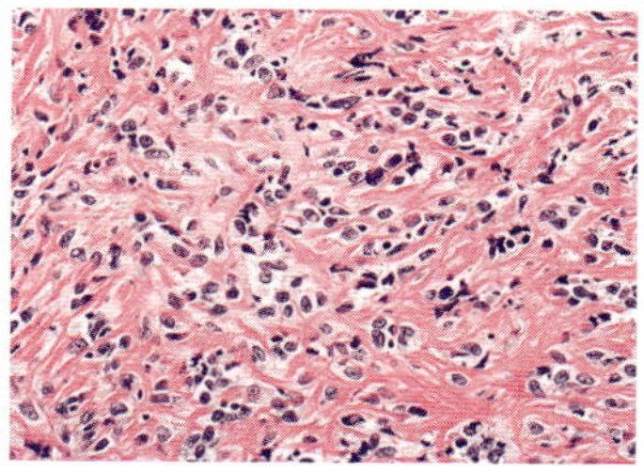
Markedly collagenized tumor with scattered nests and cords of clear cells with rounded epithelioid contours and round nuclei. Usually atypia is low with only scattered mitoses. Stroma is sclerotic to myxohyaline, sometimes with calcifications and osteochondroid metaplasia. Has same translocation as low grade fibromyxoid sarcoma, and some examples may contain areas indististinguishable from low grade fibromyxoid sarcoma. Some tumors also contain areas that mimic the herringbone fascicles of adult type fibrosarcoma. SEFS shows similar IHC staining profile as LFGMS including MUC4 reactivity.					
Incidence Note: 'Common to very common' indicates that a medium sized practice will treat at least several to dozens of patients with the lesion annually, 'Uncommon to rare' indicates the same practice size will treat one to two patients with the lesion every five years, 'Rare to very rare' indicates the same sized practice will see zero to one patient with the lesion every 20 years. Note: Cutaneous and sino-nasal tumors classified as fibroblastic/myofibroblastic are not presented in this table.					

Table 6.6 Soft tissue tumors that will most likely be re-classified as fibroblastic/myofibroblastic

Tumor	Current classification	Rationale for re-classification as fibroblastic/myofibroblastic
Intramuscular and juxta-articular myxoma	Tumor of uncertain differentiation	Tumor cells express vimentin and uncommonly CD34 consistent with fibroblast differentiation
Plexiform fibrous histiocytoma	'Fibrohistiocytic tumor'	Spindle tumor cells express smooth muscle actin but not h-caldesmon or desmin. Histiocytic cells are present and considered reactive rather than neoplastic
Deep benign fibrous histiocytoma	'Fibrohistiocytic tumor'	Spindle cell tumor with variable expression of CD34 and smooth muscle actin consistent with fibroblastic phenotype with variable differentiation to myofibroblasts
Deep 'aggressive' angiomyxoma	Tumor of uncertain differentiation	Tumor cells often express desmin and smooth muscle actin. Also commonly reactive for estrogen and progesterone receptors and may represent differentiation toward a specialized fibroblast of genital region
Angiomatoid fibrous histiocytoma	Tumor of uncertain differentiation	Tumor cells express desmin and EMA and may represent differentiation toward a specialized type of fibroblast
Pleomorphic hyalinizing angiectatic tumor (PHAT)	Tumor of uncertain differentiation	Tumor cells express CD34 and calponin consistent with fibroblasts/myofibroblasts. Some cases evolve into sarcomas indistinguishable from myxofibrosarcoma, a known fibroblastic/myofibroblastic sarcoma
Hemosiderotic fibrohistiocytic lipomatous lesion	Not classified	May represent an earlier phase of PHAT. Tumor cells express CD34 and calponin as in PHAT. This reactivity pattern is consistent with a fibroblast/myofibroblast
Phosphaturic mesenchymal tumor	Not classified	The primary tumor cell expresses fibroblast growth factor-23 (FGF23)
Pleomorphic myofibrosarcoma	Not fully characterized	Tumor is high grade and about half of the cases express actin and or desmin but are negative for h-caldesmon (a more specific marker of smooth muscle differentiation). Electron microscopy may be needed to confirm the diagnosis in cases lacking desmin and actin protein expression
Some undifferentiated high grade pleomorphic sarcomas	'Fibrohistiocytic tumor'	Some undifferentiated pleomorphic sarcomas may represent poorly differentiated fibroblastic sarcomas. The lesional cells express vimentin only
Some cutaneous tumors may also be re-classified as fibroblastic/myofibroblastic and are not presented in this table.		

RADIOLOGY

The fibroblastic and myofibroblastic tumors comprise a spectrum of benign and malignant tumors with varied appearances. With the exception of MO, these tumors show non-specific features that do not allow ready imaging diagnosis. The radiologist can only define the location of the tumor and render an estimation of the tumor's aggressiveness. Generally, biopsy or removal is commonly required for treatment and definitive diagnosis.

Nodular fasciitis

Nodular fasciitis (NF) is common in the superficial fascia or subcutaneous tissues of the upper extremity, typically the volar aspect of the forearm. They can also occur intra or inter-muscular. NF may be related to prior trauma and commonly shows rapid initial growth. The patient may have soreness and pain associated with the tumor. The MR appearance is not specific, and there is significant variation in appearance based on the cellularity, collagen and water content. Typically, the lesion is T1 iso-signal, with high signal on fluid sensitive sequences. There may be linear extensions along the fascia or adjacent to the ends of deeper lesions called the fascial tail sign that suggests the diagnosis of NF (Kransdorff 2006).

Myositis ossificans

Myositis ossificans (MO) results from ossification of a soft tissue hematoma. MO can show definitive diagnostic features because of the characteristic evolution of the lesion over several weeks, ultimately culminating in an area of soft tissue bone. However initially, there is only faint amorphous soft tissue calcification which can appear similar to osteoid, raising the specter of a possible osteosarcoma. Hopefully, a history of trauma can be elicited to corroborate the diagnosis of MO. Unfortunately, precise correlation of the location and time of trauma can be difficult. Typically, a suspected case of MO should have follow up radiographs every 2-3 weeks until a definitive appearance is evident. On radiographs, MO has denser calcification peripherally and should show a clear progression of increasing peripheral calcification, developing into corticated bone with visible internal marrow trabeculae.

If there is imaging uncertainty, CT scan can be helpful to assess if calcifications predominate in the periphery. A soft tissue calcific lesion that is denser centrally is worrisome for a sarcoma. Presumably the center of the sarcoma has had more time to develop and calcify osteoid. Alternatively, the center of a sarcoma may have necrosis or ischemic areas predisposing for dystrophic calcification. When a clear pattern of MO development is seen, then diagnosis is certain by imaging, and no biopsy should be performed. Reactive or healing bone on biopsy could potentially be misdiagnosed as malignant osteoid. It is crucial that the radiologist be accurate in their interpretation of soft tissue calcified mass so as to avoid an unnecessary biopsy of MO, and also to prevent delay in biopsy of an actual sarcoma.

Extra-abdominal fibromatosis

These are commonly poorly defined tumors with infiltrative or invasive margins despite their benign histology. The fibromatoses cannot metastasize, however, recurrence is common and aggressive management may require repeated surgery, radiation therapy or amputation. Fibromatosis can also show the fascial tail sign (along with NF). Fibromatosis shows a variable appearance on MRI likely related to the wide variation in cellularity and collagen content. Generally, the higher the collagen content, the lower the T1 and T2 signal will be. Kransdorff and Murphey (2006) make two important observations regarding MR appearance; one, the low collagen content lesions (thus high cellularity and high T2 signal) are far more likely to recur and two, positive response to radiation therapy will show decreasing MR signal as the lesion collagenization and decreases in cellularity.

Solitary fibrous tumor

Intra-thoracic solitary fibrous tumors (SFTs) are often asymptomatic despite their large size at presentation whereas SFT elsewhere in the body usually have symptoms related to the tumor's mass effect. Calcification is seen in only 9%. Avid enhancement is shown in 58%, with 79% having heterogeneous enhancement. Large feeding vessels may be seen in up to 35%, and 12% have distant metastasis at initial presentation, usually to the lung. The overall appearance of SFT is non-specific however; a large vascular tumor with large feeding vessels suggests the diagnosis.

Inflammatory myofibroblastic tumor

Previous terms for inflammatory myofibroblastic tumor (IMT) include inflammatory pseudotumor and plasma cell granuloma. IMT is most common in the lung, particularly in children but can occur anywhere. Outside the lung, abdomen and pelvis are most common, with head and neck next, and only about 4% occurring in the extremities (Coffin 1995). Patients can present with constitutional symptoms such as fever and weight loss and malaise and laboratory testing may show elevated sedimentation rate. In the lung, IMT is described as being homogeneous T1 low signal and T2 mild increased signal, with homogeneous enhancement.

Myxofibrosarcoma

These tumors contain a significant portion of myxoid material. The imaging appearance is a non-specific highly aggressive lesion with T1 low or iso-intensity and high signal on fluid sensitive sequences with heterogeneous enhancement. These tumors show heterogeneity related to the variable cellularity, hemorrhage, calcification, necrosis and areas of myxoid material.

Low grade fibromyxoid sarcoma

Low grade fibromyxoid sarcoma (LGFMS) tends to occur in the lower extremity and has a predilection for the thigh. In a retrospective series by Evans 2011, 42% of patients died of their LGFMS however, their survival ranged from 3 to 42 years. Sixty three percent of patients had recurrences which occurred on average after 3.5 years ranging up to 15 years. There is little published regarding the imaging appearance of LGFMS. Case reports indicate the MR appearance of LGFMS is of a heterogeneous mass with variable signal and enhancement depending on the fibrous and myxoid components of the tumor.

Fibromatosis colli

Although we do not have a case with histology on the benign entity of fibromatosis colli, it represents an interesting clinical and imaging diagnosis within the category of fibroblastic tumors. We present two cases with ultrasound imaging (**Figures 6.1a** through **6.1e**). Fibromatosis colli is a proliferative disorder of the sternocleidomastoid muscle in the newborn and is common cause of torticollis. The condition is usually self-limiting requiring conservative management. The etiology is uncertain but thought to be related to birth trauma and difficult delivery. The infant may present with an enlarging mass in the lower third of the sternocleidomastoid muscle. Ultrasound appearance is variable and may show diffuse

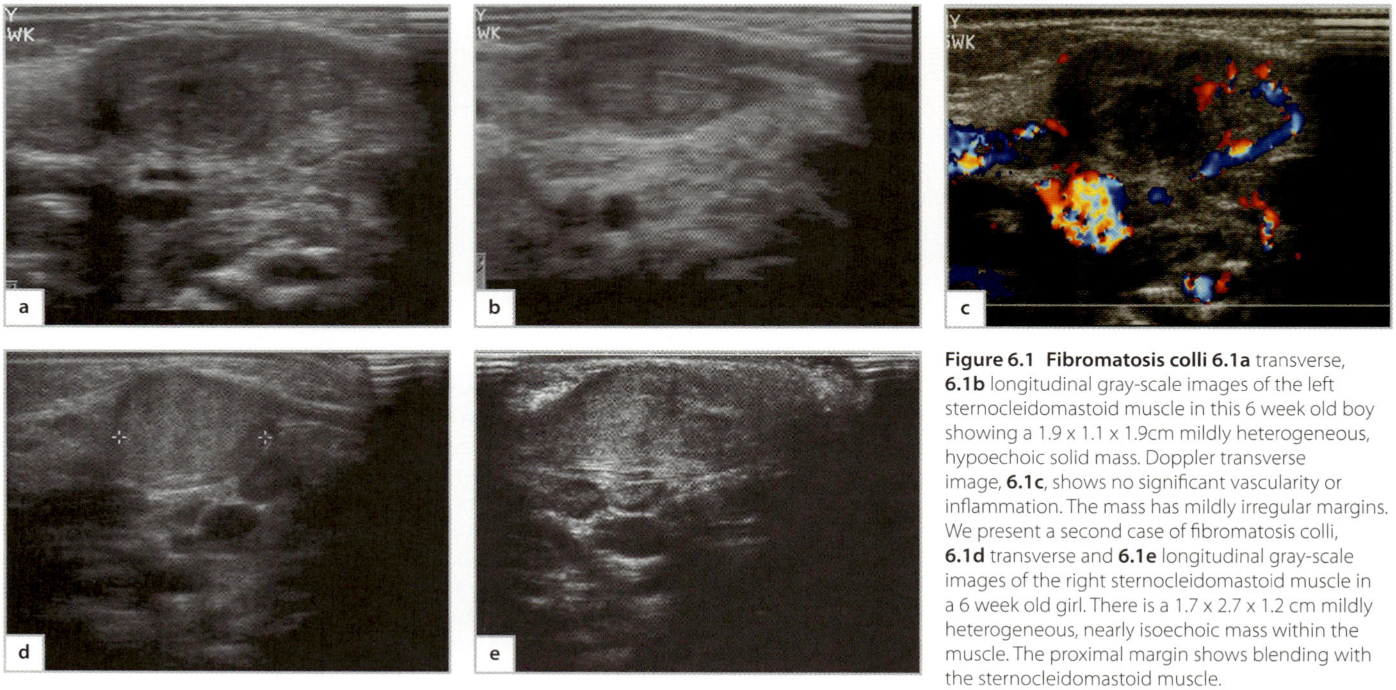

Figure 6.1 Fibromatosis colli 6.1a transverse, **6.1b** longitudinal gray-scale images of the left sternocleidomastoid muscle in this 6 week old boy showing a 1.9 x 1.1 x 1.9cm mildly heterogeneous, hypoechoic solid mass. Doppler transverse image, **6.1c**, shows no significant vascularity or inflammation. The mass has mildly irregular margins. We present a second case of fibromatosis colli, **6.1d** transverse and **6.1e** longitudinal gray-scale images of the right sternocleidomastoid muscle in a 6 week old girl. There is a 1.7 x 2.7 x 1.2 cm mildly heterogeneous, nearly isoechoic mass within the muscle. The proximal margin shows blending with the sternocleidomastoid muscle.

enlargement or a focal mass which is isoechoic or hypoechoic. The mass typically blends with the sternocleidomastoid muscle. Ultrasonography can also show the mass moves with the sternocleidomastoid muscle, (Crawford et al. 1988). On MR imaging, the mass can be isointense to normal muscle on T1 weighted images and heterogeneously high signal on T2 weighted images (Entel et al. 1997). However, MR is not typically utilized as the clinical setting and ultrasound appearance is usually diagnostic.

Dermatofibrosarcoma protuberans

Dermatofibrosarcoma protuberans (DFSP) is a malignant tumor of skin which characteristically presents as a bulky, fungating, exophytic mass. Imaging shows heterogeneous tissue with heterogeneous enhancement. The bulky nature of the clinical mass may make for dramatic imaging appearance. DFSP can have areas of fibrosarcoma in the original tumor or in the recurrence, (Mentzel et al. 1998, Connelly et al. 1992). Wide surgical margins (>3cm) apparently minimize recurrence, (Roses et al. 1986). MRI may be helpful for surgical planning by demonstrating the satellite nodules or superficial spread of the DFSP.

SURGERY

Tables 6.7 and **6.8** briefly itemize the treatment of all the WHO recognized myofibroblastic/fibroblastic tumors. In addition, treatment details are provided below for the cases presented in the second part of this chapter.

Nodular fasciitis (including ischemic fasciitis)

These lesions should be excised with a marginal margin. Recurrence is rare, even with incompletely excised lesions.

Myositis ossificans

MO is a complex, multi-factorial disorder largely beyond the scope of this text. When considering surgical management of this condition, the underlying cause of the heterotopic bone formation becomes the most important consideration. In some conditions (posttraumatic or associated with neurological injury), surgical excision may be beneficial. However, in other forms, surgery is generally ineffective and may even be detrimental, particularly in patients with genetic disorders of heterotopic ossification.

If surgery is indicated, such as in cases of ankylosis following trauma, surgery, or neurologic injury, it is generally felt that the surgery should be delayed until the heterotopic bone is 'mature' as indicated by radiographic and radionuclide studies. Various modalities have been used to decrease the incidence of recurrent ossification following resection, including NSAIDs, pre- or post-operative radiation, and post-operative use of diphosphonates, all of which have been shown to have some success.

Extra-abdominal fibromatosis (extra-abdominal desmoid)

These tumors present a substantial management problem. All present treatment modalities are associated with a high rate of local recurrence which tends to tempt excessively aggressive attempts at cure in what still represents a benign disease. Although mortality has been observed in some head, neck, and chest wall lesions, it is an exceedingly rare complication of this tumor. Radiation therapy is an effective adjuvant, but high doses are required (50-60 Gy) introducing the possibility of exchanging a lethal radiation induced sarcoma for local control of a benign diseases. Spontaneous regression or regression after biopsy appears to occur in 15% of patients. The decision about which treatment modality, or combination, should be used to treat this tumor must be carefully balanced against the potential morbidity and mortality of the treatment itself.

Table 6.7 Current treatment of predominantly to exclusively pediatric fibroblastic/myofibroblastic tumors of soft tissue

Tumor	Surgical approach	Adjuvant therapy	Comments
Fibrous hamartoma of infancy	Marginal excision	None	Recurrence rate 16%
Inclusion body fibromatosis (Infantile digital fibromatosis)	Marginal excision vs. observation	None	Recurrence rate up to 60% following excision; high rate of spontaneous regression
Fibromatosis colli	Observation	None	70% resolve by one year of age without treatment
Juvenile hyaline fibromatosis	Controversial	None	High rate of recurrence with excision
Calcifying aponeurotic fibroma	Marginal excision	None	High rate of recurrence, particularly with age <5
Calcifying fibrous tumor	Observation vs. marginal excision	None	Most regress without treatment, recurrence rare even after incomplete excision
Lipofibromatosis (infantile fibromatosis of non-desmoid type)	Wide local resection	None	Wide margins preferred due to high local recurrence rate however, due to its benign nature extent of margin needs to be considered in light of disfigurement/dysfunction
Giant cell fibroblastoma (pediatric version of DFSP)	Wide local resection	Imatinib mesylate (Gleevac) has been used in adults with DFSP. Adjuvant radiation has been used in adults with DFSP when negative margins cannot be achieved	Wide margins preferred due to 50% local recurrence rate. However, the tumor does not metastasize
Gardner fibroma	Local resection but complex options in those cases that convert to fibromatosis (desmoid tumor)	Some cases convert or transform to deep fibromatosis (desmoid tumor): these are treated as desmoid tumor (see below for desmoid type fibromatosis)	Transformation to deep fibromatosis (desmoid tumor) can occur, especially after surgery
Myofibroma/ myofibromatosis	Marginal excision for solitary lesion or watchful waiting	None	10-15% local recurrence; spontaneous regression can occur in 30-50% of lesions. Myofibromatosis with extensive visceral involvement has high mortality due to local effects
Inflammatory myofibroblastic tumor (inflammatory fibrosarcoma)	Marginal excision, consider wide margin for recurrence	Radiation therapy can be used in selected cases and has been associated with good local control	High rate of local recurrence, particularly with abdominal/ retroperitoneal tumors
Infantile fibrosarcoma (congenital fibrosarcoma)	Wide resection	Chemotherapy has reported adjuvant benefit; probably best reserved for inoperable cases	

Table 6.8 Current treatment of predominantly to exclusively adult fibroblastic/myofibroblastic tumors of soft tissue

Tumor	Surgical approach	Chemotherapy radiation therapy	Comments
Fasciitis Lesions **– Nodular fasciitis (NF)** **– Proliferative fasciitis and proliferative myositis (PFPM)** **– Ischemic fasciitis (IF) (atypical decubital fibroplasia)** **– Cranial fasciitis (CF)**	Marginal excision if clinically indicated	None	Recurrence rate extremely low for NF; low for others
Myositis ossificans (MO) and Fibroosseous pseudotumor of digits (FPD)	Marginal excision if clinically indicated	None	Recurrence rate low
Elastofibroma	Marginal excision	None	Recurrence rate low
Fibroma of tendon sheath	Marginal excision	None	Recurrence rate low
Desmoplastic fibroblastoma (collagenous fibroma)	Marginal excision	None	Recurrence rate low
Mammary-type myofibroblastoma	Marginal excision	None	Recurrence rate low
Angiomyofibroblastoma and Angiomyofibroblastoma-like tumors of male genital tract	Marginal excision	None	Recurrence rate low
Cellular angiofibroma	Marginal excision	None	Recurrence rate low
Nuchal type fibroma	Marginal excision	None	Recurrence rate low

Table 6.8: Continued from page 93

Tumor	Surgical approach	Chemotherapy/ radiation therapy	Comments
Dermatofibrosarcoma protuberans (DFSP)	Wide local excision	Imatinib mesylate may be used in large tumors or tumors not amenable to complete resection. Adjuvant radiation therapy is also helpful in these two situations	Recurrence rate low. Rare cases are fibrosarcomatous with 10-15% metastasis rate
Giant cell angiofibroma (histologic variant of solitary fibrous tumor)	Marginal excision, wide resection in malignant variants	Same as for solitary fibrous tumor	Recurrence rate low
Superficial fibromatosis (palmar fibromatosis: Dupuytren disease, plantar fibromatosis: Ledderhose disease)	Complex, refer to text	None	Recurrence rate high
Desmoid-type fibromatosis (Deep fibromatosis, aggressive fibromatosis, desmoid tumor)	Complex, refer to text	Adjuvant chemotherapy has benefit. Radiation therapy effective but should be used with caution	Recurrence rate high
Solitary fibrous tumor	Marginal excision. Wide resection with malignancy	Radiation therapy in selected cases. Adjuvant chemotherapy has been attempted but is not proven especially successful	Recurrence rate low. Tumors with some histologic features such as necrosis, nuclear crowding or pleomorphism or >4 mitoses/10 high power microscopic fields are associated with a higher risk for aggressive behavior and should be treated by wide resection if possible
Low grade myofibroblastic sarcoma (low grade myofibrosarcoma)	Wide resection	Radiation therapy in selected cases (such as inability to entirely resect tumor, some recurrences)	A high grade myofibrosarcoma also occurs that was not specifically defined in the WHO 2002 classification
Myxoinflammatory fibroblastic sarcoma (acral myxoinflammatory fibroblastic sarcoma, inflammatory myxohyaline tumor)	Wide resection	Radiation therapy in selected cases (such as inability to entirely resect tumor, some recurrences). Too few cases to define a role for chemotherapy	This tumor may be closely related to hemosiderotic fibrolipomatous tumor
Adult fibrosarcoma (fibrosarcoma, NOS)	Wide resection	Radiation therapy in selected cases (such as inability to entirely resect tumor, some recurrences)	Must exclude histologic mimics, as fibrosarcoma. NOS is a rare entity
Myxofibrosarcoma	Wide resection	Radiation therapy in most cases even with negative surgical margins (not required for amputated tumors)	Recurrence rate approaches 30%. High grade tumors have a metastasis rate of approximately 30% overall
Low grade fibromyxoid sarcoma	Wide resection	Radiation therapy in selected cases (such as inability to resect entire tumor, some recurrences). No effective chemotherapy	Recurrence rate and metastasis rate high if patients are followed long enough (over decades)
Sclerosing epithelioid fibrosarcoma	Wide resection	Radiation therapy in selected cases (such as inability to resect entire tumor, some recurrences). No effective chemotherapy	Related to low grade fibromyxoid sarcoma but more aggressive with higher short term metastasis rate and higher mortality

Wide-margin surgery has traditionally been the treatment of choice for this tumor, despite the fact that the recurrence rate is among the highest reported for any tumor typically treated with surgical resection. Because of the tendency for these tumors to invade microscopically into surrounding tissues, wide margins are difficult to achieve without extensive resection. Negative margin surgery results in a local control rate of roughly 75%, however similar rates of success have been reported following marginal resection or even margin positive surgery (Merchant et al. 1999, Nuyttens et al. 2000, Sorenson et al. 2002). The addition of radiation therapy appears to increase the local control rate to 75% with marginal surgery or positive margins and 94% with negative surgical margins (Nuyttens et al. 2000). In a study of 30 patients with >20 year follow-up, local control was obtained in all patients with a combination of surgery and radiation, however postoperative symptoms (weakness, stiffness, loss of motion, phantom pain) were related more to treatment than the disease itself (Dalen et al. 2003).

Low dose chemotherapy appears to offer a local control rate of approximately 75%, similar to surgery and radiation (alone or in combination).

Contemporary management of these tumors should include a multi-disciplinary approach beginning with treatment modalities that offer the lowest degree of permanent morbidity, or even mortality, progressing in step-wise fashion to potentially more morbid modalities only when more conservative measures fail.

CLINICAL PEARL

It is important to remember that this is a benign disease. A treatment goal of disease stability rather than cure may be satisfactory given the potential morbidity of curative surgery and the potential morbidity and even mortality which can be associated with radiation therapy, particularly in a young patient. Potentially mutilating surgery should not be considered a mainstay of treatment except perhaps in cases of multiply recurrent and progressive disease.

Solitary fibrous tumor

Because most of these tumors behave in a benign fashion, marginal resection is generally indicated as the first line of surgical treatment. Local recurrence and metastasis are each generally reported as < 10%. Indications for wide resection might include recurrent tumors and/or higher grade lesions with atypia.

Inflammatory myofibroblastic tumor

These tumors have a tendency for recurrence, probably in the 25% range, but the metastatic potential is unclear. At least a few tumors have metastasized. Wide resection is probably preferred where margins can be accomplished with low morbidity. Marginal resection with close observation, reserving more aggressive surgery for resection, is also a reasonable approach.

Myxofibrosarcoma

Wide surgical resection is indicated with this malignant tumor.

Low grade fibromyxoid sarcoma

The metastatic potential for this tumor is low over the short term (but increases with very long term follow-up), and the risk of local recurrence is high (Evans 2011). Therefore, surgical resection with wide margins is indicated.

Dermatofibrosarcoma protuberans

Wide surgical resection is generally curative for DFSP (Lemm et al. 2009, McArthur 2006). Adjuvant therapy is indicated with unresectable tumors and metastatic disease.

MEDICAL ONCOLOGY

Extra-abdominal fibromatosis (extra-abdominal desmoid)

Treatment varies dramatically and may consist of watching and waiting, complete surgical removal, amputation of the affected limb, radiation therapy, antiestrogens, NSAIDs, interferons, imatinib, or chemotherapy (Janinis et al. 2003). The classical initial treatment is surgery in the hope to cure the condition. However this concept may be challenged, as watch-and-wait or upfront hormonal treatments have been successful in treating fibromatosis (Bonvalot et al. 2008). When fibromatosis recurs after surgery, which happens in 20 to 35% of cases, the best approach is to watch and wait, as long as the pain is tolerable. NSAIDs should be used as pain medication, and opioids should be avoided given the risk of tolerance. If opioids must be used to control pain, then the patient becomes a candidate for medical therapy or radiotherapy. Medical therapy is the preferred treatment, as it has less long term life threatening side effects than radiotherapy. Most cases are sporadic, but some are associated with familial adenomatous polyposis (FAP), mainly the intra-abdominal cases (not discussed in this chapter). FAP and the Gardner syndrome both have mutations on chromosome 5q21-22, the locus for the adenomatous polyposis coli (APC) gene. Approximately 10 to 15% of individuals diagnosed with Gardner's syndrome, a type of FAP with extracolonic features, have mesenteric desmoid tumors (Nieuwenhuis et al. 2008). The genetics are linked to APC, which regulates the cellular level of a protein called β-catenin.

IHC assays performed on desmoid (n=195) and scar (n=18) identify β-catenin, cyclin D, p53, ER-β, c-Kit, EGFR, PDGFRs and PDGFs expression. Mutations of the gene encoding β-catenin are also observed in 85% to 98% of patients. Four mutations in two codons of exon 3 are identified: T41A (41%), S45F (36%), and S45P (4%), AA 45 (3%). The S45F-mutation confers a poor prognosis (PFS at 5 year, 23%, $P < 0.0001$) versus either T41A (57%) or non-mutated tumors (65%) (Lazar 2008) Nuclear β-catenin expression intensity is inversely correlated with the incidence of desmoid recurrence (Domont et al. 2008). In primary desmoids (n=81), β-catenin nuclear staining is less pronounced, but nuclear cyclin D reactivity increases in tumors which do recur. Strong nuclear p53 staining is observed in 17% of cases and also associated with increased recurrence. EGFR, c-KIT, ER-β, PDGFR α and β, and PDGF A and B reactivity do not correlate with desmoid outcome, however these proteins are used as therapeutic targets.

Desmoid tumors are more frequent in women, and the growth of desmoid tumors is accelerated during pregnancy, in premenopausal compared with postmenopausal women, and in females relative to males. A number of hormonal agents have been tried successfully. Such agents include tamoxifen and toremifene, progesterone, medroxyprogesterone acetate, prednisolone, testolactone and goserelin. The most common agent used is tamoxifen. Estrogen receptors have been demonstrated in desmoid tumors, although the receptor levels were low (Havry et al. 1982). Anti-estrogen binding sites distinct from ERs may modulate the action of anti-estrogens. Despite the lack of randomized studies conclusively proving the response to endocrine manipulation, several convincing series and case reports have documented stabilization and regression of desmoid tumors in response to hormones. Responses to tamoxifen have been observed in tumors carrying high levels of anti-estrogen binding sites but no or low estrogen receptors (Lim et al. 1986). In one series of 20 patients treated with tamoxifen or toremifene, 65% of cases had a clinical benefit from stabilization of disease to complete resolution (Brooks et al. 1992). There is no evidence that high dose tamoxifen is better than low dose administration.

Other hormonal approaches to treatment have been tried. One group used progestins and found that 8 of 11 patients significantly improved (Lanari 1983). The third series used testolactone and observed 4 responses out of 10 patients (Waddell et al. 1991). Therefore, the response rate to hormonal manipulation seems to be around 50%, but this approach is probably contraindicated in young female teenagers who are developing.

Desmoid tumors have been found to regress after exposure to indomethacin or sulindac. The mechanism of action is unclear, and ascorbic acid taken at the same time may have some synergistic properties (Waddell et al. 1980). Usually, NSAIDs are combined to a hormonal treatment. In fact in one series, the best outcome was a combination of tamoxifen at high dose (120 mg/day) and sulindac (300 mg/day), which successfully treated all desmoid tumors that were not surgically excised. Results after surgery were less impressive with only half of the patients responding (Hansmann et al. 2004).

Interferon therapy has been used in a few cases. In a series of 13 patients, 11 patients had some benefit (stabilization or regression) (Leithner et al. 2000).

The identification of CD117 and platelet-derived growth factor receptors expression in fibromatosis has prompted the study of imatinib for this disease. Two case reports treated with imatinib for recurrent disease experienced a partial response, with improved quality of life at 9 and 11 months (Mace et al. 2002). These observations prompted a phase II study which showed only a 6% response rate, but a stabilization rate around 80% at 4 months. Some responses were lasting for years. An extensive molecular correlative study of cKIT, PDGFR α&β, AKT and phospho-AKT, PTEN, phospho-FKHR, and β-catenin did not show significant correlation with outcome or response (Chugh et al. 2010).

Expression of somatostatin receptor subtype 2 has been demonstrated in some cases of desmoids. Two patients have been treated with an yttrium 90-labeled somatostatin analog with disease stabilization (De Pas et al. 2003).

The most common chemotherapy is a combination of doxorubicin and dacarbazine, which induces durable response in over 70% of cases. Of 180 patients with a histological diagnosis of desmoid tumor, only 12 patients required chemotherapy. The most common regimen was a combination of doxorubicin (60-90 mg/m^2) and dacarbazine (750-1000 mg/m^2) for a median of 5 cycles. A 66% response rate was observed with long lasting remissions (Patel et al 1993). The main danger is the long term cardiac toxicity of doxorubicin, especially when used in young patients. The weekly combination of vinblastine (5 mg/m^2/dose) and methotrexate (30 mg/m^2/dose) was tested in a phase II study was conducted within the Pediatric Oncology Group. Drugs were administered for 26 weeks then every other week for an additional 26 weeks. Of 26 assessable patients eight responded (31%) and 10 had stable disease. The median time to progression was 9.1 months (Skapek et al. 2007). Lastly, vinorelbine was used instead of vinblastine in combination with methotrexate. Neurotoxicity was significantly less with a similar or better objective response rate of 60%. Symptomatic relief, primarily of pain, occurred in 80% of patients (Weiss et al. 1999).

Solitary fibrous tumor recurrent

Most SFTs are relatively benign, localized, and treated with surgical resection, but about 5-10% will metastasize. The metastases are commonly of higher grade than the cells of the primary lesion. Frank malignant primary lesions have a much higher rate of recurrence (60%). One proposed treatment for unresectable disease is the combination of temozolomide with bevacizumab. Temozolomide 150 mg/m^2 was administered orally on days 1-7 and days 15-21 with bevacizumab 5 mg/kg intravenously on days 8 and 22, every 28 days to patients with hemangiopericytoma/SFT. Fourteen patients with measurable disease including 8 with metastatic disease were enrolled. The best response assessment using Choi criteria was a 79% partial response (PR) rate and a median progression-free interval of 6.3 months (Park et al. 2008). Otherwise, patients are candidates for clinical trials or the standard chemotherapy regimens used for undifferentiated sarcomas (see Introduction). Whenever the disease becomes resectable, an attempt at resection should be done (Robinson 2006). There is no CD34-targeted therapy available to date (Yang et al. 1998). CD34-targeted therapy could also affect the pluripotential hematopoietic stem cell, resulting in marrow aplasia.

Inflammatory myofibroblastic tumor

IMT is a rare mesenchymal neoplasm that harbors an anaplastic lymphoma kinase (ALK) gene rearrangement in many cases. Some patients present with a generalized inflammatory syndrome and fever. The majority of patients are children and young adults with solitary masses. ALK-1 positivity is present in about 50% of cases (Saab et al. 2010). Recently, crizotinib, an ALK inhibitor, has been used clinically with great efficacy in a patient who had IMT with an ALK translocation (Butrynski et al. 2010). The dose is 200 to 250 mg twice a day, orally. Maximum results were obtained with a combination of crizotinib and surgery. Further studies are necessary to determine the true impact of this targeted therapy.

Myxofibrosarcoma

Myxofibrosarcoma is one of the most common sarcoma subtypes of the elderly. The prognosis after surgery for localized disease is rather good with a 5-year overall survival of 77%. Five-year local recurrence and distant metastases rate are 18% and 15%, respectively. As with any other sarcoma, tumor size, grade, and margins are predictors of survival. A positive surgical margin is the only statistically significant prognostic factor for local relapse, and a higher histological grade correlates with distant recurrence (Sanfilippo et al. 2010). Chemotherapy for metastatic disease uses the standard regimens described in the Introduction. Recently, MET overexpression has been described in primary myxofibrosarcomas, MET overexpression is frequent; 7q gains and mRNA up regulation are observed. MET overexpression is associated with a worse outcome and could lead to the testing of targeted therapy with MET inhibitors in this patient population (Lee et al. 2010).

Low grade fibromyxoid sarcoma

Surgical resection is the treatment of choice for this sarcoma. Recurrence may occur in less than 5% of cases. Responses to chemotherapy have been poor, and with the limited experience, must be considered investigational (Folpe et al 2000).

Dermatofibrosarcoma protuberans

The t(17;22) translocation resulting in a COL1A1-PDGFB fusion protein is present in >95% of DFSP cases. In a series of 275 cases of DFSP, 13 (4.7%) have a fibrosarcomatous component, and 15% of these develop metastases. The fusion-gene is detected and expressed in all cases, both within the classical and fibrosarcomatous component, and before and after imatinib. The kinase mTOR is switched-off, despite the phosphorylation of its effectors. Phosphorylation of S6 and 4EBP1 is restricted to the fibrosarcomatous component. Thus, DFSP-derived fibrosarcoma maintains the fusion-gene and thus sensitivity to imatinib, but responses are short-lasting (Stacchiotti et al. 2011).

Imatinib mesylate is the treatment of choice for large DFSP. In a study of 25 adults with DFSP, the COL1A1-PDGFB fusion gene was detected in 21 by fluorescence in situ hybridization analysis. Imatinib, which has activity against platelet-derived growth factor receptor β, yielded a 36% response rate in these patients. The median tumor size decrease was 20.0% (range, -12.5 to 100%). Imatinib is also recommended in the neoadjuvant setting when surgery is difficult or mutilating or in nonresectable DFSP (Kérob 2010). Sixteen and eight patients with unresectable DFSP were treated with daily imatinib at 400 to 800 mg. Nine patients had a fibrosarcomatous DFSP and metastases were present in seven patients. Eleven patients (46%) had a partial response. The median time to progression was 1.7 years. And median overall survival time has not been reached with a 1-year survival rate of 87.5%. The response rates and time to progression did not differ between patients taking 400 mg or higher (Rutkowski et al. 2010).

Thus, the current treatment of choice is now imatinib at 400 mg daily when complete tumor resection is not possible or mutilating. Newer PDGFB inhibitors may become available for clinical use (Levitzki 2004).

RADIATION ONCOLOGY

Fibroblastic and myofibroblastic tumors represent a heterogeneous group of tumors for which radiation plays an important role. Radiation can be effective in preventing local recurrence in the aggressive subtypes, both malignant as well as selected benign varieties. In many of the subtypes, the role of radiation is contested. This is particularly true with heterotopic ossification prophylaxis and desmoid tumors. It is clear that radiation has a role in both these tumor subtypes, but the exact indications are disputed, often heavily. As always, the risk of radiation therapy, particularly second malignancy, has to be weighed against the benefit to local control.

Nodular fasciitis (including ischemic fasciitis)

This benign lesion has negligible risk of recurrence following surgery. Consequently, there is no role for radiation therapy.

Myositis ossificans (heterotopic ossification)

Heterotopic ossification has a broad spectrum of clinical presentations, and radiation therapy plays a role in prophylaxis against development or recurrence. The exact population that is likely to receive the best benefit is heavily disputed (Pakos et al. 2004, Vavken et al. 2009).

Extra-abdominal fibromatosis (extra-abdominal desmoid)

There is a long history of utilizing radiation in the treatment of aggressive fibromatosis or desmoid tumors. Again, the exact clinic conditions for utilization of radiation therapy are disputed. This can be seen in the multiple publications that have concluded different roles for radiation therapy (Jelinek et al. 2001, Nuyttens et al. 2000, Guadagnolo et al. 2008, Jabbari et al. 2009). It is of great importance to limit the use of aggressive local therapies that may significantly impact morbidity when the natural history of this disease can be quite indolent. In cases where further surgery would be associated with significant morbidity, radiation therapy clearly has a role.

Solitary fibrous tumor recurrent

This relatively rare entity is probably best managed by surgical excision. However, cases where surgery cannot be performed due to the location or the medical condition of the patient can be treated with radiation therapy (Bisceglia et al. 2011).

Inflammatory myofibroblastic tumor

This entity can be locally aggressive and rarely metastatic. Ideally, resection with negative margins is the treatment of choice. In patients with residual, recurrent, or unresectable disease, radiation therapy can be implemented and typically results in good local control (Kovach et al. 2006).

Myxofibrosarcoma

Typically aggressive and malignant, myxofibrosarcomas have a high rate of local recurrence and distant metastasis despite aggressive therapy. Rates of local recurrence range of 18-30%. Consequently, radiation therapy is utilized in nearly all cases (Haglund et al. 2010, Sanfilippo et al. 2011).

Low grade fibromyxoid sarcoma

The natural history of this sarcoma is quite complex. It is known to have high local recurrences and metastasis; however these recurrences can be extremely indolent (Evans 2011, Guillou et al. 2007). Consequently, appropriate treatment recommendations are highly dependent upon clinical factors with observation after resection being the standard. The role of radiation in this entity is probably relegated to palliation or to prevent recurrences that would be associated with significant morbidity.

Dermatofibrosarcoma protuberans

The mainstay of therapy is complete surgical excision with wide margins (2-3 cm preferred). However, with very large tumors not amenable to complete resection, adjuvant radiation therapy is an option (50-70 Gy).

CASES

Case 6.1 Nodular fasciitis

Clinical history and presentation

The patient is a 34 year old woman who presents with a six month history of a left elbow mass which she noted spontaneously and which has been persistent. She relates intermittent aching pain associated with the lesion. She does not feel that it has grown substantially in size over the past several months.

Physical examination reveals a 1×3 cm mass over the lateral aspect of the elbow within the substance of the brachioradialis proximally. It is mildly tender on palpation.

Surgical findings and comments

Findings at surgery reveal a dense fibrous mass. Marginal excision is performed.

Radiology findings

The MR images (**Case figs 6.1a** through **6.1c**) show a mass in the extensor muscles of the proximal forearm. This is an unusual case because it is inter-muscular and not subcutaneous. Furthermore, the forearm is the most common location for NF; however, it usually affects the volar aspect, not the radial aspect as in this case. Note the linear high signal extensions along the superior aspect (**Case fig. 6.1b**), this has been termed the fascial tail sign and is suggestive of NF. Unfortunately, no IV contrast was given preventing assessment of vascularity or necrosis.

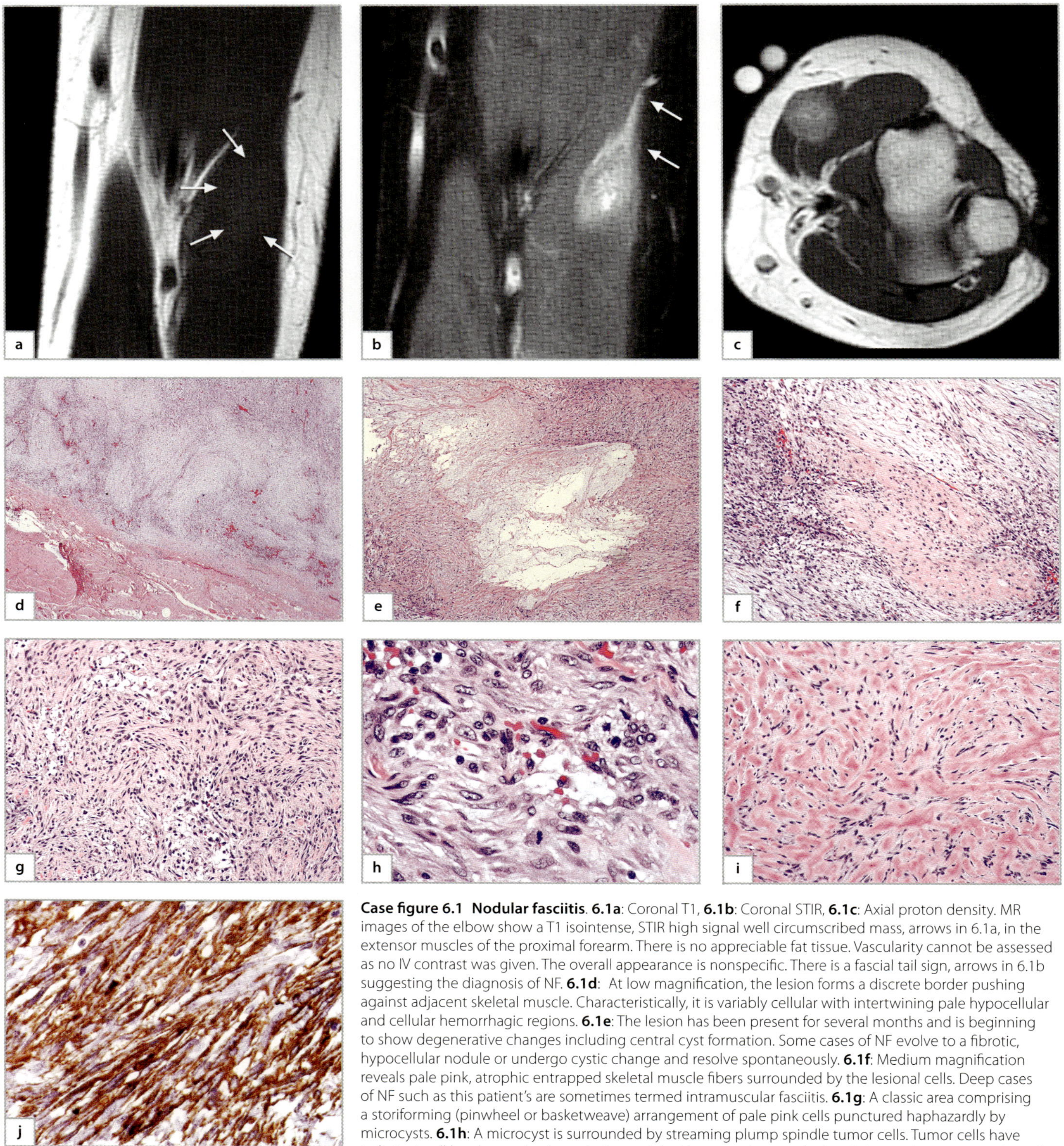

Case figure 6.1 Nodular fasciitis. **6.1a**: Coronal T1, **6.1b**: Coronal STIR, **6.1c**: Axial proton density. MR images of the elbow show a T1 isointense, STIR high signal well circumscribed mass, arrows in 6.1a, in the extensor muscles of the proximal forearm. There is no appreciable fat tissue. Vascularity cannot be assessed as no IV contrast was given. The overall appearance is nonspecific. There is a fascial tail sign, arrows in 6.1b suggesting the diagnosis of NF. **6.1d**: At low magnification, the lesion forms a discrete border pushing against adjacent skeletal muscle. Characteristically, it is variably cellular with intertwining pale hypocellular and cellular hemorrhagic regions. **6.1e**: The lesion has been present for several months and is beginning to show degenerative changes including central cyst formation. Some cases of NF evolve to a fibrotic, hypocellular nodule or undergo cystic change and resolve spontaneously. **6.1f**: Medium magnification reveals pale pink, atrophic entrapped skeletal muscle fibers surrounded by the lesional cells. Deep cases of NF such as this patient's are sometimes termed intramuscular fasciitis. **6.1g**: A classic area comprising a storiforming (pinwheel or basketweave) arrangement of pale pink cells punctured haphazardly by microcysts. **6.1h**: A microcyst is surrounded by streaming plump spindle tumor cells. Tumor cells have indistinct cell borders and pale vesicular nuclei with a granular or reticulated chromatin pattern and small nucleoli. The cytoplasm is pale eosinophilic and variably vacuolated. Notice the mitotic figure. Mitoses are common in this patient's lesion (ranging from 5-10 per 10 high power microscopic fields). **6.1i**: An area of the lesion containing dense keloidal or scar-like collagen. Such dense fibrosis is not uncommon especially in mature lesions that have persisted for several months. **6.1j**: Smooth muscle actin antibody stain. The myofibroblastic lesional cells are strongly reactive. Notice the pattern of expression: cytoplasmic with staining accentuated at the rims of the cells resulting in a 'tram track' parallel linear appearance. This tram track pattern differs from the staining pattern in smooth muscle cells which is more diffusely cytoplasmic without peripheral enhancement.

Pathology findings

Gross features

The specimen consists of portions of pale pink, rubbery soft tissue measuring in aggregate 3.0 cm. Sections reveal pale yellow, glistening firm surfaces. A small piece is placed fresh in RPMI (a type of tissue culture medium) for possible cytogenetics. The remainder is submitted for microscopic evaluation.

Microscopic features

Low magnification: The lesion is round with a pushing rather than permeative border (**Case fig. 6.1d**). At medium magnification, the tumor shows central cystic degeneration (**Case fig. 6.1e**). Although it appears sharply circumscribed at low magnification, a few atrophic skeletal muscle cells are caught up within the tumor (**Case fig. 6.1f**).

High magnification: Higher magnification discloses a cellular lesion composed of elongate to plump spindle cells arranged in both fascicles and a storiform pattern (**Case fig. 6.1g**). Additionally, multiple areas of tumor dissolution are present in which the lesional cells are pulling away from each other and thus forming microcysts. This teasing away of cells from each other in its early phase is compared to the appearance of fibroblasts in a cell culture dish or more prosaically to the stretching of taffy candy as it is pulled apart. Other characteristic features of this lesion include extravasated red blood cells notably without hemosiderin deposition, sprinkles of chronic inflammatory cells, and normal mitotic figures (**Case fig. 6.1h**). This tumor also contains areas of collagen deposition almost mimicking hypertrophic scar or keloid (**Case fig. 6.1i**). Of note, there is no necrosis, no marked cellular pleomorphism, and no atypical mitotic figures.

Special studies: Characteristic of this lesion, tumor cells diffusely and strongly express smooth muscle actin but not desmin by IHC (**Case fig. 6.1j**). The pattern of expression of smooth muscle actin is a clue to the nature of the cells, as myofibroblasts often show accentuated peripheral staining in the cell cytoplasm mimicking a tram or train track. By contrast, most smooth muscle cells express SMA in a diffuse cytoplasmic pattern. This difference is because the myofibroblasts contain fewer smooth muscle actin positive myofilaments than smooth muscle cells, and the myofilaments are peripherally placed rather than widely dispersed in the cytoplasm as in smooth muscle cells (Eyden et al. 2009).

Pathologic differential or, why isn't it one of the following?

Inflammatory myofibroblastic tumor (IMT): Both tumors contain plump to spindled myofibroblasts. One pattern of IMT closely resembles NF with cells scattered in a myxoid or edematous matrix with many inflammatory cells (lymphocytes and plasma cells primarily sometimes with a few eosinophils). However, microcysts and acute hemorrhage are usually absent in IMT. According to some experts, inflammation is more conspicuous in IMT with some tumors containing aggregates of plasma cells (Kempson et al. 2001, Fisher et al. 2011). Some IMTs contain polygonal myofibroblasts with pale nuclei and prominent nucleoli resembling ganglion cells; these cells look similar to the ganglion like cells of proliferative myositis and proliferative fasciitis. Clinically, NF usually has a rapid course with noticeable growth over a few weeks and forms a mass seldom larger than 5.0 cm. It can be sharply circumscribed from surrounding tissues while IMT is infiltrative. Some IMT are larger than fasciitis lesions (up to 17 cm in diameter). Approximately 50% of inflammatory myofibroblastic tumors express ALK that can be detected by IHC. Although not specific to IMT, this enzyme is not expressed in NF.

Spindle cell sarcoma, not otherwise specified: Most spindle cell sarcomas as cellular as NF will contain at least a few cells with nuclear pleomorphism (consisting of enlarged, hyperchromatic nuclei with coarse chromatin, irregular chromatin distribution, sharp nuclear indentations, etc). Necrosis and atypical mitoses, if present, would also distinguish spindle cell sarcoma, NOS, from NF. Finally, the microcyst formation, microhemorrhages, and tram-track smooth muscle actin reactivity are classic histopathologic features of NF that would not be evident in a high grade spindle cell sarcoma such as adult fibrosarcoma, fibrosarcoma arising in dermatofibrosarcoma protuberans, or synovial sarcoma.

Low grade myofibroblastic sarcoma (LGMS): Architecturally, this sarcoma is fascicular in most cases rather than mixed fascicular/storiform or exclusively storiform as seen in NF. It is more uniformly cellular, is infiltrative, and exhibits more prominent nuclear hyperchromasia. The microhemorrhages and microcysts of NF are absent. Most examples lack inflammation, or it is very sparse unlike in nodular fasciitis which usually contains lymphocytes, plasma cells and/or eosinophils clustered or randomly sprinkled in nearly every microscopic field. Neither LGMS nor NF expresses anaplastic lymphoma kinase (ALK) by IHC (Qiu et al. 2008).

Oncology approach

Medical oncology

This is a benign lesion with no role for chemotherapy.

Radiation oncology

As the lesion is benign and has negligible risk for local recurrence, radiation therapy is not indicated.

Patient outcome

As would be expected for this lesion, the patient is healthy with no recurrence at four years after excision.

Case table 6.1 Summary pathology findings of Case 6.1

Diagnosis	Nodular fasciitis
Size	3.0 cm in aggregate
Location	Deep forearm muscle
Margin status	Positive
Histologic grade	Not graded: benign
Pathologic stage (TNM classification)	Not staged: benign

Case 6.2 Myositis ossificans (heterotopic ossification)

Clinical history and presentation

A twenty four year old man, an active duty marine corporal, is referred because of a painful, swollen thigh that began to become symptomatic shortly after he sustained a fall on a long training run three weeks previously. The pain is constant but exacerbated by running and jumping. Physical exam reveals swelling in the middle portion of the quadriceps with tenderness to palpation. He demonstrates full range of motion accompanied by a moderate increase in pain. There is no joint effusion. Initial X-rays (see below) are consistent with soft tissue injury.

Because of continued pain with consequent limitation of activity despite conservative management including rest and anti-inflammatory agents, the patient undergoes surgical removal of the lesion 5 months after his presentation.

Surgical findings and comments

At surgery, an ovoid, firm mass is marginally excised from the quadriceps muscle.

Radiology findings

This case (**Case figs 6.2a–6.2c**) comprises a series of hip radiographs, each taken about three weeks apart. The initial film shows amorphous calcification in the anterior thigh. There is no erosion or periosteal reaction of the adjacent femur. The calcification pattern does not look like osteoid, and in fact has a peripheral predominance of calcification. Three weeks later, the calcification is clearly becoming denser peripherally and there is cortication developing on the surface of the lesion. An additional three weeks later, the lesion shows continued increasing peripheral density, and has also developed visible trabeculae indicating cancellous bone. This pattern of evolution is definitive for the diagnosis MO and no biopsy should be performed.

Pathology findings

Gross features

The specimen comprises a 6 cm oval, firm, non-compressible mass with scant attached skeletal muscle. Serial sectioning reveals a continuous, several millimeter thick shell of gritty, white tissue surrounding a soft, and tan to red interior. There is no necrosis or hemorrhage.

Microscopic features

Low magnification: Striking zonation is present. Consistent with the eggshell-like gritty rim noted on gross examination, the perimeter of the tumor comprises a narrow band of fibrous tissue with underneath a layer of mineralized woven bone (**Case fig. 6.2d**). Some of the bone is mature and closely resembles normal trabecular bone (**Case fig. 6.2e**).

High magnification: At medium magnification, some areas of tumor comprise intramembranous type bone formation (**Case fig. 6.2f**) imitating the appearance of an early fracture callus. In another region, the lesional bone contains a core of chondroid matrix simulating endochondral ossification (**Case fig. 6.2g**). The center of the lesion resembles NF and is composed of variably cellular fascicles of spindle cells with an alternating myxoid to collagenous background (**Case fig. 6.2h**). At high magnification, the elongate cells of the center feature vesicular spindle nuclei and lavender or amphophilic cytoplasm consistent with fibroblasts or myofibroblasts (**Case fig. 6.2i**). Mitoses are present but are not atypical (**Case fig. 6.2i**).

Special studies: Because the lesion exhibits classic pathologic features of zonation with reactive bone rimming a NF like center, special studies are considered unnecessary.

Pathologic differential or, why isn't it one of the following?

Osteosarcoma: Osteosarcoma can rarely occur in the soft tissues. Although it may exhibit a zonal architecture, the zones are reversed compared to MO in that the most immature cellular tissue composes the perimeter with more mature looking tissues in the center. The central part of MO can look atypical if sampled early in the course of development. However, nuclear pleomorphism, necrosis and atypical mitotic figures are absent in MO but are common in most soft tissue osteosarcomas. Radiologic correlation with gradual evolution of the lesion over several months is also reassuring that the lesion is reactive.

Fibrodysplasia ossificans progressiva (previously termed MO progressiva or Munchmeyer disease): This is a rare autosomal dominant condition leading to the formation of numerous foci of heterotopic bone throughout the soft tissues. Patients also have skeletal anomalies such as deformed toes and short thumbs. It is caused by mutation of the *ACVR1* gene (chromosome 2q23-24). Most patients are diagnosed by the age of 5 years. Biopsy should be avoided as surgical trauma stimulates more heterotopic bone formation.

Metastatic carcinoma with heterotopic bone formation: Some carcinomas metastatic to the soft tissues can elicit reactive bone formation. These tumors should feature marked pleomorphism, are usually epithelial in appearance, and should be reactive for epithelial markers such as EMA and various keratins.

Ossifying fibromyxoid tumor (OFMT): This uncommon tumor of subcutaneous tissue and muscle often forms a shell or woven or lamellar bone. The interior is strikingly different from MO and consists of bland, small round to polygonal tumor cells with sometimes a few spindle tumor cells in areas of fibrosis. There is no resemblance to NF as is notable in the central area of MO. The OFMT tumor cells are often reactive for S-100 protein and have been reported to express desmin, but reactivity for smooth muscle actin (which is positive in MO in myofibroblastic spindle cells) is unusual.

Sarcomas with metaplastic bone formation such as some examples of synovial sarcoma, myxoid liposarcoma, dedifferentiated liposarcoma, and malignant peripheral nerve sheath tumor: in practical terms, these tumors will demonstrate features of malignancy and features particular to their cell of differentiation. Such sarcomas would not be mistaken microscopically for MO.

Case fig. 6.2j illustrates the number of fibroblastic/myofibroblastic tumors resected or biopsied at the University of New Mexico Health Sciences Center for the time period 2000-2010 excluding myxofibrosarcoma. This number is representative of a medium sized academic orthopaedic surgery practice. The majority of tumors are reactive or benign.

Oncology approach

Medical oncology

This is a benign lesion with no role for chemotherapy.

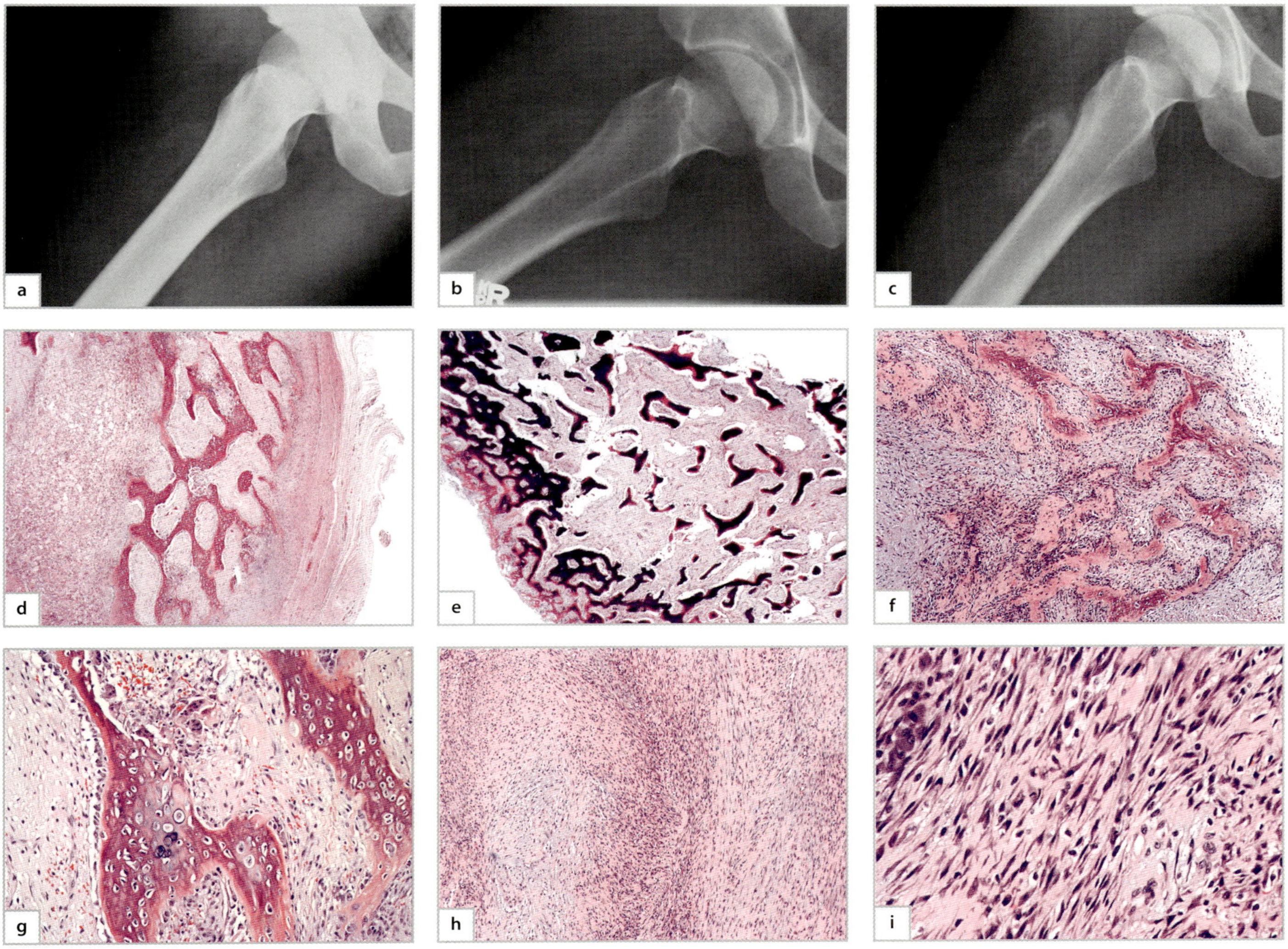

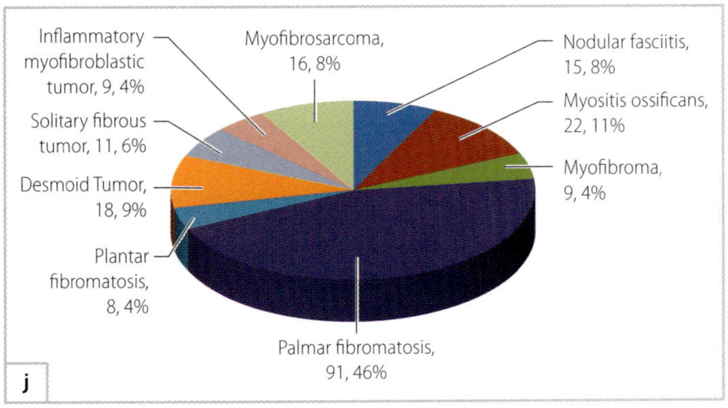

Case figure 6.2 Myositis ossificans. **6.2a**: Shows amorphous calcification in the soft tissues. These calcifications appear more coarse than osteoid and there is a suggestion of peripheral dominance to the calcification. **6.2b**: Shows increasing peripheral calcification and developing cortex. Figure 6-2c shows mature cortical bone with central trabeculae of cancellous bone. **6.2d**: Low magnification reveals the outermost fibrous capsule under which is a band of immature (woven) bone. **6.2e**: Some of the bone is mature (cancellous) and closely resembles trabecular bone. As MO evolves over several months to years, it may progressively ossify and form not only trabecular but cortical bone and bone marrow. Eventually, a few cases may completely resolve. In this photograph, marrow fat and hematopoietic elements are absent. **6.2f**: Myositis ossificans. This area of the tumor features intramembranous type bone formation. **6.2g**: Here the lesional bone mimics endochondral ossification with a residual faint blue core of what appears to be cartilage. Notice the rimming osteoblasts on one side of the new bone and the line of osteoclasts on the opposite surface consistent with reactive but lesional rather than neoplastic bone of a true monoclonal neoplasm. **6.2h**: The center of the lesion is histologically indistinguishable from NF (medium magnification). **6.2i**: At high magnification, the center of the lesion contains streams of myofibroblasts with pale lavender (amphophilic) to raggedly vacuolated cytoplasm and indistinct cell borders. Collagen is present in the background. In the upper left corner is a group of round cells with eccentric nuclei. These are myofibroblasts or osteoblasts. Two mitotic figures indicate brisk proliferative activity. **6.2j**: Common Fibroblastic/Myofibroblastic Tumors Resected at UNM HSC 2000-2010 (n= 199). The great majority of tumors are reactive or benign lesions. (This pie chart excludes myxofibrosarcoma, now considered by most pathologists a fibroblastic/myofibroblastic sarcoma.)

Radiation oncology

In this case, radiation therapy is probably not indicated. However, if the patient had a recurrence, I would consider single fraction immediate (within 48 hour) after surgical resection of the recurrence. Radiation therapy to prevent recurrence of heterotopic ossification is a well known treatment strategy. Typically this is given in the postoperative period, but alternatively can be performed preoperatively within 24 hours of the surgery. Multiple randomized trials have demonstrated that radiation therapy has a role in preventing recurrence and development of heterotopic ossification. Unfortunately, the results of these randomized studies are conflicting. In over one hundred publicized studies on prevention of heterotopic ossification following hip arthroplasty, no clear treatment strategy has been proven superior. Other therapies, namely NSAID treatments may be equally effective. Two recent meta-analyses highlight the controversy between NSAIDs and radiation therapy well (Pakos 2004, Vavken 2009). Once a heterotopic ossification develops after surgery, radiation therapy does appear to be the first choice in preventing recurrence. However, in de novo prophylaxis following surgery, controversy exists regarding indications for prophylaxis with radiation therapy. In this case, the preceding trauma likely caused the formation of the lesion, as it does not involve a joint or more importantly bone surgery in a joint, recurrence seems less likely. Consequently radiation therapy is not necessary.

Patient outcome

The patient recovers completely and has had no recurrence 3.5 years after presentation. There is a slight risk for regrowth of the lesion if it is resected in the early phase of the process. However, the patient underwent surgical excision at the appropriate time of approximately 6 months after his initiating muscle injury. Lesions removed at 6-12 months after trauma only rarely regrow.

Case table 6.2 Summary pathology findings of Case 6.2

Diagnosis	Myositis ossificans
Size	6.0 cm
Location	Quadriceps muscle
Margin status	Negative
Histologic grade	Not graded: benign
Pathologic stage (TNM classification)	Not staged: benign

Case 6.3 Inclusion body fibromatosis (infantile digital fibroma/fibromatosis)

Clinical history and presentation

The patient is an 11 month old boy with a three month history of a left toe mass which was noted spontaneously by his mother and has progressively slowly grown in size. His parents had previously brought the baby's toe mass to the attention of their pediatrician who advised biopsy. The biopsy was performed at an outlying hospital, and the patient's parents were subsequently referred to an orthopaedic oncologist.

On examination, the patient's left middle toe reveals a keloid like appearing firm mass arising from the lateral aspect. It is fixed to underlying deep tissue. The overlying skin is smooth and erythematous but nontender. The patient has no other masses or history of any other toe or finger masses.

Surgical findings and comments

A firm, small, superficial nodule is marginally excised from the lateral aspect of the left middle toe.

Radiology findings

No imaging is performed.

Pathology findings

Gross features

The specimen comprises a 1.6 cm ovoid tan-white nodule. Cross sections are homogeneous and tan to white. It is entirely submitted for microscopic review.

Microscopic features

Low magnification: At low magnification, the tumor expands the dermis and forms an elevated nodule (**Case fig. 6.3a**).

High magnification: Characteristically, the tumor entraps eccrine ducts (residual skin adnexal structures) (**Case fig. 6.3b**). The tumor is cellular and composed of short, interwoven bundles of plump spindle cells. It is cellular with a pink, slightly collagenized background. There is no necrosis and no variability in architecture. High magnification discloses characteristic round, eosinophilic inclusions in the myofibroblasts (**Case fig. 6.3c**). The inclusions are located in the cytoplasm of the plump spindle cells, and several are paranuclear. This patient has many of these inclusions readily identifiable on the standard hematoxylin and eosin stain. They are not always so prominent, and some tumors may contain only rare scattered inclusions. Consistent with fibroblasts or myofibroblasts, the nuclei of the tumor cells are pale or vesicular with fine chromatin and small nucleoli. Cytoplasm is pale pink to lavender with ill-defined cell borders, and wavy pink collagen fibers flow around the cells.

Special studies: The inclusions are highlighted glassy red on a Masson's trichrome stain (**Case fig. 6.3d**). In this field, the inclusions can be compared with red blood cells. In addition to reacting positively on a trichrome stain, the inclusions are also positive for smooth muscle actin by IHC especially after pre-treatment with hydrogen peroxide, and stain black with iron hematoxylin. They are negative on the periodic acid-Schiff (PAS) and Alcian blue stains. The tumor cells themselves express smooth muscle actin, desmin in many cases, and sometimes h-caldesmon (the last is unusual for myofibroblasts). Similar to many examples of deep and some examples of superficial fibromatosis, tumor cells may also exhibit nuclear β-catenin reactivity (Laskin et al. 2009).

Pathologic differential or, why isn't it one of the following?

The presentation in infancy in the second to fifth toe (only rarely is the great toe involved) or the second to fifth fingers (the thumb very rarely affected) and the presence of classic inclusions rarely permit any other diagnostic consideration. A few tumors in the fingers and toes of infants with the classic dermal presentation and morphology may not contain inclusions. These can still be diagnosed if all other features are present. However, the tumor can occur in older children and adults and at sites other than the hands and feet. In such instances, fibromatosis may enter the differential. In these unusual clinical circumstances, inclusion bodies must be identified to enable diagnosis. Some authors suggest that tumors with actin positive inclusion bodies in myofibroblasts that occur in adults or older children should be considered a heterogeneous group of entities and that the term, infantile digital fibroma, should be maintained as it labels a discrete specific tumor of specialized dermal myofibroblasts (Laskin et al. 2009).

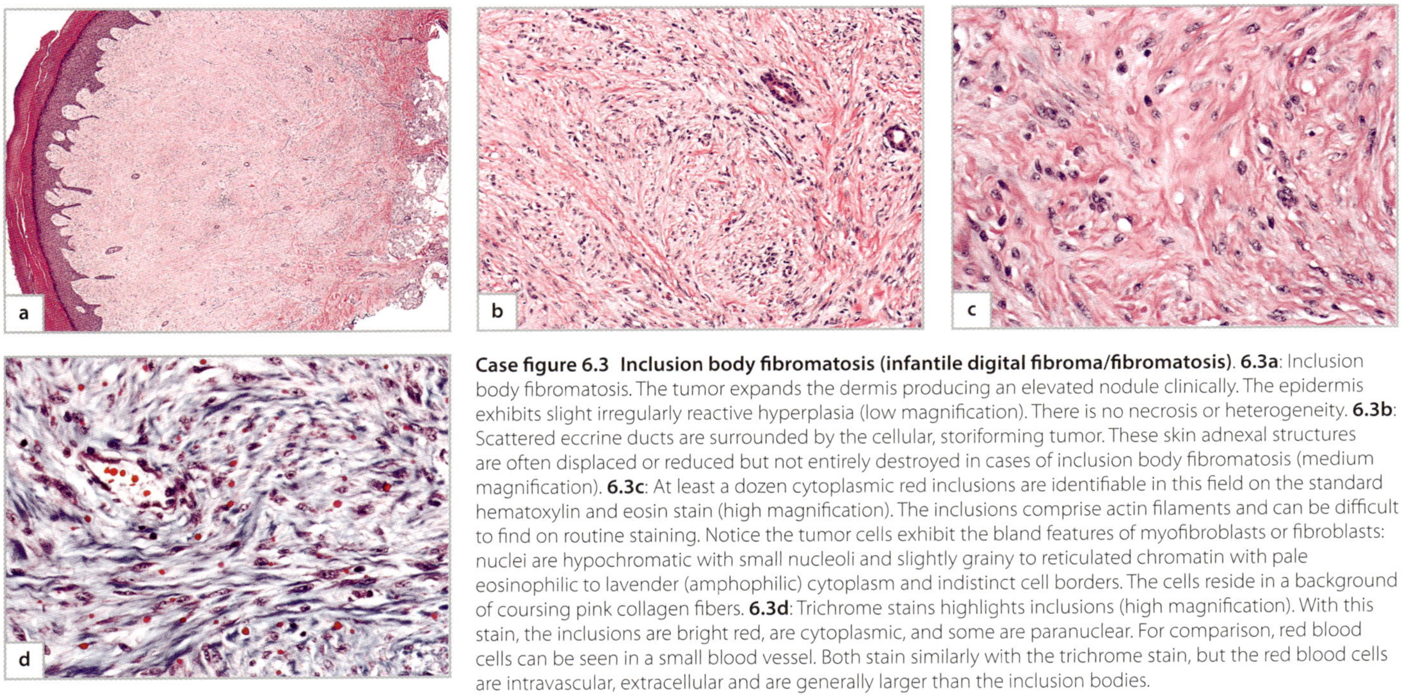

Case figure 6.3 Inclusion body fibromatosis (infantile digital fibroma/fibromatosis). **6.3a**: Inclusion body fibromatosis. The tumor expands the dermis producing an elevated nodule clinically. The epidermis exhibits slight irregularly reactive hyperplasia (low magnification). There is no necrosis or heterogeneity. **6.3b**: Scattered eccrine ducts are surrounded by the cellular, storiforming tumor. These skin adnexal structures are often displaced or reduced but not entirely destroyed in cases of inclusion body fibromatosis (medium magnification). **6.3c**: At least a dozen cytoplasmic red inclusions are identifiable in this field on the standard hematoxylin and eosin stain (high magnification). The inclusions comprise actin filaments and can be difficult to find on routine staining. Notice the tumor cells exhibit the bland features of myofibroblasts or fibroblasts: nuclei are hypochromatic with small nucleoli and slightly grainy to reticulated chromatin with pale eosinophilic to lavender (amphophilic) cytoplasm and indistinct cell borders. The cells reside in a background of coursing pink collagen fibers. **6.3d**: Trichrome stains highlights inclusions (high magnification). With this stain, the inclusions are bright red, are cytoplasmic, and some are paranuclear. For comparison, red blood cells can be seen in a small blood vessel. Both stain similarly with the trichrome stain, but the red blood cells are intravascular, extracellular and are generally larger than the inclusion bodies.

Oncology approach

Medical oncology

This is a benign lesion with no role for chemotherapy.

Radiation oncology

This is typically a self-limited disease best managed by conservative excision or simple biopsy. No role for radiation therapy has been demonstrated. Radiation therapy in this age group is to be avoided if at all possible due to effects on growth and potential second malignancy.

Patient outcome

The patient is doing well six years after presentation. Unlike some other patients with infantile digital fibromatosis, he neither presented with multiple nodules (40-60% of patients), he did not develop additional lesions (up to 20% of patients) and suffered no recurrences (~70% of patients) after simple excision of the left middle toe nodule.

Case table 6.3 Summary pathology findings of Case 6.3

Diagnosis	Infantile digital fibromatosis (inclusion body fibromatosis)
Size	1.6 cm
Location	Dermis of lateral aspect of left middle toe
Margin status	Positive
Histologic grade	Not graded: benign
Pathologic stage (TNM classification)	Not staged: benign

Case 6.4 Extra-abdominal fibromatosis (deep fibromatosis, desmoid)

Clinical history and presentation

The patient is a 58 year old man who presents with a two year history of a right arm mass. He reports initially injuring the arm when he banged it against a door. He noted no significant swelling or ecchymosis at the time of injury but noted a small soft tissue mass several weeks later that proceeded to enlarge slowly but progressively. Three months prior to presentation the mass stopped enlarging but has become increasingly symptomatic. Symptoms are described as tenderness and a constant dull ache he considers 6 out of 10 on a scale of increasing pain intensity.

Physical examination reveals a firm, deeply situated mass over the lateral aspect of the right mid arm. The limits are poorly defined on palpation. It is fixed to underlying deep tissue. It is moderately tender.

Surgical findings and comments

Because of the infiltrative nature of the tumor on imaging and physical examination, concern for malignancy is present. Open biopsy is performed with finding of a deep, infiltrative, dense fibrous soft tissue mass.

Marginal resection is performed one month following the biopsy.

One year later he is noted to have a small but symptomatic area of local recurrence. He is placed on Imatinib.

Six months following initiation of Imatinib he is noted to have slow progression of disease. Surgical excision is repeated with an attempt to obtain wider margins while retaining function and minimizing morbidity. Postoperatively, Imatinib is resumed.

One year later he remains on Imatinib. He is noted to have a small area of recurrent disease but wishes to observe and remain on Imatinib for now.

Radiology findings

The MR images (**Case figs 6.4a** through **6.4i**) show an infiltrative mass in the mid-arm that appears to partially invade the deltoid muscle. The mass has uniform intense enhancement. No fascial tail sign was seen. Although this proved to be a benign lesion, it has an overall aggressive appearance worrisome for malignancy. The very high signal on STIR sequences indicates this is a highly cellular fibromatosis and the risk of recurrence is especially high. Post-operative follow up imaging (**Case figs 6.4d** and **6.4e**) shows a fluid collection in the surgical bed with smooth, uniform thickness walls that have no nodularity or focalized enhancement. This is the typical appearance of a post-operative seroma. Subsequent follow up imaging (**Case figs 6.4f** through **6.4i**) show the seroma has resolved, but unfortunately, there is a new enhancing mass indicating recurrent disease. Note how the signal characteristics and infiltrative margins are similar to the original tumor.

Pathology findings

Gross features

The incisional biopsy specimen consists of several fragments of white, slightly rubbery tissue aggregating to 1.5 cm.

The resection specimen measures 8.7 × 6.2 × 3.2 cm and consists of tumor surfaced by scant skeletal muscle and fibroadipose tissue. Cut sections reveal a gray to white, vaguely trabeculated interior with focal hemorrhage and softening consistent with the effect of prior biopsy performed approximately one month previously (**Case fig. 6.4j**). The tumor closely approaches to within 0.1cm of the inked surgical margin.

Microscopic features

Low magnification: (The resection specimen only is described because it is histologically identical to the biopsy.) At low magnification, the tumor consists of long bundles of spindle cells that compress tumor blood vessels into thin slightly curved shapes (**Case fig. 6.4k**). In other areas, the tumor causes ectatic dilatation of the vessels (**Case fig. 6.4l**).

High magnification: At medium magnification, a less cellular area of the tumor is more fibrotic with dense collagen formation (**Case fig. 6.4m**). However, most of the tumor is more cellular and also contains scattered mast cells (**Case fig. 6.4n**). Mast cells are typical of deep fibromatosis. The tumor cells show characteristic features of fibroblasts or myofibroblasts and would in fact be interchangeable histologically with the myofibroblasts of NF or MO.

Special studies: Typical for most cases of deep fibromatosis (70-80% of adult tumors), at least some of the tumor cells aberrantly express β-catenin in the nucleus (**Case fig. 6.4o**). β-catenin is a common protein usually found in the cytoplasm but in some tumors, desmoid being one of them, abnormal nuclear accumulation is also found. One group recently reported that *lower intensity* of nuclear β catenin expression correlated with a *higher* rate of recurrence (Lazar et al. 2008).

To determine whether particular medical treatment approaches may be helpful, additional analyses are performed. Tumor cells are positive for platelet derived growth factor receptor (PDGF), negative for c-kit, and negative for estrogen receptor (all stains are immunohistochemical meaning that specific dye-tagged antibodies are applied to fixed tissue sections with appropriate controls also run).

Several large genetic studies of deep fibromatosis have reported that patients with tumors containing a mutation of the β-catenin gene, *CTNNB1*, or patients whose tumors feature trisomy 8 are at increased risk for recurrence (Lazar et al. 2008, Fletcher et al. 1995). By standard testing of losses and gains of chromosomes, a recent French analysis of 194 patients found that three quarters had genetically normal tumors at this chromosomal level of examination of the genome (Salas et al. 2010). However, 82% of patients studied at the more discriminating molecular level of individual genes had mutations of the CTNNB1 gene and 7% had mutations of the adenosis polyposis coli gene (*APC* gene), the gene involved in Gardner syndrome.

The specific mutation site on the *CTNNB1* gene may also confer greater risk for local recurrence (Lazar et al. 2008). *APC* gene mutations impede the ability of the gene's product to control β-catenin activation and represent another route to development of deep fibromatosis. Mutations of the three prime end of the *APC* gene lead to a variant presentation comprising multiple desmoid tumors without colonic polyps or other Gardner syndrome associated tumors. This form of deep fibromatosis is known as Familial infiltrative fibromatosis (FIF) or hereditary desmoid disease (HDD) (Lips et al. 2008).

Thus, current molecular analysis of a deep fibromatosis tumor can provide some information helping predict its behavior. The tumor remains a fascinating enigma, however, regarding the molecular explanation of its dual nature: marked propensity for aggressive local growth yet utter lack of ability to metastasize.

Pathologic differential or, why isn't it one of the following?

Exuberant scar: This enters the differential in a patient with a history of trauma. Unfortunately, deep fibromatosis may also occur at the site of tissue injury, making such a history less diagnostically helpful. Exuberant scars are usually smaller than deep fibromatoses. Scar tissue generally has a rounded non-permeative border with adjacent tissues, unlike fibromatosis which is permeative. Scar tissue is often more heterogeneous with areas of granulation tissue, inflammation, and marked hemorrhage. The thin, slightly curving vessels and/or ectatic vessels of desmoid tumors are not generally seen in scar tissue. Nuclear β-catenin reactivity can also be supportive, as scar myofibroblasts will show only cytoplasmic reactivity.

Superficial fibromatosis: The site of the lesion is useful, because superficial fibromatoses occur only in the hands, feet, and penis, sites that would be unusual for deep fibromatosis. Plantar and palmar fibromatosis can be hypercellular and may contain scattered multinucleated giant cells; both features are unusual for deep fibromatoses. Both superficial and deep fibromatosis can show nuclear β-catenin expression. Reportedly, only a minority of cells in superficial fibromatosis exhibit nuclear β-catenin, whereas some cases of deep fibromatosis demonstrate feature a majority of cells with nuclear staining (Miettinen 2010).

NF: A few desmoids that are hypercellular may histologically mimic NF. Both lesions can contain areas of fresh hemorrhage and both will feature cells with identical morphology. Similarly, reactivity for smooth muscle actin can be seen in both lesions. However, clinically, NF often has a rapid growth over a period of weeks, and is usually less than 4.0 cm in size. Additionally, nodular fasciitis may contain scattered osteoclast-like giant cells and scattered lymphocytes and plasma cells are common; these inflammatory cells are rare to absent in desmoid tumors. Greater collagen deposition and fewer mitoses also characterize desmoid tumors compared with the active phase of NF. Finally, approximately 70% of cases of deep fibromatosis express nuclear β-catenin; a finding not reported in NF.

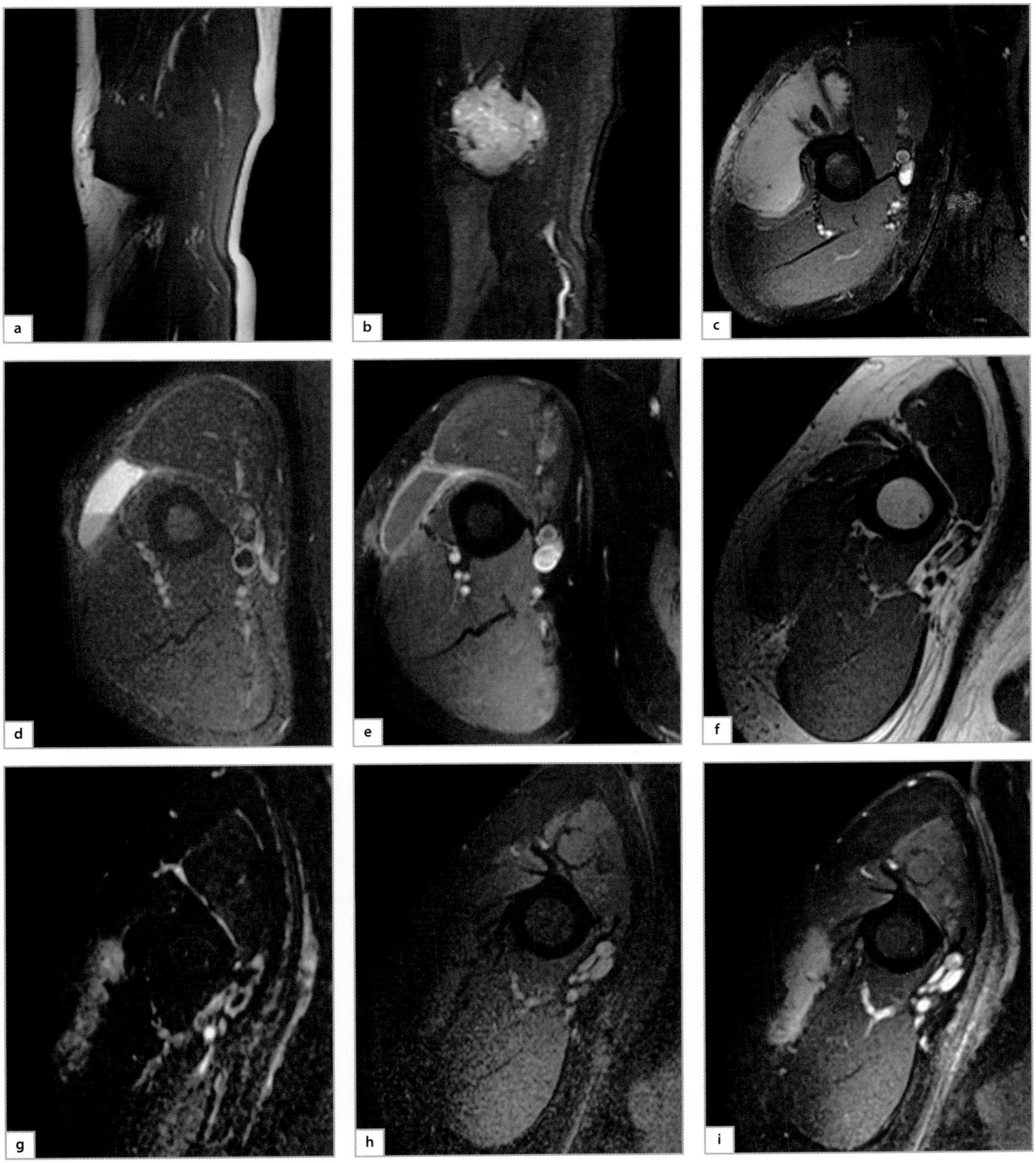

Case figure 6.4 Extra-abdominal fibromatosis (deep fibromatosis, desmoid). **6.4a**: Sagittal T1, **6.4b**: Sagittal STIR, **6.4c**: Axial T1 fat saturation post-contrast. These MR images show a T1 isointense, STIR heterogeneously high signal mass in the distal deltoid muscle of the arm. There is fairly uniform intense enhancement, no necrosis is evident. Post-operative follow up imaging with **6.4d**: Axial STIR, **6.4e**, Axial T1 fat saturation post-contrast. Images show a small rim enhancing fluid collection with fluid-fluid level. Note the wall is smooth with uniform thickness and there is no focal mass or nodular enhancing area. Findings indicate postoperative seroma. Surveillance follow-up MR imaging is performed 15 weeks later. **6.4f**: Axial T1, **6.4g**: Axial STIR, **6.4h**: T1 fat saturation, **6.4i**: T1 fat saturation post-contrast. There is now a heterogeneous mass in the surgical bed of the distal deltoid muscle consistent with recurrence. The previous seroma has resolved.

Case figure 6.4: Continued from page 105

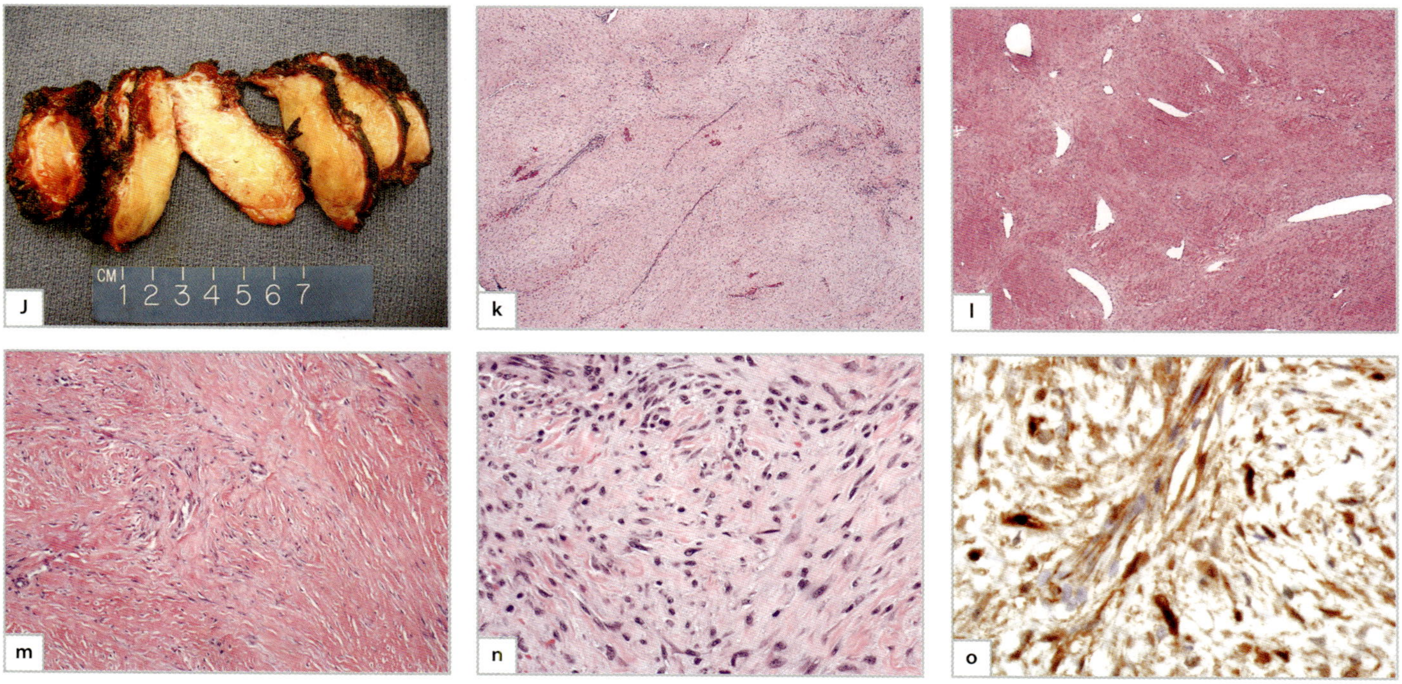

6.4J: Cut sections of tumor show a solid, trabeculated white to gray surface. **6.4k:** At low magnification, the tumor is mildly cellular with sweeps of cells compressing thin walled vessels into long, slightly angled arcs. The appearance of the squeezed vessels is a typical feature of desmoids. **6.4l**: In some areas, the tumor vessels are open and gaping instead of compressed. Such ecstatic, hemangiopericytomatous, thin walled vessels are another, less common feature of this tumor. **6.4m**: EAFs most commonly are mildly to moderately cellular but other patterns can be seen, sometimes in the same tumor. In this area, there is more prominent fibrosis and decreased cellularity (medium magnification). **6.4n**: At high magnification, the tumor cells exhibit typical features of fibroblasts/myofibroblasts: indistinct cell borders, amphophilic (lavender colored) cytoplasm, and plump spindled nuclei with fine chromatin and small nucleoli. Several mast cells are also present; these inflammatory cells are almost always seen in EAFs. The mast cells are much smaller than the tumor cells, round in shape and feature ovoid, hyperchromatic nuclei. Their distinctive granular cytoplasm cannot be appreciated in this photomicrograph. **6.4o**: Nuclear β-catenin expression is notable in several tumor cells (high magnification). Widespread cytoplasmic staining is also present. For comparison, the endothelial cell nuclei in this field are negative for β-catenin accumulation. While not specific for EAFs, nuclear β-catenin expression can be a very helpful finding when the differential diagnosis comprises exuberant scar (negative for nuclear β-catenin).

Fibrosarcoma: The uncommon hypercellular deep fibromatosis could mimic a fibrosarcoma. However, fibrosarcoma contains cells with at least mild cytologic atypia, and mitotic activity is higher (>5 mitoses per 10 high power microscopic fields). Adult type fibrosarcoma is a diagnosis of exclusion, and tumors that histologically show the fibrosarcoma herringbone pattern of spindle cells are much more likely synovial sarcoma, fibrosarcoma arising in dermatofibrosarcoma protuberans (fibrosarcoma in DFSP), or malignant peripheral nerve sheath tumor (MPNST) rather than fibrosarcoma. SS, fibrosarcoma in DFSP and MPNST express a different set of antibodies and/or feature characteristic genetic abnormalities as well as contain cells with obvious nuclear atypia (plus or minus increased mitoses and foci of necrosis).

Gardner fibroma: Gardner fibroma may evolve into extra-abdominal fibromatosis on recurrences. It is associated with Gardner syndrome. It is heavily collagenized and far less cellular then extra-abdominal fibromatosis. The lesional cells can be reactive for CD34, and a few cases display nuclear reactivity for β-catenin similar to desmoid (extra-abdominal fibromatosis) and some cases of superficial fibromatosis. A common location is back or paraspinal subcutaneous tissue, but it also can occur in the head and neck and extremities (all sites for extra-abdominal fibromatosis also). Most cases are diagnosed in childhood, sometimes before recognition that the patient has Gardner syndrome.

Nuchal type fibroma: This lesion has a striking association with diabetes mellitus in 50% of cases. The lesion occurs in an older age group than Gardner fibroma with an average age of 40 years. However, it is usually histologically indistinguishable from Gardner fibroma. Similar to Gardner fibroma, the lesional cells are CD34 reactive, and the tumor is predominantly superficial but can involve skeletal muscle in a minority of cases. Like Gardner fibroma, it is less cellular and more fibrotic than extra-abdominal fibromatosis.

Desmoplastic fibroblastoma (collagenous fibroma): This is an unusual tumor that occurs primarily in middle aged to elderly men (4:1 male to female ratio). It can be superficial or deep, is usually sharply circumscribed (unlike extra-abdominal fibromatosis), and is hypocellular with rare blood vessels. A few cases are reported to be positive for nuclear β-catenin with no reactivity for CD34. At least some cases feature a translocation also found in fibroma of tendon sheath: t(2;11)(q31;q12)(Bernal et al. 2004, Sciot et al. 1999).

Oncology approach

Medical oncology

Imatinib is administered for this patient because of persistent, symptomatic disease (the patient has pain unrelieved by NSAIDs). Because surgical resection is conservative, aiming to preserve functionality of the patient's arm, there was no attempt at complete excision at initial surgery; it is therefore not surprising that the patient has residual tumor. On a typical oral dosage of Imatinib, the patient experienced slow local recurrence. At the patient's wishes and in consultation with the surgeon and oncologist, the residual tumor is conservatively re-excised. He continues on Imatinib with slight regrowth of tumor. Currently, he is satisfied with close clinical monitoring and continued medical treatment. Imatinib has proven effective in stabilizing the growth of extra-abdominal desmoid tumors but is not universally successful (Penel et al. 2011). If the patient experiences unacceptable regrowth of the tumor, other medical options should be considered.

Radiation oncology

There are multiple studies demonstrating a role for radiation in the treatment of desmoid tumors. However, the role remains controversial. This controversy is largely due to the inconsistent natural history of the disease. Typically locally aggressive, the disease may nevertheless display long periods of stasis and rarely regress spontaneously. Consequently, evaluating the role of any therapeutic intervention is difficult. Studies have shown a potential role for radiation in cases of positive margins (Jelinek 2001, Nuyttens 2000) and unresectable disease (Guadagnolo 2008). However, current recommendations for the use of radiation therapy remain mixed as outcomes remain mixed (Gluck 2011). Radiation should be considered in aggressive cases that have positive margins or in cases of local recurrence. Even in pediatric cases, radiation should be considered as local control when with surgery alone it can be difficult to achieve (Jabbari 2009). Recommendations should be tailored to the clinical presentation reserving multi-modality treatment for aggressive cases.

Patient outcome

The patient has residual but stable disease about three years after presentation. He continues to experience flare-ups of pain; these are treated with low dose pain relievers and infrequent, local injections of corticosteroids. He continues on oral Imatinib therapy.

Case table 6.4 Summary pathology findings of Case 6.4

Diagnosis	Extra-abdominal fibromatosis (deep fibromatosis, desmoid)
Size	8.7 × 6.2 × 3.2 cm
Location	Deep tissues of right arm
Margin status	Positive
Histologic grade	Not graded: benign (but exhibits aggressive local growth)
Pathologic stage (TNM classification)	Not staged: benign (but due to aggressive local growth, can recur in 20-40% of patients and rarely can develop discontinuous tumors)

Case 6.5 Solitary fibrous tumor/hemangiopericytoma

Clinical history and presentation

The patient is a 78 year old man who presents with a two month history of a thigh mass. The mass was noted spontaneously. Over the past two weeks it appears to have grown rapidly in size and become increasingly painful.

Physical examination reveals a large, firm, tender mass in the mid-lateral aspect of the thigh.

Surgical findings and comments

Because the differential diagnosis of this lesion includes both benign and malignant entities, a formal open biopsy is performed. Following pathologic confirmation of the diagnosis, the patient is returned to the operating room on a separate date for marginal excision of the tumor. Findings at surgery reveal a large solid mass. The tumor shells out of the surrounding tissue with relative ease.

Radiology findings

The CT scan (**Case figure 6.5a**), shows a large soft tissue density mass with a few punctate calcifications. Calcifications are only seen in 9% of SFT. No bone destruction or osteoid is evident, militating against the diagnosis of various osteosarcomas. The MR images (**Case figs 6.5b** through **6.5f**), show a large mass in the vastus lateralis and intermedius muscles with T1 iso-intensity and STIR high signal. The tumor appears aggressive with infiltrative, invasive appearing margins. The tumor shows avid enhancement which is seen in the majority of SFT. Interestingly, there are several enlarged draining veins visible on MRI (**Case fig. 6.5f**) and on the blood pool image of the bone scan (**Case fig. 6.5g**) indicating this is a highly vascular tumor. Large collateral vessels are seen in 35% of SFT. The overall appearance is worrisome for a high grade sarcoma. However, the presence of large collateral vessels is somewhat unusual and suggests SFT. Nevertheless, tissue diagnosis is needed.

Pathology findings

Gross features

The biopsy comprises multiple portions of tan to focally hemorrhagic tissue aggregating to 4.5 cm. Sections are submitted fresh to cytogenetics.

The resection specimen measures 18.5 × 13 × 4.5 cm and consists of partially disrupted tumor and adjacent fibrous tissue (**Case fig. 6.5h**). Cut sections reveal a variable appearance ranging from white fibrous regions (approximately 40% of total tumor) to whorled softer tan areas (50% of tumor) to foci of golden yellow necrosis (10% of tumor). Representative tissues are taken for cytogenetics and tumor banking. The surgical margins are positive for tumor.

Microscopic features

Low magnification: The features of the biopsy specimen are identical to those of the resection; therefore, only the resection specimen is described. At low magnification, the tumor is startling for its variability. Some areas are fibrotic and hypocellular and others are highly cellular without any fibrosis (**Case fig. 6.5i**).

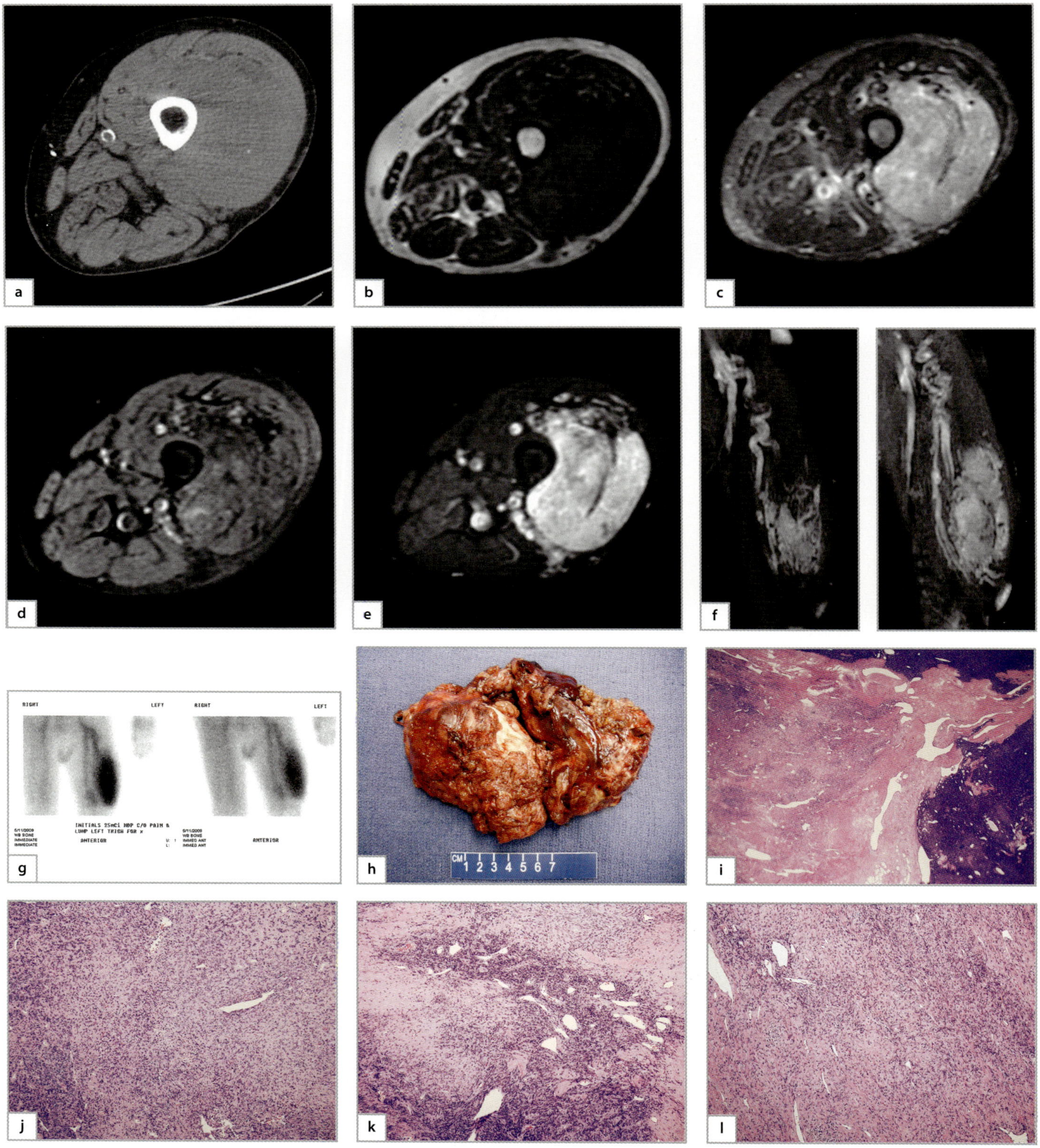

Case figure 6.5 SFT. **6.5a**: CT scan without IV contrast, **6.5b**: Axial T1, **6.5c**: Axial STIR, **6.5d**: Axial T1 fat saturation, **6.5e**: Axial T1 fat saturation post-contrast, **6.5f**: Coronal T1 fat saturation post-contrast. There is a large mass of the extensor muscles of the thigh. There is a punctate calcification seen by CT imaging. There is no appreciable fat. The mass shows non-specific T1 isointensity and STIR high signal. There is intense fairly homogeneous enhancement. Note the large draining veins extending proximally from the mass. **6.5g**: Blood pool images from Tc-99 MDP bone scan shows the significant soft tissue uptake and the large draining vein. **6.5h**: The external surface of the resection specimen shows a pink to red gyriform or bosselated tumor with adherent fresh blood clot (gross photo). The white area is fascia to which mounds of tumor are attached. The tumor bled readily during excision. Necrosis is not seen in this view.

Case figure 6.5: Continued from page 108

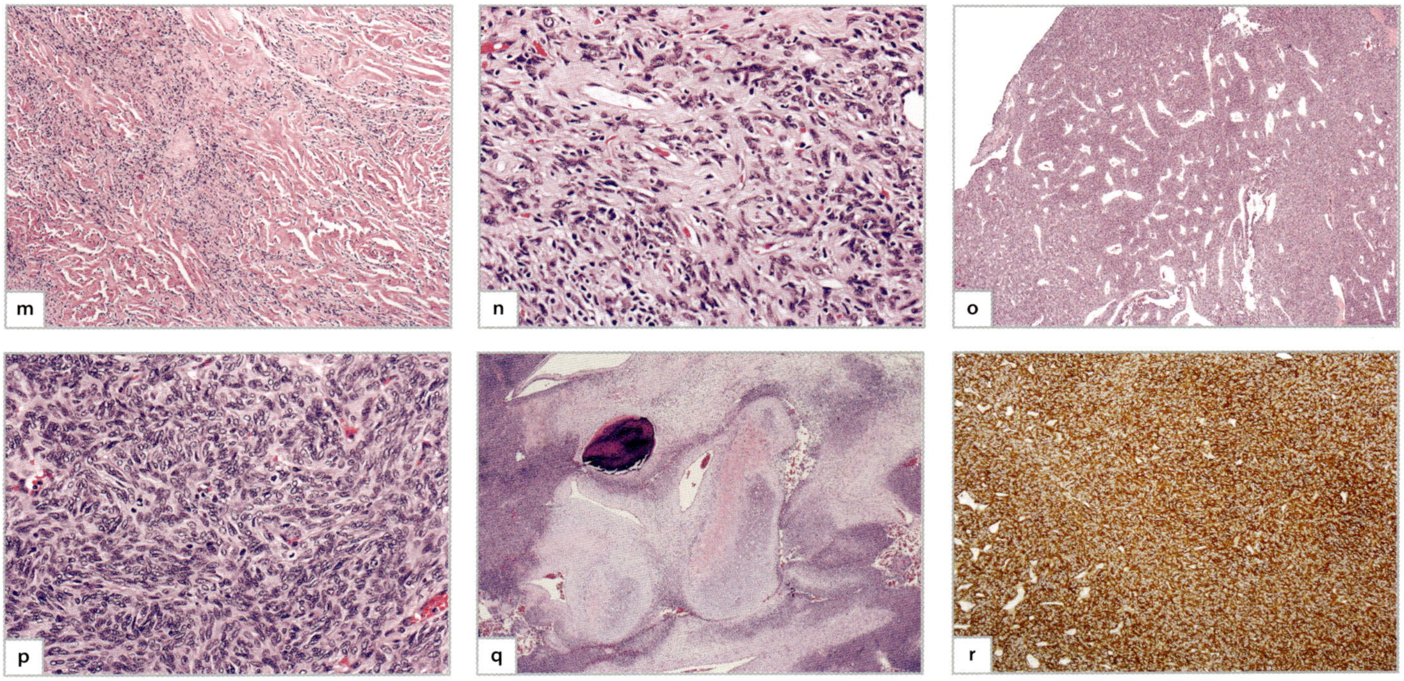

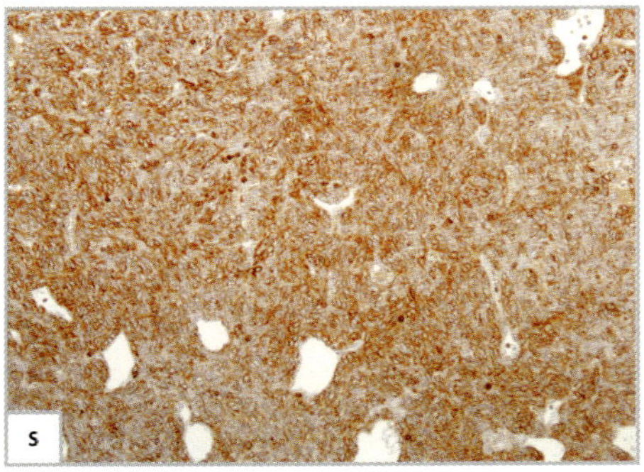

6.5i: This patient's tumor shows why SFT/HPC are considered one entity as both phases are present. The very cellular area comprises the classic hemangiopericytoma appearance, and the fibrotic, less cellular area comprises the classic solitary fibrous tumor look. In this field, the two phases abut each other and don't blend (low magnification). **6.5j:** In this field, the SFT and HPC phases blend together with a gradation in tumor cellularity and fibrosis. **6.5k**: At medium magnification, an SFT-like area shows the characteristic random variability in cellularity and fibrosis. Notice the vessels are ectatic (dilated) and vaguely 'staghorn' or 'antler horn' in shape. **6.5l**: Another SFT-like area with scattered inflammatory cells. **6.5m**: A feature commonly seen in solitary fibrous tumors is the clefting or spaces formed when the histotechnologist cuts the section (medium magnification). 6-5n Solitary Fibrous Tumor/Hemangiopericytoma. The tumor cells in the SFT-like area are jumbled with indistinct cell borders and mildly atypical, normochromatic nuclei that vary in size and shape. Marked nuclear pleomorphism is absent. Here, cell borders are indistinct. **6.5o**: The HPC portion of the patient's tumor is uniformly hypercellular with prominent 'antler horn' or 'staghorn' vascularity. **6.5p**: At high magnification, the HPC-like cells form short interlocking swirls of uniform cells with indistinct cell borders and plump, sausage shaped nuclei. Three mitotic figures can be seen; none are atypical. **6.5q**: This patient's tumor contains foci of metaplastic bone and cartilage, a rare occurrence in SFT/HPC (medium magnification). **6.5r**: Tumor cells are strongly and diffusely positive for CD34 (immunohistochemical stain; a brown color indicates positivity). **6.5s**: Tumor cells are diffusely positive for Bcl-2 (immunohistochemical stain).

High magnification: Such stark contrast is not uniform, however, and focally, a gradual blending of fibrous tumor (histologically typical of SFT), and hypercellular tumor (histologically typical of hemangiopericytoma (HPC) now termed 'cellular SFT') (**Case fig. 6.5j**) occurs. This patient's tumor superbly demonstrates the intimate relationship between SFT and what was previously called HPC. The two tumors represent poles of one entity, and the 2013 WHO classification of these tumors now labels hemangiopericytoma 'the cellular phase of SFT' (Folpe et al. 2010, Fletcher et al. 2013). Areas classic for solitary fibrous tumor are randomly fibrotic and randomly variable in cellularity (**Case figs 6.5k** and **6.5l**). This has been termed 'the patternless pattern' of SFT. Some areas contain extremely dense collagen resulting in tissue cracks during the Histology cutting process to make a section (**Case fig. 6.5m**). At high magnification, the plump spindle tumor cells in the SFT-like area are mildly atypical in nuclear size and shape with indistinct cell borders (**Case fig. 6.5n**). Marked nuclear pleomorphism is absent.

The areas in this patient's tumor that show a hemangiopericytomatous appearance are uniformly highly cellular with classic antler horn vasculature (**Case fig. 6.5o**). High magnification of these HPC-like areas reveals short swirls of uniform cells with sausage shaped nuclei and indistinct cell borders (**Case fig. 6.5p**). Mitoses are present but are not atypical. The number of mitoses averages 4 per 10 high magnification fields. An unusual feature of this patient's tumor is focal metaplastic bone and cartilage formation (**Case fig. 6.5q**).

Special studies: The tumor cells strongly and diffusely express CD34 antigen (**Case fig. 6.5r**) and are also diffusely positive for Bcl-2 (**Case fig. 6.5s**)(by IHC). SFT/HPC should be at least focally positive for CD34, and approximately 40% are reactive for Bcl-2. These proteins are not specific and unique to SFT/HPC, however, and must be interpreted in the context of the morphology to render the correct diagnosis. Some SFT/HPCs may express nuclear β catenin (perhaps up to 40% of cases) and may be focally positive for smooth muscle actin. Cytologically malignant tumors may also express keratins, and increased Ki67 (a marker of proliferating cells) (Miettinen et al. 2010).

The tumor also was examined for p53 expression which was low at less than 5% of cells reactive. A recent Italian study of 88 cases of pleural based SFTs reported that necrosis and high p53 expression were the only parameters on multivariate analysis associated with overall survival and disease free survival (Schirosi et al. 2008). This patient's tumor is necrotic.

Karyotyping reveals the following clone: 46,XY,der(10)t(1;10)(q11;p15) with the derivative chromosome resulting in a partial trisomy for chromosome 1 (+1q). SFT is a translocation specific sarcoma. The translocation occurs between two adjacent genes located on chromosome 12q13, aligning them together and results in a *NAB2-STAT6* fusion protein that functions as an abnormal transcription factor of proliferation pathways (Chmielecki et al. 2013, Robinson et al. 2013). Only a few SFTs/HPC had been previously karyotyped, and abnormalities included various translocations and other changes, none of which have been consistent. The diploid or near diploid number of chromosomes found on karyotyping is typical. The in-frame fusion of the two genes is not detectable by karyotyping.

Pathologic differential or, why isn't it one of the following?

Synovial sarcoma (SS): Generally, SS is more histologically uniform than SFT. Almost all cases contain a specific translocation, t(X;18) and even most monophasic spindle cell synovial sarcomas are positive for keratins and/or EMA. Biphasic synovial sarcoma often has a clearly identifiable epithelial component. Only a rare synovial sarcoma expresses CD34.

Malignant peripheral nerve sheath tumor (MPNST): MPNST can demonstrate intratumoral heterogeneity but cytologic atypia is usually pronounced, and atypical mitoses and necrosis are commonly present. Scattered tumor cells are reactive for S-100 protein, and most tumors will be negative for CD34 (by immunohistochemical staining).

Oncology approach

Medical oncology

The patient does not receive chemotherapy, as the tumor is entirely resected and there is no evidence of metastatic disease.

Radiation oncology

Solitary fibrous tumors are a relatively rare disease and are typically best managed by surgical excision followed by observation. These tumors can also occur in the central nervous system. In cases where surgical excision cannot be performed or is restricted to subtotal resection due to eloquence of location, stereotactic radiosurgery or fractionated external beam radiotherapy has been employed (Bisceglia 2011). In this case, observation is recommended as salvage therapy for an unlikely local recurrence has a low risk of morbidity.

Patient outcome

The patient is doing well two years following the tumor removal. Most patients with SFT are cured despite a low but unpredictable risk for

Case table 6.5a Variant features of SFT

Feature	Frequency	Comment
Pure SFT pattern of growth	Very common	'patternless pattern' of varying cellularity and fibrosis
Pure HPC pattern of growth	Uncommon	Uniformly hypercellular with short swirls and prominent 'staghorn' or pericytomatous vascular pattern
Mixed SFT and HPC patterns in one tumor	Common	Usually one pattern predominates
SFT or HPC pattern with adipose tissue	Uncommon	Previously called lipomatous hemangiopericytoma. New recommended term is 'fat-forming SFT'
Dense keloidal like collagen	Common	Rarely, stellate acellular deposits of collagen may be seen (amianthoid fibers)
Vessels with hyalinized walls	Common	Almost all SFT/HPC will exhibit a hemangiopericytomatous vascular architecture at least focally, but in many cases there are also vessels that are small and inconspicuous. Some vessels may have thick fibrotic walls (considered a degenerative change also seen in other tumors such as schwannoma).
Extensive myxoid stroma with tumor cells arranged haphazardly, in cords, or lacy, reticulated strands	Uncommon	In most cases, standard SFT is focally present
Cellular storiforming architecture with some chronic inflammation located in deep tissue and CD34 positive	Uncommon	Some cases of 'deep benign fibrous histiocytoma' may actually represent a storiforming cellular variant of SFT
Osseous or chondroid metaplasia	Rare	
Mild nuclear atypia and scattered multinucleated tumor giant cells	Relatively common	Does not increase risk for local recurrence or metastasis
Many multinucleated tumor giant cells with some bordering pseudovascular (unlined) spaces	Uncommon	Most often occurs in SFT/HPC of orbit soft tissues. Previously called giant cell angiofibroma. New recommended term is 'giant cell rich variant of SFT'
Infiltrative border, mitoses > 4 per 10 high power fields, necrosis, size > 5 cm, +/- increased cytologic atypia	Uncommon (10% of soft tissue SFT/HPC)	Indicates an increased risk for metastasis
Frank malignant features including marked pleomorphism, increased mitoses, necrosis +/- loss of CD34 expression with the malignant area showing epithelioid, round cell and/or spindle morphology	Rare	May represent dedifferentiation. Associated with greater risk for local recurrence and metastasis

metastasis. Although this patient's tumor is larger than 5 cm with necrosis, two risk factors for more aggressive behavior, he has not experienced local recurrence or metastasis. Extensive sampling of his resection showed no evidence of increased mitotic activity, marked cellular atypia or dedifferentiation, and the lack of these features may contribute to the tumor's thus far good behavior. However, patients with SFT may develop metastases many years after resection; therefore, he will be followed regularly for evidence of either local recurrence (increased risk based on the tumor size and positive margins) or metastasis.

Case table 6.5b Summary pathology findings of Case 6.5

Diagnosis	SFT
Size	18.5 × 13 × 4.5 cm
Location	Deep soft tissue of thigh
Margin status	Positive
Histologic grade	1 = well-differentiated Negative for dedifferentiation but necrosis present and large size predicts increased risk for local recurrence and metastasis
Pathologic stage (TNM classification)	T2b/NX/M0 = Stage IB

Case 6.6 Inflammatory myofibroblastic tumor

Clinical history and presentation

The patient is a 51 year old gravida 3, para 3 woman who presents with increased vaginal bleeding. Physical examination reveals a large exophytic cervical mass.

Surgical findings and comments

Biopsy of the mass is performed. Following pathologic confirmation of the diagnosis, the patient is returned to the operating room for total abdominal hysterectomy.

Radiology findings

The MR images (**Case figures 6.6a** through **6.6e**) show a lobulated T1 low signal, T2 high signal mass in the vagina with a stalk that appears to originate from the endometrium of the lower uterus. A short differential diagnosis would include a pedunculated leiomyoma, cervical tumor or endometrial tumor. The mass enhances modestly, without evidence of necrosis or matrix. There are no secondary signs of malignancy such as ascites, adenopathy or parametrial infiltration. Large uterine leiomyomas often have coarse areas of calcification which are not present. Also, leiomyomas are usually T2 low signal and appear more heterogeneous than this lesion. This is a strikingly unusual case and given the indeterminate appearance, tissue diagnosis or removal is warranted.

Pathology findings

Gross features

Two preceding biopsies comprise reddish tissue aggregating to 1.0 cm in each sample.

The subsequently resected tumor consists of multiple fragments of tan to pink, fleshy tissue measuring in aggregate 8.6 × 8.0 × 3.3 cm. The tumor is entirely resected along with the uterus, ovaries, and fallopian tubes. There is no evidence of disease other than the mass arising from the uterine cervix.

Microscopic features

Low magnification: The first biopsy is almost entirely necrotic and inflamed, and a specific diagnosis cannot be rendered. The second biopsy contains histologically viable tumor. The features are identical to those of the resection specimen, and the latter only is described. At low magnification, the tumor is cellular with a mixed fascicular and storiforming architecture (**Case fig. 6.6f**).

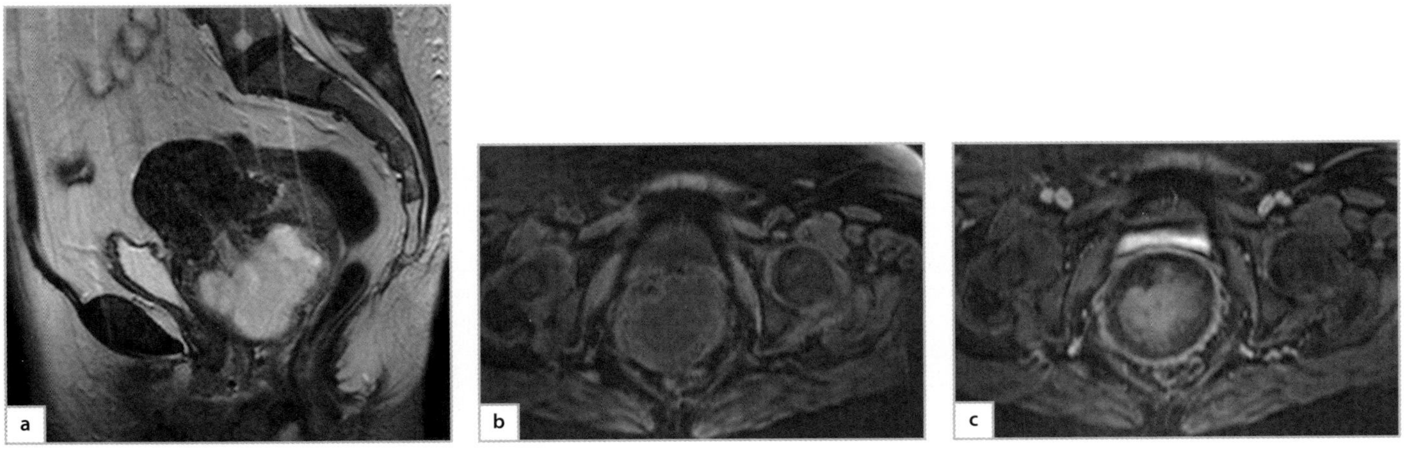

Case figure 6.6 Inflammatory myofibroblastic tumor. **6.6a**: Sagittal T2, **6.6b**: axial T1 VIBE (Volume Interpolated Breath-hold Examination - a fat suppressed 3D gradient echo sequence) **6.6c**: Axial T1 VIBE post-contrast,

Case figure 6.6: Continued from page 111

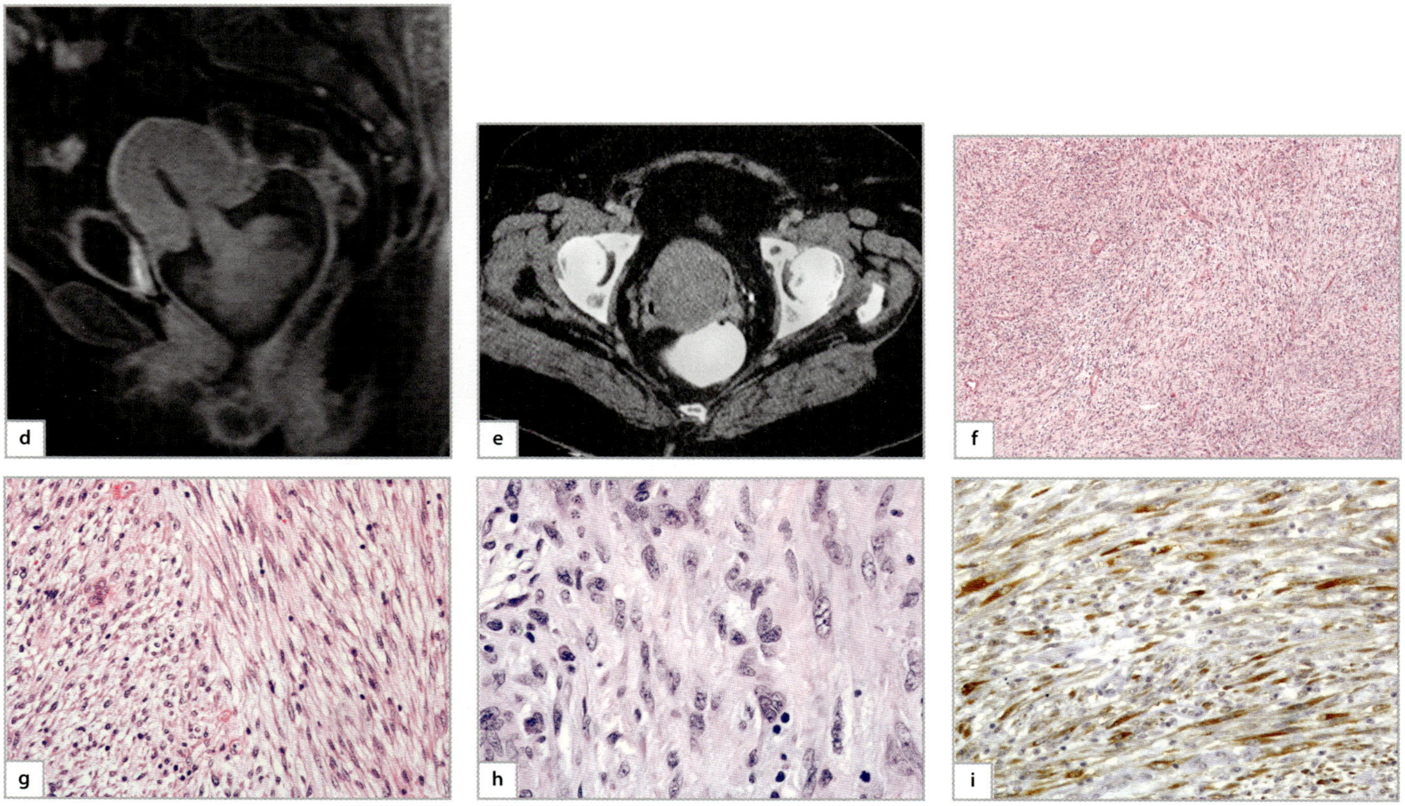

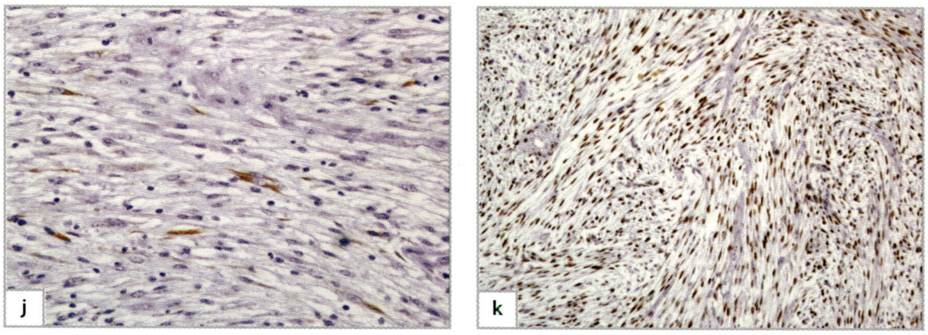

6.6d: Sagittal T1 VIBE post-contrast, **6.6e**: Axial CT scan image. The MR images show a bulky, lobulated mass in the vagina with an apparent stalk connecting it to the lower uterine segment possibly originating from the endometrium. There is moderate enhancement. CT scan shows no calcifications. **6.6f**: The tumor somewhat resembles the cellular phase of NF at low magnification. It is cellular with a fascicular and storiform architecture composed of pale plump spindle cells. **6.6g**: The spindle cells stream in intersecting fascicles. A few inflammatory cells are also scattered throughout. Clear spaces between the eosinophilic tumor cells are consistent with edema and a small amount of myxoid matrix (medium magnification). **6.6h**: At high magnification, the tumor cells fulfill the histologic expectations of myofibroblasts/fibroblasts in that the cytoplasm is pale pink to lavender (amphophilic) and the nucleus is mildly variable in size and shape but hypochromatic with reticulated chromatin and small round nucleoli. Lymphocytes and plasma cells are scattered randomly. Compare the hyperchromatic nuclei of the lymphocytes and the chunky chromatin of the plasma cells to the pale tumor cell nuclei. **6.6i**: The majority of spindle tumor cells demonstrate cytoplasmic reactivity for ALK-1 (high magnification; immunohistochemical stain). **6.6j:** Scattered tumor cells express desmin (high magnification; immunohistochemical stain). **6.6k**: Likely because this tumor is located in the female genital tract, the tumor cells are strongly and diffusely positive for estrogen receptor (medium magnification; immunohistochemical stain).

High magnification: At medium magnification, fascicles of streaming spindle tumor cells intersect at ninety degree angles (**Case fig. 6.6g**). Lymphocytes and plasma cells are scattered among the spindle tumor cells which show only mild nuclear variability. The tumor cells, whether spindled or polygonal as in **Case fig. 6.6h**, precisely conform to histologic expectations of fibroblasts/myofibroblasts: the cytoplasm is pale pink to amphophilic, and the nucleus is hypochromatic or vesicular with reticulated chromatin and small nucleoli.

Special studies: Tumor cells are reactive for anaplastic lymphoma kinase-1 (ALK-1) (**Case fig. 6.6i**). Many IMFT express anaplastic lymphoma kinase on IHC, especially those in children and young adults and those in non-soft tissues such as the uterus. The location of reactivity in the cell corresponds to the particular translocation. Only a few tumor cells express desmin (**Case fig. 6.6j**); sparse or absent reactivity is atypical of myofibroblasts. Interestingly, estrogen receptor is also expressed and may be related to the gynecologic site of the tumor (**Case fig. 6.6k**).

Pathologic differential or, why isn't it one of the following?

Case table 6.6a details the differential diagnosis of IMT. Quite a few tumors feature myofibroblastic or fibroblastic spindle cells, so the list is relatively long. Leiomyoma is also included because smooth muscle cells can somewhat resemble myofibroblasts.

Oncology approach

Medical oncology

As the tumor is completely resected, and there is no evidence of metastatic disease, chemotherapy is not a consideration. Should she have a recurrence, Crizotinib could be considered for its effect on ALK kinase.

Radiation oncology

This is a technically benign entity that can be locally aggressive and rarely metastatic. Ideally, resection with negative margins is the treatment of choice. In patients with residual, recurrent, or unresectable disease, radiation therapy can be considered.

Patient outcome

Seven years following surgery the patient is disease free.

Case table 6.6b Summary pathology findings of Case 6.6

Diagnosis	IMFT
Size	8.6 × 8 × 3.3 cm
Location	Uterine cervix
Margin status	Negative
Histologic grade	Not graded However, there are no atypical cells as have been described in some metastasizing IMFT.
Pathologic stage (TNM classification)	Not staged

Case table 6.6a Pathologic differential diagnosis of IMFT

Tumor	Architecture	Cell morphology	Immunohistochemistry	Genetics
Inflammatory myofibroblastic tumor (IMFT)	Three patterns and mixtures thereof possible: 1 Myxoid vascular pattern with edema, prominent vessels and inflammation 2 Fibrotic inflamed pattern with plate-like collagen, low cellularity, and sparse inflammation 3 Fascicular inflamed pattern Rare aggressive intra-abdominal epithelioid variant also has been described Calcifications and bone metaplasia may be present but rare Usually has an expansile or pushing border	Spindle fibroblasts or myofibroblasts with vesicular ovoid nuclei Inflammation comprises lymphocytes and plasma cells less commonly eosinophils and rarely neutrophils Ganglion like or Reed-Sternberg like cells with prominent nucleoli may be present Atypical epithelioid cells in the aggressive intra-abdominal variant	ALK-1 positive in 50% of patients (more commonly in children) Most cases show a myoid phenotype with reactivity most commonly for smooth muscle actin but also desmin and rarely caldesmon Some cases express keratins	Various translocations of ALK gene (at 2p23) with others on 1, 19, 17, 2q ,4q, and 11
Nodular fasciitis (NF)	Storiforming, cell culture or teased apart look often with microcysts Fresh hemorrhage and some inflammation Sometimes keloidal like fibrosis Sometimes fibrosis and central cystic change coincide with cellular edematous phase	Spindled to stellate cells with vesicular nuclei and small nucleoli. Inflammation usually sparse and lymphocytic	Myoid phenotype with actin positivity but only rarely expresses desmin. Actin reactivity usually is 'tram track' pattern (peripheral parallel subplasmalemmal staining). Negative for caldesmon. Negative for ALK-1	Normal karyotype in most cases
Proliferative myositis	Architecture is like NF: whorls of spindle to stellate cells May invade and spread apart skeletal muscle fibers in a 'checkerboard' pattern	Same plump spindle cells as in NF but also round ganglion like cells present with prominent nucleoli	Same as for NF Ganglion like cells can be negative for actins	Normal karyotype
Low grade myofibroblastic sarcoma	More uniform than IMFT. Fascicular and/or storiforming pattern of spindle to plump polygonal cells Inflammation is usually absent or at most sparse Prominent permeative border	Spindle cells with wavy, narrow tapered nuclei or plump vesicular nuclei. Mild nuclear atypia with a few nuclei showing moderate atypia Lymphocytes and plasma cells uncommon and focal	Negative for ALK-1 Positive for myoid markers including smooth muscle actin plus or minus desmin. Actin reactivity may be 'tram track' pattern. Caldesmon negative	Some cases may have ring chromosomes with 12p11 and 12q13 changes
Leiomyoma, conventional type	Fascicular pattern Inflammation rare	Deeply eosinophilic spindle cells Blunt ended or cigar shaped nuclei Mast cells may be present	Myoid phenotype with diffuse cytoplasmic staining for desmin (usually), smooth muscle actin (usually) and caldesmon (often). Negative for ALK-1	No specific genetic findings
Extra-abdominal fibromatosis (e-a desmoid tumor)	Fascicular to storiform pattern Hypocellular to mildly cellular Thin walled, compressed or ectatic vessels May have aggregates of lymphocytes at vessels or edge	Plump spindle to thin spindle cells with vesicular nuclei and small nucleoli Mast cells present Mitoses usually uncommon	Nuclear β-catenin expression in 70% of cases May be actin positive but usually focal not diffuse Usually desmin negative	β-catenin gene mutations (frequent) APC gene mutations uncommon in sporadic desmoids Trisomy 8 and/or20 in 10-30%

Case 6.7 Myxofibrosarcoma

Clinical history and presentation

The patient is a 72 year old woman who presents with a one year history of a posterior thigh mass which was noted spontaneously and has increased slowly but progressively in size. It is largely asymptomatic but does cause some pain with pressure while sitting.

Physical examination reveals a large, firm, deeply situated tumor in the posterior thigh. It is minimally tender. On radiologic work-up, there is no evidence of metastatic disease.

Surgical findings and comments

Biopsy of the mass is performed. One month later she is returned to the operating room for wide resection of the tumor.

Radiology findings

The MR images (**Case figs 6.7a** through **6.7d**) show a non-specific T1 low signal, STIR high signal mass with heterogeneous intense enhancement. The mass fills the flexor compartment of the thigh and abuts the sciatic nerve. This mass is highly worrisome for a sarcoma given its markedly heterogeneous appearance and enhancement. The extensive non-enhancing areas are likely due to collections of myxoid material but could also represent necrotic tumor.

Pathology findings

Gross features

The biopsy comprises mixed gray firm and amber gelatinous tissue aggregating to 3.5 cm. Some material is collected fresh for cytogenetics. The resected tumor measures 18 × 9.5 × 9.0 cm. On cut sections, it is multinodular with firm white and soft, semi-translucent gelatinous areas (**Case fig. 6.7e**). Necrosis and hemorrhage are also present. The tumor is located more than 1.0 cm from all surgical margins (this gross impression is confirmed on microscopic review).

Microscopic features

Low magnification: At biopsy, the tumor comprises a moderately cellular spindle cell neoplasm with a prominent myxoid matrix and well-defined arborizing blood vessels (**Case fig. 6.7f**). A few areas exhibit an eosinophilic background consistent with collagen deposition.

The resection specimen contains a second pattern of tumor in addition to the myxoid spindle areas noted at biopsy. The non-spindle cell area is much less cellular and consists of pleomorphic, multinucleated tumor cells floating in pools of mucin (**Case fig. 6.7g**). The entire tumor is unencapsulated and easily infiltrates between slips of skeletal muscle (**Case fig. 6.7h**).

High magnification: The spindle cell area is fascicular with hyperchromatic spindle cells coursing in a myxoid matrix (**Case fig. 6.7i**). The most atypical cells, many of them multinucleated tumor giant cells, float in a mixed mucinous and collagen stranded matrix (**Case fig. 6.7j**). Some of the tumor cells simulate lipoblasts in that the cytoplasm contains vacuoles that indent the nucleus (**Case fig. 6.7k**). These 'pseudolipoblasts' are commonly seen in myxofibrosarcoma.

Some features characteristic of myxofibrosarcoma not seen in this patient's tumor include prominent infiltrating inflammatory cells (which may be of any type) reactive immature dendritic cells; Soilleux et al. 2003), and hypercellular tumor cell condensations around slightly arcing ('curvilinear') blood vessels.

The lack of these common features merely illustrates the plasticity of tumors within a particular tumor category and the challenges this variability can pose for the reviewing pathologist.

Large areas of necrosis are present, and mitoses average 25 per 10 high power microscopic fields with some atypical division figures. Combined with cytologic pleomorphism and hypercellularity, these features establish the tumor as Grade 3 (high grade, poorly differentiated). In most studies of myxofibrosarcoma, grade predicts metastatic potential (Grade 1 rarely metastasizes), although any grade can locally recur. Low grade tumors may also convert to a higher grade on local recurrence as is the case with some other types of sarcoma.

Special studies: Both the spindle cell hypercellular regions and the hypocellular areas with giant tumor cells strongly express CD34 (**Case fig. 6.7l**). Myxofibrosarcomas fairly commonly demonstrate CD34 expression, so this is an expected result. An unexpected result is reactivity for desmin just in the tumor giant cells (**Case fig. 6.7m**). Desmin reactivity is rarely reported to occur in myxofibrosarcoma; uncommonly, the spindle tumor cells or multinucleated giant tumor cells are reactive for smooth muscle actin. This patient's tumor cells show only reactivity for desmin (in a subgroup of tumor cells) and CD34 with no reactivity for smooth muscle actin, muscle specific actin, or S-100 protein.

Cytogenetics reveals a complex aneuploid karyotype with 112-114 chromosomes and numerous structural and numerical abnormalities. Complex aneuploidy is frequently present in myxofibrosarcoma especially in intermediate and high grade tumors.

Pathologic differential or, why isn't it one of the following?

Differential diagnosis of high grade myxofibrosarcoma

Leiomyosarcoma (LMS): LMS can have extensive myxoid change, although this is much more common in uterine tumors than extremity LMS. In myxoid cases, areas characteristic of conventional leiomyosarcoma are usually also present (long streaming fascicles of eosinophilic spindle cells with cigar shape or blunt ended nuclei). Although LMS can display CD34 reactivity, the tumor cells nearly always also diffusely express at least two muscle markers such as muscle specific actin, smooth muscle actin, desmin and caldesmon. Both high grade leiomyosarcoma and myxofibrosarcoma frequently demonstrate complex aneuploid karyotypes.

Dedifferentiated liposarcoma: This type of liposarcoma is unusual in the extremities, being more common in the mediastinum or retroperitoneum. Some dedifferentiated liposarcomas will contain areas of lower grade tumor with readily identifiable adipose tissue and authentic lipoblasts. The pseudolipoblasts notable in some myxofibrosarcomas exhibit a range of resemblance to actual lipoblasts with acid mucin vacuoles causing the indentation of the nuclei. In contrast to myxofibrosarcoma, dedifferentiated liposarcoma may have tumor cells reactive for S-100 protein, and is usually CDK4 and MDM2 positive (myxofibrosarcoma may be reactive for MDM2 but should not overexpress both MDM2 and CDK4). There may be some overlapping karyotyping findings, as both tumors can contain ring or marker chromosomes containing parts of chromosome 12 in a background of complex aneuploidy.

Myxoid/round cell liposarcoma (MLPS): Areas with obvious adipose differentiation are commonly present. Tumor cells often are S-100 positive except in high grade, exclusively round cell variants.

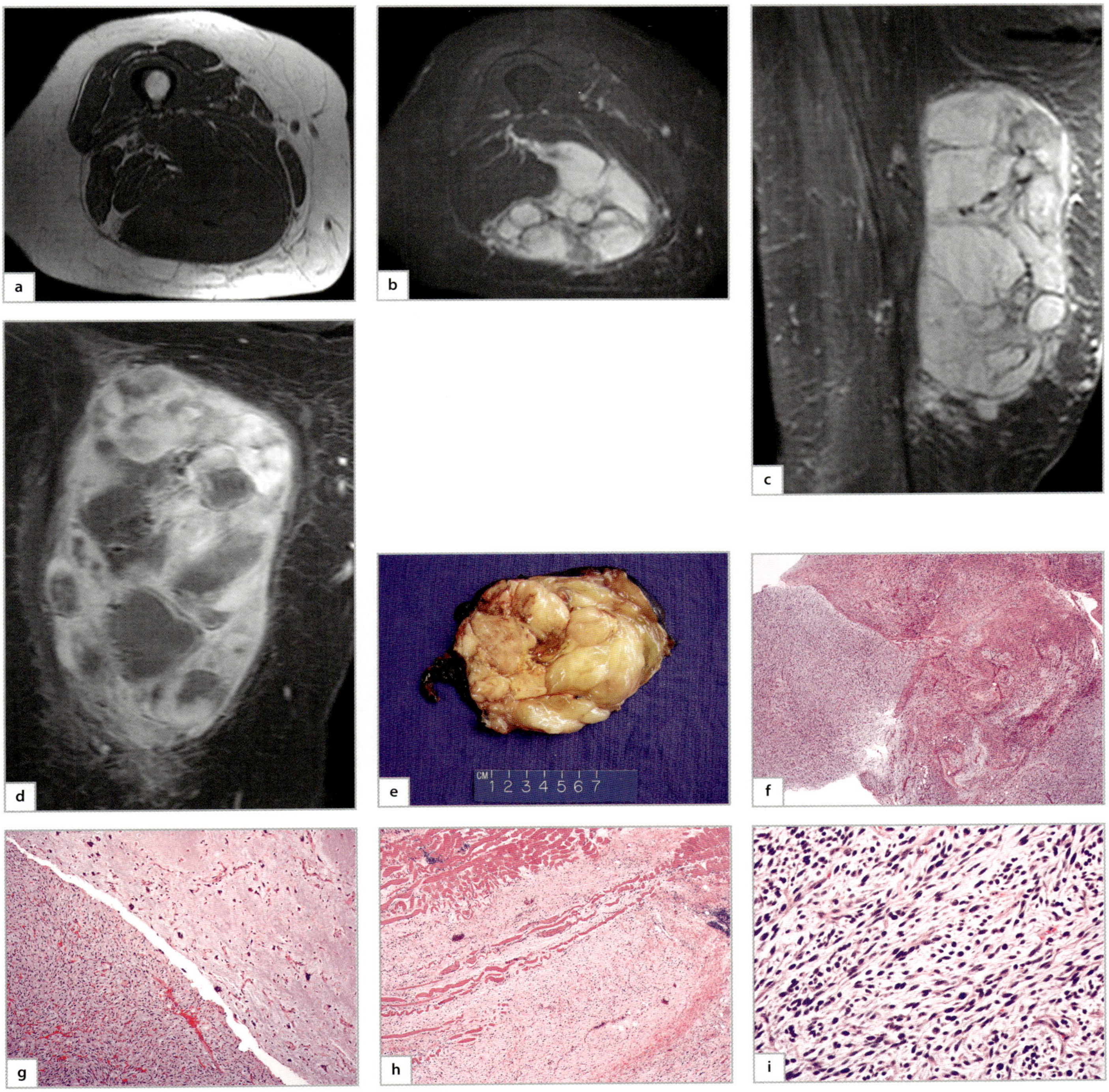

Case figure 6.7 Myxofibrosarcoma. **6.7a**: Axial T1, **6.7b**: Axial T2 fat saturation, **6.7c**: Sagittal STIR, **6.7d**: Coronal T1 fat saturation post-contract. The MR images show a large posterior thigh mass with nonspecific T1 isointensity and heterogeneous T2 high signal with intense heterogeneous enhancement. Much of the tumor does not enhance which could be due to myxoid material or necrosis. The tumor has an overall highly aggressive appearance worrisome for a high grade sarcoma. **6.7e:** The resected tumor is large and on cut sections is multinodular with semi-firm tan to soft gelatinous areas (gross photo). The center exhibits acute hemorrhage, and the pale yellow flecking tracking to the left is necrotic tumor. The black perimeter is due to inking. **6.7f**: The biopsy comprises a prominently myxoid tumor with some regions of more fibrous background. The tumor vessels form a meshwork (low magnification). **6.7g**: The resected tumor features another pattern of tumor in addition to the myxoid cellular spindle cell component. The second pattern is much less cellular and contains multinucleated tumor cells floating in pools of mucin (low magnification). **6.7h**: Most myxofibrosarcomas exhibit an infiltrative border, and this patient's tumor is no exception, as it insinuates between slips of skeletal muscle. The grade of the tumor in this field is low to intermediate. Commonly, high grade myxofibrosarcomas will contain foci of low grade tumor. **6.7i**: Higher magnification of the cellular fascicular area of the tumor discloses mildly atypical spindle cells with hyperchromatic, spindled nuclei and eosinophilic cytoplasm streaming through a myxoid matrix.

Case figure 6.7: Continued from page 115

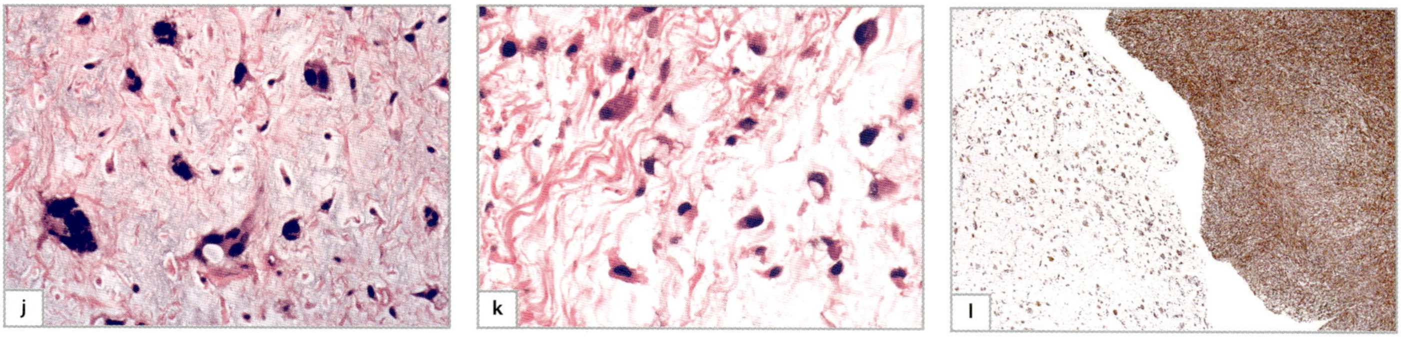

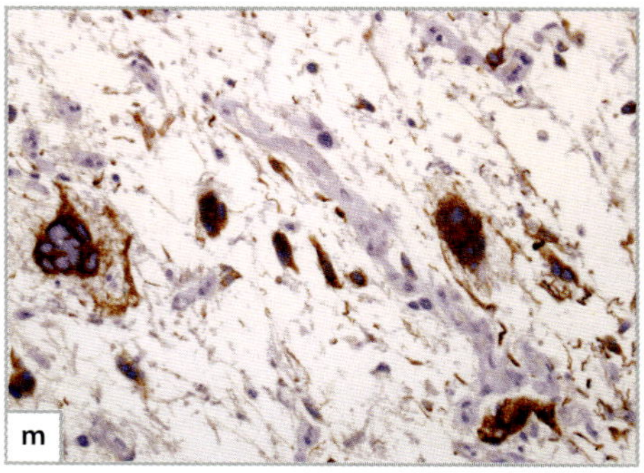

6.7j: The less cellular areas of the tumor contain the most atypical cells, many of which are multinucleated. Thin strands of collagen are scattered in the myxoid matrix (high magnification). **6.7k**: Pseudolipoblasts are a clue to the diagnosis of myxofibrosarcoma (they contain mucin rather than lipid as in real lipoblasts, and there are other minor differences). Here three such cells float among other round to polygonal tumor cells. The pseudolipoblasts contain clear vacuoles of mucin that slightly deform the nucleus or suggest a signet ring cell shape (high magnification). **6.7l**: Low magnification of the two patterns in this tumor reveals strong diffuse expression of CD34. Although not specific, this CD34 reactivity is relatively common in myxofibrosarcoma. **6.7m**: An unusual finding in this patient's tumor is expression of desmin which is limited to some of the tumor giant cells (high magnification). This has only been rarely described in myxofibrosarcoma but should not be surprising given the myofibroblastic/fibroblastic nature of the tumor cells and the sundry muscle markers these cells may express, albeit more commonly actins than desmin. Non-staining cells in this field include blood vessel endothelial cells and a few tumor cells.

Translocations specific to MLPS, namely t(12;16)(q13;p11) or t(12;22)(q13;q12 are detectable by FISH and standard karyotyping and can help differentiate the two.

MPNST: Some MPNST are myxoid, can exhibit high grade nuclear features, increased mitoses, necrosis and tumor giant cells, and approximately 25% can express CD34. However, a slim majority will also demonstrate reactivity for S-100 protein. MPNST may also show alternating bands of hypercellular and hypocellular fascicular regions, nuclear palisading, neuroid whorls, and infiltration of tumor blood vessel walls; these features are not observed in myxofibrosarcoma. Curvilinear vessels and pseudolipoblasts are absent. The MPNST spindle cells disclose nuclei that are pointy ended, wavy, or buckled in shape compared to the blunt ended, wider, straighter nuclei of the spindle cells in myxofibrosarcoma.

Undifferentiated high grade pleomorphic sarcoma: This tumor can look indistinguishable from a high grade area of myxofibrosarcoma lacking myxoid matrix. To be diagnosable as such, a high grade myxofibrosarcoma must contain at least some myxoid matrix (the percentage required for the diagnosis varies from 10% to 50% among expert soft tissue pathologists) (Folpe et al. 2010).

Differential diagnosis of LGMS

Intramuscular myxoma (IMM): The cellularity of low grade myxofibrosarcoma matches intramuscular myxoma, and both can be infiltrative into surrounding normal tissues. However, intramuscular myxoma is much less vascular than myxofibrosarcoma. Cytologic atypia including nuclear hyperchromasia can be subtle but is always present in myxofibrosarcoma and absent in IMM.

LGFMS: See Case 6.8.

Differential diagnosis of rare epithelioid variant of myxofibrosarcoma

Metastatic melanoma: Melanoma is rarely myxoid. However, it often comprises round cells with discrete borders and nucleoli mimicking an epithelioid neoplasm. Approximately one third of metastatic melanomas contain melanin pigment. Immunohistochemically, most but not all metastatic melanomas are reactive for antibodies to S-100 protein, Melan A, and/or HMB45; these proteins are not expressed in epithelioid variant myxofibrosarcoma. Most cases of epithelioid variant myxofibrosarcoma contain classic areas of myxofibrosarcoma e.g., myxoid matrix supporting spindle and polygonal cells with curvilinear vessels, perivascular concentrations of cells, and pseudolipoblasts. Clinical history can be helpful.

Metastatic carcinoma: Metastatic carcinomas should be reactive for a variety of epithelial markers such as keratins, epithelial membrane antigen (EMA), carcinoembryonic antigen (CEA) and others depending on the particular tumor. Diagnostically helpful again are classic myxofibrosarcoma areas present in most epithelioid variant myxofibrosarcoma.

Other epithelioid appearing sarcomas such as epithelioid sarcoma and epithelioid variants of leiomyosarcoma, liposarcoma, and malignant peripheral nerve sheath tumor. If the classic areas of myxofibrosarcoma are absent or scarce, prudent use of IHC and in some cases genetic tests should discriminate between these tumors.

Oncology approach

Medical oncology

Because the tumor is completely resected with adequate margins and there is no evidence of metastatic disease, chemotherapy is not proposed.

Radiation oncology

The patient declines adjuvant radiation therapy. Intermediate and high grade myxofibrosarcomas have a high rate of local recurrence despite aggressive local therapy. Thirty four cases reviewed from Harvard had a local recurrence rate of 30%, despite wide or radical resection and radiation therapy in a majority of cases (Haglund 2010). Similarly, the Italians reviewed their experience and also found high local recurrence rates, 18% (Sanfilippo 2011). In these cases, I recommend adjuvant/neoadjuvant radiation therapy unless an amputation is performed. This recommendation is largely based on the high rate of local recurrence.

Patient outcome

Two years postoperatively, the patient has normal function and no evidence of local recurrence or metastatic disease. This good outcome is not unexpected, because even high grade myxofibrosarcomas exhibit a relatively low metastatic rate of 30-35% compared with other high grade sarcomas (Dei Tos 2006). However, the patient will be followed regularly on an annual basis to exclude local recurrence and metastasis.

Case table 6.7 Summary pathology findings of Case 6.7

Diagnosis	Myxofibrosarcoma
Size	18 × 9.5 × 9 cm
Location	Deep soft tissue of thigh
Margin status	Negative; all greater than 1.0 cm
Histologic grade (FNCLCC grading system)	3 = poorly differentiated
Pathologic stage (TNM classification)	T2b/NX/M0 = Stage III

Case 6.8 Low grade fibromyxoid sarcoma

Clinical history and presentation

The patient is a 46 year old woman who presents with a four year history of an arm mass which has been asymptomatic and stable until four weeks ago when it rapidly enlarged and became painful. It was previously evaluated by her primary care physician and was felt to be a lipoma.

Physical examination reveals a large, firm, deeply situated tumor in the lateral aspect of the arm. It is tender on palpation.

Surgical findings and comments

Biopsy of the mass is performed. Two weeks later she is returned to the operating room for wide resection of the tumor.

Radiology findings

The MR appearance (**Case figs 6.8a** through **6.8c**), shows a non-specific T1 low signal, STIR high signals mass in the subcutaneous tissues. There is heterogeneous intense enhancement. This lesion appears less aggressive and varied than the myxofibrosarcoma (see Case 6-7). However, the degree of heterogeneity still is worrisome for a sarcoma and tissue diagnosis is needed.

Pathology findings gross features

The biopsy comprises gray soft tissue portions aggregating to 2 × 1.5 × 0.8 cm. A small amount is submitted fresh for karyotyping. The resection consists of a well-circumscribed, gray to mucoid mass measuring 4.9 × 4.8 × 3.8 cm. It closely approaches surgical margins. A sample is submitted fresh to Cytogenetics.

Microscopic features

Low magnification: Since the biopsy and resection are histologically similar, only the resection is described. The tumor at low mag is predominantly fibrous but dappled by pale areas (**Case fig. 6.8d**).

High magnification: Medium magnification of a fibrotic area reveals characteristic fingerprint-like whorls of collagen with embedded neoplastic fibroblasts (**Case fig. 6.8e**). The tumor cells have indistinct cell borders, and the oval to spindled nuclei is normochromatic with fine chromatin. In addition to the fibrotic areas, two other areas are noted, myxoid and cellular regions. The myxoid areas contain a gray myxoid matrix in addition with reduced collagen fibers (**Case figs 6.8f**). Most of the fibrous regions contain identical cells as seen in the myxoid areas (**Case fig. 6.8g**). However, the third region in this patient's tumor is more cellular with slightly increased nuclear atypia (**Case fig. 6.8h**). The whorling pattern is preserved, and a few cells are more rounded with perceptible cell borders.

Special studies: By IHC, the tumor cells focally express CD34 and smooth muscle actin with equivocal weak expression of EMA (epithelial membrane antigen). There is no reactivity for desmin, caldesmon, S-100 protein or nuclear β-catenin. The proliferation rate measured by Ki-67 antibody staining is less than 5%. This case was not assessed for expression of the transmembrane glycoprotein, MUC4, which may be a very sensitive and relatively specific IHC marker of LGFMSs and its high grade, more aggressive relative, sclerosing epithelioid fibrosarcoma (Doyle et al. 2011).

Both specimens submitted for karyotyping grow successfully. Many LGFMS contain a translocation t(7;16)(q34;p11) which creates the following fusion gene, *FUS-CREB3L2* (a *FUS-CREB3L1* translocation has also been reported resulting in t(11;16)). This patient's two karyotypes reveal a clonal translocation: t(7;16) helping to confirm the diagnosis.

Pathologic differential or, why isn't it one of the following?

Low grade myxofibrosarcoma: Older individuals are usually affected. Tumors are often multinodular, especially the superficial cases. In contrast to low grade fibromyxoid sarcoma, myxofibrosarcoma is predominantly myxoid Oda et al. 2004). Less myxoid areas are generally hypercellular and more atypical with storiforming pleomorphic

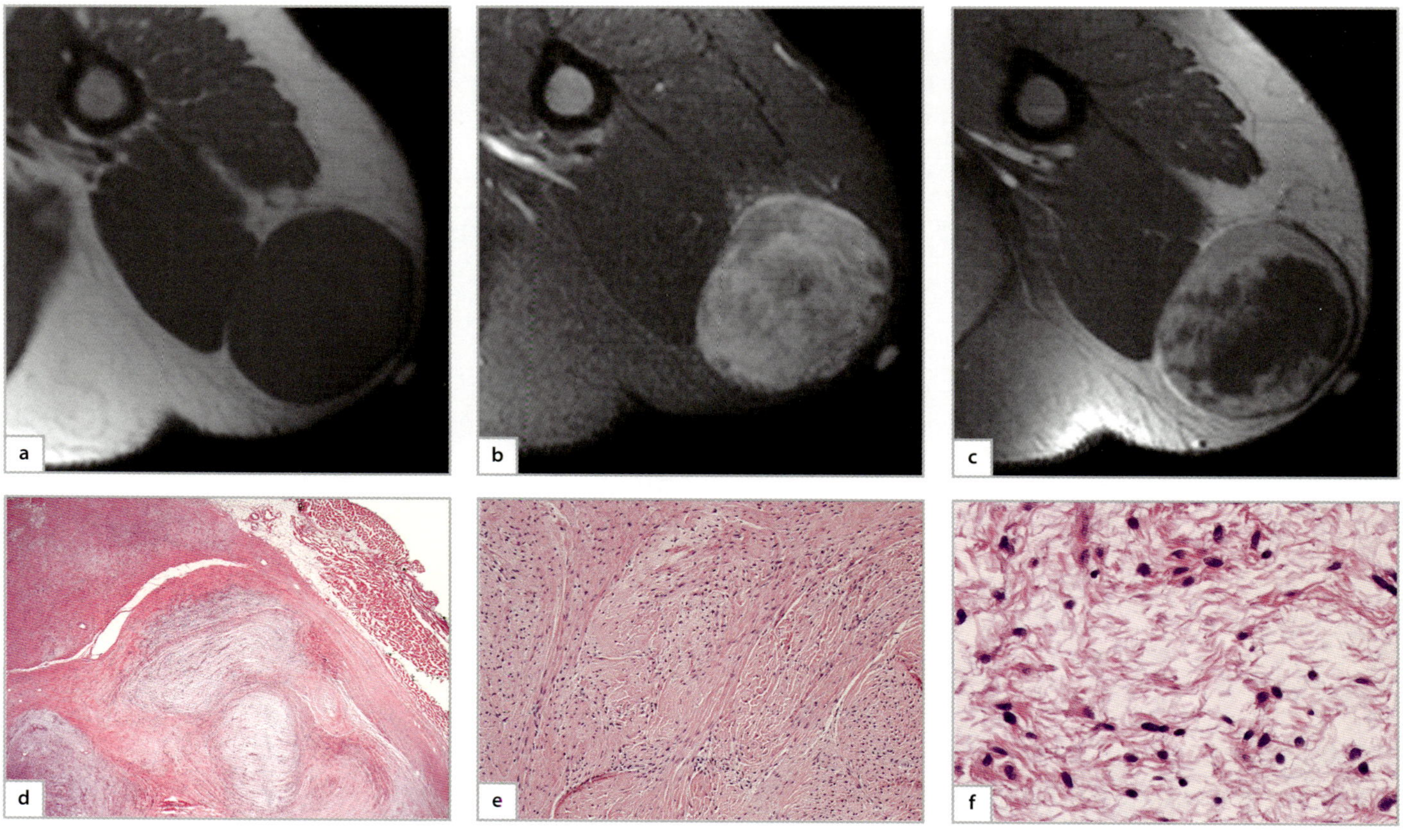

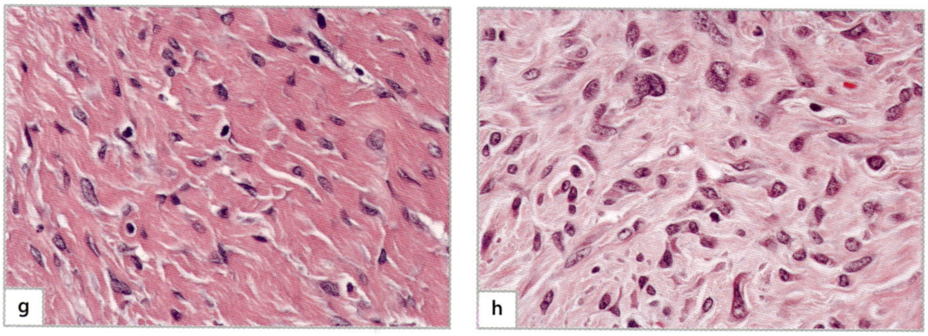

Case figure 6.8 LGFMS. **6.8a**: Axial T1, **6.8b**: Axial STIR, **6.8c**: Axial T1 fat saturated post-contrast. The MR images show a T1 low signal, STIR high signal fairly homogeneous mass in the subcutaneous tissues of the shoulder. There is heterogeneous intense enhancement with central non-enhancing areas likely from necrosis. The overall appearance is not specific. **6.8d**: The resection consists of fibrous pink areas with intermixed pale regions (low magnification). **6.8e**: A fibrotic region is composed of intersecting sheafs of spindle cells with indistinct cells borders in association with abundant pink collagen. **6.8f**: A more myxoid area of the tumor contains a gray myxoid matrix in addition to splayed collagen fibers and bland spindle cells with indistinct cell borders (high magnification). **6.8g**: At high magnification, the spindle cells have indistinct cell borders and oval to spindle nuclei with fine chromatin. The background contains collagen fibers produced by the fibroblastic tumor cells. **6.8h**: This area of the tumor is more cellular, with slightly more pleomorphism. However, nuclei remain pale, and mitotic figures are rare and not atypical (high magnification).

spindle and giant cells. The mesh of curvilinear vessels in myxofibrosarcoma is eye-catching particularly in the less cellular regions. The vascular arrangement of LGFMS is less obtrusive except in some markedly myxoid areas. Often the tumor cells of myxofibrosarcoma will condense around vessels, and inflammatory cells, primarily lymphocytes and plasma cells but also eosinophils and neutrophils, may be conspicuous. These features are absent in LGFMS. Pseudolipoblasts (tumor cells with cytoplasmic mucin droplets mimicking lipoblasts) are commonly seen in low grade myxofibrosarcoma. Even in low grade tumors, at least some cells will exhibit significant nuclear atypia with enlarged, hyperchromatic nuclei. It is uncommon for LGFMS to exhibit nuclear atypia with recurrences more likely to do so. CD34 can be strongly positive in low grade myxofibrosarcoma and is rarely so in LGFMS. MUC4 is absent (thus far in one paper) in low grade myxofibrosarcoma.

Soft tissue perineurioma: This tumor is usually fibrotic but may have myxoid areas. Tumor cells are long and slender and arranged in fascicles, storiforming whirls, and sometimes meningothelial like balls. Usually, the tumor cells are EMA, GLUT-1, and claudin-1 reactive; unfortunately, LGFMS also exhibits reactivity for these proteins. Abrupt transitions from myxoid to fibrous areas are absent in perineurioma. Perineurioma is negative for MUC4 (Doyle et al. 2011; 40 examples tested). Cytogenetically, perineurioma displays abnormalities of chromosome 22 including monosomy 22 and mutations in the NF2 gene, while LGFMS shows FUS translocations. Recurrent abnormalities and translocations involving 10q22q24 have also been reported (Brock et al. 2005).

Intramuscular myxoma (IMM): Most IMMs are uniformly myxoid and hypocellular with widely scattered simple shaped vessels.

Uncommonly, an example may be slightly more cellular and vascular with mild fibrosis. Abrupt transitions between markedly fibrotic and markedly myxoid areas are absent. The vascular arcades of some LGFMS are absent. CD34 can be strongly positive; such reactivity is rare in LGFMS. MUC4 is not reported to be reactive in IMM (20 cellular myxomas tested; Doyle et al. 2011). Myxoma is negative for FUS-CREB translocations.

Myxoid desmoid tumor: A few desmoids may be focally or rarely wholly myxoid. Most will contain conventional areas of mild to moderately cellular, parallel aligned fibroblasts/myofibroblasts in sweeping fascicles. Thin walled, compressed, non-arcing vessels, lymphocyte congeries at vessels and tumor edge, and interspersed mast cells are features not observed in LGFMS. Nuclear β-catenin reactivity is present in 70% of cases and is rare in LGFMS. Desmoids do not express EMA or MUC4 (20 desmoids assessed, Doyle et al. 2011). Desmoids exhibit mutations of the β catenin or APC genes and trisomies of chromosomes 8 and/or 20 (minority of cases) or uncommonly complex karyotypes (De Wever et al. 2000), while LGFMS features FUS-CREB translocations.

Solitary fibrous tumor: Most SFTs lack myxoid areas. Both SFT and LGFMS contain fibrous regions. The often prominent fingerprint like whorls and abrupt transitions from fibrous to myxoid regions of LFGMS are absent in the 'patternless' pattern of SFT in which random fibrotic and more cellular regions intermix. The vessels of SFT are often hyalinized and do not form arcades. Hemangiopericytomatous vessels may be seen in both tumors. By IHC, most SFT are strongly reactive for CD34 and bcl-2 and uncommonly reactive for EMA. SFT does not appear to express MUC4 (Doyle et al. 2011; 20 cases examined).

The translocation in SFT is that of *NAB2-STAT6* and not a *FUS-CREB* translocation.

Oncology approach

Medical oncology

Chemotherapy is not administered, as the patient has no evidence of metastasis. Furthermore, there is no effective chemotherapy for low grade fibromyxoid sarcoma (as of 2011).

Radiation oncology

The natural history of this sarcoma is quite complex. It is known to have high local recurrences and frequent metastasis (Evans 2011, Guillou 2007). However, the progression of the disease is typically quite slow with recurrence and metastases occurring many years after diagnosis and treatment. Due to the indolent nature of this disease, appropriate treatment recommendations will be highly dependent upon clinical

Case table 6.8a Variant features of LGFMS

Feature	Frequency	Comment
Sharply demarcated fibrous and myxoid regions with fibrous areas predominating	Very common	This is the classic appearance of LGFMS
Arcades of vessels	Very common	Can resemble the curvilinear vessels of myxofibrosarcoma in the myxoid areas
Fingerprint-like whorls of spindle cells	Very common	This may be most apparent in the transition from fibrous to myxoid areas
Focal herringbone architecture	Uncommon	This is never the predominant pattern
Hemangiopericytoma like vessels	Uncommon	When present occurs in the fibrous areas and can mimic solitary fibrous tumor
Giant collagen rosettes	Uncommon	Acellular hyalinized collagen center surrounded by a band of epithelioid fibroblasts. The cuffing fibroblasts may express S-100 protein. Previously termed: 'hyalinizing spindle cell tumor with giant rosettes' this is now known to be a variant pattern of LGFMS with no difference in behavior
Marked hypercellularity	Uncommon	May be present focally de novo or may occur in recurrences
Epithelioid tumor cells	Uncommon	May be associated with increased cellularity
Nuclear pleomorphism	Rare	More common in recurrences than de novo tumor
Keloidal or scar like collagen	Rare	
Tigroid pattern of strips of back to back fibrous and myxoid areas	Rare	This rare pattern was described by the pathologist who originally recognized LGFMS as a distinct entity, Harry Evans, M.D. (Evans 2011)
Osseous metaplasia	Rare	Noted by Dr Evans
Cell clusters, strands, palisades or retiform network of cells	Rare	Noted by Dr Evans
Cystic degeneration	Rare	Noted by Dr Evans
Foci of sclerosing epithelioid fibrosarcoma	Rare	If this is the majority of the tumor, the better diagnosis is sclerosing epithelioid fibrosarcoma, a more aggressive tumor
EMA reactivity	Common	Nonspecific but seen in 40% or more of cases
MUC4 reactivity	Very common	According to one recent 2011 series of 49 cases (Doyle et al. 2011); diagnostically helpful
Translocation t(7;16)(q34;p11) or t(11;16)(p11;p11)	Very common	Presence of one or the other translocation may become a requirement for the diagnosis (Moller et al. 2011)

factors with observation after resection being the standard. The role of radiation in this entity is not well understood, and should only be performed for palliation or to prevent recurrences that would be associated with significant morbidity.

Patient outcome

Five and one-half years later, the patient has normal function and no evidence of local recurrence or metastatic disease. However, the patient will be followed carefully indefinitely, as LFGMS is associated with recurrences and metastases up 45 years after initial presentation (Evans 2011).

Case table 6.8b Summary pathology findings of Case 6.8

Diagnosis	LGFMS
Size	4.9 × 4.8 × 3.8 cm
Location	Superficial: subcutaneous tissue of upper arm
Margin status	Negative but close at 0.1 cm with a fascial plane
Histologic grade (FNCLCC classification)	1 = low grade
Pathologic stage (TNM classification)	T1a/N0/MO = Stage IA

Case 6.9 Dermatofibrosarcoma protuberans with areas of fibrosarcoma

Clinical history and presentation

The patient is a 74 year old woman who presents with a five month history of weight loss and weakness. Two months prior to presentation she notes a mass in the back.

Physical examination reveals a cachectic elderly female with the lesion seen in **Case fig. 6.9a**.

A biopsy is performed and the pathologic diagnosis confirms dermatofibrosarcoma protuberans (DFSP) with fibrosarcomatous transformation.

Surgical findings and comments

Due to the extensive nature of the tumor and poor nutritional status of the patient, Imatinib is begun in an effort to stabilize or shrink the tumor while the patient's nutritional status is corrected. Little change in the tumor is observed over the ensuing three months.

Surgical resection is performed with attempted wide margins. Wide surgical margins are obtained around most of the tumor except where it enters the retroperitoneum unilaterally. In this area, a marginal margin is obtained. A wound vac is applied. Despite the massive size of the tissue defect resulting from the resection, the wound vac accomplishes a complete wound closure over a period of approximately six months.

Radiology findings

The MR images in **Case figs 6.9b** through **6.9f** show the typical appearance of a DFSP. There is a bulky exophytic mass of the skin with heterogeneous signal and enhancement. This case has deep invasion of the paraspinal muscles. The mass shows superficial irregularity from ulceration.

Pathology findings

Gross features

The tumor is received as one large lobulated mass that protrudes outwardly from the skin surface (**Case fig. 6.9g**). Most of the tumor has ulcerated through the skin. The tumor surface is focally necrotic and purulent. Cross sections are very firm but not gritty, pale pink to white, and vaguely whorling (**Case fig. 6.9h**). Necrosis is less than 5%.

Microscopic features

Low magnification: DFSP usually involves both the dermis and subcutis, and that prevails for this patient's tumor (**Case fig. 6.9i**). Unusually however, it also focally penetrates the fascia and extends into skeletal muscle.

High magnification: Realizing that such a large tumor may be heterogeneous, the pathologist's assistant carefully cuts many sections for microscopic review. Only a few areas exhibit the classic storiform growth pattern of typical DFSP (**Case figs 6.9j** and **6.9k**). Instead, 90% of the submitted sections reveal a higher grade spindle cell sarcoma which has lost the storiform growth pattern, is more cellular with more atypical, 'plumper' nuclei, and more mitotically active than the conventional DFSP areas (**Case figs 6.9l** through **6.9n**). The deep aspect of the tumor infiltrates the subcutaneous fat in a classic layering or honeycomb manner, preserving islands and bands of adipocytes (**Case fig. 6.9k**). In some high grade areas, a herringbone growth pattern is apparent (**Case fig. 6.9o**) with malignant cells aligned in long thin, sharply intersecting bands. This pattern is often seen in the 10% of DFSP tumors containing fibrosarcomatous or higher grade areas.

Special studies: The tumor is strongly positive for CD34 by IHC, even in most of the higher grade areas (**Case fig. 6.9p**). About half of DFSP tumors harboring fibrosarcomatous transformation will exhibit loss of CD34 in the higher grade regions. In this patient's tumor, higher grade areas exhibit an approximately 30% nuclear positivity rate for Ki-67, a proliferation marker indicating a cell is actively engaged in the cell cycle and not in the resting phase (**Case fig. 6.9q**).

Cytogenetic karyotyping is performed, and the tumor contains two related abnormal cell lines with extensive structural and numerical abnormalities including giant marker chromosomes. Such giant marker or ring chromosomes contain amplified regions of 17 and 22 encompassing the collagen type I gene α on chromosome 17q and the platelet-derived growth factor β on chromosome 22q.

Pathologic differential or, why isn't it one of the following?

Deep benign fibrous histiocytoma (DBFH): This tumor also shows focally to diffusely a storiform component. However, it tends to be less monotonous in appearance with some herringbone or diffuse growth and often contains additional cell types such as macrophages, multinucleated osteoclast-like giant cells and more commonly exhibits a hemangiopericytomatous growth pattern. The layering

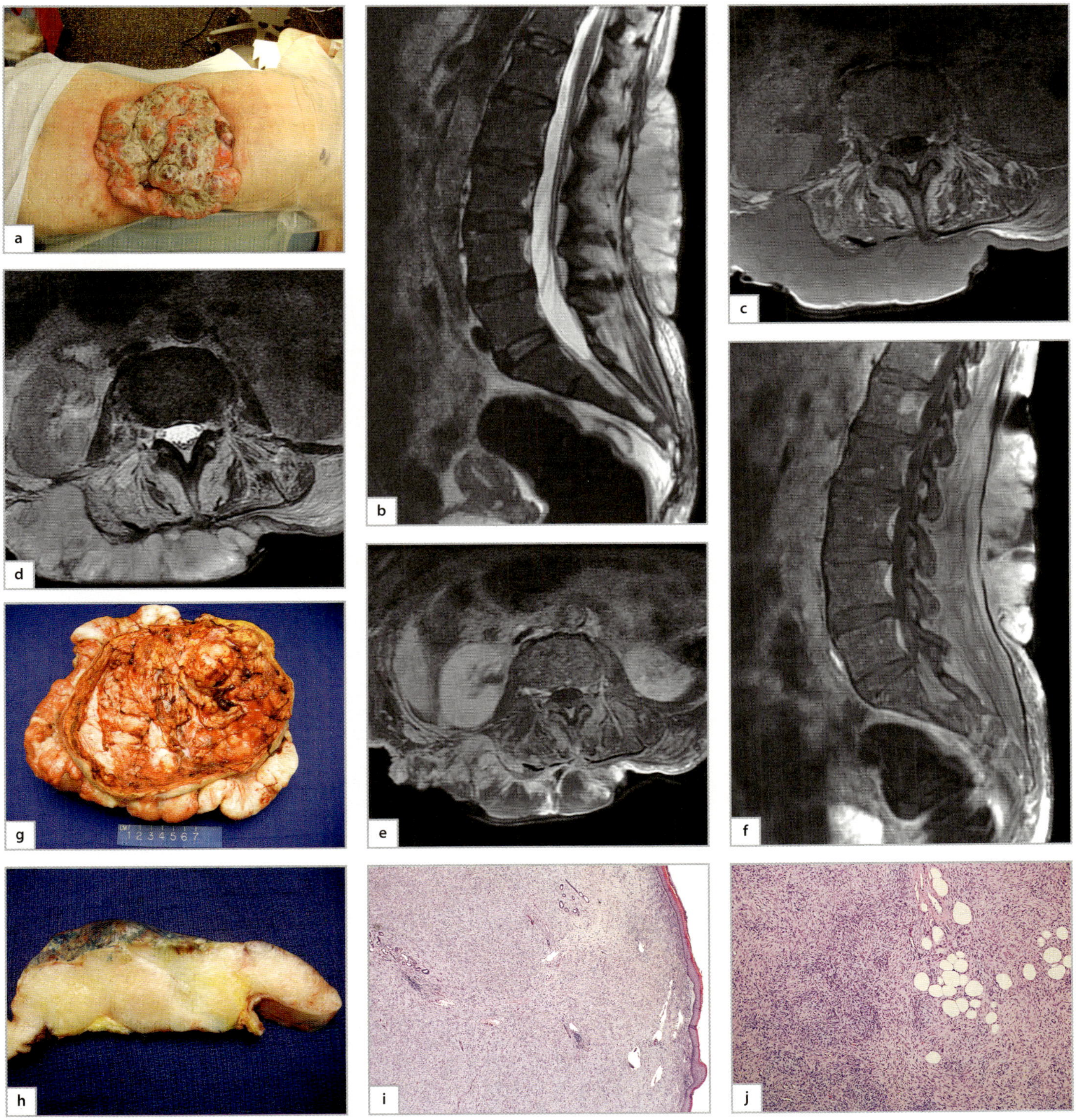

Case figure 6.9: Dermatofibrosarcoma protuberans. 6.9a: DFSP, patient at presentation. The tumor is massive but not necrotic and not super-infected. **6.9b**: Sagittal T2 MR image. **6.9c**: Axial T1 MR image. **6.9d**: Axial T2 MR image. **6.9e**: Axial T1 fat saturated post-contrast. **6.9f**: Sagittal T1 fat saturated post-contrast. Images show a bulky exophytic mass of the skin. This DFSP shows deep invasion lateral to the paraspinal musculature. The lesion has heterogeneous enhancement and surface irregularity from ulceration. Note the overhanging margin inferiorly as seen in sagittal 6.9f. **6.9g**: Gross photo of resection. The tumor is massive (24cm) and forms a single exophytic lobulated mass with areas of superficial necrosis and purulence. **6.9h**: Gross photo of a sample cross section of tumor. The tumor is firm with a whorled pink to white cut surface. **6.9i**: Low magnification. The tumor involves the dermis and extends to just below the base of the epithelium. **6.9j**: Medium magnification. Approximatley 10% of the tumor shows a storiform or cartwheel pattern of short intersecting clusters of plump spindle cells. This storiform architecture is typical of DFSP.

Case figure 6.9: Continued from page 121

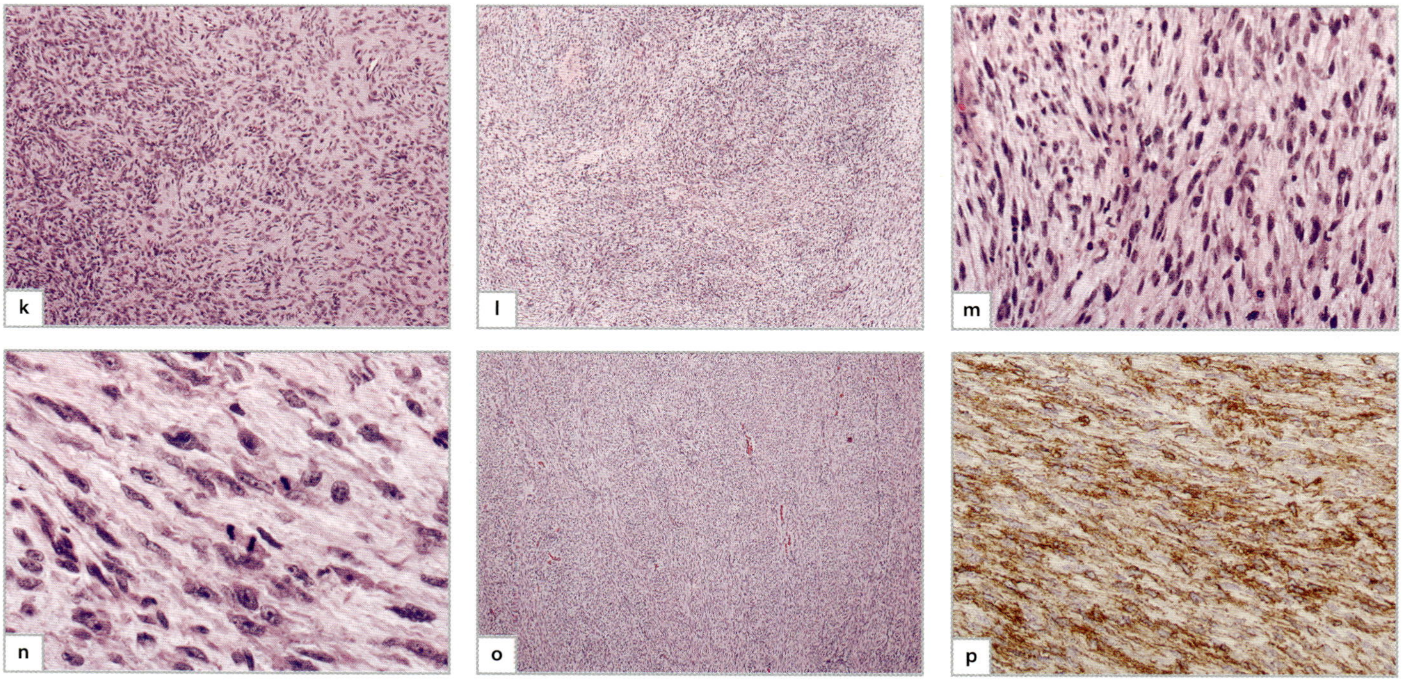

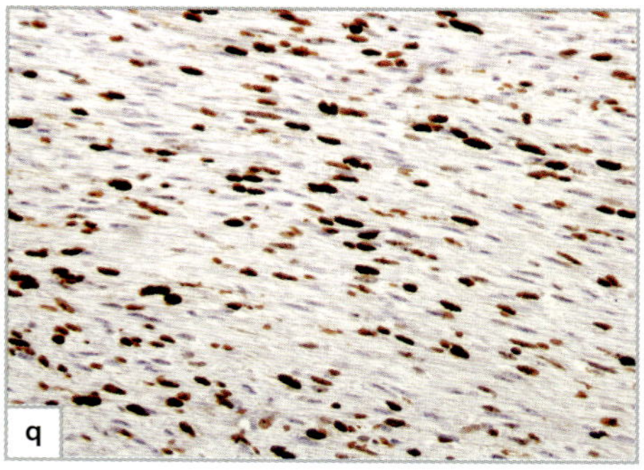

6.9k: High magnification. Classic storiform pattern of short intersecting bundles or whorls of plump spindle cells with indistinct cell borders. **6.9l**: Low magnification. Ninety percent of this patient's tumor consists of higher grade spindle cell sarcoma that loses the storiform architecture. **6.9m**: Medium magnification of higher grade area. The tumor cells are arranged in long thin fascicles and feature hyperchromatic, slender spindled nuclei. **6.9n**: High magnification of high grade area. Mitoses are more common in the higher grade area (two are present in this field). **6.9o:** Medium magnification of higher grade area. Some of the higher grade areas of this patient's tumor exhibit a herringbone growth pattern identical to that seen in fibrosarcoma. **6.9p**: Medium magnification of higher grade area. CD34 is expressed throughout the patient's tumor, even in most of the higher grade areas (immunohistochemical stain: brown is a positive reaction). **6.9q**: Medium magnification of higher grade area. Correlating with the higher mitotic rate in the fibrosarcomatous areas, Ki-67, a proliferation marker expressed in the nuclei of cells engaged in the cell cycle, is relatively markedly elevated with a 30% tumor cell positive rate. By contrast, only approximately 5-10% of the tumor nuclei in the conventional areas are positive (photo not shown).

or honeycomb infiltration into subcutaneous fat typical of DFSP is absent. Deep benign fibrous histiocytoma can be reactive for CD34 but usually only focally unlike conventional DFSP which is diffusely positive. Two other proteins are reportedly detectable in DFSP and not DBFH: low-affinity nerve growth factor receptor, p75 and apolipoprotein D (Fanburg-Smith et al. 2001, West et al. 2004). FISH or RT-PCR can also be used to confirm the DFSP translocation t(17;22)(q22;q13).

Leiomyosarcoma: Leiomyosarcoma enters the differential because it can form a spindle cell tumor in the dermis and subcutis. It usually affects older patients, however. The tumor cells are distinctly eosinophilic with blunt ended, 'cigar-shaped' or 'train car-shaped' nuclei. A storiform pattern is usually absent. The tumor cells are strongly and diffusely positive for muscle markers such as smooth muscle actin (SMA) and desmin (DFSP is negative for only focally positive for SMA generally in myoid areas). Examination for the DFSP translocation can be useful.

Spindle cell carcinoma or sarcomatoid carcinoma: This tumor usually affects older patients than those with DFSP and is unusual outside the head and neck (DFSP can occur in the head and neck but only in approximately 15% of cases). Spindle cell carcinoma does not grow in a uniform storiform pattern, often shows marked cytologic atypia, and will be negative for CD34 and usually positive at least focally for epithelial markers (by IHC).

Oncology approach

Medical oncology

Imatinib is the recommended neoadjuvant treatment when surgery is difficult or mutilating or in nonresectable DFSP (Kérob et al. 2010). The partial response rate is almost 50%, with a median time to progression of about 1.7 years and a 1-year survival rate of 87.5%. The response rates and time to progression do not differ between patients taking 400 mg or higher doses (Rutkowski et al. 2010).

Hence, the recommended starting dose is 400 mg daily when complete tumor resection is not possible or mutilating. Newer PDGFB inhibitors may become available for clinical use soon (Levitzki et al. 2004).

Radiation oncology

DFSP is a radioresponsive disease. Retrospective series show that radiation therapy should be considered for residual disease after surgery

Case table 6.9a Range of histologic findings in DFSP

DFSP histologic feature	Frequency
Storiform (cartwheel or basket weave) architecture	Almost always (it may be lost in recurrences with transformation to fibrosarcoma and there are rare superficial fibrosarcomas that exhibit the same translocation as DFSP but lack a storiform architecture)
Fibrosis	Relatively common, at least focally within one tumor; consists of collagen deposition between tumor cells
Herringbone fascicular architecture	Uncommon; occurs with fibrosarcomatous transformation; present initially or develops in recurrences of approximately 10% of patients with DFSP
Pleomorphic undifferentiated sarcoma pattern and cytology	Rare, less common than fibrosarcomatous transformation, may be associated with more aggressive course
Myxoid change	Uncommon, only rarely is it diffuse
Myoid nodules	Uncommon, they comprise myointimal proliferation of the walls of tumor blood vessels
Scattered pigmented cells containing melanin	Uncommon, called the Bednar or pigmented variant of DFSP
Granular cell change	Rare; does not affect behavior or prognosis
Pseudovascular spaces lined by multinucleated irregular shaped tumor giant cells often with collagenized matrix	Uncommon, usually occurs in childhood or adolescent cases, called giant cell fibroblastoma or juvenile DFSP; adults may show this pattern or mixed patterns of typical DFSP and giant cell fibroblastoma

especially in cases in which repeat surgery would be difficult. Doses as low as 60Gy are effective in controlling microscopic disease. Radiation therapy is an option in this case if further surgery is contraindicated to treat the recurrence.

Patient outcome

Postoperatively, the patient is continued on Imatinib. MRI performed six months postoperatively reveals a local recurrence in the area of the marginal margin. The patient dies of unrelated medical causes shortly thereafter.

Case table 6.9b Summary pathology findings of Case 6.9

Diagnosis	DFSP with transformation to fibrosarcoma
Size	24.5 × 24 × 3.5 cm
Location	Predominantly superficial (90%) but with extension through fascia into skeletal muscle (10%)
Margin status	Tumor extends to inked deep surgical margins
Histologic grade (FNCLCC system)	2 (intermediate grade) due to fibrosarcomatous transformation; conventional DFSP is grade 1
Pathologic stage (TNM classification)	T2b/N0/M0 by pathologic and clinical staging = Stage IIB

REFERENCES

Alaggio R, Barisani D, Ninfo V, et al. Morphologic overlap between infantile myofibromatosis and infantile fibrosarcoma: a pitfall in diagnosis. Pediatr Dev Pathol 2008;11:355–362.

Bernal K, Nelson M, Neff J, et al. Translocation (2;11)(q31;q12) is recurrent in collagenous fibroma (desmoplastic fibroblastoma). Cancer Genet Cytogenet 2004;149:161–163.

Bisceglia M, Galliani C, Giannatempo G, et al. Solitary Fibrous Tumor of the Central Nervous System: A 15-year Literature Survey of 220 Cases (August 1996-July 2011). Adv Anat Pathol 2011;18(5):356–392.

Bonvalot S, Eldweny H, Haddad V, et al. Extra-abdominal primary fibromatosis: Aggressive management could be avoided in a subgroup of patients. Eur J Surg Oncol 2008;34(4):462–8.

Brooks MD, Ebbs SR, Colletta AA, et al. Desmoid tumors treated with triphenylethylenes. Eur J Cancer 1992;28A:1014–1018.

Butrynski JE, D'Adamo DR, Hornick JL, et al. Crizotinib in ALK-rearranged inflammatory myofibroblastic tumor. N Engl J Med 2010;363(18):1727–33.

Carretto E, Dall'Igna P, Alaggio R, et al. Fibrous hamartoma of infancy: an Italian multi-institutional experience. J Am Acad Dermatol 2006;54:800–3.

Chmielecki J, Crago AM, Rosenberg M, O'Connor R et al. Whole-exome sequencing identifies a recurrent *NAB2-STAT6* fusion in solitary fibrous tumors. Nature Genetics 2013;45(2):131–132.

Chugh R, Wathen JK, Patel SR, et al. Efficacy of Imatinib in Aggressive Fibromatosis: Results of a Phase II Multicenter Sarcoma Alliance for Research through Collaboration (SARC) Trial. Clin Cancer Res 2010;16: 4884.

Coffin CM, Hornick JL, Zhou H, et al. Gardner fibroma: a clinicopathologic and immunohistochemical analysis of 45 patients with 57 fibromas. Am J Surg Pathol 2007;31:410–416.

Coffin CM, Watterson J, Priest JR, et al. Extrapulmonary inflammatory myofibroblastic tumor (inflammatory pseudotumor). A clinicopathologic and immunohistochemical study of 84 cases. Am J Surg Pathol 1995;19(8):859–72.

Connelly JH, Evans HL. Dermatofibrosarcoma protuberans. A clinicopathologic review with emphasis on fibrosarcomatous areas. Am J Surg Pathol Oct;16(10):921–925.

Crawford SC, Harnsberger HR, Johnson L, et al. Fibromatosis Colli of Infancy: CT and Sonographic Findings. AJR Dec 1988;151:1183–1184.

Dalen BP, Bergh PM, Gunterberg BU. Desmoid tumors: A clinical review of 30 patients with more than 20 years' follow-up. Acta Orthop Scand 2003;74:455–459.

De Pas T, Bodei L, Pelosi G, et al. Peptide receptor radiotherapy: a new option for the management of aggressive fibromatosis on behalf of the Italian Sarcoma Group. Br J Cancer 2003;88: 645–647.

De Wever I, Dal Cin P, Fletcher CDM, et al. Cytogenetic, clinical, and morphologic correlations in 78 cases of fibromatosis: a report from the CHAMP Study Group. Mod Pathol 2000;13(10):1080–85.

Domont J, Bénard J, Lacroix L, et al. Detection of β-catenin mutations in primary extra-abdominal fibromatosis (EAF): An ancillary diagnostic tool. J Clin Oncol 2008;26: (May 20 suppl; abstr 10518)

Doyle LA, Möller E, Dal Cin P, et al. MUC4 is a highly sensitive and specific marker for low-grade fibromyxoid sarcoma. Am J Surg Pathol 2011;35:733–741.

Elco CP, Marino-Enriquez A, Abraham JA et al. Hybrid myxoinflammatory fibroblastic sarcoma/hemosiderotic fibrolipomatous tumor: report of a case providing further evidence for a pathogenetic link. Am J Surg Pathol 2011;34:1723–1727.

England DM, Hochholzer L, McCarthy MJ. Localized benign and malignant fibrous tumors of the pleura: A clinicopathologic review of 223 cases. Am J Surg Pathol 1989;13:640–658.

Entel RJ, Carolan FJ. Congenital muscular torticollis: magnetic resonance imaging and ultrasound diagnosis. J Neuroimaging Apr 1997;7(2):128–130.

Erickson-Johnson MR, Chou MM, Evers BR, Roth CW et al. Nodular fasciitis: a novel model of transient neoplasia induced by *MYH9-USP6* gene fusion. Lab Invest 2011;91:1427–1433.

Evans HL. Low-grade fibromyxoid sarcoma: a clinicopathologic study of 33 cases with long-term follow-up. Am J Surg Pathol 2011;35(10):1450–62.
Fanburg-Smith JC, Miettinen M. Low-affinity nerve growth factor receptor (p75) in dermatofibrosarcoma protuberans and other nonneural tumors: a study of 1,150 tumors and fetal and adult normal tissues. Hum Pathol 2001;32(9):976–83.
Fisher C, Montgomery EA, Thway K. Biopsy Interpretation of Soft Tissue Tumors.. Wolters Kluwer/Lippincott Williams and Wilkins: Philadelphia, 2011.
Fisher, C. Myofibroblastic malignancies. Adv Anat Pathol 2004;11:190–201.
Fletcher CDM, Krishnan Unni K, Mertens F (Eds). World Health Organization Classification of Tumours. Pathology and Genetics of Tumours of Soft Tissue and Bone. Lyon: IARC Press, 2002.
Flucke U, Han J, van Krieken JM, et al. Cellular angiofibroma: analysis of 25 cases emphasizing its relationship to spindle cell lipoma and mammary-type myofibroblastoma. Mod Pathol 2011;24:82–89.
Folpe AL, Inwards CY (eds). Bone and Soft Tissue Pathology. A volume in the series: Foundations in Diagnostic Pathology. Goldblum JR (series ed). Philadelphia: Elsevier Saunders, 2010.
Folpe AL, Lane KL, Paull G, et al. Low-grade fibromyxoid sarcoma and hyalinizing spindle cell tumor with giant rosettes: a clinicopathologic study of 73 cases supporting their identity and assessing the impact of high-grade areas. Am J Surg Pathol 2000;24(10):1353–60.
Gluck I, Griffith KA, Biermann JS, et al. Role of radiotherapy in the management of desmoid tumors. Int J Radiat Oncol Biol Phys 2011;80(3):787–92.
Gold JS, Antonescu CR, Hajdu C, et al. Clinicopathologic correlates of solitary fibrous tumors. Cancer 2002;94:1057–68.
Guadagnolo BA, Zagars GK, Ballo MT. Long-term outcomes for desmoid tumors treated with radiation therapy. Int J Radiat Oncol Biol Phys 2008;71(2):441–7.
Guillou L, Benhattar J, Gengler C, et al. Translocation-positive low-grade fibromyxoid sarcoma: clinicopathologic and molecular analysis of a series expanding the morphologic spectrum and suggesting potential relationship to sclerosing epithelioid fibrosarcoma: a study from the French Sarcoma Group. Am J Surg Pathol 2007;9:1387–402.
Haglund K, Chandrajit PR, Nascimento AF, et al. Recurrence Patterns and Survival for Patients with Intermediate and High Grade Myxofibrosarcoma. Int J Radiat Oncol Biol Phys 2012;82(1):361–7.
Hajibashi S, Wang WL, Lazar AJF, et al. The desmoid tumor proteome; identifying molecular markers using a clinically annotated tissue microarray. CTOS Abstract #34885, 2008
Hansen T, Katenkamp K, Brodhun M, et al. Low-grade fibrosarcoma--report on 39 not otherwise specified cases and comparison with defined low-grade fibrosarcoma types. Histopathol 2006;49:152–160.
Hansmann A, Adolph C, Vogel T, et al. High-dose tamoxifen and sulindac as first-line treatment for desmoid tumors. Cancer 2004;100(3):612–20.
Havry P, Reitamo JJ, Vihko R et al. The desmoid tumor. III. A biochemical and genetic analysis. Am J Clin Pathol 1982;77:681–685.
Jabbari S, Andolino D, Weinberg V, et al. Successful treatment of high risk and recurrent pediatric desmoids using radiation as a component of multimodality therapy. Int J Radiat Oncol Biol Phys 2009;75(1):177–82
Janinis J, Patriki M, Vini L, et al. The pharmacological treatment of aggressive fibromatosis: a systematic review. Ann Oncol 2003;14(2):181–190.
Jelinek JA, Stelzer KJ, Bruckner CE, et al. The efficacy of radiotherapy as postoperative treatment for desmoid tumors. Int J Radiat Oncol Biol Phys 2001;50(1):121–5.
Jha P, Moosavi C, Fanburg-Smith JC. Giant cell fibroblastoma: an update and addition of 86 new cases from the Armed Forces Institute of Pathology, in honor of Dr. Franz M. Enzinger. Ann Diagn Pathol 2007;11(2):81–8.
Kempson RL, Fletcher CDM, Evans HL, et al. Atlas of Tumor Pathology – Tumors of the Soft Tissues. Bethesda: AFIP Press 2001.
Kérob D, Porcher R, Vérola O, et al. Imatinib mesylate as a preoperative therapy in dermatofibrosarcoma: results of a multicenter phase II study on 25 patients. Clin Cancer Res 2010;16(12):3288–95
Kovach SJ, Fischer AC, Katzman PJ, et al. Inflammatory myofibroblastic tumors. J Surg Oncol. 2006; 94(5):385–91.
Kransdorf MJ, Murphey MD. Imaging of Soft Tissue Tumors, 2nd ed. Baltimore: Lippincott Williams and Wilkins, 2006:486.
Lanari A. Effect of progesterone on desmoid tumors (aggressive fibromatosis). N Engl J Med 1983; 309:1523.
Laskin WB, Miettinen M, Fetsch JF. Infantile digital fibroma/fibromatosis: a clinicopathologic and immunohistochemial study of 69 tumors with long-term follow-up. Am J Surg Pathol 2009; 33:1–13.
Lau PP, Lui PC, Lau GT, et al. EWSR1-CREB3L1 gene fusion: a novel alternative molecular aberration of low grade fibromyxoid sarcoma. Am J Surg Pathol 2013;37:734–738.
Lazar AJ, Tuvin D, Hajibashi S, et al. Specific mutations in the {β}-catenin gene (CTNNB1) correlate with local recurrence in sporadic desmoid tumors. Am J Pathol 2008;173(5):1518–27.
Lee JC, Li CF, Fang FM, et al. Prognostic implication of MET overexpression in myxofibrosarcomas: an integrative array comparative genomic hybridization, real-time quantitative PCR, immunoblotting, and immunohistochemical analysis. Mod Pathol 2010;23:1379–1392.
Leithner A, Schnack B, Katterschafka T et al. Treatment of extra-abdominal desmoid tumors with interferon-α with or without tretinoin. J Surg Oncol 2000;73:21–25.
Lemm D, Mugge LO, Mentzel T, et al. Current Treatment Options in Dermatofibrosarcoma Protuberans. J Cancer Res Clin Oncol 2009;135:653–665.
Levitzki A. PDGF receptor kinase inhibitors for the treatment of PDGF driven diseases. Cytokines and Growth Factor Reviews 2004;15(4):229–235.
Liegl B, Fletcher CDM. Ischemic fasciitis: analysis of 44 cases indicating an inconsistent association with immobility or debilitation. Am J Surg Pathol 2008;32:1546–1552.
Lim CL, Walker MJ, Mehta RR, et al. Estrogen and antiestrogen binding sites in desmoid tumors. Eur J Cancer Clin Oncol 1986;22(5):583–7.
Lips DJ, Barker N, Clevers H, et al. The role of APC and β-catenin in the aetiology of aggressive fibromatosis (desmoid tumors). EJSO 2009;35:3–10.
Mace J, Sybil Biermann J, Sondak V, et al. Response of extraabdominal desmoid tumors to therapy with imatinib mesylate. Cancer 2002;95:2373–2379.
Marino-Enriquez A, Wang W-L, Roy A, et al. Epithelioid inflammatory myofibroblastic sarcoma: an aggressive intra-abdominal variant of inflammatory myofibroblastic tumor with nuclear membrane or perinuclear ALK. Am J Surg Pathol 2011;35:135–144.
Matthews MR, Cockerell CJ. An historic perspective of infantile myofibromatosis. Advances in Dermatology 2006;22:279–305.
McArthur G. Dermatofibrosarcoma protuberans: recent clinical progress. Ann Surg Oncol 2007;14(10):2876–2886.
Mentzel T, Calonje E, Wadden C, et al. Myxofibrosarcoma: clinicopathologic analysis of 75 cases with emphasis on the low grade variant. Am J Surg Pathol 1996;20:391–405.
Mentzel T, Dry, S, Katenkamp D, et al. Low grade myofibroblastic sarcoma: analysis of 18 cases in the spectrum of myofibroblastic tumors. Am J Surg Pathol 1998;22:1228–1238.
Merchant NB, Lewis JJ, Woodruff JM, et al. Extremity and trunk desmoids tumors: A multifactorial analysis of outcome. Cancer 1999; 86:2045–2052.
Mentzel T, Beham A, Katenkamp D, et al. Fibrosarcomatous ('high-grade') dermatofibrosarcoma protuberans: clinicopathologic and immunohistochemical study of a series of 41 cases with emphasis on prognostic significance. Am J Surg Pathol 1998;22(5):576–687.
Miettinen M, Modern Soft Tissue Pathology Tumors and Non-Neoplastic Conditions. Cambridge: Cambridge University Press 2010.
Möller E, Hornick JL, Magnusson L, et al. FUS-CREB3L2/L1-positive sarcomas show a specific gene expression profile with upregulation of CD24 and FOXL1. Clinical Cancer Research 2011;17:2646–2656.
Nascimento A, Ruiz R, Hornick JL, et al. Calcifying fibrous 'pseudotumor': clinicopathologic study of 15 cases and analysis of its relationship to inflammatory myofibroblastic tumor. Int J Surg Pathol 2002;10:189–196.
Nascimento AF, Bertoni F, Fletcher CDMF. Epithelioid variant of myxofibrosarcoma: expanding the clinicomorphologic specrtum of myxofibrosarcoma in a series of 17 cases. Am J Surg Pathol 2007;31:99–105.
Nieuwenhuis MH, De Vos Tot Nederveen Cappel W, Botma A, et al. Desmoid tumors in a Dutch cohort of patients with familial adenomatous polyposis. Clin Gastroenterol Hepatol 2008;6(2):215–9.
Nuyttens JJ, Rust PF, Thomas CR Jr, et al. 3rd. Surgery versus radiation therapy for patients with aggressive fibromatosis or desmoid tumors: A comparative review of 22 articles. Cancer 2000;88(7):1517–23.
O'Brien KP, Seroussi E, Dal Cin P, et al. Various regions within the α-helical domain of the COL1A1 gene are fused to the second exon of the PDGFB gene in dermatofibrosarcomas and giant-cell fibroblastomas. Genes Chromosomes Cancer 1998;23(2):187–93.
Oda Y, Takahira T, Kawaguchi K, et al. Low-grade fibromyxoid sarcoma versus low-grade myxofibrosarcoma in the extremities and trunk. A comparison

of clinicopathological and immunohistochemical features. Histopathol 2004;45:29–38.

Pakos EE, Ioannidis JP. Radiotherapy vs. nonsteroidal anti-inflammatory drugs for the prevention of heterotopic ossification after major hip procedures: a meta-analysis of randomized trials. Int J Radiat Oncol Biol Phys 2004;60(3):888–95.

Park MS, Patel SR, Ludwig JA, et al. Combination therapy with temozolomide and bevacizumab in the treatment of hemangiopericytoma/malignant solitary fibrous tumor. J Clin Oncol 2008;26(S):10512.

Patel SR, Evans HL, Benjamin RS. Combination chemotherapy in adult desmoid tumors. Cancer 1993;72(11):3244–7.

Penel N, Le Cesne A, Bui BN et al. Imatinib for progressive and recurrent aggressive fibromatosis (desmoid tumors): an FNCLCC/French Sarcoma Group Phase II trial with long-term follow up. Ann Oncol 2011;22:452–457.

Qiu X, Montgomery E, Sun B. Inflammatory myofibroblastic tumor and low grade myofibroblastic sarcoma: a comparative study of clinicopathologic features and further observations on the immunohistochemical profile of myofibroblasts. Hum Pathol 2008;39:846–856.

Robinson LA. Solitary fibrous tumor of the pleura. Cancer Control 2006;13:264–9.

Rose B, Tamvakopoulos GS, Dulay K, et al. The clinical significance of the FUS-CREB3L2 translocation in low-grade fibromyxoid sarcoma. J Orthop Surg Res 2011;6:15.

Roses DF, Valensi Q, LaTrenta G, et al. Surgical treatment of dermatofibrosarcoma protuberans. Surg Gynecol Obstet 1986;162(5):449–452.

Rutkowski P, Van Glabbeke M, Rankin CJ, et al. Imatinib mesylate in advanced dermatofibrosarcoma protuberans: pooled analysis of two phase II clinical trials. J Clin Oncol 2010;28(10):1772–9.

Saab ST, Hornick JL, Fletcher CD, et al. IgG4 plasma cells in inflammatory myofibroblastic tumor: inflammatory marker or pathogenic link? Mod Pathol 2010;24:606–612.

Salas S, Chibon F, Noguchi T, et al. Molecular characterization by array comparative genomic hybridization and DNA sequencing of 194 desmoid tumors. Genes Chromosomes Cancer 2010;49:560–568.

Sanfilippo R, Miceli R, Grosso F, et al. Myxofibrosarcoma: prognostic factors and survival in a series of patients treated at a single institution. Ann Surg Oncol 2011;18(3):720–5.

Skapek SX, Ferguson WS, Granowetter L, et al. Pediatric Oncology Group. Vinblastine and methotrexate for desmoid fibromatosis in children: results of a Pediatric Oncology Group Phase II Trial. J Clin Oncol 2007;25(5):501–6.

Sorensen A, Keller J, Nielsen OS, et al. Treatment of aggressive fibromatosis: A retrospective study of 72 patients followed for 1–27 years. Acta Orthop Scand 2002;73:213–219.

Stacchiotti S, Pedeutour F, Negri T, et al. Dermatofibrosarcoma protuberans-derived fibrosarcoma: Clinical history, biological profile and sensitivity to imatinib. Int J Cancer 2011;129(7):1761–72.

Surveillance, Epidemiology, and End Results (SEER) Program (www.seer.cancer.gov) SEER*Stat Database: Incidence - SEER 13 Regs Research Data, Nov 2010 Sub (1992–2008) <Single Ages to 85+, Katrina/Rita Population Adjustment> - Linked To County Attributes - Total U.S., 1969–2009 Counties, National Cancer Institute, DCCPS, Surveillance Research Program, Cancer Statistics Branch, released April 2011, based on the November 2010 submission.

Surveillance, Epidemiology, and End Results (SEER) Program (www.seer.cancer.gov) SEER*Stat Database: Incidence - SEER 17 Regs Research Data + Hurricane Katrina Impacted Louisiana Cases, Nov 2010 Sub (1973–2008 varying) - Linked To County Attributes - Total U.S., 1969–2009 Counties, National Cancer Institute, DCCPS, Surveillance Research Program, Cancer Statistics Branch, released April 2011, based on the November 2010 submission.

Tassano E, Nozza P, Tavella E, et al. Cytogenetic characterization of a fibrous hamartoma of infancy with complex translocations. Cancer Genet Cytogenet 2010;201:66–69.

Vallat-Decouvelaere AV, Dry SM, Fletcher CD. Atypical and malignant solitary fibrous tumors in extrathoracic locations: evidence of their comparablility to intra-thoracic tumors. Am J Surg Pathol 1998;22(12):1501–1511.

Vavken P, Castellani L, Sculco TP. Prophylaxis of heterotopic ossification of the hip. Clin Orthop Relat Res 2009;467:3283–3289.

Waddell WR, Gerner RE. Indomethacin and ascorbate inhibit desmoid tumours. J Surg Oncol 1980;15:85–90.

Waddell WR, Kirsch WM. Testolactone, sulindac, warfarin, and vitamin K1 for unresectable desmoid tumors. Am J Surg 1991;161:416–421.

Wang XL, DeSchepper AMA, Vanhoenacker F, et al. Nodular fasciitis: correlation of MRI findings and histopathology. Skeletal Radiol Jan 2002;31:155–161.

Weiss AJ, Horowitz S, Lackman RD. Therapy of desmoid tumors and fibromatosis using vinorelbine. Am J Clin Oncol 1999;22(2):193–5.

West RB, Harvell J, Linn SC, et al. Apo D in soft tissue tumors: a novel marker for dermatofibrosarcoma protuberans. Am J Surg Pathol 2004;28(8):1063–9.

Wignall OJ, Moskovic EC, Thway K, et al. Solitary fibrous tumors of the soft tissues: review of the imaging and clinical features with histopathologic correlation. Am J Roentgenol 2010;195(1):w55–62.

Yang Q, Mamounas M, Yu G, et al. Human Gene Therapy 1998;9(13):1929–1937.

FURTHER READING

Hosalkar HS, Torbert JT, Fox EJ, et al. Musculoskeletal desmoid tumors. J Am Acad Orthop Surg 2008;16:188–198.

Kaplan FS, Glaser DL, Hebela N, et al. Heterotopic ossification. J Am Acad Orthop Surg 2004;12:116–125.

Chapter 7 So-called fibrohistiocytic tumors and undifferentiated/unclassified sarcomas of soft tissue

OVERVIEW

The category 'fibrohistiocytic tumors' has been disintegrating since the mid-1980s driven by advances in laboratory testing. When pathologists applied antibodies to some of the purported malignant tumors of this group, a large percentage of the sarcomas showed differentiation along non-'fibrohistiocytic' lines, including smooth muscle, adipose tissue, and peripheral nerve sheath (Fletcher 1992).

It is not surprising that a classification of tumors proposed in 1963 should prove less than stable over the ensuing decades. The archetypal malignant tumor of this category, pleomorphic- storiform malignant fibrous histiocytoma (MFH), was characterized by cell culture studies showing tumor cells performing histiocyte functions and then elongating like fibroblasts (Ozzello et al. 1963, Matushansky et al. 2009). These cells were termed 'facultative fibroblasts'. Further support for this unique cell accrued when the tumor cells were shown to express antigens thought to be specific for histiocytes including α-1-antitrypsin, lysozyme and others (Kempson et al. 2001). Through the 1970s, the MFH category expanded into five subtypes that accounted for the majority of adult soft tissue sarcomas diagnosed in the 1980s and into the 1990s.

The standing of MFHs (and benign tumors that also seemed to show features of histiocytes and fibroblasts) crumbled under the onslaught of more sophisticated laboratory analyses which also indicated that cell culture studies could be misleading, electron microscopy findings non-specific, and histiocytic enzyme production broadly present in many cell types. Additionally, many tumors that appeared histiocytic actually in fact did have a histiocytic component albeit one consisting of an influx of benign histiocytes responding to signals released by the actual neoplastic non-histiocytic cells. With new specific antibodies and genomic profile analysis, it has come to be understood that most tumors initially considered MFHs or other types of fibrohistiocytic tumors actually are not histiocytic in origin and represent a diverse group of neoplasms that happen to appear histologically similar. What were once the most common sarcomas of adults, MFHs, are now diagnoses of exclusion. Moreover, the term 'malignant fibrous histiocytoma' is in the process of disappearing, due to efforts of expert soft tissue pathologists.

The disappearance of the primary malignant tumor in the category of 'fibrohistiocytic tumors', MFH has affected the other category tumor members leading to ongoing reclassification into other types of soft tissue tumors: "unavoidably, the fall of the progenitor affected its progeny" (Al-Agha et al. 2008). Certainly, there are true tumors of histiocytes: reticulohistiocytoma and xanthoma, among others. However, the 'facultative fibroblast' the putative cell of origin of these tumors, does not exist. In this transitional period of dissolution of 'fibrohistiocytic' tumors of soft tissue, there are still some mesenchymal neoplasms that by virtue of history and cytologic appearance are placed in this category with a caveat that they may be shortly transferred to other, more substantiated tumor groups. Because the term 'malignant fibrous histiocytoma' is so clinically prevalent, its demise is still ongoing. To confuse matters more, a common superficial tumor, benign fibrous histiocytoma, shows no signs of name change. Despite these obstacles, expert pathologists officially introduced a new nomenclature for the MFHs (the malignant versions of the fibrohistiocytic tumors of soft tissue category) in 2002. **Table 7.1** provides the 2013 World Health Organization (WHO) classification of fibrohistiocytic tumors of soft tissue. It's a motley lot in which the members are united by exhibiting "a poorly defined morphological descriptor of histiocytic differentiation" (Fletcher et al. 2002). Also included in this chapter are the undifferentiated/unclassified sarcomas of soft tissue, as these were historically termed 'malignant fibrous histiocytomas'.

CLASSIFICATION

Currently, the WHO recognizes five tumors all of which have a propensity for local recurrence with a low risk of metastasis. Notably this is an assortment of tumors some of which may be of synovial cell differentiation (giant cell tumor of tendon sheath and diffuse-type giant cell tumor of tendon sheath and diffuse-type giant cell tumor) others fibroblastic or myofibroblastic (such as plexiform fibrohistiocytic tumor), and others fibroblastic or myofibroblastic. (such as plexiform fibrohistiocytic tumor and deep benign fibrous histiocytoma).

DEMOGRAPHICS

As might be expected for a conglomerate of probably unrelated tumors, there is a broad age range for these lesions from pediatric to elderly. In most cases, with the exception of tenosynovial giant cell tumors, males and females are approximately equally affected. There are no known genetic germ line predispositions for any of these tumors, and no specific risk factors have been identified.

PATHOGENESIS

The only common thread linking these tumors is histological: a storiform growth pattern with or without a complement of cells with 'histiocytic' features. The causes of these tumors are unknown. Some of these tumors are relatively rare, and therefore genetic information is absent to very sparse (this pertains to plexiform fibrohistiocytic tumor, deep benign fibrohistiocytoma, and giant cell tumor of soft tissue (low malignant potential)). Some of the tumors are characterized by complex karyotypes (the undifferentiated pleomorphic sarcomas) (Kresse et al. 2010). Others have characteristic and specific defined cytogenetic

Table 7.1 WHO classification of so-called fibrohistiocytic tumors of soft tissues (2013)

Tumor	Behavior	Additional comments
Giant cell tumor of tendon sheath (localized tenosynovial giant cell tumor)	Benign	Recurrences occur in 4-30% of cases. Treated by simple conservative re-excision
Diffuse type giant cell tumor (diffuse tenosynovial giant cell tumor, pigmented villonodular synovitis [PVNS])	Intermediate	Locally aggressive with frequent local recurrence (30%). Exceptional tumors metastasize
Plexiform fibrohistiocytic tumor	Intermediate	Local recurrences in 12-37%. Rarely metastasizes to regional lymph nodes and/or lungs
Deep benign fibrous histiocytoma	Intermediate	Recurrence rate is low if completely excised; otherwise it is ~20%. Rare tumors may metastasize
Giant cell tumor of soft tissue (low malignant potential)	Intermediate	Metastasis is a rare event. Transformation to high grade sarcoma may rarely occur.
Tumors which are now considered 'undifferentiated' or 'unclassified' (previously termed malignant fibrous histiocytomas)		
Undifferentiated pleomorphic high grade sarcoma	Malignant	Previously termed 'pleomorphic/storiform malignant fibrous histiocytoma'. This is not a tumor of histiocytes
Undifferentiated pleomorphic sarcoma with giant cells	Malignant	Previously termed 'giant cell malignant fibrous histiocytoma'. This is not a tumor of histiocytes
Undifferentiated pleomorphic sarcoma with prominent inflammation	Malignant	Very rare. Previously termed 'inflammatory malignant fibrous histiocytoma'. This is not a tumor of histiocytes
Benign: does not recur or recurs non-aggressively and does not metastasize; Intermediate: can aggressively recur and/or rarely metastasizes (~5%); Malignant: can recur and commonly metastasizes.		

findings such as for tenosynovial giant cell tumor. **Table 7.2** highlights the genetic findings of this scatter-shot group of tumors. As is the case with many other tumors described in this text, genetic specifics have not been entirely elucidated, and much work is ongoing.

In terms of the nature of the malignant versions of these tumors (the undifferentiated pleomorphic sarcomas; dwindingly known as the MFH tumors), several theories currently are propounded. They can be divided into four main proposals that are not necessarily mutually exclusive:

1. *Final common pathway of dedifferentiation:* The undifferentiated pleomorphic sarcomas represent a final common pathway for specific sarcomas equivalent to dedifferentiation. An example of evidence to support this includes a recent 2009 comparison of eighteen extremity leiomyosarcomas with age matched and stage matched extremity undifferentiated pleomorphic sarcomas (n = 31). In this genomic profiling study using gene expression profiling and specific arrays, the authors determined that only the expression of nine genes differed between leiomyosarcoma of the extremity and undifferentiated pleomorphic sarcoma suggesting that these tumors are closely related with the latter dedifferentiating from the former (Carnerio et al. 2009).
2. *Origin from mesenchymal stem cells:* A second possible origin for these undifferentiated sarcomas is malignant transformation of mesenchymal stem cells (primitive, pleuripotential soft tissue cells). Evidence to support this idea derives from gene expression profiles indicating a close genetic relationship between MFH type tumors and mesenchymal stem cells (Matushansky et al. 2009).
3. *Unrecognized specific differentiation along known tumor types:* It is also possible that some of these undifferentiated pleomorphic sarcomas may actually represent very early stages of differentiation of specific other tumor types such as malignant peripheral nerve sheath tumor and leiomyosarcoma. For this theory, it is stated that current levels of scientific investigation are not sensitive enough to identify their line of differentiation, but that future advances may be able to assign lines of differentiation (Matushansky et al. 2009).
4. *Unrecognized differentiation to new unique tumor types:* A fourth possibility is that a small subset of these pleomorphic sarcomas is differentiating along a pathway that hasn't been fully characterized. For example, this small subset could evolve similar to the gastrointestinal stromal tumors (GIST) in which years were required before it was determined that these tumors differentiate toward the phenotype of Interstitial Cells of Cajal.

One emphatic fact is that these undifferentiated high grade sarcomas occasionally still erroneously labeled as MFHs (much to the consternation of some experts) are not in any way related to true histiocytes. One of the former categories of MFH, myxofibrosarcoma (known previously as myxoid MFH) is now considered a tumor of fibroblastic differentiation. It thus represents one of the first MFH variants to be assigned a specific line of differentiation. As noted above, the other undifferentiated sarcomas may sort out to include tumors that are just poorly differentiated progressed sarcomas of specific subtypes that can no longer be recognized as a specific subtype but could become recognized as specific sarcomas with advances in testing, they may include tumors that are just undifferentiated end-stage sarcomas that have shed all specific markers of differentiation, they may include tumors that are closely related to mesenchymal stem cells but with malignant transformation, and a small subset may actually differentiate to a type of mesenchymal cell that has not yet been characterized (the last possibility is least likely).

PATHOLOGY

Table 7.3 lists the so-called fibrohistiocytic tumors of soft tissue and the undifferentiated/unclassified sarcomas of soft tissue. It should be noted that tenosynovial giant cell tumors are most likely synovial cell in differentiation, plexiform fibrohistiocytic tumors are most likely myofibroblastic or fibroblastic attracting a large influx of histiocytes, deep benign fibrohistiocytoma is related to superficial fibrohistiocytoma and again is more likely fibroblastic in differentiation, the pleomorphic high grade sarcomas represent a mixture of possible types of tumors, and giant cell tumor of soft tissue (low malignant potential) may also represent a tumor of fibroblasts. Thus it is anticipated that most tumors currently labeled as so-called fibrohistiocytic will be transferred to the category of fibroblastic/myofibroblastic tumors in the next version of the WHO. classification of soft tissue tumors.

Table 7.2 Genetics of so-called fibrohistiocytic tumors of soft tissue and undifferentiated/unclassified tumors of soft tissue

Tumor	Chromosomal abnormality	Genes involved	Percentage of tumors with abnormality
Giant cell tumor of tendon sheath (localized tenosynovial giant cell tumor)	t(1;2)(p11;q36–37) Other translocations of 1p11 with 3q21, 5q31, 11q11. Also translocations involving 16q24	CSF1 (at 1p11) = colony stimulating factor 1 CO6A3 (at 2q36–37) = collagen type 6 promotor	> 50% have clonal abnormalities
Diffuse type tenosynovial giant cell tumor (pigmented villonodular synovitis)	As above. Also, can show trisomies of chromosomes 5 and 7 more commonly than localized form	As above. The translocation t(1;2) (p11;q36–37) results in inundation of the tumor by histiocytes	>80% have clonal abnormalities
Deep benign fibrous histiocytoma	One case only with t(16;17)(p13.3;q21.2)	Unknown	May be isolated case; additional six cases tested were negative for this translocation
Plexiform fibrohistiocytic tumor	No consistent abnormalities	Unknown	Unknown
Giant cell tumor of soft tissue	Unknown (UNM patient has a complex aneuploid karyotype but also has unconventional high grade sarcomatous areas)	Unknown	Unknown
Undifferentiated high grade pleomorphic sarcoma	Complex aneuploid karyotype: Gains of 1p areas, 1q and 20q in ~55%. Losses of 10q, 13q, 2q, 1q and 16q (50–64%)	Unknown consistent findings. Some may have p53, HRAS, KRAS and NRAS mutations	Most have complex aneuploidy
Undifferentiated pleomorphic sarcoma with giant cells	Complex aneuploid karyotype as above	Unknown	Most have complex aneuploidy
Undifferentiated pleomorphic sarcoma with prominent inflammation	Complex aneuploid karyotype	Unknown	Most have complex aneuploidy

Tenosynovial giant cell tumors

Giant cell tumors of the tenosynovial type occur as a localized or diffuse type of tumor. Based on recent similarity of the neoplastic cells immunohistochemically to normal synovial cells, the current speculation is that these tumors are derived from or differentiating towards synoviocytes (Boland et al. 2009). There are behavioral differences between the localized and diffuse tenosynovial giant cell tumors that may be secondary to a number of factors including the propensity for the diffuse form to involve large joints and the localized form to affect small joints of the hands and feet, epigenetic differences between the tumors and possibly genetics, although both tumors share common karyotype features and translocations (the diffuse type more frequently harbors trisomies).

Although both tumors may recur, the diffuse type displays a more aggressive local growth more difficult to control with conservative surgery, and synovectomy is often required. A somewhat synonymous term for the diffuse type of tenosynovial giant cell tumor is pigmented villonodular synovitis (PVNS). This older term reflected the thinking that this lesion was a reactive and not neoplastic process. The current concept of these tumors is that they are neoplastic with consistent cytogenetic abnormalities.

Rarely, the diffuse type of giant cell tumor of tendon sheath may metastasize; sometimes these particular metastasizing tumors have increased cytologic atypia, mitoses, and necrosis (Li et al. 2008).

Interestingly, the tenosynovial giant cell tumors are characterized by large numbers of infiltrating histiocytes and often scattered osteoclast-like giant cells both of which hone in on sites with overexpression of CSF-1. The CSF-1 gene is usually translocated (located in chromosome 1p13) and often diffusely expressed in these tumors (West et al. 2006). CSF-1 is an inflammatory mediator that recruits macrophages and can stimulate the formation of osteoclast-like giant cells. Its diffuse expression in the neoplastic cells of tenosynovial giant cell tumors may actually represent a possible target for creation of therapeutic agents in cases refractory to conventional therapy (Cupp et al. 2007).

Plexiform fibrohistiocytic tumor

Plexiform fibrohistiocytic tumor generally occurs in young adults and children, although a broad age range may be affected. It was originally specifically described by Franz Enzinger and Renyuan Zhang in 1988 (Moosavi et al. 2007). It is rare, and the cytogenetics have not been fully characterized. Although many cells in the lesion comprise recruited histiocytes, the actual neoplastic cells are considered to be fibroblastic or myofibroblastic. Most plexiform fibrohistiocytic tumors behave only with a risk of local recurrence; however a very small minority may metastasize and cause patient death (Moosavi et al. 2007).

Deep benign fibrous histiocytoma

Like the MFH category of tumors, many tumors diagnosed as deep benign fibrous histiocytomas have now been reassessed. Based on current diagnostic criteria, it is probable that many formerly diagnosed deep benign fibrous histiocytom (deep MFH) actually represented solitary fibrous tumors (Miettinen et al. 2010). Even so, a small number of tumors that resemble superficial fibrous histiocytomas and which arise in the subcutaneous tissues and deep soft tissue still fulfill strict histologic criteria for deep benign fibrous histiocytoma. A recent review of 69 such cases states that these tumors must demonstrate a classic storiform pattern of growth that at least focally, contain intermixed lymphocytes, and often share other features with the cutaneous type of benign fibrous histiocytoma. However, unlike cutaneous benign fibrous histiocytoma, they also can express CD34 and feature hemangiopericytomatous vasculature similar to solitary

Table 7.3 So-called fibrohistiocytic tumors of soft tissue and undifferentiated/unclassified tumors of soft tissue grouped by behavior

Tumor	Incidence	Age and sex distribution	Body site	Histopathology including IHC: Medium magnification	Histopathology including IHC: High magnification
Benign: does not recur aggressively and does not metastasize					
Giant cell tumor of tendon sheath (localized tenosynovial giant cell tumor)	Common to very common	Adults F > M	Most common in hands, then feet; rarely in tendons around knee and other joints	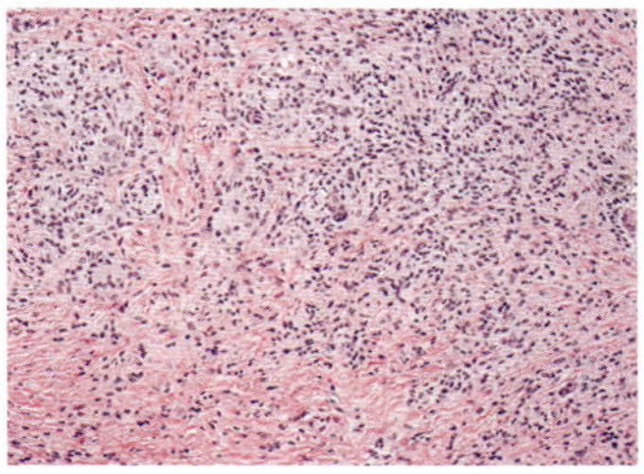	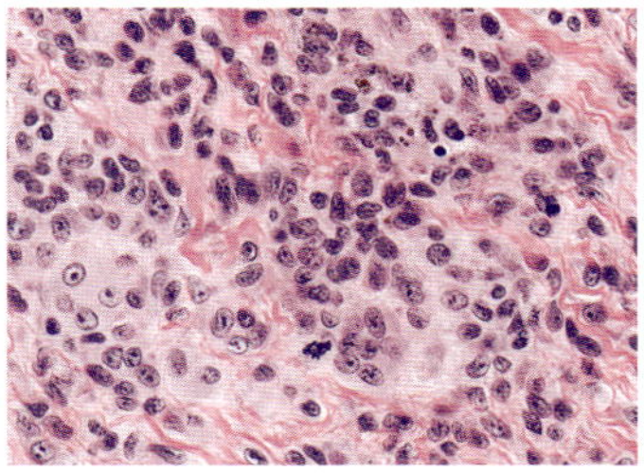
Cellular nodule of mixed cell types including larger epithelioid cells, smaller histiocytes, spindle cells, and osteoclast-like giant cells. Nuclei are pale and not atypical. Mitoses can be numerous but not abnormal. The background is variably fibrotic. Xanthomatous macrophages and hemosiderin can be present. Usually less than 4 cm and located in a tendon. The true lesional cells (larger epithelioid cells) show scattered positivity for desmin and more uniform positivity for clusterin.					
Diffuse type giant cell tumor (diffuse tenosynovial giant cell tumor, also known as PVNS)	Uncommon to rare	Most common in young adults. F > M	Large joints: knee, hip, ankle, elbow; unusual location is temporal-mandibular joint; rarely occurs only in soft tissue without joint involvement	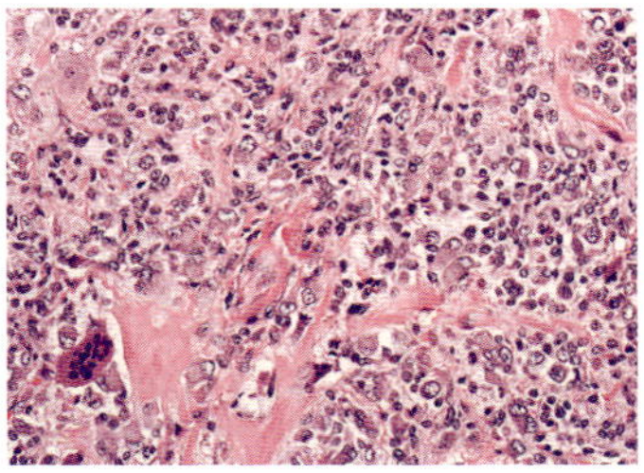	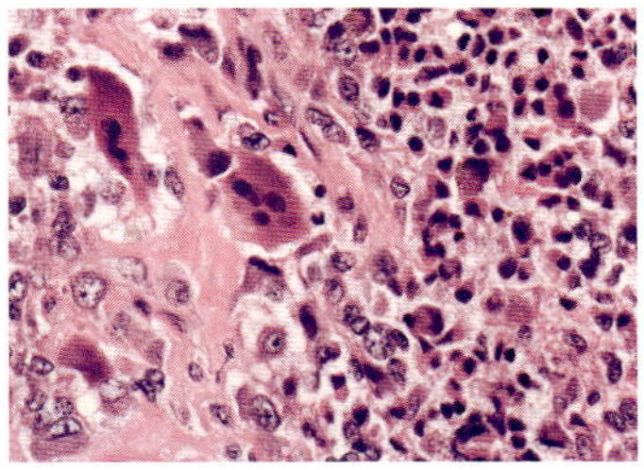
Same complement of cells as for the giant cell tumor of tendon sheath except that the epithelioid cells may be more numerous and more commonly contain hemosiderin. By definition, the tumor grows diffusely in the joint space; many also extend into surrounding soft tissues. Rarely, it is totally extra-articular. IHC staining is similar to localized form.					
Deep benign fibrous histiocytoma	Rare to extremely rare	Broad age range including children but most patients are in 30s-40s. Males may be slightly more commonly affected	Extremities, then head and neck, then trunk. Most are subcutaneous but can be deep	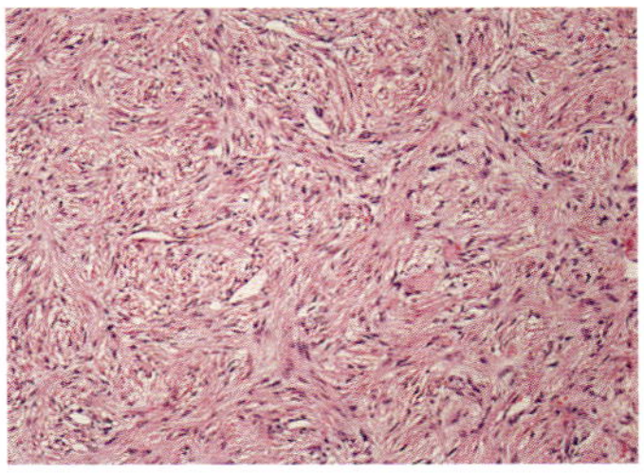	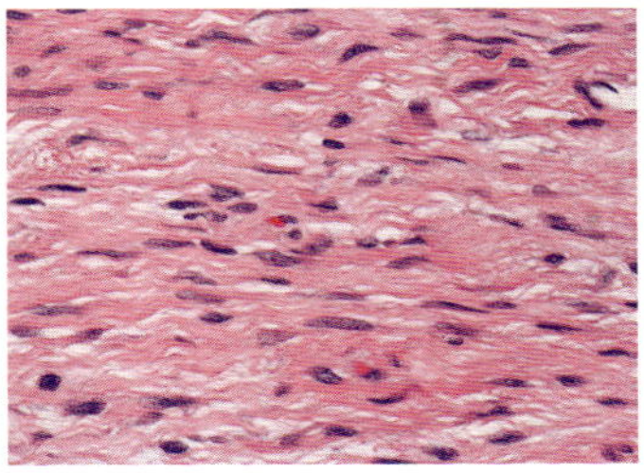
Well-circumscribed tumor with at least some areas showing a tight or loose storiform growth pattern formed by bland ovoid and spindle cells with intermixed lymphocytes. A few tumors contain scattered more atypical cells. Other findings include multinucleated tumor cells and osteoclast-like cells, foam cells, "staghorn" vessels, fibrosis, collarette of lymphyocytes, and metaplastic bone. IHC: ~50% of cases positive for CD34 and smooth muscle actin; rarely positive for desmin.					
Intermediate: can aggressively recur and/or rarely (~5%) metastasizes					
Plexiform fibrohistiocytic tumor	Uncommon to rare	Broad age range but most are young adults and children. M = F	Most in upper extremity and head and neck. Most are located at dermal-subcutaneous border but can be entirely dermal or extend to skeletal muscle	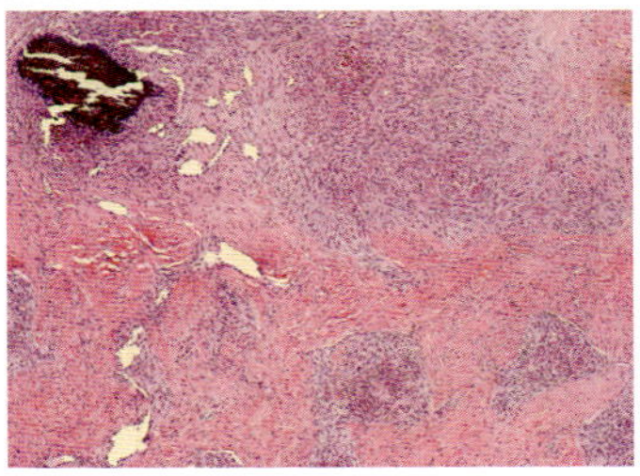	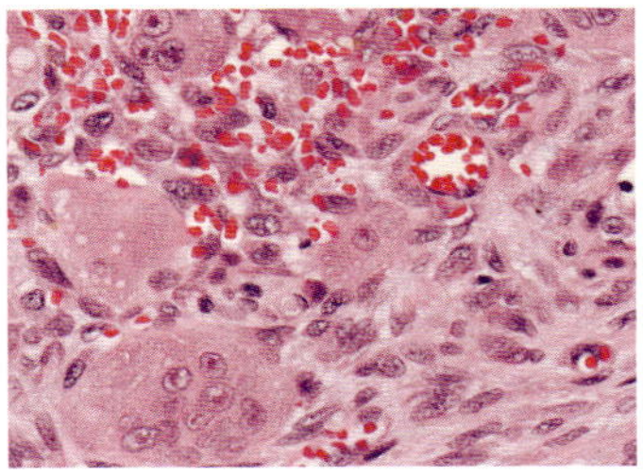
Three growth patterns occur: 1) multiple dispersed nodules containing round or spindle cells with osteoclast-like giant cells, hemorrhage, and chronic inflammation, 2) fibroblastic with mats of spindle cells arranged in scattered (plexiform) foci with the appearance of desmoid tumor, 3) mixed pattern combining both prior patterns. Normal mitoses can be seen. Unusual findings include: metaplastic bone, myxoid change, cytologic atypia, fibrous tissue replacement. IHC: CD68 stains the histiocytes and osteoclast-like giant cells; the spindle to ovoid cells can be smooth muscle actin, muscle specific actin, and calponin.					

Table 7.3: Continued from page 129

Tumor	Incidence	Age and sex distribution	Body site	Histopathology including IHC Medium magnification	 High magnification
Giant cell tumor of soft tissue (low malignant potential)	Extremely rare	Broad age range from children to elderly; most are middle aged. M > F	Proximal extremities, trunk, rarely hands/feet and intra-abdominal. 60% subfascial; 40% subcutis or dermis	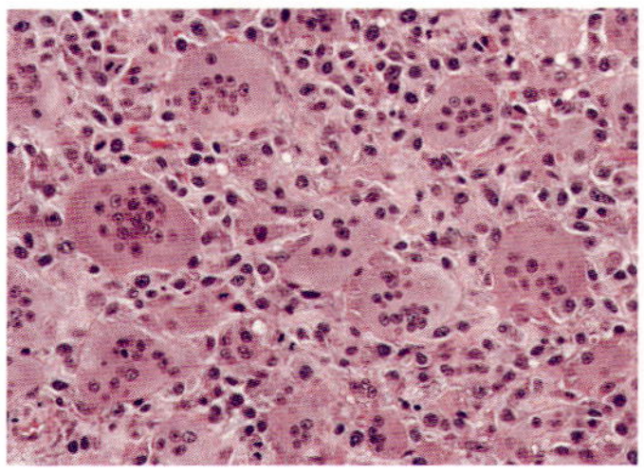	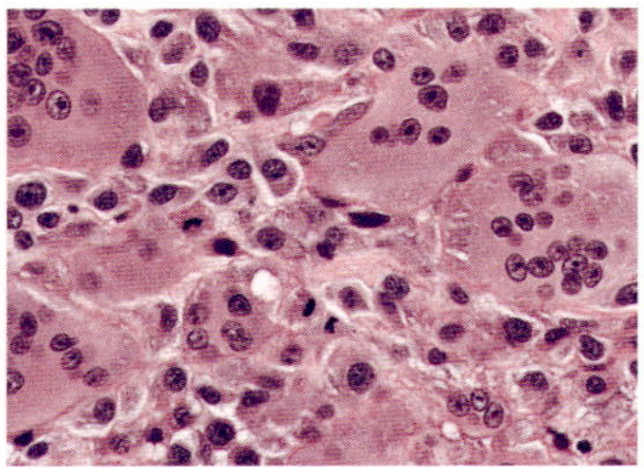
Mulinodular or multilobular tumor comprising evenly distributed multinucleated osteoclast-like giant cells in a background of ovoid, round and spindle cells. Mitoses can be numerous. Other findings: rim of metaplastic bone, hemorrhage, cystic change, fibrosis, foamy macrophage. Basically, the tumor looks like giant cell tumor of bone +/- ABC change. IHC: CD68 positive in histiocytes and osteoclast-like cells; SMA in mononuclear tumor cells. Possibly p63 in mononuclear tumor cells.					
Malignant: can recur and commonly metastasizes					
Undifferentiated high grade pleomorphic sarcoma	Common to very common	Older adults (6th decade and beyond) M = F	Lower extremity, trunk, head and neck. Deep location	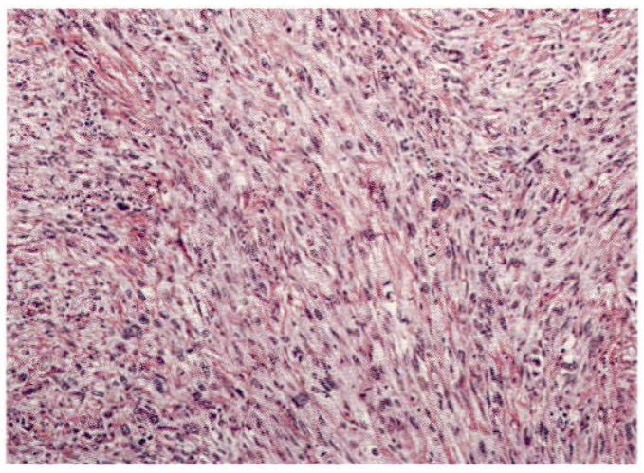	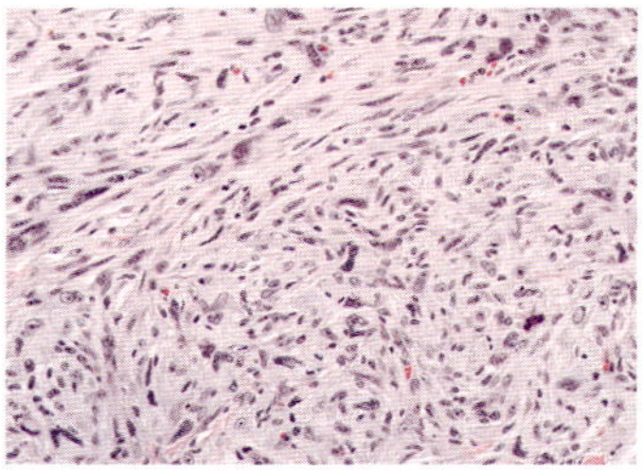
Cellular storiforming and fasciular tumor often with widespread hemorrhage and necrosis. Tumor cells are spindled, polygonal and epithelioid (can be mixed in one tumor) with marked nuclear pleomorphism including tumor giant cells. Mitoses are numerous and often abnormal. Other findings include: myxoid change, fibrosis, and chronic inflammation. IHC: There should not be diffuse reactivity for any specific markers of differentiation. Smooth muscle actin, desmin and keratins can be positive but only focally.					
Undifferentiated pleomorphic sarcoma with giant cells	Uncommon to rare	Older adults. M = F	Extremities, trunk. Deep location predominantly but can occur in subcutis	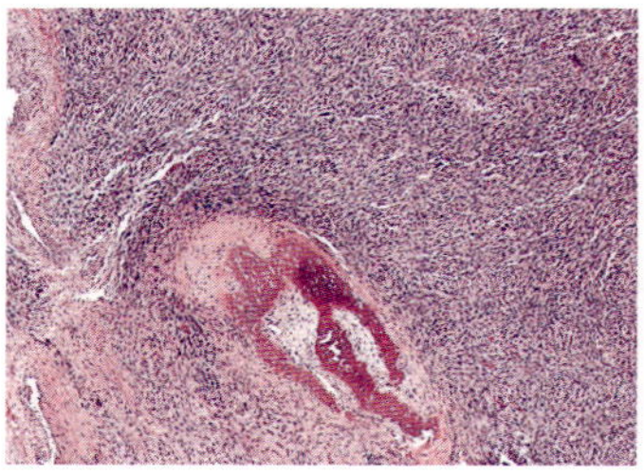	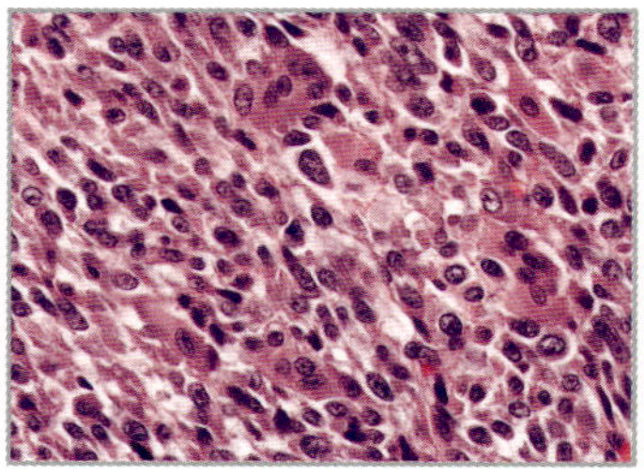
The tumor is similar to undifferentiated high grade pleomorphic sarcoma except that it also contains prominent osteoclast-like giant cells. It can also more commonly contain foci of metaplastic bone and hemorrhage can be prominent.					
Undifferentiated pleomorphic sarcoma with prominent inflammation	Uncommon to rare	Older adults. M = F	Retroperitoneal; rare in deep soft tissues of extremities	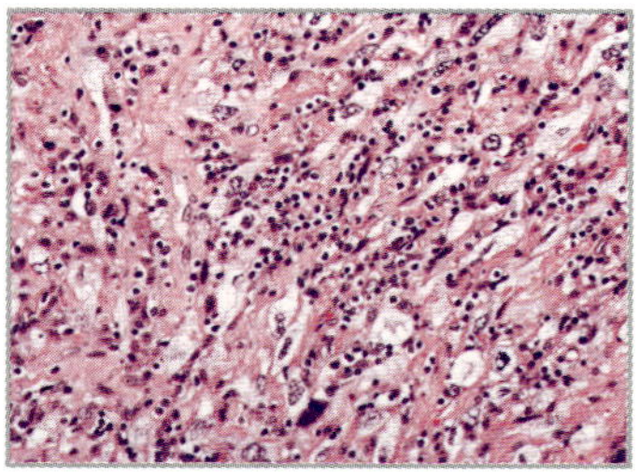	
This is a rare tumor now diagnosed only after exclusion, in particular, of dedifferentiated liposarcoma. The inflammatory cells can markedly outnumber the atypical epithelioid to spindle neoplastic cells. The inflammation is usually neutrophilic but also can compose xanthomatous histiocytes and lymphocytes.					
'Common to very common' indicates that a medium sized practice will treat at least several to dozens of patients with the lesion annually, 'Uncommon to rare' indicates the same practice size will treat one to two patients with the lesion every five years, 'Rare to very rare' indicates the same sized practice will see zero to one patient with the lesion every 20 years. M: male, F: female. IHC: immunohistochemistry.					

fibrous tumor. Differences from solitary fibrous tumor are detailed in the Cases section of this chapter. The local recurrence rate is reported at 20% especially if the lesion is inadequately excised. Tumors may rarely metastasize and lead to patient death (Gleason et al. 2008).

Giant cell tumor of soft tissue (low malignant potential)

This rare tumor was previously lumped with 'undifferentiated high grade pleomorphic sarcoma with giant cells' as a sarcoma of soft tissues infiltrated by numerous osteoclast-like giant cells. However, by definition, giant cell tumor of soft tissues (low malignant potential) should contain areas of low grade tumor that look histologically indistinguishable at high magnification from giant cell tumor of bone even to the extent of occasionally containing secondary cystic changes similar to aneurysmal bone cyst as occurs in some giant cell tumors of bone. One histologic difference of giant cell tumor of soft tissue from giant cell tumor of bone is that most of these tumors have a multinodular architecture with separation of the nodules by fibrous septae. Even though it is a soft tissue tumor, giant cell tumor of soft tissue produces metaplastic bone in approximately 50% of cases generally rimming the exterior of the multiple nodules. This bone is histologically bland rather than showing marked cytologic atypia as would be seen in extraosseous osteosarcoma.

The genetics of giant cell tumor of soft tissue are not known, as it is an unusual tumor. Consistent with its name, giant cell tumor of soft tissue (low malignant potential) only rarely metastasizes. It is considered a member of the fibrohistiocytic tumors of soft tissue perhaps because of its large number of multinucleated osteoclast-like giant cells in association with small histiocytes that inundate the lesion.

Undifferentiated pleomorphic sarcomas

Undifferentiated high grade pleomorphic sarcoma, undifferentiated pleomorphic sarcoma with giant cells, and undifferentiated pleomorphic sarcoma with prominent inflammation represent the three tumors are MFH variants that have been more appropriately renamed. Two other previous members of the MFH group, myxofibrosarcoma (myxoid MFH) and angiomatoid fibrous histiocytoma (angiomatoid MFH) have been reassigned to other categories (fibroblastic tumors and tumors of uncertain differentiation, respectively). As previously discussed, undifferentiated pleomorphic high grade sarcoma may encompass several types of histologically similar sarcomas including undifferentiated sarcoma arising from a more differentiated specific type of sarcoma such as leiomyosarcoma, a malignant mesenchymal stem cell sarcoma, a differentiating tumor that is not recognized as a differentiating tumor due to limitations of current methodology, or possibly a sarcoma that differentiates along a pathway that is currently not characterized (these are not mutually exclusive possibilities). All three of the undifferentiated pleomorphic sarcomas are tumors of exclusion that can look identical on standard histology review to other specific tumor types such as leiomyosarcoma, melanoma, dedifferentiated liposarcoma, and sarcomatoid carcinoma, among others.

Although it is ideal to try to identify specific lines of differentiation in a high grade pleomorphic sarcoma, the effort to do so may sometimes be considerable. For example, a recent study examining tumors that looked otherwise like pleomorphic high grade undifferentiated sarcoma of the retroperitoneum required at least 40 paraffin tissue blocks to find a few areas of these retroperitoneal tumors that clinched the diagnosis of liposarcoma (Al-Agha 2008). Therefore, faced with a high grade pleomorphic malignancy located in the soft tissue, opportunity and means must apply to extensively sample and perform immunohistochemical staining, not to mention genetic analysis. Winnowing those tumors with specific differentiation from the truly undifferentiated pleomorphic sarcomas can be important in predicting prognosis. For example, tumors that have muscle or myofibroblast differentiation may be more aggressive than undifferentiated high grade pleomorphic sarcoma. Eventually, with further sophistication in evaluating gene expression panels and consequent development of more targeted therapies, it will become critical to exactly classify sarcomas just as with other types of cancer.

RADIOLOGY

As noted in the preceding Pathology section, so-called fibrohistiocytic tumors comprise a diverse group of soft tissue lesions. Some have useful or characteristic imaging features. The remainder has non-specific features that could represent benign or malignant pathology, not necessarily indicative of a 'fibrohistiocytic' lesion. The radiologist is often limited to only describing the lesion and its location.

Giant cell tumor of tendon sheath is an uncommon, painless, benign tumor that occurs in association with the tendon sheath. They occur more frequently in the hand but can occur in the feet. Eighty percent involve the volar aspect of the first three digits (Llauger 1999). Williams, 2010, showed there was a 12.7% local recurrence rate of hand lesions followed for an average of 51 months. Given the suggestive clinical presentation, imaging workup is sometimes limited. Radiographs may show a soft tissue density mass. Calcification and periosteal reaction are rare. Pressure type erosion of the adjacent bone may develop in 20%. MRI may show T1 iso-intensity to muscle with T2 heterogeneous and low signal, and strong homogeneous enhancement (Llauger 1999).

PVNS is a rare proliferative disorder closely related to GCTTS histologically. PVNS is a monoarticular process usually affecting a large joint of the lower extremity. The knee is involved in about 80% of cases (Llauger 1999). PVNS occurs in a focalized form, also called Localized Giant Cell Tumor of Tendon Sheath, or in the more common diffuse form where the proliferative tissues involve the entire joint. Surgical resection can be frustrated by recurrences in 18–45% (Schnirring-Judge 2011). Treatment options include external beam radiation, as well as, synoviorthesis – the intra-articular injection of a radioisotope (Yttrium 90, Dysprosium 165 or Rhenium 186) to achieve synovectomy.

PVNS typically presents with periarticular chronic appearing erosions (with corticated margins) and preservation of joint space. Eighty percent of patients have joint pain and 79% may have an effusion (Ottaviani 2010). MRI classically shows lobulated and confluent areas of mixed signal tissue with variable enhancement. The tissue characteristically has irregular areas that are low signal on all sequences related to hemosiderin deposition. Gradient echo sequences will show these dark areas to 'bloom' and appear larger due to signal dephasing from the iron in the hemosiderin. The radiologist can play an important role in preoperative planning and the careful follow-up surveillance for recurrence.

The plexiform histiocytic tumor is a rare lesion for which there is little imaging literature describing its appearance. These tumors may show infiltrative margins and the lesion may be quite extensive. The tumor may appear to invade by insinuating between tissues rather than destroying or displacing them. Hence there may be little mass effect for the size of the tumor.

The remaining tumors in this group of fibrohistiocytic tumors of soft tissue and undifferentiated/unclassified tumors of soft tissue have a non-specific appearance. Thus, the high grade pleomorphic sarcoma, giant cell tumor of soft tissue and deep benign fibrous histiocytoma all typically have heterogeneous signal with irregular margins and show heterogeneous enhancement. Interestingly, the giant cell tumor of soft tissue is a benign entity yet appears indistinguishable from many malignant lesions. Although this is a rare lesion, it lends hope for the patient that there may be a benign histology discovered on biopsy for what appears on imaging to be an aggressive sarcoma.

SURGERY

Giant cell tumor of tendon sheath

These tumors should be excised with a marginal margin. Persistent tumor may do substantial damage to the associated tendon, and may occasionally lead to (or even present with) tendon rupture. Recurrence following marginal excision is rare (Adelani et al. 2008, Tyler et al. 2006).

Diffuse-type giant cell tumor (pigmented villonodular synovitis)

Although the biologic behavior of this entity may vary considerably, recurrence is common, satisfactory excision is difficult, and persistence of the lesion and/or multiple recurrences may lead to severe damage of the associated articular cartilage, which in turn may lead to advanced degenerative arthritis.

Complete synovectomy is the treatment of choice for this condition. Even with complete synovectomy, recurrence rates have ranged from 8–50% (Adelani et al. 2008, Mendenhall et al. 2006, Tyler et al. 2006).

The recurrence rate is higher in the presence of damage to the articular surface. Additionally, symptoms are less likely to be alleviated by synovectomy alone when there is significant co-existing cartilage damage. With advanced degenerative arthritis, total joint arthroplasty results in better alleviation of symptoms and a lower risk of recurrence than synovectomy alone.

Damage to the articular cartilage may be progressive even in those patients who undergo successful synovectomy without recurrence.

Deep benign fibrous histiocytoma

Marginal excision of these tumors generally results in a very low rate of local recurrence. Deep tumors that are also multinodular, infiltrative, or located in difficult areas (orbit) have a higher recurrence rate, but this is probably a reflection of increased difficulty obtaining satisfactory removal of the primary tumor.

Plexiform fibrohistiocytic tumor

Resection with wide margins is the treatment of choice for this tumor (Taher and Pushpanathan 2007).

CLINICAL PEARL

Aspiration of an involved joint characteristically returns blood.

CLINICAL PEARL

Gross inspection at surgery typically reveals a rust colored lesion secondary to extensive hemosiderin pigmentation. When a sample of the tumor is placed in a bowl of saline it characteristically exhibits a pattern of 'ferning.'

GRAY AREA

Equivalent recurrence rates have been reported in the literature for both arthroscopic and open synovectomy. Complete synovectomy is technically difficult by either approach, particularly in the knee and elbow. Arthroscopic synovectomy may result in a higher rate of local recurrence when the disease is associated with bony cysts or large associated soft tissue masses.

GRAY AREA

Whether the recurrence rate is lower following joint arthroplasty because the procedure facilitates a better synovectomy or whether removal of the articular cartilage removes a stimulus for tumor recurrence remains controversial.

Giant cell tumor of soft tissue (with dedifferentiation)

Representing a variation of a low grade soft tissue sarcoma, wide surgical margins are indicated.

Undifferentiated pleomorphic sarcoma (three variants)

Resection with wide surgical margins is the treatment of choice for these sarcomas.

MEDICAL ONCOLOGY

There is no medical oncology intervention for the following diagnoses: giant cell tumor of tendon sheath, PVNS, deep benign fibrous histiocytoma, and plexiform fibrohistiocytic tumor. However in lesions expressing receptor activator of nuclear factor κ B (RANK) (usually an osteoclastic origin), inhibitors of the pathway might theoretically have some efficacy.

Giant cell tumor of soft tissue with dedifferentiation

The giant cell tumor of soft tissue (GCTST) has to be differentiated from undifferentiated high-grade pleomorphic sarcoma (UHPS) with giant cells because of its more benign behavior. Dedifferentiated tumors may metastasize, but this happens in less than 10% of cases and the treatment is then the same as for UHPS (Oliveira 2000, O'Connell 2000). Because of some similarity of the undifferentiated pleomorphic sarcoma with giant cells to giant cell tumor of the bone (Lau 2005), the use of denosumab may be considered. Denosumab inhibits the ligand for RANK, a type I membrane protein expressed on the surface of osteoclasts and involved in their activation upon ligand binding (Thomas 2010).

Undifferentiated high-grade pleomorphic sarcoma

Adjuvant chemotherapy

There is some evidence from various meta-analyses that adjuvant chemotherapy, especially the combination of doxorubicin and ifosfamide, improves overall survival in patients with high grade soft tissue sarcoma.

The Cochrane Controlled Trials Register, UKCCCR Register of Cancer Trials, Physicians Data Query, EMBASE, MEDLINE and CancerLit were searched for randomized trials of adjuvant chemotherapy after local treatment in adults with localized resectable soft tissue sarcoma, with accrual completed by December 1992.

Fourteen trials of doxorubicin-based adjuvant chemotherapy involving 1568 patients were included. Median follow-up was 9.4 years. Overall recurrence-free survival was better after adjuvant chemotherapy (Hazard ratio of 0. 75 (95% CI 0.64–0.87)). For overall survival, the hazard ratio of 0.89 (95% CI 0.76–1.03) was not significant but potentially represented an absolute benefit of 4% (95% CI -1 to 9) at 10 years. There was no consistent evidence of a difference in effect according to age, sex, stage, site, grade, and histology, extent of resection, tumor size, or exposure to radiotherapy. However, the strongest evidence of a beneficial effect on survival was shown in patients with sarcoma of the extremities (Cochrane Database 2000). In an updated analysis, this data was confirmed. Four additional trials were identified representing now 18 trials with 1953 patients. The odds ratio for local recurrence was 0.73 [95% confidence interval (CI) 0.56–0.94; P =0.02] in favor of chemotherapy. For overall survival, doxorubicin alone had an odd ratio of 0.84 (95% CI, 0.68–1.03; P = 0.09), which was not statistically significant. However, the combination of doxorubicin with ifosfamide had an odd ratio of 0.56 (95% CI, 0.36–0.85; P = 0.01) in favor of chemotherapy (Pervaiz 2008). The French Sarcoma Group database is a prospective database of 1513 adult patients with non-metastatic soft tissue sarcomas. The cases of 420 patients treated with adjuvant chemotherapy from 1980 to 1999 were reviewed. The median follow-up was 9 years. While young age, non-well-differentiated liposarcoma histology, deep location, bone and/or neurovascular invasion and grade 2 or 3 were significantly associated with a higher likelihood to receive adjuvant chemotherapy. Improved metastasis-free survival {5-year MFS: 58% versus 49%, hazard ratio (HR) 0.7 [95% confidence interval (CI) 0.6–0.9], P = 0.01} and overall survival (OS) [5-year OS: 58% versus 45%, HR 0.6 (95% CI 0.5–0.8), P = 0.0002] were noted in grade 3 patients (Italiano 2010). Data are expected from the Sarcoma mUlti-Center Clinical Evaluation of the Efficacy of riDaforolimus (SUCCEED) study, in which patients were randomized to either maintenance oral ridaforolimus or placebo. The preliminary analysis favors ridaforolimus. The full report is pending.

These meta-analyses, registry analysis, and randomized clinical trial favors adjuvant chemotherapy in patients with high grade soft tissue sarcoma, whether it is a biological agent (mTOR inhibitor), or a doxorubicin-based regimen. However, the absolute benefit is limited First line chemotherapy for recurrent or metastatic disease.

No particular treatment has been shown superior in terms of survival. One approach in patients with oligometastases is to induce tumor shrinkage to facilitate resection of the remaining lesions. This strategy has been used especially for lung metastases, with a success rate of up to 45% (Billingsley 1999).

Single agent

The standard of care remains the anthracyclines, specifically doxorubicin as a single agent (see Chapter on Chemotherapy).

Trabectedin is a marine derived alkaloid that inhibits the nucleotide excision repair pathway and also causes transcriptional interference. The response to single agent therapy in the first line setting parallels that of the combination of doxorubicin and ifosfamide (Yovine 2004). In 36 patients with metastatic STS, trabectedin was given at a dose of 1.5 mg/m^2 as a 24-hour continuous infusion. The majority of these patients had never received chemotherapy before, and the predominant histologies were LMS and liposarcoma. Objective response rate was 17.1%. Recombination DNA repair pathways were studied in 113 patients with advanced sarcomas, which were enrolled in trabectedin studies. High expression of the common allele (aspartic acid at codon 1104) of ERCC5, high expression of ERCC1, and BRCA1 haplotype were significantly associated with improved PFR, PFS, and OS. These SNPs may represent a potential DNA repair signature that could be used for the prediction of clinical response to trabectedin in patients with soft tissue sarcomas (Italiano 2011). Grade 3 and 4 toxicities were most commonly hematological or due to a reversible transaminitis that usually occurred 3 - 4 days after drug administration. This transaminitis can be attenuated with the use of prophylactic dexamethasone (Paz-Ares 2010). Trabectedin is also a vesicant that can cause extravasation reactions and is best administered through a central catheter.

Combination chemotherapy

As with single agent chemotherapy, survival is no different than after treatment with any chemotherapy combination. However, if the goal is to shrink the tumors to improve the symptoms, combination chemotherapies will induce a better response rate. Two combinations of chemotherapy are interchangeably used.

1. The combination of doxorubicin and ifosfamide is frequently used in the United States as front line chemotherapy in the treatment of metastatic STS. However, this combination can have significant toxicities. The anthracycline doxorubicin has the potential to cause cardiotoxicity in a minority of patients (Schein 1975). Prevention of cardiomyopathy involve change in drug administration, administration of dexrazoxane, a chelating agent that interferes with iron-mediated free radical generation thought to be at least partially responsible for anthracycline induced cardiomyopathy (Seifert 1994), and monitoring of the cardiac ejection fraction by multigated cardiac imaging (MUGA). Ifosfamide, an alkylating agent, has the potential to cause hemorrhagic cystitis, neurotoxicity and renal tubular acidosis (Cohen 1975). Ifosfamide is usually contraindicated in elderly patients and in those with pre-existing renal impairment. More recently, a stabilized active metabolite of ifosfamide, palifosfamide, that does not degrade into acrolein (responsible for the bladder toxicity) or chloroacetaldehyde (responsible for the neurotoxicity), is being studied in a phase III trial in combination with doxorubicin, following a successful randomized phase II trial of doxorubicin single agent versus doxorubicin and palifosfamide (without MESNA). In this phase II of 62 patients, a response rate of 23% was observed versus 9% for doxorubicin single agent. The hazard ratio for progression free survival (PFS) was 0.427 favoring the combination arm (p-value = 0.0190. No episodes of encephalopathy or hemorrhagic cystitis were seen. The trial results are expected in 2014 (Verschraegen 2010).
2. Activity of the combination of gemcitabine and docetaxel was first reported in the setting of patients with advanced LMS yielding a 53% response rate (Hensley 2002). Gemcitabine is given at 900 mg/m^2 over 90 minutes on days 1 and 8 of a 21 day cycle. Docetaxel was given on day 8 only at a dose of 100 mg/m^2. The use of this combination in other sarcoma subtypes has shown response rates between 23 and 43% (Maki 2007, Leu 2004) with responses seen in high-grade undifferentiated pleomorphic sarcomas. A modification of this combination was tested in a phase IB study in 35 assessable patients with chemotherapy-naïve STS. Gemcitabine was given at 1500 mg/m^2 every 2 weeks, docetaxel was given at 50 mg/m^2 and bevacizumab at 5 mg/kg also every 2 weeks. The overall response rate was 30.1%, with an additional 47% achieving stable

disease for a median of 6 months. Best responses were observed in patients with undifferentiated pleomorphic sarcomas and angiosarcoma with confirmed complete pathological responses. No grade 3 or 4 hematologic toxicity was observed. Grade 3 and 4 adverse events were all attributed to bevacizumab, which was concerning as the benefit of bevacizumab in this study is unclear (Verschraegen 2008).

Second line treatments

The recommendation is to offer a clinical trial to eligible patients.

Trabectedin: It is approved in Europe for patients who have failed prior anthracycline therapy.

mTOR inhibitors: Activating mutations in growth factor receptors lead to activation of the phospatidylinositol 3′ kinase (PI3k)-Akt-mammalian target of rapamycin (mTOR) pathway (Wan 2007). This pathway is involved in cell cycle progression, proliferation and angiogenesis (Wullschleger 2006). The cytoplasmic tuberous sclerosis complex (TSC) 1 and 2 proteins normally act as tumor suppressor genes and inhibit mTOR activity. If these regulators are absent or abnormal, mTOR activity increases, leading to the development of various tumors (Italiano 2010). PTEN, which regulates PI3K activation, is the most frequently deleted tumor suppressor gene in various cancers including STS. PI3K in turn activates AKT which activates mTOR, leading to increased cell proliferation and reduction of apoptotic mechanisms. STS (160 LMS and various pleomorphic undifferentiated tumors) with complex genomics were studied by array comparative genomic hybridization and transcriptome analysis. Five groups were identified, corresponding to well-differentiated LMS (Group A) or to poorly differentiated sarcomas groups (B–E). Genes of interest included loss of PTEN, especially in groups A, C, and D (Gibault 2011).

Several mTOR inhibitors have been studied in the setting of advanced sarcoma. In a phase II study of ridaforolimus (AP23573; Ariad Pharmaceuticals) in advanced refractory bone and STS, 193 patients were evaluable (Chawla 2005). The study drug was given at 12.5 mg/day intravenously daily for 5 days every 2 weeks. The most significant side effects were mucositis, rash, hyperlipidemia, fatigue and thrombocytopenia. There were five partial responses and a clinical benefit rate of 28%. Another study looked at temsirolimus (CCI-779; Wyeth Pharmaceuticals) given at 25 mg/week for 3 weeks out of four in advanced STS. Forty-one patients were evaluable, with one partial response in a patient with fibrosarcoma that lasted 36 weeks (Okuno 2006). The lack of significant objective responses seen in these studies may reflect two specific concepts. The first being that targeted agents may not generate a typical response per RECIST criteria therefore re-emphasizing that stable disease may be a valid endpoint in the management of metastatic sarcoma. On the other hand, identifying resistance mechanisms to mTOR inhibition may help improve therapeutic responses, as mTOR acts as an axis for sarcoma cell growth.

RADIATION ONCOLOGY

So-called fibrohistiocytic tumors of soft tissue are subclassified into several specific pathologic entities ranging from low grade to high grade. Complete surgical excision is the preferred treatment for all types of fibrohistiocytic tumors. The use of radiation therapy has been reported in the literature for most types of fibrohistiocytic tumors. In general, radiation in certain circumstances may be used effectively for low grade lesions in cases of residual disease after surgery, while radiation is used routinely as an adjuvant treatment after surgery for high grade lesions.

Giant cell tumor of tendon sheath and PVNS are low grade fibrohistiocytic tumors which are usually treated with surgical excision alone. Nonetheless, radiation has been used for some tumors in cases of residual disease. Whether or not radiation should be used routinely for residual disease is controversial. This decision should be based on factors such as difficult location for further surgery. This is particularly true for diffuse-type giant cell tumor which tends to occur in locations in which complete surgical excision is difficult. In cases in which radiation is used for residual disease, relatively low doses of radiation in the range of 20 to 35 Gy have been found to be effective for high rates of local control. A Stanford University series showed a local control rate of 75% (Horoschak et al. 2009).

Several retrospective studies have looked at the use of radiation for intermediate risk tumors formerly called fibrohistiocytic tumors such as dermatofibrosarcoma protuberans. Radiation has also been reportedly used for giant cell tumor of soft tissues. Due to the rarity of giant cell tumor of soft tissues, most of the radiation experience with this specific pathologic entity involves the potentially related entity, giant cell tumor of bone. In rare cases of residual disease after surgery, radiation has been used for giant cell tumors of bone, and moderate doses of at least 50 Gy have been shown to be extremely effective. Higher doses of at least 60 Gy have been used for dermatofibrosarcoma protuberans. Ballo reported an actuarial local control rate of 95% at 10 years for dermatofibrosarcoma protuberans (Ballo et al. 1998). Therefore, the authors conclude that radiation should be considered as a treatment option in DFSP cases of positive margins or unresectable disease.

High grade undifferentiated/unclassified sarcomas should be treated as any other high grade sarcoma. Complete surgical resection remains the standard of care. This is then followed by routine adjuvant radiation even in cases with negative margins except in unusual circumstances. In the randomized study of the use of adjuvant radiation in the treatment of soft tissue sarcoma, the actuarial local failure rate at 10 years is 22% for patients not receiving radiation versus 0% for those receiving radiation (Yang et al. 1998).

CASES

Case 7.1 Giant cell tumor of tendon sheath

Clinical history and presentation

The patient is a 54-year-old woman who presents with a one year history of a mass over the radial aspect of the index finger. She relates slow growth of the mass and mild pain with pressure.

Physical examination reveals a soft, minimally tender mass over the radial aspect of the index finger. The mass is fixed to underlying deep tissue.

Surgical findings and comments

Surgical exploration reveals a rust colored soft tissue lesion adherent to the flexor tendon sheath. The mass displaces but does not invade the neurovascular bundle. Because this tumor has a characteristic gross visual appearance, it is removed with a marginal margin without formal biopsy.

Radiology findings

The two radiographic views, (**Case figs 7.1a** and **7.1b**) show a focal soft tissue mass along the radial aspect of the proximal phalanx of the index finger. There is mild focal pressure erosion with a smooth corticated intact margin. There is no soft tissue calcification and no evidence for tophus. Extra-articular erosions can also be seen in gout but are associated with episodes of pain. Also, the erosions of gout will have indistinct, destructive margins, sometimes with overhanging edges, not corticated pressure type erosions as seen with GCTTS. **Case figs 7.1c** and **7.1d** represent an additional case of GCTTS which has more prominent focal soft tissue swelling but no bone erosion.

Pathology findings

Gross features

The specimen comprises a lobulated ovoid mass of gray to white, firm soft tissue measuring 1.6 cm in maximum dimension. The cut surface is also gray to white and firm.

Microscopic features

Low magnification: The tumor is sharply circumscribed but unencapsulated. It is heterogeneous with cellular and fibrotic (eosinophilic or pink) areas (**Case fig. 7.1e**).

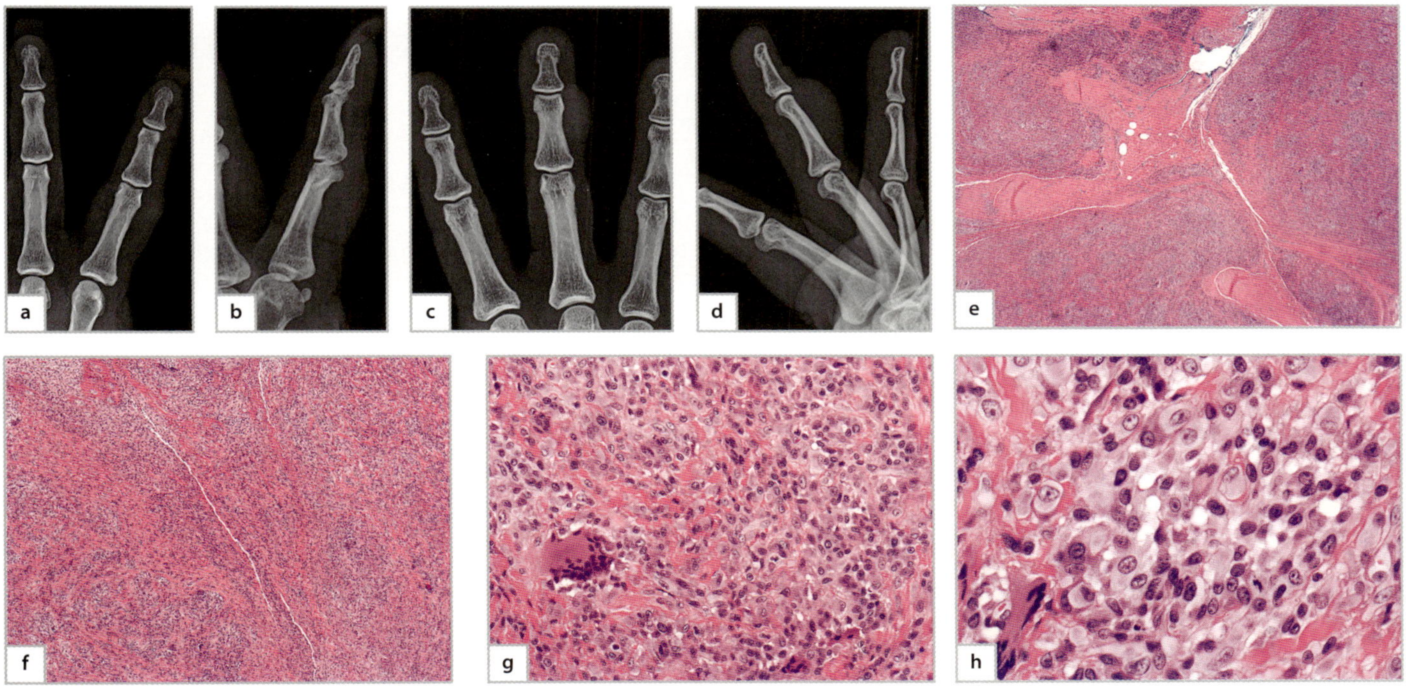

Case figure 7.1 Giant cell tumor of tendon sheath. 7.1a: Postero-anterior radiograph, **7.1b**: Oblique radiograph of the index finger. There is a soft tissue density mass along the radial side of the index finger, just proximal to the proximal interphalangeal joint. Note the pressure erosion of the proximal phalanx with intact cortex visible on the oblique view. **7.1c**: Postero-anterior radiograph and **7.1d**: Lateral radiograph of an additional patient with GCTTS show a soft tissue tumor along the ulnar aspect of the long finger, adjacent to the middle phalanx. This case does not show bone erosion. **7.1e**: Low magnification. The tumor is solid and variably cellular with fibrotic collagenized areas (pink or eosinophilic regions) and cellular areas. **7.1f**: Medium magnification. Tumor cells do not form distinct patterns such as fascicles, storiform growth or a cell culture appearance. The background stroma is rich in collagen. **7.1g**: A mixed population of cells (polymorphous) characterizes the tumor including histiocytes, other inflammatory cells, multinucleated osteoclast-like cells, and rare actual neoplastic cells. **7.1h**: High magnification. The neoplastic cells of both giant cell tumor of tendon sheath and diffuse tenosynovial giant cell tumor are larger than histiocytes with a round or reniform (kidney shaped) nucleus and moderate amounts of amphophilic (lavender colored) cytoplasm. These cells form the minority of the tumor cells.

High magnification: Higher magnification reveals swirls of cells embedded in a fibrotic (collagenized) stroma. There is no distinct architectural pattern such as fascicular or storiform growth (**Case fig. 7.1f**). Some fields contain multinucleated osteoclast-like giant cells mixed with the mononuclear tumor cells (**Case fig. 7.1g**). At highest magnification, the tumor cells comprise multiple types: small round cells consistent with histiocytes, larger, sparser, pale round (epithelioid) cells with round or kidney-bean shaped nuclei and none to a small amount of cytoplasmic hemosiderin (**Case fig. 7.1h**), true macrophages containing hemosiderin pigment (known as siderophages), and the osteoclast-like giant cells. Additionally, a few lymphocytes course among the tumor cells but don't aggregate. Mitoses are present and number up to 3 per high power microscopic field, but no atypical mitotic figures are identified. The overall mitotic rate is approximately 5 per 10 high power fields (400x magnification). Necrosis and nuclear pleomorphism are absent.

Special studies: Because this is a classic clinical presentation and classic histology, no special stains are performed. However, less classic examples (tumors with uniform hypercellularity or no osteoclast-like giant cells, for example) could be examined for expression of desmin and clusterin (Boland et al. 2009). The large, epithelioid tumor cells are uniformly reactive for clusterin (a glycoprotein) while a subset of these cells are usually (in about 70% of case) also reactive for desmin. Interestingly, these large cells share the same immunohistochemical profile as normal synoviocytes: scattered desmin reactivity, diffuse clusterin reactivity, and strong membranous positivity for podoplanin (D2-40). Two prominent soft tissue expert pathologists, Andrew Folpe and Jason Hornick, speculate that giant cell tumor of tendon sheath and its relative, diffuse type tenosynovial giant cell tumor (also called PVNS when confined to the joint space) represent neoplasms of synovial cells and not histiocytes (Boland et al. 2009). This is an example of future erosion of the category of fibrohistiocytic tumors.

PATHOLOGY PEARL

Antibodies do not determine the diagnosis! Antibody reactions are helpful in securing a diagnosis, but since no single antibody is specific for one tumor and usually stains multiple different tumors and normal tissues, a pathologist must integrate antibody results with the lesion's morphology, genetic results and the clinical and radiologic findings to render the correct diagnosis.

Genetics was not performed on this tumor. However, a majority of both the localized and diffuse types of tenosynovial giant cell tumor (remember, giant cell tumor of tendon sheath is the localized form) contain translocations involving the CSF1 gene on chromosome 1p13 with other partners such as *COL6A3* on chromosome 2q35 (Cupp et al. 2007).

Pathologic differential or, why isn't it one of the following?

Fibroma of tendon sheath: This also forms a nodular mass in or attached to a tendon and is also most common in the hands and feet of young to middle aged adults similar to GCTTS. Both are circumscribed but not encapsulated. Whereas giant cell tumor of tendon sheath contains histiocytes and larger epithelioid cells, siderophages, and osteoclast-like giant cells, fibroma of tendon sheath is a myofibroblastic tumor formed by cytologically bland plump spindle cells. Both tumors may feature areas of fibrosis. Fibroma of tendon sheath characteristically contains slit-like, thin-walled arcing vessels. While often reactive for smooth muscle actin (as myofibroblasts) the tumor cells of fibroma of tendon sheath are negative for desmin and clusterin. The genetics of fibroma of tendon sheath have not been clearly defined. However, one case report described a translocation t(2;11) (Dal Cin et al. 1988).

Nodular fasciitis (NF): NF rarely occurs in the hands and feet. When it does, it comprises myofibroblastic and fibroblastic spindle cells streaming in a myxoid to fibrotic stroma. The classic 'tissue culture' teased apart look of the spindled cells as well as acute hemorrhage and infiltrates of lymphocytes distinguish it from giant cell tumor of tendon sheath. GCTTS often contains siderophages and the large epithelioid tumor cells may also contain the pigment; hemosiderin deposition is rare in NF. Immunohistochemically, nodular fasciitis tumor cells are reactive for smooth muscle actin and only rarely expresses desmin, a pattern of expression the lesion shares with fibroma of tendon sheath. In fact, some investigators propose that fibroma of tendon sheath represents a site specific variant of nodular fasciitis (Folpe et al. 2010).

Palmar or plantar fibromatosis (superficial fibromatosis): These lesions are more superficial in location than GCTTS, occurring in the fascia and surrounding subcutaneous fat and sometimes extending to the dermis. Although cellularity varies from high to low with concomitant fibrosis, the constituent cells are plump to elongate spindle cells. The large epithelioid cells of GCTTS (presumed the true neoplastic cells of the tumor and most likely synovial in differentiation) are absent. The spindle cells stream together in linear or curving arrays. Because the tumor cells are fibroblasts, myofibroblasts, and mature fibrocytes, they react variably for smooth muscle actin but are nonreactive for clusterin and only rarely reactive for desmin. Some cases my show nuclear β-catenin reactivity similar to deep fibromatosis (desmoid tumor). Nuclear β-catenin reactivity is not described in tenosynovial giant cell tumors (either localized or diffuse type).

Oncology approach

Medical oncology

As this is a benign lesion, the medical oncology department is not consulted.

Radiation oncology

Historically, giant cell tumor of tendon sheath has a high rate of local recurrence of up to 45% after surgery alone. This high rate of recurrence has been attributed to location in which complete excision is often difficult. Nonetheless, complete resection is the treatment of choice. In cases where complete resection is not possible, radiation therapy may be used. Generally, lower doses such as 20 Gy have been found to be effective.

Patient outcome

The patient has had no recurrence one year after the procedure.

Case table 7.1 Summary pathology findings of Case 7.1

Diagnosis	Giant cell tumor of tendon sheath (localized tenosynovial giant cell tumor)
Size	1.6 × 1 × 0.8 cm
Location	Tendon of index finger
Margin status	Negative; closest margin is 0.1 cm
Histologic grade	Not graded: benign
Pathologic stage (TNM classification)	Not staged: benign

Case 7.2 PVNS (tenosynovial giant cell tumor, diffuse type)

Clinical history and presentation

The patient is a 39-year-old woman who presents with a one and one-half year history of elbow pain that began after a minor trauma. Although episodes of both pain and swelling occur with periodic exacerbation, she has noted a slowly progressive increase in overall pain, swelling, and frequency of symptomatic episodes.

Imaging findings and history are felt to be consistent with PVNS.

Surgical findings and comments

The extensive nature of the disease was felt to preclude arthroscopic synovectomy, therefore an extensive open synovectomy is performed through a medial approach. Operative findings reveal the typical, and extensive, rust-colored synovial proliferation characteristic of this disease. Early degeneration of the cartilage surfaces is visualized along with bony erosions at multiple areas of capsular insertion.

Radiology findings

Case figs 7.2a and **7.2b** show lobulated soft tissue mass postero-medial to the elbow on radiographs. There is a large apparent elbow effusion. Note the chronic appearing erosions of the anterior aspect of the distal humeral cortex seen on the lateral view. There is also chronic erosion of the lateral aspect of the proximal ulna seen on the oblique view. The joint space is preserved and there are no calcified bodies seen. The differential diagnosis for the findings of joint effusion, chronic erosions and joint space preservation includes PVNS and synovial osteochondromatosis. The absence of calcified bodies in this case favors PVNS. The MR images in **Case figs 7.2c** through **7.2f** show lobulated mixed signal masses filling the joint. The tissue extends into the bone erosions and expands into the soft tissues. There are also the characteristic irregular areas of low signal on all sequences caused by hemosiderin. The lesions show only modest enhancement.

Pathology findings

Gross features

The tumor comprises multiple soft, compressible nodules (**Case fig. 7.2g**). On cross sectioning, the largest nodule reveals a gelatinous variegated yellow opaque to semitranslucent cut surface (**Case fig. 7.2h**).

Strictly speaking, PVNS refers to the exclusively intra-articular variant of diffuse tenosynovial giant cell tumor, whereas a tumor located either in the soft tissue and joint space or in the soft tissue alone is more correctly termed diffuse type tenosynovial giant cell tumor. However, many cases of PVNS disclose minor extra-articular involvement, while cases of predominantly extra-articular tumor may slightly extend into the joint, so the strict categorization in terms of title generally belies the commonly mixed sites of involvement. It might be more accommodating and practical to suggest that PVNS refer to exclusively intra-articular diffuse tenosynovial giant cell tumors OR to those tumors with predominantly intra-articular involvement and only minor soft tissue extension outside the joint.

In this patient, both the joint space and surrounding soft tissues are approximately equally involved.

Microscopic features

Low magnification: The tumor is multinodular and cellular at low magnification interspersed by streaks of less cellular fibrosis (**Case fig. 7.2i**). It also forms villous projections in portions taken from the joint space synovium. The majority of the tumor (90%) is cellular.

High magnification: At medium magnification, the tumor characteristically comprises multiple cell types. The majority of the cells are not neoplastic but recruited into the tumor, and these include inflammatory cells (histiocytes, siderophages, and xanthomatous histiocytes, lymphocytes, and plasma cells) and osteoclast-like giant cells (**Case fig. 7.2j**). The actual neoplastic cells, typically partially obscured by recruited normal reactive cells, consists of the relatively large, pale epithelioid round cells described previously in Case 7.1. In fact, there is little appreciable difference in the microscopic features of the localized (see Case 7.1) versus the diffuse type of tenosynovial giant cell tumor (see Case 7.2). **Case fig. 7.2k** captures the mixed cell population at high magnification: xanthomatous histiocytes (bubbly clear cytoplasm) mixed with scattered hemosiderin-tinged epithelioid tumor cells, smaller histiocytes, and a few lymphocytes. The proportion of cells varies from field to field with dispersed multinucleated osteoclast-like giant cells (**Case fig. 7.2l**) and areas dominated by histiocytes (**Case fig. 7.2m**). Mitoses are present averaging up to 2 per 10 high power microscopic fields but are not atypical, and there is no worrisome nuclear atypia (hyperchromasia, coarse granular chromatin, irregular distribution of chromatin, sharply angulated nuclei).

Special studies: Scattered epithelioid cells are positive for desmin by IHC as is reported in both the diffuse and localized variants of tenosynovial giant cell tumor. No further studies are performed.

Pathologic differential or, why isn't it one of the following?

Localized tenosynovial giant cell tumor (giant cell tumor of tendon sheath): These two lesions cannot be reliably distinguished microscopically, as the diffuse form of tenosynovial giant cell tumor may form nodules also, and the types of cells present are the same. Irregular infiltration into adipose tissue or skeletal muscle is limited to the diffuse type. Reportedly, the diffuse type is often more cellular and less fibrotic than localized tenosynovial giant cells tumor, and pigmented tumor cells and cyst formation are also considered more common. Cytogenetically, both tumors feature translocations of the CSF1 gene at chromosome 1p11, but the diffuse tumors may more often also contain trisomies of chromosomes 5 and 7 (Mietttinen 2010). While both tumors show a predilection for young adult females, the diffuse form often involves large joints (most commonly the knee) while the localized form prefers the hands and feet.

Hemosiderotic synovitis: This inflammatory condition of the synovium is caused by repeated bouts of intra-articular bleeding. Like PVNS, it manifests as a villous hyperplasia with hemosiderin deposition and includes a mixed population of synovial cells, macrophages and scattered multinucleated giant cells. The large joints may be affected, and patients may also have an underlying bleeding disorder (hemophilia, for example) or arthritis. Desmin positive cells have not been reported in hemosiderotic synovitis; however, these cells may be few in number in PVNS and may not be represented in a biopsy. A recent study of the giant cells in PVNS and hemosiderotic synovitis suggests that the immunophenotype of these cells differs in a diagnostically helpful manner. According to these investigators, the giant cells of PVNS exhibit the properties and phenotype of osteoclasts (CD51+, CD14- and HLA-DR-) while the histologically identical giant cells of hemosiderotic synovitis express proteins consistent with a macrophage phenotype (CD51-,

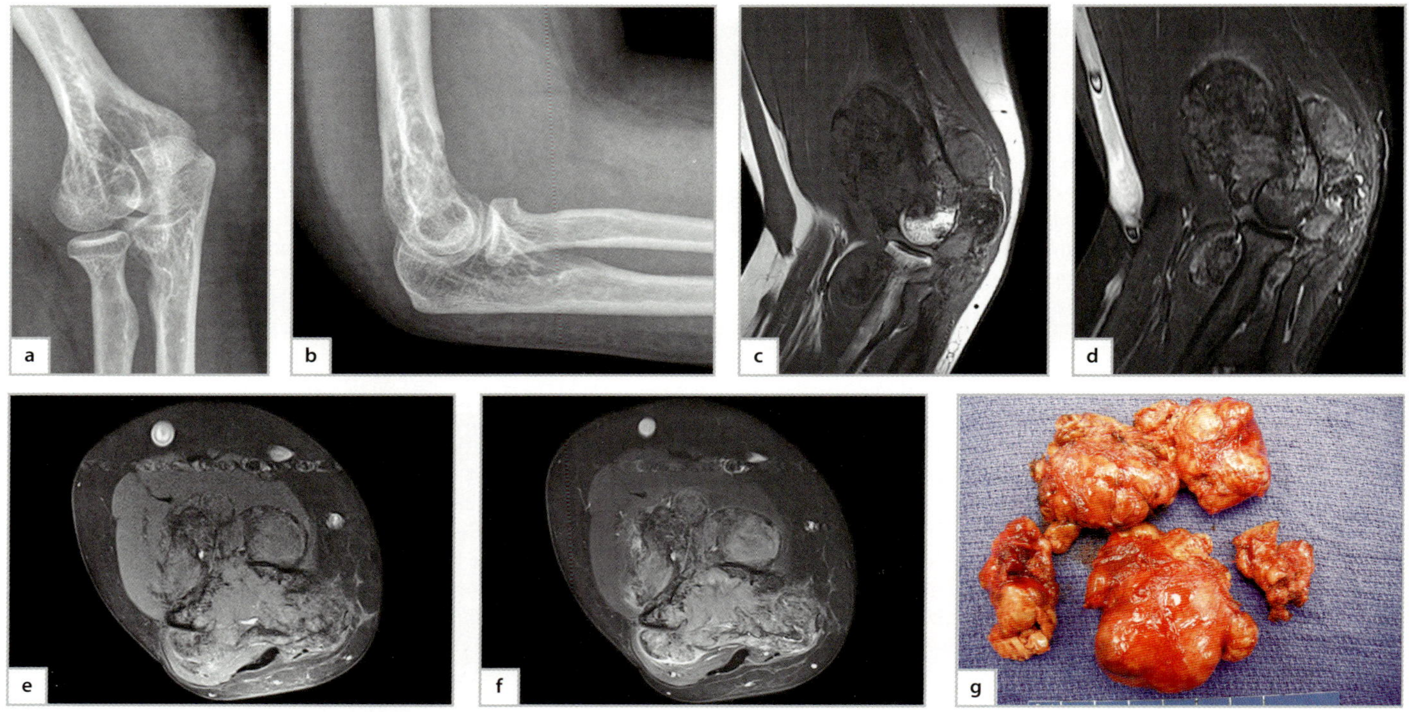

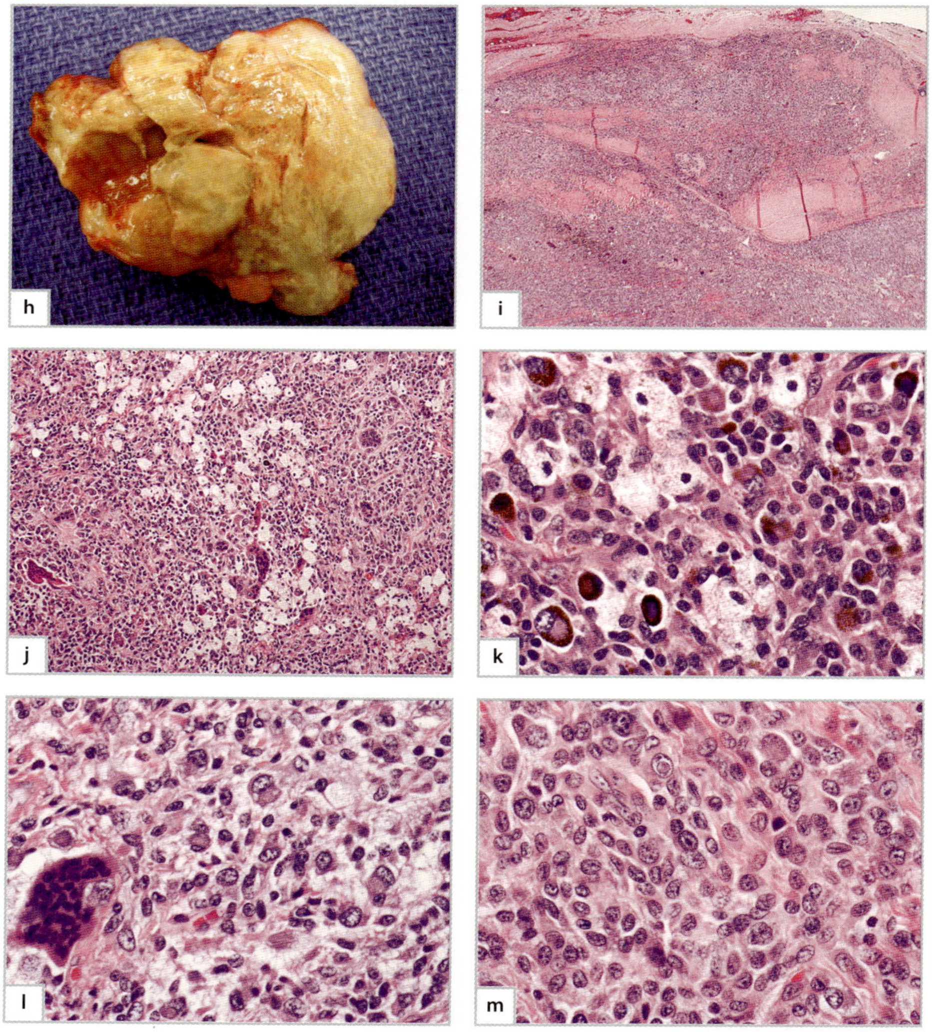

Case figure 7.2 PVNS (tenosynovial giant cell tumor, diffuse type) 7.2a: Oblique radiograph. **7.2b**: Lateral radiograph show erosions of the proximal ulna with large effusion related to the soft tissue mass of PVNS. **7.2c**: Sagittal T1 MR image. **7.2d:** Sagittal STIR MR image. **7.2e:** Axial T1 fat saturation pre-contrast MR image. **7.2f**: Axial T1 fat saturation post-contrast MR image. MR images show bulky, lobulated heterogeneous masses filling the elbow joint. Note areas that appear dark on all sequences related to hemosiderin deposition. There are erosions of the distal humerus. PVNS shows variable heterogeneous enhancement. **7.2g**: Resected tumor. The tumor comprises multiple compressible nodules. **7.2h**: Cross section of tumor nodule. The tumor exhibits a splotchy appearance with striated yellow and mucoid areas intermixed. Golden brown foci are consistent with pigment (hemosiderin). **7.2i**: low magnification. Just like the localized form of tenosynovial giant cell tumor, the diffuse form is variably cellular with areas of prominent fibrosis. **7.2j**: Medium magnification. A cellular area comprises a mixture of cells including xanthomatous histiocytes (the clear cells percolating down the center of the field). **7.2k**: High magnification. The intimate intermixing of different cell types is a characteristic feature of both the localized and diffuse types of tenosynovial giant cell tumor. Four cell types are present in this field: the clear xanthomatous histiocytes, smaller histiocytes, lymphocytes, and the actual neoplastic cells which in the area contain peripheral cytoplasmic rims of brown granular hemosiderin pigment. **7.2l**: High magnification. A multinucleated osteoclast like giant cell swirls among the neoplastic cells and inflammatory cells. **7.2m**: High magnification. Another 400x field shows primarily histiocytes with a few intermingled neoplastic tumor cells. Variation from field to field is typical of these tumors.

CD14+ and HLA-DR+)(Mahendra et al. 2010). Thus, in difficult small biopsies of hemosiderin laden, inflamed and hyperplastic synovium, immunohistochemical staining with these markers, in concert with desmin and clusterin staining, may improve diagnostic accuracy.

Giant cell tumor of soft tissue (giant cell tumor of low malignant potential): This is an unusual tumor of the soft tissues that histologically remarkably resembles giant cell tumor of bone. The lesion is usually superficial extending to the deep dermis and comprises a multinodular mass formed by histiocytes, spindle cells, and osteoclast-like giant cells. Areas of fibrosis, reactive bone formation (and rarely cartilage) and cysts containing blood suggestive of aneurysmal bone cyst are common. PVNS involves the joint space (including tumors with predominantly extra-articular growth), does not form a peripheral rim of reactive bone, often contains neoplastic cells and histiocytes with intracytoplasmic hemosiderin, and spindled lesional cells are rare. Immunohistochemically, tenosynovial giant cell tumors contain tumor cells that are variably desmin positive and reportedly diffusely clusterin positive. This reactivity pattern has not been described in giant cell tumor of soft tissue. Cytogenetically, PVNS features the CSF1 gene translocation, which has also not been reported in giant cell tumor of soft tissue (admittedly, reports of the genetics of giant cell tumor of soft tissue are few).

Malignant diffuse tenosynovial giant cell tumor: Malignant behavior consisting of lymph node and distant metastses is exceptional in diffuse type tenosynovial giant cell tumor (and does not occur at all in the localized form). Some of these tumors exhibit increased cellularity, marked cytologic atypia sometimes including a malignant spindle cell component, necrosis, and an increased mitotic rate with atypical mitotic figures (Li et al. 2008). Prior radiation may be causative in some reported cases. A very rare diffuse tenosynovial giant cell tumor with conventional histology and proliferative rate will behave malignantly. **Case figs 7.2n** and **7.2o** compares the diffuse and localized types of tenosynovial giant cell tumor resected at the University of New Mexico Health Science Center from 2000 to 2010. These numbers reflect those of a medium sized academic oncologic orthopedic practice. Consistent with the literature, the localized form is much more common in the hands and feet; the reverse is true for the diffuse form. The diffuse form also is most common in slightly younger adults. Females outnumber males for the localized form, while the distribution is more equal in the diffuse form.

Case table 7.2 Summary pathology findings of Case 7.2

Diagnosis	Diffuse tenosynovial giant cell tumor (PVNS)
Size	9 × 3 × 2 cm
Location	Elbow joint with extension into surrounding soft tissues
Margin status	Positive focally in soft tissue component
Histologic grade	Not graded: benign
Pathologic stage (TNM classification)	Not staged: benign

Oncology approach

Medical oncology

Because this lesion is benign although locally aggressive, there is no role for medical oncology.

Radiation oncology

Radiation therapy has been used for PVNS in cases of residual disease or recurrence after initial surgical resection. Retrospective studies examining the role of postoperative radiation have been performed. A series of patients from Stanford University showed high rates of local control (75%) with low rates of toxicity (Horoschak et al. 2009). Therefore, radiation may be used for residual disease. A dose of 35 Gy is commonly used. Alternatively, intraarticular radioisotope therapy has been used effectively. In this case, radiation therapy may be considered if the patient has residual disease after surgery or continues to have recurrences despite further surgery.

Patient outcome

Six months following the resection, the patient has signs of early recurrence on follow-up MRI and repeat synovectomy is planned. Radiation therapy will be held in reserve.

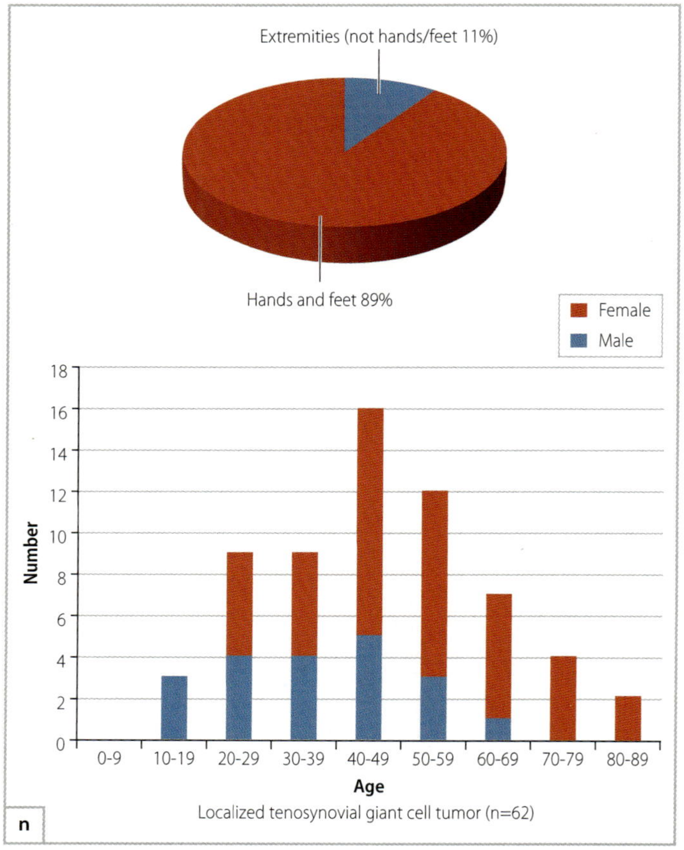

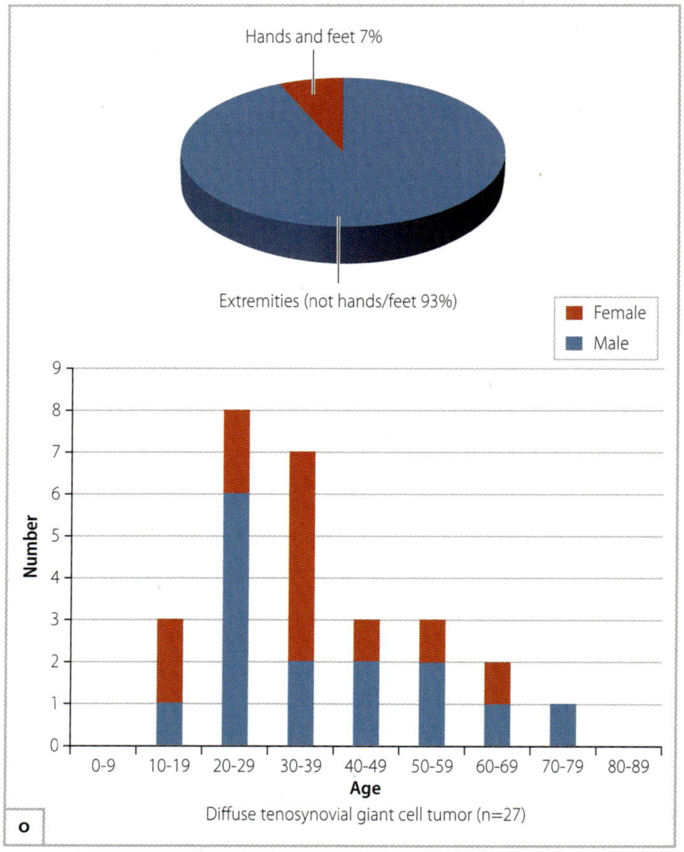

Case figure 7.2n and **7.2o** Localized and diffuse tenosynovial giant cell tumors resected at UNM HSC 2000-2010.

Case 7.3 Deep benign fibrous histiocytoma

Clinical history and presentation

The patient is a 54-year-old man who presents with an eight year history of a slowly enlarging, painless buttock mass first noted following a work-related injury.

Physical examination reveals a large, firm, nontender mass with the gluteus maximus. The mass is adherent to the surrounding muscle.

Surgical findings and comments

Because the differential diagnosis includes both benign and malignant entities, a formal open biopsy is performed. Following pathologic confirmation of the diagnosis, the patient is returned to the operating room on a separate date for marginal excision of the tumor. Findings at surgery reveal a large solid mass consisting of dense fibrous type tissue. The tumor shells out of the surrounding tissue with relative ease.

Radiology findings

The images in this case, (**Case figures 7.3a** through **7.3c**), show a left buttock mass with T1 low signal and STIR high signal. There is a rim of fairly intense enhancement and a focal nodule along the posterior wall of the mass. This tumor might reasonably be considered a high grade malignancy with extensive central necrosis warranting tissue diagnosis, fortunately for this patient, the diagnosis was benign.

Pathology findings

Gross features

The resected tumor consists of an 11 cm firm mass with a white cut surface and a central hemorrhagic cavity consistent with prior biopsy. The tumor focally extend to the deep inked surgical margin.

Microscopic features

Low magnification: The tumor exhibits alternating cellular and fibrotic regions. A cartwheel or storiform (short interwoven swirling fascicular pattern) architecture is appreciable at intermediate magnification (**Case fig. 7.3d**). The storiform pattern is a requirement for the diagnosis of deep benign fibrous histiocytoma (Gleason et al. 2008).

High magnification: Cellular areas feature cells without marked atypia, and there is no necrosis (**Case fig. 7.3e**). Scattered blood vessels are slightly ectatic and staghorn shaped (**Case fig. 7.3f**) a feature common to deep benign fibrous histiocytoma (seen in 40% of a recent critical review of 69 cases) (Gleason et al. 2008). At highest magnification (**Case fig. 7.3g**), the tumor cells are pink with indistinct cell borders. Tumor nuclei are hypochromatic (pale) with fine chromatin and scattered intranuclear pseudoinclusions.

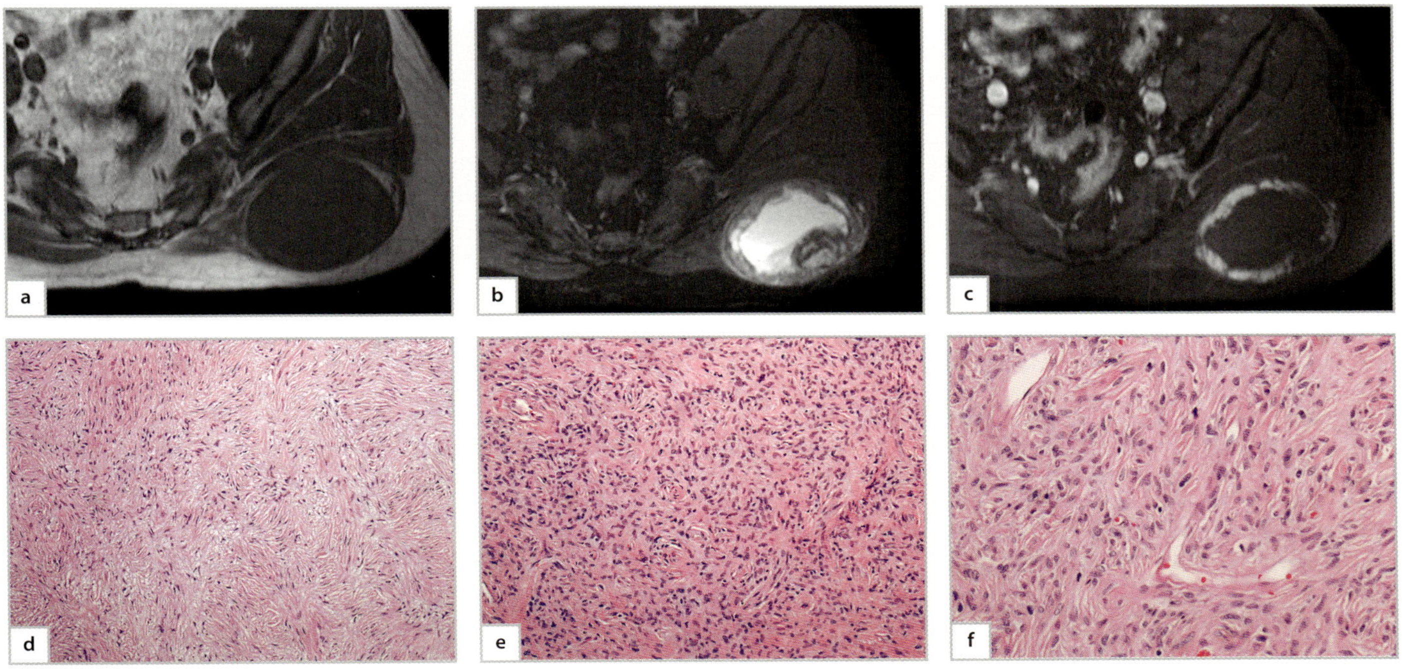

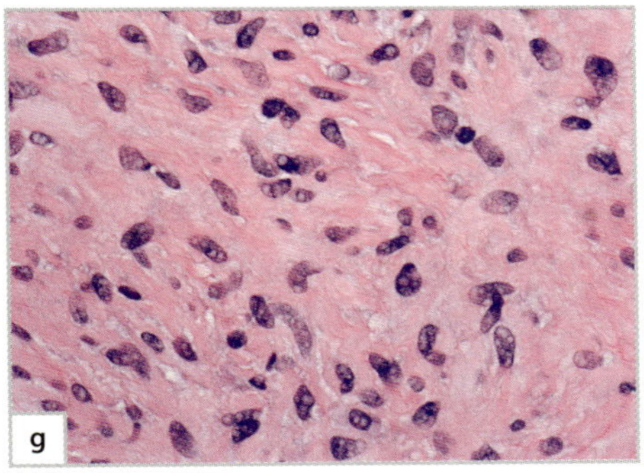

Case figure 7.3 Deep benign fibrous histiocytoma. 7.3a: Axial T1 MR image. **7.3b**: Axial STIR MR image. **7.3c**: Axial T1 fat saturated post-contrast MR image. There is a predominantly T1 low signal, STIR high signal mass with moderate heterogeneity in the gluteus maximus muscle. The mass has intense rim enhancement. **7.3d**: At low magnification, the tumor exhibits a cartwheel or storiforming growth pattern, even in a relatively fibrotic hypocellular region. **7.3e**: A cellular area consists of a single cell type without necrosis. **7.3f**: Thin-walled, ectatic blood vessels consistent with 'staghorn' vasculature is present focally (seen in about 40% of deep benign fibrous histiocytomas and not a specific finding). **7.3g**: High magnification reveals eosinophilic tumor cells with inconspicuous cell borders and oval to spindle hyperchromatic nuclei. Some nuclei contain nuclear pseudo-inclusions, also not a specific finding in deep benign fibrous histiocytoma.

Special studies: Because the above description could match multiple mesenchymal tumors, predominantly those that are fibroblastic and/or myofibroblastic or nerve sheath in differentiation, a battery of immunohistochemical stains are applied to a representative block of tumor. The tumor cells generally are non-reactive but disclose scattered cells positive for Factor XIIIa. There is no reactivity to the following antibodies: CD34, smooth muscle actin, muscle specific actin, desmin, EMA, broad-spectrum keratins, S-100 protein, c-kit, and CD68 (controls are appropriately reactive). Cytogenetic karyotyping is successful and reveals two clones: one with an interstitial deletion of the long arm of chromosome 15 (del(15)(q15q22) and the second with a translocation t(7;16)(q10;q10). Neither of these abnormalities are characteristic of a particular soft tissue tumor [the t(7;16) of low grade fibromyxoid sarcoma and sclerosing epithelioid fibrosarcoma involves different genes at 7q34(*CREB3L2*) and 16p11 (*FUS*)].

Pathologic differential or, why isn't it one of the following?

Solitary fibrous tumor/hemangiopericytoma (SFT/HPC): The histologic features of solitary fibrous tumor/hemangiopericytoma overlap with those seen in this tumor. However, the patient's tumor features a more uniform storiform pattern of growth than is usual for SFT/HPC. Usually, SFT/HPC is positive for CD34 by immunohistochemical staining. Up to forty percent of deep benign fibrous histiocytomas are also reactive for this protein, so in some cases, CD34 reactivity cannot distinguish the two entities.

Myopericytoma: This tumor is usually not so storiforming and instead classically demonstrates concentric swirling of plump spindle cells around prominent small vessels. However, in occasional cases, a more broadly fascicular and less angiocentric growth dominates and could resemble this patient's tumor. Both tumors usually occur in the subcutaneous tissues of the extremities of young to middle-aged adults. However, myopericytomas are positive for smooth muscle actin, usually diffusely. By contrast, most deep benign fibrous histiocytomas are negative or only focally positive for smooth muscle actin (by immunohistochemical staining).

Peripheral nerve sheath tumor such as perineurioma or neurofibroma: The mixture of cell types consistent in neurofibroma is absent in this patient's tumor. Furthermore, this tumor is negative for both CD34 and S-100 protein both of which are present in the cells of neurofibroma. Perineurioma is a diagnostic possibility as it comprises one cell type arranged in storiform and fascicular patterns (perivascular whorling is also seen). However, perineurial cells are generally more slender with bipolar processes (conspicuous on vimentin staining). The cells of perineurioma also express EMA, often CD34, claudin-1 and GLUT1 in contrast to deep benign fibrous histiocytoma, which is sometime CD34 positive but negative for EMA (information on claudin-1 and GLUT1 expression in deep benign fibrous histiocytoma is not available). Karyotyping may be helpful, as perineuriomas exhibit abnormalities of chromosome 22 (usually involving the NF2 tumor suppression gene) (Fisher et al. 2011).

Low grade fibromyxoid sarcoma (LGFMS): Low grade fibromyxoid sarcoma seldom occurs in a suprafascial location. Myxoid regions with arcades of vessels transition to fibrous hypocellular regions. A storiform pattern of growth is uncommon. Similar to perineurioma, the tumor cells may be EMA and claudin-1 reactive. A specific translocation t(7;16)(q34; p11) combining the *FUS* gene with *CREB3L2* or *CREB3L1* appears to be specific for LGFMS (and its higher grade 'relative', sclerosing epithelioid fibrosarcoma).

Dermatofibrosarcoma protuberans (DFSP): DFSP is a classic storiforming tumor that arises in the dermis and extends into the subcutaneous adipose tissue. It usually affects young adults on the trunk and upper extremities. The monotony of the storiform growth (except in cases with fibrosarcomatous change) and the layered infiltrative growth into subcutaneous fat are dissimilar to the patient's tumor which has a circumscribed border and variegated hypercellular and fibrotic regions. DFSP is usually strongly diffusely positive for CD34, and karyotyping or FISH reveals specific translocations (the most common being t(17;22)(q22;q13) but also t(2;17) and t(9;22)).

Oncology approach

Medical oncology

There is no indication for a medical oncology consultation as the tumor is almost undoubtedly going to behave in a benign fashion.

Radiation oncology

Deep benign fibrous histiocytoma is a rare and poorly recognized entity. Its clinical behavior is not fully understood and published data on the use of radiation therapy for this particular entity is nonexistent. Therefore, the effectiveness of radiation is not known. The largest published series reports rates of local recurrence in excess of 20%. Fortunately, this patient undergoes proper surgical therapy and has not recurred.

Patient outcome

The patient is disease free 5 years following the tumor removal.

Case table 7.3 Summary pathology findings of Case 7.3

Diagnosis	Deep benign fibrous histiocytoma
Size	11 × 8 × 4 cm
Location	Subcutaneous fat
Margin status	Focally positive at deep margin
Histologic grade	Not graded: benign*
Pathologic stage (TNM classification)	Not staged: benign*

* The majority of deep benign fibrous histiocytomas behave in a benign fashion with a relatively low rate of local recurrence (~25%). However, two of 69 patients (3%) developed metastatic disease and died of tumor in a recent series (Gleason et al. 2008).

Case 7.4 Plexiform fibrohistiocytic tumor

Clinical history and presentation

The patient is a 3-year-old boy who was noted to have a 'pea-sized' mass in the axilla at birth which has grown rapidly in size.

Open biopsy is performed at another institution with a pathologic diagnosis of congenital fibrosarcoma. He is treated with a 6 week course of chemotherapy but is switched to somatostatin due to tumor progression. The tumor has been radiographically stable but involves the brachial plexus resulting in complete loss of motor and sensory function of the upper extremity except the shoulder and biceps muscles.

Surgical findings and comments

Surgical resection with a goal of wide margins is indicated. Because the patient has essentially a flail upper extremity with extensive involvement of the neurovascular structures at the level of the brachial plexus and concomitant involvement of the chest wall, forequarter amputation with partial chest wall resection is performed.

Radiology findings

This unusual case, **(Case figs 7.4a** through **7.4d)** shows an infiltrative tumor with little mass effect despite its extensive size. The lesion has nonspecific T1 low signal and STIR high signal with intense enhancement. Note how the tumor insinuates between structures without displacing them. This case shows a small posterior satellite lesion with an apparent feeding vessel. A typical sarcoma would be more focalized with a dominant mass that pushes or destroys adjacent structures. An angiomatous lesion such as hemangioma or lymphangioma could have a similar infiltrative pattern without mass effect. However, hemangiomas may be identifiable by the presence of fat tissue, phleboliths or feeding vessels. Lymphangiomas should not have significant enhancement.

Pathology findings

Gross features

The amputation specimen comprises the left arm and shoulder. In the soft tissues of the upper arm and axilla is an ill-defined firm white tumor that tracks along neurovascular bundles. The mass is approximately 7 cm in length and 1.5 cm in width, but it is difficult to measure its boundaries precisely because it merges subtly with surrounding fibrous tissue. A section of tumor is taken under sterile conditions for karyotyping.

Microscopic features

Low magnification: Congruent with the tumor's name, the lesion comprises multiple discreet but unencapsulated nodules in the deep

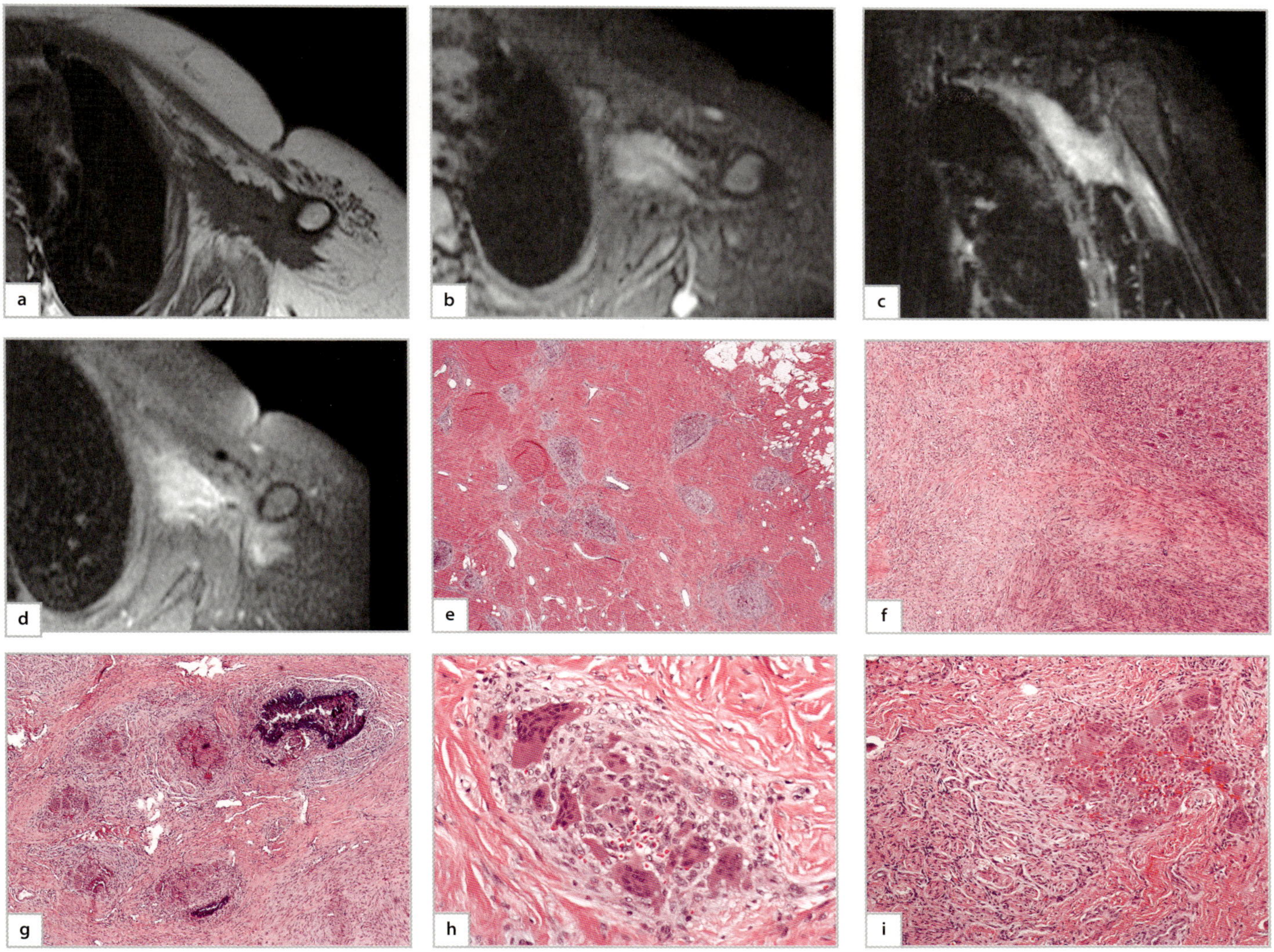

Case figure 7.4 Plexiform fibrohistiocytic tumor. 7.4a: Axial T1 MR image. **7.4b**, axial STIR MR image. **7.4c**, coronal STIR MR image. **7.4d**: axial T1 fat saturation post-contrast. MR images show an infiltrating T1 low signal, STIR high signal mass with intense uniform enhancement. The lesion is infiltrating and quite extensive spanning from the lung apex to the mid arm. Note the minimal mass effect. **7.4b**: shows a small posterior satellite lesion with an apparent feeding vessel. **7.4e**: Low magnification. The tumor at low power forms multiple small nodules in the deep dermis. The surrounding stroma in which the round to ovoid nodules reside is also abnormal. **7.4f**: Low magnification. Tumor stroma is cellular with a pink or eosinophilic hue due to collagen deposition. **7.4g**: Medium magnification. A cluster of the discrete tumor nodules demonstrate two features described in this tumor: central hemorrhage in a nodule (common) and metaplastic bone formation (rare). **7.4h**: Higher magnification. The fibrohistiocytic portion of the tumor consists of oval to round nodules formed by histiocytes. As is usual, multinucleated giant cells aggregate in the nodules, possibly attracted to the hemorrhage. This particular nodule does not contain metaplastic bone. **7.4i**: Medium magnification. A minority of plexiform fibrohistiocytic tumors will display perineural growth. This patient's tumor is exceptional in that the histiocytic nodules preferentially form in close association with neurofibromas (this patient also has NF1). Neurofibromatous area is on the left.

dermis and subcutaneous fat (plexiform growth) (**Case fig. 7.4e**). However, the small to medium sized nodules (several millimeters in diameter) visible at low magnification are also associated with larger, diffusely cellular areas composed of uniform spindle cells (**Case fig. 7.4f**). A few of the discrete, small nodules contain foci of metaplastic bone (**Case fig. 7.4g**). Osteoid formation is a rare feature of plexiform fibrohistiocytic tumor. Some of the nodules display central hemorrhage (**Case fig. 7.4g**), also commonly seen in this tumor (Moosavi et al. 2007).

High magnification: A representative section through one of the discrete small nodules shows a mixture of mononuclear histiocytic cells and several osteoclast-like giant cells (**Case fig. 7.4h**). A minority of plexiform fibrohistiocytic tumors exhibit perineural growth; this patient's tumor may be unique in that it colonizes several neurofibromas in a collision manner (**Case figs 7.4i and 7.4j**). The patient has in fact recently been diagnosed with neurofibromatosis Type I, and the gross appearance of involvement of neurovascular bundles represents plexiform neurofibroma rather than plexiform fibrohistiocytic tumor, which usually forms nodules of a size not so readily apparent on gross examination.

Special studies: Some of the nodules show an affinity for the patient's neurofibromas (**Case fig. 7.4k**) with plexiform

Case figure 7.4: Continued from page 143

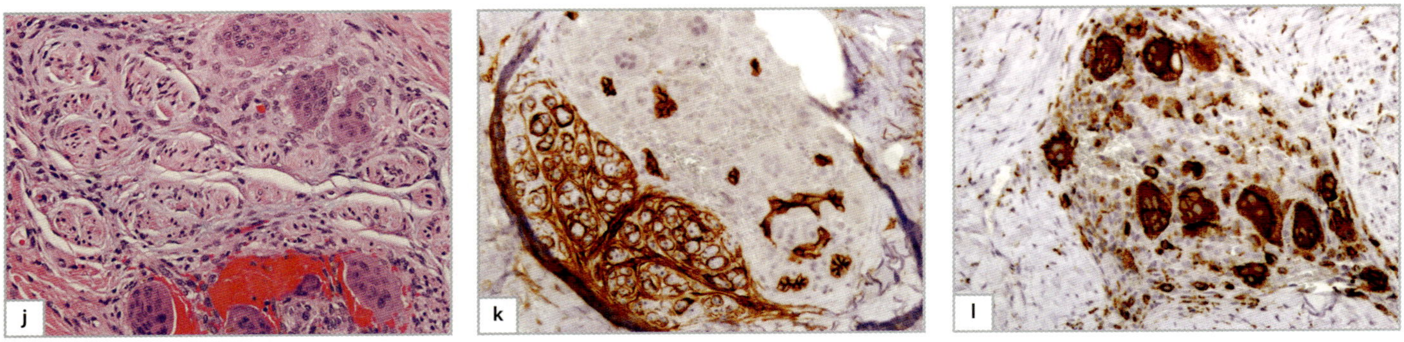

7.4j: Higher magnification. A fibrohistiocytic nodule (upper right portion of photomicrograph) encroaches on a neurofibroma (lower left). **7.4k**, Antibody to S-100 protein reveals nerve tissue (brown positive ball like clusters lower left) partly enveloped by a histiocytic nodule of the tumor. **7.4l**, CD68 reactivity. CD68 antibody stains histiocytes and multinucleated giant cells in the fibrohistiocytic nodule of the tumor (brown color; hematoxylin counterstain).

fibrohistiocytic tumor partially surrounding neurofibroma highlighted on an S-100 protein immunohistochemical stain (neurofibroma S-100 protein positive and plexiform fibrohistiocytic tumor S-100 protein negative). Consistent with histiocytic differentiation, the multinucleated osteoclast-like giant cells are CD68 reactive as well as smaller mononuclear cells (**Case fig. 7.4l**). Spindled cells growing diffusely around the discrete tumor nodules are reactive for smooth muscle actin.

Pathologic differential or, why isn't it one of the following?

Fibrous hamartoma of infancy: Like PFHT, fibrous hamartoma of infancy is a tripartite tumor that occurs in the dermis and subcutaneous tissue. However, the three components are: 1) adipose tissue, 2) primitive pale spindle cells arranged in loose nodules, and 3) fibroblastic/myofibroblastic spindle cells spreading throughout the lesion as fibrous trabeculae. Unlike PFHT, fibrous hamartoma of infancy does not occur after puberty but only in early childhood, and osteoclast-like giant cells and a plexiform growth pattern are rare.

Cellular neurothekeoma: Based on overlap in age, body site location and tissue depth, morphology, and immunohistochemistry reactivity (including positivity for antibodies to NKI-C3 and MiTF), some expert soft tissue pathologists suggest that cellular neurothekeoma and PFHT are closely related if not the same tumor (Fisher et al. 2011, Moosavi et al. 2007). Cellular neurothekeoma differs from PFHT in being more commonly confined to the dermis, comprising discrete nodules without an additional diffuse fibroblastic/myofibroblastic stromal accompaniment, more frequently showing slight cytologically atypia, more frequently exhibiting myxoid change, more commonly lacking multinucleated giant cells, and being associated with an excellent prognosis without reports of metastasis to lymph nodes or lungs.

Myofibroma: In some cases of PFHT, the diffuse myofibroblastic/fibroblastic pattern can dominate. Such tumors resemble myofibroma which is also a diffuse myofibroblastic/fibroblastic tumor occurring in infancy through the elderly but most commonly affecting children to 2 years of age in the head and neck. While most myofibromas are solitary, some are multifocal, and the tumor can occur in deep soft tissues, bone, and the viscera (a spectrum of involvement more expansive than PFHT). Somewhat distinct from PFHT is the zonation of cell types that occurs in myofibroma (some cells are pale with slender bipolar uniform nuclei) and some are rounder with less cytoplasm akin to the cells of glomus tumors. A hemangiopericytomatous growth pattern may be conspicuous with ectatic 'staghorn' vessels, and tumor cells may whorl around vessels. Although giant cells may be present, they are usually scattered throughout the tumor, not aggregating as in PFHT into discrete histiocytic nodules around fresh hemorrhage. Myofibroma also features secondary changes that are rare in PFHT such as calcification, necrosis and stromal hyalinization. Both tumors express SMA with no expression of desmin and h-caldesmon, so immunohistochemistry does not help distinguish the two tumors.

Giant cell tumor of soft tissue (low malignant potential): This rare tumor most commonly occurs in middle-aged adults, but children can be affected, and it is usually subcutaneous like PFHT and forms multiple discreet nodules. However, the nodules of giant cell tumor of soft tissue are larger than in PFHT, and a second diffuse background growth of myofibroblastic/fibroblastic cells characteristic of PFHT is lacking. Immunohistochemically, the giant cells of both tumors are positive for CD68, and cells in both tumors can express smooth muscle actin. There is little known of the genetics of giant cell tumor of soft tissue and PFHT, so ancillary molecular testing is not currently diagnostically helpful.

Lipofibromatosis: This is a rare pediatric tumor (most patients are less than 2 years old) that preferentially involves the hands and feet. It occurs in the dermis and subcutaneous fat predominantly and closely resembles fibrous hamartoma of infancy except that it lacks the primitive spindle cell component consisting instead of adipose tissue separated by bands of myofibroblasti/fibroblastic pink spindle cells. Fibrohistiocytic nodules with osteoclast-like giant cells and a plexiform growth pattern are absent. The spindle cells express smooth muscle actin variably, and may also be positive for CD34, BCL2 and S-100 protein (Miettinen 2010).

Case table 7.4 Summary pathology findings of Case 7.4

Diagnosis	Plexiform fibrohistiocytic tumor
Size	Difficult to determine due to intermixed neurofibroma; possibly 7 cm in greatest dimension
Location	Dermis and subcutaneous adipose tissue
Margin status	Negative by greater than 1.0 cm
Histologic grade	Not graded; mild atypia may occur but does not have significance
Pathologic stage (TNM classification)	T2a/N0/M0 by pathologic and clinical staging = Stage IB

Oncology approach

Medical oncology

There is no role for medical oncology in this patient who has miniscule risk for developing metastases.

Radiation oncology

Surgery with negative margins is the preferred treatment. Radiation therapy has no known role for the treatment of this disease.

Patient outcome

The patient is disease free 6 years following the operative procedure.

Case 7.5 Giant cell tumor of soft tissue with transformation to high grade sarcoma

Clinical history and presentation

The patient is an 82-year-old man who presents with a buttock mass discovered incidentally after a CT scan performed for gastrointestinal complaints one month previously. Since then he has noted the presence of a palpable painless mass.

Physical examination reveals a large firm buttock mass. It is nontender and fixed to surrounding tissue.

Needle biopsy is performed which is consistent with a high grade sarcoma. Work-up reveals no metastatic disease.

Surgical findings and comments

Wide resection of the tumor is performed, removing a portion of the gluteus maximus muscle for margin.

Radiology findings

Giant cell tumor of soft tissue is a rare entity as demonstrated in (**Case fig. 7.5a)** CT scan image. The mass has mild peripheral enhancement. There is marked increased metabolic activity seen on positron emission tomography (**Case fig. 7.5b).** The mass has an overall nonspecific appearance that could be seen with many soft tissue sarcomas. A radiologist encountering this mass would reasonably raise the specter of this being a malignant tumor.

Pathology findings

Gross features

The wide resection comprises skeletal muscle and a large tumor measuring 11 cm in maximum dimensions. The tumor is greater than 1.0 cm from all margins including a separately submitted 'true deep margin.' Cross sections of the predominantly circumscribed tumor reveal a heterogeneous interior composed of tan relatively firm tissue, yellow soft necrotic areas, and gelatinous regions. A central cystic cavity is also present (**Case fig. 7.5c**).

Microscopic features

Low magnification: At low magnification, most of the tumor is markedly cellular with interspersed areas of abrupt necrosis. There is no evidence of multilobulation or multinodularity as is present in ~85% of giant cell tumors of soft tissue of uncertain malignant potential. Of the histologically viable tumor, there are two distinct areas at low magnification, one comprising numerous evenly scattered multinucleate osteoclast-like giant cells (**Case fig. 7.5d**) and the other comprising an intersecting fascicular growth of spindle cells without giant cells (**Case fig. 7.5e**).

High magnification: At higher magnification, the two regions described above abut each other but do not intermingle. The lower grade portion consists of mononuclear round cells evenly infiltrated by multinucleate giant cells (**Case figs 7.5f** and **7.5g**). The giant cells appear histologically identical to osteoclasts with distinct cell borders, pale eosinophilic cytoplasm, and randomly arranged, uniform, small, round hypochromatic nuclei. Both regions of tumor exhibit mitotic activity, and up to 60 mitoses per 10 high power microscopic fields are counted. The fascicular spindle cell foci (**Case figs 7.5h** and **7.5i**) do not contain the osteoclastic giant cells, show moderate nuclear atypia including hyperchromaticity and range in size, and atypical mitoses are easily spotted. Some of the high grade tumor discloses myxoid features (**Case fig. 7.5j**) possibly matching the gelatinous areas noted grossly. Vascular invasion is identified, interestingly comprising lower grade, giant cell rich tumor implants (**Case fig. 7.5k**). Such invasion is commonplace in pure giant cell tumor of soft tissue (low malignant potential).

Special studies: Both the low grade and spindle cell high grade areas exhibit foci of nuclear reactivity for p63 (by immunohistochemistry) (**Case fig. 7.5l**). Interestingly, giant cell tumor of bone is also positive for p63. A small portion of the high grade tumor is strongly reactive for desmin (**Case fig. 7.5m**) and some of the spindle cells also express S-100 protein and smooth muscle actin (a mixed profile not diagnostic of any particular differentiation). There is no reactivity for neurofilaments, GFAP (both can be positive in malignant peripheral nerve sheath tumor), pan-keratins (marker of carcinoma and rare sarcomas) and TLE-1 (nuclear positivity is reportedly fairly specific for synovial sarcoma). (All antibody positive and negative controls are appropriately reactive.)

Karyotyping reveals hyperdiploidy (~63–70 chromosomes) with extensive structural and numerical abnormalities. These findings are consistent with a high grade sarcoma and are not specific. It is not possible to determine if the sample sent for cytogenetics consisted of low grade or high grade tumor.

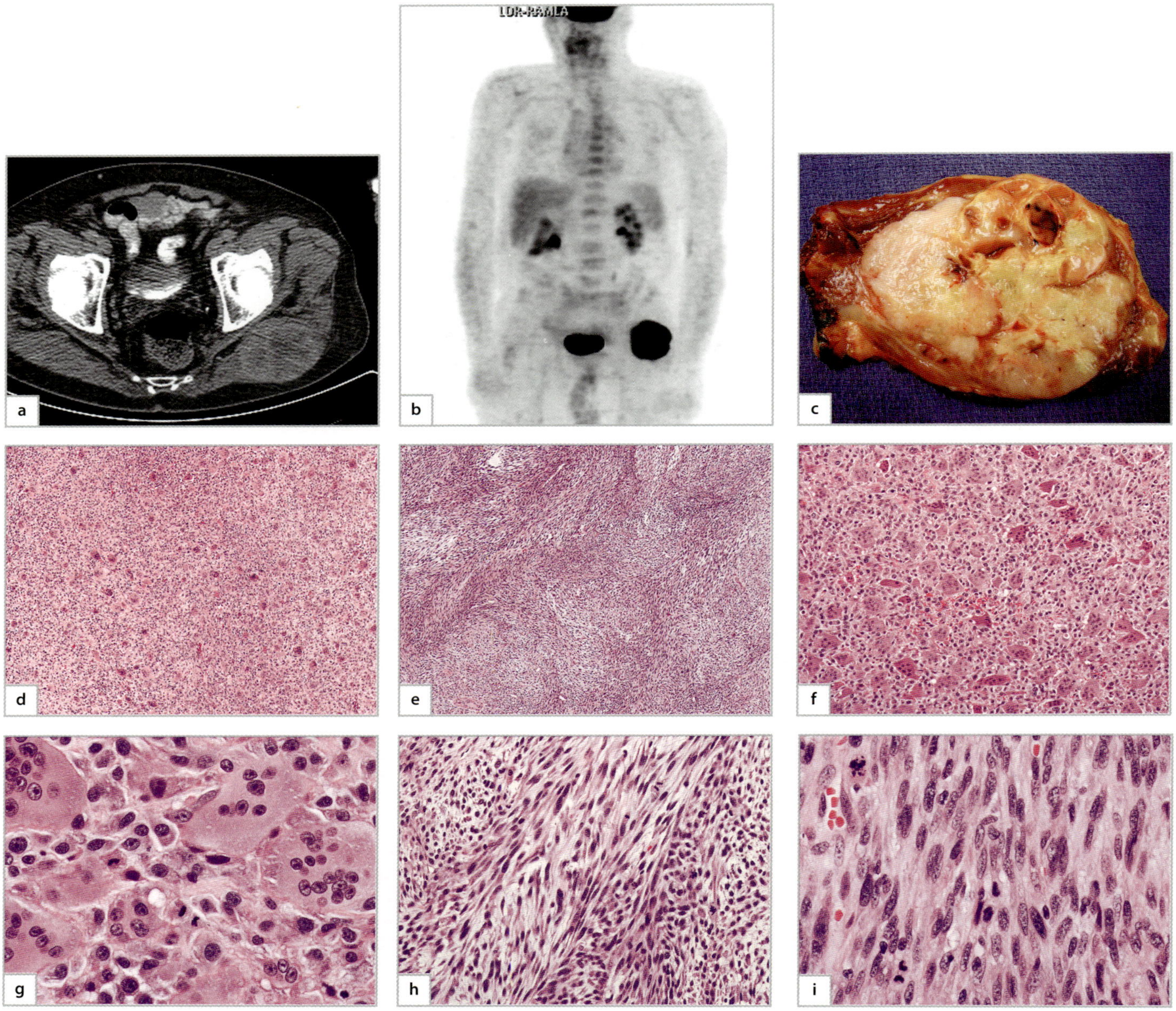

Case figure 7.5 Giant cell tumor of soft tissue with transformation to high grade sarcoma. 7.5a: Computed tomography image post-contrast, **7.5b**: Positron emission tomogram. These show a heterogeneous density mass with modest peripheral enhancement centered in the gluteus maximus muscle. The mass shows marked increased metabolic activity on PET imaging. **7.5c**: Gross photo. The tumor on cross section is heterogeneous with firm white 'fish-flesh' areas, yellow soft necrosis, and regions of gelatinous change. This variable appearance with obvious necrosis strongly suggests malignancy. The center is cystic with hemorrhage, and this cavity may be secondary to prior biopsy. **7.5d**: Low magnification. The low grade area of the tumor looks identical to giant cell tumor of bone with osteoclast-like giant cells evenly scattered among mononuclear round cells. **7.5e**: Low magnification. In contrast with the low grade regions, the high grade sarcoma comprises intersecting fascicles of spindle cells. **7.5f**: Medium magnification. This area is histologically consistent with giant cell tumor of soft tissue (low malignant potential). Importantly, there is no significant cytologic atypia in the non-giant cell population. **7.5g**: High magnification. Mitotic figures are present among the mononuclear cells in this low grade giant cell rich portion of the tumor. Like giant cell tumor of bone, the nuclei of the mononuclear cells resemble those of the osteoclast-like giant cells. **7.5h**: Intersecting fascicles of spindle cells comprise the high grade portion of this patient's unusual tumor. In appearance, it mimics adult type fibrosarcoma. **7.5i**: Moderate nuclear atypia is present in the high grade spindle cell regions, and atypical mitoses (one is noted in this field) are confined to only the high grade spindle cell areas.

Case figure 7.5: Continued from page 146

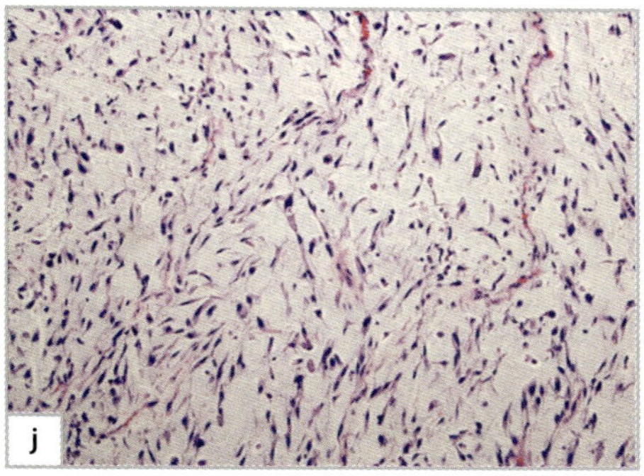

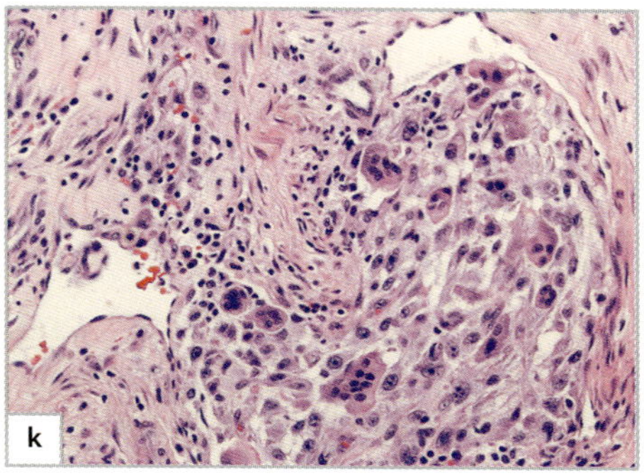

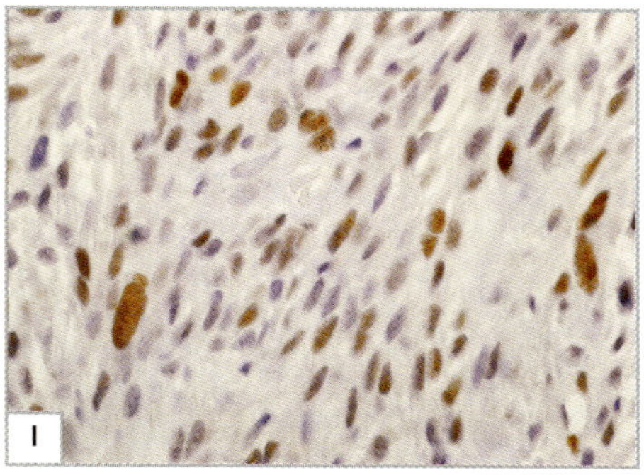

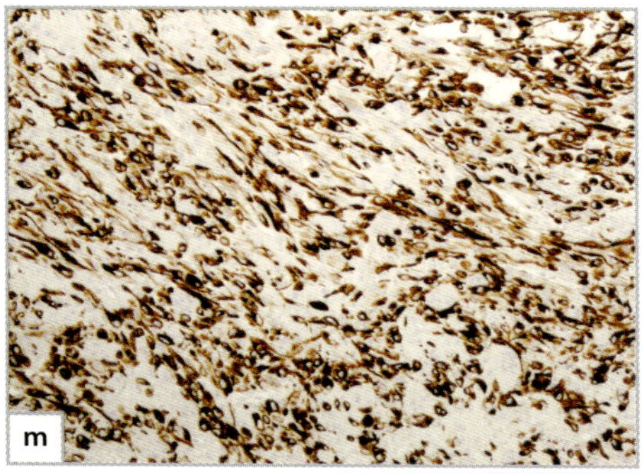

7.5j: Medium magnification. Some of the high grade spindle areas show myxoid change possibly accounting for some of the gelatinous regions noted grossly. **7.5k**: Higher magnification. Vascular invasion is present and occurs as plugs of low grade, giant cell rich tumor distending thin-walled channels. **7.5l**: High magnification. Tumor nuclei in the high grade spindle cell sarcoma region are positive for p63 by immunohistochemistry. Nuclear p63 expression is also present in the low grade areas. **7.5m**: Medium magnification. The high grade spindle cell component is variably positive for desmin (positive in approximately 10% of the high grade sampled tumor). High grade cells also variably express smooth muscle actin and S-100 protein.

Pathologic differential or, why isn't it one of the following?

Undifferentiated pleomorphic sarcoma with giant cells: This is the correct term for what was previously called giant cell subtype of MFH. Few tumors meet this classification currently, as many tumors with pleomorphic mononuclear cells and intermixed osteoclast-like giant cells (with or without multinucleated pleomorphic tumor giant cells) can be slotted into the categories below based on immunohistochemistry and the finding of more typical tumor areas such as smooth muscle fascicle growth (for leiomyosarcoma), tumor osteoid (for osteosarcoma), and gland or keratin production (anaplastic carcinoma). Only after immunohistochemistry and thorough review can a tumor is designated 'undifferentiated pleomorphic sarcoma with giant cells.' Although both tumors by definition are infiltrated by osteoclast-like tumor giant cells, unlike giant cell tumor of soft tissue (low malignant potential), undifferentiated pleomorphic sarcoma with giant cells is replete with markedly atypical mononuclear and sometimes multinucleated tumor cells and should not contain areas that resemble giant cell tumor of soft tissue. This patient's tumor is more appropriately diagnosed as a giant cell tumor of soft tissue (low malignant potential) that has developed a subclone of high grade sarcoma, admittedly a rare event. However, the areas of the tumor that resemble giant cell tumor of bone (characteristic of giant cell tumor of soft tissue, low malignant potential), perhaps even the p63 nuclear reactivity, and the abrupt transition to spindle cell sarcoma support an interpretation of a progression from a lower grade giant cell tumor of soft tissue.

Leiomyosarcoma with osteoclast-like giant cells: Areas of leiomyosarcoma infiltrated by osteoclast-like giant cells should also exhibit atypia in the stromal cells the latter of which are usually spindle in shape. Often, there are foci of conventional leiomyosarcoma which are usually diffusely positive for multiple muscle markers including desmin, smooth muscle actin, and caldesmon (this patient's tumor exhibits strong but only focal desmin and smooth muscle actin reactivity; caldesmon staining was not performed). Cytogenetically, leiomyosarcoma of soft tissue commonly displays an aneuploid karyotype that would be indistinguishable from this patient's.

Osteosarcoma primary to the soft tissue: Some osteosarcomas contain many osteoclast-like giant cells interspersed among the tumor cells. However, neoplastic bone formed by cytologically atypical cells is also present and intimately intermingled with tumor cells. Fifty percent of giant cell tumors of soft tissue (low malignant potential) also contain bone. However, it is metaplastic, not associated with cytologically atypical osteoblasts, and generally forms perimeter rings around nodules of tumor.

Anaplastic carcinoma with giant cells metastatic to the soft tissues: This is an unlikely diagnosis for this patient as he has not history of carcinoma or masses elsewhere. Most anaplastic carcinomas with osteoclast-like giant cells are uniformly high grade and would not harbor foci identical to giant cell tumor of bone. Moreover, this patient's tumor is reactive for desmin and smooth muscle actin, with no reactivity for a panel of keratins. Glandular or squamous differentiation as might be seen focally in anaplastic carcinoma is also absent.

Oncology approach

Medical oncology

As there is no evidence for metastatic disease at the time of work-up and surgery, chemotherapy is held in reserve for possible use once evidence of metastases occurs. Should the disease recur, the patient would become a candidate for standard chemotherapy with single agent doxorubicin, given his age. The metastatic lesions or the local recurrence should be re-biopsied to assess the presence of giant cells. If these are still present, a therapeutic trial of subcutaneous denosumab could be considered, at a biweekly dose of 120 mg for one month, then monthly, prior to the initiation of chemotherapy.

Case table 7.5 Summary pathology findings of Case 7.5

Diagnosis	Giant cell tumor of soft tissue (low malignant potential) with transformation to high grade spindle cell sarcoma
Size	11.0 × 8.5 × 7.5 cm
Location	Deep, intramuscular
Margin status	Negative; all by greater than 1.0 cm
Histologic grade (FNCLCC system)	3 (high grade)
Pathologic stage (TNM classification)	T2b/N0/M0 by pathologic and clinical staging = Stage III at time of wide resection

Radiation oncology

The treatment of choice is complete surgical excision for giant cell tumor of soft tissue. In cases of incomplete resection, radiation therapy should be considered. High local control rates are reported with the use of radiation therapy for giant cell tumors. In this particular case, the giant cell tumor transformed into a high grade sarcoma. Therefore, radiation therapy is indicated despite negative margins. The patient successfully undergoes a complete course of radiation therapy.

Patient outcome

Six months after surgery and having completed radiation therapy, the patient is well with no evidence of disease.

Case 7.6 Undifferentiated pleomorphic sarcoma (a morphologic pattern of undifferentiated/unclassified sarcoma)

Clinical history and presentation

A 55-year-old man presents with a one-year history of an arm mass noted spontaneously. The mass is subsequently noted to progressively increase in size. It is minimally symptomatic.

Physical examination reveals a large, firm, deep soft tissue mass in the area of the biceps.

Open biopsy is performed, with a diagnosis of high grade sarcoma. Staging CT scan is negative for metastatic disease.

Surgical findings and comments

Wide resection of the tumor is performed.

Radiology findings

The MR appearance of this undifferentiated high grade pleomorphic sarcoma (formerly termed MFH, pleomorphic storiform variant) is typical of many sarcomas. The MR images in **Case figs 7.6a** through **7.6d** show a fairly uniform T1 low signal mass with heterogeneous T2 high signal and heterogeneous enhancement. The appearance is not specific, however, clearly represents an aggressive sarcoma with non-enhancing areas of necrosis or matrix. This particular patient had a postoperative seroma develop as seen in **Case figs 7.6e** through **7.6h**. This shows a fluid-fluid level and a low signal intensity rind. The rind likely has hemosiderin and fibrous healing tissue causing its low signal. The T1 high signal of the anterior fluid fraction likely represents blood degradation products such as met-hemoglobin and other proteinaceous material. This seroma was followed with routine MR imaging and decreased in size over months. Note there is no nodule or focal enhancing portion as might be seen with tumor residual or recurrence.

Pathology findings

Gross features

The biopsy comprises a 2.2 × 2 × 1 cm aggregate of tan and hemorrhagic soft tissue.

The resection specimen consists of a large ovoid resection of adipose tissue and muscle with an ellipse of attached skin containing a well-healed incision. Cross sections of the specimen reveal a single 7.8 × 7 × 5.1 cm myxoid to yellow-tan mass that is unencapsulated, 70% fibrous, 20% gelatinous and 10% cystic and hemorrhagic. Most margins are greater than 1.0 cm from the gross tumor edge, but the deep is close at 0.2 cm.

Wedge resection of the lower right lung (performed 13 months after initial diagnosis) reveals a 3.2 cm nodule of metastatic sarcoma histologically identical to that arising in the patient's left arm. The parenchymal margin is negative for tumor and it does not breach the pleura. The nodule is approximately 25% necrotic.

Microscopic features

Low magnification: The biopsy is diagnosed as high grade sarcoma, not otherwise specified as it consists of pleomorphic spindle cells arranged in intersecting fascicles. Mitotic figures are numerous (up to 20 per 10 high power microscopic fields with atypical forms) and necrosis affects 50% of the tumor.

The resection specimen features similar histology to the biopsy except in two respects: 1) approximately 5% of the tumor consists of intermediate grade tumor identical to myxofibrosarcoma (**Case fig. 7.6i**), and 2) some areas of the tumor are infiltrated by inflammatory cells and contain tumor cells with clear or vacuolated cytoplasm (**Case fig. 7.6j**). These areas of inflammation and clear cell change track closely with serpinginous regions of necrosis (**Case fig. 7.6k**).

High magnification: Areas away from necrosis comprise broad fascicles of spindle to polygonal cells with moderate nuclear atypia (**Case fig. 7.6l**). Regions of clear cell change, again primarily located adjacent to abrupt necrosis and possibly representing degenerative changes, are polygonal to epithelioid (rounded) with marked variation in nuclear shape, number of nuclear lobes, and many mitotic figures (**Case figs 7.6m** and **7.6n**).

Special studies: Immunohistochemistry performed on the biopsy reveals no specific line of differentiation, as there is less than 5% reactivity for smooth muscle actin and desmin and no reactivity for antibodies to mixed keratins, S-100 protein, CD34, myogenin, caldesmon, and HMB-45 (controls are appropriately reactive).

Karyotyping performed on a portion of the biopsy finds three of 20 cells with a t(13;20)(p11.2;q11.2) which is not known to be specific for any particular sarcoma and may represent an artifact of long term in situ culture. Two more attempts at karyotyping are performed, one which yields a normal male karyotype (collected from the wide resection specimen) and the last showing a near triploid male chromosome complement (of 67–72 chromosomes) with extensive

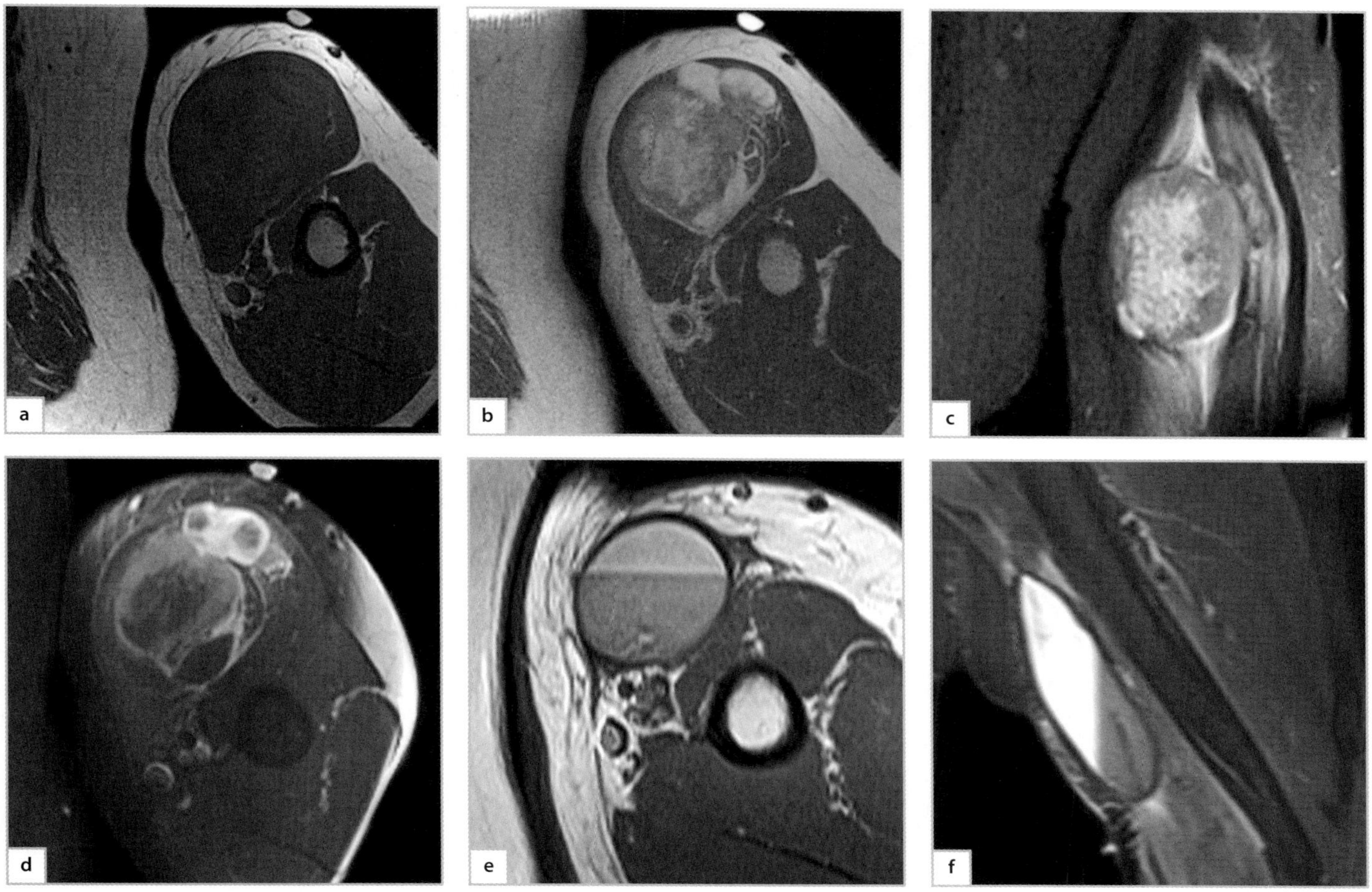

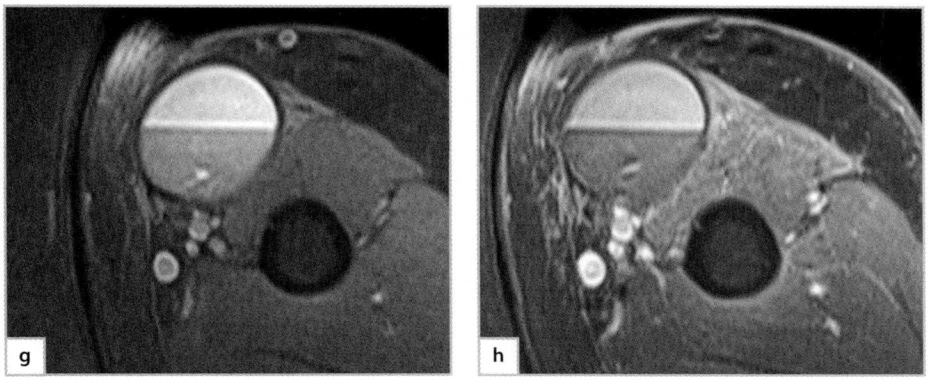

Case figure 7.6 Undifferentiated pleomorphic sarcoma (a morphologic pattern of undifferentiated/unclassified sarcoma) 7.6a: Axial T1 MR image. **7.6b**: Axial T2 MR image, **7.6c**: Coronal STIR MR image, **7.6d**: Axial T1 fat saturated post-contrast MR image. MR imaging shows a T1 isointense, T2 and STIR high signal intensity heterogeneous mass in the biceps muscle of the arm. The mass has heterogeneous intense enhancement. Postoperative Seroma. **7.6e**: Axial T1 MR image. **7.6f**: Sagittal STIR MR image, **7.6g**: Axial T1 fat saturated, **7.6h**: Axial T1 fat saturated post-contrast. This seroma lies in the surgical bed of the biceps muscle. There is an obvious fluid level. The fluid has variable appearance, but often is T1 high signal due to protein and blood degradation products. **7.6i**: Low magnification. Up to 5% of the patient's tumor exhibits morphology indistinguishable from an intermediate grade myxofibrosarcoma.

structural and numerical abn ormalities in all cells examined (collected from the lung metastasis). This last karyotype, aneuploid with many non-specific abnormalities, is most consistent with the diagnosis of undifferentiated pleomorphic sarcoma, high grade.

Pathologic differential or, why isn't it one of the following?

Myxofibrosarcoma, high grade: Some soft tissue expert pathologists might designate this tumor as a Grade 4 myxofibrosarcoma because a small component is histologically consistent with that diagnosis. However, other experts require that at least 10% to up to 50% of the tumor comprise myxoid regions with curvilinear vessels before rendering the diagnosis. In practical terms, deep Grade 4 myxofibrosarcoma has a similar prognosis to undifferentiated high grade pleomorphic sarcoma, and treatment is the same.

Leiomyosarcoma, high grade (LMS- HG): High grade leiomyosarcoma usually contains areas of typical fascicular malignant smooth muscle cells with eosinophilic cytoplasm and blunt ended to cigar shaped nuclei. Clear cell change may occur, however, and undifferentiated

Case figure 7.6: Continued from page 149

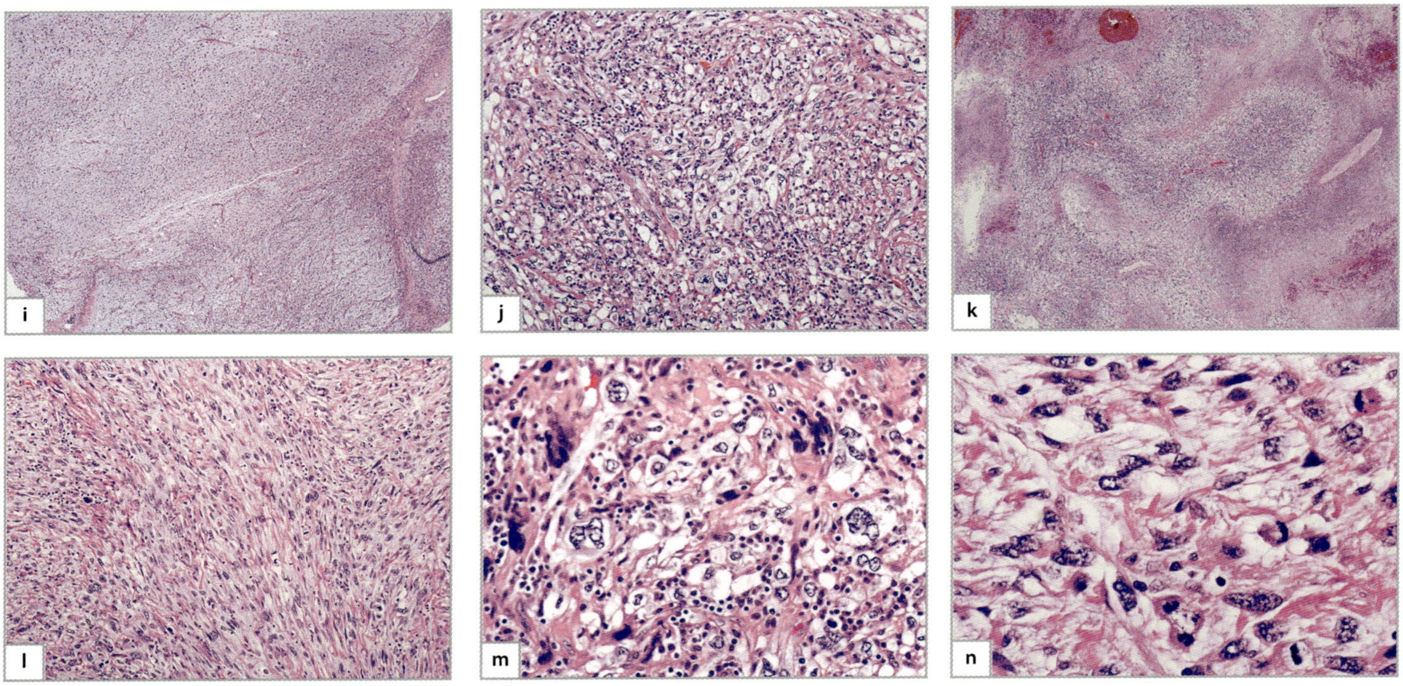

7.6j: Undifferentiated pleomorphic sarcoma, high grade, medium magnification. Some tumor cells show vacuolated or clear cytoplasm. Notice the intermingled inflammatory cells (lymphocytes and plasma cells predominantly). **7.6k**: Undifferentiated pleomorphic sarcoma, high grade, low magnification. Areas of viable tumor form bands around tumor blood vessels. Tumor cells beyond reach of adequate oxygenation show abrupt necrosis. The outermost, histologically viable cells (cells with preserved nuclear features including well-defined rather than smudgy chromatin) show cytoplasmic vacuolation or clearing, a possible ischemia-induced degenerative change. **7.6l**: Undifferentiated pleomorphic sarcoma, high grade, medium magnification. Tumor far from necrosis is more spindled with cells arranged in broad interweaving fascicles. **7.6m**: Undifferentiated pleomorphic sarcoma, high grade, medium magnification. Morphologically, the tumor varies; in this area, it is reminiscent of undifferentiated pleomorphic sarcoma with prominent inflammation (UPSPI). However, in most cases of UPSPI the inflammatory component consists of neutrophils and eosinophils rather than in this patient's tumor in which the infiltrating inflammatory cells are predominantly lymphoplasmacytic (lymphocytes and plasma cells). **7.6n**: Undifferentiated pleomorphic sarcoma, high grade, high magnification. In this field, the tumor cells exhibit clear cytoplasm, moderate nuclear atypia and mitotic figures.

pleomorphic sarcomas may also contain eosinophilic cells. Immunohistochemistry can be very helpful, as LMS-HG will diffusely express at least some muscle markers (most commonly desmin and smooth muscle actin). By definition, undifferentiated high grade pleomorphic sarcoma does not demonstrate diffuse reactivity for muscle markers or any other proteins pointing to a specific line of differentiation.

Dedifferentiated liposarcoma: Dedifferentiated liposarcoma (DDLPS) may contain areas of lower grade adipocytic tumor with well-defined adipocytes and lipoblasts; such areas are not seen in this patient's tumor. CDK4 and MDM2 staining were not performed on the patient's tumor because at the time this patient presented, the antibodies had not yet been characterized as useful in diagnosing liposarcomas. It would be reasonable to use those antibodies as part of panel in future cases such as this patient's. This patient's karyotype does not show evidence of amplification of 12q in the form of giant marker or ring chromosomes classic for dedifferentiated liposarcoma.

Malignant peripheral nerve sheath tumor, high grade: Malignant peripheral nerve sheath tumor (MPNST) is heterogeneous microscopically and could resemble this tumor. However, it commonly also harbors areas of spindle cells with buckled or wavy, pointed nuclei arranged in long fascicles that at low power can impart a distinctive striped appearance. Tumor cells can also particularly aggregate around

Case table 7.6 Summary pathology findings of Case 7.7

Diagnosis	Undifferentiated high grade pleomorphic sarcoma
Size	7.8 × 7.0 × 5.1 cm
Location	Deep
Margin status	Negative: all > 1.0 cm except deep at 0.2 cm
Histologic grade (FNCLCC system)	Grade 3 (mitoses > 20/10 hpf; < 50% necrosis, and areas of marked nuclear atypia)
Pathologic stage (TNM classification)	T2b/N0/M0 at time of original resection = Stage III

blood vessels. These features are not appreciated in this patient's tumor. Moreover, MPNST usually will demonstrate some reactivity for neural markers by immunohistochemistry even if focally. These markers (of varying specificity and sensitivity) include S-100 protein, neurofilaments, and GFAP of which S-100 protein is most commonly expressed and in a patchy pattern. There is no expression of S-100 protein in this patient's tumor. Both tumors are associated with a complex aneuploid karyotype, so standard karyotyping is not helpful in discriminating between the two tumors.

Perivascular epithelioid cell tumor, malignant: An unusual tumor that rarely arises in soft tissue and is more common in women but a possibility given the epithelioid clear cells and spindle cells present. Perivascular epithelioid cell tumors express melanocytic and myoid markers, and those markers are absent in this patient's tumor.

Oncology approach

Medical oncology

Nine months postoperatively, CT scan of the chest reveals metastatic disease with only two lesions. The patient receives a four month neoadjuvant regimen consisting of gemcitabine and docetaxel which yields a minor remission. A bronchoscopy and right video-assisted wedge resection of the right lower lobe is then performed with resection of two solitary pulmonary metastases. However, the disease recurs in the lungs within one month of surgery. The patient is enrolled on a clinical trial with weekly irinotecan and temsirolimus but does not tolerate the chemotherapy and asks to be referred to hospice. He succumbs to metastatic disease six months later.

Radiation oncology

Undifferentiated high grade pleomorphic sarcoma, being high grade, may benefit from adjuvant radiation in order to enhance local control. Even with negative margins after resection, the local recurrence rate is expected to be high. This patient receives radiation therapy to the primary site. Unfortunately, he develops metastatic disease but the primary site is locally controlled.

Patient outcome

The patient succumbs to metastatic disease approximately two years after wide resection of his tumor, with treatment also including postoperative radiation therapy, resection of pulmonary nodules, and trials of chemotherapy.

REFERENCES

Adelani MA, Wupperman RM, Holt GE. Benign synovial disorders. J Am Acad Orthop Surg 2008;16:268–275.

Billingsley KG, Burt ME, Jara E, et al. Pulmonary metastases from soft tissue sarcoma: analysis of patterns of diseases and postmetastasis survival. Ann Surg 1999;229(5):602–10; discussion 610–2.

Chawla SP SK, Chua V, Menendez LR, et al. A phase II study of AP23573 (an mTOR inhibitor) in patients (pts) with advanced sarcomas. American Society of Clinical Oncology: American Society of Clinical Oncology, 2005.

Cohen MH, Creaven PJ, Tejada F, et al. Phase I clinical trial of isophosphamide (NSC-109724). Cancer Chemother Rep 1975;59:751–5.

Gibault L, Perot G, Chibon F, et al. New insights in sarcoma oncogenesis: a comprehensive analysis of a large series of 160 soft tissue sarcomas with complex genomics. J Pathol 2011;223:64–71.

Hensley ML, Maki R, Venkatraman E, et al. Gemcitabine and docetaxel in patients with unresectable leiomyosarcoma: results of a phase II trial. J Clin Oncol 2002;20:2824–31.

Italiano A, Delcambre C, Hostein I, et al. Treatment with the mTOR inhibitor temsirolimus in patients with malignant PEComa. Ann Oncol 2010;21(5):1135–7.

Italiano A, Delva F, Mathoulin-Pelissier S, et al. Effect of adjuvant chemotherapy on survival in FNCLCC grade 3 soft tissue sarcomas: a multivariate analysis of the French Sarcoma Group Database. Ann Oncol 2010;21(12):2436–41.

Italiano A, Laurand A, Laroche A, et al. ERCC5/XPG, ERCC1, and BRCA1 gene status and clinical benefit of trabectedin in patients with soft tissue sarcoma. Cancer 2011;117(15):3445–56.

Lau YS, Sabokbar A, Gibbons CL, Giele H, Athanasou N. Phenotypic and molecular studies of giant-cell tumors of bone and soft tissue. Hum Pathol 2005;36(9):945–54.

Leu KM, Ostruszka LJ, Shewach D, et al. Laboratory and clinical evidence of synergistic cytotoxicity of sequential treatment with gemcitabine followed by docetaxel in the treatment of sarcoma. J Clin Oncol 2004;22:1706–12.

Liegl-Atzwanger B, Hofmann G, Leithner A, et al. Undifferentiated high-grade pleomorphic sarcoma (UHPS): Diagnostic criteria, differential diagnosis, and treatment. An attempt to erasure the misnomer "MFH". Eur Surg 2009;41/4:143–149.

Llauger J, Palmer J, Roson N, et al. Pigmented villonodular synovitis and giant cell tumors of the tendon sheath: radiologic and pathologic features. AJR 1999;172:1087–1091.

Maki RG, Wathen JK, Patel SR, et al. Randomized phase II study of gemcitabine and docetaxel compared with gemcitabine alone in patients with metastatic soft tissue sarcomas: results of sarcoma alliance for research through collaboration study 002 [corrected]. J Clin Oncol 2007;25:2755–63.

Mendenhall WM, Mendenhall CM, Reith JD, et al. Pigmented Villonodular Synovitis. Am J Clin Oncol 2006;29:548–550.

O'Connell JX, Wehrli BM, Nielsen G P, et al. Giant cell tumors of soft tissue: a clinicopathologic study of 18 benign and malignant tumors. Am J Surg Pathol 2000;24(3):386–95.

Okuno SH, Bailey HH, Adkins DR, et al. A multicenter phase 2 consortium (P2C) study of the mTOR inhibitor CCI-779 in advanced soft tissue sarcomas (STS). In: ASCO. Atlanta, Georgia; 2006.

Oliveira AM, Dei Tos AP, Fletcher CD, et al. Primary giant cell tumor of soft tissues: a study of 22 cases. Am J Surg Pathol 2000;24(2):248–56.

Ottaviani S, Ayral X, Dougados M, et al. Pigmented villonodular synovitis: a retrospective single-center study of 122 cases and review of the literature. Seminars in Arthritis and Rheumatism, Sep 2010.

Paz-Ares L, Lopez-Pousa A, Poveda A, et al. Trabectedin in pre-treated patients with advanced or metastatic soft tissue sarcoma: a phase II study evaluating co-treatment with dexamethasone. Invest New Drugs 2012;30(2):729–40.

Pervaiz N, Colterjohn N, Farrokhyar F, et al. A systematic meta-analysis of randomized controlled trials of adjuvant chemotherapy for localized resectable soft-tissue sarcoma. Cancer 2008;113(3):573–81.

Sarcoma Meta-analysis Collaboration (SMAC) Adjuvant chemotherapy for localised resectable soft tissue sarcoma in adults. Cochrane Database Syst Rev 2000; (2 and 4):CD001419.

Schein PS, Winokur SH. Immunosuppressive and cytotoxic chemotherapy: long-term complications. Ann Intern Med 1975;82:84–95.

Schnirring-Judge M, Lin B. Pigmented villonodular synovitis of the ankle – radiation therapy as a primary treatment to reduce recurrence: a case report with 8 year follow-up. The Journal of Foot and Ankle Surgery 2011;50(1):108–116.

Seifert CF, Nesser ME, Thompson DF. Dexrazoxane in the prevention of doxorubicin-induced cardiotoxicity. Ann Pharmacother 1994;28:1063–72.

Taher A, Pushpanathan C. Plexiform fibrohistiocytic tumor: a brief review. Arch Pathol Lab Med 2007;131:1135–1138.

Thomas D, Henshaw R, Skubitz K, et al. Denosumab in patients with giant-cell tumour of bone: an open-label, phase 2 study. Lancet Oncol 2010;11(3):275–80.

Tyler WK, Vidal AF, Williams RJ, et al. Pigmented Villonodular Synovitis. J Am Acad Orthop Surg 2006;14:376–385

Verschraegen C, Chawla S, Mita M, et al. PICASSO Study Investigators. A phase II, randomized, controlled trial of palifosfamide plus doxorubicin versus doxorubicin in patients with soft tissue sarcoma (PICASSO).J Clin Oncol 2010;28:15 (suppl;abstr 10004).

Verschraegen C, Quinn R, Rabinowitz I, et al. Phase Ib study of docetaxel (D), gemcitabine (G), and bevacizumab (B) in patients (pts) with advanced or recurrent soft tissue sarcoma (STS). 2012;23(3):785–90.

Wan X, Helman LJ. The biology behind mTOR inhibition in sarcoma. Oncologist 2007;12:1007–18.

Williams J, Hodari A, Janevski P, et al. Recurrence of giant cell tumors in the hand: a prospective study. J Hand Surg Am 2010;35(3):451–456.

Wullschleger S, Loewith R, Hall MN. TOR signaling in growth and metabolism. Cell 2006;124:471–84.

Yovine A, Riofrio M, Blay JY, et al. Phase II study of ecteinascidin–743 in advanced pretreated soft tissue sarcoma patients. J Clin Oncol 2004;22:890–9.

Chapter 8 Muscle tumors of soft tissue

OVERVIEW

Tumors in this group differentiate in the direction of smooth muscle or skeletal muscle (with exceptional tumors showing dual differentiation). Well-differentiated sarcomas and benign muscle tumors resemble normal smooth muscle or skeletal muscle cells to a remarkable degree that is easily appreciable on standard histology review. Poorly differentiated (high grade) leiomyosarcomas and rhabdomyosarcomas may mimic other sarcomas, and ancillary studies are required for accurate classification.

The role of ancillary testing is increasing in soft tissue and bone tumor pathology, and muscle tumors are no exception. For example, confirmatory molecular genetics diagnosis of alveolar rhabdomyosarcoma is now a requirement for patient entry into various national treatment protocols. It is vital to distinguish between A-RMS and embryonal rhabdomyosarcoma (E-RMS) because of therapeutic and prognostic differences. Some E-RMS are indistinguishable from A-RMS on routine pathology review; the finding of specific gene translocations associated exclusively with alveolar rhabdomyosarcoma can resolve diagnostic dilemmas.

Advances in molecular diagnostic tools have been accompanied by efforts to identify additional genetic prognostic and predictive biomarkers. The pace of research in this area comprises several reports annually that detail new insights into the molecular pathogenesis of muscle sarcomas. Winnowing these results to those useful for diagnosis, prognosis and treatment decisions requires large scale enrollment of patients into carefully monitored clinical trials. In the US, nearly all pediatric patients with E-RMS and A-RMS are on such trials. However, adults with muscle sarcomas (including the rare adult cases of embryonal and alveolar rhadomyosarcoma), with the exception of uterine leiomyosarcoma, do not have the option of enrolling in a specific muscle sarcoma trial but may participate in trials enrolling patients with multiple types of sarcoma.

The 2013 classification of muscle tumors by the World Health Organization (WHO) includes a new type of muscle sarcoma: spindle cell/sclerosing rhabdomyosarcoma.

CLASSIFICATION

The WHO classification of muscle tumors of soft tissue is presented in **Table 8.1**.

DEMOGRAPHICS

Smooth muscle tumors of soft tissue include benign superficial tumors located in the subcutaneous fat or dermis (pilar type leiomyoma, a rare skin tumor not further discussed, and angioleiomyoma, also known as angiomyoma), the extremely rare leiomyoma of (deep) soft tissue, and the rare leiomyosarcoma (LMS) of deep soft tissue and more common atypical smooth muscle tumor/leiomyosarcoma of dermis/subcutis, respectively. Uterine leiomyomas and leiomyosarcomas are excluded from this group by virtue of location, and because they exhibit estrogen and progesterone hormone receptor expression. It is necessary to briefly discuss them, however, as occasional Müllerian type smooth muscle tumors venture into the territory of orthopaedic surgeons.

Uterine leiomyomas are extremely common and greatly outnumber all types of soft tissue smooth muscle tumors. For example, for the period 2000-2010 at the University of New Mexico Health Sciences Center, 1400 patients had uterine leiomyomas (in many cases, more than one each) removed compared to 29 patients with excision of smooth muscle tumors of soft tissue: > 98% of all leiomyomas surgically excised were of uterine origin. Uterine leiomyomas, many retroperitoneal smooth muscle tumors in women and a few other variants of leiomyomas such as benign metastasizing leiomyoma are Müllerian derived and differ from soft tissue leiomyomas in reactivity for progesterone and estrogen receptors, WT-1 reactivity and genetic findings (Patil et al. 2011, Nucci et al. 2007).

Table 8.1 WHO classification of muscle tumors of soft tissue (2013)

Tumor	Behavior	Additional comments
Angioleiomyoma	Benign	Superficial tumor of subcutis or dermis
Leiomyoma of deep soft tissue	Benign	Rare with strict histologic requirements so as not to under diagnose leiomyosarcoma
Leiomyosarcoma	Malignant	Uncommon in soft tissue with several histologic variants
Rhabdomyoma	Benign	Most common in the heart Soft tissue versions include adult type, pediatric type, and genital type
Embryonal rhabdomyosarcoma Variants include spindle cell RMS (pediatric), botryoid RMS, and anaplastic RMS	Malignant	Most common type of rhabdomyosarcoma
Alveolar rhabdomyosarcoma Variant includes solid alveolar RMS	Malignant	Genetic confirmation is required for the diagnosis
Pleomorphic Rhabdomyosarcoma	Malignant	Almost exclusively seen in adults
Spindle cell/sclerosing rhabdomyosarcoma	Malignant	Occurs in both children and adults with male predilection. Outcome is significantly better in pediatric patients

Benign: does not recur or does not recur aggressively and does not metastasize. Intermediate: can recur aggressively locally and/or rarely metastasizes (<5%)

Malignant: can recur and commonly metastasizes. RMS: rhabdomyosarcoma

However, a few Müllerian type leiomyomas will present as inguinal soft tissue masses and thus be excised by an orthopaedic or general surgeon (Patil et al. 2011). Rarely, inguinal leiomyosarcomas in women will express hormone receptors; these may represent Müllerian type leiomyosarcomas rather than LMS of soft tissue.

Soft tissue leiomyomas include a specific subset occurring in the male external genitalia. These are rare, occur generally in older men, and may exhibit cytologic atypia worrisome for malignancy. The degree of atypia mimics that seen in some benign uterine tumors and importantly, is not associated with mitotic activity. Distinct, location-specific criteria must be used to accurately determine malignancy in a smooth muscle tumor (Hornick et al. 2003, Weiss 2002). Location in the body plays a paramount role in smooth muscle tumor classification and behavior. A pathologist must be very careful in assessing smooth muscle neoplasms of the deep soft tissue: any mitotic activity, even without cytologic atypia, likewise any necrosis, or atypia alone should prompt strong consideration that the tumor may behave malignantly (Hornick et al. 2003). Referral of such cases to a soft tissue pathologist expert may be prudent. Combinations of any of the three histologic parameters: 1) mitotic activity, 2) necrosis, and 3) cytologic atypia, should result in a diagnosis of leiomyosarcoma in a subfascial soft tissue smooth muscle tumor.

An unusual group of smooth muscle tumors occurs in immunocompromised patients in association with Epstein-Barr virus infection. Affected patients include those with HIV/AIDS, individuals on organ transplant immunosuppressive therapy and patients on steroids, among others. Patients may develop multiple tumors, the tumors may contain primitive round cell appearing areas, and a lymphocytic inflammatory infiltrate is always present (Deyrup et al. 2006). Most occur in the lungs and liver or other visceral sites, but soft tissues are sometimes involved and can be the presenting finding in HIV/AIDS patients.

In contrast to smooth muscle tumors, benign and malignant skeletal muscle tumors (with the exception of pleomorphic rhabdomyosarcoma and spindle cell/sclerosing rhabdomyosarcoma) show a predilection for children and adolescents. Spindle cell/sclerosing RMS occurs in both children and adults with a 6:1 male to female ratio (Fletcher et al. 2013).

The Surveillance Epidemiology and End Results (SEER) data for leiomyosarcomas and rhabdomyosarcomas diagnosed in the United States and registered in several SEER sites for the years 1994 to 2008 are provided in histogram and text format (these numbers do not encompass all US patients with these sarcomas but a sampling of ~20% of the population).

The research database of the SEER program (13 registries) was used to review the characteristics of the following rhabdomyosarcoma subtypes (their associated ICD-O-3 histology codes are in parentheses): mixed (8902/3), embryonal (8910/3), alveolar (8920/3), spindle cell (8912/3), pleomorphic (8901/3), and not otherwise specified (NOS) (8900/3). Leiomyosarcomas were evaluated as well: epithelioid (8891/3), myxoid (8896/3), and NOS (8890/3). All cases were limited to connective, subcutaneous and other soft tissues (ICD-O topography codes = C49.0 - C49.9).

Rhabdomyosarcomas are rare, with average annual age-adjusted incidence rates per million of 0.4 for alveolar, 0.3 for embryonal, 0.2 for pleomorphic and NOS, and 0.0 for mixed type and spindle cell subtypes during the selected 15-year period, 1994-2008. Leiomyosarcomas are also rare, with average annual age-adjusted incidence rates per million of 0.1 for epithelioid, and myxoid, and 3.6 for NOS. Generally, leiomyosarcomas occur more frequently in females compared to males because a large percentage of these tumors are of uterine origin. However, when anatomic site is restricted, as seen in this chapter, leiomyosarcomas are diagnosed more often in males than in females.

The number of SEER cases per rhabdomyosarcoma and leiomyosarcoma subtypes arising in soft tissues is shown in **Figures 8.1** and **8.2**, respectively.

Overall, rhabdomyosarcomas of the connective, subcutaneous, and other soft tissues are diagnosed more frequently in the lower limb, hip and pelvis. Most tumors in the head, face and neck are of the alveolar and embryonal subtypes. **Figure 8.3** depicts the RMS subtypes by anatomic site. Spindle cell cases are separated into two groups by age category; pediatric cases are less than 20 years old, and adult cases are 20 years old and older.

Most rhabdomyosarcoma subtypes are diagnosed in children, with pediatric spindle cell rhabdomyosarcoma having the youngest mean age at diagnosis (5.0 years). Pleomorphic rhabdosarcoma is defined as an adult disease in the SEER database, and is largely seen in an older population (mean = 60.9 years) but with a wide age range. However, embryonal and alveolar RMS occurs in adults and actually account for ~60% of cases (compared to pleomorphic RMS) (Stock et al. 2009). **Figure 8.4** shows the age distribution by subtype.

Leiomyosarcomas, in contrast to rhabdomyosarcomas, are much

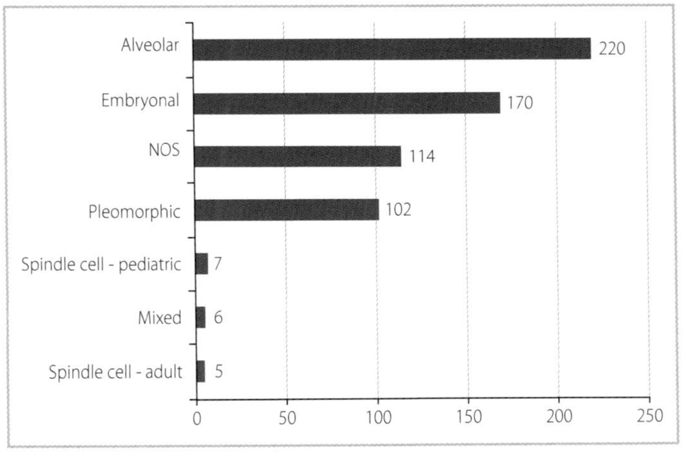

Figure 8.1 Frequency of rhabdomyosarcoma subtypes in 13 SEER registries between the years 1994 and 2008.

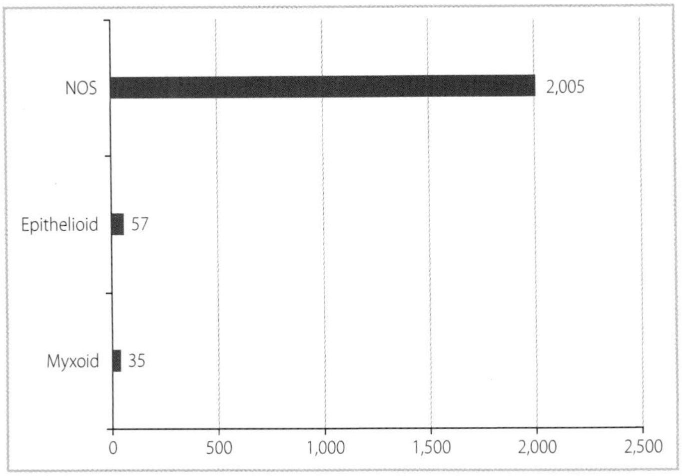

Figure 8.2 Frequency of leiomyosarcoma subtypes in 13 SEER registries between the years 1994 and 2008.

Rhabdomyosarcoma subtype	Connective, subcutaneous, and other soft tissues: Head/face/neck	Upper limb/shoulder	Lower limb/hip	Thorax	Abdomen	Pelvis	Trunk	Overlap*	NOS
Alveolar	51	40	49	15	9	43	4	2	7
Embryonal	53	8	17	8	19	58	3	2	3
NOS	18	8	35	7	17	18	2	1	7
Pleomorphic	5	11	46	12	9	13	9	1	1
Spindle cell (pediatric)	0	1	1	2	2	0	1	0	0
Mixed	0	1	0	0	0	2	3	0	0
Spindle cell (adult)	3	1	1	0	0	0	0	0	0
Total	130	70	149	43	51	134	23	6	18

* "A tumor that overlaps the boundaries of two or more subcategories and whose point of origin cannot be determined." (Fritz et al., 2000).
Figure 8.3 depicts the subtypes by anatomic site. Spindle cell cases are separated into two groups by age category; pediatric cases are less than 20 years old, and adult cases are 20 years old and older.

Figure 8.3 Rhabdomyosarcoma subtype by soft tissue site for cases in 13 SEER registries diagnosed between 1994 and 2008.

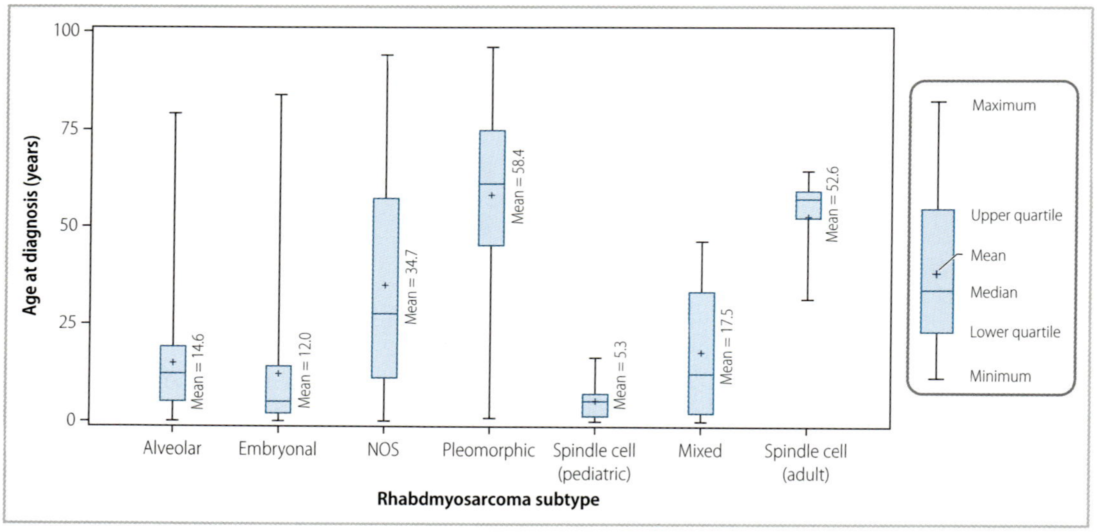

Figure 8.4 Age distribution by rhabdomyosarcoma subtype for cases in 13 SEER registries diagnosed between 1994 and 2008 (N=624).

more likely to occur in adults than children. The mean age at diagnosis for leiomyosaroma is very similar across subtypes (58.3 to 61.2 years) as seen in **Figure 8.5**. **Figure 8.6** shows the distribution of soft tissue leiomyosarcoma morphologic subtype according to body site. Most occur in the lower limbs/hip.

PATHOGENESIS/ETIOLOGY

As with other soft tissue tumors, most tumors of muscle have an unknown etiology. However, it is likely for most tumors that genetic aberrations account for both the etiology and pathogenesis. For those tumors that occur predominantly in the pediatric age group, abnormal growth factor signaling or differentiation could also contribute to pathogenesis. In general, however, cancer (including sarcomas) is fundamentally a genetic or, less often, an epigenetic disease. **Table 8.2** lists the genetic findings found thus far in muscle tumors of soft tissue.

Smooth muscle tumors

Most patients with leiomyosarcomas are middle aged or older; thus, accumulation of environmental stresses, accruing unrepaired mutations, and diminished immune regulation occurring with aging most likely collaborate in tumor creation.

Unusually, an infectious etiology occurs in one type of smooth muscle tumor that is initiated by a combination of patient immunosuppression and infection (possibly multiple re-infections) by Epstein-Barr virus.

The great majority of smooth muscle tumors comprise those of gynecologic origin. These tumors are so common that they may almost be considered a normal occurrence in the uterus of a middle

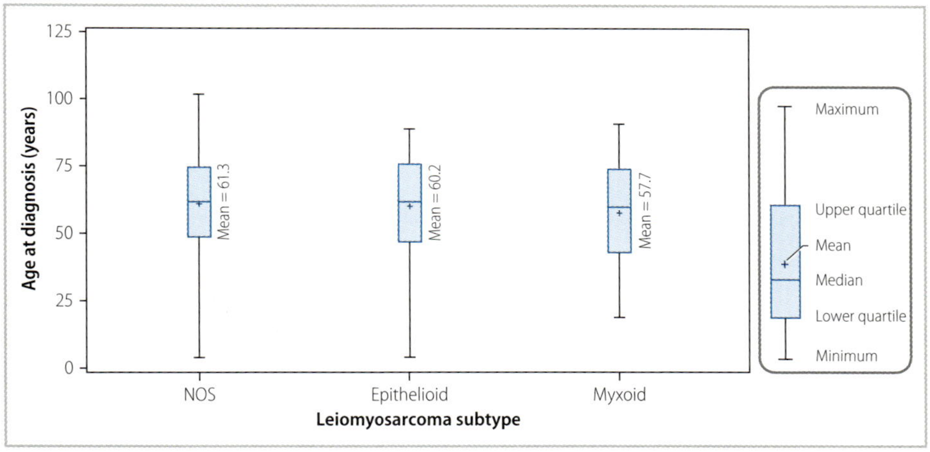

Figure 8.5 Age distribution by leiomyosarcoma subtype for cases in 13 SEER registries diagnosed between 1994 and 2008 (N=2,097).

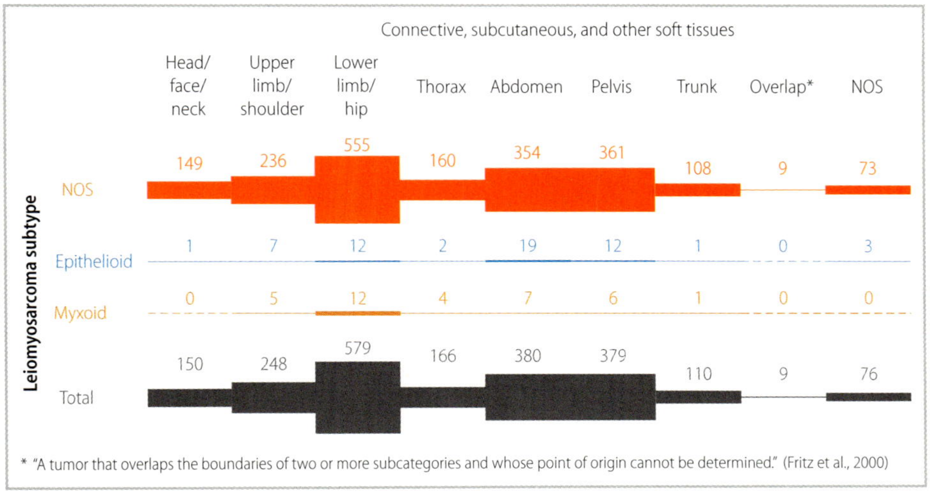

Figure 8.6 Leiomyosarcoma subtype by soft tissue site for cases In 13 SEER registries diagnosed between 1994 and 2008.

Table 8.2 Genetics of muscle tumors of soft tissue

Tumor	Chromosomal abnormality	Genes involved	Percentage of tumors with abnormality
Angioleiomyoma	No consistent abnormalities found. Translocations include t(X;10)(q22;q23.3), t(X;11)(p11.4;p15), t(4;5)(p12;q33) and various deletions (loss of 22 most commonly) and additions (gain at Xq most commonly)	Unknown	Unknown
Leiomyoma of soft tissue	Unknown	Unknown	Unknown
Leiomyoma of scrotum	t(12;14)(q15;q24) in one case report	*HMGA2*	Unknown
Müllerian type leiomyoma of inguinal canal	Multiple different findings including trisomy 12, t(12;14), rearrangements of 6p, 10q, 12q15 13q and deletions of 7q, 3q and 1p	*HMGA2* [involved in the t(12;14)]	Unknown but may be similar to uterine leiomyomas of which 40% have abnormal karyotypes
EBV-associated smooth muscle tumors	The tumors are clonal and most patients with multiple tumors have new clones at each site No other information available at this time	Interaction of EBV with genome in unknown manner.	Unknown
Leiomyosarcoma of soft tissue	Complex aneuploid karyotypes with some preferential losses (any one of these seen in no more than 20% of cases) of 3p21-p23, 8p21-pter, 13q12-13, 13q32-qter, 1q42-qter, 2p15pter, 18p11, 1p36, 11q23-qter, 10q23-qter and most frequent gain at 1q12-q31		Majority have complex aneuploidy

Table 8.2: Continued from page 155

Tumor	Chromosomal abnormality	Genes involved	Percentage of tumors with abnormality
Embryonal rhabdomyosarcoma	Complex aneuploid karyotype but a subset have mild hyperdiploidy (tetraploidy is rare) Gain of 8q, 1q and 20q and 19 fairly common Loss of 3 or part of 3 fairly common LOH of 11p and 11q common with amplification of retained alleles Allelic imbalance fairly common of 10q, 10p, 6q and 4q	*FGFR1* gained in (30%) *CDK4* amp & O-E *MYCN* amp & O-E *MYC* amp & O-E *RB1* altered (50%)	Majority have complex aneuploidy Percentage with specific gene abnormalities varies but is not 100%
Alveolar rhabdomyosarcoma	t(2;13)(q35;q14)	*PAX3-FOXO1A* fusion (60-75% of fusion positive cases)	Specific translocations involving FOX01 gene may become a requirement for the diagnosis of A-RMS
	t(1;13)(q36;q14)	*PAX7-FOXO1A* fusion (20-25% of fusion positive cases)	
	t(X;2)(q13;q35)	*PAX3-AFX1* fusion (<1% of A-RMS)	*PAX3-FOXO1A* imparts a uniformly poor prognosis
	t(2;2)(q35;p23)	*PAX3-NCOA1* fusion (<1% of A-RMS)	*PAX7-FOXO1A* may impart a relatively better prognosis (for A-RMS)
	t(2;8)(q35;q13)	*PAX3-NCOA2* fusion (rare)	
	t(8;13;9)(p11.2;q14;q32)	*FOXO1-FGFR1* fusion (rare)	
	FUSION NEGATIVE A-RMS	25% of histologically classic A-RMS. Gene expression profiles are heterogeneous and overlap with E-RMS	
	12q13-q14 amplified (usually in *PAX3-FOXO1* cases) LOH and amplification of 11p, especially in fusion negative cases. LOH of 4q and 1q in some cases. Some cases show tetraploid karyotypes	*CDK4* and others amp *MYCN* amp & O-E *MYOG* amp & O-E *TFAP2* (6p24), *CDH3* (16q22.1), *CNR1* (6q14-15) O-E *RB1* altered (15%)	
Pleomorphic rhabdomyosarcoma	Complex aneuploid karyotype. More common findings include -2, -13, -14, -15, -16 and -19	Unknown	Majority have complex aneuploidy
Spindle cell/ sclerosing rhabdomyosarcoma	Complex aneuploid karyotype including gains and losses of whole and partial chromosomes	Unknown	Majority have complex aneuploidy

LOH: loss of heterozygosity. O-E: over expressed. Amp: amplified. See References for papers pertaining to this table. This static list of genetic abnormalities must be viewed in the context of continuing discovery and refinement of genetic findings.

aged woman, as they are found in ~75% of hysterectomy specimens (Mills et al. 2009). These Müllerian smooth muscle tumors may be responsive to hormones such as estrogen and progesterone which may play a significant role in promoting their development. Orthopaedic and general surgeons may encounter these Müllerian smooth muscle tumors when these tumors occur in the inguinal soft tissues of women.

Some deep seated and cutaneous smooth muscle tumors arise from the walls of blood vessels. In addition, rarely, patients with combined pilar type leiomyomas (leiomyomas arising from the arrector pili smooth muscles of skin) and uterine leiomyomas carry a germline mutation in the fumarate hydratase gene located on chromosome 1q. These individuals are also at risk for papillary renal cell carcinoma. It is unknown why this mitochondrial protein causes this odd triplet of tumors.

Leiomyosarcomas usually display a complex aneuploid karyotype. There are no characteristic, universal karyotypic abnormalities. Losses and gains of whole chromosomes or partial chromosomes are common. A review of 45 cases of conventional and pleomorphic leiomyosarcomas suggested that losses at 1p36 and 8p21-pter may increase the risk of metastasis (Mandahl et al. 1999). Mutations in the p53 gene on 17p are frequent as in many other malignant solid tumors. Decreased expression of p16 protein, in some cases through hypermethylation of the gene promoter, has been reported in ~30% of soft tissue leiomyosarcomas and may independently confer a worse prognosis (Yang et al. 2009). Multiple genes have been reported to be mutated or show increased or decreased expression in LMS, but breakthrough discoveries enabling tailored therapy have not yet been reported.

Skeletal muscle tumors

Fetal rhabdomyoma may occur sporadically or in the setting of nevoid basal cell carcinoma syndrome (caused by mutations of PTCH, a tumor suppressor gene) (Mietinnen et al. 2010). Adult rhabdomyoma is not associated with any syndromes. It does not occur outside the head and neck and has been proposed to arise from muscles of the branchial arches (Mietinnen et al. 2010). A third type of rhabdomyoma, the genital type, usually occurs in the vagina or cervix. Recently, a novel new type of rhabdomyoma, 'sclerosing paratesticular rhabdomyoma' has been described in four patients aged 19-42 years (median 25.5 years) (Jo et al. 2013 [abstract only]).

The pediatric predominance of most rhabdomyosarcomas is striking. In fact, rhabdomyosarcoma is the most common soft tissue sarcoma in children (see **Figure 8.4** for the age distribution of rhabdomyosarcomas according to SEER data). However, pleomorphic RMS is more common in adults. The spindle cell/sclerosing RMS may represent two different entities, as adult cases have a much worse prognosis than pediatric cases. Rhabdomyosarcoma may also occur as a component in another type of sarcoma (such as malignant peripheral nerve sheath tumor, dedifferentiated liposarcoma, dedifferentiated chondrosarcoma, and others) and can even form a part of a non-sarcomatous tumor such as in a germ cell tumor, Wilm's tumor, pleuropulmonary blastoma, and primary brain tumor (medulloblastoma). Thus, although overall a rare tumor, rhabdomyosarcoma in general affects a broad age group, a broad set of locations from soft tissue to bone to viscera and brain, and it can develop as a minor, or rarely major, component in another malignancy.

A few syndromes are associated with an increased risk of rhabdomyosarcoma. They are: Li Fraumeni syndrome, neurofibromatosis type 1, familial pleuroblastoma (PPB)-predisposition syndrome, Noonan syndrome, Costello syndrome, Beckwith-Wiedemann syndrome, and Multiple Endocrine Neoplasia Type 2a among others (Smith et al. 2001, Kuroiwa et al. 2009, Ahmadi et al. 2010). The incidence of RMS in patients with these syndromes is generally low; however, one should be aware that the patients are at increased risk for development of these tumors. Genetic abnormalities are being explored to determine the myriad mangled pathways involved in RMS pathogenesis in these patients. Such work may also shed light on the much more prevalent sporadic rhabdomyosarcoma. **Table 8.3** lists the predisposition syndromes associated with rhabdomyosarcoma (Xia et al. 2002).

The subdivision of rhabdomyosarcoma into embryonal, alveolar and spindle cell/sclerosing types was based initially on histologic differences noted at microscope review. Importantly, these types (and their subtypes) are also associated with distinct genetic differences. Alveolar RMS is characterized by specific translocations of the

Table 8.3 Syndromes associated with muscle differentiated tumors

Syndrome	Germline genetic abnormality	Patient characteristics	Tumor or tumors involved
Reed Syndrome (multiple cutaneous and uterine leiomyomatosis)	Fumarate hydratase gene mutations on 1q43.	Younger women with multiple small skin leiomyomas and symptomatic uterine leiomyomas (>50% have hysterectomy by 30 years)	Cutaneous leiomyomas, uterine leiomyomas
Hereditary leiomyomatosis and renal cell cancer	Fumarate hydratase gene mutations on 1q43.	Younger adult women, very rare	Uterine leiomyomas and Type II papillary RCC or collecting duct carcinoma of kidney
Li Fraumeni familial cancer syndrome	*p53* (17p13.1) and CHK2 genes inactivated	100% of women with classic syndrome develop cancer under age 45 years 75% of men with classic syndrome develop cancer under age 45 years	Breast, adrenocortical carcinoma, leukemia, soft tissue and bone sarcomas including rhabdomyosarcoma, among others
Hereditary retinoblastoma	*RB1* gene (13q12-14) altered	Infants to young children with bilateral retinoblastomas or unilateral retinoblastoma + family history	Surviving patients at risk for osteosarcoma and rhabdomyosarcoma
Beckwith-Wiedemann syndrome	Methylation abnormalities on 11p15 including *IGF-II* (insulin-like growth factor II) and H19	Specific phenotype includes macroglossia, prominent eye, organomegaly, hemihypertrophy etc.	Wilms tumor, hepatoblastoma, rhabdomyosarcoma and others
Familial pleuroblastoma (PPB)-predisposition syndrome	*DICER1* germline mutation	30% of kindreds in which a child has been diagnosed with pleuropulmonary blastoma have this predisposition syndrome	Various benign and malignant tumors including pleuropulmonary blastoma, soft tissue sarcomas, cystic nephroma, ciliary body medulloepithelioma etc
Noonan syndrome	Genetically heterogeneous 60% have mutations of the *RAS/MAPK* pathway	Physical features include particular facial features, short stature, pectus deformity	RMS is very rare (may be incidental)
Multiple endocrine neoplasia syndrome type 2a (MEN 2a)	*RET* proto-oncogene (10q11.2) activating mutations	MEN 2a is 55% of MEN 2 cases	Medullary thyroid carcinoma, pheochromocytoma, parathyroid tumors and others; RMS rarely reported
Costello syndrome	*HRAS* mutations	Set of physical features and moderate mental retardation among others	Embryonal rhabdomyosarcoma
Nijmegen breakage syndrome	*NBS1* truncating mutation	Set of physical features and mental retardation among others Increased sensitivity to ionizing radiation or mutagens that produce double stranded DNA breaks	Increased risk for various cancers including breast, prostate, melanoma, lymphoma, and sarcoma Rare reported case of RMS
Rubinstein-Taybi syndrome	*CREBBP* and *EP300* mutations	Skeletal abnormalities, glaucoma, cardiac and renal defects, etc	Rare reported case of RMS (may be incidental)
Roberts syndrome	*ESC02* mutations	Extremely rare, phenotype mimics that of Fanconi anemia patients	Rare reported case of RMS (may be incidental)
Duchenne muscular dystrophy	*DMD* (Xp21.1) mutations, usually deletions	X-linked so predominantly affects boys. Characteristic muscle weakness clinically apparent by age 5 years	RMS develops very rarely (may be incidental)
Neurofibromatosis type 1	*NF1* (neurofibromin) inactivated	Suite of clinical features can be used to make diagnosis (axillary freckling, iris Lisch nodules, multiple café au lait spots, neurofibromas, etc.)	Variety of benign and malignant peripheral nerve sheath tumors and other tumors; RMS reported to occur in 1.5-6% of patients

PAX3 or PAX7 genes with additional changes also common, while embryonal RMS and spindle cell/sclerosing RMS show complex aneuploid changes without specific translocations (Bridge et al. 2011, Folpe et al. 2002). Some of the genes involved in the pathogenesis of RMS beyond the characteristic alveolar RMS translocated genes include p53, MDM2, ARF, CDKN2A/B, IGF2, GPC5, RAS, MYCN and deltaNp73 (O'Brien et al. 2012). The genes involved may be mutated, amplified, deleted, alternatively spliced, or overexpressed. Some genes are involved in embryonal RMS, some in alveolar RMS, and some are implicated in both tumors.

PATHOLOGY

The pathologic features of the muscle tumors of soft tissue are synopsized in **Tables 8.4** and **8.5** with representative photomicrographs. Most common body sites involved by the various malignant muscle tumors are depicted in **Figure 8.3** (determined by SEER data).

Histologic grading

Benign tumors are not graded. Some sarcomas, and especially RMS, show only residual differentiated components persisting or maturing after neoadjuvant therapy. Thus, grading should only be performed on non-treated specimens.

Although not part of the grading systems used for sarcomas, margin status and presence or absence of lymphatic channel and vascular invasion must be reported, as these impact patient prognosis. The distance from margins must be stated precisely if less than 1.0 cm. Of course, adequate sampling of the tumor in Pathology is essential with a minimum of 1 section taken per centimeter maximum diameter of the tumor.

Smooth muscle tumors

Leiomyosarcomas are graded according to the degree of differentiation (how closely the tumor resembles normal smooth muscle), the mitotic rate, and presence or absence of necrosis. The estimate of necrosis in some cases may need to be based on radiologic features, as it can be under sampled at pathologic sectioning. Tumor should be fixed rapidly to preserve histologic features. Mitotic figures especially can degenerate due to delayed fixation leading to a falsely low count. Before rapid fixation, the tumor should be sampled for tumor banking and cytogenetics. Also, because some molecular tests require fresh frozen tumor, it is important to plan ahead in the pathology dissection suite to triage the tumor specimen efficiently and appropriately. Most pathologists use the French Federation of Cancer Centers (FNCLCC) grading system which has prognostic value and is reproducible among pathologists. The majority of soft tissue LMS are at least intermediate grade.

Skeletal muscle tumors

The benign skeletal muscle tumors are not graded. Rhabdomyosarcomas vary in cellularity from myxoid hypocellular tumors to crowded hypercellular alveolar RMS. The degree of differentiation to skeletal muscle also is highly variable. The range comprises primitive, small round blue cells found in alveolar RMS and some E-RMS to mature cells that form cross-striations and myotubules (multinucleated elongate eosinophilic cells with peripherally aligned nuclei parallel to long axis of the cell). Primitive stellate cells or round cells may dominate with more differentiated rhabdomyofibroblasts interspersed (these are cells with bright eosinophilic cytoplasm and well-preserved nuclei). A few cases will only contain primitive cells, and immunohistochemistry is required to identify the skeletal muscle nature of the tumor. Even with identifiable rhabdomyoblasts or myotubules, IHC is compulsory.

Some pediatric RMS exhibit marked cellular pleomorphism which can be as pronounced as in adult type pleomorphic RMS. It can occur in both embryonal and alveolar tumors. The pleomorphism, termed 'anaplasia' is defined as: 'large lobate hyperchromatic nuclei at least 3 times the size the neighboring nuclei with our without large atypical (obvious multipolar) atypical mitotic figures' (Qualman et al. 2008).

Occasional tumors will appear to be composed of a mixture of embryonal and alveolar RMS.

A new type of rhabdomyosarcoma has only been recently described, spindle cell/sclerosing RMS (Mentzel et al. 2000). This tumor may histologically mimic fibrosarcoma or leiomyosarcoma when entirely composed of spindle cells, and may contain densely fibrotic areas resembling osteoid or chondroid. The dense hyalinized areas may cause clefting in the tumor cells suggesting malignant vessel formation. Some investigators suggest that spindle cell/sclerosing RMS is closely related to pleomorphic RMS, as some tumors feature hybrid morphologies (Stock et al. 2009).

Behavior

In general, sarcomas composed of muscle differentiated cells behave aggressively. However, the botryoid type and pediatric spindle cell types of embryonal RMS have an excellent five year survival rate. The International Classification of Rhabdomyosarcoma is presented in **Table 8. 6**.

Grade and stage currently are the mainstays of determining patient prognosis. However, that will soon change. For example, in leiomyosarcoma, immunohistochemical expression of at least three of five markers (smooth muscle γ actin, calsequestrin 2, human muscle cofilin2, myosin light chain kinase, and sarcolemmal membrane associated protein) may identify a subset of LMS with a better prognosis. This expression profile is independent of histologic grade and can also be seen in ~20% of leiomyomas (Mills et al. 2011).

Patients with alveolar RMS have a worse outcome than those with embryonal RMS. However, patients whose tumors exhibit a classic alveolar morphology but are negative for A-RMS translocations ('fusion negative' A-RMS) may experience the same, relatively better outcome as embryonal rhabdomyosarcoma (Williamson et al. 2010).

Rare rhabdomyosarcomas exhibit a mixed pattern of embryonal and alveolar RMS. A case presenting this mixed histology should be tested for specific alveolar RMS gene fusions to determine whether the tumor's behavior and biology is more likely to emulate A-RMS or E-RMS (Wexler et al. 2010).

Risk stratification for rhabdomyosarcomas is undergoing continuing refinement. Features portending a worse outcome in nonmetastatic RMS identified by the Intergroup Rhabdomyosarcoma Study Group/Children's Oncology Group include: age <1 year or > or equal to 10 years, A-RMS type, tumor >5 cm in diameter, tumor invasiveness, nodal involvement, higher clinical group and unfavorable primary site (Huh et al. 2010). For high risk RMS patients, additional poor prognostic features comprise: two or more sites of metastases, bone or bone marrow involvement, age < 1y or >/= 10 years, and unfavorable primary tumor site (Huh et al. 2010). Diffuse myogenin reactivity (greater than 80% nuclear reactivity) is just one tissue based finding that may also predict more aggressive behavior (Heerema-McKenney et al. 2008).

Table 8.7 compiles the survival data for patients with LMS and RMS (SEER data).

Five-year relative survival for rhabdomyosarcoma subtypes range from 38.8% to 66.8%, with 'mixed' type and embryonal cases having the best prognosis, and NOS and pleomorphic cases the worst

Table 8.4 Predominantly pediatric muscle tumors of soft tissue grouped by behavior

<table>
<tr><th rowspan="2">Tumor</th><th rowspan="2">Incidence</th><th rowspan="2">Age and sex distribution</th><th rowspan="2">Body site (in order of occurrence)</th><th colspan="2">Histopathology description including IHC</th></tr>
<tr><th>Medium magnification</th><th>High magnification</th></tr>
<tr><td colspan="6">Benign: does not recur or recurs non-aggressively and does not metastasize</td></tr>
<tr><td>Fetal rhabdomyoma</td><td>Rare</td><td>Children but also rarely in adults.
M > F</td><td>Almost all occur in head and neck</td><td>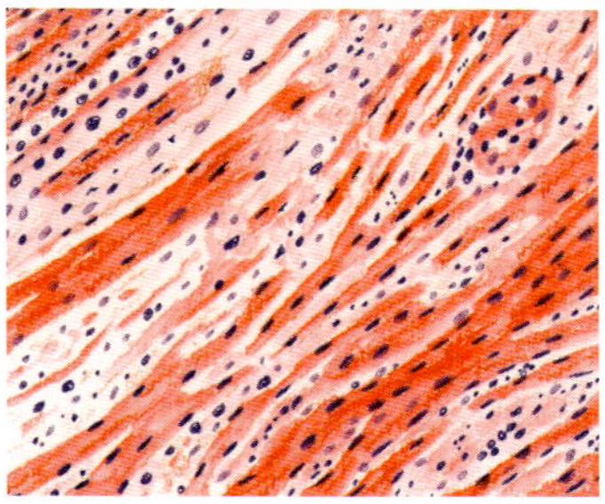</td><td>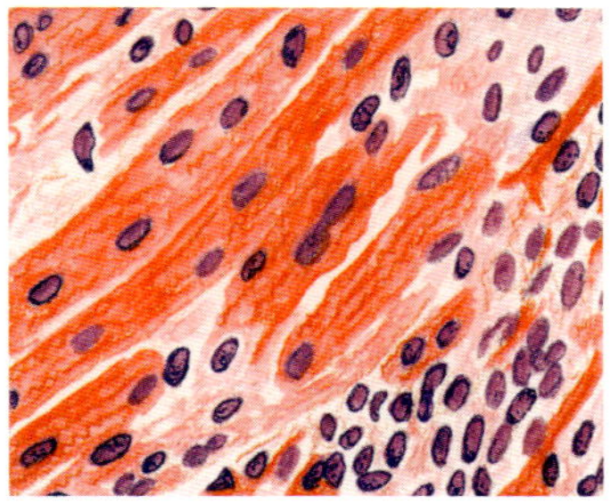</td></tr>
<tr><td colspan="6">Bundles of spindled rhabdomyoblasts with a myxoid background. Some cases are more cellular with strap-like or ganglion-like tumor cells. Cross striations may be seen in some cells. No necrosis or atypia and only rare normal mitotic figure. IHC: Tumor cells express myoglobin but are also reactive for desmin and muscle specific actin. S-100 and SMA may also be positive.</td></tr>
<tr><td>EBV-associated leiomyosarcoma and leiomyoma</td><td>Rare</td><td>Children and young adults most commonly</td><td>Visceral and peripheral sites, often with more than one tumor simultaneously</td><td>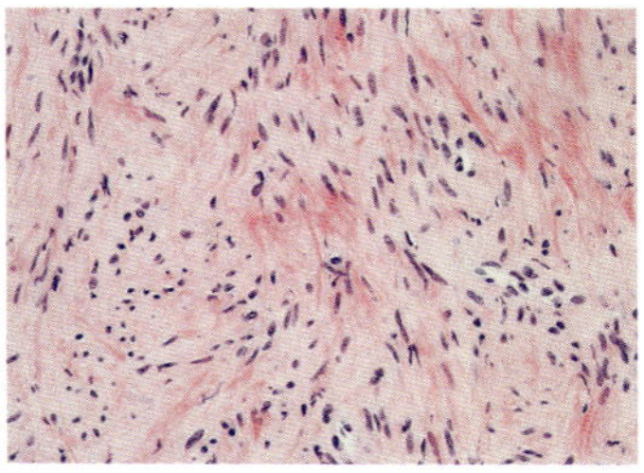</td><td>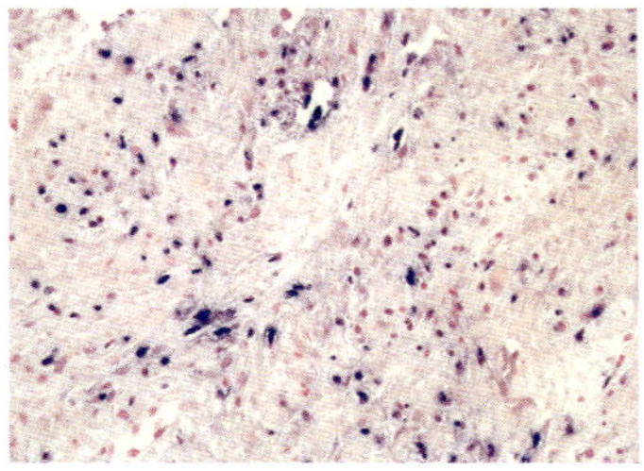</td></tr>
<tr><td colspan="6">May be fasciculated and spindled like conventional LM but can be partly or entirely composed of ovoid cells. Usually there is minimal atypia and few to no mitoses. IHC: SMA is positive; EBV ia usually strongly positive. Desmin often negative.</td></tr>
<tr><td colspan="6">Malignant: can recur aggressively and/or commonly metastasizes</td></tr>
<tr><td>Embryonal rhadomyosarcoma</td><td>Common</td><td>Most common rhabdomyosarcoma (60-70% of all RMS). Generally occurs in children <5 years. Rare adult cases.
M slightly > F</td><td>Head and neck including parameningeal and orbit, genitourinary tract, retroperitoneum/ trunk; minority in</td><td>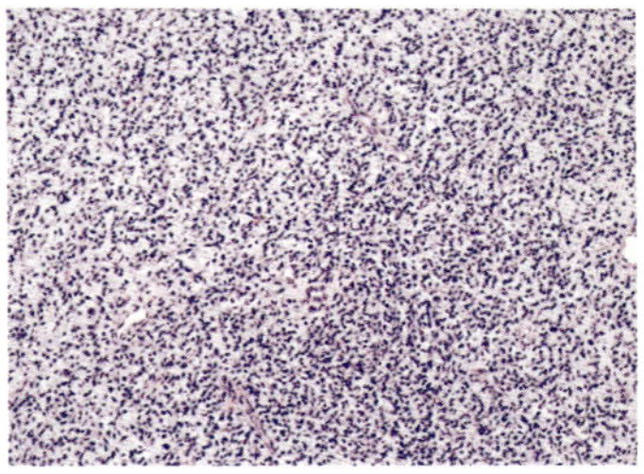</td><td>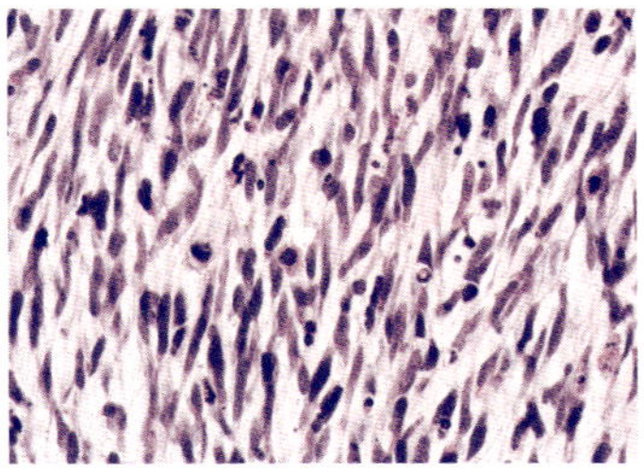</td></tr>
<tr><td colspan="6">Many cases recapitulate the appearance of embryonal skeletal muscle: spindle to stellate primitive cells set in a myxoid background with hypercellular zones more likely than the myxoid areas to contain differentiated rhabdomyocytes with cross striations. Some fascicle or sheet like growth is common. A few, densely cellular E-RMS fall into the histologic differential of small round blue cell tumor. Some cases have eosinophilic spindle cells and 1/3rd contain highly differentiated cells with cytoplasmic cross striations. Mitoses may be scarce to numerous. Cellularity can vary within a single tumor. After neoadjuvant therapy, the tumor cells may be very well differentiated with bright eosinophilic cytoplasm. IHC: 90% are positive for myogenin (nuclear reactivity) and MSA while desmin is usually positive. MyoD1 is also positive in the majority of cases. Not uncommonly, some tumors show focal S-100 protein, keratin, EMA, and CD99 reactivity.</td></tr>
<tr><td>E-RMS pediatric spindle cell variant</td><td>Common</td><td>Older children.
M > F</td><td>Paratesticular; a few in head and neck and extremities</td><td>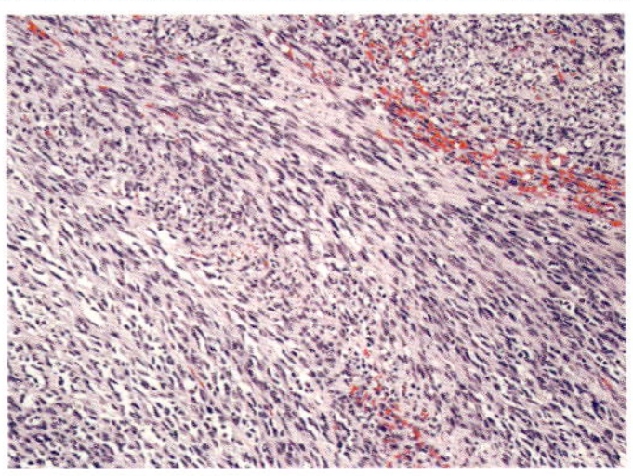</td><td>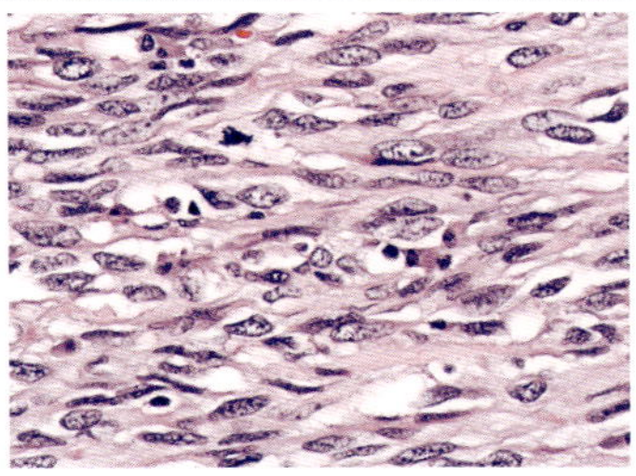</td></tr>
<tr><td colspan="6">Crowded fascicles of spindle cells that can mimic fibrosarcoma or leiomyosarcoma.
Tumor cells may have bright eosinophilic cytoplasm and cross striations are almost always seen in at least a few cells. Fibrotic (collagenized) background is common.
Can have a focal component of conventional embryonal RMS.</td></tr>
</table>

Table 8.4: Continued from page 159

Tumor	Incidence	Age and sex distribution	Body site (in order of occurrence)	Histopathology description including IHC Medium magnification	High magnification
E-RMS botryoid variant	Common	Young children M slightly > F	Bladder, vagina, bile ducts, uterus; rarely pharynx, cheek, gingivae, conjunctiva, ear	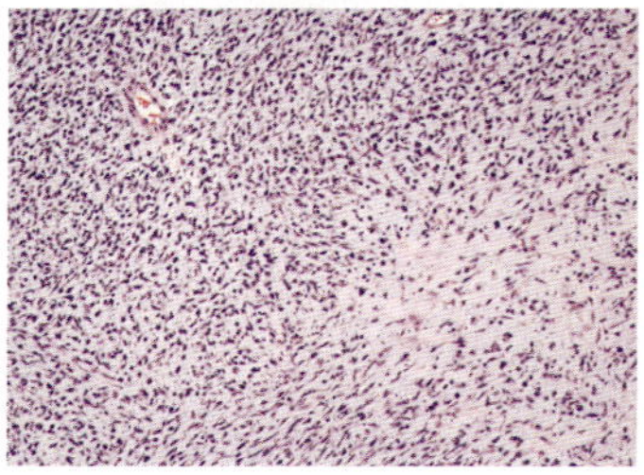	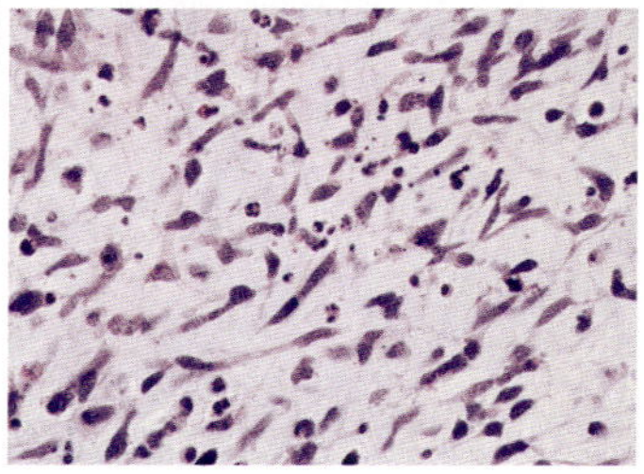
This variant occurs in association with an epithelium and is not seen in the soft tissues. It features stellate to spindle cells set in a myxoid matrix with hypercellular zone beneath the epithelium ('cambium layer'). Mature rhabdomyoblasts may be present.					
E-RMS anaplastic variant	Rare	Young children	Same distribution as for typical E- RMS	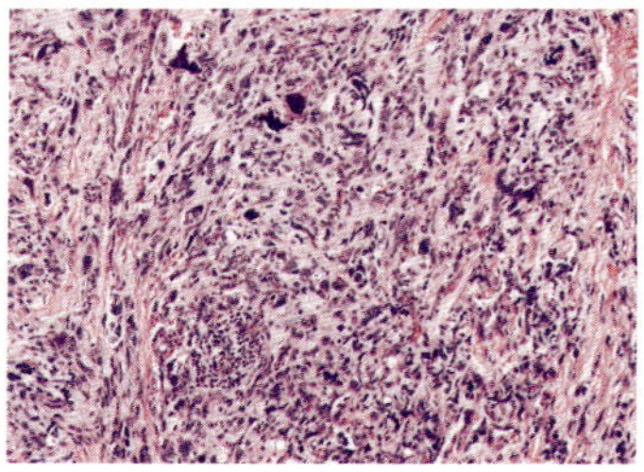	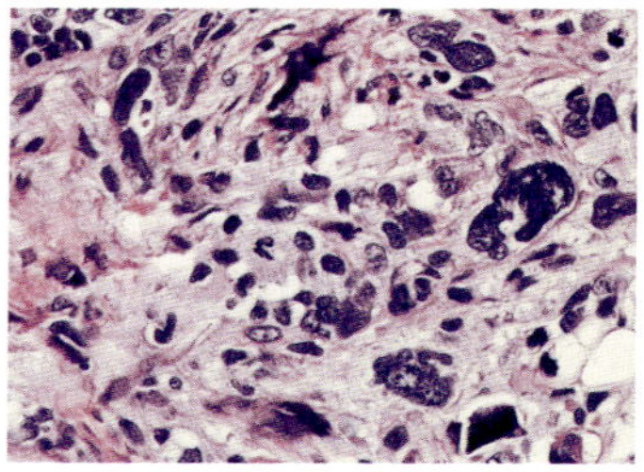
Multifocal or diffuse areas of markedly pleomorphic tumor cells with nuclei 'three times or greater the diameter' of nuclei of surrounding typical E-RMS cells. Atypical mitotic figures are common. IHC: Tumor cells are positive for myogenin and MyoD1 (less sensitive) with only 60% positive for desmin. Anaplastic E-RMS is rare.					
Alveolar rhabdomyosarcoma	Common	Older children and adolescents (average age of 12 years)	Extremities, parameningeal and sinuses. Rarely can present with diffuse bone marrow involvement and no known primary site	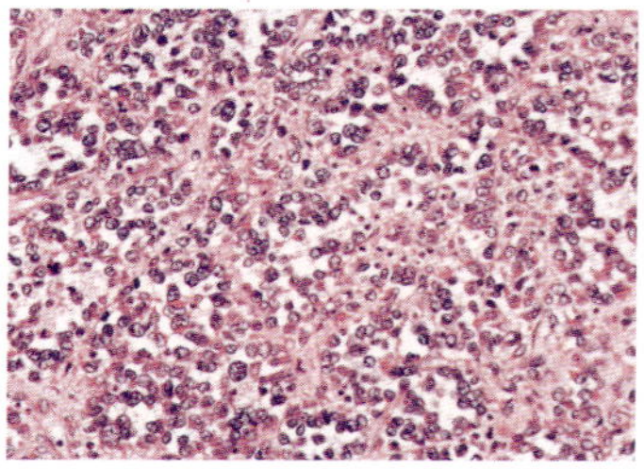	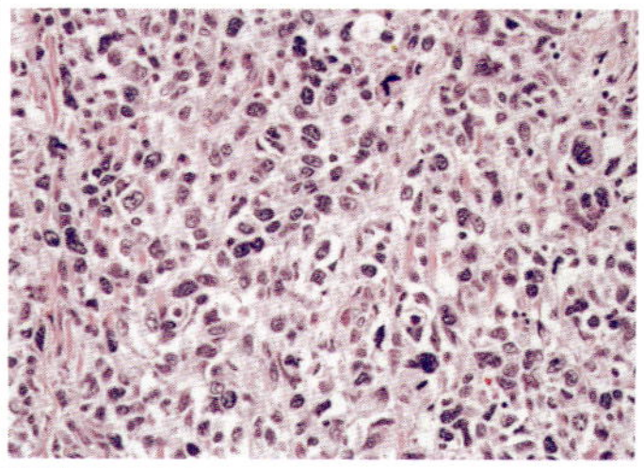
Nests of cells with central dropout mimicking the appearance of lung alveoli. Tumor cells are round to popcorn shaped with a high nuclear to cytoplasmic ratio and can mimic lymphoma or Ewing sarcoma. Scattered multinucleated tumor giant cells ('wreath cells') may be present. Mitoses and necrosis common. IHC: Myogenin is often more diffusely positive than in embryonal RMS. Rhabdomyoblasts (tumor cells with bright eosinophilic cytoplasm and sometimes cross-striations) are sometimes scattered throughout. Anaplasia as defined above for E-RMS can also occur in alveolar RMS.					
A-RMS solid variant	Rare	As above	As above	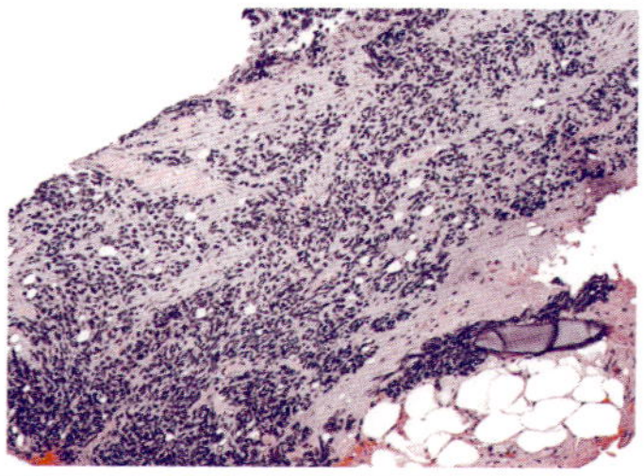	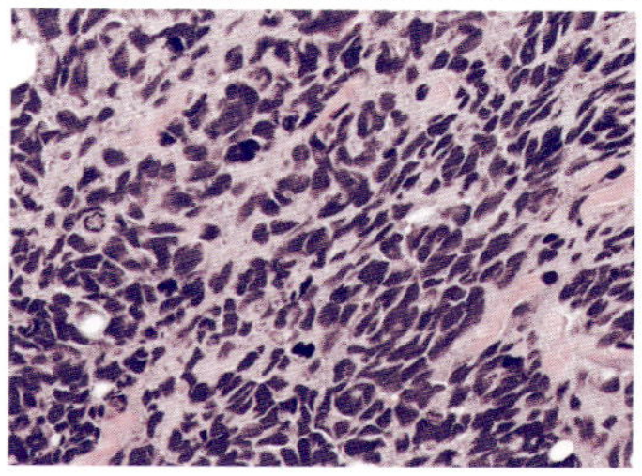
Solid sheets of small round blue cells often with scattered wreath cells and rhabdomyoblasts. IHC: As with typical A-RMS, most cases are positive for myogenin diffusely and desmin. May have aberrant keratin, EMA, S-100 protein, CD99 and synaptophysin reactivity.					
Incidence note: 'Common to very common' indicates that a medium sized practice will treat at least several to dozens of patients with the lesion annually, 'Uncommon to rare' indicates the same practice size will treat one to two patients with the lesion every five years, 'Rare to very rare' indicates the same sized practice will see zero to one patient with the lesion every 20 years.					
RMS: rhabdomyosarcoma, LM: leiomyoma, LMS: leiomyosarcoma, A-RMS: alveolar RMS, E-RMS: embryonal RMS, IHC: immunohistochemistry.					
SMA: smooth muscle actin. MSA: muscle specific actin. Note: Cutaneous and gynecologic tumors classified as muscle tumors are not presented in this Table.					

Table 8.5 Predominantly adult muscle tumors of soft tissue grouped by behavior

Tumor	Incidence	Age and sex distribution	Body site (in order of occurrence)	Histopathology description including IHC	
				Medium magnification	High magnification
Benign: does not recur or recurs non-aggressively and does not metastasize					
Angioleiomyoma (vascular leiomyoma)	Common	30s to 60s most common but broad age range F > M for solid variant	Subcutis or deep dermis of extremities and head (especially venous variant)	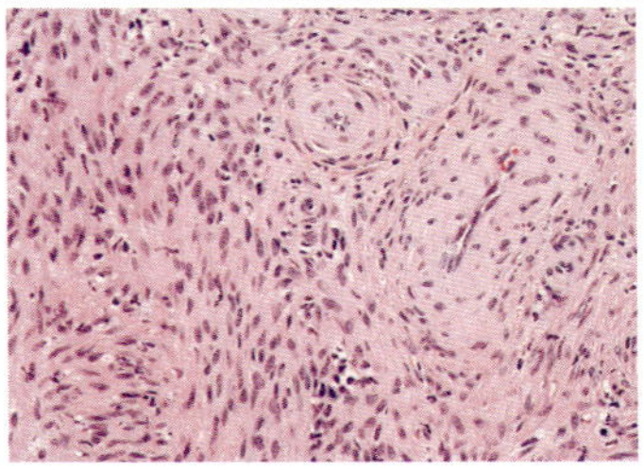	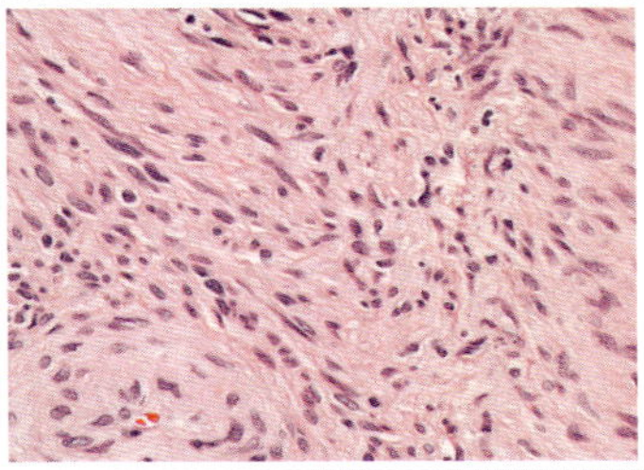
Three variants (solid, venous and cavernous) all composed of uniform smooth muscle cells merging with vessels (thin walled in 'solid' variant, thick walled in 'venous' variant, and ectatic and thin walled in 'cavernous' variant). Myxoid change, calcifications, and hyalinization common. Tumor cells are positive for actin and caldesmon with variable reactivity for desmin.					
Leiomyoma of scrotum	Rare	40s and older men	Scrotum Paratestis soft tissue	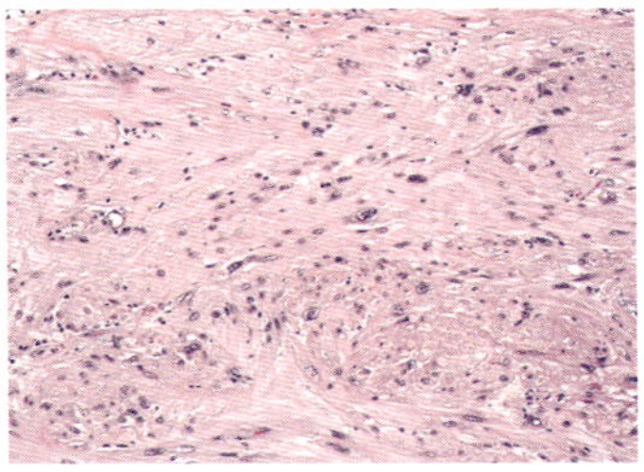	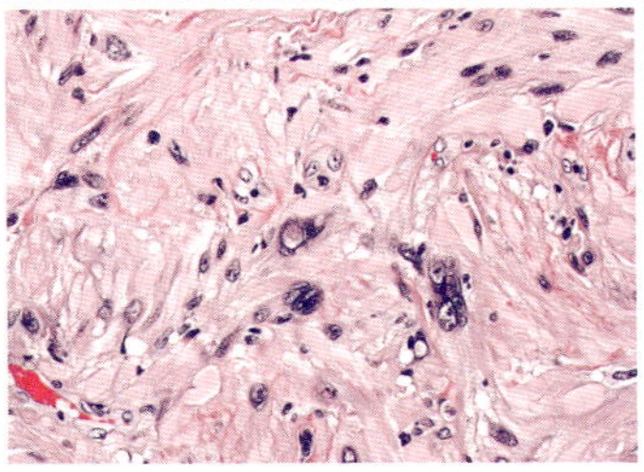
May look like conventional leiomyoma: sweeping fascicles of plump to thin spindle cells with blunt ended or cigar shaped nuclei. A few cases show symplastic features: cytologic atypia including multinucleation, nuclear enlargement and nucleoli. Some of the atypical nuclei appear degenerated but the atypia is not indicative of malignancy. These cases are called 'bizarre' or 'atypical' LM of scrotum. No mitotic activity. May be positive for androgen receptors.					
Mullerian type leiomyoma of inguinal canal	Rare	Adult women	Inguinal canal soft tissues	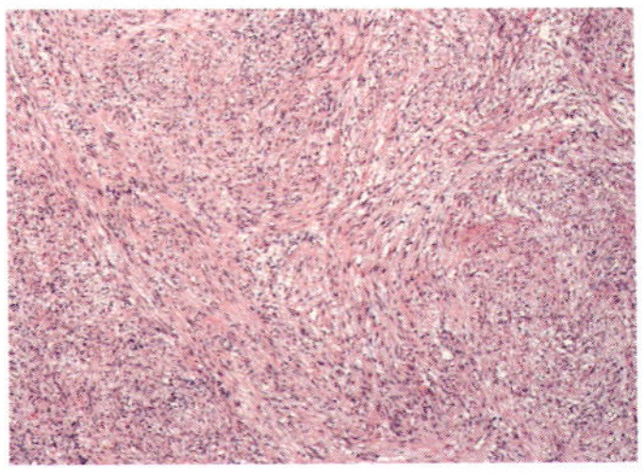	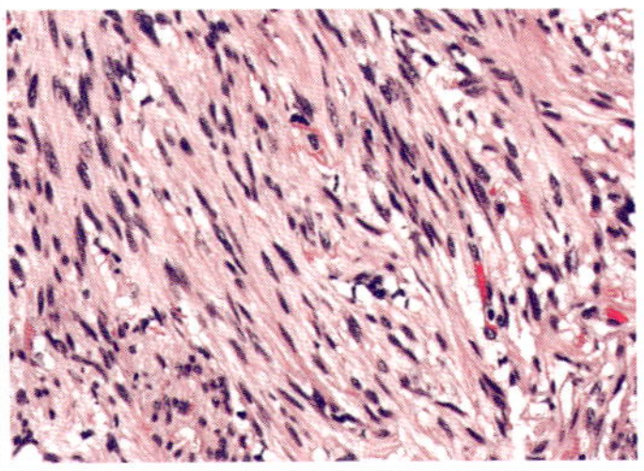
Resembles a conventional uterine leiomyoma. Also, like uterine LM, it is positive for estrogen and progesterone receptors in contrast to nearly all soft tissue leiomyomas and soft tissue LMS.					
EBV-associated smooth muscle tumors	Rare	Immunocompromised Adults (often post-transplant) and children with EBV infection	Viscera most common but can occur in soft tissues.	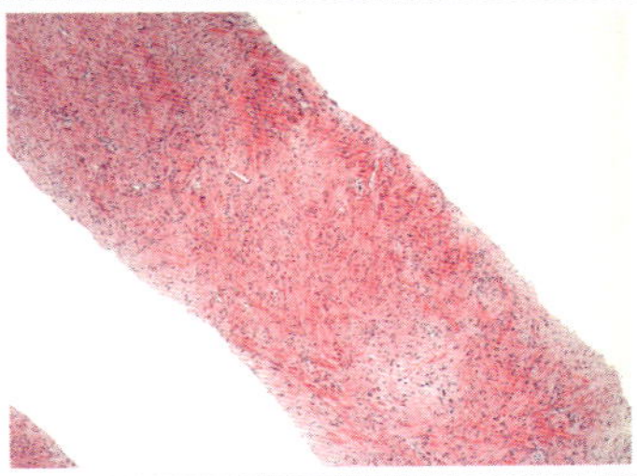	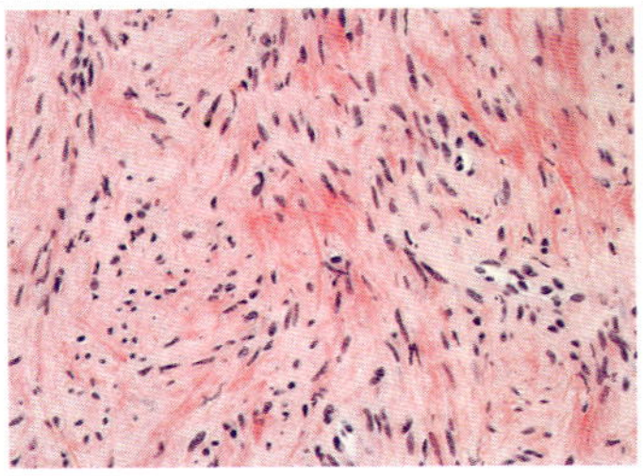
May be fasciculated and spindled like conventional LM but can be partly or entirely composed of ovoid or primitive round cells. Lymphocyte infiltrates are common. Usually, there is minimal atypia and few to no mitoses. SMA is positive; EBV is usually strongly positive. Desmin is often negative.					
Leiomyoma of deep soft tissue	Very rare	Adults, young to middle aged M = F	Extremities	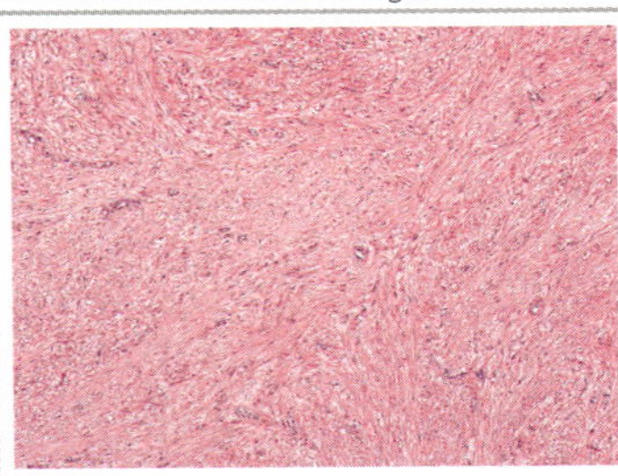	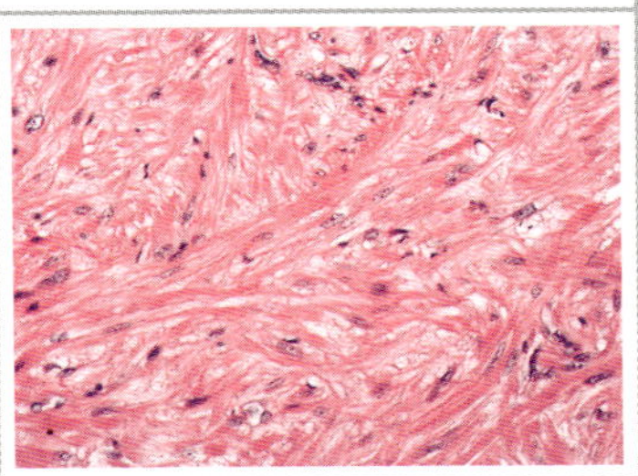
Intersecting fascicles of spindle shaped smooth muscle cells. Tumor cells have cigar shaped or train car shaped nuclei, eosinophilic cytoplasm, and sometimes paranuclear vacuoles. Myxoid change, calcifications, and hyalinization can occur. Necrosis, mitoses > 1/50hpf and nuclear atypia are absent. Tumor cells often positive for more than one muscle marker such as desmin, SMA, HHF-actin, calponin, and caldesmon.					

Table 8.5: Continued from page 161

Tumor	Incidence	Age and sex distribution	Body site (in order of occurrence)	Histopathology description including IHC Medium magnification	High magnification
Adult rhabdomyoma	Rare	Middle aged adults but broad age range including rarely children. M > F	Head and neck ST. 20% are multifocal	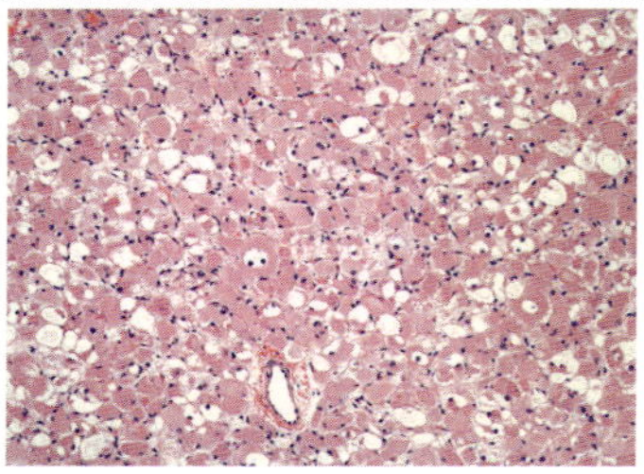	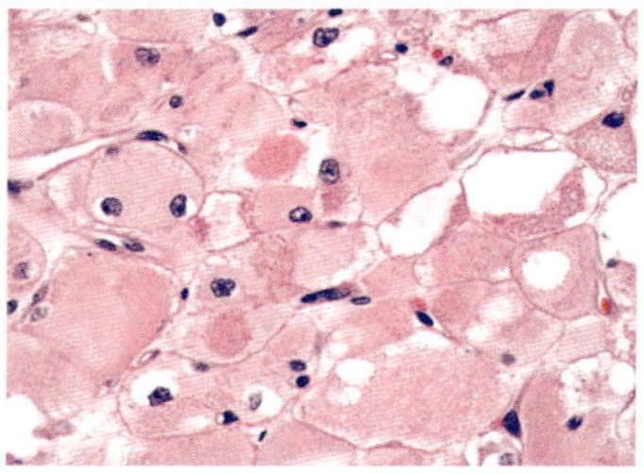
Sheets of large round to polygonal cells with clear and deeply eosinophilic cytoplasm. Nuclear are small and generally eccentrically located. Cross striations may be seen in some cells. There is no atypia, no mitotic activity, and no necrosis. Positive for MSA, desmin, myoglobin. May be positive for S-100 protein.					
Malignant: can recur aggressively and/or commonly metastasizes					
Leiomyosarcoma	Uncommon	Middle aged and older adults. F > M in retroperitoneum M > F for deep soft tissue. M = F in cutaneous and subcutaneous sites	Extremities, retroperitoneum, Can be dermal only, (termed 'atypical smooth muscle tumor') extend into subcutis, subcutis only, or in deep ST. Some cases initially occur in viscera and then metastasize to soft tissue	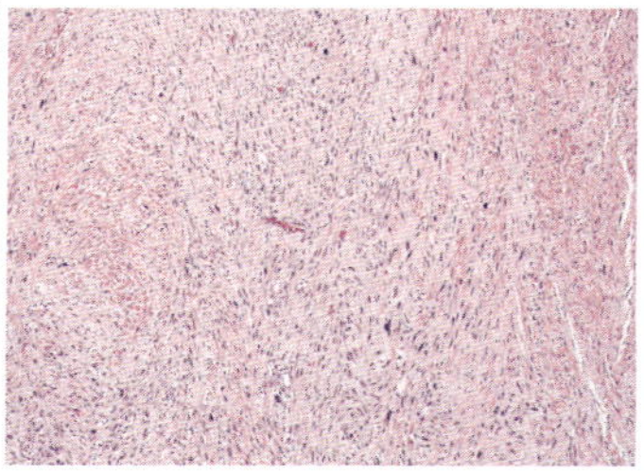	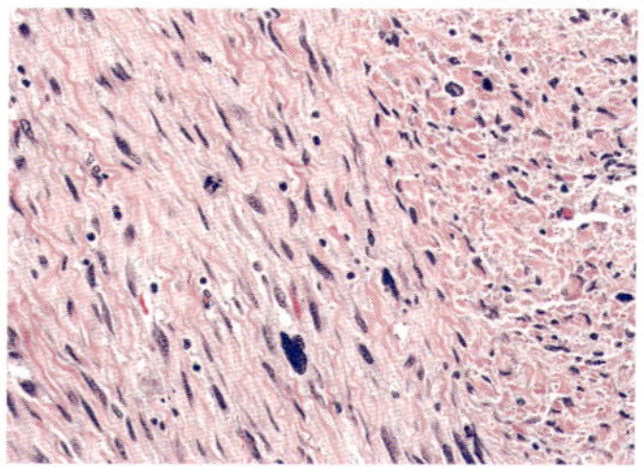
Many cases comprise intersecting long fascicles of spindle cells with eosinophilic cytoplasm and blunt ended or cigar shaped nuclei. Low grade tumors have scattered more atypical cells. High grade tumors may mimic pleomorphic spindle cell sarcoma, NOS. Some cases have myxoid change, some have epithelioid appearing cells, and rarely inflammation is prominent. A few cases have scattered osteoclast-like giant cells. By definition, muscle markers must be positive. This includes SMA, MSA, desmin caldesmon. 10-20% are reactive for keratins, more for EMA, rarely diffusely and strongly. Negative for myogenin. Negative for c-kit.					
Pleomorphic rhabdomyosarcoma	Rare	Middle aged and older adults. Exceptional in children (in pediatric age group it may be the same as or related to RMS with diffuse anaplasia)	Extremities, head and neck, trunk, and rarely elsewhere	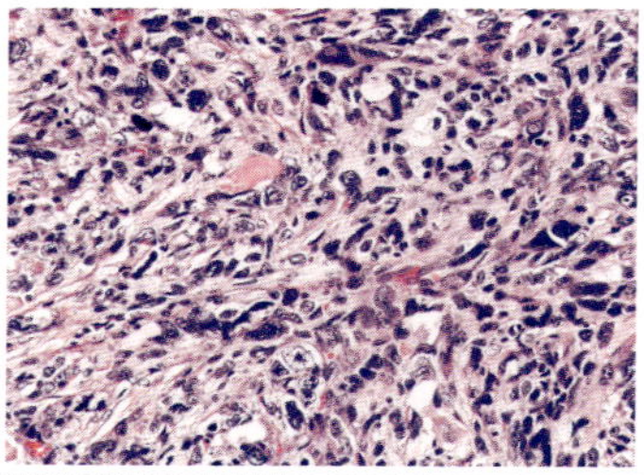	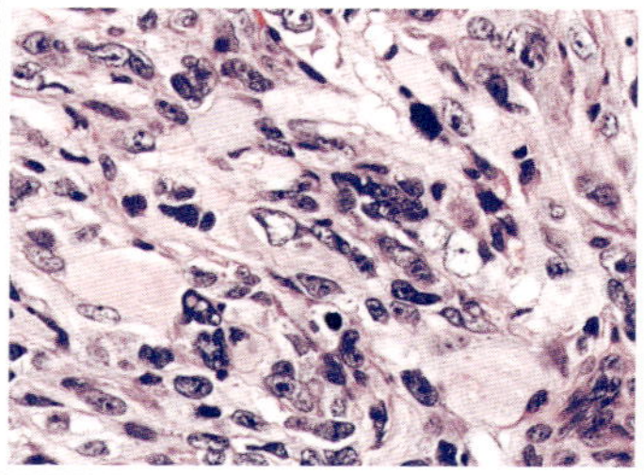
Sheets and fascicles of markedly pleomorphic spindle cells and tumor giant cells. A few cells may have marked eosinophilia consistent with rhabdomyoblasts, but IHC is necessary for the diagnosis. Tumor cells should be positive for myogenin or MyoD1 but rarely are negative. These cases can only be diagnosed on ultrastructural examination which is seldom conducted. Most cases are desmin reactive.					
Adult spindle cell/sclerosing/ pseudovascular Rhabdomyosarcoma	Rare	Adults, usually middle aged and older	Extremities, head and neck, trunk and rarely elsewhere	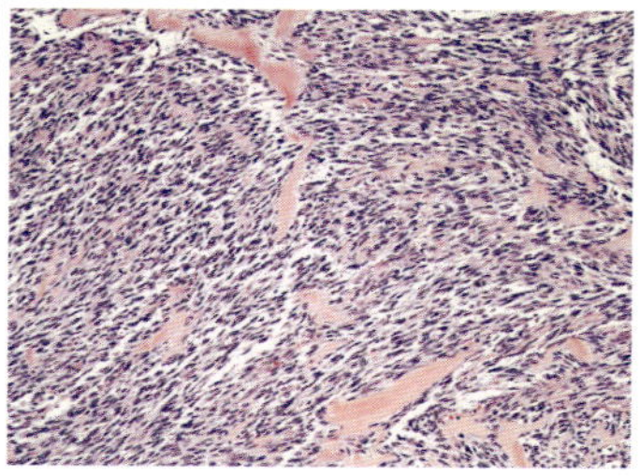	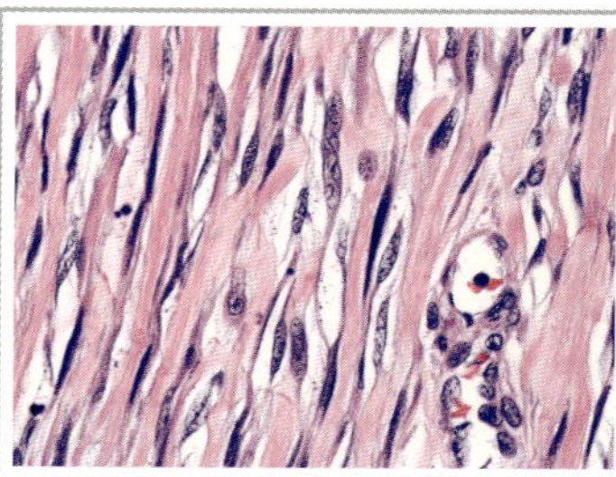
This type of RMS may form a spectrum with pleomorphic RMS and both may be labeled 'adult type RMS'. It consists of fascicles of thin to plump atypical spindle cells with or without pseudovascular spaces, dense collagen deposition mimicking chondroid or osteoid, and markedly pleomorphic areas. All cases are positive for myogenin (may be focal in less than 10% of cells), desmin, and many cases are also positive for SMA. Keratins and EMA may also be positive.					
Incidence note: 'Common to very common' indicates that a medium sized practice will treat at least several to dozens of patients with the lesion annually, 'Uncommon to rare' indicates the same practice size will treat one to two patients with the lesion every five years, 'Rare to very rare' indicates the same sized practice will see zero to one patient with the lesion every 20 years.					
RMS: rhabdomyosarcoma, LMS: leiomyosarcoma. SMA: smooth muscle actin.					
Note: Cutaneous and gynecologic tumors classified as muscle tumors are not presented in this Table.					

Table 8.6 International classification of rhabdomyosarcoma

Tumor	Prognosis
Botryoid rhabdomyosarcoma	Superior
(Pediatric) spindle cell rhabdomyosarcoma	Superior*
Embryonal rhabdomyosarcoma**	Intermediate
Alveolar rhabdomyosarcoma	Poor
Undifferentiated sarcoma	Poor

* Prognosis may be intermediate for pediatric spindle cell RMS located outside the paratesticular soft tissue.

**Embryonal rhabdomyosarcoma with anaplasia and adult type spindle cell rhabdomyosarcoma have a poor prognosis.

Superior prognosis: > 90% long term survival

Intermediate prognosis: ~70% long term survival

Poor prognosis: ~45% long term survival

Table 8.7 Five-year relative survival rate* by rhabdomyosarcoma and leiomyosarcoma subtype in 13 SEER registries for years 1994 and 2008, percent survival (SE=standard error).

Sarcoma type	Percent survival (SE)
Rhabdomyosarcoma	
Alveolar	47.4% (3.8%)
Embryonal	61.0% (4.1%)
NOS	38.8% (5.3%)
Pleomorphic	45.1% (6.3%)
Mixed	66.8% (27.3%)
Spindle cell (adults)	0.0% (0.0%)
Spindle cell (pediatric)	57.2% (25.0%)
Leiomyosarcoma	
NOS	64.2% (1.5%)
Epithelioid	54.3% (9.8%)
Myxoid	44.9% (9.9%)

* Five-year survival was the chosen instead of 10 year survival due to small numbers in a few of the subtypes.

(38.8% and 45.1%, respectively). Adult spindle cell/sclerosing RMS may be particularly aggressive, but as only five cases were cataloged by SEER, caution is warranted in predicting its behavior. Similarly, of cases diagnosed with leiomyosarcomas, 44.9% to 64.2% are still alive 5 years after diagnosis, relative to the general population of corresponding sex and age.

Additional laboratory testing

Immunohistochemistry

Immunohistochemistry plays a key and indeed required role in diagnosing muscle differentiated tumors. The most important muscle markers are: desmin, smooth muscle actin (SMA), muscle specific actin (MSA), caldesmon, myogenin, MyoD, and myoglobin. Smooth muscle tumors are most often reactive for SMA and MSA with approximately 80% of cases reactive for desmin and caldesmon. Reactivity for SMA and/or MSA is a requirement. However, because these markers can also be seen in non-muscle tumors including myofibroblastic tumors, correlation with histologic features and clinical presentation is mandatory.

Skeletal muscle tumors are also often reactive for desmin and MSA with only subsets of tumors such as spindle cell/sclerosing RMS reactive for smooth muscle actin. Myogenin, myoglobin, and MyoD are expressed only in skeletal muscle differentiated tumors. Myoglobin is produced only in more mature tumor cells and thus is not very useful in rhabdomyosarcomas which are usually composed predominantly of less differentiated cells. By definition, RMS must express myogenin or MyoD. Myogenin and MyoD reactivity must be nuclear, and some cases are only focally positive in RMS, staining fewer than 10% of tumor cells. The MyoD antibody can be challenging to optimize in the pathology laboratory; therefore, antibodies to myogenin are much more commonly used in the clinical setting.

Other markers that can label muscle related tumors include CD5 (a glycoprotein receptor normally present on T-lymphocytes and some B-lymphocytes), p63, and WT-1 as well as a new set of molecularly derived markers that may have prognostic significance in LMS (smooth muscle γ actin, calsequestrin 2, human muscle cofilin2, myosin light chain kinase, and sarcolemmal membrane associated protein) (Mills et al. 2009). A small pilot study evaluating CD5 expression in muscle related tissue reported strong diffuse cytoplasmic staining in normal muscle with absent expression in rhabdomyomas and high grade LMS and RMS (McNab et al. 2009). If this reactivity pattern is verified in additional studies, it could be useful in distinguishing between residual mature tumor and intermixed atrophic normal muscle in post-chemotherapy specimens. Another preliminary study reported that p63 (a member of the p53 family with broad expression in multiple normal tissues and tumors) intensifies the appearance of cross striations in skeletal muscle cells and in SM differentiated tumors in a manner superior to desmin (Martin et al. 2011). It could thus be useful in subtle RMS cases (smooth muscle is also stained with p63 antibody, so it is not exclusive to skeletal muscle tumors). Reactivity for WT-1 is relatively non-specific and usually not helpful.

Importantly, some antigens are expressed in muscle tumors that may cause diagnostic confusion. For example, keratins (CAM5.2 and AE1/AE3) and EMA were expressed in 26 to 44% respectively, in a study of 100 leiomyosarcomas but only rarely with diffuse reactivity (Iwata et al. 2000). Likewise, skeletal muscle tumors can also express keratins and EMA. Especially when occurring in the head and neck, reactivity for CD56 and synaptophysin can falsely suggest a diagnosis of neuroendocrine carcinoma. In such cases, reactivity for myogenin or MyoD and genetic results will lead to the correct diagnosis (Yasuda et al. 2009).

One final tricky aspect of IHC usage in leiomyosarcomas is the loss of expression of muscle markers in dedifferentiated areas. This can make the diagnosis difficult to impossible if this is the only area biopsied as definitional muscle marker expression is absent (such as with a needle core sample) (Nicolas et al. 2010, Oda et al. 2001).

Routine cytogenetics

Karyotyping is not particularly useful in the diagnosis of leiomyosarcoma other than to exclude tumors with specific chromosomal changes detectable at the Giemsa banding level. Most leiomyosarcomas exhibit a complex aneuploid karyotype without specific consistent abnormalities. E-RMS, pleomorphic RMS, and spindle cell/sclerosing RMS also feature complex aneuploidy. E-RMS has preferential gains and losses of chromosomal material at certain points in the genome, but this is not helpful diagnostically and is often not detectable except by comparative genomic hybridization (Miettinen et al. 2010).

Molecular genetics

A-RMS requires FISH or rtPCR to detect the two most common translocations: t(2;13)(q35;q14) and t(1;13)(p36;q14). Refer to **Table 8.2** for more details. Molecular geneticists are discovering aberrations that may be amenable to targeted therapy and or have prognostic/predictive potential. As noted previously, careful prospective evaluation of the new findings will be necessary and entail multicenter patient participation.

RADIOLOGY

We will focus on the leiomyoma of skin and the soft tissues which can be divided by depth of location. Skin lesions include piloleiomyomas, angioleiomyomas (vascular leiomyomas), and genital leiomyomas. These skin leiomyomas rarely receive imaging and tend to present clinically. The deeper lesions may become quite large before discovery. The superficial lesions do not typically have visible calcification on radiography, but imaging experience is limited. Vascular angioleiomyomas tend to occur in the hand and feet and appear as a well-defined oval mass superficial to the fascia. They have an overall non-specific T1 low signal and T2 or STIR high signal appearance, with a variable enhancement. However, (Gupte et al. 2008), describe a linear or branching hyperintense pattern on fluid sensitive sequences. The deeper lesions may show different calcification patterns, fleck or sand like calcifications, plaque like calcification or coarse mulberry calcifications as seen with uterine leiomyomas (Kransdorf et al. 2006).

Cutaneous atypical smooth muscle tumors have a better prognosis and tend not to require imaging. However, leiomyosarcoma (LMS) arising in the subcutaneous tissues tend to present as larger tumors and have a worse prognosis. The soft tissue LMS can be clinically divided by retroperitoneal or peripheral location. Retroperitoneal tumors are more common in women, presenting larger in size and having greater chance of metastatic disease. LMS is the second most common primary retroperitoneal tumor of adults. Soft tissue LMS of the extremities are more common in men and can be more aggressive tumors. LMS of vessels is quite rare and predominantly affects the veins with the IVC being most common site. Patients can present with venous thrombosis related to their tumor. LMS can also involve arteries, in which case the pulmonary arteries are most commonly affected. LMS most commonly metastasizes to lung, however, liver is the second most common site seen in 47% of cases (Shmookler et al. 1983). Although skin metastasis is rare, LMS is the most common sarcoma to metastasis to the skin, with the scalp being the most common location of deposition (Wang et al. 2011).

Embryonal rhabdomyosarcoma (RMS) tends to occur in the first decade of life and involve the orbit, head and neck regions as well as the genitourinary tract. Alveolar RMS occurs in all ages but tends to affect adolescents and young adults. Alveolar RMS tumors tend to arise in muscles of the extremities. The pleomorphic subtype occurs in older adults involving the extremities and is an aggressive sarcoma (Parham et al. 2006).

Leiomyosarcoma and rhabdomyosarcomas tend to have non-specific MR imaging features with T1 low signal and high signal on T2 or STIR sequences. There is usually heterogeneous enhancement. Calcification with LMS is not common, (McLeod et al. 1984). Hemorrhage and necrosis is common with LMS (Harman et al. 1992). Rhabdomyosarcomas have local bone invasion in 24% of cases at presentation (Simmons et al. 1978).

SURGERY OF MUSCLE TUMORS OF SOFT TISSUES

Leiomyoma

These are benign tumors with a low rate of local recurrence. Marginal excision is the primary treatment of choice. Resection with wider margins might be considered in the rare case of a multiply recurrent tumor.

Leiomyosarcoma

These tumors should be resected with wide margins. Adjuvant therapy should be strongly considered in addition to surgery.

Rhabdomyosarcoma

Although successful treatment of rhabdomyosarcoma requires systemic chemotherapy, surgery can be a helpful adjunct. Surgical resection with wide margin is considered the treatment of choice in those tumors where complete and adequate resection can be performed without an unacceptable loss of function or cosmetic result. Tumors most amenable to surgical resection are typically in the trunk and extremities. Tumors that cannot be resected without severe loss of function are usually best treated with radiation therapy rather than surgery. Debulking is not generally beneficial with the possible exception of embryonal tumors in the retroperitoneum. Rhabdomyosarcoma is somewhat unusual as soft tissue sarcomas go in that wide resection of the tumor prior to the initiation of chemotherapy results in a down-staging to a lower clinical group which offers a more favorable prognosis. Therefore, if an initial procedure consists of a biopsy or marginal excision, wide re-excision is generally preferred, in those patients who are surgical candidates, prior to initiation of chemotherapy.

In patients with tumors that are considered unresectable at presentation, neoadjuvant use of chemotherapy and/or radiation therapy may shrink the tumor enough to make the patient a surgical candidate.

MEDICAL ONCOLOGY

Leiomyoma of soft tissue and rhabdomyoma

As these are benign lesions, chemotherapy is not warranted. This includes the EBV-virus associated smooth muscle tumors that occur in immunocompromised patients.

Leiomyosarcoma

Leiomyosarcoma is a cancer of the smooth muscle and arises anywhere in the body. Treatment depends in part on the anatomical localization. Benign and low grade tumors might be sensitive to hormones, especially when they originate from the uterus. High grade tumors however should be treated according to the general principles of multidisciplinary treatment (see Chapter 1). Leiomyosarcoma has a tendency to widely metastasize (liver, lungs, brain, and bones), including to unusual places, such as soft tissues, skin, or other muscles.

Chemotherapy generalities

Two studies have looked at large scale chemotherapy data for soft tissue sarcomas, and in both, leiomyosarcoma had a poorer response to anthracycline-based chemotherapy than most other soft tissue subtypes. The first study is a meta-analysis conducted by the European Organization for Research and Treatment of Cancers (EORTC) (van Glabbeke et al. 1999) (**Table 8.8**). Patients treated on 7 randomized studies that were all anthracycline-based (doxorubicin or epirubicin) were pooled for the analysis.

The overall survival for leiomyosarcoma was 52 weeks and the overall response rate was 22%. The response rate decreases significantly when patients are diagnosed with liver metastases. Therefore, the lower probability of response to chemotherapy in leiomyosarcoma patients might be linked to the increased frequency of liver metastases in these patients. Correlation of these two factors could be a result of the high proportion of abdominal leiomyosarcoma cases in this series, which have a greater propensity for liver metastases.

Table 8.8 EORTC meta-analysis of leiomyosarcoma patients treated with an anthracycline-based chemotherapy regimen

Total no. of leiomyosarcoma patients (7 studies)	No. of deaths	1 year survival (%)	2 year survival (%)	Median survival time (weeks)	P (comparison with all soft tissue sarcomas)
540	449	49	20	52	NS
No. of leiomyosarcoma patients treated with anthracycline regimen	**No. of responders**	**Response rate (%)**			**P**
492	110	22			.002

The second study examined response and survival after first line chemotherapy treatment for advanced STS. Most regimens were anthracycline based, with 299 patients treated with single agents versus 189 treated with a combination. Ninety-five patients did not receive an anthracycline as the first treatment. A 33% overall response rate was seen with 22% having disease stabilization. The overall survival was 12 months. Interestingly, this study also demonstrated that patients treated with combination chemotherapy experienced longer survival than those treated with a single agent. A non-significant trend for improved survival was found for STS patients who had locally advanced disease (15 months) compared with those who had either localized metastatic disease (13 months) or disseminated metastases (9 months) ($P < 0.06$). Patients with leiomyosarcoma had similar survival (11 months) and response to chemotherapy than those seen with other STS (Karavasilis et al. 2008).

These results show the lack of specificity of anthracycline-based chemotherapy for the treatment of leiomyosarcoma. More recently the combination of gemcitabine and docetaxel was reported to be more efficacious for leiomyosarcoma than for other sarcomas. The combination of these two drugs yielded a 53% overall remission rate with 20% stable disease (SD) in patients with leiomyosarcoma and an overall survival of 17.9 months in one study (Hensley et al. 2002) and an 18.4% overall remission rate (24.2% for the leiomyosarcoma subtype), and an overall survival of 12.1 months in the other study (Bay 2006). In this combination, gemcitabine is administered intravenously on days 1 and 8 at 900 mg/m^2 over 90 min and docetaxel on day 8 at 100 mg/m^2. Treatment is repeated every 21 days until progression of disease (PD). The combination may be superior to gemcitabine alone (Maki et al. 2007). Grade 3 and 4 adverse events are common and granulocyte-colony stimulating factor necessary to alleviate side effects of neutropenia. In an alternate 2 week schedule, leiomyosarcoma did not seem more sensitive to this combination (Verschraegen et al. 2011).

Treatment according to histologic type

Medical treatment of leiomyosarcoma follows the chemotherapy principles described above. However, if the tumor is hormone receptor positive (seen in some primary LMS of gynecologic origin), a trial of hormonal therapy with GnRH agonist or SPRM might be helpful. The first line chemotherapy should be the combination of gemcitabine and docetaxel given on the every 3 week schedule. If patients have progression of disease an anthracycline-based regimen remains indicated. Participation in a clinical trial, especially if specific to leiomyosarcoma is indicated. Chemotherapy agents being tested are trabectedin and ixabepilone. Biological agents being studied include bevacizumab, pazopanib, axitinib, and temsirolimus.

Cytogenetics anomalies include overexpression of CD97. CD97 is the founding member of a small subfamily within the adhesion class called EGF-TM7 family. In vitro, CD97 increases single cell random motility and directed migration and invasion. It is strongly expressed in smooth muscle cells. It can be detected when it is glycosylated, which is the case in about 25% of leiomyosarcomas. Betulinic acid might inhibit CD97 function (Mustafa et al. 2004).

Other chromosome anomalies target genes that control groups of high motility proteins, HMGIC (high mobility group protein isoform I-C) and HMGA2 (high mobility group AT-hook 2). These proteins interfere with DNA and DNA repair process. There are currently no inhibitors of high mobility group protein (Miao et al. 2008).

Rhabdomyosarcoma

Rhabdomyosarcoma can exist as a de novo original tumor, or as a heterologous element in another soft tissue sarcoma, particularly in some uterine sarcomas. When it is a heterologous element, the patient is treated according to the primary sarcoma, discounting the rhabdomyosarcoma differentiation. When rhabdomyosarcoma is the original histologic diagnosis, then the treatment is as described below. In adults, the median age at diagnosis is the mid twenties. Hence, in adults, rhabdomyosarcoma is exceedingly rare.

In a study of 39 adults with rhabdomyosarcoma treated between 1973 and 1996, 26 had localized/locoregional disease and 13 patients had metastatic disease at presentation. The overall 5- and 10-year survival rates were 31% and 27%, respectively. Five-year survival rates for patients with tumors less than 5 cm, 5 to 10 cm, and more than 10 cm were 60%, 14%, and 0%, respectively. Metastatic disease at presentation and poor response to chemotherapy were independent predictors of death on multivariate analysis. Age, location, nodal status, and histologic subtype were not associated with survival in adults with rhabdomyosarcoma, but the small number of patients might confound the data.

Treatment of patients with metastatic disease is palliative at best. They should enroll in a clinical study whenever feasible.

Most patients with loco-regional disease could be treated preoperatively and all should receive post-operative chemotherapy unless it is a < 5 cm embryonal lesion that has been resected with a wide margin, where the use of chemotherapy might not always be beneficial. The intergroup rhabdomyosarcoma study group has been studying various regimens in children over the years (Crist et al. 2001). There are no randomized studies in adults. The most common chemotherapy combination are VAC (vincristine, actinomycin-D, and cyclophosphamide), VAI (vincristine, actinomycin-D, and ifosfamide), or VIE (vincristine, ifosfamide, and etoposide). **Table 8.9** shows the various regimens. All regimens are given in blocks of 8 weeks (one pulse) for 5 times with a rest between pulses. Radiotherapy is given during the second pulse, except for VA (vincristine, actinomycin-D given for good prognosis cases), when it is during the first pulse. All these are equally active in children. The second most common combination includes doxorubicin and ifosfamide (plus mesna) with or without dacarbazine (AI or MAID). Vincristine-based regimens might be superior to doxorubicin-based regimens.

The overall response rate is around 80%, with a complete response rate of 40 to 50%. Females might do better than males. The 5-year survival rates are better for head and neck tumors than for deep tumors, such as genitourinary. This might be related to the size at diagnosis.

Table 8.9 Chemotherapy regimens for rhabdomyosarcomas

Regimens	Drugs	Doses	Administration	Schedule
VA	Vincristine	1.5 mg/m^2; maximum dose, 2 mg	IV	Weekly
	Actinomycin-D	0.015 mg/kg; maximum dose, 0.5 mg	IV	Daily × 5, every 3 weeks
VAC	Vincristine	1.5 mg/m^2; maximum dose, 2 mg	IV	Weekly
	Actinomycin-D	0.015 mg/kg; maximum dose, 0.5 mg	IV	Daily × 5, every 3 weeks
	Cyclophosphamide	2.2 g/m^2	IV	Day 1, every 3 weeks
	Mesna	2.2 g/m^2	IV	Day 1, every 3 weeks
VIE	Vincristine	1.5 mg/m^2; maximum dose, 2 mg	IV	Weekly
	Ifosfamide	1.8 g/m^2/d	IV	Days 1 to 5, every 3 weeks
	Mesna	1.8 g/m^2/d	IV	Days 1 to 5, every 3 weeks
	Etoposide	100 mg/m^2/d	IV	Days 1 to 5, every 3 weeks
Comments	Radiation therapy given concomitantly with chemotherapy for 5 to 6 weeks, but etoposide and actinomycin-D are then omitted			
AI, every 3 weeks	Doxorubicin	25mg/m^2/d	Continuous infusion	Days 1, 2, and 3
	Ifosfamide	1.5 to 2.5 g/m^2/d	IV	Days 1 to 4
	Mesna	1.5 to 2.5 g/m^2/d	IV	Days 1 to 4
MAID, every 3 weeks (Antman, 1993)	Doxorubicin	15 mg/m^2/d	Continuous infusion	Days 1, 2, 3, and 4
	Dacarbazine	250 mg/m^2/d	Continuous infusion	Days 1, 2, 3, and 4
	Ifosfamide	2.0 g/m^2/d	IV	Days 1 to 3
	Mesna	2.0 g/m^2/d	IV	Days 1 to 4
VAC also called VDC [not to be confused with actinomycin-D containing VAC], every 3 weeks (Palumbo R, 1998)	Vincristine	Maximum dose of 2 mg	IV	Day 1
	Doxorubicin (=adriamycin)	70 mg/m^2	IV	Day 1
	Cyclophosphamide	600 mg/m^2	IV	Day 1
Supportive care	Granulocyte colony-stimulating factor	5 μg/kg/d	SC	As needed between chemotherapies
IV = intravenous; mg = milligrams, m = meter				

Approximately 60% of A-RMS cases express PAX3-FKHR and thus contain the t(2;1), 20% express PAX7-FKHR and thus contain the t(1;13), and 20% are fusion-negative. These fusion proteins function as tumorigenic aberrant transcription factors, causing the cells to divide (Ahn et al. 2006). New inhibitors are being searched for. For example, transcriptional activity of PAX3/FKHR can be inhibited by the kinase inhibitor PKC412 (Amstutz et al. 2008)

RADIATION ONCOLOGY

Radiation therapy has no role in the treatment of leiomyomas. On the other hand, leiomyosarcomas require complete resection, if possible. Unless the estimated risk of recurrence is low, post operative radiation is indicated in most cases of extremity leiomyosarcoma. Leiomyosarcomas occur at other locations besides the extremities such as the gastrointestinal tract and uterus. Data on the use of radiation therapy to treat the gastrointestinal variant is limited, but radiation therapy is commonly used to treat uterine sites. The largest retrospective study of the use of radiation therapy for uterine sarcomas included 529 leiomyosarcomas. Adjuvant radiation resulted in a statistically significant improvement in the 5-year local-regional failure-free survival (98% vs. 84%) compared to the surgery alone group (Sampath et al. 2010).

Treatment recommendations for embryonal and alveolar rhabdomyosarcoma have evolved from IRS studies and most patients are still treated on these clinical trials. If possible, tumors are removed surgically. Radiation therapy is used almost all of the time to treat the primary site of disease even after complete removal. The only exception in which radiation therapy is not used is for embryonal tumors after complete resection. In addition, radiation therapy is used for metastatic sites of disease. Doses to the primary site range from 3600 cGy to 5040 cGy depending on completeness of surgical resection and lymph node involvement. Rhabdomyosarcoma in adults occurs rarely. Radiation therapy is usually prescribed, but due to the scarcity of cases, results are not well defined.

CASES

Case 8.1 Angioleiomyoma (vascular leiomyoma, angiomyoma)

Clinical history and presentation

The patient is an otherwise well 53 year old man with a chief complaint of an intermittently painful lump in his foot that is uncomfortable to walk on. He believes he has had it for several years and has not noticed any changes in size or pain intensity. Examination reveals a firm nodule in the posterior portion of his left heel that is non-tender to palpation.

Surgical findings and comments

Because of the benign appearance radiologically, clinical history consistent with a benign tumor and superficial location, a marginal excision is performed.

Radiology findings

The MR images (**Case figs 8.1a** through **8.1c**) show a subcutaneous mass with moderately irregular boarders. The mass is remarkable for the extensive areas of low signal on all sequences that suggest either hemosiderin or calcification. Unfortunately, no radiograph is available to assess for calcification. Likewise, no contrast is given to assess for fluid, necrosis or matrix components. The overall appearance is non-specific, and the radiologist might suggest an indolent lesion given the probable calcification and the absence of adjacent edema.

Pathology findings

Gross features

The small, nodular tumor is excised with overlying skin. It measures 1.5 × 1.5 × 1.0 cm and exhibits a white, semi-translucent, gritty, partially calcified cut surface. It extends 0.3 cm from the skin and focally abuts the resection margin. A small portion of tumor is taken fresh for cytogenetics.

Microscopic features

Low magnification: The tumor is remarkable for large nodular calcifications (**Case fig. 8.1d**). It is primarily located in the dermis but also extends into the subcutaneous fat. It exhibits a pushing rather than permeative margin.

High magnification: The tumor is uniformly hypocellular with interspersed thin walled, curving vessels (**Case fig. 8.1e**). Tumor cells are brightly eosinophilic with indistinct cell borders and blunt ended, vesicular nuclei without atypia (**Case fig. 8.1f**). Calcifications form abruptly and don't elicit an inflammatory reaction (**Case fig. 8.1g**). Necrosis and mitotic activity are absent.

Special studies: CD34 immunohistochemical staining discloses numerous slit like, curving blood vessels characteristic of the solid or capillary type of angioleiomyoma (**Case fig. 8.1h**). As expected, the tumor cells are strongly and diffusely positive for smooth muscle actin with uniform staining throughout the cytoplasm (**Case fig. 8.1i**). Desmin expression is also strong and diffuse. A karyotype of the tumor is officially 46, XY. Interestingly, however, four of six non-clonal aberrations show alterations of chromosomes that have been described to occur with increased frequency in uterine type leiomyoma (rearrangements of chromosomes 1,3, and 13)(Hodge et al. 2007).The non-clonal aberrations of this patient's tumor include: 46,XY,t(13;20)(q14;p13), 46,XY,t(9;17)(q34;q21), 46,XY,t(3;5)(q11.1;p13), 46,XY,add(9)(q13), 46,XY,t(1;3;5)(q32;q21;p15) and 46,XY, t(13;17)(p13;q25).

Pathologic differential or, why isn't it one of the following?

Leiomyoma of deep soft tissue: Leiomyoma of deep soft tissue commonly contains calcifications and by definition has no mitotic activity and absent to minimal atypia as in this patient's tumor. However, this patient's tumor is superficial, and the vascular pattern of slightly curving slit-like capillaries is consistent with the solid or capillary variant of angioleiomyoma. Leiomyoma of deep soft tissue is a rarely made diagnosis of exclusion.

Glomus tumor: Like angioleiomyoma, glomus tumors tend to form small dermal or subcutaneous tumors that can be painful. However, glomus tumors contain glomus type cells that are rounded with distinct

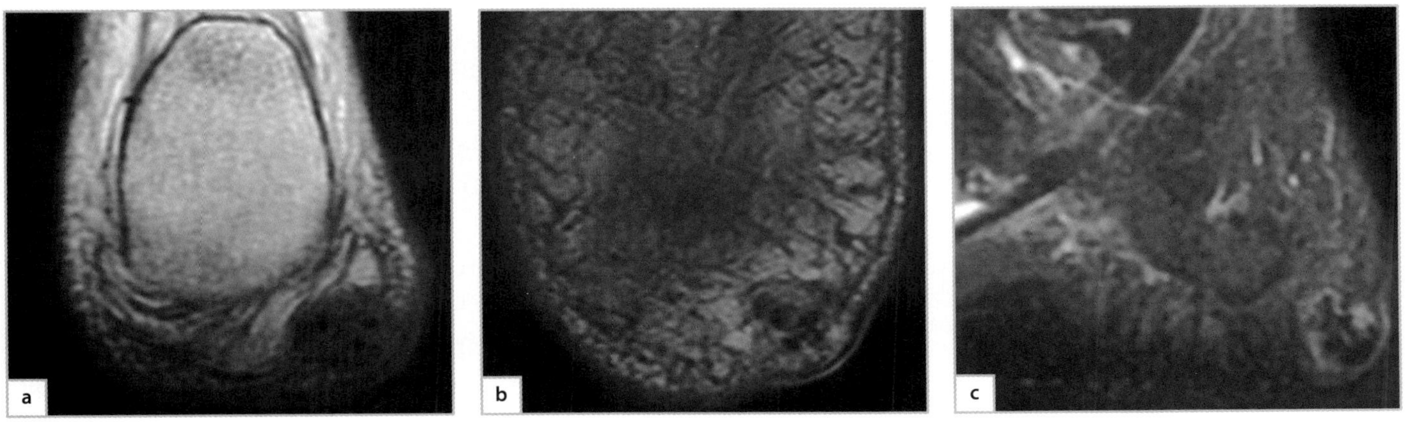

Case figure 8.1 Angioleiomyoma of soft tissue. 8.1a: Coronal T1 MR image. **8.1b**: Axial T2 fat saturated MR image. **8.1c**: Sagittal STIR MR image. There is a 1.5 × 1.4 × 1.5 cm heterogeneous signal mass in the subcutaneous tissues of the heel. Lobulated areas of low signal on all sequences suggest hemosiderin or calcification. There is no adjacent edema. Vascularity cannot be assessed because contrast was not given.

Case figure 8.1: Continued from page 167

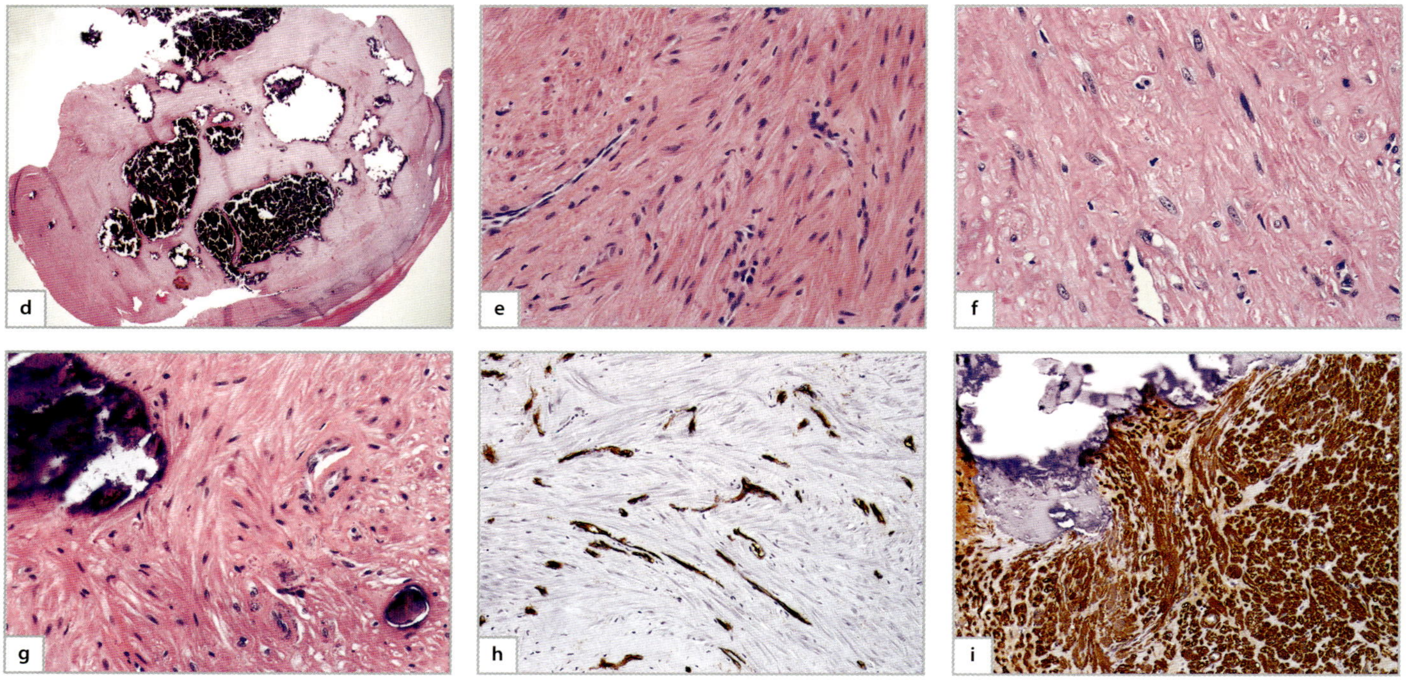

8.1d: Low magnification. The tumor is striking for large nodular aggregates of calcium. It is located close to the skin surface and in other sections also involves the subcutaneous fat. **8.1e**: High magnification. Tumor cells are brightly eosinophilic with indistinct cell borders. Slit-like, capillary sized vessels are characteristic of the solid or capillary variant. Cells in the upper left show mild cytoplasmic clumping similar to contraction bands of smooth muscle cells. **8.1f**: High magnification. Tumor cell nuclei are not atypical and exhibit the cigar or train car shape typical of smooth muscle differentiated cells. Nuclei are hypochromatic with small nucleoli. **8.1g**: High magnification. Calcifications in the tumor elicit no inflammatory response. **8.1h**: CD34 immunostain. CD34 antibody highlights the numerous, slightly curving, slit-like capillaries characteristic of the solid or capillary type of angioleiomyoma. **8.1i**: Smooth muscle actin immunostain. In this field, which includes a calcification, the tumor cells are strongly and diffusely positive for smooth muscle actin. The reactivity is evenly sustained throughout the cytoplasm of the tumor cells in contrast to the subplasmalemmal 'tram-track' accentuation evident in myofibroblastic tumors.

cell borders and small, uniform nuclei. A variant of glomus tumor contains a smooth muscle component, glomangiomyoma, but that tumor features large vascular spaces and still contains some glomus cells. Except for the glomangiomyoma subtype, glomus tumors are negative for desmin expression and up to 30% express CD34. This patient's tumor is strongly positive for desmin and negative for CD34. It has been reported that desmin reactivity is less often present in the venous and cavernous variants of angioleiomyoma (Matsuyama et al. 2007).

Low grade leiomyosarcoma: Low grade leiomyosarcoma exhibits more cytologic atypia with moderate variation in nuclear size and shape and some nuclear hyperchromasia and often demonstrates mitotic activitiy.

Pilar leiomyoma (piloleiomyoma): This is a rare entity that usually presents clinically as a single or multiple skin nodules. Histologically, it comprises swatches of smooth muscle disposed haphazardly in the dermis and embedded in collagenized stroma. The bundles of smooth muscle resemble enlarged arrector pili smooth muscle. This patient's tumor is a solid dermal and subcutaneous tumor with a solid growth and with prominent calcifications.

Case table 8.1: Summary pathology findings of Case 8.1

Diagnosis	Leiomyoma of soft tissue
Size	3.0 cm
Location	Subcutaneous fat of heel of foot
Margin status	Negative
Histologic grade (FNCLCC grading system)	Not graded: benign
Pathologic stage (AJCC tnm classification)	Not staged: benign

Oncology approach

Medical oncology

This is a benign tumor with no role for chemotherapy.

Radiation oncology

This is a benign tumor with no role for radiation therapy.

Patient outcome

The patient is doing well ten years after resection without recurrence.

Case 8.2 Leiomyosarcoma

Clinical history and presentation

The patient is a 79 year old male who presents with a three month history of a right groin mass. The mass was noted spontaneously and was initially felt to represent an inguinal hernia.

Physical examination reveals a large, firm mass in the inguinal region of the right groin. It is firmly adherent to surrounding structures. Mild tenderness is elicited on palpation.

Surgical findings and comments

Open biopsy of the mass is performed. Pathologic results are consistent with leiomyosarcoma.

Wide resection of the tumor is performed. Wide margins are obtained with no compromise to surrounding vital structures.

Radiology findings

The MR images (**Case figs 8.2a** through **8.2c**) of this 79 year old man show a nonspecific T1 low signal, STIR high signal 9.8 × 9.9 × 10 cm mass with intense enhancement worrisome for a sarcoma. This leiomyosarcoma did not show gross necrosis or hemorrhage on imaging. Interestingly, this patient's initial recurrence did not occur in the typical locations of lung or liver, but rather he developed paraspinal muscle metastasis discovered on his 2.5 year follow up CT (**Case fig. 8.2d**).

Pathology findings

Gross features

The open biopsy comprises multiple fragments of tan to red tissue. The wide resection specimen consists of a small ellipse of skin overlying an oblong portion of soft tissue that on cross sectioning reveals a 14.5 × 10.1 × 9 cm grossly circumscribed tumor. Serial sections of the tumor show a tan to white whorled interior without necrosis, hemorrhage, or calcifications. Tissue is collected fresh for tissue banking and cytogenetics.

The paraspinal soft tissue mass found 2.5 years after initial presentation is sampled by needle core biopsy under CT guidance. Several tan cylinders of tissue 0.1 cm wide and up to 1.0 cm long are submitted for standard processing.

Microscopic features

Since the open biopsy histologically matches the wide resection specimen, only photographs from the resection are presented.

Low magnification: The resection reveals a cellular tumor composed of long sweeping fascicles oriented perpendicularly to one another (**Case fig. 8.2e**). There is no necrosis or hemorrhage other than at the prior biopsy site.

High magnification: At higher magnification, the tumor cells are spindled with pale eosinophilic cytoplasm and ovoid, hyperchromatic nuclei that vary from blunt ended to pointy ended or tapered (**Case fig. 8.2f**). Scattered among the spindled cells are prominent, highly atypical cells with larger, pleomorphic nuclei. Some of the spindle tumor cells exhibit ragged cytoplasmic clumping and clearing approximating the more regular contraction bands of benign smooth muscle cells (**Case fig. 8.2g**). The mitotic rate averages 10 per 10 high magnification fields, and atypical mitoses are easily found (again, **Case fig. 8.2f**). In some areas, wiry collagen fibrils stream alongside the tumor cells. The tumor, although circumscribed grossly, infiltrates and destroys skeletal muscle (**Case fig. 8.2h**). Based on the moderate degree of atypia, the mitotic rate of 10-19 mitoses/10 HPF, and the lack of necrosis, the tumor is graded as intermediate according to the FNCLCC system.

The needle core biopsy of the paraspinal metastatic tumor shows the same fascicular spindle cell features as the initial biopsy and resection (**Case fig. 8.2i**).

Special studies: Immunohistochemically, the tumor cells strongly express smooth muscle actin (SMA) diffusely in the cytoplasmic distinctly different from the 'tram track' or subplasmalemmal accentuated pattern of reactivity noted in myofibroblastic tumors. Approximately 20% of the tumor cells also express h-caldesmon. Unusually, the tumor is negative for desmin (it is absent in ~12% of leiomyosarcomas). Interestingly, however, the tumor cells in the paraspinal metastasis sampled approximately 18 months later are strongly reactive for desmin (**Case fig. 8.2j**) and negative for actin,; the reverse of the original staining pattern. It is not uncommon for tumors to evolve and demonstrate variable IHC results upon metastasis; in this patient's tumor, the cells continue to exhibit a muscle phenotype although with different markers.

A sample of tumor from the main resection specimen yields a complex aneuploid karyotype with extensive structural and numerical

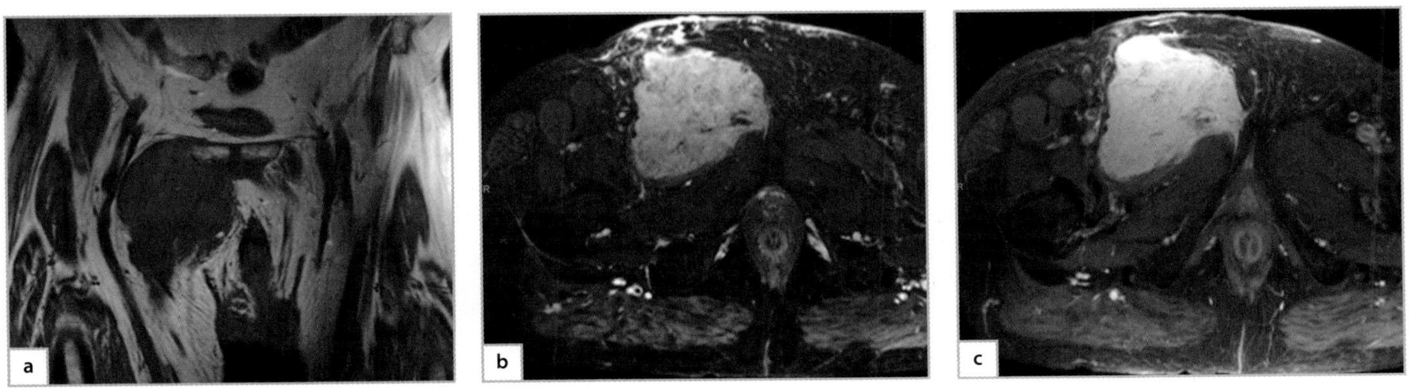

Case figure 8.2: Leiomyosarcoma radiology images. 8.2a: Coronal T1 MR image. **8.2b**: Axial STIR MR image. **8.2c:** Axial T1 fat saturation post-contrast MR image. The MR images show a nonspecific large mass in deep soft tissues of the right groin region. This does not clearly originate from a vessel. The mass has nonspecific T1 isointensity to adjacent muscle, STIR high signal and intense diffuse enhancement.

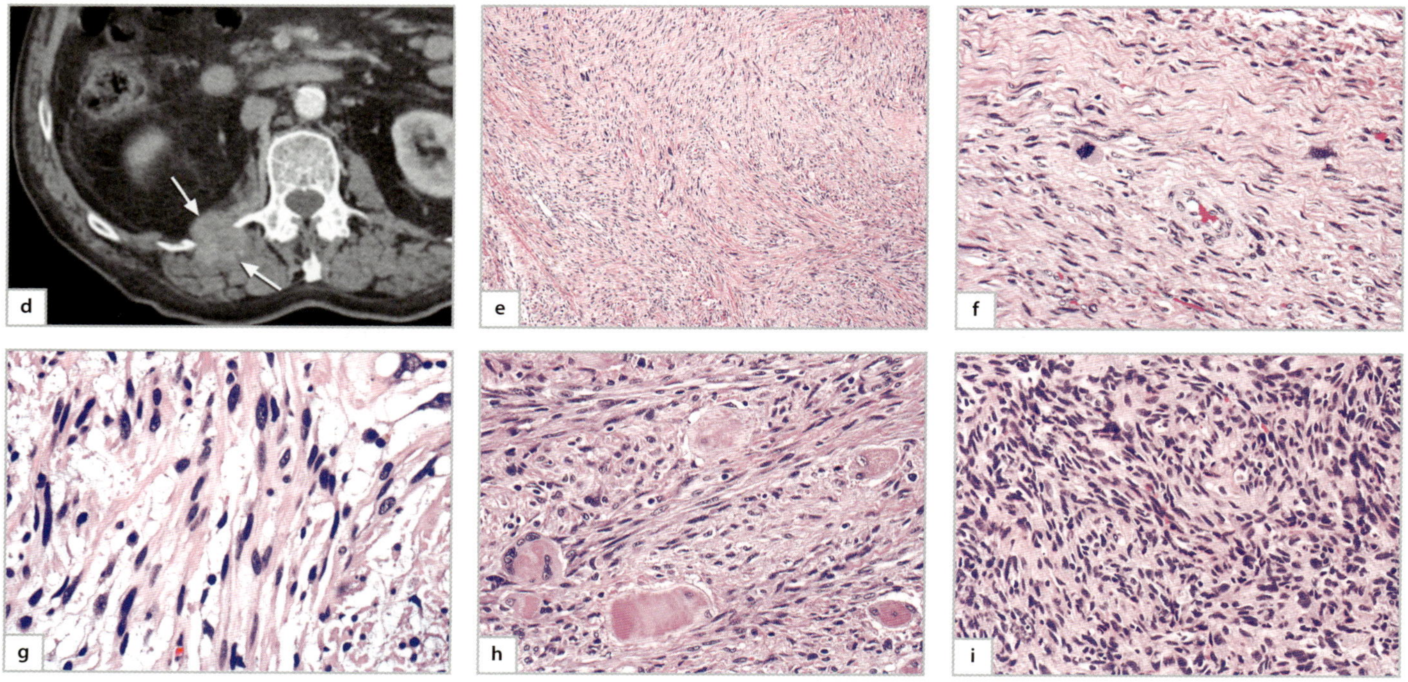

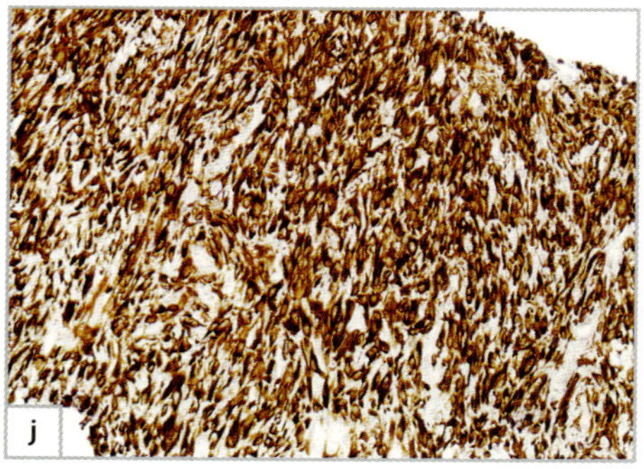

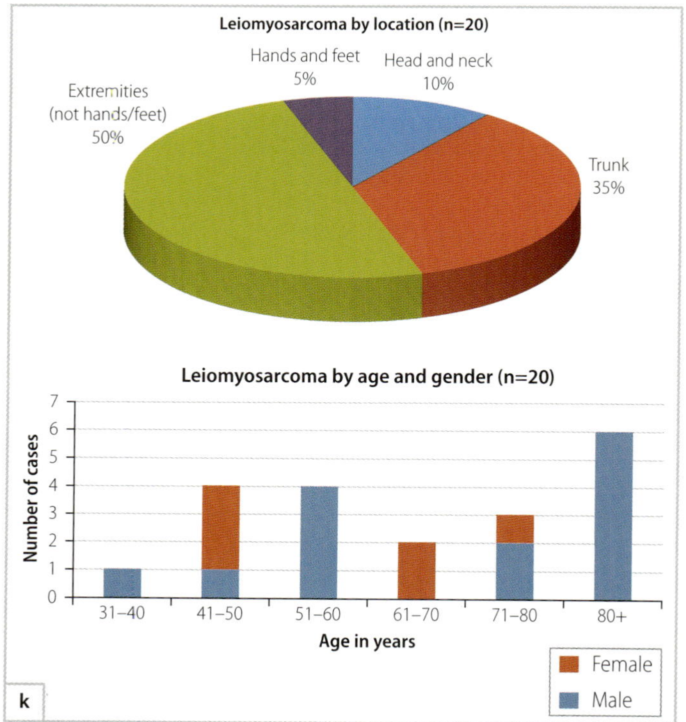

8.2d: Axial post-contrast CT scan image obtained 2.5 years later shows a slightly hyperdense mass (arrows) in the right paraspinal muscles. There is no appreciable calcification. **8.2e**: Lower magnification reveals sweeping bundles or fascicles of spindle cells. The tumor is cellular, and even at low magnification, a few cells stand out with larger, darker nuclei. **8.2f**: Higher magnification. Tumor cells are primarily spindled with blunt ended to pointy ended, tapered or fusiform nuclei. A mitotic figure is seen in this field. Wiry collagen fibers run parallel to the tumor cells. **8.2g**: High magnification. The neoplastic smooth muscle cells exhibit ragged cytoplasmic clearing and contraction of cytoplasm reminiscent of contraction bands of normal smooth muscle. This is a common feature that can provide a clue to the smooth muscle nature of the tumor. Two mast cells are also present, another common but nonspecific occurrence in smooth muscle tumors. **8.2h**: High magnification. The spindled tumor cells infiltrate and destroy skeletal muscle here seen as large multinucleated rounded cells. **8.2i**: Medium magnification. The needle core biopsy of the metastatic paraspinal mass reveals a cellular spindle cell neoplasm that does not show specific features of smooth muscle differentiation such as brightly eosinophilic cytoplasm, contraction bands, or blunt ended nuclei. However, it is histologically identical to some areas of the original tumor. **8.2j**: Medium magnification. The paraspinal tumor contains areas that strongly express desmin (immunohistochemical stain with DAB chromogen). **8.2k**: Soft tissue leiomyosarcomas resected at UNM Health Sciences Center 2000-2010 abnormalities including marker and ring chromosomes of unknown origin. Ring chromosomes are rare in leiomyosarcoma, but the complex karyotype is otherwise typical of LMS.

The tumor karyotype is: 44~48,X,-Y,add(5)(p15),-9,add(9)(q34),add(17)(q25),add(19)(q13.4),+1~6mar,+1~2r[cp11]

The gains of 5p15, portion of 17 and portion of 19 with loss of one chromosome 9 have been previously reported in leiomyosarcoma (Yang et al. 2009).

Pathologic differential or, why isn't it one of the following?

Leiomyoma of deep soft tissue: Leiomyoma of deep soft tissue is a very rare tumor that can only be diagnosed using strict, narrow criteria. Cytologic atypia combined with even a rare mitotic figure would exclude this diagnosis. This patient's tumor has moderate nuclear atypia and moderate numbers of mitotic figures including atypical forms. Thus, it meets the criteria for malignant smooth muscle tumor rather than leiomyoma. The complex karyotype is also consistent with LMS.

Myofibroblastic sarcoma: Like LMS, this tumor is characteristically composed of long fascicles formed by streaming spindle cells (a few sheet like and storiforming areas may also be present). The degree of nuclear atypia ranges from mild to moderate and would overlap with the atypia of this patient's tumor. Since myofibroblasts are related to smooth muscle cells, there is also considerable overlap immunohistochemically. Both tumors commonly express smooth muscle actin, and muscle specific actin, but desmin is less often positive in myofibroblastic sarcoma than in LMS (Eyden et al. 2008). Importantly, myofibroblastic sarcoma located in soft tissue is negative for h-caldesmon, and this patient's tumor is positive. Additionally, the reactivity for actins is diffusely cytoplasmic instead of linear and subplasmalemmal ('tram trak') as is generally the case in myofibroblastic sarcoma. Low to intermediate grade myofibrosarcoma is associated with genetic abnormalities including ring chromosomes and abnormalities of 12p11 and 12q13-q22, but these are not consistent findings. This patient's tumor does feature ring chromosomes which is rare in LMS. However, the additional gains and losses are consistent with the diagnosis of leiomyosarcoma.

Dedifferentiated liposarcoma: Dedifferentiated liposarcoma can contain heterogeneous areas including malignant smooth muscle. However, often a lower grade liposarcoma component is present with lipoblasts. In addition, all areas of tumor should show strong reactivity for MDM2 and CDK4. This patient's tumor does not contain any lipoblasts, and it is negative for MDM2 and CDK4 by immunohistochemical staining.

Figure 8.2k totals the number of soft tissue leiomyosarcomas resected or biopsied at the University of New Mexico Health Sciences Center from 2000-2010. In this small series, males predominate, there are no pediatric patients, and 80% are older than 50 years. Hand and feet and head and neck are uncommon sites of origin. The University of New Mexico Health Sciences Center is representative of a moderately sized academic orthopaedic oncology practice.

Oncology approach

Medical oncology

Chemotherapy is initiated when the patient develops metastatic disease. He tolerates a combination of gemcitabine and docetaxel. However, there is only a transient, minimal response. The patient's advanced age and co-morbidities limit his subsequent therapeutic options, and the patient agrees to palliative care.

Radiation oncology

Post-operative radiation therapy is generally recommended for extremity leiomyosarcoma in order to improve local control. Doses are

Case table 8.2a Variant histologic features of leiomyosarcoma of deep soft tissue

Feature	Frequency	Comment
Myxoid change	Uncommon	Most commonly, the myxoid change is focal and typical areas of LMS ((long sweeping fascicles of eosinophilic spindle cells with blunt ended, variably pleomorphic nuclei and interspersed prominently atypical large nuclei) are also present. Pure myxoid LMS can have three patterns: fascicular, reticular/microcystic, or multinodular. Nuclear grade in pure myxoid LMS is usually low to intermediate
Inflammation	Uncommon	Rarely, the inflammation can almost obscure the tumor cells. It is usually composed of lymphocytes and/or plasma cells
Metaplastic bone	Rare	Reactive appearing bone without cytologic atypia
Malignant bone	Rare	Osteoid and mineralized bone with markedly atypical osteoblasts. This would be consistent with dedifferentiation
Malignant cartilage	Rare	Hyaline cartilage matrix with atypical chondrocytes and chondroblasts. This finding is consistent with dedifferentiation
Highly pleomorphic areas resembling high grade pleomorphic sarcoma, nos	Rare	This is considered 'dedifferentiated' LMS. Usually, it forms a minority of the tumor. Rarely, it may comprise the majority of the tumor, and multiple sections will be required to confirm the muscle phenotype. Dedifferentiated areas are negative for muscle markers
Verocay bodies	Uncommon	Alignment of the tumor cells in a fence or palisade pattern. This is more typical of schwannoma, but can be seen also in smooth muscle tumors
Storiform architecture	Uncommon	This can be seen focally in LMS and may be especially prominent in more myxoid examples
Pointy ended nuclei	Uncommon	Even classic LMS may harbor a few tumor cells with pointy ended nuclei that resemble the nuclei of schwann cells. When present, this type of nucleus is usually a minority component
Epithelioid cells	Rare	Rare soft tissue LMS will contain foci of epithelioid tumor cells (round cells with distinct cell borders). Exceptionally, this is the main or sole cell type in soft tissue LMS. When the epithelioid cells are negative for muscle markers in the setting of other areas typical of LMS, they can be considered consistent with dedifferentiation
Rhabdoid cells	Rare	These are small to medium sized round cells with brightly eosinophilic cytoplasm. They are negative for skeletal muscle markers but otherwise resemble rhabdomyoblasts. Their presence in a LMS is consistent with dedifferentiation
Osteoclast like giant cells	Uncommon	These may be prominent and evenly dispersed throughout the tumor
Pseudolipoblasts	Rare	These mimic true lipoblasts, but the cytoplasmic vacuoles do not indent the nucleus, and the cells are S-100 protein negative.

LMS = leiomyosarcoma. This list may not capture all possible variant features, especially those reported in individual case reports.

Case table 8.2b: Summary pathology findings of Case 8.2

Diagnosis	Leiomyosarcoma
Size	14.5 cm
Location	Deep soft tissue of groin
Margin status	Negative
Histologic grade at initial diagnosis (FNCLCC grading system)	Tumor differentiation score of 2 = moderately differentiated but considered high grade for treatment and prognosis purposes
Pathologic stage at initial diagnosis (AJCC TNM classification)	Stage III = T2b/N0/M0 (deep tumor greater than 5.0 cm with negative lymph nodes and no metastases)

similar to those used for other soft tissue sarcomas, which is usually at least 60 Gy. This patient does undergo post-operative radiation therapy and experiences excellent local control. Unfortunately, he later develops metastatic disease.

Patient outcome

After surgical resection, chemotherapy, and radiation the patient develops multiple, progressing metastases. Two years following the appearance of the metastases (3.5 years after his initial presentation) the patient dies of widespread metastatic disease. This outcome is unfortunately not unexpected given the aggressive nature of soft tissue leiomyosarcoma.

Case 8.3 Embryonal rhabdomyosarcoma

Clinical history and presentation

The patient is a ten month old baby boy who presents with marked calf enlargement and pain causing him to refuse to stand on his leg. He had been previously diagnosed as having a 'greenstick fracture,' but his leg progressively became more painful, and his parents became concerned at the firmness of his calf leading them to seek a second opinion.

Physical examination reveals the presence of a large, ill-defined and deeply situated, firm soft tissue mass involving the entirety of the left calf.

Surgical findings and comments

Open biopsy is performed revealing embryonal rhabdomyosarcoma. The extensive nature of the tumor precludes the possibility of limb salvage surgery, therefore below knee amputation is performed which is two years later revised without complications.

The patient eventually develops metastatic tumor in the left thigh approximately three years after his initial presentation. This is first biopsied and then removed without intent for wide margins.

Radiology findings

The MR images (**Case figs 8.3a** through **8.3c**) show a non-specific mass with T1 low signal, and high signal on T2 and STIR sequences. The mass measures 7.5 × 3.7 × 4.5 cm and occupies much of the posterior calf. There is pressure erosion of the posterior cortex of the tibia. Although a quarter of rhabdomyosarcomas can have bone invasion at presentation, this case had not yet developed bone invasion or destruction.

Pathology findings

Gross features

The initial incisional biopsy consists of 1.0 cm in aggregate fragments of gray to white glistening soft tissue. A portion is sent for karyotyping. Bone marrow biopsies performed several days later are negative for tumor.

The below the knee amputation specimen contains a large tumor embedded in the posterior, lateral and anterior muscle compartments of the calf. Cross sections of the 8.5 × 4.5 × 4.5 cm mass reveal a firm, multinodular tan mass with areas of yellow necrosis and hemorrhage. Grossly, it abuts the fibula but does not invade it. Amputation margins are widely negative for tumor. Simultaneously with the amputation, five lymph nodes are also removed from the groin measuring 0.3 to 0.5 cm in maximum dimension. Fresh tumor is again submitted for karyotyping, as the first specimen yielded only a normal karyotype.

Approximately three years after amputation, a biopsy of a new left thigh mass comprises yellow to tan to focally hyperemic soft tissue aggregating to 2.0 cm. Repeat bilateral bone marrow biopsies are negative for tumor. The left thigh mass is excised and comprises a 4.5 cm in diameter semi-firm ('fish flesh' consistency) tan mass that abuts grossly surgical margins. An additional single, non-enlarged groin lymph node is also removed.

As he grows, the patient also undergoes amputation stump revision (which reveals no tumor on microscopic examination).

Microscopic features

The original biopsy, amputation specimen and metastatic tumor are histologically identical and show a similar pattern of muscle marker reactivity. Only photomicrographs from the resection specimen are provided.

Low magnification: Examining many sections of tumor reveals a 30% cellular spindle cell component and 70% high grade, markedly pleomorphic component. The spindle cells are arranged in fascicles or a basket-weave (storiform) pattern (**Case fig. 8.3d**). The majority of the tumor is diffusely anaplastic apparent even at relatively low magnification (**Case fig. 8.3e**). The anaplastic areas comprise vaguely fasciculated to solid sheets of pleomorphic cells.

High magnification: At higher magnification, the spindle cell areas of tumor look similar to LMS even with irregular cytoplasmic clearing (**Case fig. 8.3f**). The background is collagenized. Pure pediatric spindle cell RMS (which has been considered a less aggressive type of embryonal RMS) often contains many cells with cross striations indicative of advanced differentiation. This patient's tumor, however, does not contain any spindle cells with cross striations and more closely resembles the spindle cell/sclerosing RMS seen in adults. The anaplastic areas easily meet the definition of anaplasia in RMS: hyperchromatic tumor nuclei at least three times the size of adjacent tumor nuclei at their narrowest diameter (**Case fig. 8.3g**). Necrosis is

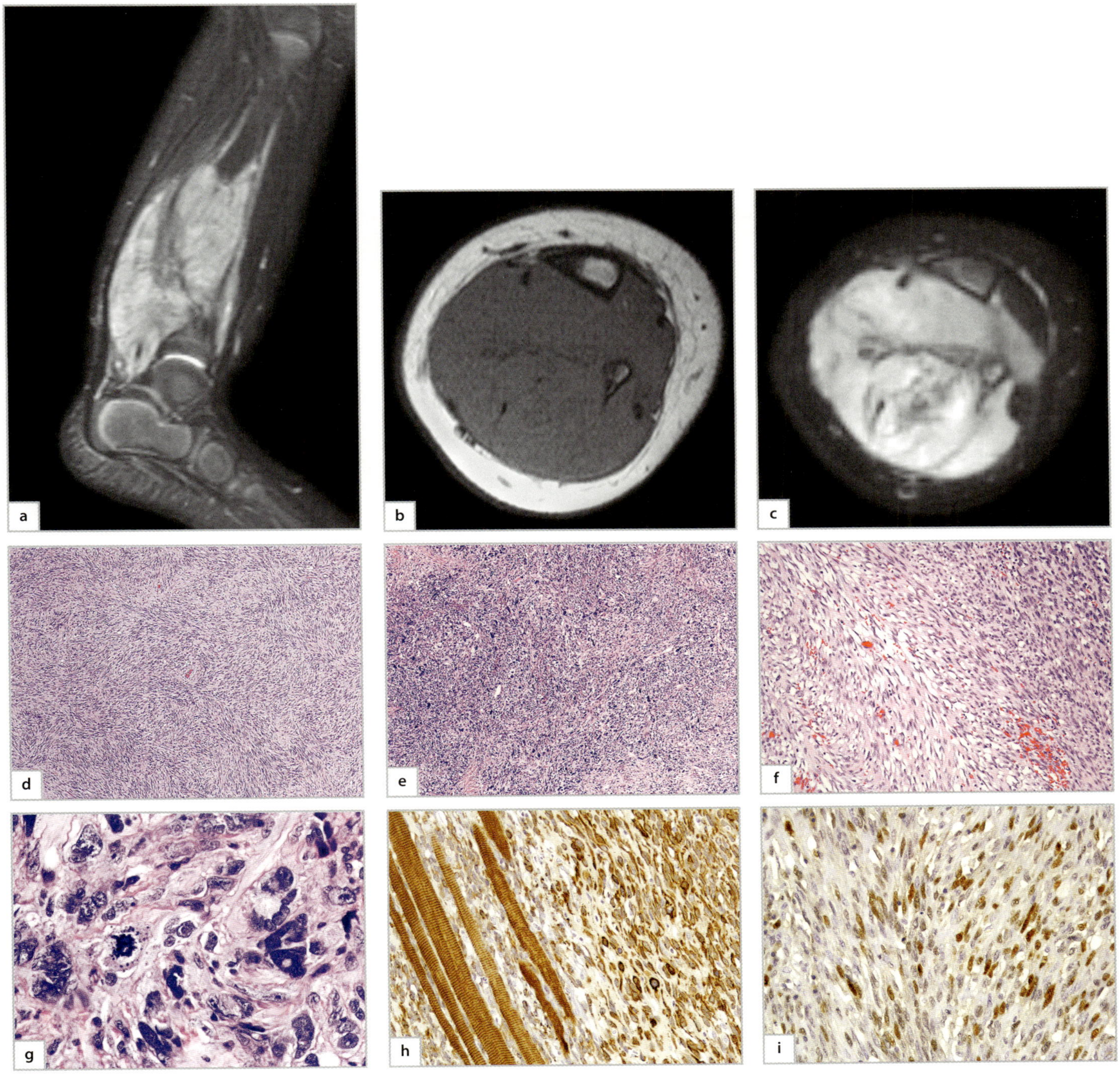

Case figure 8.3 Embryonal rhabdomyosarcoma radiology images. 8.3a sagittal STIR MR image. **8.3b** axial T1 MR image. **8.3c** axial T2 fat saturated MR image. The MR images show a large nonspecific appearing mass of the distal calf. The mass is T1 isointense to muscle and high signal on STIR and T2 fat saturated images. The mass has caused mild pressure erosion of the posterior tibia without marrow edema or destruction of cortex. Vascularity cannot be assessed as no IV contrast was given. **8.3d**: Low magnification. A minority of the tumor consists of cellular spindle cells arranged in a storiform or fascicular pattern (storiform pattern shown here). **8.3e**: Low magnification. The majority of the tumor shows diffuse anaplasia characterized by clusters of large, markedly pleomorphic tumor cells. Diffuse anaplasia (rather than focal anaplasia) may be associated with a more aggressive course. **8.3f**: Spindle cell region. Some embryonal RMS are entirely composed of fascicles of spindle cells as seen in this photomicrograph. This is an area of the patient's tumor that is lower grade. **8.3g**: High magnification, anaplastic area. Anaplasia may be focal (widely scattered pleomorphic cells) or diffuse (clusters of cells). The nuclei must be hyperchromatic and at least three times larger than adjacent tumor nuclei at their narrowest diameter. Here the nuclei are not only large and hyperchromatic but variable in shape. A mitotic figure is also present. **8.3h**: Desmin IHC stain. Desmin stains both the residual normal skeletal muscle fibers, nicely highlighting the cross striations (left), and also is strongly expressed in the surrounding tumor cells. Desmin is commonly expressed in both smooth muscle tumors and skeletal muscle tumors. **8.3i**: Myogenin IHC stain. Myogenin stains approximately 15% of the tumor nuclei in this field of the spindle cell component of the tumor. In contrast to desmin which is expressed also in smooth muscle cells, myogenin nuclear reactivity is seen exclusively in skeletal muscle tumors.

widespread, and mitotic figures number up to 25 per 10 high magnification microscopic fields. Atypical mitoses are present. There is no lymphovascular invasion. All lymph nodes are negative for tumor.

Central review of the tumor by the Children's Oncology Group confirms the diagnosis of embryonal rhabdomyosarcoma with diffuse anaplasia.

Special studies: Tumor cells are strongly and diffusely reactive for desmin (**Case fig. 8.3h**). Myogenin nuclear reactivity is variable, with some areas of anaplasia showing diffuse expression and spindle cell areas demonstrating nuclear reactivity in a lower proportion of tumor cells (**Case fig. 8-3i**). In addition, tumor cells are negative for smooth muscle actin and diffusely reactive for muscle specific actin. One of three karyotypes obtained over the course of the patient's treatment is abnormal with the following findings: 46,XY, t(7;9)(q32;p22) in seven cells, 47,XY,r(11)(p15q25)+mar in four cells, and 46,XY,del(13)(q11;q21) in three cells. These results could be representative of the tumor or due to secondary changes occurring in long term *in situ* culture.

Pathologic differential or, why isn't it one of the following?

Alveolar rhabdomyosarcoma: A-RMS exhibits an alveolar or solid growth of small round cells with a high N/C ratio which can resemble lymphoma or Ewing sarcoma. Scattered rhabdomyoblasts with bright eosinophilic cytoplasm and multinucleated giant tumor cells with peripherally placed nuclei ('wreath cells') are commonly present. Although diffuse anaplasia does occur in A-RMS, it is relatively uncommon compared with its incidence in E-RMS. Finally, in this patient, there is no evidence of t(1;13), t(2;13) or the other translocations described in fusion positive A-RMS.

Spindle cell variant of E-RMS: This variant of RMS is usually located in the paratesticular region then head and neck; extremity location is infrequent. Most of the tumor should comprise eosinophilic spindle cells, and cytoplasmic cross striations should be evident in some. Diffuse anaplasia is exceptional in spindle cell E-RMS and focal anaplasia is also rare (Qualman et al. 2008, Parham 2006). Spindle cell/sclerosing RMS however, may show nuclear atypia.

Pleomorphic rhabdomyosarcoma: This type of RMS occurs only rarely in children. In pediatric patients with pleomorphic RMS, foci of conventional embryonal RMS may be identified (Parham, 2006). Distinguishing between pleomorphic RMS and embryonal RMS with anaplasia may be challenging. Cytogenetic findings are not helpful in most instances, as both tumors often demonstrate a complex aneuploid karyotype without broadly consistent changes. Pleomorphic RMS exhibits extreme diffuse atypia, while anaplastic E-RMS should have significant areas of typical E-RMS present. A-RMS with anaplasia can be distinguished from pleomorphic RMS by areas of residual alveolar or solid small round blue cell morphology; most importantly, molecular results showing gene fusions typical of A-RMS are very helpful.

Case table 8.3a Variant histologic features of embryonal and alveo ar rhabdomyosarcoma and possible novel RMS types

Feature	Frequency	Type of RMS involved	Comment
Anaplasia	10%	E-RMS A-RMS	May be associated with a worse outcome. Defined as large hyperchromatic nuclei at least 3x as large as adjacent tumor nuclei at their narrowest diameter
Mixed pattern combining E-RMS and A-RMS	Rare	N/A	The U.S. Children's Oncology Group (COG) requires at least 50% alveolar pattern to diagnose the tumor as A-RMS. However, these cases are best assessed by molecular genetics to look for A-RMS fusions. Fusion negative cases may behave similarly to E-RMS
Clear cell change	Rare	Not known, possibly only E-RMS	The cells have vacuolated clear cytoplasm due to glycogen or lipid droplets. Tumor cells may mimic lipoblasts. Clear cell change is relatively common as a focal finding in RMS but in pure form is rare
Epithelioid cell change	Rare	May be a distinct variant of RMS. May also be seen focally in A-RMS	Recently reported series of 16 adults (predominantly older) with epithelioid, fairly uniform tumor cells diffusely positive for desmin and reactive for myogenin. The histology mimics melanoma or carcinoma. Aggressive course. Several cases also featured rhabdoid cells. Epithelioid cells may also be seen focally in alveolar RMS
Sclerosis	Uncommon	Can be seen in E-RMS and A-RMS May also represent a distinct type of RMS related to adult spindle cell RMS or pleomorphic RMS	Dense sclerosis is described in a few cases of E-RMS and A-RMS (including fusion positive cases). In adults, most examples may be part of the spectrum of adult spindle cell RMS or pleomorphic RMS
Rhabdomyoma like RMS	Very Rare	Uncertain relationship to E-RMS	Strongly resembles rhabdomyoma with clusters of more differentiated cells amidst primitive cells. Features consistent with RMS rather than rhabdomyoma include: increased mitoses, atypical mitoses, anaplastic cells, cambium layer, and capsular penetration or permeative invasion
Rhabdoid cells	Rare	A-RMS Pure rhabdoid RMS	Can be seen focally In A-RMS. May be difficult to distinguish from rhabdoid tumor of ST. INI-1 and myogenin reactivity may be helpful in excluding rhabdoid tumor. Unknown whether pure rhabdoid tumor is a variant of A- or E-RMS
Ectomesenchymoma	Very Rare	E-RMS, pediatric spindle cell RMS, A-RMS	Defined as RMS containing neoplastic neurons and/or neuroblasts with or without ganglion cells. Behave similarly to RMS
Hemophagocytosis	Very Rare	A-RMS	Tumor cells ingest red blood cells, white blood cells and cellular debris. May be associated with hemophagocytic syndrome

RMS: rhabdomyosarcoma, E-RMS: embryonal RMS, A-RMS: alveolar RMS. This list does not capture all possible variant features, especially those described in individual case reports.

Oncology approach

Medical oncology

Chemotherapy is initiated postoperatively according to a specific Pediatric Oncology Group protocol. This consists of vincristine, actinomycin-D, and Cytoxan × 47 weeks. He also periodically receives G-CSF, dexamethasone, mesna, and ondansetron. The patient tolerates chemotherapy well with minimal side effects. Upon cessation of therapy, the patient is followed regularly with office visits, repeat chest CT scan, and MRI.

Three years later, the patient is noted to have a new, 'pea-sized' mass in the left groin that rapidly grows over a period of two weeks. Biopsy confirms metastatic rhabdomyosarcoma. Staging workup then reveals a metastatic deposit in the right upper lung with right hilar adenopathy. The patient is then placed on Children's Oncology Group (COG) chemotherapy protocol ARST-0121 consisting of doxorubicin and cyclophosphamide with alternating ifosfamide and etoposide. He tolerates the new regimen of chemotherapy well with transient mild nausea, vomiting and weakness. However, despite aggressive chemotherapy, he develops progressive pulmonary metastases and dies of disease five years after initial presentation.

Radiation oncology

Since this patient had embryonal rhabdomyosarcoma which was completely resected with widely negative margins, no post-operative radiation therapy was recommended. The primary site is well controlled, but he later develops a regional failure and distant metastatic disease years later. Palliative radiation therapy is an option for metastatic disease.

Case table 8.3b Summary pathology findings of Case 8.3

Diagnosis	Embryonal rhabdomyosarcoma with diffuse anaplasia
Size	8.5 × 4.5 × 4.5 cm
Location	Deep skeletal muscle of left distal lower extremity
Margin status	Widely negative (amputation specimen)
Histologic grade (FNCLCC grading system)	Grade 3 = high grade
Pathologic stage (AJCC TNM classification)	III = T2b high grade tumor with negative lymph nodes and distant metastasis
Clinical group staging for RMS	I = localized disease, completely resected

Patient outcome

The patient succumbs due to pulmonary metastases five years after initial presentation.

Case 8.4 Alveolar rhabdomyosarcoma

Clinical history and presentation

The patient is a 14 year old, morbidly obese teenage boy who presents with a three month history of diffuse pain in his extremities and muscles, increasing weakness and more recently the development of a left foot mass, fevers, and night sweats. He reports recent weight loss of 30 pounds. Serological studies conducted at an outside hospital suggest recent CMV and EBV infections.

Over the course of his three months of symptoms, his weakness progressed and foot mass continued to enlarge prompting a repeat visit to his primary care provider who then ordered a battery of serological tests. These revealed elevations of LDH, creatinine kinase including MB isoenzyme, C-reactive protein, and a mildly elevated white blood cell count with normal red blood cell indices.

Because of the abnormal laboratory findings and newly developed left foot mass, the patient is then referred for evaluation to the pediatric oncology clinic at the University Hospital. Physical examination reveals 'peg' shaped lower extremities from the knee down with a somewhat shiny and smooth look. He is very sensitive even to light touch along the lateral aspects of the legs across their entire length. His pain is worse with deep palpation. A 5 × 5 cm round, firm, tender but non-erythematous mass is present on the lateral aspect of the left foot over the metatarsals. Additional findings include morbid obesity and pain in a band across the lumbar spine area, and the patient's lumbar spine is tender to moderately deep palpation and percussion.

Given the patient's left foot mass and relatively long duration of symptoms out of proportion to an EBV or CMV related infection, the patient is considered to have a possible inflammatory paraneoplastic syndrome and he is admitted for a full work-up.

Subsequent physical examination by the orthopaedic oncologist reveals a large mass on the plantar aspect of the left foot as well as diffuse mild weakness throughout both lower extremities.

Surgical findings and comments

Biopsy of the foot mass is performed revealing alveolar rhabdomyosarcoma.

Further work-up reveals metastatic disease to the lumbar spine and bone marrow involvement by tumor.

Radiology findings

The MR images (**Case figs 8.4a** through **8.4c**) show an expansile, intensely enhancing 6.9 × 4.5 × 4 cm mass of the foot surrounding the fourth metatarsal. The soft tissue portion shows non-specific T1 low signal and STIR high signal. The 4th metatarsal marrow shows abnormal T1 low signal and STIR high signal indicating edema or cellular invasion. The abnormal marrow signal with enhancement in the 4th metatarsal marrow indicates frank bone invasion. The coronal image (**Case fig. 8.4c**) shows cortical erosion. The uniform, intense enhancement indicates the tumor does not have appreciable matrix and it has

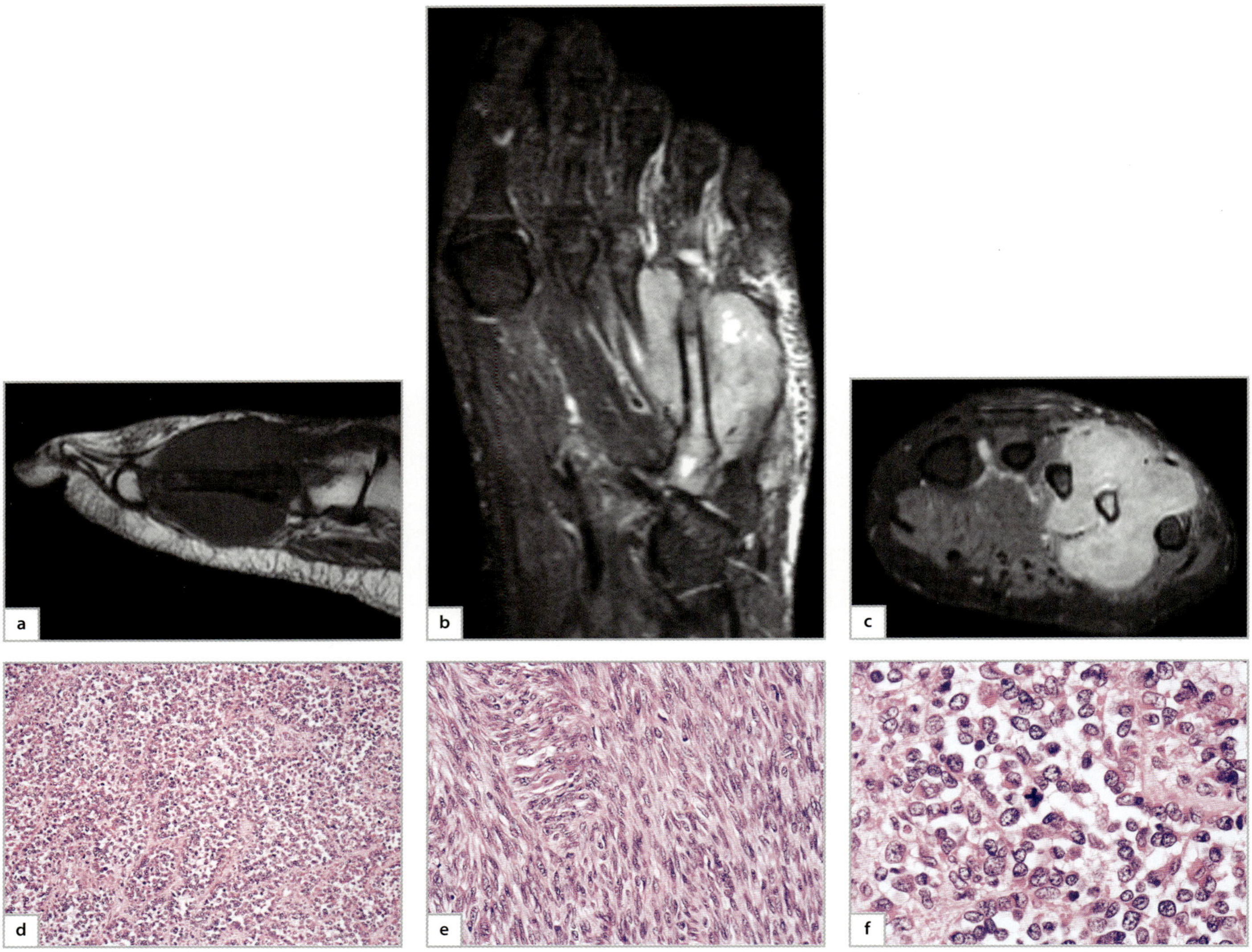

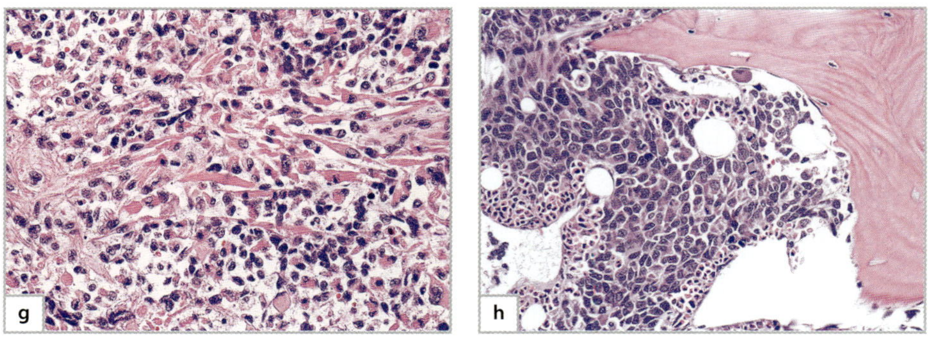

Case figure 8.4 Alveolar rhabdomyosarcoma radiology images. **8.4a** Sagittal T1 MR image. **8.4b**: Axial STIR MR image. **8.4c**: Coronal T1 fat saturated post-contrast MR image. MR images show a nonspecific mass of the forefoot with T1 isointensity, STIR high signal, and fairly uniform intense enhancement. The tumor surrounds the fourth metatarsal with areas of cortical bone erosion, and the marrow has abnormal signal with enhancement indicating bone invasion. **8.4d**: Low magnification. Classic alveolar pattern of A-RMS consists of nests of tumor cells with central dyscohesion and cell dropout leading to an appearance mimicking pulmonary alveoli. **8.4e**: Medium magnification. A minority of this patient's tumor demonstrates a fascicular spindle cell appearance resembling embryonal RMS. **8.4f**: High magnification. The alveolar areas feature round tumor cells with eosinophilic cytoplasm and a high N/C ratio. Some of the nuclei exhibit multilobulation described sometimes as 'popcorn' like. This is a nuclear trait more often seen in A-RMS than E-RMS. **8.4g**: Higher magnification. Scattered strap cells with cross striations are identified (microscope condenser is out to highlight the banded cytoplasm). **8.4h**: Bone marrow at high magnification. At presentation, bilateral bone marrow biopsies demonstrate paratrabecular aggregates of tumor. Notice the tumor cells are larger than the adjacent hematopoietic cells.

Case figure 8.4: Continued from page 176

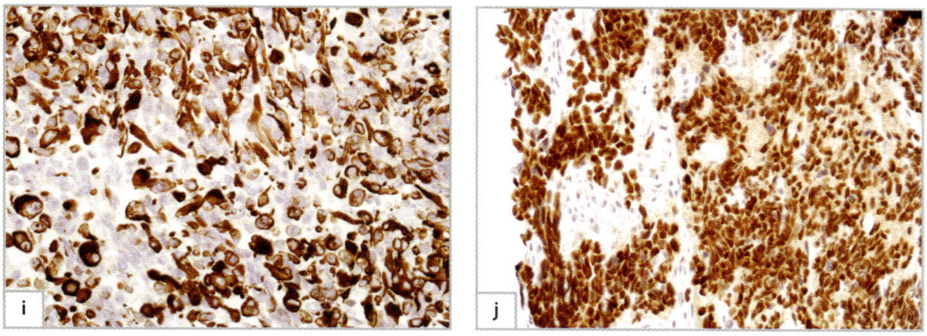

8.4i: Desmin IHC stain. Tumor cells are diffusely positive for desmin. **8.4j**: Myogenin IHC stain. The majority of the patient's tumor cells disclose strong nuclear staining for myogenin antibody. A-RMS often exhibits diffuse myogenin reactivity.

not yet developed gross necrosis. Given the age and extremity location, rhabdomyosarcoma is a likely diagnosis.

Pathology findings

Gross features

The biopsy comprises fragmented tan to white fleshy tumor fragments aggregating to 2 cm. A sample is sent fresh to Cytogenetics. Because the patient is Stage IV at presentation, resection of the tumor is not performed. Bone marrow biopsies are also obtained one week after the foot mass was sampled. The patient's forehead tumor biopsied approximately three years after initial presentation consists of two 1.0 cm fragments of tissue a portion of which is held for possible cytogenetic study.

Microscopic features

Low magnification: The majority of the patient's foot mass consists of interconnected nests of loosely cohesive tumor cells that dissect through fibromuscular tissue (**Case fig. 8.4d**). A few areas demonstrate a fascicular, spindle cell growth pattern (**Case fig. 8.4e**). These spindle cell areas comprise less than 10% of the tumor.

High magnification: The nested areas of tumor are formed by round cells with a high nuclear to cytoplasmic ratio. Simulating lung alveoli, the clear spaces result from central cellular dyscohesion and dropout (**Case fig. 8.4f**). This is the classic appearance of A-RMS. Rhabdomyoblasts with cross-striations are scattered among the less differentiated cells (**Case fig. 8.4g**). Necrosis is present that is geographic (involves broad areas) but also affects individual cells. Mitotic figures are numerous at more than 10/10 high magnification fields, and atypical forms are identified.

Both bone marrow biopsies reveal metastatic tumor (**Case fig. 8.4h**).

Central review of the initial tumor biopsy by the Children's Oncology Group confirms the diagnosis of alveolar rhabdomyosarcoma.

Special studies: The tumor in the foot and the soft tissue metastasis are strongly diffusely positive for desmin (**Case fig. 8.4i**) and myogenin (**Case fig. 8.4j**). More than 80% of nuclei express myogenin, a level of high reactivity more common in A-RMS than E-RMS. There is no reactivity for S-100 protein, WT-1, synaptophysin, NSE, or chromogranin. Staining with CD99 antibody is cytoplasmic rather than membranous.

Unfortunately, specimen sent to Cytogenetics is necrotic, and consequently karyotyping is unsuccessful.

Pathologic differential or, why isn't it one of the following?

Embryonal rhabdomyosarcoma: The classic alveolar pattern present in more than 50% of the tumor supports the diagnosis of alveolar RMS. Mixed E-RMS/A-RMS occur and are currently determined to be alveolar if that component comprises >50% of the tumor. The patient's tumor is only biopsied, however, and sampling may have over-represented the alveolar component. Clinically, however, the patient's age at presentation (14 years) and site (extremities) are more consistent with alveolar than embryonal RMS. In addition, the diffuse myogenin reactivity, and involvement of the bone marrow are more often seen in A-RMS than E-RMS.

Malignant Triton tumor (MTT): This is a malignant peripheral nerve sheath tumor with a rhabdomyoblastic component. It is often associated with neurofibromatosis type 1, and the mean age of presentation is in the 30s. Unlike this patient's tumor, the malignant skeletal muscle component in MTT does not show an alveolar RMS histology but is composed of spindled rhabdomyoblasts.

Ectomesenchymoma: This tumor primarily consists of RMS (spindle, embryonal, or alveolar types) with scattered neuroblasts or neurons and sometimes ganglion cells. It is rare and behaves similarly to RMS. Immunohistochemistry is often required to confirm the presence of neoplastic neural cells. This patient's tumor has no neural appearing cells, and there is no reactivity for S-100 protein, neuron specific enolase, or synaptophysin (antibodies which can identify neuroblasts or neurons and ganglion cells).

Oncology approach

Medical oncology

Chemotherapy is initiated along with radiation therapy to the lumbar spine. The patient is placed on COG Protocol ARST0431 for newly diagnosed, high risk metastatic rhabdomyosarcoma. The regimen consists of a combination of intense dose chemotherapy with vincristine, irinotecan, ifosfamide, etoposide, doxorubicin , cyclophosphamide, and dactinomycin with radiotherapy. This clinical trial started in mid-2006 with a completion date of 2010. The patient also receives emergency palliative radiation to the right psoas muscle and LS spine to 4500 cGy because of acute nerve root compression with severe pain. Subsequent to his radiation therapy (to foot and spine) and his chemotherapy, the patient is considered to have partial response with diffuse metastatic bone disease. He is able to ambulate and has no pain but persists with slight bilateral lower limb weakness.

Over the course of the next two years, the patient continues to progress with development of new metastases. He is given a course of chemotherapy including cyclophosphamide, vinorelbine, and bevacizumab. The patient is currently alive with widely metastatic disease to the bone including a new site in the skull three years after initial presentation.

Radiation oncology

Since the patient has alveolar rhabdomyosarcoma, radiation therapy is indicated for treatment of the primary site in all instances. Furthermore, patients with metastatic disease usually receive radiation therapy to all metastatic sites. Whole lung irradiation is prescribed for patients with more than one lung metastases. If possible, surgical resection for the primary site as well as the metastatic site may be performed prior to radiation therapy.

Patient outcome

Surgery, radiation therapy and two courses of aggressive chemotherapy have enabled the patient to survive three years post presentation of Stage IV alveolar rhabdomyosarcoma. The patient is alive with widespread disease and reduced ability to ambulate.

Case table 8.4 Summary pathology findings of Case 8.4

Diagnosis	Alveolar rhabdomyosarcoma
Size	6.9 × 4.5 × 4.0 cm
Location	Deep (subfascial) tissue of foot
Margin status	N/A as the tumor is biopsied only because Patient is Stage IV at presentation
Histologic grade (FNCLCC grading system)	Grade 3 = High grade
Pathologic stage (AJCC TNM classification)	T2b/N0/M1 = Stage IV
Clinical group staging for RMS	Clinical Group IV (any size primary tumor with or without regional lymph node involvement, with distant metastases, without respect to surgical approach to primary tumor)

Case 8.5 Adult spindle cell/sclerosing rhabdomyosarcoma

Clinical history and presentation

The patient is a 45 year old man who presents with a three month history of an enlarging mass in the left forearm. Fifteen years prior to presentation, the patient was involved in a motor vehicle collision suffering a complex fracture of the forearm requiring open reduction and internal fixation. Although the fractures healed, he developed a pseudarthrosis of the elbow.

Physical examination reveals prior healed scars. The elbow joint is ankylosed at the neutral position. There is a large mass involving the mid-portion of the forearm circumferentially.

Surgical findings and comments

Neoadjuvant chemotherapy is initiated without benefit. Due to the extensive nature of the tumor, history of prior complex surgery, and the ankylosed elbow, limb salvage surgery is not felt to be feasible. Above elbow amputation is performed.

Radiology findings

The images (**Case figs 8.5a** through **8.5e**) show a large aggressive tumor of the flexor compartment in this 45 year old man with remote previous fractures and fixation hardware. The MR appearance is non-specific with T1 low signal, STIR high signal, and heterogeneous intense enhancement. There are no distinguishing features such as calcifications. Although the tumor surrounds the radius, it does not appear to originate in the radius as there is no destruction or erosions of bone. The radiologist can only ascertain this is an aggressive tumor and suggest a sarcoma.

Additional radiologic imaging studies performed during the patient's initial workup reveal several small pulmonary nodules possibly consistent with metastatic disease.

Pathology findings

Gross features

The incisional biopsy of the tumor consists of 6 cm in aggregate of gray to white firm to soft sticky tumor fragments. A portion is submitted fresh to Cytogenetics.

The left forearm amputation shows a large tumor 5 cm proximal to the olecranon (**Case fig. 8.5f**). Cross sections reveal a fleshy, lobulated white to tan 19.5 × 13.5 × 7.5 cm mass abutting the ulna and radius without gross invasion of the bones. The mass is focally gritty and hemorrhagic but no areas of necrosis are grossly discernable (**Case fig. 8.5g**).

Microscopic features

Since the biopsy and the resected tumor are histologically identical, only photomicrographs of the resected tumor are provided.

Low magnification: The tumor is irregularly heterogeneous with three patterns. The most prevalent (about 60%) consists of cellular spindle areas with minimal sclerosis (or collagenization)(**Case fig. 8.5h**). Approximately 30% of the tumor is densely sclerotic (**Case fig. 8.5i**). The third pattern is myxoid and resembles hypocellular areas of classic embryonal RMS. The three patterns also feature numerous foci of obvious rhabdomyoblasts, best appreciated in the sclerotic regions. The three components intermingle to varying extent throughout the tumor sections.

High magnification: At higher magnification, heavily collagenized areas form narrow clefts lined by tumor cells that somewhat mimic vascular channels or microalveoli (**Case fig. 8.5j**). Rhabdomyoblasts cluster conspicuously, especially in sclerotic fields (**Case fig. 8.5k**). Strap cells with cross striations are readily identified (**Case fig. 8.5l**). Myxoid areas suggestive of classic E-RMS contain more primitive appearing stellate to spindle cells (**Case fig. 8.5m**). Markedly pleomorphic tumor cells are lacking, and the neoplastic spindle cells exhibit only mild nuclear atypia (**Case fig. 8.5n**). Necrotic tumor comprises 30% of the total volume, and mitoses number average 10/10 high magnification fields. Lymphovascular invasion is not identified. Two lymph nodes are negative for tumor.

Special studies: Consistent with the diagnosis of rhabdomyosarcoma, the tumor cells are diffusely strongly positive for desmin

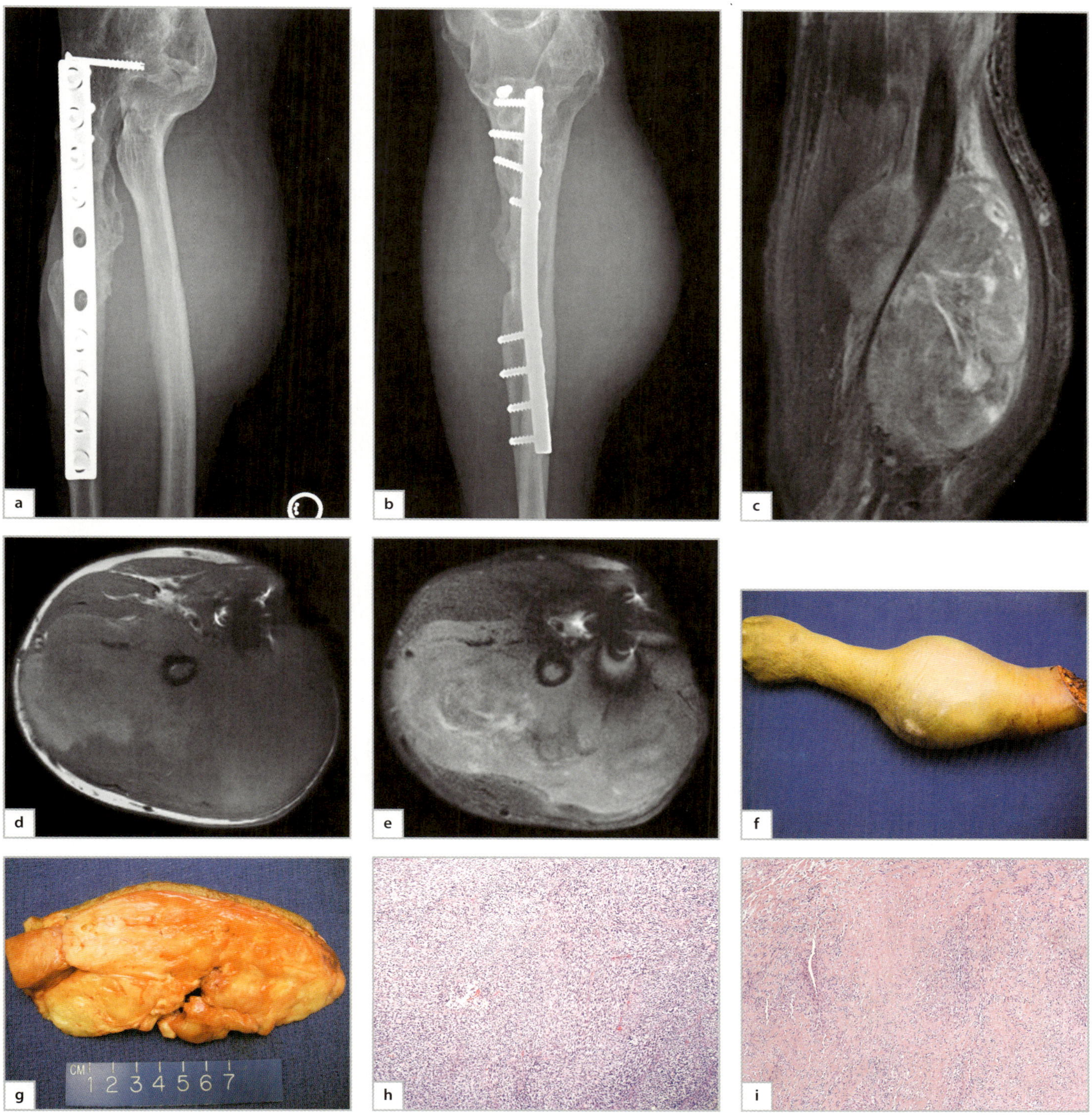

Case figure 8.5 Adult spindle cell rhabdomyosarcoma radiology images. **8.5a** and **8.5b**: Anteroposterior and lateral radiographs of the forearm. **8.5c**: Coronal STIR MR image. **8.5d**: Axial T1 MR image. **8.5e**, Axial T1 post-contrast MR image. The radiographs show a large soft tissue mass without calcification or bone erosion. The ulnar hardware was placed for remote previous fracture fixation and causes metallic artifact. The MR images show a mass measuring 10.4 × 12 × 7.3 cm in the flexor compartment of the proximal forearm. The mass has nonspecific T1 low signal with STIR high signal and shows heterogeneous intense enhancement. **8.5f**: Gross photo of forearm amputation. The tumor forms a large mass just distal to the elbow. **8.5g**: Gross photo of representative cross section of tumor. Typical of a sarcoma, the tumor is vaguely lobulated and fleshy with small chalky white areas suggestive of necrosis. **8.5h**: Low magnification. Sixty percent of the tumor comprises interweaving short fascicles of fairly uniform spindle cells. **8.5i**: Low magnification. Thirty percent of the tumor is densely sclerotic with heavy collagen deposition.

Case figure 8.5: Continued from page 179

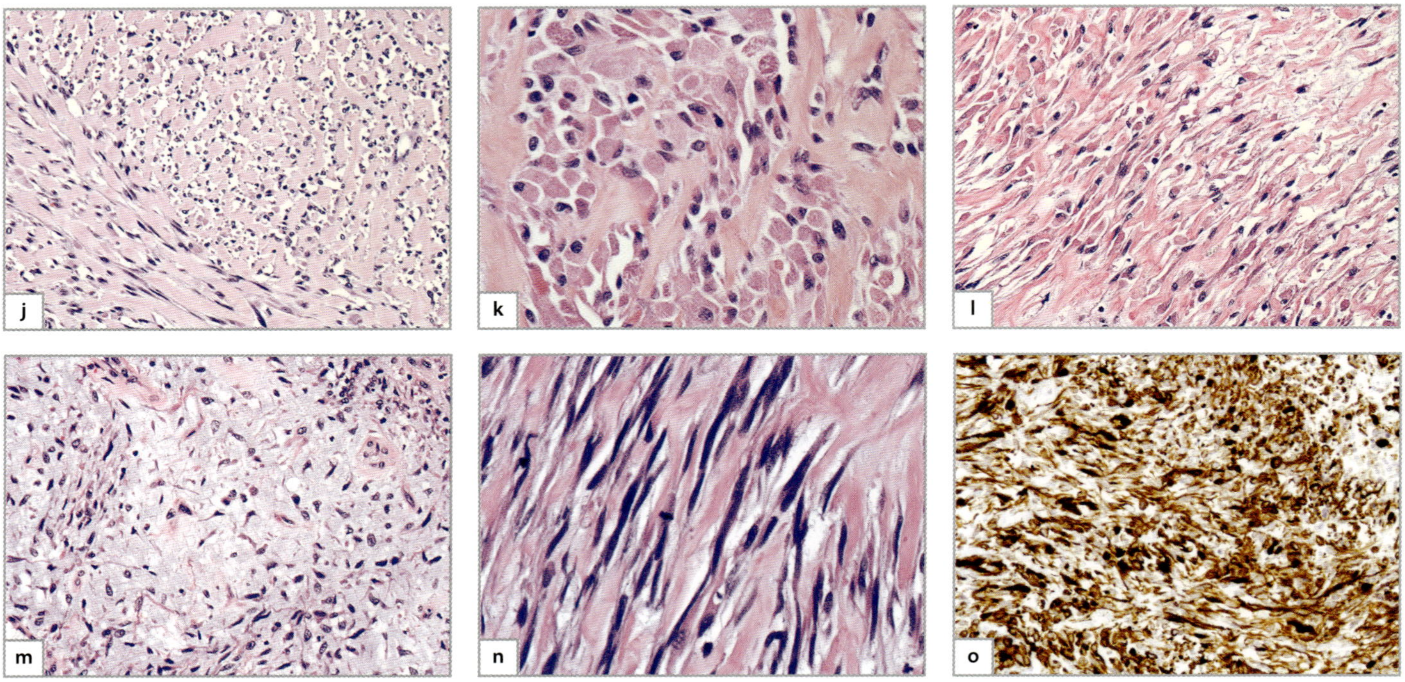

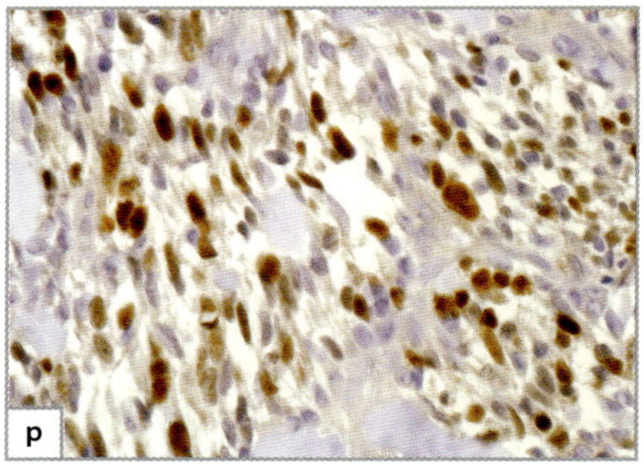

8.5j: Higher magnification. Some of the sclerotic areas feature narrow clefts lined by tumor cells. This has been described as a pseudovascular or microalveolar pattern. **8.5k**: High magnification. Rhabdomyoblasts are a key clue to the diagnosis of RMS, and this patient's tumor contains abundant clusters of the brightly eosinophilic cells with characteristic clumpy cytoplasm. **8.5l**: High magnification, condenser out. Removing the condenser of the microscope helps accentuate cross-striations in some of the rhabdomyoblasts. **8.5m**: High magnification. Ten percent of the patient's tumor resembles embryonal RMS: myxoid hypocellular areas containing primitive stellate and spindle cells. **8.5n**: High magnification. The spindle tumor cells are uniform with pointy ended, slightly hyperchromatic nuclei. A mitotic figure is evident. A nonspecific field such as this could easily be seen in leiomyosarcoma, low grade myofibroblastic sarcoma or even sarcomatoid carcinoma, among others. **8.5o**: Desmin IHC. Tumor cells are diffusely strongly positive for desmin, an intermediate filament protein that usually is expressed in muscle tumors. **8.5p**: Myogenin IHC. A minority of tumor cells express myogenin, a specific skeletal muscle marker. Adult spindle cell/sclerosing RMS may show only focal myogenin reactivity in contrast to most A-RMS which commonly diffusely express this transcriptional regulator.

(**Case fig. 8.5o**). Approximately 10% of tumor cells express myogenin (variable reactivity is reported in adult spindle cell RMS)(**Case fig. 8.5p**). Tumor cells show multifocal expression of smooth muscle actin (30% of tumor cells reactive).

The tumor karyotype is complex with two related and evolving cell lines and multiple numerical and structural abnormalities: 45~46,-10,t(11;14)(p13;q11.2),-16,add(17)(p13),+1~2mar [cp10]/46,XY,t(1;7)(q21;q36),-10,add(10)(q22),t(11;14)(p13;q11.2),-16,del(22)(q12),+2mar[6]/46,XY[4]. There are few reports of the karyotype of adult spindle cell/sclerosing RMS. Findings include complex aneuploidy that is more commonly hyperdiploid (but tetraploidy has also been reported), encompassing +2,+7, +8, +9, +11,+12,+14,+16,+18,+19 and +21, and loss of 3, parts of 12, Y and 10q22 without consistency across cases (Wang et al. 2008).

Pathologic differential or, why isn't it one of the following?

Leiomyosarcoma: Although LMS can exhibit the storiforming cellular spindle cell areas, myxoid areas, and sclerosing areas of this patient's tumor; it does not contain rhabdomyoblasts which are relatively abundant in this tumor. LMS also does not express myogenin, which, although only labeling 10% of tumor cells, is sufficiently positive in this tumor to confirm skeletal muscle differentiation.

Myofibroblastic sarcoma: The storiforming spindle cell areas and relatively low nuclear grade could be consistent with low grade myofibroblastic sarcoma. However, rhabdomyoblasts are inconsistent with the diagnosis. Myogenin reactivity is not reported in myofibroblastic sarcoma.

Sclerosing epithelioid fibrosarcoma: Sclerosing epithelioid fibrosarcoma (SEFS) may contain areas spindle cell areas as are present in this patient's tumor. The sclerotic regions are highly reminiscent of SEFS at low magnification. However, once again, rhabdomyoblasts and myogenin nuclear expression exclude that diagnosis. SEFS often discloses a t(7;16)(q34;p11) (FUS-CREB3L2) translocation on genetic analysis. This patient's tumor lacks the translocation.

Oncology approach

Medical oncology

The patient is placed on a course of neoadjuvant chemotherapy comprising vincristine, dactinomycin and cyclophosphamide every three weeks × 3 courses. He tolerates chemotherapy well with only a small gastrointestinal bleed. However, no benefit occurs, and he is switched to doxorubicin and ifosfamide plus vincristine × 1 course. While on the new regiment, the tumor enlarges slightly. Four months after initial biopsy, the patient undergoes amputation of the forearm tumor.

Radiation oncology

Adult type rhabdomyosarcomas are known to be much more aggressive than the pediatric variety. They are also less common in adults than children. Post-operative radiation is usually prescribed, but guidelines are not well defined due to the lack of case series reported in the literature.

Patient outcome

After the amputation, the patient's pulmonary nodules grow, and CT scans also reveal an enlarged left axillary lymph node and multiple peritoneal and omental nodules. Additionally, in just a few months, a painful soft tissue mass of his left chest attains a size of 15 cm. The patient requests supportive care only and is followed by a local oncologist close to his small home town easing significant travel stress for the patient and his family. He succumbs to the effects of widely metastatic disease approximately one year after his initial presentation.

Case table 8.5 Summary pathology findings of Case 8.5

Diagnosis	Adult spindle cell rhabdomyosarcoma
Size	19.5 × 13.5 × 7.5 cm
Location	Deep soft tissue of forearm
Margin status	Widely negative (amputation performed)
Histologic grade (FNCLCC grading system)	Grade 3
Pathologic stage (AJCC TNM classification)	At least stage III (high grade tumor >5.0 cm in deep soft tissue). Possibly Stage IV because of small pulmonary nodules (two measuring 0.6 and 0.8 cm)

REFERENCES

Ahmadi N, Harley E. Costello syndrome and its importance in cancer screening. Arch Otolaryngol Head Neck Surg 2010;136:1029–1029.

Ahn EH, Barr FG. PAX3 (paired box gene 3 (Waardenburg syndrome 1)). Atlas Database: July 2006. http://AtlasGeneticsOncology.org/Genes/PAX3ID70ch2q35.html

Amstutz R, Wachtel M, Troxler H, et al. Phosphorylation regulates transcriptional activity of PAX3/FKHR and reveals novel therapeutic possibilities. Cancer Res 2008;68:3767–76.

Antman K, Crowley J, Balcerzak SP, et al. An intergroup phase III randomized study of doxorubicin and dacarbazine with or without ifosfamide and mesna in advanced soft tissue and bone sarcomas. J Clin Oncol 1993;11:1276–1285.

Balat O, Balat A, Verschraegen C. Sarcoma botryoides of the uterine endocervix: long-term results of conservative surgery. Eur J Gynaecol Oncol 1996;17(5):335–7.

Barr FG, Duan F, Smith LM, et al. Genomic and clinical analysis of 2p24 and 12q13-q14 amplification in alveolar rhabdomyosarcoma: a report from the children's oncology group. Genes Chromosomes Cancer 2009;48:661–672.

Bay JO, Ray-Coquard I, Fayette J, et al. Docetaxel and gemcitabine combination in 133 advanced soft-tissue sarcomas: a retrospective analysis. Int J Cancer 2006;119:706–711.

Cavazzana AO, Schmidt D, Ninfo V, et al. Spindle cell rhabdomyosarcoma. A prognostically favorable variant of rhabdomyosarcoma. Am J Surg Pathol 1992;16(3):229–35.

Chiles MC, Parham DM, Qualman SJ, et al. Sclerosing rhabdomyosarcomas in children and adolescents: a clinicopathologic review of 13 cases from the Intergroup Rhabdomyosarcoma Study Group and Children's Oncology Group. Pedriatr Dev Pathol 2004;7:583–594.

Chwalisz K, DeManno D, Garg R, et al. Therapeutic potential for the selective progesterone receptor modulator asoprisnil in the treatment of leiomyomata. Semin Reprod Med 2004;22(2):113–9.

Crist WM, Anderson JR, Meza JL, et al. Intergroup rhabdomyosarcoma study-IV: results for patients with nonmetastatic disease. J Clin Oncol 2001;19(12):3091–102.

Davicioni E, Anderson MJ, Finckenstein FG, et al. Molecular classification of rhabdomyosarcoma- genotypic and phenotypic determinants of diagnosis. A report from the Children's Oncology Group. Am J Pathol 2009;174:550–564.

Deyrup A, Lee VK, Charles E, et al. Epstein-Barr virus associated smooth muscle tumors are distinctive mesenchymal tumors reflecting multiple infection events: a clinicopathologic and molecular analysis of 29 tumors from 19 patients. Am J Surg Pathol 2006;30:75–82.

Esnaola NF, Rubin BP, Baldini EH, et al. Response to chemotherapy and predictors of survival in adult rhabdomyosarcoma. Ann Surg 2001;234(2):215–223.

Folpe AL, McKenney JK, Bridge JA, et al. Sclerosing rhabdomyosarcoma in adults: report of four cases of a hyalinizing, matrix-rich variant of rhabdomyosarcoma that may be confused with osteosarcoma, chondrosarcoma, or angiosarcoma. Am J Surg Pathol 2002;29:1175–1183.

Fritz A, Percy C, Jack A, et al. (Eds). International Classification of Diseases for Oncology, 3rd ed. Geneva: World Health Organization, 2000;45.

Gorunova L, Bjerkehagen B, Heim S. Paratesticular leiomyoma with a der(14) t(12;14)(q15;q24). Cancer Genetics 2011;204:465–468.

Gupte C, Butt SH, Tirabosco R, et al. Angioleiomyoma: magnetic resonance imaging features in ten cases. Skeletal Radiol 2008;37(11):1003–9.

Hartman DS, Hayes WS, Choyke PL, et al. From the archives of the AFIP. Leiomyosarcoma of the retroperitoneum and inferior vena cava: radiologic-pathologic correlation. Radiographics 1992;12(6):1203–20.

Heerema-McKenney A, Wijnaendts LCD, Pulliam JF, et al. Diffuse myogenin expression by immunohistochemistry is an independent marker of poor survival in rhabdomyosarcoma: a tissue microarray study of 71 primary tumors including correlation with molecular phenotype. Am J Surg Pathol 2008;32:1513–1522.

Hensley ML, Maki R, Venkatraman E, et al. Gemcitabine and docetaxel in patients with unresectable leiomyosarcoma: results of a phase II trial. J Clin Oncol 2002;20:2824–2831.

Hodge JC, Morton CC. Genetic heterogeneity among uterine leiomyomata: insights into malignant progression. Hum Mol Genet 2007;16:R7–R13.

Hu WW, Skapek SX. Childhood rhabdomyosarcoma: new insights on biology and treatment. Curr Oncol Rep 2010;12:402–410.

Jo Vy, CDM Fletcher CDM. Sclerosing paratesticular rhabdomyoma: A morphologically distinct variant mod. Pathol 2013;26 Suppl 2:1A-534A.

Jo VY, Marino-Enriquez A, Fletcher CDM. Epithelioid rhabdomyosarcoma: clinicopathologic analysis of 16 cases of a morphologically distinct variant of rhabdomyosarcoma. Am J Surg Pathol 2011;35:1523–1530.

Karavasilis V, Seddon BM, Ashley S, et al. Significant clinical benefit of first-line palliative chemotherapy in advanced soft-tissue sarcoma. Retrospective analysis and identification of prognostic factors in 488 patients. Cancer 2008;112(7):1585–1591.

Kransdorf MJ, Murphey MD. Imaging of Soft Tissue Tumors, 2nd edn. Baltimore: Lippincott Williams & Wilkins. 2006.

Kransdorf MJ. Malignant soft-tissue tumors in a large referral population: distribution of diagnoses by age, sex and location. Am J Roentgenol 1995;164(1):129–34.

Kuroiwa M, Sakamoto J, Shimada A, et al. Manifestations of alverclar rhabdomyosarcoma as primary cutaneous lesions in a child with Beckwith-Wiedemann syndrome. J Pediatr Surg 2009;44:e31–35.
Li G, Ogose A, Kawashima H, et al. Cytogenetic and real-time quantitative reverse-transcriptase polymerase chain reaction analyses in pleomorphic rhabdomyosarcoma. Cancer Genet Cytogenet 2009;192:1–9.
Liu J, Guzman MA, Pezanowski D, et al. FOXO1-FGFR1 fusion and amplification in a solid variant of alveolar rhabdomyosarcoma. Mod Pathol 2011;24:1327–1335.
Maki RG, Wathen JK, Patel SR, et al. Randomized phase II study of gemcitabine and docetaxel compared with gemcitabine alone in patients with metastatic soft tissue sarcomas: results of sarcoma alliance for research through collaboration study 002. J Clin Oncol 2007;25:2755–2763.
Mandahl N, Flether CDM, Dal Cin P, et al. Comparative cytogenetic study of spindle cell and pleomorphic leiomyosarcomas of soft tissues: a report from the CHAMP Study Group. Cancer Genet Cytogenet 2000;116:66–73.
Martin SE, Temm CJ, Goheen MP, et al. Cytoplasmic p63 immunohistochemistry is a useful marker for muscle differentiation: an immunohistochemical and immunoelectron microscopic study. Mod Pathol 2011;24:1320–1326.
Matsuyama A, Hisaoka M, Hashimoto H. Angioleiomyoma: a clinicopathologic and immunohistochemical reappraisal with special reference to correlation with myopericytoma. Hum Pathol 2007;38:645–651.
McLeod AJ, Zornoza J, Shirkhoda A. Leiomyosarcoma: computed tomographic findings. Radiology 1984;152(1):133–136.
Mentzel T, Katenkamp D. Sclerosing, pseudovascular rhabdomyosarcoma in adults. Clinicopathologic and immunohistochemical analysis of three cases. Virchows Arch 2000;436(4):305–311.
Mentzel T. Spindle cell rhabdomyosarcoma in adults: a new entity in the spectrum of malignant mesenchymal tumors of soft tissues. Pathologe 2010;31(2):91–6.
Miao Y, Cui T, Leng F, et al. Inhibition of high-mobility-group A2 protein binding to DNA by netropsin: a biosensor-surface plasmon resonance assay. Anal Biochem 2008;374(1):7–15.
Mills A, Beck AH, Montgomery KD, et al. Expression of subtype-specific group 1 leiomyosarcoma markers in a wide variety of sarcomas by gene expression analysis and immunohistochemistry. Am J Surg Pathol 2011;35:583–589.
Missiaglia E, Selfe J, Hamdi M, et al. Genomic imbalances in rhabdomyosarcoma cell lines affect expression of genes frequently altered in primary tumors: an approach to identify candidate genes involved in tumor development. Genes Chromosomes Cancer 2009;48:455–467.
Mustafa T, Gimm O, Chen Z, et al. Betulinic acid is an effective CD97 inhibitor in the human medullary thyroid carcinoma cell line MTC-SK. Proceedings American Association Cancer Research 2004;45:A4238.
Nicolas MM, Tamboli P, Gomez JA, et al. Pleomorphic and dedifferentiated leiomyosarcomas: clinicopathologic and immunohistochemical study of 41 cases. Hum Pathol 2010;41:663–671.
Nieman LK, Blocker W, Nansel T, et al. Efficacy and tolerability of CDB-2914 treatment for symptomatic uterine fibroids: a randomized, double-blind, placebo-controlled, phase IIb study. Fertil Steril 2011;95(2):767-72.e1–2.
Nishio J, Iwasaki H, Ohjimi Y, et al. Chromosomal imbalances in angioleiomyomas by comparative genomic hybridization. Inter J Mol Med 2004;13:13–16.
Nucci MR, Drapkin R, Dal Cin P, et al. Distinctive cytogenetic profile in benign metastasizing leiomyoma: pathogenetic implications. Am J Surg Pathol 2007;31:737–743.
Oda Y, Miyajima K, Kawaguchi K, et al. Pleomorphic leiomyosarcoma: clinicopathologic and immunohistochemical study with special emphasis on its distinction from ordinary leiomyosarcoma and malignant fibrous histiocytoma. Am J Surg Pathol 2001;25:1030–1038.
Palumbo R, Palmeri S, Gatti C, et al. Combination chemotherapy using vincristine, adriamycin, cyclophosphamide (VAC) alternating with ifosfamide and etoposide (IE) for advanced soft tissue sarcomas: a phase II study. Oncol Rep 1998;5(1):69.
Parham DM, Ellison DA. Rhabdomyosarcomas in adults and children: an update. Arch Pathol Lab Med 2006;130(10):1454–65.
Patil DT, Laskin WB, Fetsch JF, et al. Inguinal smooth muscle tumors in women – a dichotomous group consisting of Mullerian-type leiomyoma and soft tissue leiomyosarcoma: an analysis of 55 cases. Am J Surg Pathol 2011;35:315–324.
Qualman S, Lynch J, Bridge J, et al. Prevalence and clinical Impact of anaplasia in childhood rhabdomyosarcoma. A report from the Soft Tissue Sarcoma Committee of the Children's Oncology Group. Cancer 2008;113:3242–3247.
Saikawa Y, Tone Y, Ikawa Y, et al. Hemophagocytic alveolar rhabdomyosarcoma. J Clin Oncol 2008;24:5783–5784.
Sampath S, Schultheiss TE, Ryu JK, et al. The role of adjuvant radiation in uterine sarcomas. Int J Radiat Oncol Biol Phys 2010;76(3):728–734.
Shmookler BM, Lauer DH. Retroperitoneal leiomyosarcoma. A clinicopathologic analysis of 36 cases. Am J Surg Pathol 1983;7:269–80.
Simmons M, Tucker AK. The radiology of bone changes in rhabdomyosarcoma. Clin Radiol 1978;29(1):47–52.
Smith AC, Squire JA, Thorner P, et al. Association of alveolar rhabdomyosarcoma with the Beckwith-Wiedemann syndrome. Pediatr Dev Pathol 2001;4:550–8.
Stock N, Chibon F, Binh MBN, et al. Adult-type rhabdomyosarcoma: analysis of 57 cases with clinicopathologic description, identification of three morphologic patterns, and prognosis. Am J Surg Pathol 2009;33:1850–1859.
Surveillance, Epidemiology, and End Results (SEER) Program (www.seer.cancer.gov) SEER*Stat Database: Incidence - SEER 13 Regs Research Data, Nov 2010 Sub (1992-2008) <Single Ages to 85+, Katrina/Rita Population Adjustment> - Linked To County Attributes - Total U.S., 1969-2009 Counties, National Cancer Institute, DCCPS, Surveillance Research Program, Cancer Statistics Branch, released April 2011 (updated 10/28/2011), based on the November 2010 submission.
Svarvar C, Bohling T, Berlin O, et al. Clinical course of nonvisceral soft tissue leiomyosarcoma in 225 patients from the Scandinavian Sarcoma Group. Cancer 2007;109(2):282–91.
Van Glabbeke M, van Oosterom AT, et al. Prognostic factors for the outcome of chemotherapy in advanced soft tissue sarcoma: an analysis of 2,185 patients treated with anthracycline-containing first-line regimens. A European Organization for Research and Treatment of Cancer Soft Tissue and Bone Sarcoma Group Study. J Clin Oncol 1999;17:150–157.
Verschraegen CF, Arias-Pulido H, Lee SJ, et al. Phase IB study of the combination of docetaxel, gemcitabine, and bevacizumab in patients with advanced or recurrent soft tissue sarcoma: the Axtell regimen. Ann Oncol 2012;23(3):785-90.
Wang J, Tu X, Sheng W. Sclerosing rhabdomyosarcoma: a clinicopathologic and immunohistochemical study of five cases. Am J Clin Pathol 2008;129:410–415.
Wang WL, Bones-Valentin RA, Prieto VG, et al. Sarcoma metastases to the skin: A clinicopahologic study of 65 patients. Cancer 2012;118(11):2900–4.
Welborn J, Fenner S, Parks R. Angioleiomyoma: a benign tumor with karyotypic alterations. Cancer Genetics Cytogenet 2010;199:147–148.
Wexler LH, Ladanyi M. Diagnosing alveolar rhabdomyosarcoma: morphology must be coupled with fusion confirmation. J Clin Oncol 2010;28:2126–2128.
Williamson D, Missiaglia E, de Reyniès A, et al. Fusion gene-negative alveolar rhabdomyosarcoma is clinically and molecularly indistinguishable from embryonal rhabdomyosarcoma. J Clin Oncol 2010;28:2151–2158.
Yang J, Du X, Chen K, et al. Genetic aberrations in soft tissue leiomyosarcoma. Cancer Lett 2009;275:1–8.
Yu Z, Kelsey A, Alaggio R, et al. Clinical utility gene card for: alveolar rhabdomyosarcoma. Eur J Hum Genet 2011;e1–e4.

FURTHER READING

Ferrari A, Dileo P, Casanova M, et al. Rhabdomyosarcoma in adults: a retrospective analysis of 171 patients treated at a single institution. Cancer 2003;98(3):571–580.
Hayes-Jordan A, Andrassy R. Rhabdomyosarcoma in children. Curr Opin Pediatr 2009;21(3):373–378.
Paulino AC, Okcu MF. Rhabdomyosarcoma. Curr Probl Cancer 2008;32(1):7–34.
Fletcher CDM, Bridge JA, Hogendoorn P, Mertens F (eds). World Health Organization Classification of Tumours of Soft Tissue and Bone, 4th Ed. Lyon: IARC Press, 2013.

Chapter 9 Pericytic/perivascular tumors

OVERVIEW

Pericytic/perivascular tumors comprise glomus tumors, myopericytoma including myofibroma, and angioleiomyoma (World Health Organization [WHO] 2013 classification).

Nearly all glomus tumors and myopericytic tumors are benign, but rare, aggressive, malignant variants occur. Additionally, glomus tumors include a well defined 'glomus tumor of uncertain malignant potential.' Even when benign, both tumors (but more commonly glomus tumors) may present with a remarkable degree of pain and cold sensitivity. Similarly, angioleiomyoma also presents with pain or cold sensitivity in more than half of cases. Following simple excision for sporadic solitary glomus tumor, myopericytoma and angioleiomyoma, local recurrence does not exceed 10%.

The cell of differentiation for glomus tumors and myopericytoma is described as a perivascular myoid cell, myopericyte, microvascular pericyte, or pericyte. This is a cell that exhibits varying differentiation towards smooth muscle but also has specific features due to an intimate geographic and functional relationship to vascular endothelial cells. This results in close apposition of tumor cells to blood vessels that manifests as cuffs and swirls of lesional cells encircling small vessels in an onion skin pattern, compressive bulging into vessel lumens, or even true vascular invasion which is without clinical consequence in an otherwise histologically benign tumor. By constrast, angioleiomyomas are composed of smooth muscle cells of which some are specialized perivascular, desmin-negative cells. Glomus cells are absent in angioleiomyoma.

A tumor that one might surmise is a pericytic or perivascular tumor based on its former name, soft tissue hemangiopericytoma, actually represents a 'cellular SFT,' an unrelated neoplasm. In contrast to glomus tumors and myopericytoma, the hemangiopericytoma/solitary fibrous tumor (HPC/SFT) does not express muscle markers and instead commonly shows CD34 and BCL-2 reactivity. By electron microscopy, SFT tumor cells are closely related to fibroblasts and are not pericytes. However, similar to perivascular/pericytic tumors, SFT/HPC tumor cells hug thin-walled intralesional vessels distorting their shapes to mimic staghorns or antler horns and sometimes also markedly bulge against the vessel walls imitating invasion. This describes the architecture, which, unfortunately, is not specific to pericytic/perivascular tumors and SFT/HPC but may also be commonly observed in synovial sarcoma, mesenchymal chondrosarcoma, infantile fibrosarcoma, and less commonly in leiomyosarcoma, malignant peripheral nerve sheath tumor, liposarcoma, and undifferentiated sarcoma, among a few others (Gengler et al. 2006). As usual, accurate, specific diagnosis of soft tissue tumors relies not just on histomorphology but also integrates the immunohistochemistry (IHC) profile, genetic data, and clinical and radiologic findings.

CLASSIFICATION

Table 9.1 lists the pericytic/perivascular tumors of soft tissues classified by the WHO in 2013.

DEMOGRAPHICS

Glomus tumors

Glomus tumors are relatively uncommon. Nearly all are benign, and most occur in young adults with either sex equally affected except in the subungual area in which case the tumor occurs much more commonly in women. A particular subvariant, glomangioma (also

Table 9.1 WHO classification of pericytic/perivascular tumors of soft tissue (2013)

Tumor	Behavior	Additional comments
Glomus tumors [includes solid glomus tumor, glomangioma (glomuvenous malformation), glomangiomyoma, glomangiomatosis, symplastic glomus tumor, glomus tumor of uncertain malignant potential, and glomangiosarcoma]	Benign in almost all cases	1% of glomus tumors are malignant (malignant glomus tumor or glomangiosarcoma) 10% are multiple Rare cases are familial
Myopericytoma (includes tumors with a component of myofibroma or glomus tumor) **Myofibroma** (as a pure histologic pattern) is now also included in this category	Benign in almost all cases	Rare myopericytomas are malignant (malignant myopericytoma) Some cases are multiple May be associated with EBV infection in some patients
Angioleiomyoma	Benign	This tumor is also considered by some experts a smooth muscle tumor. However, it does present with similar symptoms (pain and cold sensitivity) and is histologically closely associated with blood vessels similar to glomus tumors and myopericytomas
Benign: does not recur or recurs non-aggressively and does not metastasize. Intermediate: can recur aggressively and/or rarely metastasizes (<5%). Malignant: can recur and commonly metastasizes.		

known as glomuvenous malformation) occurs with greater frequency in children. Most tumors are cutaneous or subcutaneous, although deeper and visceral tumors occur also. The superficial tumors present as small nodules, or in the case of the subungual lesion, as a discoloration under the nail bed.

Malignant glomus tumor and malignant myopericytoma are exceedingly rare; whether the rarity is due to genuine lack of these sarcomas or due in part to misclassification is unknown. Surveillance, Epidemiology and End Results (SEER) data were evaluated from 13 registries during a 15 year period (1994–2008) focusing on glomangiosarcoma (ICDO-3 code is 8710/3) and malignant glomus tumors (ICDO-3 code is 8711/3). The data presented here is restricted to connective, subcutaneous, and 'other' soft tissue. The average annual incidence rate for both glomangiosarcoma and malignant glomus tumors is 0.0 per million. There was 1 glomangiosarcoma case and 8 malignant glomus tumor cases reported in 13 SEER registries for the designated time period. The mean age at diagnosis for patients with malignant glomus tumors is 40.3 years (median = 42.5 years, range = 9.0–61.0 years). Based on the selection criteria, the site of malignant glomus tumors were found in the shoulder, hip and thorax.

Myopericytoma

Myopericytomas are rare lesions, although the rarity may be partially attributable to a lack of identification of this tumor by pathologists, as it is a relatively newly described entity that can exhibit overlapping features with other tumors such as glomus tumor, angioleiomyoma, infantile HPC (preferably termed the cellular variant of myofibroma) and myofibroma. In reality, myopericytoma sits in the center of a spectrum of inter-related myopericytic tumors (see **Figure 9.1**).

Most myopericytomas are painless and occur as a solitary lesion in adults, typically in the superficial tissue of the distal extremities. Any age can be affected, however, without a strong gender predilection. Less than 10% occur as multiple tumors, usually but not always confined to one general area (such as lower leg)(Mentzel et al. 2006).

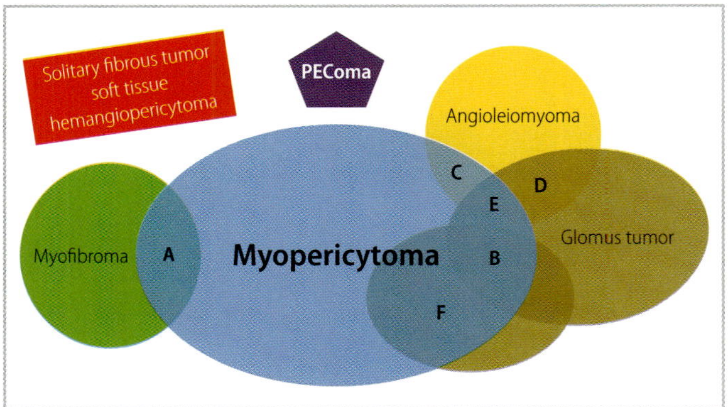

Figure 9.1 Inter-relationship of pericytic/perivascular tumors. Note that HPC/SFT and pecoma (perivascular epithelioid cell tumors) are not related to each other or to the pericytic/perivascular tumor. However, they commonly exhibit a perivascular or hemangiopericytic architecture and could be mistaken for a pericytic/perivascular tumor. A: Myopericytoma with myofibromatous component; B: Myopericytoma with glomus cell component; C: Myopericytoma with angioleiomyomatous component; D: Glomangiomyoma; E: Myopericytoma with glomus cell and angioleiomyomatous component; F: Myopericytoma with HPC-like glomus cell pattern (glomangiopericytoma)

Rarely, myopericytoma displays malignant histologic features. In these cases, the tumor behaves aggressively with a high local recurrence rate, significant risk for metastasis (>40%), and grim five year prognosis matching that of high grade, deep soft tissue leiomyosarcoma (McMenamin et al. 2002). However, tumors confined to the subcutaneous tissue may behave better (Mentzel et al. 2006) concordant with other sarcoma types limited to superficial soft tissue.

Angioleiomyoma

This benign superficial tumor is fairly common and occurs most frequently in young to middle aged adults. Lower extremity lesions occur more often in females while the reverse is true for other body sites.

PATHOGENESIS/ETIOLOGY

The etiologies of glomus tumors, myopericytic tumors and angioleiomyoma are not known. As with other soft tissue and bone tumors, a combination of environmental factors (including EBV infection in rare myopericytomas in AIDS patients), genetic alterations, and possibly epigenetic changes are presumed to be causal.

A few glomus tumors are familial and show truncating mutations of the glomulin gene at chromosome 1p21-22 (Gombos et al. 2008). This gene may also be involved in the more common sporadic glomus tumor.

Glomangiomatosis may be a congenital malformation rather than true neoplasm given its similarity to angiomatosis.

Several cases of myopericytoma have been reported with a t(7;12)(p21-22;q13-15) translocation which fuses the *ACTB* gene (β-actin; 7p21-22) to the *GLI* gene (glioma-associated oncogene homologue 1; 12q13-15) resulting in activation of the *GLI* oncogene (Dahlen et al. 2004). For both the described abnormality of the glomulin gene at 1p21-22 in glomus tumors and the *ACTB-GLI* fusion reported in myopericytoma, the percentage of these tumors bearing these abnormalities is unknown. Tumors (possibly most commonly located in the tongue) showing a hemangiopericytomous architecture without onion skin layering of tumor cells around vessels as in the typical myopericytoma may be more likely to contain the *ACTB-GLI* fusion gene (Dahlen et al. 2004).

Recently, myopericytomas with diffuse expression of Epstein-Barr virus encoded RNAs have been reported in four patients with acquired immunodeficiency syndrome. The tumors exhibited typical morphology or primarily myofibromatous histology, were often located in the viscera, two were multifocal, and two showed increased cellular atypia and/or mitoses (Calderaro et al. 2008, Lau et al. 2009, Ramdial et al. 2011). However, despite alarming features including brain lesions in two individuals, long term survival was observed (at least four years; one patient was lost to follow-up). This behavior matches that of visceral smooth muscle tumors occurring in AIDS patients and which are also EBV associated.

Angioleiomyomas may also occur with increased frequency in EBV infected, immunocommpromised patients, but most are found in patients without these conditions.

PATHOLOGY

The pericytic/perivascular tumors can be bewildering because of terminology similarity, because some tumors contain areas resembling another pericytic/perivascular tumor, and because subvariant morphology and degenerative changes can partially mask classic, more readily diagnosable features. In reality, all perivascular/pericytic tumors are closely related. **Figure 9.1** illustrates this continuum in a Venn diagram fashion. Myopericytoma can be visualized as the central, bridging tumor flanked on either side of the spectrum by myofibroma and glomus tumor. The perivascular epithelioid cell tumor or Pecoma is not related to these tumors, as it features cells with mixed smooth muscle and melanocytic marker expression. Likewise, as previously discussed, solitary fibrous tumor/hemangiopericytoma is not a pericytic/perivascular tumor but a fibroblastic tumor.

Consistent with a specialized myoid phenotype, the pericytic/perivascular tumors express actins and variably express caldesmon and desmon. There is no expression of melanocytic or epithelial markers. Angioleiomyoma is primarily a smooth muscle tumor and lacks glomus cells. **Table 9.2** describes the incidence, body site locations, histologic features and IHC of pericytic/perivascular tumors.

Table 9.2 Pericytic/perivascular tumors of soft tissues

Tumor	Incidence	Age and sex distribution	Body site (in order of frequency)	Histopathology description including IHC	
				Medium magnification	High magnification
Benign: does not recur or does not recur aggressively and does not metastasize					
Solid glomus tumor and variants	Common	All ages but young adults most commonly. M = F except subungual variants in which F > M	Superficial Upper extremity especially fingers/hand/wrist, trunk, lower extremity (may also occur in viscera); may rarely occur in muscle	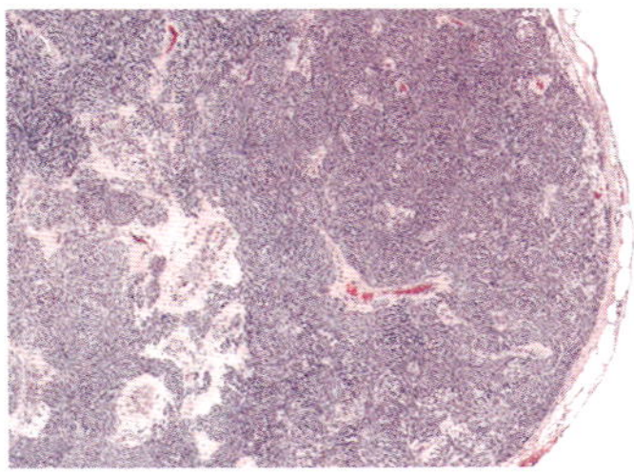	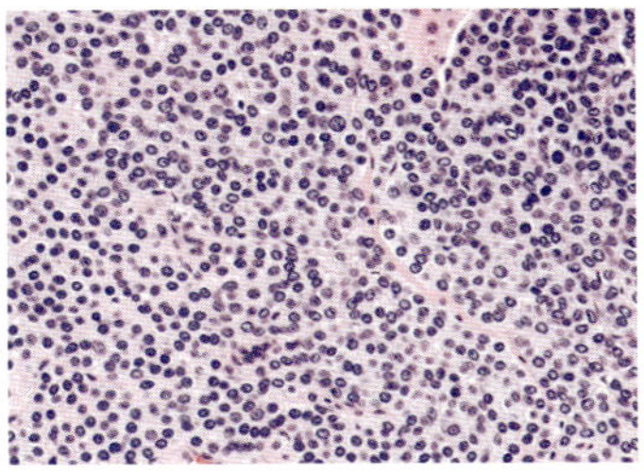
Solid type: most common, circumscribed nodule (up to 3 cm) of uniform round cells with crisp cell borders, round nuclei, rare mitoses, no necrosis or pleomorphism *Glomangioma:* Cells as above with component of dilated thin walled vessels. *Glomangiomyoma:* Cells as above with dilated vessels and also slips of spindled smooth muscle cells. All tumors may focally cluster around vessels in adjacent normal tissue and may show vascular invasion. IHC: All glomus tumors are reactive for SMA, MSA, and may be reactive for caldesmon. Collagen IV shows sharp membranous staining. Negative for S-100 and keratins; desmin rarely focally positive, and CD34 sometimes positive, especially in myxoid cases.				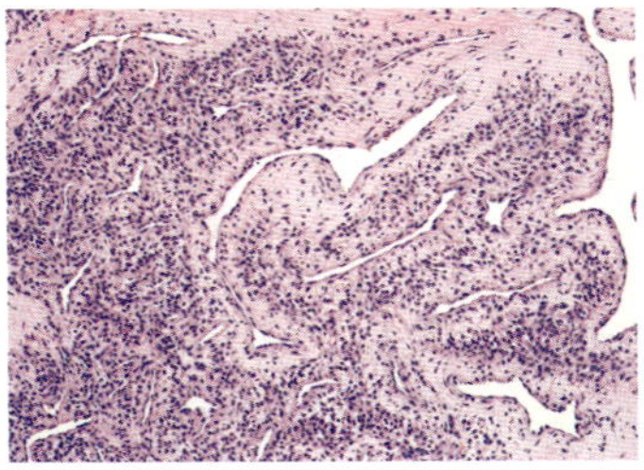	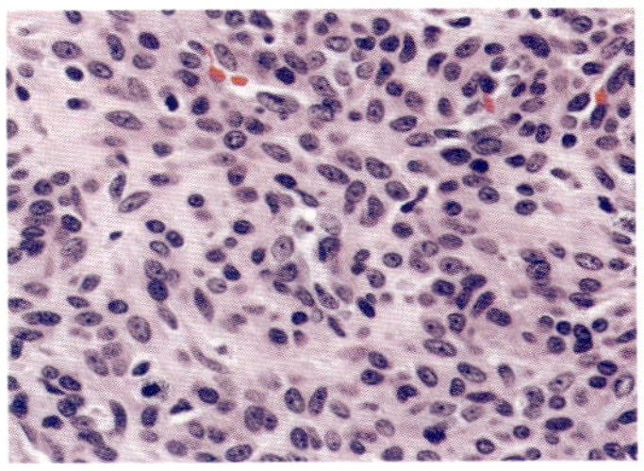
Glomangiomatosis	Very rare	More common in children but young adults also affected (rarely presents in middle age). May be familial (autosomal dominant inheritance). Possibly F > M	Extremities, trunk	No photo available due to rarity of glomangiomatosis	
Very rare pattern of multiple glomus tumors associated with vessels and secondary adipose tissue (looks like angiomatosis with addition of bands and nests of perivascular glomus cells). No cytologic atypia or mitotic activity. Infiltrative growth pattern.					
Symplastic glomus tumor	Very rare	Same age as for solid glomus tumor and variants	Same distribution as for solid glomus tumor and variants	No photo available due to rarity of symplastic glomus tumor	
Glomus tumor with scattered pleomorphic tumor cells showing nuclear hyperchromasia, nuclear enlargement and often multinucleation. Considered a type of benign degenerative atypia. Absent to only rare normal mitoses and no necrosis. Small size and circumscribed.					
Myopericytoma	Rare	Primarily middle aged adults but any age may be affected. M may be slightly > F	Dermis or subcutis of extremities, trunk, head and neck	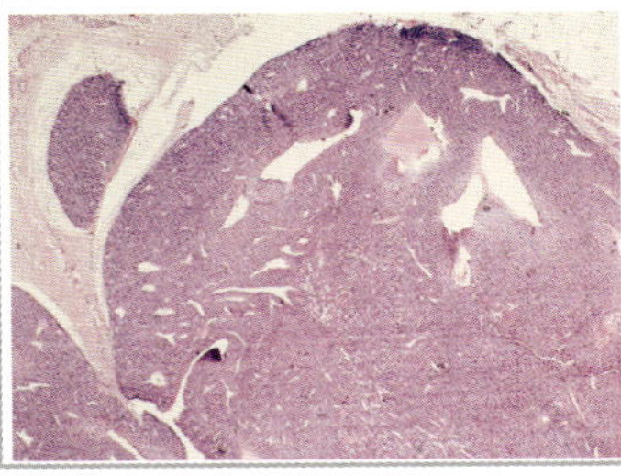	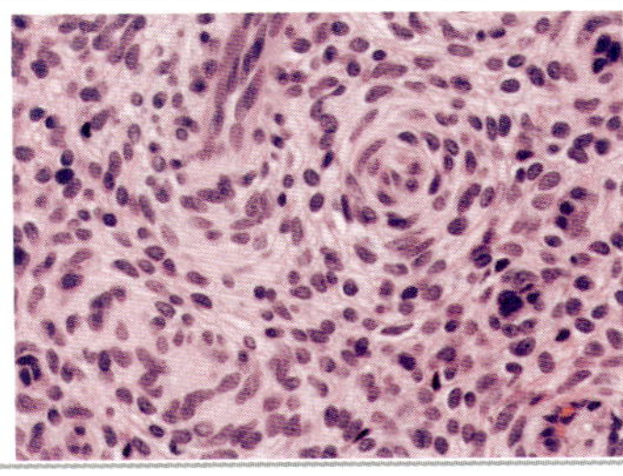
Classic tumor shows concentrically arranged, ovoid to spindle shape myoid appearing cells swirling around small intratumoral vessels in an onion skin pattern. Tumor cells may also replace the muscularis of medium sized vessels. Tumors are usually circumscribed but adjacent vessels may show cuffing by tumor cells and peripheral rim of ectatic, thin-walled vessels. Tumors may also have fascicular and fibrotic regions with compressive bulging into vein walls (resembling myofibroma). Other tumors may contain foci resembling glomus tumor and/or angioleiomyoma. Mitoses are sparse, and there is no necrosis. IHC: Positive for SMA, MSA, caldesmon with rare reactivity for desmin. Negative for S-100 and keratins					

Table 9.2: Continued from page 185

Tumor	Incidence	Age and sex distribution	Body site (in order of frequency)	Histopathology description including IHC	
				Medium magnification	**High magnification**
Myofibroma (as a pure histologic pattern)	Uncommon to rare (myofibromatosis)	Birth to 2 years but any age may be affected. M > F	Superficial tissues of head and neck including oral cavity but can occur anywhere including viscera. Can be multicentric but solitary form much more common	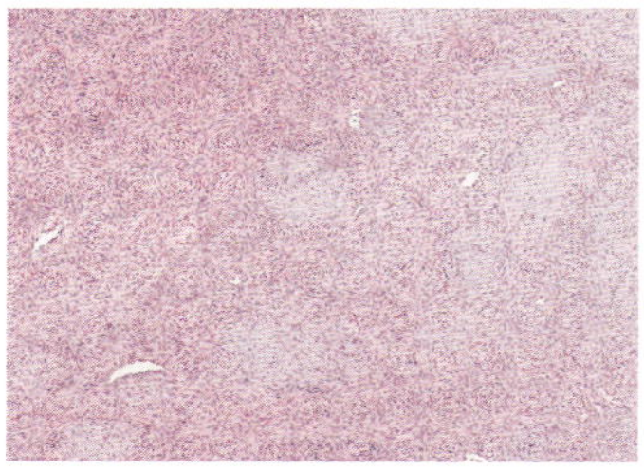	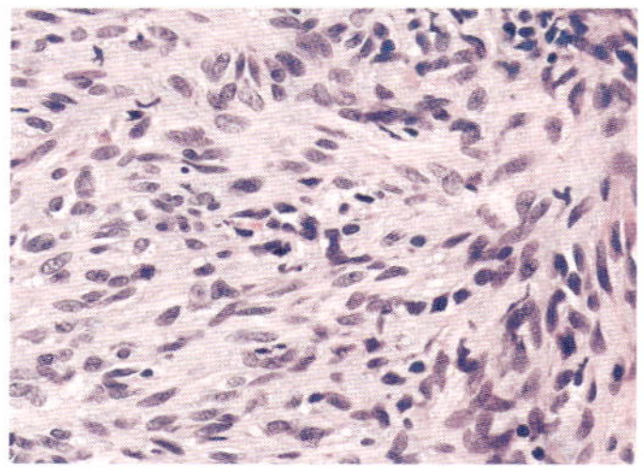
Usually biphasic growth of 1) nodules of mature elongate myofibroblasts distributed in pink matrix, 2) cellular, more primitive fibroblastic areas in between the less cellular pale pink myofibroblastic nodules. Component 2 can have ectatic, 'antler-horn' vessels (HPC vascular pattern). Calcifications, necrosis, fibrosis, and intravascular growth common. IHC: Positive for smooth muscle actin (in myoid nodules) and CD34 in primitive fibroblastic areas (latter may also express MSA)					
Angioleiomyoma	Common	Young to middle aged adults most commonly but broad age range. F > M for solid variant. F > M in lower extremities	Subcutis or deep dermis of extremities and head and neck	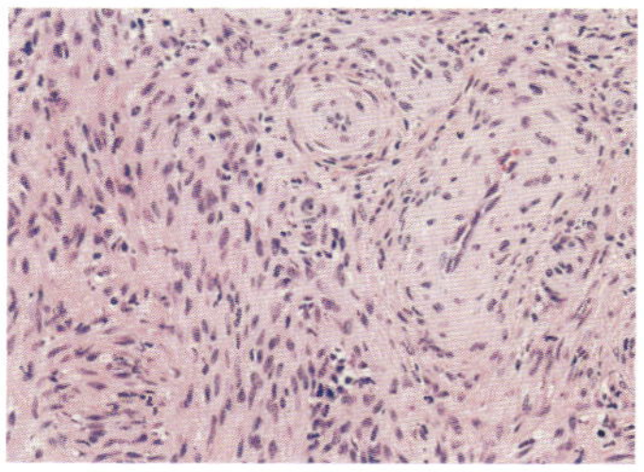	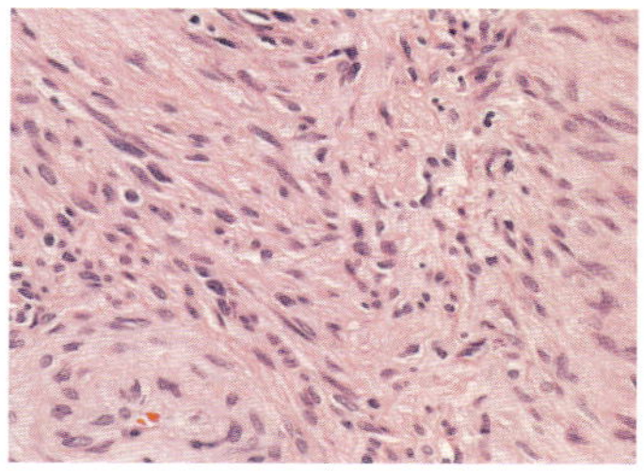
Three variants: solid, venous and cavernous. All composed of smooth muscle cells merging with vessels (thin walled in 'solid' variant, thick walled in 'venous' variant, and dilated and thin walled in 'cavernous' variant). Myxoid change, calcifications and hyalinization common. Most cases <3 cm. IHC: SMA, MSA, positive with variable reactivity for caldesmon and desmin.					
Intermediate: can recur aggressively and/or rarely metastasizes (<5%)					
Glomus tumor of uncertain malignant potential	Rare	Broad age range but primarily young to older adults. M = F	Lower extremity, trunk, upper extremity	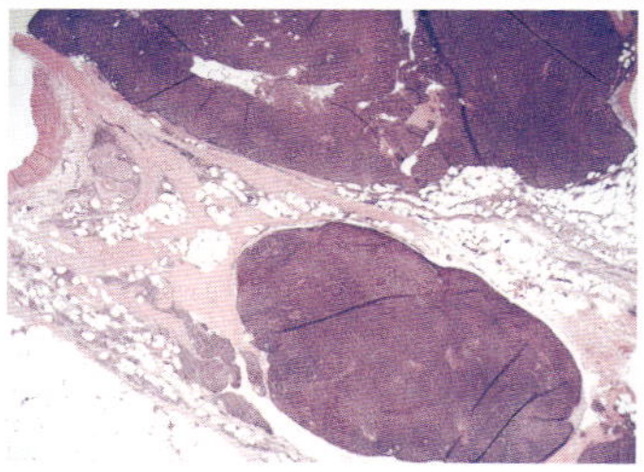	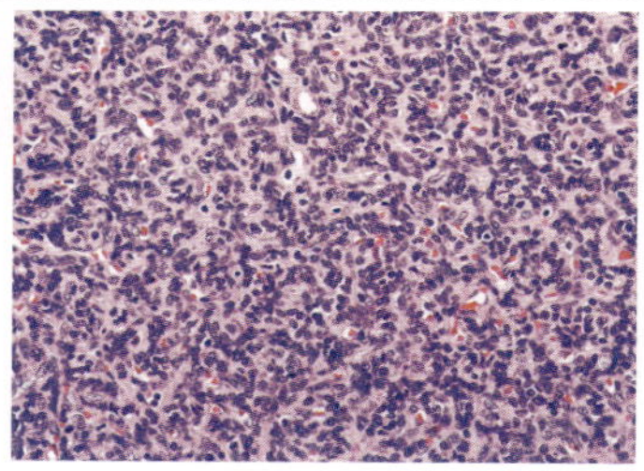
Subset of glomus tumors with atypical features not sufficient to outright consider malignant. Nuclear grade is low to moderate but not high grade. Examples: size >2cm and deep location or superficial location with increased but normal mitoses. May contain a benign glomus tumor component.					
Malignant: can recur and commonly metastasizes					
Glomangiosarcoma (malignant glomus tumor)	Very rare	Primarily adults including elderly. M = F	Lower extremity, upper extremity, and trunk. Can occur in hands and feet but far less commonly than benign glomus tumor. May be superficial or deep	No photo available due to rarity of glomangiosarcoma	
Sarcoma composed of glomus cells that may be round or spindled or both. Newest criteria for malignancy are: 1) atypical mitotic figures and/or 3) marked nuclear atypia and mitotic activity (5 or more mitoses/50 hpf). Tumors are usually > 2 cm. Benign glomus tumor component may be present. IHC: Collagen IV membranous staining may be especially helpful in differential dx. Tumors also positive for SMA, MSA, and variably for caldesmon.					

Table 9.2: Continued from page 186

Malignant Myopericytoma	Very Rare	Middle aged and elderly adults most commonly. Not reported in children	Deep soft tissues of extremities including hands/ feet; H&N, trunk	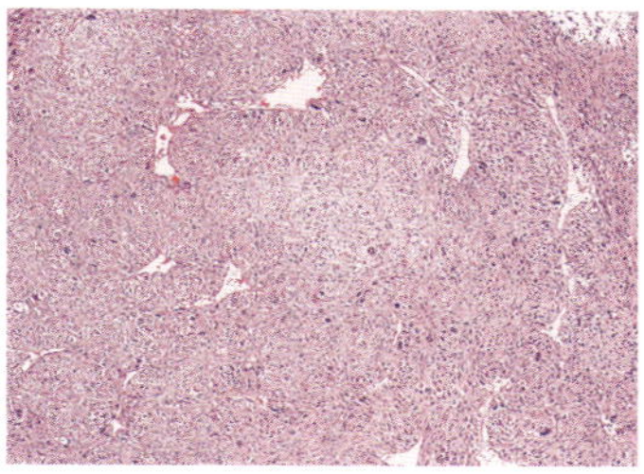 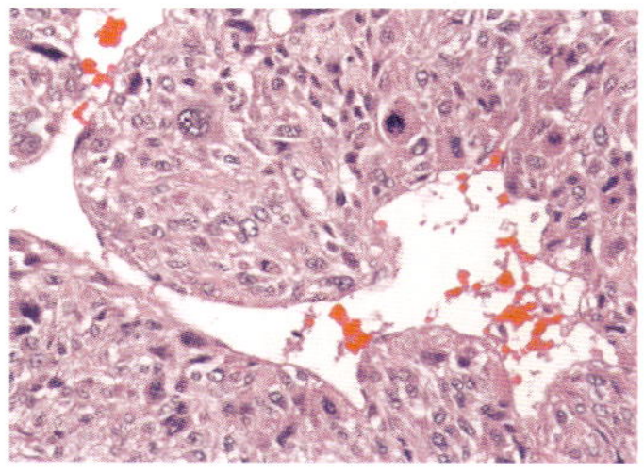
Infiltrative tumor comprising cells ranging from plump, spindled myoid to elongate spindled or glomus cell like. Concentric perivascular growth usually present. May show compressive bulging into veins, replacement of muscularis of medium-sized veins, and perivascular involvement of non-tumoral vessels. Features nuclear atypia, increased mitoses, and necrosis. IHC: SMA, MSA positive; may be caldesmon positive. Usually negative for keratins, EMA, desmin. S-100 negative.				

M: male, F: female. SMA: smooth muscle actin, MSA: muscle specific actin.

Incidence Note: 'Common to very common' indicates that a medium sized practice will treat at least several to dozens of patients with the lesion annually, 'Uncommon to rare' indicates the same practice size will treat one to two patients with the lesion every five years, 'Rare to very rare' indicates the same sized practice will see zero to one patient with the lesion every 20 years

Histologic grading

Glomus tumors

Nearly all glomus tumors are histologically and behaviorally benign and closely resemble glomus cells of the normal glomus body that regulates tissue temperature by adjusting blood flow in the extremities. Rare, otherwise typical glomus tumors may exhibit nuclear atypia without an appreciable mitotic rate (less than 1/50 hpf); these symplastic glomus tumors contain some cells with enlarged, often irregularly shaped nuclei with hyperchromasia and smudgy chromatin and scattered, multinucleated, tumor giant cells.

In 2001 Folpe and colleagues reviewed 52 atypical glomus tumors for the purpose of identifying histologic features that would predict behavior. Their initial criteria for malignancy were as follows: deep (subfascial) tumor greater than 2 cm, or superficial or deep tumor with atypical mitoses or moderate to high nuclear grade with greater than or equal to 5 mitoses per 50 hpf (Folpe et al. 2001). In many tumor examples, several of these features coincided. According to the authors, low nuclear grade comprises cells that look like normal glomus cells with small regular nuclei and indistinct nucleoli, moderate nuclear grade comprises cells with increased nuclear variability and scattered prominent nucleoli, while high nuclear grade is typified by cells with nuclei two to three types the size of normal glomus cell nuclei, marked nuclear variability, and diffuse, prominent nucleoli.

In their review of 52 cases of atypical glomus tumors, the authors also created a category of 'glomus tumor of uncertain malignant potential' characterized by superficial tumors with increased mitoses (>5/50 hpf), or large size only (>2 cm) or deep location only. When stratifying the atypical and malignant glomus tumors in this fashion, the authors found that metastasizes occurred in approximately 40% of malignant tumors and not in any of the other tumors (mean follow-up of 5.5 years) (Folpe et al. 2001). Using these aforementioned criteria, glomangiomatosis lacks features of glomangiosarcoma or glomus tumor of uncertain malignant potential and shows diffuse growth akin to angiomatosis but with the addition of increased glomus cells surrounding the proliferation of small or large blood vessels.

More recently, with study of additional cases, it has become clear that deep location or large size alone (>2 cm) does not indicate malignancy. Currently, a malignant glomus tumor is diagnosed based on marked nuclear atypia and/or atypical mitotic figures. Tumors with at least one atypical feature (such as large size, or deep location) are now considered glomus tumors of uncertain malignant potential (Folpe et al. 2010; Fletcher et al. 2013).

Clearly, the histologic criteria predicting malignant behavior are complicated. This is understandable given the rarity of the tumors that behave aggressively, as there are few of these tumors to study in a statistically significant manner.

Myopericytoma

The vast majority of myopericytomas are benign. An extremely rare malignant variant has been described which exhibits permeative growth, marked nuclear atypia, an elevated mitotic rate, and areas of necrosis (McMenamin et al. 2002, Fischer et al. 2011). There is no 'myopericytoma of uncertain malignant behavior' category.

Angioleiomyoma

Angioleiomyomas are benign and are not graded. Mitotic activity may be present, however, and it is important to not confuse such examples with leiomyosarcoma or atypical smooth muscle tumor of soft tissue.

Behavior

As noted previously, most glomus tumors and myopericytomas are benign tumors. Ten percent of glomus tumors are multiple, 10% are at risk for local recurrence, and approximately 1% are malignant. The rare malignant cases thus far reported appear to behave aggressively.

Similarly, myopericytomas exhibit a low rate of local recurrence with complete conservative excision. Some patients present with metachronous tumors usually involving one body site such as the foot. The very rare malignant myopericytoma appears to behave aggressively with early metastasis and short survival time (McMenamin et al. 2002). Patients with superficial tumors entirely resected at low stage may have a better outcome (Mentzel et al. 2006).

It is possible that in exceptional circumstances, benign glomus tumors and myopericytomas may transform to glomangiosarcoma or malignant myopericytoma, respectively, because these sarcomas not uncommonly contain foci identical to their benign counterpart.

Additional laboratory testing

As might be expected given their close relationship, the immunohistochemical profile of glomus tumor and myopericytoma is nearly identical. Both express muscle actins (smooth muscle actin and muscle specific or HHF-actin) and both commonly also express caldesmon. Potentially, specific antibodies may be developed in the future that could readily distinguish glomus tumors from myopericytoma.

In general, distinguishing between a glomus tumor and a myopericytoma with focal glomoid features may sometimes present a challenge. Fortunately, this diagnostic conundrum does not incur clinical significance. The same holds true for solitary myofibroma versus myopericytoma, as some myopericytomas contain fields of tumor histologically identical to myofibroma. Myopericytomas that do contain regions simulating related tumors also contain fields of classic myopericytoma; these latter regions lead to the correct diagnosis.

IHC

Glomus tumors diffusely express smooth muscle actin and (and usually) caldesmon and show membranous (actually pericellular) Type IV collagen reactivity. Desmin expression is commonly absent or at most focal except in the variant containing smooth muscle, the glomangiomyoma . CD34 is usually negative except in glomus tumors with secondary myxoid change in which case CD34 may be expressed. Tumor cells are negative for keratins and S-100 protein.

Myopericytoma shares a similar immunohistochemical expression profile with glomus tumor comprising diffuse reactivity for smooth muscle actin, HHF-actin (muscle specific actin), collagen IV and caldesmon. Some tumors show patchy reactivity for calponin. In most cases, desmin is not expressed. Tumor cells are negative for EMA, CD34, and pankeratins. Malignant myopericytoma, however, has been reported to focally express EMA and keratins (McMenamin et al. 2002).

Angioleiomyomas express smooth muscle antigens including smooth muscle actin, muscle specific actin and calponin with variable expression of h-caldesmon. Desmin is usually also expressed except in areas of concentric swirling of tumor cells around vessels (Fletcher et al. 2013).

Routine cytogenetics

In general, glomus tumors are not karyotyped because classic histologic features, IHC expression profile and clinical presentation enable the correct diagnosis.

In rare instances, routine cytogenetics may be helpful in the diagnosis of myopericytoma, because karyotyping may reveal the potentially characteristic translocation t(7;12)(p21-22;q13-15). However, this translocation may be more specific to tumors showing a dominant HPC pattern of growth (Dahlen et al. 2004).

Angioleiomyomas are usually diploid. No consistent genetic findings have been reported.

Molecular genetics

PCR or fluorescence in-situ hybridization can be performed to identify the t(7:12) translocation.

Malignant glomus tumor and malignant myopericytoma have not been examined for targetable cell pathway aberrations as is ongoing for other sarcomas. The extreme rarity of these sarcomas limits specimen access for such studies.

RADIOLOGY OF PERICYTIC/ PERIVASCULAR TUMORS

Glomus tumor is a relatively rare tumor arising from the glomus body. These usually occur in the subungual region of the finger tips. They can present with the clinical triad of pain, point tenderness and cold sensitivity. Radiographs are often normal or may show a sharply circumscribed lucent lesion with sclerotic margins. MR usually shows very high signal on fluid sensitive sequences and commonly has intense uniform enhancement (Glazebrook et al. 2011). A differential for distal phalanx lucent lesion includes enchondroma and epidermal inclusion cyst. Enchondromas are usually not calcified in the digits and are medullary in location and may have mild endosteal scalloping. Epidermal inclusion cyst is usually asymptomatic.

Malignant glomus tumors, or glomangiosarcomas are quite rare and usually only show local invasion. Distant metastasis can occur however, this is thought to be extremely rare. Unfortunately, we do not have a case with imaging. Case reports indicate the tumors are hypervascular and well defined with modest PET uptake (Rodriguez-Justo et al. 2001, Kleontas et al. 2010).

Myopericytoma is a benign tumor of the skin occurring in the distal extremities of adults. Less common locations include the head and neck and trunk (Terada 2010). They present as a firm mass that is usually painless, (Paek et al. 2011). There is little published of the imaging appearance of myopericytoma. Roh et al. 2011, describes intense enhancement on CT with marked hypervascularity of power Doppler ultrasound imaging.

SURGERY OF PERICYTIC/ PERIVASCULAR TUMORS

Glomus tumor benign variants

Marginal excision of these tumors results in a very low (<10%) rate of recurrence. Recurrences occur more commonly with incompletely excised tumors or with rare diffuse or infiltrative tumors.

Glomus tumor of uncertain malignant potential

Conservative surgery results in a low incidence of recurrence. Despite its nomenclature, metastases have not been reported if the tumor is classified correctly.

Glomangiosarcoma (Malignant glomus tumor)

This is a rare sarcoma that should be treated with aggressive surgical resection.

Myopericytoma

Most myopericytomas are benign lesions and can be treated conservatively. A few recurring and malignant cases have been reported. Recurrence, particularly multiple, would warrant more aggressive surgical resection.

Angioleiomyoma

Simple excision is curative.

MEDICAL ONCOLOGY OF PERICYTIC/PERIVASCULAR TUMORS

Glomus tumors

Most glomus tumors are benign, and up to 25% are transmitted in an autosomal dominant manner, with incomplete penetrance (Calvert et al. 2001, Simi et al. 2005, Tran et al. 1994). Only offspring of males possessing the disease gene develop tumors through genomic imprinting. Deletions in the glomulin gene have been discovered in affected families (Brouillard et al. 2002, Hoekzema et al. 2010).

The typical benign solitary lesion is small, rarely exceeding 1.0 cm in greatest dimension. It usually forms a bulging unencapsulated mass with an irregular, nodular dark red-bluish surface. When multiple, the tumors are usually 0.1–0.3 cm in diameter, but lesions up to 3.0 cm have been reported (Chen et al. 1995, Fornage 1988, Schopp et al. 2009). Symptoms include excruciating pain out of proportion to size, localized tenderness, and cold sensitivity. The lesion is characteristically solitary with a benign clinical behavior and arises in anatomic location rich in glomus bodies, such as under the nails, under the skin of the palm and soles, but could be found anywhere in any soft tissue. The average age at presentation is between 30 and 50 years of age, but these tumors can occur at any age. They are usually solitary and small. Solitary glomus tumors of the digit are more frequent in adult women.

Glomus tumors account for 1–4.5 % of tumors in the hand. Finger tumors are usually painful, and the pain is exacerbated by cold. The pain can be intense and radiate into the arm and elbow. Although patients seek medical attention early, the mass is frequently too small to be identified on physical examination (Koc et al. 2007), thus years may elapse from onset of symptoms to correct diagnosis. Sometimes, a small blue spot can be seen at the base of the nail.
In 10% of cases, multiple tumors may develop and this happens usually 10–15 years earlier than the development of a solitary lesion. About one third of multiple glomus tumors occur in children.

Multiple tumors should not be confused with metastases of a malignant glomus tumor. Malignant glomus tumors or glomangiosarcomas are rare (Folpe et al. 2001). Metastases from glomus tumors occur in very few cases due to the rarity of the malignant version (De Chiara et al. 2003, Lancerotto et al. 2012). Metastases are found in lungs, lymph nodes, liver, vertebrae, ribs, and spleen.

Myopericytoma

Most myopericytomas are benign. Related tumors include infantile-type myofibromatosis, solitary myofibroma, infantile haemangiopericytoma, and glomangiopericytoma (Granter et al. 1998).

Multiple myopericytomas may occur (Mentzel et al. 2006). Treatment is surgical only. Local recurrences are uncommon. Malignant myopericytoma is extremely rare and appears to behave aggressively (from the small number of cases reported to date).

Medical oncology of glomangiosarcoma and maligannt myopericytoma

There is no specifically defined treatment for malignant metastatic glomus tumor or myopericytoma. They should be considered sarcoma and treated with generic sarcoma chemotherapy. Palliative measures should be initiated early in the metastatic process.

RADIATION ONCOLOGY OF PERICYTIC/PERIVASCULAR TUMORS

As a group, pericytic and perivascular tumors are typically uncommon to rare and usually benign. Most common management is surgical resection only. In cases of recurrent, aggressive, or incompletely excised lesions, radiation therapy can be considered for local control. In cases where surgery is associated with significant morbidity, radiation therapy could also be considered. Given these tumors are typically identified in the distal extremities; radiation therapy has not played a large role in the treatment of this tumor type.

CASES

Case 9.1 Glomus tumor

Clinical history and presentation

The patient is a 24-year-old female who relates an approximately one year history of progressive pain along the radial aspect of her long finger. She states that approximately 2 years ago, she had an injury to this finger when she slammed it in a car door sustaining a partial nail injury. Symptoms began approximately one year ago. Within the past 6 weeks the pain has become more intense and is now excruciating. She describes the pain as sharp needle-like pain that begins under her nail and radiates proximally. Pain has been refractory to treatment with amitriptyline. It does wake her up at night and soaking it under hot water helps mildly. Her hand has been sensitive to cold. However, she denies any swelling or drainage at the nail.

Examination of the patient's left hand reveals no swelling or signs of infection at the long finger distal interphalangeal joint or nail. There is no surrounding erythema. There is no drainage. She is exquisitely point tender to the radial aspect of her long finger distal to the distal interphalangeal joint and around the nail. She does have full range of motion at the distal interphalangeal joint and proximal interphalangeal joint with no discoloration or palpable mass. She is otherwise neurologically intact throughout the hand, and sensation is intact to light touch along the left long finger.

Radiology findings

The case (**Case figs 9.1a** through **9.1f**) shows a subtle erosive lesion of the distal phalanx of the 3rd finger. On MRI, the mass is quite small perhaps accounting for the only modest enhancement and STIR high signal seen. Typically, glomus tumors are higher signal on STIR and T2 images with strong enhancement. The location is typical; along the medial or lateral margins of a distal phalanx.

The additional case of glomus tumor shown in radiographs (**Case figs 9.1g** and **9.1h**) has the more typically seen sharply defined erosion, with smooth, sclerotic margins. Often MR imaging is not needed given the typical radiographic appearance and clinical presentation.

Surgical findings and comments

At surgery, a fleshy tumor is encountered deep to the nail bed and is curetted.

Pathology findings

Gross features

The specimen consists of multiple tissue fragments aggregating to 1.5 cm. Ink is applied to a larger fragment that contains a tan solid nodule measuring 0.5 cm maximally.

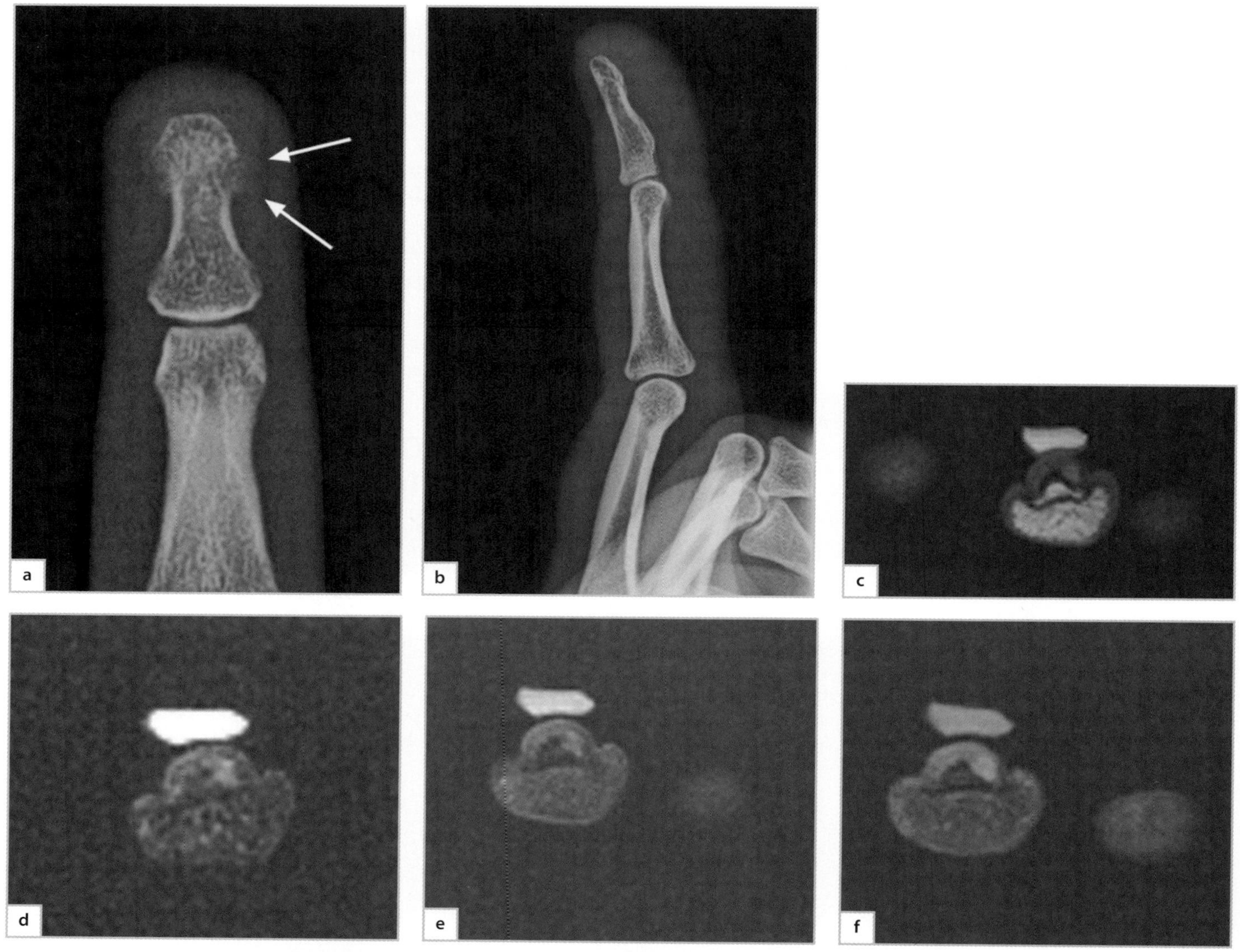

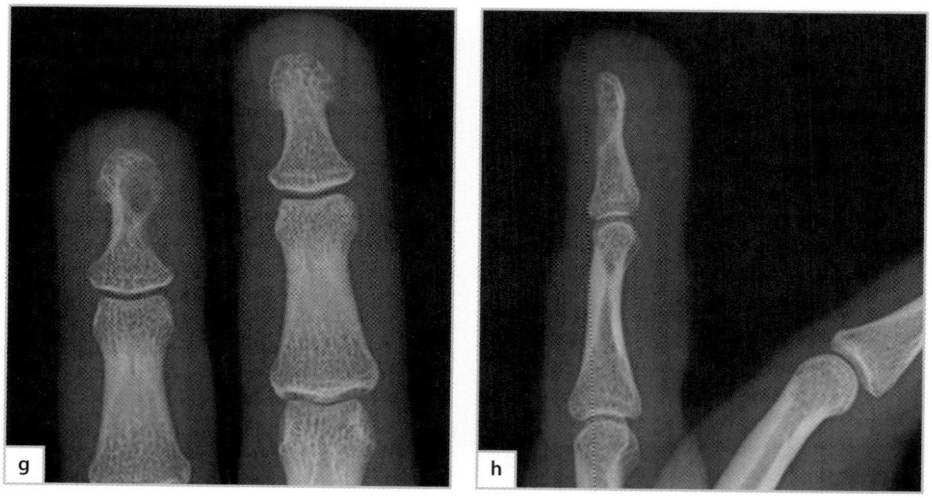

Case figure 9.1 Glomus tumor.
9.1a: Anteroposterior, **9.1b:** lateral radiographs show a subtle lucent lesion of the radial aspect of the 3rd finger distal phalanx. **9.1c:** Axial T1, **9.1d:** Axial STIR, **9.1e:** Axial T1 fat saturation pre-contrast and **9-1f** axial T1 fat saturation post-contrast MR images show a small mass (2.7 × 5.6 × 2.6 mm) with mild T1 high signal and moderate STIR high signal in the unguis of the 3rd finger. The lesion shows minimal enhancement. Note the subtle scalloping of the cortex, best seen on axial images with normal marrow. We present an additional case of glomus tumor. **9.1g:** Anteroposterior, **9.1h:** Lateral radiographs showing a lucent sharply defined defect of the radial aspect of the 4th distal phalanx. There is mild soft tissue swelling. The margins are mildly sclerotic and smooth.

Case figure 9.1: Continued from page 190

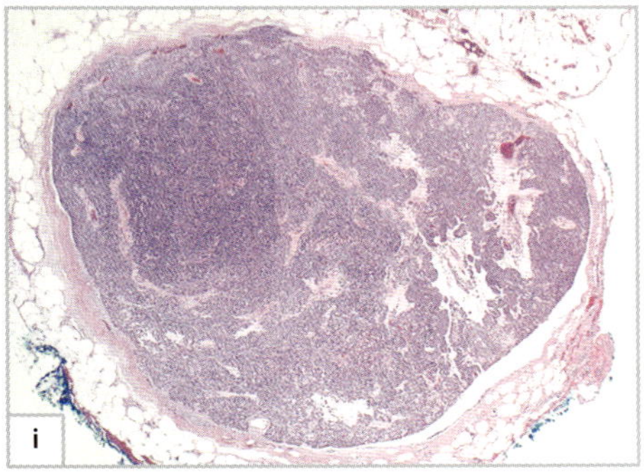
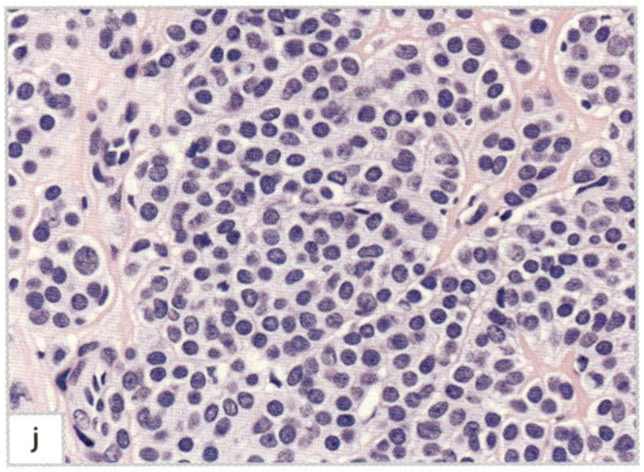
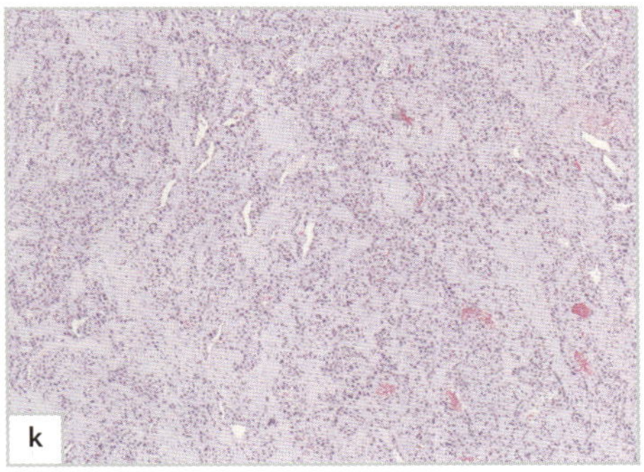
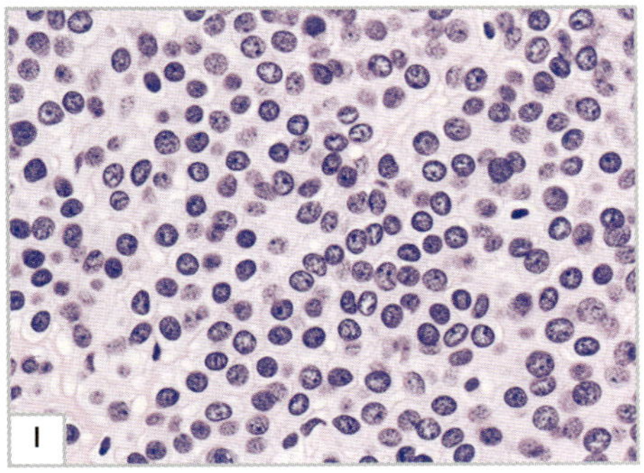

9.1i: Solid variant, low magnification. The patient's tumor is small, located in subcutaneous tissue, and encapsulated. Although small vessels are numerous in the tumor, it is termed the solid variant because large cavernous veins are absent (the glomangioma variant). **9.1j:** Solid variant, medium magnification. In this field, the tumor is nested or organoid. Other areas comprise more sheet like growth interrupted by frequent small vessels. The scant background matrix is hyalinized. **9.1k:** Solid variant with prominent myxoid matrix. Some glomus tumors feature a prominent myxoid matrix as is the case with this example (not the patient's tumor). Myxoid glomus tumors are more likely to express CD34 than non-myxoid cases. **9.1l:** Solid variant, high magnification. Classic glomus cell features are present including evenly spaced round tumor cells with famously uniform round nuclei without hyperchromasia or macronucleoli (the nuclei appear punched out from a single mold). Fine pink strands of basement membrane encase each cell; this would appear as membranous Collagen IV expression by IHC. Not every field in the patient's tumor is so well organized (cells elsewhere are jumbled without so much basement membrane), but areas like this clinch the diagnosis.

Microscopic features

Low magnification: The single small tumor is small, encapsulated and cellular (**Case fig. 9.1i**). Many solitary glomus tumors exhibit a pushing or discrete margin and some, as in this case, feature a true capsule. Even encapsulated tumors may involve adjacent vessels with increased glomus cells clustered against walls of small veins. This patient's tumor does not show this extension beyond the tumor.

High magnification: Medium magnification reveals nests of uniform, round cells embedded in a hyalinized matrix (**Case fig. 9.1j**). Glomus tumors may also contain a myxoid matrix (**Case fig. 9.1k**). Interestingly, myxoid glomus tumors are more likely to express CD34 than non-myxoid examples. High magnification shows the classic features of glomus cells: uniform round cells with sharply defined cell borders. The nuclear to cytoplasmic ratio is typically moderate meaning there is relatively scant cytoplasm (**Case fig. 9.1l**). The round to slightly oval tumor cell nuclei are normochromatic with evenly distributed chromatin and inconspicuous to small nucleoli. Necrosis and mitotic activity are absent. Thin strands of basement membrane material encircle every cell.

Special studies: This case is classic in presentation, location and histologic features, so special stains or studies are not performed. However, if performed, the tumor cells would diffusely express smooth muscle actin, and Collagen IV antibody would highlight the pericellular basement membrane matrix.

Pathologic differential or, why isn't it one of the following?

Myopericytoma: Although some myopericytomas contain areas indistinguishable from glomus tumor, other areas would feature plump myoid spindle cells swirling around tumor blood vessels in a concentric, onion skin pattern. Such areas are absent in this tumor. Glomus tumors and myopericytoma share a similar IHC expression pattern, so IHC would not distinguish the two lesions. Both occur most commonly in superficial tissues in adults. However, glomus tumor more commonly causes intense, episodic pain, and the nail bed is a common site in adult women.

Angioleiomyoma (angiomyoma, ALM): A glomangiomyoma (GAM, a variant of glomus tumor) would be more difficult to distinguish from angioleiomyoma than this patient's solid variant glomus tumor, as both ALM and GAM contain large, dilated or cavernous veins invested by tumor cells. Glomangiomyoma contains recognizable glomus cells in addition to smooth muscle cells; while angioleiomyoma is devoid of glomus cells, consisting only of smooth muscle cells in intimate association with dilated veins. Angioleiomyoma contains many cells reactive for desmin, while glomangiomyoma has only scattered foci of desmin positive, spindled smooth muscle cells.

Skin appendage tumor such as hidradenoma: A solid variant glomus tumor appears similar to an epithelial tumor because of nests and sheets of epithelial appearing cells. The most likely epithelial entities in the differential are the dermally located sweat gland tumors. These usually form duct structures and will express keratins and EMA and not SMA; the opposite of glomus tumor IHC reactivity.

Intradermal melanocytic nevus: Intradermal melanocytic nevus enters the differential when a glomus tumor is superficial and unencapsulated. Cytoplasmic melanin pigment and reactivity for melanocytic markers with no reactivity for SMA (reactivity is exceptional in melanocytic tumors) help distinguish nevus from glomus tumor. Glomus tumors usually also exhibit membranous appearing (but pericellular) Collagen IV expression that is absent in dermal nevi.

Case table 9.1a Histologic variants and variant features of sporadic benign glomus tumors

Feature or variant	Frequency	Comments
Solid glomus tumor	Common (80%)	Solid nodules of typical glomus cells with inconspicuous but numerous small capillary sized blood vessels
Extra-tumoral perivascular sheathing by neoplastic glomus cells	Common	Normal vessels outside the tumor attract nests and bands of tumor cells. No clinical significance except may be related to 10% local recurrence rate
Glomangioma	Uncommon (15%)	Large ectatic veins with bands of glomus cells
Glomangiomyoma	Uncommon (5%)	Typical glomus cells present but also patches of spindled smooth muscle cells (the latter are often desmin positive)
Multiple glomus tumors	Uncommon (10%)	Glomangioma is most common variant to present as multiple nodules
Glomus tumor with marked HPC vessels	Uncommon	This HPC like pattern, if prominent and associated with classic glomus cells, has been termed 'glomangiopericytoma'
Glomus tumor with epithelioid cells	Rare	
Glomus tumor with oncocytes	Rare	Tumor cells contain granular eosinophilic cytoplasm
Symplastic glomus tumor	Rare	Scattered tumor cells have enlarged hyperchromatic nuclei of various shapes and some multinucleation. No increased mitotic activity. No clinical significance
Glomus tumor with extensive myxoid change	Rare	Background is markedly myxoid This variant may be more commonly CD34 reactive
Vascular invasion in otherwise benign tumor	Rare	No clinical significance
Glomangiomatosis	Very rare	Angiomatosis decorated with perivascular nodules or bands of glomus cells. May be a malformation and not true neoplasm. Dominant feature is the abnormal vessels, usually large ectatic veins of variable wall thickness

Table 9.1a lists the histologic variants and variant features of the sporadic glomus tumors.

Oncology approach

Medical oncology and radiation oncology

This is a benign lesion with no role for medical or radiation oncology.

Patient outcome

Two years postoperatively the patient has no symptoms and no evidence of recurrence.

Case table 9.1b Summary pathology findings of Case 9.1

Diagnosis	Glomus tumor, solid variant
Size	0.5 cm
Location	soft tissue deep to nail bed of left long finger
Margin status	Negative
Histologic grade (FNCLCC grading system)	Benign (not graded)
Pathologic stage (AJCC TNM classification)	Benign (not graded)

FNCLCC: Fédération Nationale des Centres de Lutte contre le cancer (French Federation of Cancer Centers). AJCC: American Joint Committee on Cancer

Case 9.2 Glomus tumor of uncertain malignant potential

Clinical history and presentation

The patient is a 54-year-old woman with a lifelong history of multiply recurrent glomus tumors involving the right foot. She is status post resections one, two, 28, and 32 years prior to presentation. She is significantly disabled at the present time requiring a wheelchair. Past medical history is also significant for hypertension and adult onset diabetes mellitus.

Examination of the right foot reveals multiple healed scars with a pes planovalgus deformity. She has diffuse and substantial tenderness on palpation.

Due to the extensive and recurrent nature of her disease, in addition to substantial scarring from prior surgery and the diffuse nature of her pain, it is felt that amputation is the only procedure likely to minimize recurrence and return the patient to a functional condition.

Surgical findings and comments

Right below knee amputation is performed.

Radiology findings

Because of the patient's long history, imaging is not performed at the time of amputation. Prior images are not available for review.

Pathology findings

Gross features

The amputation specimen is carefully sectioned to reveal multiple (12) dermal, subcutaneous and subfascial pink to red nodules in the anterior and posterior right calf and ankle (**Case fig. 9.2a** shows one such nodule on cut section). The nodules appear grossly circumscribed and are located 2–8 cm apart from each other. The closest nodule to the resection margin is located 11 cm distal to it. Eleven nodules range in size from 0.2–3 cm. However, the largest, deepest tumor measures 12 × 3.5 × 2 cm and runs proximally to distally along the anterior tibial periosteal surface. Multiple sections are taken for routine histology, some tissue is collected for tumor banking, and some tumor is submitted for cytogenetic analysis.

Microscopic features

Low magnification: Although apparently circumscribed on gross examination, neoplastic cells infiltrate surrounding tissue adjacent to the grossly apparent tumor nodules (**Case fig. 9.2b**). This is a common phenomenon in glomangiomatosis, and benign and malignant glomus tumors, so by itself does not indicate aggressive behavior. Sections of the largest, deep tumor confirm the periosteal-based location presumed on gross examination (**Case fig. 9.2c**).

High magnification: Sections of the larger nodules are similar and reveal a markedly hypercellular tumor with scattered thin-walled ectatic vessels (**Case fig. 9.2d**). Necrosis is absent. Fibrotic regions or alternating hypercellular and hypocellular areas are not identified. At higher magnification, the tumor continues to appear very uniform. A subtle crescentic alignment of some tumor nuclei is appreciable (**Case fig. 9.2e**). There is an impression of high vascularity based on slit like spaces filled with red blood cells. Cytologic atypia is absent. Only rare, normal mitotic figures are identified (approximately 1/50 high magnification microscopic fields).

Special studies: Antibody to CD31 verifies the marked vascularity of the tumor (**Case fig. 9.2f**). Many of the branching small vessels assume a 'staghorn' or 'antler horn' appearance created by tumor cells pressing and deforming capillary and vein shapes. This HPC pattern is not specific but is typical of many pericytic/perivascular tumors including glomus tumors and myopericytoma. Smooth muscle actin is expressed by tumor cells consistent with glomus cells (**Case fig. 9.2g**). Tumor cells do not express desmin, S-100 protein, or CD34. Karyotyping is unsuccessful, as the tumor cells fail to grow in culture.

Pathologic differential or, why isn't it one of the following?

Multiple myopericytomas: Myopericytomas can present as metachronous or synchronous multiple tumors, but this happens much less frequently than in glomus tumors. A HPC pattern as is present in this patient's lesions, is often seen in myopericytoma. However, common to nearly all myopericytomas are small and/or medium sized veins

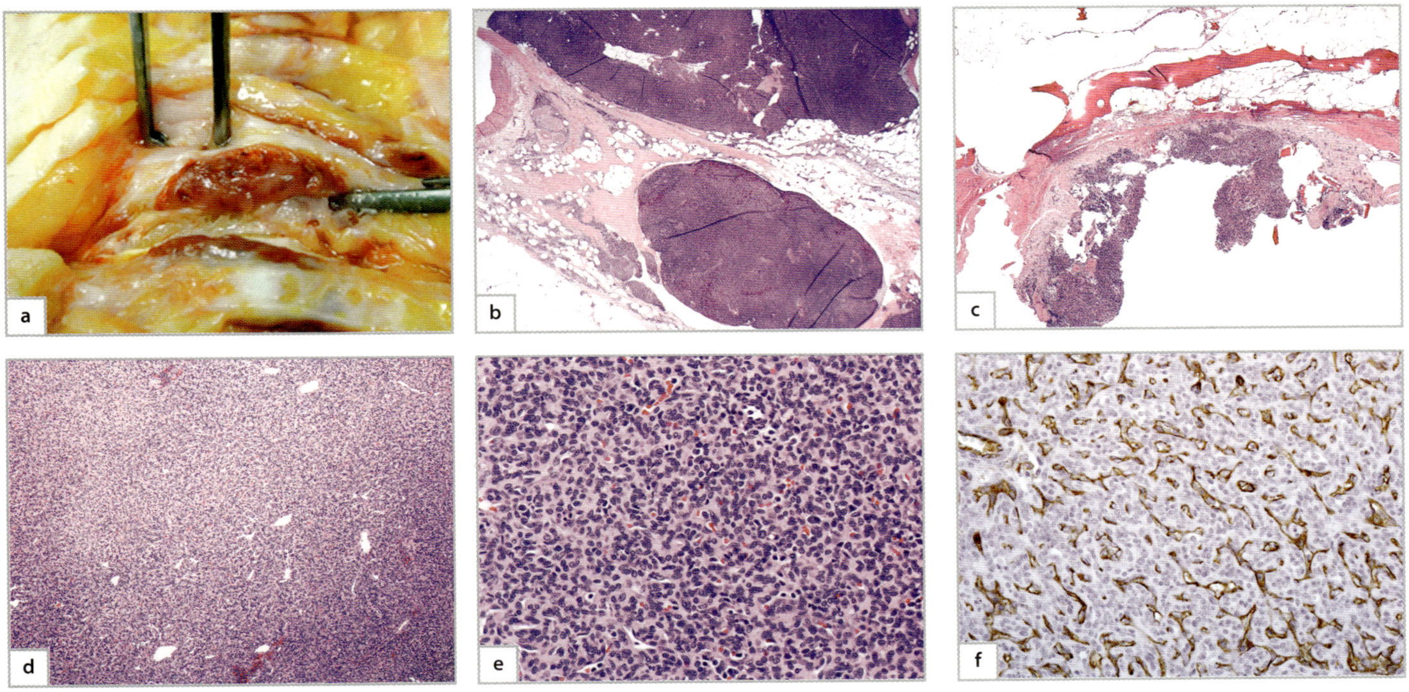

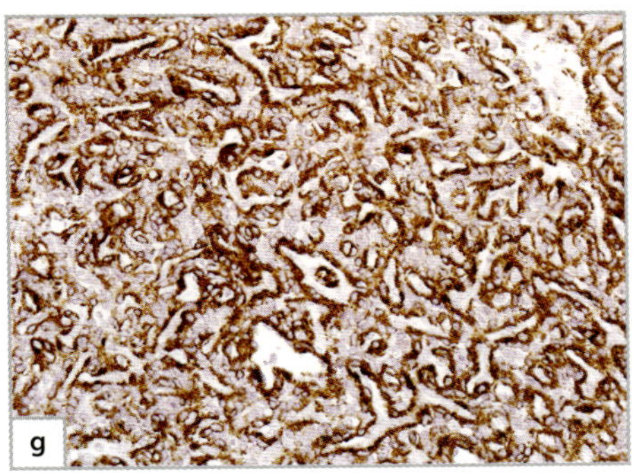

Case figure 9.2 Glomus tumor of uncertain malignant potential. **9.2a:** Gross photo of tumor in situ. A representative cross section of a subfascial tumor reveals a grossly circumscribed pink to red tumor with an uneven cut surface. On the right just above and behind the right forceps is a second tumor nodule. **9.2b:** Low magnification. Although grossly circumscribed, the neoplastic glomus cells creep into fibroadipose tissue adjacent to larger tumor nodules. Such infiltration is common in both benign and malignant glomus tumors. **9.2c:** Low magnification. The largest tumor in this patient is deep and adherent to periosteum of the tibia. **9.2d:** Medium magnification. A representative section of a larger tumor nodule reveals cellular whorls of cells tightly adherent to thin-walled, ectatic vessels (HPC architecture). **9.2e:** High magnification. The tumor is highly cellular but uniform. Slit-like vessels are inconspicuous but numerous. **9.2f:** CD31 antibody stain. The exuberantly vascular nature of the tumor is clearly seen (CD31 brown chromagen dyes the abundant branching small vessels). Notice the tumor cells push against and deform the vessels leading to the classic 'staghorn' or 'antler horn' HPC appearance. **9.2g:** Smooth muscle actin antibody stain. Both the smooth muscle cells of the vessels and many tumor cells express smooth muscle actin. Glomus tumors of all types always express smooth muscle actin.

with an eye-catching, concentric, 'onion skin' perivascular array of tumor cells. Additionally, at least some myopericytic tumor cells, which can be plump, spindled or ovoid, should exhibit a more myoid appearance with a lower N/C ratio than neoplastic glomus cells. This is because of a greater volume of eosinophilic cytoplasm than is found in glomus cells. The onion skin pattern and more myoid appearing cells of myopericytoma are not identified in this patient's tumor.

Glomangiomatosis: This entity is basically angiomatosis with extra bands or sashes of glomus cells. In other words, consistent with its name, the primary driving component of glomangiomatosis is the vascular element which usually consists of large, ectatic, malformed veins (less commonly, the vessels are capillary sized with a larger feeder vein). This patient's lesion is one of separate, hypercellular tumors without a dominating vascular component. The patient's periodic cropping of new, spatially discrete lesions over a thirty year time span is much more consistent with multiple glomus tumors than glomangiomatosis. Moreover, glomangiomatosis is extremely rare with fewer than 12 reported cases. By contrast, 10% of patients with glomus tumors have multiple lesions; certainly not a common event but not exceptional like glomangiomatosis.

Glomangiosarcoma (malignant glomus tumor): According to some soft tissue pathology experts, glomangiosarcoma is not synonymous with malignant glomus tumor (Fisher et al. 2011). Some consider them two types of malignant glomus tumor (Folpe et al. 2010). The criteria defining malignancy in glomus tumors have also evolved (Folpe et al. 2001, Folpe et al. 2010). By the current criteria, malignant glomus tumor must demonstrate high nuclear grade and mitotic activity or atypical mitoses. One subtype consists of a high grade spindle cell sarcoma arising from a benign glomus tumor (what others have termed glomangiosarcoma), while the other comprises a mitotically active, round cell sarcoma (usually without a benign element) with nuclear pleomorphism and expression of smooth muscle actin and pericellular collagen IV without desmin, keratin or S-100 protein expression. By these new criteria (2010), glomus tumor of uncertain malignant potential has at least one atypical feature other than nuclear pleomorphism, such as large size and deep location without cellular atypia or mitotic activity. This patient's tumor thus fits into the category of glomus tumor of uncertain malignant potential.

Case table 9.2 Summary pathology findings of Case 9.2

Diagnosis	Glomus tumor of uncertain malignant potential arising from a background of multiple glomus tumors
Size	12 × 3.5 × 2 cm
Location	Subfascial soft tissue of calf
Margin status	Widely negative (amputation performed)
Histologic grade (FNCLCC grading system)	Not graded
Pathologic stage (AJCC tnm classification)	Not staged

FNCLCC = Fédération Nationale des Centres de Lutte contre le cancer (French Federation of Cancer Centers). AJCC = American Joint Committee on Cancer

Oncology approach

Medical oncology

In this case, the tumor is entirely resected and there is no need for a medical oncology treatment.

Radiation oncology

There is no known role for radiation therapy in this type of tumor, especially following an amputation.

Patient outcome

Two years postoperatively the patient is an independent ambulatory with a below-knee prosthesis. There is no evidence of recurrent or metastatic tumor.

Case 9.3 Malignant myopericytoma

Clinical history and presentation

The patient is a 51-year-old woman who noticed a mass on her right upper back six weeks prior to presentation. The mass was noted spontaneously. It is asymptomatic.

On the right upper back, the patient has a 12 × 12 cm, firm, superficial mass noted. There is an approximately 3-cm incision with sutures in place, consistent with the previous incisional biopsy. The patient has no tenderness to palpation and no erythema or signs of infection.

Surgical findings and comments

Open biopsy is performed at an outside facility prior to referral. Pathology from the biopsy is interpreted at the outside facility as representing a malignant spindle cell neoplasm. Review by pathology at the referral center revises the diagnosis to myopericytoma with features of malignancy. Wide resection is performed.

Radiology findings

The CT and MR images (**Case fig. 9.3a** through **9.3e**) show a nonspecific heterogeneous mass in the subcutaneous tissues. Myopericytomas are described as being most common in the skin of distal extremities. Although there is only modest enhancement on CT and MRI, the overall heterogeneity leaves the impression of an aggressive tumor. There is no appreciable fat tissue seen on the T1 images. The radiologist can only suggest a worrisome tumor such as sarcoma and await tissue diagnosis.

Pathology findings

Gross features

The incisional biopsy is performed at an outside institution and consists of fleshy tan tumor fragments aggregating to 2.5 cm in maximum diameter.

The resection specimen consists of a 12 × 10 × 7 cm portion of soft tissue with muscle attached at the deep margin and a superficial skin ellipse. The specimen is differentially inked according to specific margins, and serial sections reveal a 9.5 × 8 × 7 cm firm, yellow to white tumor with a central cystic cavity consistent with prior biopsy site (**Case fig. 9.3f**). Multiple areas are hemorrhagic or congested. Margins appear grossly free of tumor. Fifteen cassettes of tumor are prepared, and tumor is collected fresh for cytogenetics and tumor banking.

Microscopic features

Only the resection specimen is described, as the initial biopsy is histologically identical.

Low magnification: The tumor is highly cellular and 80% comprises a HPC appearance at low magnification (**Case fig. 9.3g**). Twenty percent consists of fascicles and solid sheets of spindle cells with large areas of necrosis and fibrosis.

High magnification: The tumor cells abut and bulge into the lumens of thin-walled vessels, a pattern that is not specific but is described in malignant myopericytoma (**Case fig. 9.3h** and **9.3i**)(McMenamin et al. 2002). Additional patterns noted in this tumor and also reported in myopericytoma include a microcystic pattern of tumor cell dissolution (**Case fig. 9.3j**) and focal fascicular growth. Despite numerous sections, a classic onion skin concentric rimming of tumor cells around vessels is not identified. However, the combination of HPC and myofibromatous patterns supports the diagnosis of malignant myopericytoma. Tumor cells are spindled to polygonal with pale eosinophilic or amphophilic cytoplasm, marked nuclear pleomorphism, and numerous mitotic figures are present (>20/hpf) including atypical forms (**Case fig. 9.3k**). Inflammation is absent. Individual apoptotic cells are numerous.

Special studies: Immunohistochemical staining is performed and reveals the following: moderate expression of smooth muscle actin (**Case fig. 9.3l**), weaker expression of muscle specific actin (**Case fig. 9.3m**), and no reactivity for: desmin, caldesmon, calponin, S-100 protein, mixed keratins, EMA, p63, myogenin, CDK4 and MDM2. CD31 and CD34 are expressed only in vessels and highlight the intimate relationship of tumor to blood vessels with tumor cells protruding into vessel walls (**Case fig. 9.3n**).

The karyotype is complex and hypertriploid with extensive structural and numerical abnormalities: Identifiable breakpoints are located at 1q12, 2p23, 2q31, 3q21, 4p14, 4p16, 5p15, 5q31, 6p23, 6q21, 7p22, 11p11.2, 12p12, 16p11.2, and 17p11.2 (some breakpoints cannot be identified). Notably, a breakpoint at 7p22 is the same breakpoint previously reported in several cases of myopericytoma in which the β-actin gene at 7p21-22 is fused to the GLI gene at 12q13-15)(Dahlen et al. 2004).

Pathologic differential or, why isn't it one of the following?

Leiomyosarcoma (LMS): LMS may occur in the subcutaneous tissue of the trunk of a patient this age. Moreover, it can be high grade. However, most cases do not show such prominent HPC growth or marked protrusion into blood vessel lumens as is the case here. Some high grade LMS will contain lower grade classic fascicular areas of eosinophilic spindled cells with blunt ended or cigar shaped nuclei and cytoplasmic clearing suggestive of contraction bands. Such areas and cells are absent in this patient's tumor. By IHC both LMS and malignant myopericytoma are reactive for SMA and muscle specific actin (HHF-35). Both may be positive for caldesmon. Desmin is usually absent in myopericytomas (including the malignant version), while approximately 90% of LMS express desmin. This patient's tumor is negative for desmin. Up to 40% of LMS also express keratins. There is

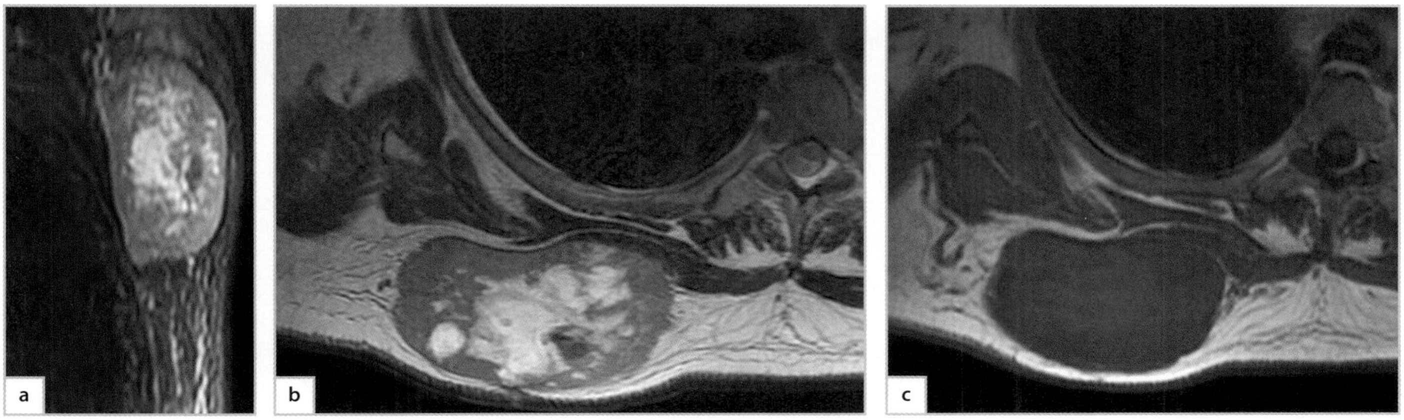

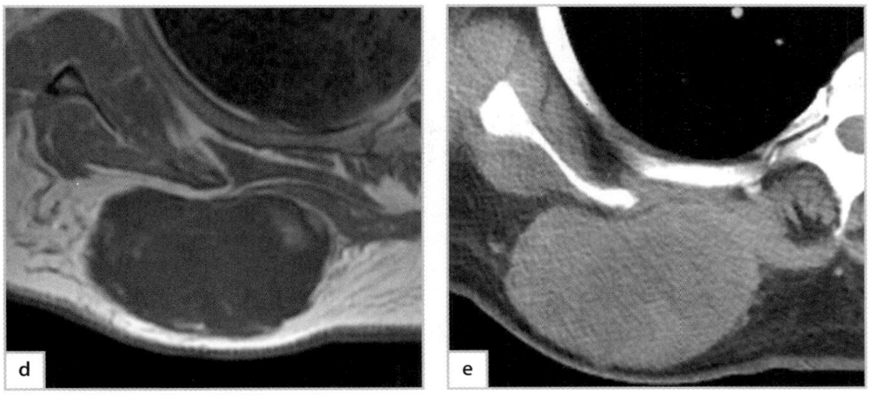

Case figure 9.3 Malignant myopericytoma. **9.3a**: Sagittal STIR MR image, **9.3b**: Axial T2 MR image, **9.3c**: Axial T1 MR image, **9.3d**: Axial T1 post-contrast MR image, **9.3e**: Axial CT image post IV contrast. The CT image shows a homogeneous isodense mass in the subcutaneous tissues without appreciable enhancement. There is no calcification or apparent necrosis. The MR images show a heterogeneous mass measuring 8.9 × 4.5 × 8.7 cm with minimal peripheral nodular enhancement. Note the intact plane of separation between the mass and the adjacent deep rhomboid musculature as seen on fig. 9.3b. The T2 high signal areas without enhancement may represent matrix or necrotic tissue. The overall appearance is not specific, but the heterogeneity is worrisome for an aggressive lesion such as a sarcoma.

Case figure 9.3: Continued from page 195

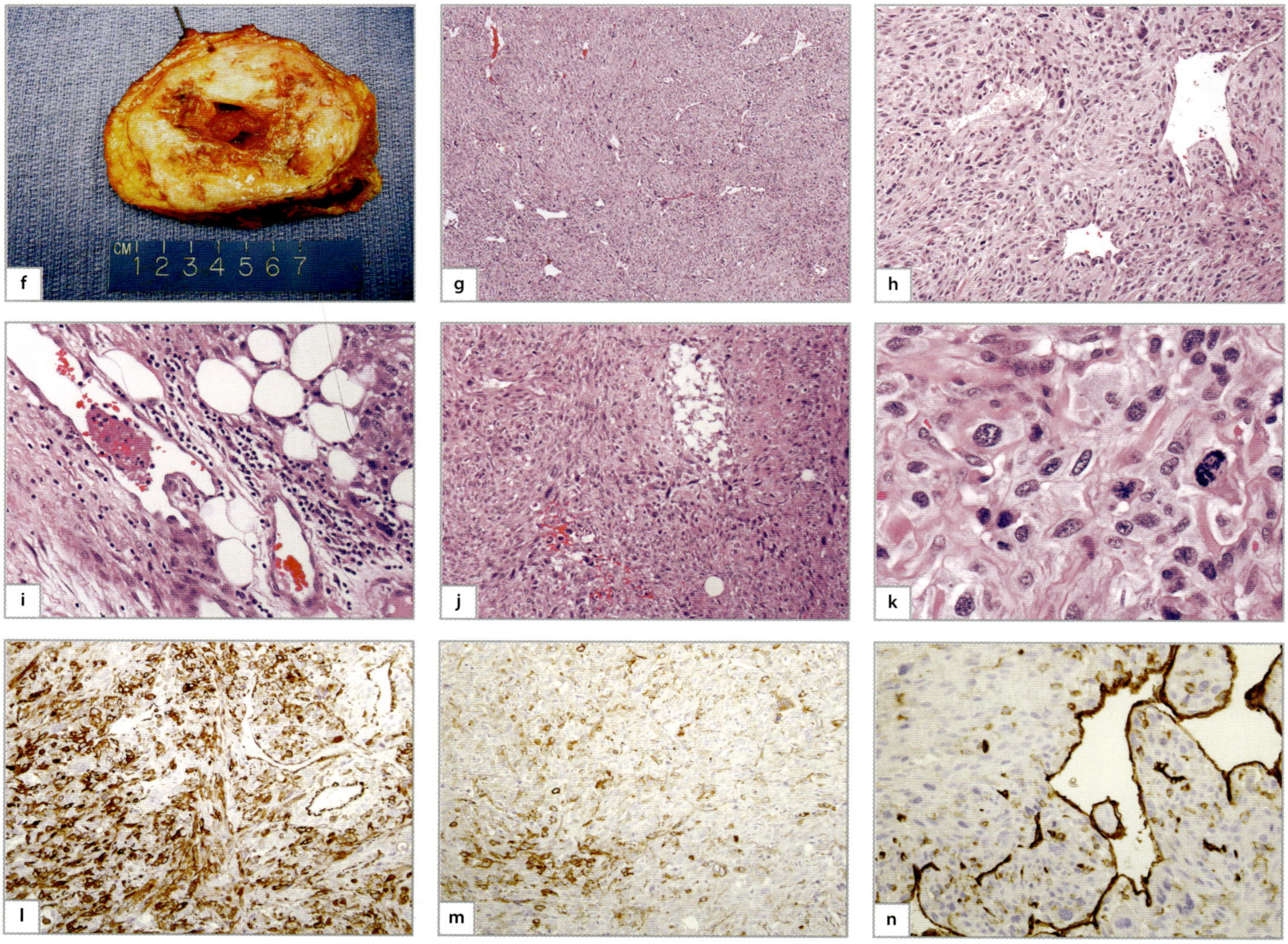

9.3f: Gross specimen cross section. The tumor is large and mostly circumscribed, although a slip of adipose tissue is engulfed on the right side. A central cystic hemorrhagic cavity is consistent with recent prior biopsy. Hemorrhagic foci are also noticeable away from the biopsy site. **9.3g:** Lower magnification. The tumor presents a heterogeneous growth pattern, but 80% comprises a cellular vaguely nodular arrangement of tumor cells with interspersed compressed, angulated 'staghorn', thin walled vessels (HPC architecture). The HPC pattern is not specific to myopericytoma but commonly seen in both benign and malignant forms. **9.3h:** Medium magnification. Intratumoral veins are distorted by undermining tumor cells. **9.3i:** Medium magnification. A thin walled vein next to the tumor shows subendothelial protrusion of tumor cells and thrombus formation. This honing in on vessels outside the main tumor is a feature common to benign and malignant perivascular/pericytic tumors. **9.3j:** Medium magnification. Sprinkled throughout the HPC areas are microcysts and foci of acute hemorrhage. These may represent remnants of destroyed, ruptured blood vessels. Such microcyst formation has been described in malignant myopericytoma. **9.3k:** High magnification. In this field, the tumor cells are polygonal with amphophilic cytoplasm and marked nuclear pleomorphism. Atypical mitotic figures reinforce the high grade nature of the sarcoma. Strands and thicker bands of pink material are consistent with basement membrane or collagen. Pericellular collagen deposition can be seen in myopericytoma as well as glomus tumors. **9.3l:** Smooth muscle actin antibody stain. About 50% of tumor cells show cytoplasmic expression of this muscle marker. Two cross sections of a medium sized vein in the upper right corner possibly exhibit a subtle radial arrangement of tumor cells. **9.3m:** Muscle specific (HHF) actin antibody stain. Expression of HHF actin is generally less intense and diffuse than for smooth muscle actin. **9.3n:** CD31 antibody stain. Tumor cells form bulbous protrusions into this vein, distorting and compressing it. If there was a muscular wall in this vessel, it has been effaced by tumor cell invasion.

no reactivity for keratins in this patient's tumor. Thus, based on the overall morphology and IHC pattern, malignant myopericytoma is the strongly favored diagnosis.

Dermatofibrosarcoma protuberans: The subcutis of the shoulder is a perfect location for dermatofibrosarcoma protuberans (DFSP). However, this tumor is much more pleomorphic than classic DFSP which exhibits a storiforming architecture of plump spindle cells. Some DFSP undergo sarcomatous transformation: the resulting high grade component resembles adult type fibrosarcoma in most cases. DFSP is CD34 reactive in most cases and usually does not express SMA or MSA or at most only focally. DFSP harbors a specific translocation fusing the collagen 1A1 gene to the platelet derived growth factor β gene: t(17;22)(q21;q13). This patient's tumor is non-reactive for CD34 and there is no evidence of a *COL1A1-PDGFB* translocation by karyotype.

High grade spindle cell sarcoma, not otherwise specified: This patient's tumor discloses a substantial degree of muscle marker expression. It therefore cannot be considered a high grade undifferentiated sarcoma. Sarcomas expressing muscle markers may behave particularly aggressively; therefore, it is important to note this finding in the pathology report.

High grade or poorly differentiated SFT: SFT commonly manifests a HPC pattern of growth but the extreme degree of subendothelial bulging into vascular spaces as is seen in this patient's tumor has not been described in SFT. SFT should express CD34 and often Bcl-2 and membranous CD99 with at most focal expression of SMA or muscle specific actin. This patient's tumor is negative for CD34 and shows prominent muscle marker expression.

Malignant glomus tumor: Malignant glomus tumor is characterized by two patterns: 1) high grade spindle cell sarcoma arising in the background of benign glomus tumor, 2) high grade round cell tumor with appropriate IHC expression consistent with glomus cell differentiation. Neither of these two types applies to this patient's tumor: it does not contain a benign glomus tumor element, and it is not a malignant round cell tumor.

Tables 9.3a and **9.3b** list the histologic variants and variant features of myopericytoma and malignant myopericytoma, respectively. As is obvious, the range of morphologic features is very broad but thematically similar: all patterns but one (leiomyomatous) entail an intimate association of tumor cells with vessels. In most cases, at least some of the cells have a spindled myoid appearance, but some cases comprise only cells that resemble glomus cells ('glomoid' cells: rounded cells but with more eosinophilic cytoplasm and slightly less uniformly round nuclei than true glomus cells). Other tumors contain foci of actual glomus cells with monotonous round nuclei, sharply defined cell borders and pericellular basement membrane material. Tumors need to be extensively sampled in order to identify the characteristic pericytomatous pattern. The finding of multiple patterns in one tumor supports the notion that myofibroma, glomus tumor, angioleiomyoma and myopericytoma (pure pericytomatous pattern) are inter-related.

Oncology approach

Medical oncology

There is no standard chemotherapy for malignant myopericytoma. Because the margins of resection are negative and the work-up does not reveal metastases, no adjuvant chemotherapy is offered. The patient is referred to radiation therapy for a consultation.

Case table 9.3a Variants and variant histologic features of myopericytoma

Histologic variant or feature	Frequency	Comment
Pericytomatous pattern	Most common pattern. May comprise the entire tumor	Pink, plump ovoid or spindle tumor cells encircle tumor vessels in an onion skin, concentric manner and may swirl off into surrounding stroma, cartwheel like
Mixed architectural patterns	Common	Most myopericytomas are composed of mixtures of the patterns listed in this table
HPC pattern	Common pattern. Usually combined with pericytomatous pattern	Hypercellular comprising pink, plump ovoid or spindle tumor cells compressing small vessels into 'staghorn' or 'antler horn' shapes Often may form the periphery of a tumor with central pericytomatous pattern
Glomangiomatous pattern	Uncommon. Must be combined with pericytomatous pattern.	Tumor cells are rounded with round nuclei and scant cytoplasm identical to glomus cells and aggregate around large, dilated blood vessels
Myofibromatous pattern	Uncommon. Must be combined with pericytomatous pattern	Alternating zones of hypercellular small basophilic spindle cells and myoid spindle cells (cells with a larger amount of cytoplasm that is eosinophilic). Myoid zones may show collagenization. Myoid nodules bulge or protrude into larger thin-walled vessels. The bulging nodules are often hypocellular myxoid or fibrotic
Angioleiomyomatous pattern	Uncommon. Must be combined with pericytomatous pattern	Smooth muscle bundles course around prominent dilated blood vessels
Leiomyomatous pattern	Common. Must be combined with pericytomatous pattern	Fascicles of eosinophilic spindle cells that resemble myofibroblasts or smooth muscle cells
Secondary hemorrhage, fibrosis, calcification	Common in larger or longstanding tumors	Secondary fibrosis is more diffuse and not zonal like myofibromatosis pattern. It does not form bulbous nodules protruding into vessels. Rarely, metaplastic bone may also develop as a secondary change
Involvement of peritumoral vessels	Common	Cords and rings of tumor cells involve vessels outside the main tumor mass. This also occurs commonly in glomus tumors
Symplastic changes	Uncommon	Scattered cells show degenerative nuclear atypia without increased mitotic activity similar to symplastic glomus tumors
Extensive myxoid stromal change	Uncommon	
Multiple tumors	Uncommon	Occurs less frequently for myopericytoma than glomus tumor. Can be metachronous or synchronous and usually but not always confined to one body site such as lower leg or hand
EBV associated myopericytoma	Rare	Reported thus far in AIDS patients. Tumors show all possible myopericytomatous patterns. May be multifocal. Behavior may be indolent, even with nuclear atypia
Intravascular location	Rare	Tumor may be entirely located with a vein lumen
Immature cellular variant	Rare	Hypercellular comprising short spindle cells with scant basophilic cytoplasm and uniform ovoid nuclei encircling blood vessels in a pericytomatous pattern
Hypocellular fibroma-like variant	Rare	Hypocellular but with prominent fibrotic stroma and pericytomatous pattern of perivascular swirling

Case table 9.3b Variants and variant histologic features of malignant myopericytoma (only a few cases have been reported; so frequency of features is tentative)

Histologic variant or feature	Frequency	Comment
Pericytomatous pattern	Always	This may be subtle or focal in high grade tumors
Cords of perivascular tumor cells well away from leading edge of tumor	Common	Similar cord like extension along adjacent vessels occurs in benign myopericytoma and in glomus tumors
Fascicular pattern of spindle cells	Common	Resembles the fascicles of myofibroma but with more atypia
HPC pattern	Common	Mitoses and atypia present
Tumor necrosis	Common	Includes geographic and apoptotic necrosis
Microcysts	Common	Tumor cells fall away from each other; often near areas of necrosis
Hypocellular fibrotic regions	Uncommon	Dispersed atypical tumor cells embedded in fibrous stroma
Subendothelial proliferation of tumor cells	Common	Tumor cells bulge or telescope into vessel lumens similar to myofibroma (part of the myofibromatous pattern)
Foci of glomus type cells	Uncommon	Pericytomatous pattern is also present as well as atypia and mitotic figures
Tumor is composed of undifferentiated round to oval cells	Uncommon	Not as much cytoplasm and more nuclear variability
High mitotic rate	Common	Higher than 10/10 hpf
Atypical mitotic figures	Common	May be scattered and few in any given tumor

Case table 9.3c Summary pathology findings of Case 9.3

Diagnosis	Malignant myopericytoma
Size	9.5 × 8 × 7 cm
Location	Subcutaneous tissue of posterior shoulder
Margin Status	Negative; closest margin is 0.2 cm with all others >/= 1 cm
Histologic grade (FNCLCC grading system)	High grade
Pathologic stage (AJCC tnm classification)	Stage III = T2a (superficial tumor > 5 cm) and high grade (grade 3) with no nodal or distant metastases

FNCLCC: Fédération Nationale des Centres de Lutte Contre le Cancer (French Federation of Cancer Centers Sarcoma Group). AJCC: American Joint Committee on Cancer

Radiation oncology

Due to the rarity of this tumor type and recent reclassification, it is difficult to determine indications for radiation therapy. With the high grade nature of this tumor and close margins, radiation therapy is likely indicated, as I believe it is not unreasonable to classify this as a high grade soft tissue sarcoma. However, with this particular histological description, there is no literature describing outcomes and indications for radiation therapy. In general, gross total resection is associated with the best outcomes.

Patient outcome

One year postoperatively the patient has no signs of local recurrence or metastasis.

REFERENCES

Brouillard P, Boon LM, Mulliken JB, et al. Mutations in a novel factor, glomulin, are responsible for glomuvenous malformations ('glomangiomas'). Am J Hum Genet 2002;70:866–74.

Calderaro J, Polivka M, Gallien S, et al. Multifocal Epstein Barr virus (EBV)-associated myopericytoma in a patient with AIDS. Neuropathol Appl Neurobiol 2008;34(1):115–7.

Calvert JT, Burns S, Riney TJ, et al. Additional glomangioma families link to chromosome 1p: no evidence for genetic heterogeneity. Hum Hered 2001;51:180–2.

Chen WC, Lee TS, Ku MC, et al. Glomus tumors of the upper extremity: experience with twelve cases. Zhonghua Yi Xue Za Zhi (Taipei) 1995;55: 163–7.

Dahlén A, Mertens F, Mandahl N, et al. Molecular genetic characterization of the genomic ACTB-GLI fusion in pericytoma with t(7;12). Biochem Biopys Res Commun 2004;325(4):1318–23.

De Chiara A, Apice G, Mori S, et al. Malignant glomus tumour: a case report and review of the literature. Sarcoma 2003;7:87–91.

Dray MS, McCarthy SW, Palmer AA, et al. Myopericytoma: a unifying term for a spectrum of tumours that show overlapping features with myofibroma. A review of 14 cases. J Clin Pathol 2006;59(1):67–73.

Fisher C, Mentzel T, Montgomery EA, et al (Eds). Diagnostic Pathology Soft Tissue Tumors. Salt Lake City: AMIRSYS, 2011.

Folpe AL, Fanburg-Smith JC, Miettinen M et al. Atypical and malignant glomus tumors: analysis of 52 cases, with a proposal for the reclassification of glomus tumors. Am J Surg Pathol 2001;25(1):1–12.

Fornage BD. Glomus tumors in the fingers: diagnosis with US. Radiology 1988;167:183–5.

Gengler C, Guillou L. Solitary fibrous tumour and haemangiopericytoma: evolution of a concept. Histopathology 2006;48:63–74.

Glazebrook KN, Laundre BJ, Schiefer TK, et al. Imaging features of glomus tumors. Skeletal Radiol 2011;40(7):855–862.

Gombos Z, Zhang PJ. Glomus tumor. Arch Pathol Lab Med 2008;132(9):1448–52.

Granter SR, Badizadegan K, Fletcher CD. Myofibromatosis in adults, glomangiopericytoma, and myopericytoma: a spectrum of tumors showing perivascular myoid differentiation. Am J Surg Pathol 1998;22(5):513–25.

Hoekzema R, Zonneveld IM, van der Wal AC. Type 2 segmental glomangiomas. Dermatol Online J 2010;16:8.

Jalali M, Netscher DTJ, Connelly JH. Glomangiomatosis. Ann Diag Pathol 2002;6(5):326–328.

Kleontas A, Barbetakis N, Asteriou C et al. Primary glomangiosarcoma of the lung: A case report. J Cardiothorac Surg 2010;5:76.

Koc O, Kivrak AS, Paksoy Y. Subungual glomus tumour: magnetic resonance imaging findings. Australas Radiol 2007;51 Spec No.:B107–9.

Lancerotto L, Salmaso R, Sartore L et al. Malignant Glomus Tumor of the Leg Developed in the Context of a Superficial Typical Glomus Tumor. Int J Surg Pathol 2012;20(4):420–4.
Lau PPL, Wong OK, Lui PCW, et al. Myopericytoma in patients with AIDS: A new class of Epstein-Barr Virus-associated tumor. Am J Surg Pathol 2009;33(11):1666–1672.
McMenamin ME, Fletcher CDM. Malignant myopericytoma: expanding the spectrum of tumours with myopericytic differentiation. Histopathology 2002;41(5):450–460.
Mentzel T, Dei Tos A, Sapi Z, et al. Myopericytoma of skin and soft tissues: clinicopathologic and immunohistochemical study of 54 cases. Am J Surg Pathol 2006;30(1):104–113.
Park EA, Hong SH, Choi JY, et al. Glomangiomatosis: magnetic resonance imaging findings in three cases. Skeletal Radiol 2005;34(2):108–11.
Paek JO, Kang HS, Yeo KY, et al. A case of myopericytoma of the lower leg. Ann Dermatol 2011;23(2):201–204.
Ramdial PK, Sing Y, Deonarain J, et al. Periampullary Epstein-Barr virus-associated myopericytoma. Human Pathol 2011;42(9):1348–1354.
Rettig AC, Strickland JW. Glomus tumor of the digits. J Hand Surg Am 1997;2:261–5.
Rodriguez-Justo M, Aramburu-Gonzalez JA, Santonja C. Glomangiosarcoma of abdominal wall. Virchows Arch 2001;438(4):418–420.
Roh BH, Lee SK, Kwon SY. Myopericytoma of the neck: Sonographic appearance and sonographically guided needle biopsy. J Clin Ultrasound 2011;39(8):469–472.
Schopp JG, Sra KK, Wilkerson MG. Glomangioma: a case report and review of the literature. Cutis 2009;83:24–7.
Simi L, Sestini R, Ferruzzi P, et al. Phenotype variability of neural crest derived tumours in six Italian families segregating the same founder SDHD mutation Q109X. J Med Genet 2005;42:e52.
Terada T. Minute myopericytoma of the neck: a case report with literature review and differential diagnosis. Pathol Oncol Res 2010;16(4):613–616.
Tran LP, Velanovich V, Kaufmann CR. Familial multiple glomus tumors: report of a pedigree and literature review. Ann Plast Surg 1994;32:89–91.

FURTHER READING

Fisher C, Montgomery EA, Thway K. Biopsy Interpretation Series: Biopsy Interpretation of Soft Tissue Tumors. Philadelphia: Walters Kluwer/Lippincott Williams and Wilkins, 2011.
Hornick JL, ed. Practical Soft Tissue Pathology: A Diagnostic Approach. Philadelphia: Elsevier Saunders, 2013.

Chapter 10 Vascular tumors of soft tissues

OVERVIEW

This chapter concerns vascular tumors of the deep (subfascial) soft tissue and/or the subcutis. Vascular tumors that occur exclusively in the skin (dermis) are not discussed, as the orthopaedic surgeon seldom deals with these lesions, and radiologic studies are generally not performed. However, some vascular tumors typically centered in the dermis are described, as they may involve deeper tissue and thus come to the attention of the orthopaedist and radiologist. A few vascular tumors reviewed in this chapter may also develop in viscera such as the liver, spleen, thyroid gland, etc. Vascular tumors of bone are presented in Chapter 24.

As with most soft tissue tumor categories, the benign and intermediate vascular tumors outnumber the malignant varieties by types and incidence. This is fortunate, as angiosarcoma is an aggressive sarcoma with a particularly poor prognosis overall. Complete surgical excision was and continues to be the mainstay of treatment, augmented by radiation therapy to help control local disease. Historically, chemotherapy has not been beneficial. However, with new insights into the molecular pathobiology of angiosarcoma, targeted therapies are forthcoming. These have the promise of greatly improving survival of angiosarcoma patients.

Importantly, today, 20% of angiosarcoma patients presenting with metastatic disease achieve long term survival (Fayette et al 2007). Thus, curative rather than palliative therapy should be strongly considered in individuals with advanced disease.

CLASSIFICATION

The classification of vascular tumors of soft tissue is provided in **Table 10.1**: World Health Organization (WHO) Classification of Vascular Tumors of Soft Tissue (2013).

The pediatric age group presents with abundant vascular lesions, and distinguishing between a malformation and a hemangioma may not be possible histologically. Non-neoplastic vascular ectasias may cause significant morbidity and sometimes death (Klippel-Trenaunay syndrome, Sturge-Weber syndrome, port wine stain, etc). These are not discussed in detail in this text.

DEMOGRAPHICS

Hemangiomas rival lipoma as the most common soft tissue tumor. They far outnumber lipoma if one includes superficial hemangiomas such as cherry angioma which affects a majority of the elderly.

Orthopaedic surgeons may be consulted for pediatric and adult hemangiomas when the lesions extensively involve the subcutaneous or deeper tissues. These can include rapidly growing capillary hemangiomas in children (known as juvenile hemangioma) and newly described non-involuting and rapidly involuting congenital hemangioma (abbreviated as NICH and RICH, respectively). Close clinical correlation is required to enable the correct diagnosis, as surgical intervention is contraindicated in some cases.

Tables 10.3 and **10.4** provide information on the incidence of those vascular tumors that may be evaluated by an orthopaedist. These include tumors that are seldom subfascial but can form bulky subcutaneous masses.

For the malignant vascular tumors of soft tissue, Surveillance, Epidemiology, and End Results (SEER) data were evaluated from 13 registries during a 15 year period (1994-2008). This section focuses on 5 malignant histologic types (with the ICDO-3 code presented parenthetically): hemangiosarcoma (angiosarcoma) (9120), malignant hemangioendothelioma (9130), malignant epithelioid hemangioendothelioma (9133), Kaposi sarcoma (9140), and lymphangiosarcoma (9170). All tumors presented arise in the soft tissue (connective and subcutaneous).

The average annual incidence rate is 0.8 per million for hemangiosarcoma, 0.2 per million for Kaposi sarcoma, 0.1 per million for malignant epithelioid hemangioendothelioma, and 0.0 per million for malignant hemangioendothelioma and lymphangiosarcoma. Males have higher rates of hemangiosarcoma (1.0 per million) and Kaposi sarcoma (0.3 per million) of the soft tissue compared to females (0.8 per million and 0.0 per million, respectively). There are no differences in incidence rates of malignant epithelioid hemangioendothelioma, malignant hemangioendothelioma, and lymphangiosarcoma between males and females.

The number of cases reported in 13 SEER registries is shown in **Figure 10.1**. These registries encompass approximately ~20% of the U.S. population.

The mean ages for the selected vascular tumors of the soft tissue are similar among patients diagnosed with malignant hemangioendothelioma (mean = 50.0 years), malignant epithelioid hemangioendothelioma (mean = 50.2 years), and Kaposi sarcoma (mean = 51.9 years). The oldest group of patients were diagnosed with lymphangiosarcoma (mean = 70.0 years). **Figure 10.2** depicts the age distribution of vascular tumors of the soft tissue.

PATHOGENESIS/ETIOLOGY

Hemangiomas

The specific causes of most types of hemangiomas are unknown. As with other diseases, a multifactorial etiology combining environmental and genetic events is suspected for both neoplastic vascular tumors and vascular malformations.

Spindle cell hemangioma, when occurring in the setting of Maffucci syndrome, is often associated with mutations of the *IDH1* or *IDH2* genes (Pansuriya et al, 2011).

It has been variously proposed that epithelioid hemangioma (previously termed angiolymphoid hyperplasia with eosinophilia) is reactive and arises in the setting of a traumatized normal medium-sized vessel, that it is lymphatic rather than vascular, and that it is a neoplasm. There are no reports of the genetic findings of epithelioid hemangioma except one case evaluated with other vascular tumors and vascular malformations. This case was noted to have a mutation of the *TEK* gene which encodes for an endothelial cell tyrosine kinase receptor, TIE2 (Ye et al. 2011). Notably, mutations of this gene have also been reported in other hemangiomas including juvenile hemangioma and in vascular malformations (Ye et al. 2011, Limaye et al. 2008). In fact, multiple studies confirm that somatic genetic mutations play a role in

Table 10.1 WHO classification of vascular tumors of soft tissue (2013)

Tumor	Behavior	Additional comments
Hemangiomas **Synovial hemangioma** **Intramuscular hemangioma** **Venous hemangioma** **Spindle cell hemangioma**	Benign*	*Intramuscular angioma (intramuscular hemangioma) may recur in up to 50% of cases Some hemangiomas may actually represent vascular malformations
Epithelioid hemangioma	Benign*	Distinctive histology warrants separate classification from other hemangiomas *May locally recur in 33% of cases
Angiomatosis	Benign*	Must involve multiple tissue types or multiple muscles *High local recurrence or persistence rate (50-90%)
Lymphangioma	Benign*	*May locally recur or persist
Kaposiform hemangioendothelioma	Intermediate	May be associated with Kasabach-Merritt syndrome (consumptive coagulopathy; especially retroperitoneal examples) Locally aggressive but does not metastasize
Retiform hemangioendothelioma	Intermediate	Rarely metastasizes
Papillary intralymphatic angioendothelioma	Intermediate	Locally recurrent Rarely metastasizes (and only to lymph nodes)
Composite hemangioendothelioma	Intermediate	Up to 15% metastasis rate (usually to regional lymph nodes only) 50% local recurrence rate May be associated with lymphedema, Kasabach-Merritt syndrome, or Maffucci syndrome (one case reported in a patient with NF2) No deaths due to disease reported
Pseudomyogenic (epithelioid sarcoma-like) hemangioendothelioma	Intermediate	Rarely metastasizing Rare and usually multifocal
Kaposi sarcoma	Intermediate	Rarely metastasizing in most cases
Epithelioid hemangioendothelioma (EHE)	Malignant	EHE metastasizes in 20-30% and causes death in 10-20% (if one includes cases with anaplastic or high grade features) EHE with low grade, classic features has 3% death rate and 17% metastasis rate
Angiosarcoma of soft tissue	Malignant	Five year overall survival of 40-50%
Benign: does not recur or if it does, is treated conservatively and does not metastasize. Intermediate: can locally recur aggressively (usually treated with wide excision) and/or only rarely (<2-5%) metastasizes. Malignant: can locally recur aggressively and commonly metastasizes.		

Table 10.2 Predominantly pediatric vascular tumors of soft tissue grouped by behavior

Tumor	Incidence	Age and sex distribution	Body site (in order of occurrence)	Histopathology description including IHC	
				Medium magnification	High magnification
Benign: does not recur or recurs non-aggressively and does not metastasize					
Juvenile hemangioma (common infantile hemangioma, strawberry nevus)	Common	Infants and young children, most commonly	Skin most common site Rarely exclusively involves subfascia	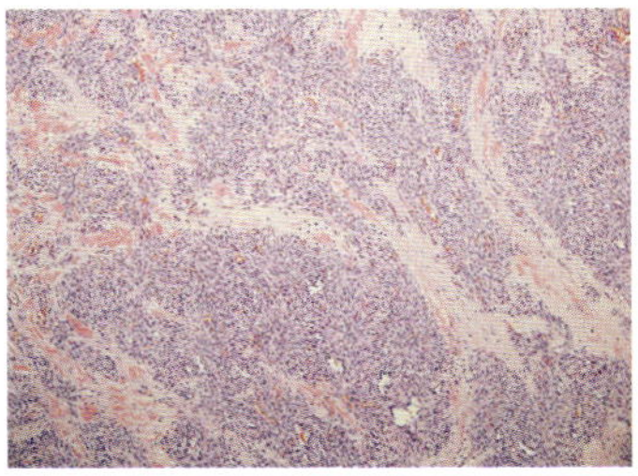	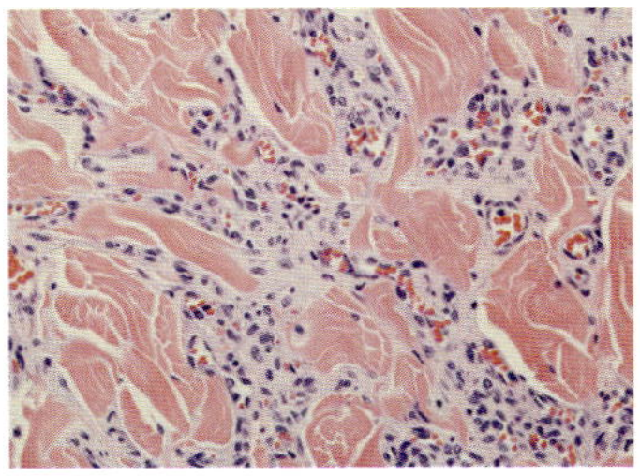
Lobulated, non-infiltrative cellular tumor composed of bland endothelial cells forming capillaries. The vessel lumens may be compressed centrally and appear to form solid growth. Reticulin and muscle actin stains can highlight vessel formation centrally. Mitotically active but no atypical mitoses. Positive for GLUT-1 expression and typical vascular markers (CD31 and CD34).					
Cavernous hemangioma	Uncommon	Infants and young children	Skin, deep soft tissue, viscera such as liver Blue rubber bleb nevus syndrome = multiple skin and GIT cavernous hemangiomas	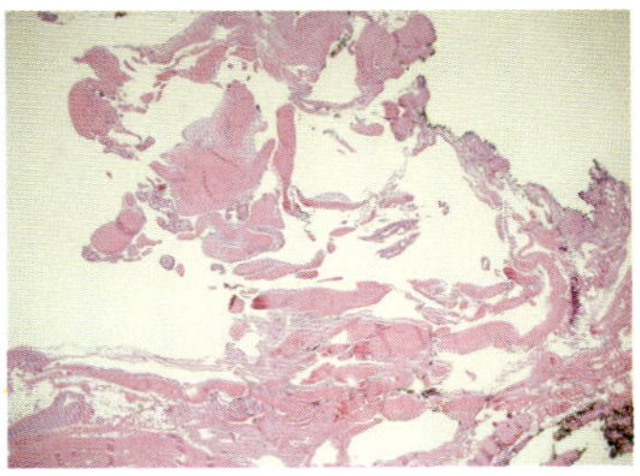	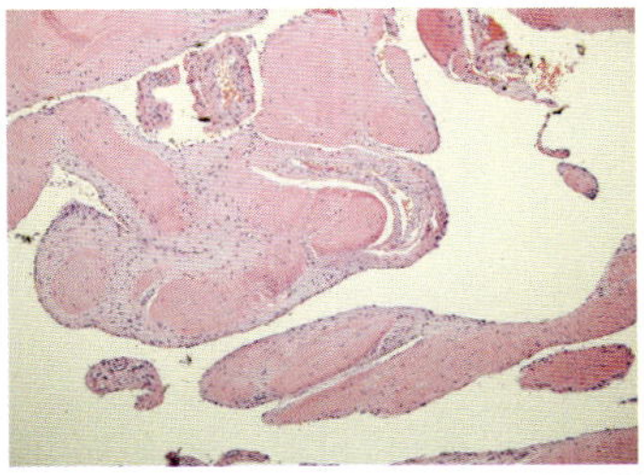
Large dilated vessels form a spongy anastomosing network looking like a sieve. Lining endothelial cells are flattened and inconspicuous. Can have thrombosis, calcifications, and osseous metaplasia. Vessel walls are often fibrotic. Periphery is well-circumscribed. No cytologic atypia or mitotic activity. Sinusoidal hemangioma is probably a histologic variant.					

Table 10.2: Continued from page 201

Tumor	Incidence	Age and sex distribution	Body site (in order of occurrence)	Histopathology description including IHC Medium magnification	High magnification
Rapidly involuting congenital hemangioma (RICH)	Rare	Congenital (spontaneously regresses in the first year of life)	Skin but may form bulky subcutaneous lesion	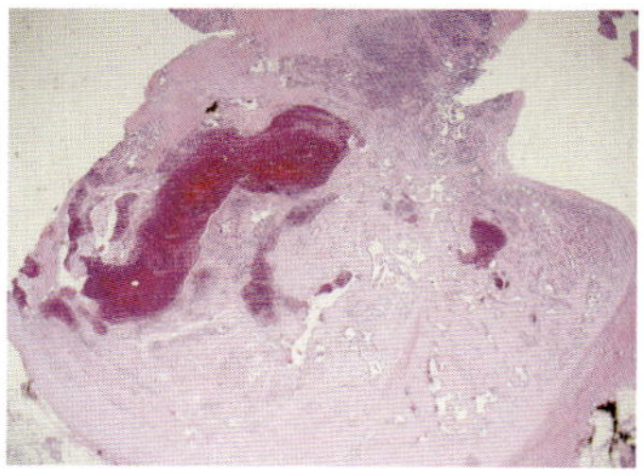	
Circumscribed lobules of capillaries that can undergo fibrosis, thrombosis and calcification. May have prominent central draining vessels in each lobule. Center first becomes fibrotic as lesion involutes. Negative for GLUT-1 in almost all cases. Positive for vascular markers CD31 and CD34.					
Non-involuting congenital hemangioma (NICH)	Rare	Congenital (does not regress)	Skin but may form bulky subcutaneous lesion	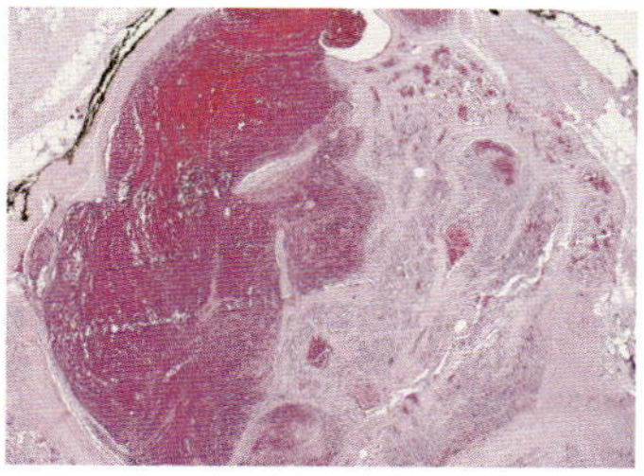	
Lobules of larger and often thicker walled vessels than in RICH. Interlobular stroma usually contains arteries, abnormal veins and AV or arteriolobular fistulae. May represent a vascular malformation. Negative for GLUT-1 and positive for vascular markers. NICH excised at age 2-4 years may resemble RICH, so the two are related.					
Cutaneovisceral angiomatosis with thrombocytopenia (multifocal lymphangioendo-theliomatosis with thrombocytopenia or infantile hemorrhagic angiodysplasia)	Very rare	Congenital with new lesions cropping up in childhood	Multiple skin papules, macules and plaques with involvement also of GIT, lung, liver, spleen, bone, muscle, and synovium	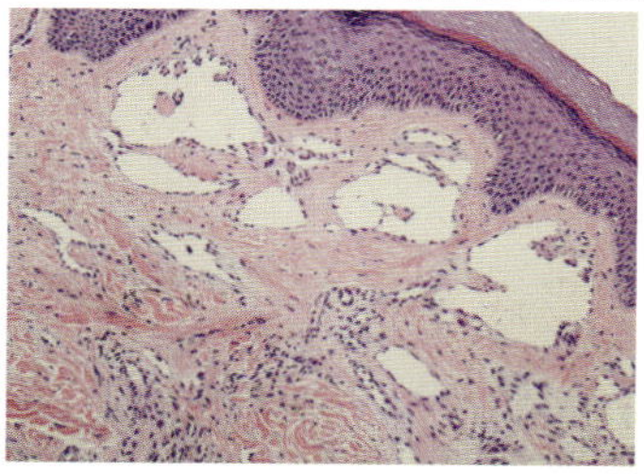	
Clustered, thin-walled, dilated vascular channels wind through the dermis and subcutaneous tissues. Some of the bland endothelial cells 'hobnail' (round nuclei protrude into the lumen) or form intraluminal papillary projections with fibrotic cores. Can look similar to hobnail hemangioma and lymphangioendothelioma, but these two lesions do not have extracutaneous involvement or thrombocytopenia.					
Synovial hemangioma	Very rare	Children or adolescents; adults very rarely	Synovium of knee, elbow, hand	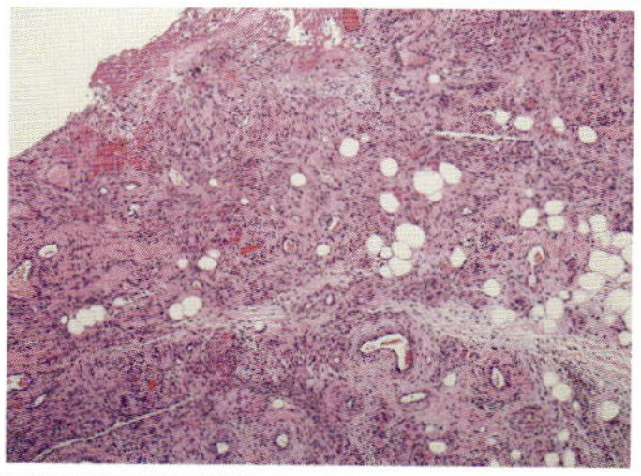	
Circumscribed or diffuse. Can look like a cavernous hemangioma with multiple, thin-walled vein sized vessels or a capillary hemangioma. Located immediately below synovial surface. Often associated with hemosiderin and fibrous or myxoid stroma. May cause reactive synovial hyperplasia. May be a malformation.					
Lymphangioma	Common	Congenital to young childhood most commonly	Head and neck, groin, trunk, limbs, intra-abdominal	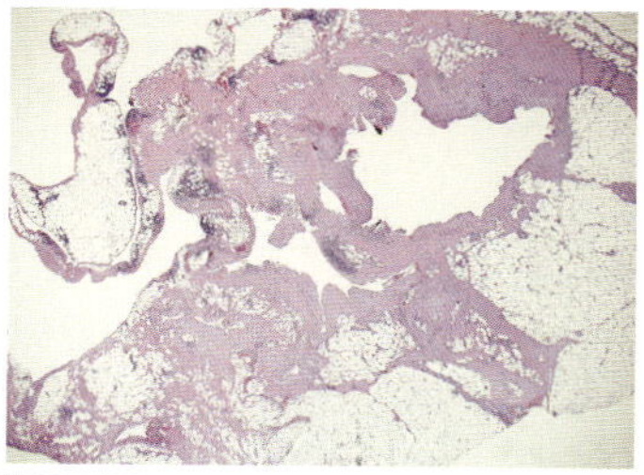	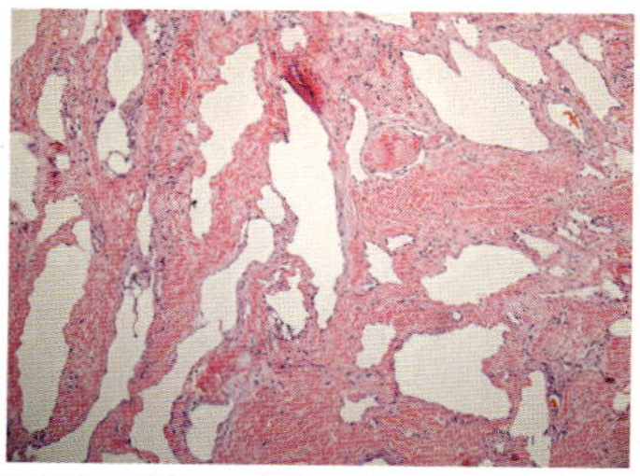
Non-circumscribed collection of dilated, thin-walled lymphatic channels with flattened lining cells. May have fibrosis, mast cells, and lymphoid aggregates in surrounding tissue. Vessels contain proteinaceous material, a few red blood cells, or are empty. Some larger vessels may have a muscular wall. No atypia or necrosis. Congenital neck lymphangioma ('cystic hygroma') can be associated with Turner syndrome (monosomy X).					

Table 10.2: Continued from page 202

Tumor	Incidence	Age and sex distribution	Body site (in order of occurrence)	Histopathology description including IHC	
				Medium magnification	High magnification
Angiomatosis	Common	All ages but children to young adults most commonly; rare after 40 years	Leg, trunk, and arm. Must involve multiple tissue planes such as skin, subcutis muscle and bone or multiple contiguous muscles	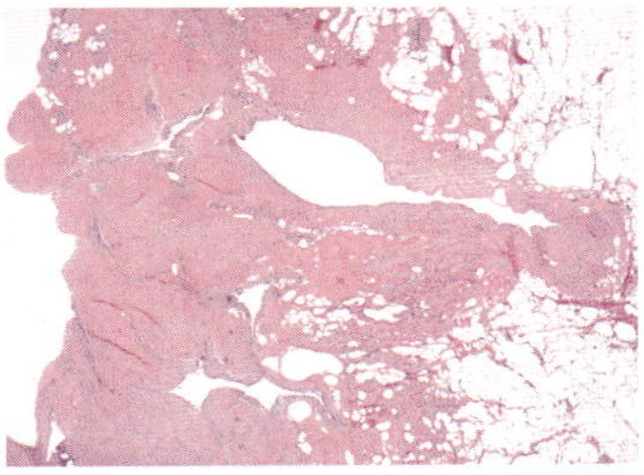	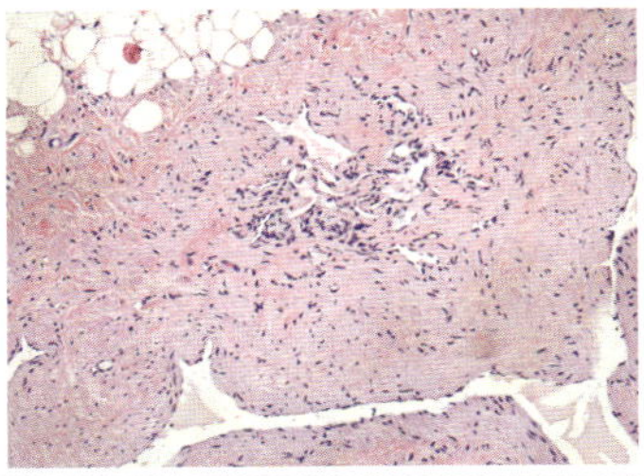
Non-circumscribed. Most common histology is various vessel sizes and calibers from capillary to large ectatic veins embedded in mature adipose. Less commonly, the tumor can appear like a non-circumscribed capillary hemangioma embedded in fat. (Basically, most look exactly like an intramuscular hemangioma.) Rarely, glomus cells are prominent: *glomangiomatosis+. Some cases have distinctive pattern of small vessels cascading from the walls of the larger vessels. No atypia, absent to rare mitoses, and no necrosis. Negative for GLUT-1.					
Intermediate: can recur locally aggressively and/or may rarely metastasize (<5%)					
Kaposiform hemangioendothelioma	Rare	Infancy to early childhood most common, but can occur in adults	Skin, soft tissues of extremities then trunk, retroperitoneum	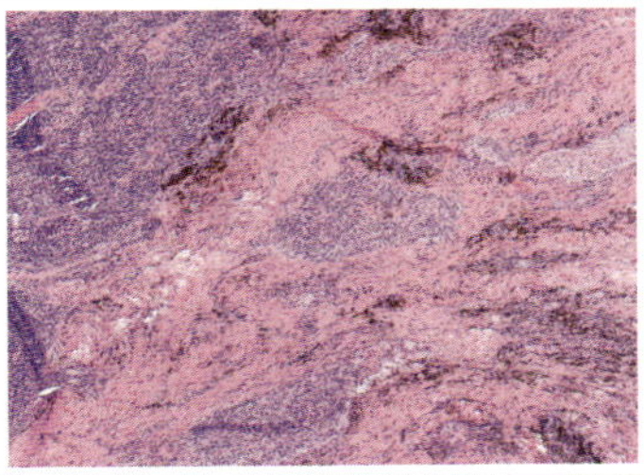	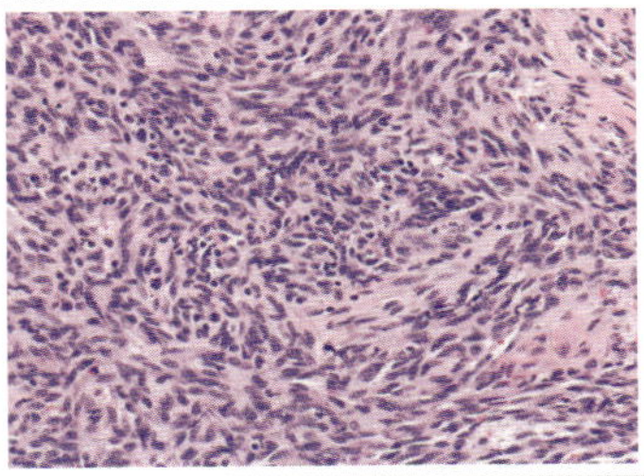
Infiltrative. Nodules and fascicles of streaming to swirling spindle cells with interspersed slit-like vascular spaces and capillaries. Other common findings include a lymphangioma-like periphery of dilated, thin-walled lymphatic channels and glomeruloid groups of more rounded cells with or without fibrin thrombi. Entire tumor is CD31 CD34 and FLI-1 reactive. D2-40 is distinctly expressed in spindle cells but not glomeruloid foci. Some SMA positivity in pericytes. No atypia, no atypical mitoses. Negative for HHV8 expression. Closely related to tufted angioma of skin.					
Papillary intralymphatic angioendothelioma (Dabska tumor)	Very rare	Children most commonly, but also young adults F slightly > M	Skin including subcutis of distal extremities; rarely occurs elsewhere including viscera	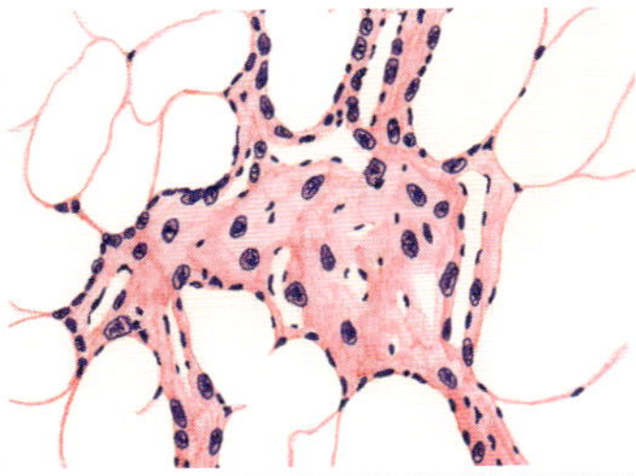	
Non-circumscribed, Infiltrative tumor of dilated, thin-walled lymphatic channels that contain free-floating and ball-like papillae. The papillae are covered by endothelial cells with bulging hyperchromatic nuclei (hob nailing). Papillary cores are fibrous or hyalinized. Surrounding stroma may be sclerotic, may have lymphangioma-like changes, and often has lymphocytic inflammation. Probably closely related to retiform hemangioendothelioma.					

M: male, F: female. OS: osteosarcoma. IHC: immunohistochemistry, ABC: aneurysmal bone cyst.

Incidence note: 'Common to very common' indicates that a medium sized practice will treat at least several to dozens of patients with the lesion annually, 'uncommon to rare' indicates the same practice size will treat one to two patients with the lesion every five years, 'Rare to very rare' indicates the same sized practice will see zero to one patient with the lesion every 20 years.

Table 10.3 Predominantly adult vascular tumors of soft tissue grouped by behavior

Tumor	Incidence	Age and sex distribution	Body site (in order of occurrence)	Histopathology description including IHC	
				Medium magnification	High magnification
Benign: does not recur or recurs non-aggressively and does not metastasize					
Capillary hemangioma	Very common	All ages	Skin	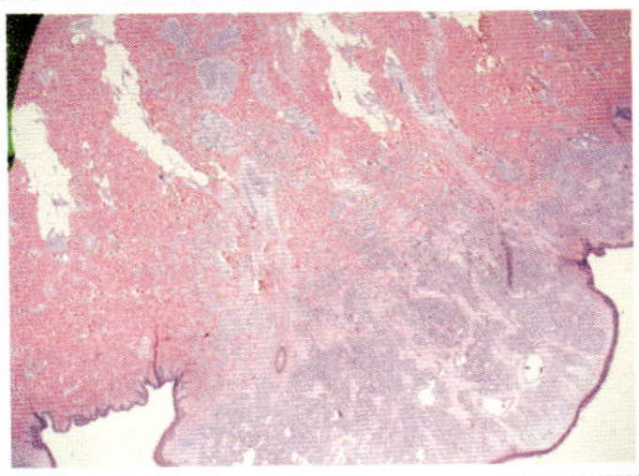	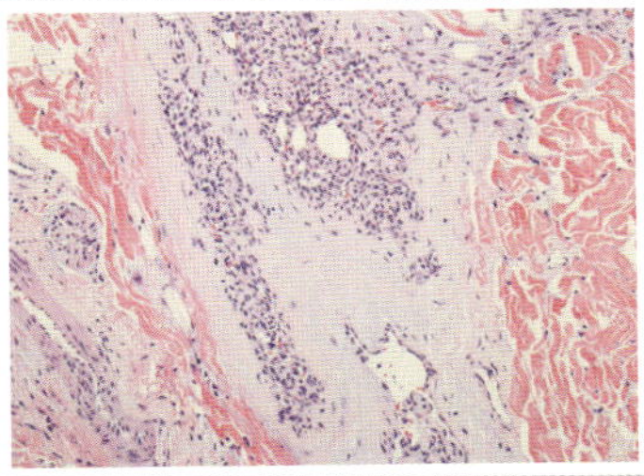
Sharply circumscribed, non-infiltrative lobules of capillary-sized vessels. No cytologic atypia and no atypical mitoses. Older lesions may have fibrosis with scattered, single ectatic vessels. Positive for routine vascular markers.					

Table 10.3: Continued from page 203

<table>
<tr><th rowspan="2">Tumor</th><th rowspan="2">Incidence</th><th rowspan="2">Age and sex distribution</th><th rowspan="2">Body site (in order of occurrence)</th><th colspan="2">Histopathology description including IHC</th></tr>
<tr><th>Medium magnification</th><th>High magnification</th></tr>
<tr><td>Intramuscular hemangioma</td><td>Common</td><td>All ages but adolescents and young adults most commonly</td><td>Intramuscular lesion of thigh, lower leg, head and neck and trunk
M = F</td><td>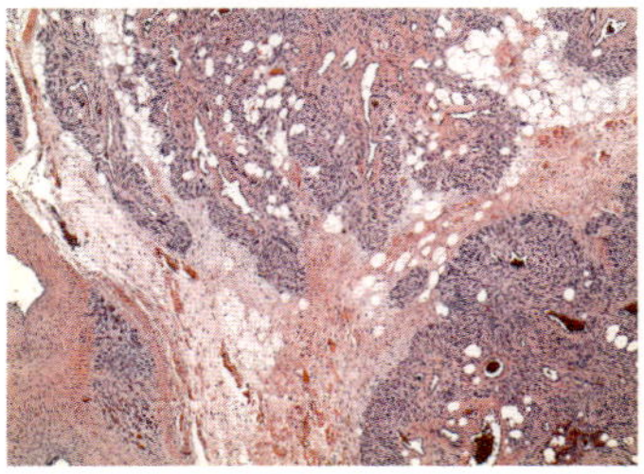</td><td>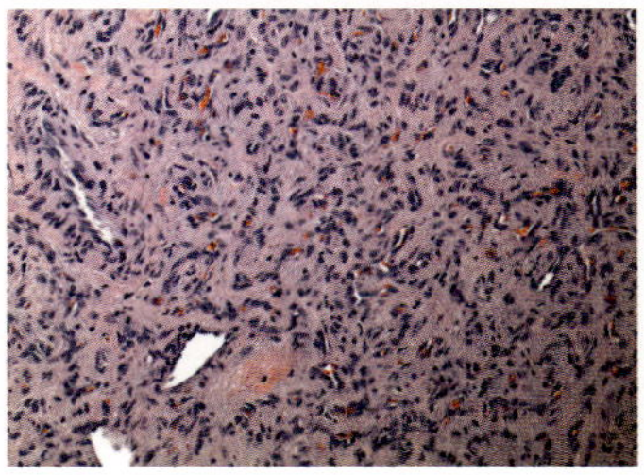</td></tr>
<tr><td colspan="6">Non-circumscribed proliferation of vessels embedded in mature adipose tissue +/- atrophic skeletal muscle fibers. Most commonly, the vessels are mixed caliber, but lesions resembling capillary hemangioma also occur. May have lymphatic like channels also. Secondary thrombosis, calcification, and metaplastic ossification can occur. Confined to one muscle. No cytologic atypia. Some cases may be malformations.</td></tr>
<tr><td>Venous hemangioma</td><td>Rare</td><td>Adults and rarely children</td><td>Subcutaneous or deep</td><td>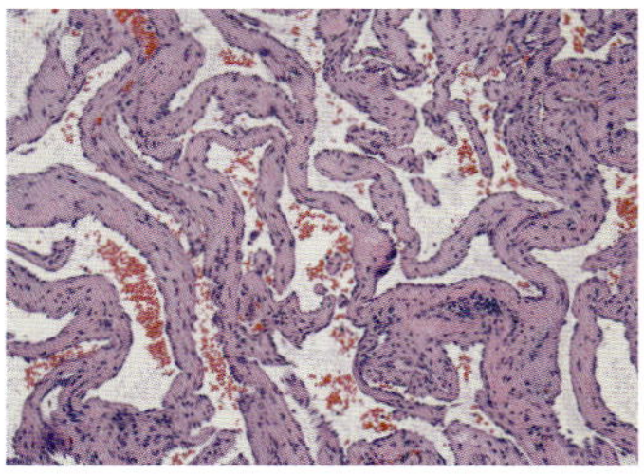</td><td></td></tr>
<tr><td colspan="6">Non-circumscribed collection of thick-walled veins often with calcifications and thrombosis. Some veins may be very dilated. Elastic stains show lack of internal elastic lamina consistent with veins rather than arteries.</td></tr>
<tr><td>Spindle cell hemangioma</td><td>Rare</td><td>Young adults most commonly
M = F</td><td>Skin including subcutis</td><td>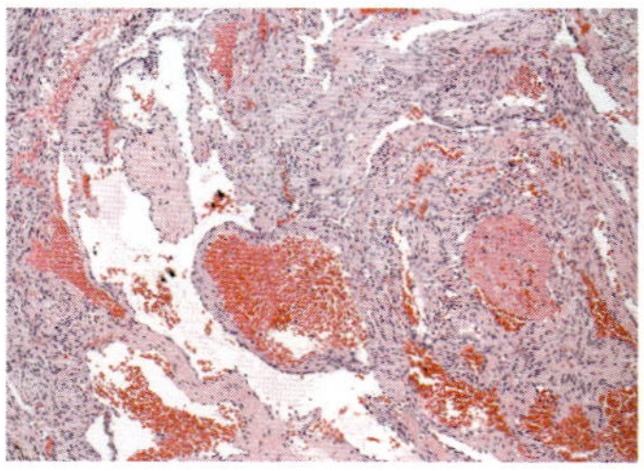</td><td>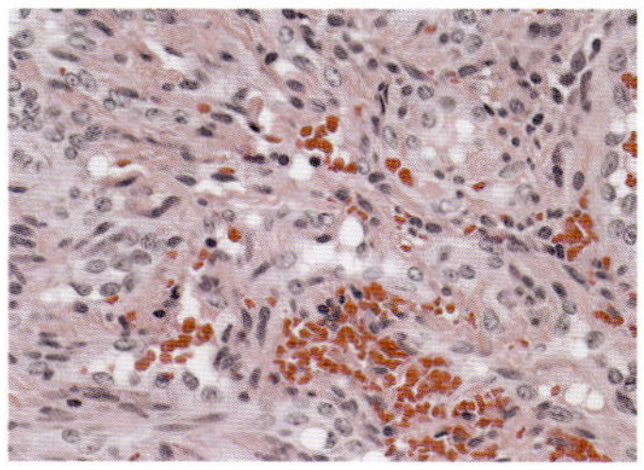</td></tr>
<tr><td colspan="6">Usually circumscribed lesion composed of 1) cavernous hemangioma like area and 2) spindle cell areas that feature slit-like vascular lumens. May have intravascular component. Some endothelial cells are highly vacuolated and look like fat cells. No necrosis, atypia, or inflammation. Mitoses may be present but without atypical forms. Tumor cells comprise endothelial cells (CD31, CD34 positive) and pericytic cells (SMA positive). Negative for GLUT-1 and HHV8. 5% of patients have Maffucci syndrome (multiple enchondromas and vascular tumors).</td></tr>
<tr><td>Epithelioid hemangioma (angiolymphoid hyperplasia with eosinophilia)</td><td>Rare</td><td>Young to middle aged adults; children rarely</td><td>Skin including subcutis; deep soft tissue (including bone) uncommonly</td><td>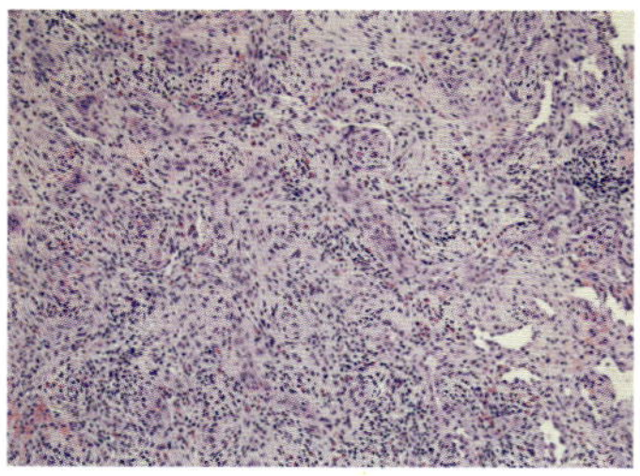</td><td>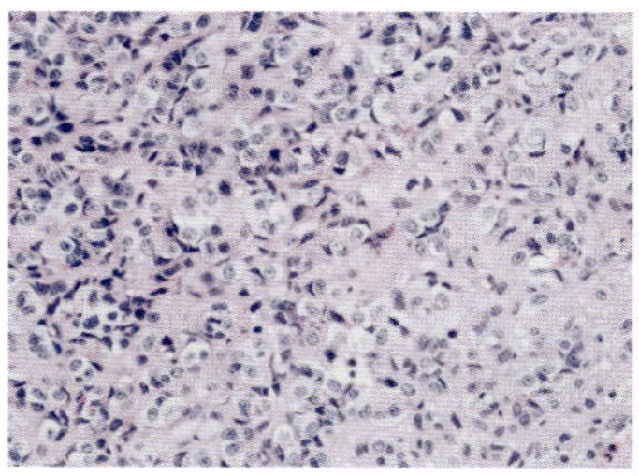</td></tr>
<tr><td colspan="6">Cellular proliferation of epithelioid (large round eosinophilic cells with distinct cell borders) endothelial cells. The cells can form solid areas, but vessels and pericytes can often be identified in the 'solid' areas by reticulin and SMA staining. Capillary type vessels lined by epithelioid endothelial cells are present at least focally. Half of cases have a central, damaged artery infiltrated by tumor cells. Stroma often contains numerous eosinophils and lymphocytes. No significant nuclear atypia and no atypical mitoses. May be positive for low molecular weight keratins (keratins 8 and 18). Positive for vascular markers such as CD31, CD34 and FLI-1.</td></tr>
</table>

Table 10.3: Continued from page 204

Tumor	Incidence	Age and sex distribution	Body site (in order of occurrence)	Histopathology description including IHC: Medium magnification	High magnification
Intermediate: can recur locally aggressively and/or may rarely metastasize (<5%)					
Retiform hemangioendothelioma (retiform)	Rare	Middle aged adults most commonly, but also children. F > M	Skin including subcutis	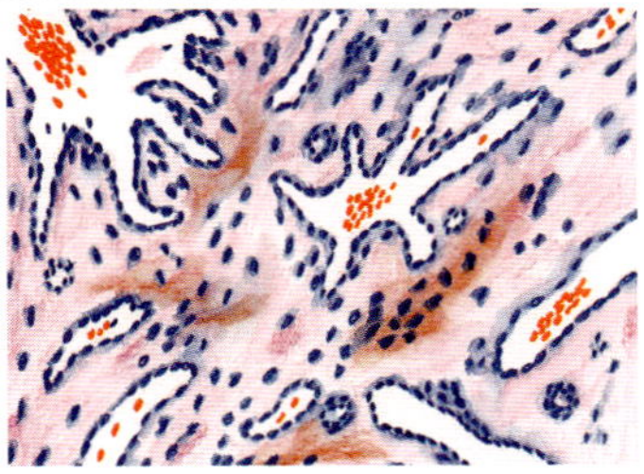	
Non-circumscribed, infiltrative proliferation of layered, connecting, thin walled-vascular channels reminiscent of rete testis architecture. Endothelial cell nuclei are hyperchromatic and 'hobnail' into vessel lumens. Some cases have papillary balls like Dabska tumor (and retiform HE is probably related to Dabska tumor). Prominent lymphocytic inflammation present in stroma in most cases. Mitoses rare but not atypical. Positive for CD31 and CD34 but negative in most cases for D2-40. Negative for HHV8 expression.					
Composite hemangioendothelioma	Very rare	Young adults most commonly but also children	Skin including subcutis of extremities including foot/ ankle and hands, but also head and neck	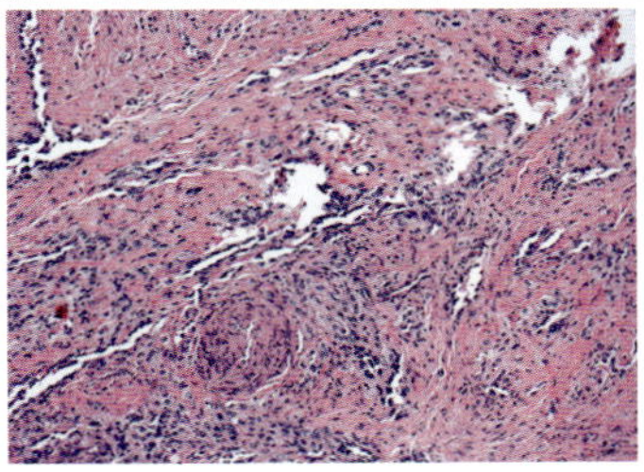	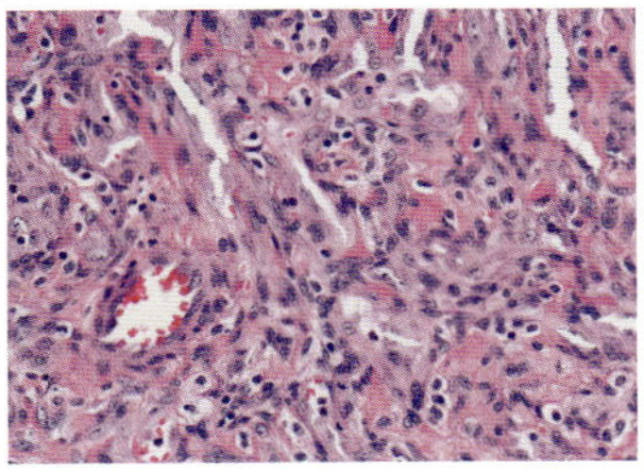
Infiltrative. Characterized by a mixture of other vascular tumor patterns from benign to intermediate to malignant. Most common combinations are epithelioid HE and retiform HE. Other patterns can include angiosarcoma (low grade most commonly), Kaposiform HE, spindle cell hemangioma, epithelioid hemangioma, and AV malformation. The components involved don't predict behavior even with high grade angiosarcoma pattern present. HHV8 negative and positive for CD31, CD34, and FLI-1. One series of four cases reported D2-40 reactivity in KHE component.					
Pseudomyogenic hemangioendothelioma (PM-HE) [Epithelioid sarcoma-like hemangioendothelioma (ESL-HE)]	Very rare	Young adults most commonly M = F	Superficial and deep soft tissues most commonly of extremities but also chest wall and head and neck. May be multifocal	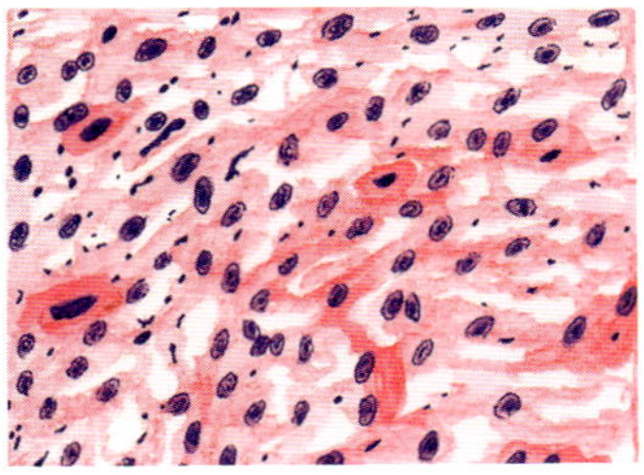	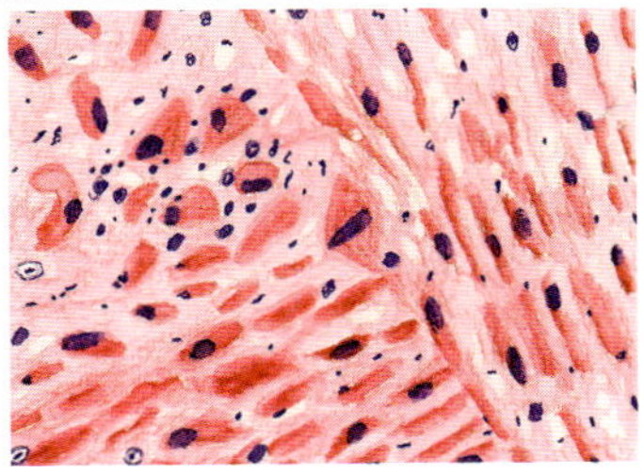
		Young adults most commonly. M >> F	Dermis (31%), subcutis (20%) muscle (34%), bone (14%). 66% multifocal including multiple tissue planes. Most commonly extremities including hands and feet but also H&N, trunk		
Rare, recently described tumor. ESL-HE was first described in 2003 with 7 cases. PM-HE was first described in 2011 with 50 cases and proposed to be the same as ESL-HE. Behavior: local recurrence, low risk for regional LN metastasis, and very low risk for distant metastasis. ESL-HE: Sheets, nodules, and fascicles of predominantly rounded, eosinophilic (epithelioid) cells set in a desmoplastic stroma. Some areas of spindled tumor cells. No vascular channel formation and no hemorrhage. 50% had cells with cytoplasmic vacuoles consistent with early vascular lumen formation. Low mitotic rate. No necrosis. Mild cytologic atypia. Positive for CD31, FLI-1, keratins. Negative for CD34. PM-HE: fascicles and sheets of plump eosinophilic spindle cells with focal, more epithelioid cells. Vesicular nuclei with variably prominent nucleoli. Low grade in nearly all cases; a few with high grade foci. Low mitotic rate. Necrosis rare. Neutrophil infiltrate prominent in few cases. AE1/AE3 keratins and FLI-1 positive. Variably positive for CD31. Negative for CD34.					

Table 10.3: Continued from page 205

Tumor	Incidence	Age and sex distribution	Body site (in order of occurrence)	Histopathology description including IHC	
				Medium magnification	High magnification
Kaposi sarcoma	Uncommon	1. classic indolent KS: Mediterranean elderly men 2. endemic African KS: African children and middle-aged adults 3. iatrogenic KS: solid organ transplant patients or patients on corticosteroids 4. AIDS-associated KS	Skin and lymph nodes most commonly but also soft tissue and viscera. Bone only extremely rarely	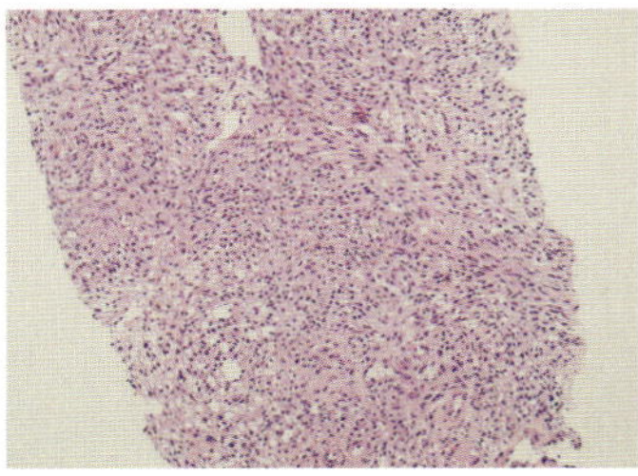	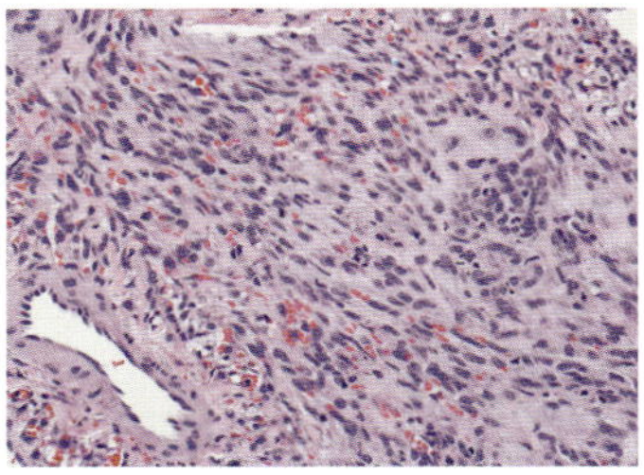
Infiltrative fascicular proliferation of myoid (eosinophilic) spindle cells with interspersed slit-like vascular spaces. Extracellular hyaline globules, extravasated red blood cells, hemosiderin and chronic inflammation common. (Earliest stage, 'patch' stage, has fewer spindle cells and more ectatic small vessels.) Cytologic atypia is minimal except in endemic African form. Tumor cells express CD31, CD34, and FLI-1 and can be positive for D2-40. Most importantly, all cases are reactive for HHV8 antibody. HIstologic variants include tumors resembling lymphangioma or cavernous hemangioma.					
Epithelioid hemangioendo-thelioma (EHE)	Uncommon	Adults of all ages; rare in children F > M	Subcutis and deep ST of extremities, head and neck, trunk Rarely occurs in dermis Visceral locations include liver, spleen, lungs	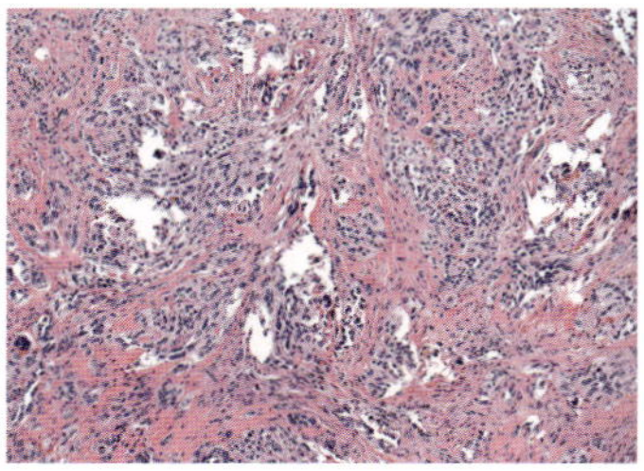	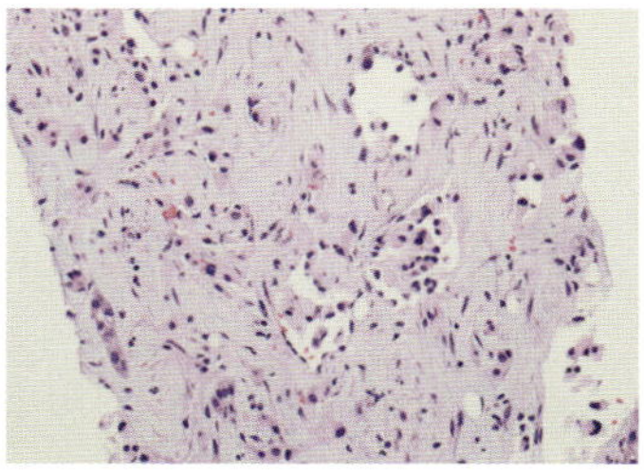
Infiltrative cords, strands, nests and single cells set in a myxoid, myxochondroid, or collagenous-hyaline matrix. Most of the cells are epithelioid (round with distinct cell borders, moderate N/C ratio, and round nuclei). A few cells may be more spindled. Cells with intracytoplasmic lumens (appear like vacuoles) commonly seen. Well- formed vessels are absent to rare. Intraluminal growth in small to medium sized vessels is common. I/3rd show increased atypia with prominent nucleoli, nuclear variation, increased mitoses, solid growth, and necrosis. These high grade or 'malignant EHE' may behave more aggressively. Almost all are positive for CD31 and FLI-1, 60-90% positive for CD34. May be positive for low molecular weight keratins and D2-40.					
Angiosarcoma of soft tissue	Rare			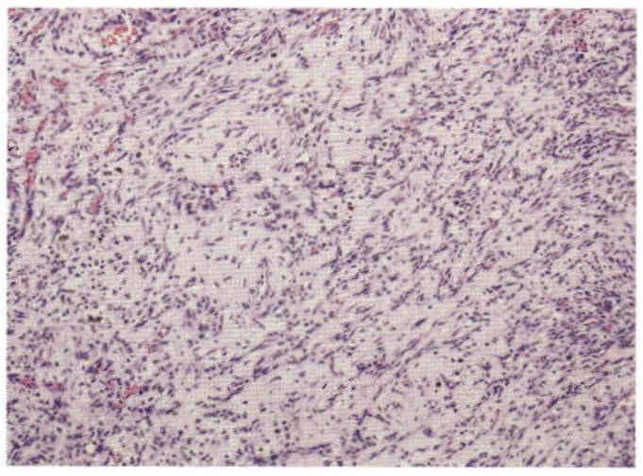	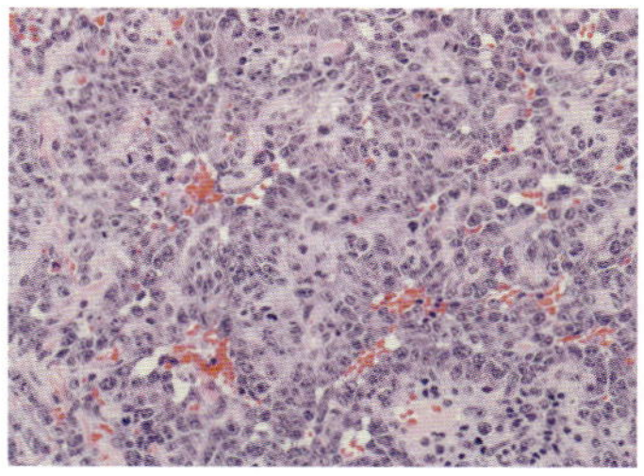
Infiltrative tumor with four main appearances: Low grade vascular tumor with vessels of low cytologic atypia infiltrating normal tissue. Intermediate grade tumors with mixture of vessel formation and spindle or epithelioid solid growth with moderate nuclear atypia. High grade spindle cell tumors with only rare or few tumor vessels or slit-like vascular spaces mimicking a spindle cell sarcoma. Epithelioid angiosarcoma with only rare or few tumor vessels or slit-like vascular spaces mimicking carcinoma or melanoma. Tumor cells are positive for CD31, FLI-1, CD34 in varying proportions. Also may be positive for D2-40 and low molecular weight keratins. Negative for HHV8 expression.					

M: male, F: female. IHC: immunohistochemistry

Incidence note: 'Common to very common' indicates that a medium sized practice will treat at least several to dozens of patients with the lesion annually, 'Uncommon to rare' indicates the same practice size will treat one to two patients with the lesion every five years, 'Rare to very rare' indicates the same sized practice will see zero to one patient with the lesion every 20 years.

Table 10.4 Ten-year relative survival rate in 13 SEER registries for years 1994 and 2008, % survival (SE=standard error).

Vascular tumor type*	Percent survival (SE)
Hemangiosarcoma	22.8% (3.9%)
Kaposi sarcoma	50.7% (8.1%)
Malignant epithelioid hemangioendothelioma	55.6% (10.5%)
Malignant hemangioendothelioma	62.1% (11.3%)

* Due to a small number of cases, 10 year survival could not be calculated for lymphangiosarcoma.

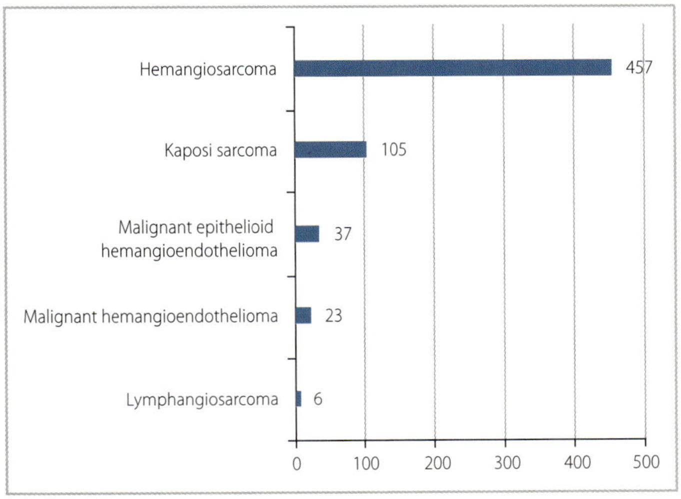

Figure 10.1 Frequency of vascular tumors of the soft tissue in 13 SEER registries between the years 1994 and 2008.

sporadic and inheritable vascular malformations, and at least some of these mutations may also be seen in vascular neoplasms (Duffy 2010).

Hemangioendotheliomas

Epithelioid hemangioendothelioma has a t(1;3)(p36;q25) in the majority of cases analyzed (Tanas et al. 2011, Errani et al. 2011). This translocation fuses the WWTR1 gene (3q25), a transcription regulator, with the CAMTA1 gene (1p36), a transcription activator. The time from first publication of two cases of this translocation in EHE to identification of the genes involved spanned 10 years (Mendlick et al. 2001). The t(1;3)(p36;q25) translocation appears to be unique for the classic histologic variant of EHE, both low and high grade forms, and is present in the majority of cases thus far tested. It was not found in the epithelioid sarcoma-like variant of HE (Errani et al. 2011). A possible potentiating role of Bartonella bacterial infections in epithelioid hemangioendothelioma has been suggested based on analysis of three patients (Mascarelli et al. 2011).

The other, long-establshed types of hemangioendothelioma, retiform HE, composite HE, and Kaposiform HE, lack the t(1;3)(p36;q25). A newly described variant of hemangioendothelioma, pseudomyogenic hemangioendothelioma, may show a non-random t(7;19)(q22;q13) translocation involving unknown genes (Trombetta et al. 2011). A third new type of epithelioid hemangioendothelioma lacking the t(1;3)(p36;q25) translocation and characterized by unusual histologic features has been proposed which exhibits TFE3 gene rearrangements (Antonescu et al. 2013).

Papillary intralymphatic angioendothelioma may develop in some cases from a pre-existing lymphangioma.

Kaposi sarcoma

Human herpes simplex virus 8 is implicated in all forms of Kaposi sarcoma. This includes classic KS of elderly men of Mediterranean

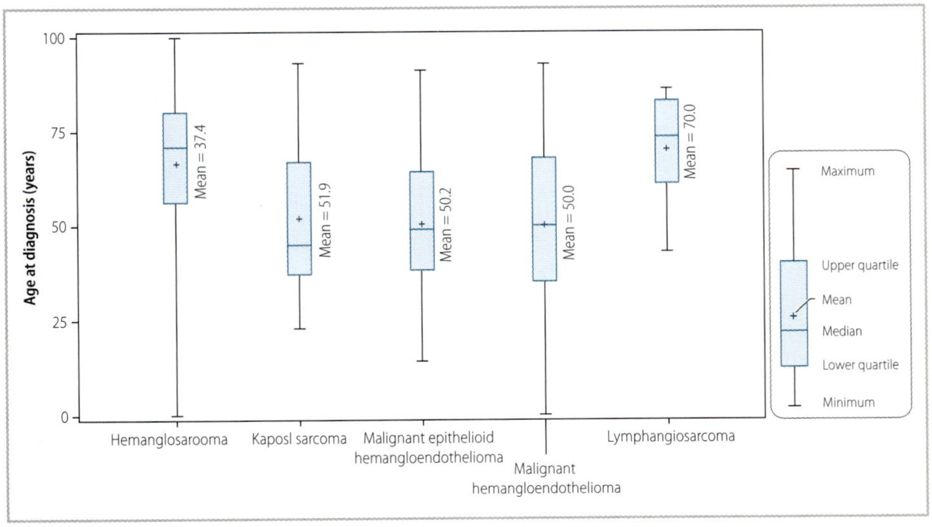

Figure 10.2 Age distribution of vascular tumors of the soft tissue among cases in 13 SEER registries during the time period 1994-2008 (N=628).

and African origin, endemic KS of African men and children, epidemic KS of HIV/AIDS, and iatrogenic KS in immunocompromised patients, non-HIV related.

Angiosarcoma

Angiosarcoma is associated with a panoply of risk factors. These include familial or genetic syndromes (Klippel-Trenaunay syndrome, Maffucci syndrome, NF-1, familial retinoblastoma, xeroderma pigmentosum and possibly mutated BRCA1 or BRCA2), exposures (anabolic steroids, Thorotrast, arsenic in pesticides, radium, and vinyl chloride), lymphedema (as in Stewart-Treves syndrome), solar radiation, persistent foreign bodies (synthetic mesh, orthopedic prostheses, retained surgical gauze, bullets or shrapnel, etc), and certain tumors (benign vascular lesions, nerve sheath tumors, germ cell tumors, and leiomyoma)(Abraham et al. 2007, Young et al. 2010).

There are no specific consistent genetic findings in angiosarcoma. The gamut of changes ranges from normal karyotype to aneuploid karyotype with extensive numerical and structural alterations. Most high grade tumors display a complex aneuploid karyotype. The most common findings are trisomy 5, deletion of 7p, and abnormalities of 8, 20 and 22 (Young et al. 2010).

The molecular genetic analysis of angiosarcoma is in its early phases. Pathways implicated include those of the VEGF group (vascular endothelial growth factor) and the corresponding receptors, RAS, WT-1, Galectin-3, p53 and ETS1 as well as others. The possible promoting roles of stromal cells and reactive inflammatory cells are also being investigated.

PATHOLOGY

Refer to **Tables 10.2** and **10.3** for brief descriptions and representative photomicrographs and medical illustrations of vascular tumors that can involve the subcutaneous and deeper soft tissues. The intermediate and malignant tumors are uncommon to rare, and thus refinements of classification are ongoing as more cases are examined. New entities have also been described including pseudomyogenic hemangioendothelioma, epithelioid-sarcoma like hemangioendothelioma and epithelioid hemangioendothelioma with TFE3 rearrangement.

When evaluating a potential vascular tumor, the pathologist must contend with: rare new tumor types, features that overlap with vascular malformations, reactions to infectious agents that can mimic a vascular tumor (bacillary angiomatosis), and confusing secondary changes superimposed on a tumor that are themselves vascular (papillary endothelial hyperplasia and exuberant granulation tissue).

The rarity of some tumors should prompt a cautious diagnostic approach, especially in instances of major clinical treatment differences depending on the diagnosis rendered. Prudence is highly recommended and in some cases, referral to a national expert soft tissue pathologist may be in the patient's best interest. Of course, experts also have access to the latest accessory diagnostic tools including esoteric antibodies, PCR and FISH probes and direct sequencing. Such referrals may also advance the field of vascular tumor classification by enabling accrual of more cases for detailed analysis.

Histologic grading

Benign vascular tumors are not histologically graded. Most appear cytologically uniform with normochromatic nuclei and no atypical mitotic figures. Occasional hemangiomas may exhibit degenerative atypia, and these have been termed 'symplastic hemangioma.' These hemangiomas contain cells with enlarged hyperchromatic nuclei with smudgy chromatin and are analogous to the benign but degenerative atypia found in 'ancient schwannoma' or 'ancient neurofibroma.' There is no coarse granular hyperchromasia or irregular distribution of chromatin as in true nuclear atypia, and abnormal mitotic figures are not identified. In addition, fibrosis, fibrin deposition, and hemosiderin deposits may be present suggestive of prior injury.

Epithelioid hemangioendothelioma and other hemangioendotheliomas

Epithelioid hemangioendothelioma is not formally graded, although one third of cases display high grade features of necrosis, increased mitotic activity with atypical division figures, enlarged, pleomorphic nuclei, prominent nucleoli and solid growth. Some experts have labeled EHE with these findings: 'malignant or 'high grade' EHE. It is controversial whether these atypical features predict more aggressive behavior (Folpe et al. 2010, Deyrup et al. 2008).

Composite hemangioendothelioma, considered an intermediate behaving tumor by the WHO, may contain high grade areas histologically consistent with high grade angiosarcoma. Based on only a few tens of cases, tumors with high grade regions do not behave differently than those with low grade elements (Tsai et al. 2011).

Retiform HE, kaposiform HE, and papillary intralymphatic angioendothelioma display mild to at most modest nuclear atypia (hyperchromasia of hobnailing endothelial cell nuclei) and are considered intermediate behaving by the WHO They are not formally graded using the FNCLCC or other system.

Kaposi sarcoma

Kaposi sarcoma is not formally graded using the FNCLCC or other system. Histologically, however, most cases display mild to moderate cytologic atypia. High grade nuclear pleomorphism and prominent mitotic activity are more common in the African endemic cases (Folpe et al 2010).

Angiosarcoma

Angiosarcomas range from low grade (FNCLCC Grade 1) to high grade (FNCLCC Grades 2 and 3) tumors. Not uncommonly, one tumor will contain both low and high grade regions. Grade 1 tumors are characterized by well-formed vessels that permeate normal tissues, have a low mitotic rate and minimal nuclear atypia. High grade tumors are poorly differentiated with spongy or sieve-like areas, necrosis, mitotic activity, and solid areas with or without interspersed, slit-like vascular spaces. Some high grade angiosarcomas closely resemble a fascicular spindle cell sarcoma. Others appear epithelioid suggesting metastatic carcinoma, melanoma, or another type of sarcoma with epithelioid cells such as proximal type epithelioid sarcoma. A careful search usually discloses vasoformative areas (slit-like vascular spaces or abortive vessels lined by atypical malignant endothelial cells). Immunohistochemistry is essential in cases where the malignant vessel formation is scant or absent.

SEER data for the years 1994-2008 indicate the most common body sites for SEER-tracked malignant vascular tumors are the head and neck and lower extremity (**Figure 10.3**).

Behavior

Hemangiomas

Hemangiomas are benign. Some have a tendency to regress spontaneously (RICH and some juvenile hemangiomas), some may present as crops of lesions, some may pose cosmetic problems, and some are painful. A few are associated with significant local morbidity, recurrence or persistence (such as intramuscular hemangioma, spindle cell hemangioma, lymphangioma and angiomatosis).

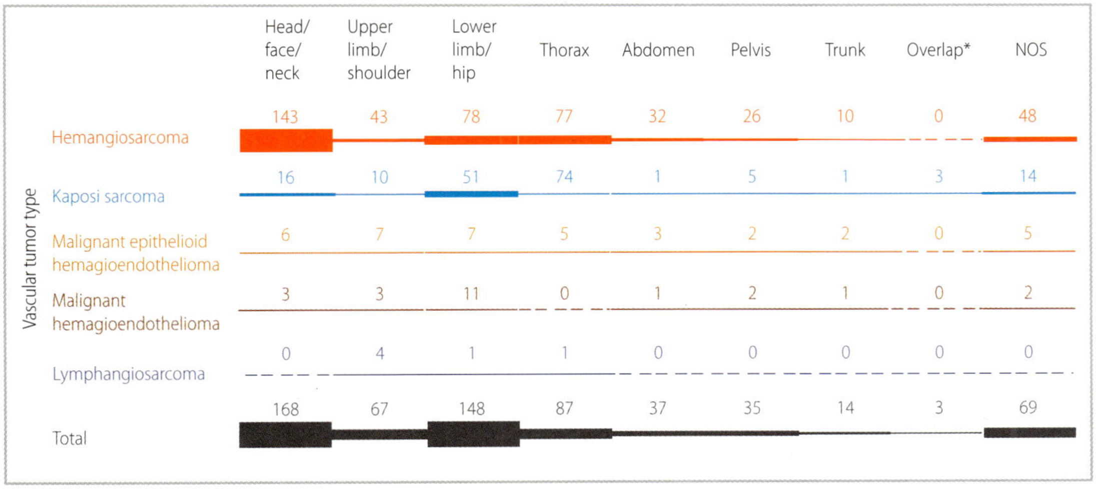

Figure 10.3 Vascular tumors of the soft tissue by site for cases in 13 SEER registries diagnosed between 1994 and 2008.

Epithelioid hemangioendothelioma and other hemangioendotheliomas

All of the hemangioendotheliomas may locally recur. Metastasis risk is very low (<5%) for retiform HE, Kaposiform HE, composite HE, and papillary intralymphatic angioendothelioma. By contrast, there is a substantial risk for metastasis and death in patients with epithelioid hemangioendothelioma (20-30% metastasis; 10-20% mortality)(Fisher et al. 2011). Risk factors for more aggressive behavior in EHE include tumors greater than 3 cm in diameter and tumors with greater than 3 mitotic figures/50 high magnification microscopic fields (Deyrup et al. 2008). Some authors also suggest that anaplastic features (high nuclear grade, many mitoses, necrosis, and sheet-like growth) behave more aggressively (Folpe et al. 2010).

Kaposiform HE (and possibly also composite HE) may be associated with Kasabach-Merritt syndrome which resolves upon complete excision of the tumor.

Two new variants of hemangioendothelioma, epithelioid sarcoma-like hemangioendothelioma and pseudomyogenic hemangioendothelioma have the capacity to recur locally and uncommonly regionally metastasize but only rarely metastasize to a distant site (Hornick et al. 2011; Billings et al. 2003). Relatively few cases of these new hemangioendotheliomas have been reported, and it is possible that they represent a histologic spectrum of one new hemangioendothelioma subtype. A variant of epithelioid hemangioendothelioma associated with TFE3 gene rearrangement is too newly described to predict behavior.

Kaposi sarcoma

The behavior of KS depends in part on the clinical form. Classic KS of elderly Mediterranean, African and central European men is typically indolent, spares the viscera, and is a multifocal dermal process. KS associated with iatrogenic causes (such as use of steroids or other immunosuppressive drugs in patients with solid organ transplants) improves with cessation of the causative therapy. African or endemic KS ranges from indolent to aggressive behavior. Finally, epidemic KS generally behaves aggressively without treatment.

Angiosarcoma

Overall, soft tissue angiosarcoma portends a poor outcome (five year overall survival ~40%). High histologic grade and epithelioid morphology may be particularly ominous (Fayette et al. 2007, Abraham et al. 2007). Additional negative prognostic factors include size > 5 cm, old age, metastases at presentation, poor performance status, visceral site (especially heart) and tumor associated with radiation or lymphedema (Young 2010, Abraham et al. 2007).

From SEER data (1994-2008), ten-year relative survival (or relative to the general population of corresponding sex and age) for vascular tumors of the soft tissue ranges from 22.8% to 62.1%, with hemangiosarcoma cases having the worst prognosis, and malignant hemangioendothelioma cases the best (**Table 10.4**)

Additional laboratory testing

Immunohistochemistry

Selected antibody use empowers the pathologist. However, this use must be discerning, as the number of antibodies 100% sensitive and 100% specific for a particular tumor are very few out of thousands commercially available. A 'shotgun' approach to antibody selection will result in a diagnosis full of holes. Antibodies should be selected that can support or refute the pathologist's rational, honed histologic differential that is aligned with the clinical and radiologic findings.

The most common antibodies used to identify vascular tumors are CD34 (generally the most sensitive except for angiosarcoma), CD31 (more specific than CD34), FLI-1 (sensitive and relatively specific compared to CD34) and ERG. FLI-1 and ERG have the advantage of crisp nuclear staining. In most histologic differentials, it is important to use more than one of these antibodies. For example, epithelioid sarcoma, which can look like EHE occasionally, is often CD34 reactive and keratin expressing like EHE. It is negative for CD31 and FLI-1, however.

Not just vascular tumors express these 'vascular markers'. Rare carcinomas express CD34 or CD31, and CD31 antibody also stains histiocytes and plasma cells (usually in a grainy cytoplasmic manner rather than in a membranous pattern as in many vascular tumors). In general, in a high grade tumor, CD31 with or without FLI-1, ERG or CD34 reactivity is more convincing for vascular differentiation than a tumor with only CD34 expression. FLI-1, however, is usually positive in Ewing sarcoma/PNET, some lymphoblastic lymphomas and a few other carcinomas and rare sarcomas, and those entities would need to be excluded by integrating clinical presentation, histomorphology and additional markers (Mhawech-Fauceglia et al. 2007).

Podoplanin (D2-40 antibody) is another protein that can be expressed in vascular and lymphatic channel tumors. However, its broad spectrum of reactivity with other tumors including carcinomas, mesothelioma, and other sarcomas limits its usefulness. It is controversial whether D2-40 reactivity specifically denotes lymphatic rather than vascular differentiation in angiosarcomas.

Antibody to GLUT-1 can be useful in evaluating a cellular, vasoformative pediatric tumor. In this setting, it is very sensitive and specific for juvenile (congenital infantile) hemangioma.

Epithelioid hemangiomas, epithelioid hemangioendotheliomas, and some angiosarcomas, especially epithelioid angiosarcomas, often express keratins and/or EMA (epithelial membrane antigen). This could lead to an erroneous diagnosis of carcinoma unless careful attention is paid to vasoformative areas, and a panel of antibodies is used that includes the other vascular markers.

Wilms tumor antigen-1 may be useful in the context of distinguishing a vascular malformation from a true vascular neoplasm. Staining is generally absent to very focal in malformations and diffuse in most vascular tumors (Dhaybi et al. 2010, Lawley et al. 2005, Trindade et al. 2011). However, WT1 is also expressed in reactive proliferating endothelium and normal endothelium, so it does not distinguish between a neoplasm and exuberant organizing thrombus.

Because many benign and low grade vascular tumors contain neoplastic pericytes as well as endothelial cells, smooth muscle actin will be expressed in these tumors in pericytes that cuff the endothelial cells. Recall also that any traumatized tumor may have SMA-positive reactive, non-neoplastic myofibroblasts; these should not be mistaken for tumor cells.

Other contenders for use in vascular tumor diagnosis include antibodies to Prox1, VEGFR3, and Claudin-5, among others (Miettinen et al. 2011, Huu et al. 2010). As sophisticated proteome and transcriptome data accumulate, more antibodies will be developed of greater specificity and sensitivity.

Table 10.5 lists the antibody reactivity patterns reported for vascular tumors of soft tissue and subcutis.

Table 10.5 Immunohistochemistry profiles of vascular tumors of subcutaneous tissues and deep soft tissues

Tumor or lesion	Vascular markers	Other markers	Comments
Vascular malformation (VM)	CD31, CD34, FLI-1 positive	D2-40 may be positive WT-1 is usually absent	Lack of WT-1 reactivity may be useful in guiding treatment choice
Rapidly involuting congenital hemangioma (RICH)	CD31, CD34, FLI-1 positive	WT-1 positive	Antibody staining not necessary except where VM is in differential
Non-involuting congenital hemangioma (NICH)	CD31, CD34, FLI-1 positive	WT-1 positive	Antibody staining not necessary except in cases where VM is in differential
Cutaneovisceral angiomatosis with thrombocytopenia	CD31, CD34, FLI-1 positive	D2-40 may be positive	Antibody staining not necessary
Juvenile (congenital infantile) hemangioma	CD31, CD34, FLI-1 positive	GLUT-1 is almost always positive	GLUT-1 is sensitive and specific for juvenile hemangioma
Intramuscular hemangioma and angiomatosis	CD31, CD34, FLI-1 positive	WT-1 positive in intramuscular hemangioma	WT-1 staining may be useful in guiding treatment choice
Spindle cell hemangioma	CD31, CD34, FLI-1 positive in endothelial cells	Negative for GLUT-1 and HHV8 Positive for SMA in spindle cells Positive for Prox1	Juvenile hemangioma and KS may be in the histologic differential
Lymphangioma	May be focally or weakly CD31 and CD34 positive	D2-40 positive WT-1 negative	Antibody staining not necessary
Epithelioid hemangioma	CD31, CD34, FLI-1 positive	WT-1 positive SMA positive in neoplastic pericytes Keratins (AE1/AE3) may be positive	May have obscuring inflammation composed of lymphocytes +/- eosinophils Vascular markers and SMA highlight compressed vessels in cellular, solid-appearing areas
Papillary intralymphatic angioendothelioma (PILA)	CD31, CD34, FLI-1 positive	Prox1 positive (n=1) D2-40 usually positive	
Retiform hemangioendothelioma	CD31, CD34, FLI-1 positive	D2-40 usually negative Prox1 usually positive	PILA and retiform HE may be related although D2-40 reactivity reportedly differs
Kaposiform hemangioendothelioma	CD31 and CD34 positive (especially in glomeruloid foci)	Prox1 positive in spindle cells D2-40 positive in spindle cells HHV8 negative GLUT-1 negative	Differential is most commonly between Kaposi sarcoma and juvenile hemangioma
Composite hemangioendothelioma	CD31, CD34 and FLI-1 positive	D2-40 may be positive	<75 cases reported in the literature
Pseudomyogenic hemangioendothelioma (epithelioid sarcoma-like hemangioendothelioma)	CD31, ERG and FLI-1 positive CD34 negative	Keratin positive (AE1/AE3) SMA may be positive INI-1 positive (intact) Prox1 negative (n=1)	Differential diagnosis is smooth muscle tumors (would be SMA and usually desmin, caldesmon positive; negative for CD31, FLI-1) and epithelioid sarcoma (usually CD31 and FLI-1 negative; often INI-1 negative)
Epithelioid hemangioendothelioma	CD31, ERG C-terminus directed and FLI-1 almost always positive CD34 commonly positive	Keratins positive in 25% (keratins 7,8) to 100% (keratin 18), EMA may be weakly positive Prox1 positive in 50% D2-40 may be positive	

Table 10.5: Continued from page 210

Tumor or lesion	Vascular markers	Other markers	Comments
Kaposi sarcoma	CD31, CD34, ERG C-terminus directed, and FLI-1 positive	HHV8 always positive Prox1 positive D2-40 often positive	Early plaque phase and lymphangioma like cases may be subtle; HHV8 stain especially helpful
Angiosarcoma NOS	CD31 positive, FLI-1 almost always positive, CD34 variable	Keratins positive (keratins 7,8, 18 or 19, included in AE1/AE3 cocktail) in ~50% D2-40 may be positive SMA may be positive in a few cases Prox1 usually negative in deep AS c-kit positive in ~50%	Histologic differential depends on morphology of the angiosarcoma Different antibody panels are required for AS looking like spindle cell sarcoma, AS looking like carcinoma or melanoma, and AS looking like epithelioid sarcoma
Epithelioid angiosarcoma	CD31 positive, FLI-1 almost always positive, CD34 variable	Keratins positive (keratins 7,8, 18 or 19; AE1/AE3) in ~90%	Need to histologically exclude carcinoma, melanoma or epithelioid sarcoma

Routine cytogenetics

Karyotyping is not of great utility in specifically identifying most vascular tumors. When EHE is in the differential, classic cytogenetics may reveal the t(1;3)(p36;q25) now considered specific and sensitive for the diagnosis. The translocation may also be identified by FISH and PCR techniques. TFE3 gene rearrangements may be the hallmark of a new proposed subtype of epithelioid hemangioendothelioma (Antonescu et al. 2013).

Molecular genetics

Currently, other than for EHE diagnosis, the role of molecular genetic analysis of vascular tumors is limited. Undoubtedly, that will change.

Radiology of vascular tumors of soft tissues

The vascular tumor chapter comprises a spectrum of benign and malignant lesions with broadly varied appearance. The benign vascular lesions include intramuscular hemangioma and soft tissue angiomatosis. Intramuscular hemangioma is confined to a single muscle, whereas soft tissue angiomatosis extends across tissue planes to involve multiple muscles or muscles and dermis. These are otherwise similar appearing and generally show heterogeneous T1 low signal, and have T2 or STIR high signal on MR images. They typically show no capsule and have irregular or infiltrating margins. In other tumors, an irregular or infiltrative margin is a highly worrisome feature indicating tumor aggressiveness. However, with these tumors there is often a striking lack of mass effect or only minimal expansion of a compartment and distortion of adjacent structures.

Also, these vascular tumors have a unique pattern of spread which appears as gentle insinuation into and between adjacent tissues, as opposed to the destructive invasion seen with most sarcomas. These lesions enhance variably with contrast sometimes showing delayed enhancement due to the large vascular spaces which fill by slow leaking of contrast. Occasionally, there are large feeding and draining vessels which may present a hemorrhage risk during surgery or biopsy. Also, there may be small rounded calcified foci visible in the soft tissues on radiographs indicating phleboliths within a hemangioma.

Unfortunately, not all of vascular lesions have the unique features described. However, when a radiologist encounters an ill-defined tumor, without much mass effect, that appears to insinuate across tissue compartments without destruction or displacement, hemangioma and angiomatosis should be strongly considered.

Angiosarcoma is a rare vascular malignancy with variable appearance that can occur in several unique clinical settings. Angiosarcoma is the most common primary malignancy of the heart. Angiosarcoma is also one of the potential secondary sarcomas that can occur after radiation therapy. Stewart-Treves syndrome describes the rare complication of angiosarcoma arising from long standing lymphedema. Although many causes of chronic lymphedema may result in Stewart-Treves syndrome, such as trauma, filariasis, congenital, it is most commonly seen after radical mastectomy.

More recently, Stewart-Treves syndrome is being seen in the setting morbidly obesity. Shon 2011 describes five obese patients with massive localized lymphedema who then develop cutaneous angiosarcomas. Superficial angiosarcomas are nonspecific appearing tumors demonstrating skin thickening and nodularity but usually no enlarged vessels. A patient with previous mastectomy and radiation therapy who presents with skin changes and a mass may erroneously be thought to have breast cancer recurrence and not a secondary angiosarcoma.

Deep soft tissue angiosarcomas also have the nonspecific appearance of an aggressive tumor, however, they are more likely to show enlarged, tortuous vessels and usually show intense enhancement.

SURGERY

Although these tumors are rare in reference to their cutaneous counterparts, they can represent one of the most frustrating musculoskeletal neoplasms from a treatment standpoint, particularly extensive lesions such as angiomatosis.

Intramuscular hemangioma

Asymptomatic tumors may be simply observed. Many of these tumors, particularly those presenting in childhood, will involute over time. Small tumors may be excised with marginal or wide margins, and will often provide a satisfactory result in terms of outcome and recurrence. Large tumors, which are most likely to be associated with symptoms and cosmetic deformity, can prove challenging, and often impossible, to treat. Operating on large tumors can be associated with extensive hemorrhage and high rates of recurrence. Embolization can be used preoperatively to decrease hemorrhage associated with surgery. Embolization (used in high-flow lesions) and sclerotherapy (used in low-flow lesions) have been used with mixed success in the actual treatment of these lesions.

Recurrence rates following surgery range from 10-50%. The rate of local recurrence is lower (probably less than 10%) for wide margin surgery than for marginal excision (probably in the range of 25%).

Soft tissue angiomatosis

Recurrence rates following resection for these extensive tumors can approach 90%. Although these lesions can be symptomatic, disabling, and disfiguring, cure is difficult to accomplish and these patients should be treated as conservatively as possible.

Lymphangioma

Lymphangiomas are less likely to spontaneously involute than hemangiomas and also are more likely to require treatment. Cystic lymphangiomas are often well circumscribed and can be treated with marginal excision with a relatively low recurrence rate. Cavernous lymphangiomas tend to be more invasive and may require wider margins for complete excision and have a higher incidence of local recurrence. Extensive lesions may require a staged surgical excision.

Epithelioid hemangioendothelioma

Because these tumors represent an intermediate grade malignancy with high potential recurrence rate and possibility of metastasis, wide surgical resection is indicated.

Angiosarcoma

Wide surgical resection is the treatment of choice for this malignancy.

MEDICAL ONCOLOGY

Infantile hemangioma

Hemangioma is the most common tumor of infancy, occurring in about 10% of babies and in up to 22% of preterm babies weighing less than 1000 g. The female-to-male ratio is 3–1.8. Most hemangiomas appear after birth and proliferate for 8 to 18 months before regressing over the next 5–8 years, leaving a 'port-wine stain.' The 2 most anatomical areas are the nape of the neck and the bottom of the spine. Small capillary port-wine stains are treated with laser therapy. However, big vascular hemangioma complications include obstruction of the airway or impairment of vision. A large hemangioma could divert a considerable volume of blood and cause high-output heart failure. The Kasabach–Merritt syndrome is a consumption coagulopathy associated with giant hemangioma. Thus, proliferating infantile hemangioma can compress vital structures or cause systemic symptoms leading to a >50% mortality. These big proliferative lesions require intervention.

The classical treatment is oral and intralesional corticosteroids during the growth phase of the hemangioma, with a 30-50% success rate (Weber, et al. 1990).

In 1992, Folkman et al proposed treatment with interferon α, which is effective during and after the proliferation phase. Daily subcutaneous injections of interferon alfa-2a (IFNa) (up to 3 million IU/m^2) in 20 infants with life-threatening or vision-threatening hemangiomas who had failed corticosteroid therapy induced a >50% regression in 18 patients over an average of 8 months (range, 2–13 months). IFNa also stabilized an associated consumptive coagulopathy in 3 of these patients within 7 days (Ezekowitz, et al. 1992). Side effects of IFNa include fever, chills, rarely necrosis of the overlying skin of the hemangioma. IFNa should be used only if steroid, β-blocker, and other potentially less toxic therapies fail. The current recommended treatment of infantile hemangioma is a β-blocker (propranolol at of 2–3 mg/kg/d in 2–3 divided doses, acebutolol, or topical timolol) (Leaute-Labreze, et al. 2008). Duration of therapy lasts from 2–10 months. The effect is almost immediate with softening and discoloration of the lesion. Most continue to improve until nearly flat and with significantly diminished color. Because of side effects, treatment must be closely monitored at the start of therapy (cardiorespiratory monitoring and glycemia). β-Blockers are contraindicated when there are concomitant cerebrovascular anomalies. Once treatment is completed a gradual taper is necessary.

Imiquimod cream which works by stimulation of toll-like receptor 7 (TLR-7) and increase in local interferon α and γ secretion has induced involution of infantile hemangiomas (Welsh, et al. 2004).

Klippel–Trenaunay–Weber syndrome and Sturge–Weber syndrome are 2 congenital phakomatoses causing osteoangiomatosis, involving extremities, and cerebral angiomatosis, respectively (Garzon, et al. 2007). The first condition can be treated symptomatically with compression stockings, or surgically with sclerosis or debulking. The presence of an arteriovenous fistula within the angiomatosis can lead to high output cardiac failure, and treatment should then be more aggressive. Unfortunately, these lesions have a tendency to recur locally. The Sturge–Weber syndrome is an angioma affecting the cerebral hemisphere in newborns, causing seizures and mental retardation. Often a port wine stain is present on the face. These diseases might overlap as part of a family of phakomatoses pigmentovascularis. There is no role for medical oncology in these syndromes.

Lymphangioma

Lymphangioma is a benign tumor which does not regress with time. Complications can be extremely serious, and include chronic infections, compression of airway, or feeding problems. Surgical excision is usually not complete and carries a complication rate of 10–30%, with a recurrence rate of 15–50%. Laser therapy can be used for localized lymphangiomas.

Sclerosing therapy started with the injection of chemotherapy such as bleomycin (Tanigawa, et al. 1987). An alcoholic solution (Ethibloc) has been tried with a 60% success rate, but final esthetic results might not be optimal (Herbreteau, et al. 1993). OK-432 (Picibanil), a lyophilized incubation mixture of group A *Streptococcus pyogenes* of human origin, was first used in Japan and yielded promising results (Ogita, et al. 1994). The technique has been widely reproduced with a similar success rate and has become a treatment of choice. Results are excellent in lymphangioma of the macrocystic type (88% success rate) and satisfactory in microcystic and mixed type lesions (60% success rate) (Luzzatto, et al. 2000). Adverse effects of OK-432 are mild and disappear quickly. A risk of anaphylactic reaction is possible in patients with allergic reactions to penicillin. Late side effects are almost insignificant. OK-432 could also be used in a neoadjuvant fashion prior to surgical resection (Poldervaart, et al. 2009).

Kaposi sarcoma

The classic Kaposi sarcoma (KS) was first described by a Hungarian dermatologist, Moritz Kaposi, in 1872. Prior to the AIDS epidemic, KS remained a rare tumor seen usually on the lower legs of elderly men of Mediterranean or African origin. An endemic KS was also described in prepubescent children in Africa. Patients receiving immunosuppressive therapy can also be affected (Penn 1979). These varieties are less lethal than the epidemic KS, a disseminated fulminant form (Antman, et al. 2000). KS is an AIDS defining illness (http://www.cdc.gov/mmwr/preview/mmwrhtml/00018871.htm) .

In 1994, a novel herpes virus, human herpesvirus-8 (HHV-8) was found in all forms of KS, but infection with the virus appears to be necessary but not sufficient for the development of KS (Chang, et al. 1994). KS behavior ranges from indolent to fulminant and behavior affects the choice of treatment. While the incidence peaked in the early 1990s, the cases of Kaposi's sarcomas have dramatically declined with the advent of highly active anti-retroviral therapy (HAART) (Rouhani, et al. 2008).

Presentation

Often the disease presents in the skin as violaceous papules, but oral, visceral, or nodal KS are also common and may precede cutaneous involvement. An excision biopsy is needed for definitive diagnosis. Differential diagnoses include bacillary angiomatosis, non-Hodgkin lymphoma, melanoma, and some cutaneous fungal or bacterial infections. Oral lesions are common and a mouth examination should always be done.

Another common site for KS lesions is the gastrointestinal tract (>40% of AIDS cases). Observation is sufficient until lesions become symptomatic, because asymptomatic lesions do not alter the prognosis of AIDS. Endoscopy is the best diagnostic method. Other sites include the pulmonary tract, lymph nodes, liver, spleen, heart, pericardium, bone, and bone marrow. Besides symptoms related to the location of the lesions, lymphedema is a frequent complication and might be caused by lymphatic involvement by the KS.

Treatment

Because HAART enables KS regression and control of the disease into a more indolent clinical problem, it is essential for the Medical Oncologist to partner with the infectious disease specialist. The first step is to optimize HAART therapy to increase the immune defenses of the patient (Cattelan, et al. 2005, Tam, et al. 2002). Once HAART is optimized, lesions causing problems, such as bleeding or pain, should be treated. For patients on immunosuppressive therapy, discontinuation or reduction of the immunosuppressants is recommended.

Localized disease can be treated by ablative procedures such as cryotherapy, intralesional injections of chemotherapy, alitretinoin gel, radiotherapy, topical immunotherapy (imiquimod), or surgical excision. Since KS is caused by a viral agent, studies are also evaluating the effects of anti-viral drugs (Cattamanchi et al. 2011).

Extensive cutaneous disease or internal disease requires intravenous chemotherapy only for symptomatic control of the lesions. The addition of chemotherapy to HAART does not improve survival (Mosam, et al. 2012). A randomized trial of HAART alone or HAART and chemotherapy in treatment-naïve AIDS patients with KS, who had no symptomatic lesions, showed a 39% response rate with HAART arm and 66% after the addition of chemotherapy, but an identical survival of 77% at 12 months. HAART consisted of stavudine, lamivudine and nevirapine and chemotherapy was a combination of bleomycin, doxorubicin, and vincristine every 3 weeks or oral etoposide. **Table 10.6** shows the active chemotherapy agents for KS

Epithelioid hemangioendothelioma

Epithelioid hemangioendotheliomas (EHE) present in middle age mainly in bone, liver and lung (Lau, et al. 2011). They are equivalent to low-grade angiosarcoma, but can metastasize via the lymphatic system to the liver, lung, or bone. Treatment is usually surgical with wide excision and lymph-node dissection. Liver transplantation has also been performed. There is no role for medical oncology, unless the disease has metastasized, in which case treatment is the same as with angiosarcoma (See next section).

Angiosarcoma

Angiosarcoma is a cancer of the endothelial cell and could arise anywhere in the body. The most common organs where angiosarcomas originate are the skin, in particular the scalp, and the breast. Angiosarcoma arising from a chronic lymphedema is a syndrome named for Stewart and Treves. The cause of the lymphedema might not be relevant, but in oncology many cases are seen after breast cancer therapy. There are different types of angiosarcoma depending on the cell of origin. Histologically, a vascular type (CD34 positive D2-40 negative), a mixed type (CD34 positive D2-40 positive), and a lymphatic type (CD34 negative D2-40 positive) have been proposed (Kamo, et al. 2011). **Table 10.7** shows predisposing conditions for angiosarcoma.

Biology

Molecularly, angiosarcomas, a cancer derived from endothelial cells, are a group of diseases with various patterns, and clinical behavior varies with the site of origin (Fayette, et al. 2007). Various mutations in molecules of the VEGFR pathway have been described. Thus inhibitors of the VEGF pathway are now studied to target these cells. Other molecular pathways are also being described (**Table 10.8**).

Presentation

The clinical presentation of angiosarcoma depends on the site of origin. Cutaneous angiosarcoma are initially flat, resembling a bruise

Table 10.6 Chemotherapy agents for Kaposi sarcoma

Drugs	Dose	ORR	Reference
Pegylated liposomal doxorubicin	20 mg/m² every 2-4 weeks	38% to 58%	(Northfelt, et al. 1997, Stewart, et al. 1998)
Liposomal daunorubicin	40 mg/m² every 2 weeks	25%	(Gill, et al. 1996)
Paclitaxel	100 mg/m² iv over 3 hrs every 2 weeks	59%	(Gill, et al. 1999)
Docetaxel	25 mg/m² every week × 8 wks, then every other week	42%	(Lim, et al. 2005)
Doxorubicin, bleomycin, & vinblastine (ABV)	40 mg/m² day 1 15 U/m² days 1, 15 6 mg/m² day 1 every 4 weeks	28% to 84%	(Gill, et al. 1996, Laubenstein, et al. 1984)
Oral etoposide	50 mg/day for 7 days every other week	36% to 70%	(Evans, et al. 2002)
Vinorelbine	30 mg/m² every 2 weeks	43%	(Nasti, et al. 2000)
Bleomycin & Vincristine	15 IU/m² & 2 mg every 3 weeks × 6	23%	(Stewart, et al. 1998)
Interferon α	3 to 20 million units subcutaneously, daily to 3 times a week	25 to 50%	(Dezube 2002)

Table 10.7 Conditions associated with angiosarcomas

Conditions	Causes	Comments	Reference
Toxic exposure	Radiation, arsenic, vinyl chloride, thorium dioxide, foreign bodies	Mainly in liver	(Bosetti, et al. 2003, Jennings, et al. 1988)
Chronic lymphedema	Post-surgical or radiotherapy	Also called 'secondary angiosarcoma' or Stewart-Treves syndrome	(Ron 2003, Styring, et al. 2010)
	Infectious	Filariasis	(Krishnamoorthy, et al. 2012)
	Congenital	Milroy's syndrome (VGFR3 mutation)	(Connell, et al. 2009)
		Meige's syndrome	(Andersson, et al. 1995)
Congenital conditions	Maffucci syndrome	Multiple enchondromas and hemangiomas/ lymphangiomas	(Perkins, et al. 1996)
	Klippel-Trenaunay syndrome	See Angiomatosis (above in this chapter)	
	Neurofibromatosis NF-1 and non-congenital schwannomas		(McMenamin, et al. 2001, Riccardi, et al. 1984)
	Mutated BRCA1 or BRCA2		(West, et al. 2008)
Vascular conditions	Arteriovenous-fistula	In immunosuppressed patients after renal transplant	(Ahmed, et al. 2002)

Table 10.8. Described genetic changes in angiosarcomas

Pathway	Genetic alteration	Comment	References
VEGFR	VEGFR2 mutations	Radiation breast angiosarcoma	(Antonescu, et al. 2009)
	VEGFR3 mutations	Lymphangiosarcoma, Milroy's syndrome	(Connell, et al. 2009)
	Loss of VGFR2	Worse prognosis	(Itakura, et al. 2008)
RAS and downstream pathways	Activation of the pathway after toxic exposure	Liver Heart	(Garcia, et al. 2000, Weihrauch, et al. 2002)
Myc	Amplification	Secondary angiosarcoma	(Fernandez, et al. 2012)
Transcription factor ETS1	Overexpression	Metastatic behavior	(Naito, et al. 2000)
Others	Wilms' tumor-1 Galectin-3 Fascin Prox1	Lymphangiosarcoma and cutaneous angiosarcoma	(Dim, et al. 2007, Johnson, et al. 2007, Miettinen, et al. 2012, Ueda, et al. 2003)

until a purple papule arise. The lesions are usually multifocal in a 'tentacle pattern'. Unattended, they grow quickly, and unfortunately they often are diagnosed after ulceration causes bleeding. In case of cutaneous origin, imaging might not show an initial thin plaque of tumor, and in this case, the diagnosis is clinical and must be confirmed with a skin biopsy. In soft tissue or visceral angiosarcoma, tumors present often because they have become bulky and painful or the patient is bleeding. A staging work-up is necessary, because angiosarcomas eventually become metastatic in most patients. Metastases can spread anywhere with liver, pleural and peritoneal cavities, and lungs being common sites. Prognosis is grimmer than with other soft tissue sarcomas with a 30-40% survival at 5 years and a median survival of 7 to 12 months (Fury, et al. 2005, Rouhani, et al. 2008).

Treatment

Surgical excision alone is inadequate and a multidisciplinary approach is necessary. Because the tumor infiltrates beyond the visible disease in cutaneous angiosarcoma, margins are contaminated despite an attempt at radical surgery.

Historically, treatment was a combination of radiation and surgery. More recently, with the introduction of paclitaxel and antiangiogenic agents, chemotherapy is now added to this multimodality therapy. There are no randomized trials to guide best therapeutic approach. Some prospective phase II studies have been published, but none have differentiated subtypes of angiosarcoma.

Neoadjuvant and adjuvant chemotherapy: Adjuvant chemotherapy for soft tissue sarcoma might have a minimal role in improving survival (Cochrane 2000). There are no specific data for angiosarcoma. However, some data on neoadjuvant chemotherapy are now being collected because of the availability of angiogenic inhibitors. In one series of 15 patients with periorbital angiosarcoma treated with neoadjuvant chemotherapy over 23 years in the hope to preserve eye function. Fourteen had a complete clinical response. Thus, definitive surgery was unnecessary in 9 patients. The median disease-free interval for the neoadjuvant chemotherapy group was about 12 months with 9 recurrences (DeMartelaere, et al. 2008). In another prospective trial of gemcitabine, docetaxel, and bevacizumab in patients with soft tissue sarcoma, all four patients with angiosarcoma had a response (3 complete responses and 1 partial response). Two patients with visceral angiosarcoma who had a pathological complete response are alive 4 years later. One patient with a breast angiosarcoma who had a partial response is also alive today without disease and the only patient with a facial angiosarcoma who had a complete clinical response, recurred 1 year later and did not survive (Verschraegen, et al. 2012). Thus the use of neoadjuvant chemotherapy should be considered for the treatment of newly diagnosed angiosarcoma. There are case reports of success with the combination of liposomal doxorubicin with radiation therapy (Holloway, et al. 2005). Clinical trials are sorely needed.

Treatment of metastatic disease:Doxorubicin based regimens were the main option until the 1990's. Very few patients with angiosarcoma were enrolled in these large randomized trials, making assessment difficult (Budd 2002). With doxorubicin as a single agent, median progression-free survival (PFS) is about 5 months and median overall survival (OS) less than one year (Italiano, et al. 2011). Doxorubicin-based regimens induce better responses without improved survival. Liposomal doxorubicin has similar outcomes (Skubitz, et al. 2005). Interferon-α alone or in combination with chemotherapy might stabilize angiosarcoma (Burns, et al. 2002).

Taxanes have been tried with more success, however as single agents, they are not curative. **Table 10.9** shows one study and all series with greater than 5 patients. There are many other case reports of success. Head and neck cutaneous angiosarcomas are responding better to taxanes. In combination with radiotherapy, durable responses have been described, but the average survival remains less than 1 year with this class of agent.

Biological therapy has focused on anti-angiogenic agents, either VEGF inhibitors or VEGF receptor inhibitors (**Table 10.10**). As single agents, responses are seen; but there is no prolongation of survival. In combination with chemotherapy or radiation therapy, prolonged remissions are observed.

Further trials are ongoing (**Table 10.11**) to better define the role of anti-angiogenic agents with chemotherapy or radiation therapy.

Table 10.9 Taxanes for advanced angiosarcoma

Drug	Dose	Outcome	References
Weekly paclitaxel	60-90 mg/m^2	ORR 43%	(Italiano, et al. 2011)
Weekly paclitaxel*	80 mg/m^2 on days 1, 8, 15 every 4 weeks	ORR 18%	(Penel, et al. 2008)
Paclitaxel	Weekly or every 3 weeks	ORR 62%	(Penel, et al. 2012)
Paclitaxel	140 mg/m^2 by continuous infusion over 7 days every 4 weeks	ORR 62%	(Skubitz, et al. 2005)
Docetaxel	25 mg/m^2 weekly for 8 weeks	ORR 66%	(Nagano, et al. 2007)

*The only prospective study

Table 10.10 Studies of anti-angiogenic agents for angiosarcomas

Drug	Number of patients	Outcome	References
Bevacizumab + radiotherapy	2	CR	(Koontz, et al. 2008)
Bevacizumab + docetaxel & gemcitabine	4	3 CR and 1 PR	(Verschraegen, et al. 2012)
Bevacizumab	26	ORR 12%	(Agulnik, et al. 2009)
Sorafenib	37	ORR 14%	(Maki, et al. 2009)
Sorafenib	9	ORR 11%	(Ryan, et al. 2008)
Sunitinib	2	No response	(George, et al. 2009)

Table 10.11 Open studies for angiosarcoma (2012)

Drug	Trial	Condition
Chemotherapy	Paclitaxel in treating patients with locally advanced or metastatic soft tissue angiosarcoma or lymphangiosarcoma that cannot be removed by surgery	Unresectable & metastatic
Bevacizumab	Bevacizumab in treating patients with angiosarcoma	Unresectable & metastatic
Sorafenib	Sorafenib in treating patients with angiosarcoma that is locally advanced, metastatic, or unable to be removed by surgery	Unresectable & metastatic
Pazopanib	Phase II study evaluating the role of pazopanib in angiosarcoma	Unresectable & metastatic
	Pazopanib hydrochloride followed by chemotherapy and surgery in treating patients with soft tissue sarcoma	Neoadjuvant window of opportunity
Axitinib	A study of axitinib in patients with advanced angiosarcoma and other soft tissue sarcomas	Unresectable & metastatic
Chemotherapy and anti-angiogenic agent combination	Paclitaxel + bevacizumab (Avastin) for the treatment of metastatic or unresectable angiosarcoma	Unresectable & metastatic
	Efficacity of weekly paclitaxel in association or not with bevacizumab in metastatic or locally advanced angiosarcomas	Unresectable & metastatic
	Gemcitabine and docetaxel with bevacizumab in selected sarcoma subtypes	Unresectable & metastatic
	Gemcitabine hydrochloride with or without pazopanib hydrochloride in treating patients with refractory soft tissue sarcoma	Unresectable & metastatic
	Pazopanib with gemcitabine and docetaxel for the neoadjuvant chemotherapy treatment of high risk (tumors > 5 cm, high grade) soft tissue sarcomas – A Phase 1B study	Neoadjuvant prior to surgery

Source: Clinicaltrials.gov

RADIATION ONCOLOGY

Vascular tumors of soft tissue can vary from benign disease such as hemangiomas to malignant cancers at high risk for relapse and death. Overall, surgical management is the mainstay of curative treatment. RT largely plays an adjuvant role to optimize local control, and is usually reserved for high grade tumors, such as angiosarcoma. However, depending on tumor size and location, radiation can be the primary treatment modality, such as for vulvar lymphangioma circumscriptum. Kandil et al., report local control of thoracic lymphangiomas treated with RT alone (Kandil et al. 1997). RT has been successful in treatment of congenital vulvar lymphangioma circumscriptum (Yildiz et al. 2008). RT has also been shown to be highly effective as monotherapy for treatment of Kaposi's sarcoma.

Angiosarcoma of the breast can occur after curative radiation doses are delivered for treatment of breast adenocarcinoma. Primary management is surgical, and local and distant relapse is high even with R0 resection (Seinen et al. 2012). Local control is improved with combined modality therapy (surgery and RT) combined to either alone (Guadangnolo et al. 2011). In the setting of re-irradiation, the University of Florida experience favors hyperfractionation to minimize late tissue complications, with a total dose of 60 Gy (Scott et al. 2012). Doses can range from 60-70 Gy, with 5 year local control rates of approximately 50-60%.

CASES

Case 10.1 Intramuscular hemangioma

Clinical history and presentation

The patient is a 16 year old boy who presents with a one year history of a left shoulder mass. The mass was noted spontaneously and was initially asymptomatic but has grown progressively in size and has become increasingly symptomatic. The mass increases in size and symptoms with activity and decreases with rest.

Physical examination reveals a prominent mass over the anterior aspect of the left shoulder, which has a soft consistency and is mildly tender. There are overlying skin striations.

Surgical findings and comments

Wide resection is chosen as the procedure of choice, as it can be accomplished with minimal added morbidity over a marginal resection and should lead to a lower recurrence rate. The procedure is performed as planned. Blood loss is measured at 600cc.

Radiology findings

The MR images (**Case figures 10.1a** through **10.1e**) show a striking example of a vascular tumor with numerous serpentine dilated vessels confined to the pectoralis major muscle. The mass is heterogeneous with irregular infiltrative margins. Interestingly, the anterior half of the mass is less T2 hyperintense and has less enhancement perhaps indicating less perfusion and edema in this portion of the tumor. The mass shows relatively little mass effect despite its large size, a herald feature of hemangiomas. Likewise, it appears to insinuate into adjacent tissues without displacement as seen by the subtle blending of the tumor with the pectoral muscle along its anteromedial margin. There is a lack of destruction evidenced by the preservation of the subcutaneous fat and the pectoralis tendon.

On careful examination of the cross sectional image stacks, the engorged vessels could be traced back to the subclavian artery and vein. Given the size of the vessels, intra-operative bleeding risk is a concern. Although not employed in this case, interventional radiology can perform pre-operative embolization therapy to mitigate potential hemorrhage risk.

Pathology findings

Gross features

The specimen consists of a 9 × 8 × 6.5 cm unoriented portion of muscle. Sectioning reveals an unencapsulated but relatively circumscribed, intramuscular, 6.5 × 4.5 × 2.5 cm tumor composed of numerous tortuous vessels embedded in a gray to pink stroma. There is no necrosis. The margins are close (0.5 cm in one area) but grossly uninvolved. Multiple representative sections are submitted.

Microscopic features

Low magnification: Multiple sections reveal a lesion remarkably histologically similar to lobular capillary hemangioma (LCH) except there may be a few more large vessels present than are typically noted in LCH (**Case fig. 10.1f**).

High magnification: At medium magnification, the capillary sized vessels form lobules in association with a dilated vein similar to a 'feeder vessel' noted in some LCH (**Case fig. 10.1g**). High magnification of a lobule demonstrates a scattered mitotic figure. There is no necrosis or nuclear atypia (**Case fig. 10.1h**).

Special studies: Because the lesion is histologically compatible with intramuscular hemangioma and matches the clinical and radiologic impressions, no special studies are performed. If performed, the lesional cells would strongly express the vascular markers, CD31, CD34, ERG and FLI-1. There would be no reactivity for GLUT-1 (expressed in juvenile hemangioma) and no reactivity for D2-40 (usually limited to lymphatic channels in well-differentiated tumors).

Pathologic differential or, why isn't it one of the following?

Angiomatosis: Angiomatosis and intramuscular hemangioma are usually histologically indistinguishable. Both lesions typically comprise a collection of medium sized, ectatic vessels often embedded in reactive adipose tissue. A histologic feature reported to be more common in angiomatosis consists of congeries of smaller vessels spilling out from the muscularis of a larger vessel. That is not present in this case which instead represents an uncommon morphologic variant of intramuscular hemangioma mimicking lobular capillary hemangioma. Since the tumor is located exclusively in one muscle rather than involving multiple muscles or tissue planes, it fits the definition of intramuscular hemangioma rather than angiomatosis.

Lymphangioma: Deep lymphangioma consists of a mix of smaller and large ectatic, generally thin-walled channels that may contain lymph

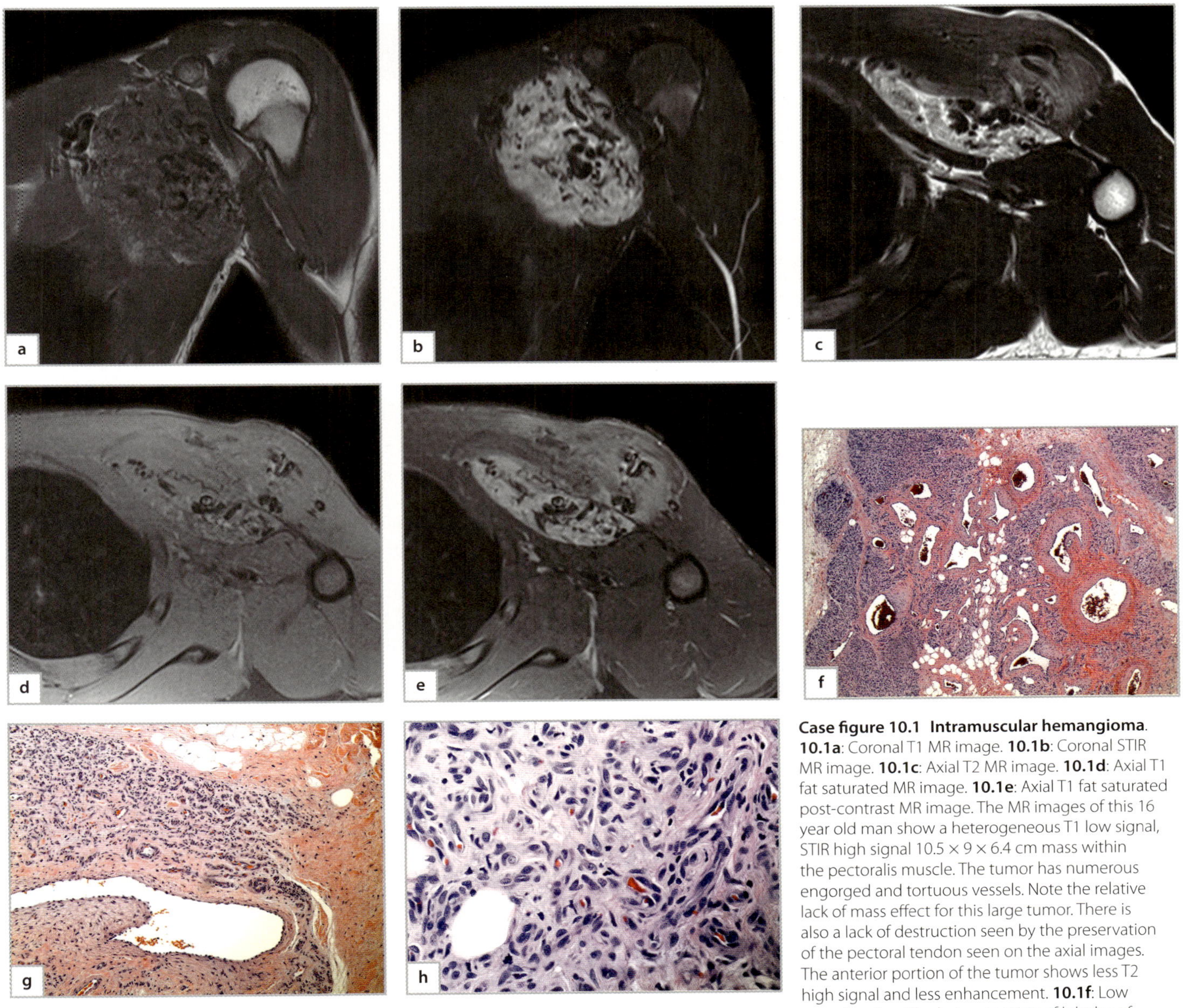

Case figure 10.1 Intramuscular hemangioma. **10.1a**: Coronal T1 MR image. **10.1b**: Coronal STIR MR image. **10.1c**: Axial T2 MR image. **10.1d**: Axial T1 fat saturated MR image. **10.1e**: Axial T1 fat saturated post-contrast MR image. The MR images of this 16 year old man show a heterogeneous T1 low signal, STIR high signal 10.5 × 9 × 6.4 cm mass within the pectoralis muscle. The tumor has numerous engorged and tortuous vessels. Note the relative lack of mass effect for this large tumor. There is also a lack of destruction seen by the preservation of the pectoral tendon seen on the axial images. The anterior portion of the tumor shows less T2 high signal and less enhancement. **10.1f**: Low magnification. The lesion consists of lobules of capillaries intermixed with dilated veins. **10.1g**: Medium magnification. This patient's lesion is histologically similar to a lobular capillary hemangioma with larger, 'feeder' vessels. **10.1h**: High magnification. The lesion is cellular where it forms lobules of capillaries. A mitotic figure is present . However, there is no nuclear atypia or necrosis.

fluid or a few red blood cells or appear empty. A scattered vessel may have a partial muscularis, but most vessels will consist only of a single layer of luminal lining cells. The stroma may be fibrotic, and lymphoid aggregates are common. Lymphangiomas should express D2-40 in addition to variable expression of CD31 and CD34.

Angiosarcoma: Angiosarcoma is very rare in this age group. It would feature a permeative proliferation of cytologically atypical cells attempting, with varying success, to form vessels.

Oncology approach

Medical oncology

This is a benign lesion with no role for medical oncology.

Case table 10.1 Summary pathology findings of Case 10.1

Diagnosis	Intramuscular hemangioma
Size	6.5 × 4.5 × 2.5 cm
Location	Pectoralis muscle
Margin status	Negative (closest margin is 0.5 cm)
Histologic grade (FNCLCC grading system)	Benign (not graded)
Pathologic Stage (AJCC TNM classification)	Benign (not staged)

FNCLCC: Fédération Nationale des Centres de Lutte Contre le Cancer
AJCC: American Joint Committee on Cancer

Radiation oncology

There is no definitive role for radiotherapy (RT) in the management of this disease. RT has been shown to be efficacious in treatment of cavernous sinus hemangiomas.

Patient outcome

One year postoperatively the patient is doing well with a normal shoulder and no evidence of recurrence.

Case 10.2 Soft tissue angiomatosis

Clinical history and presentation

The patient is a 28 year old man with a right posterior thigh mass first noted approximately 12 years ago. The mass was noted spontaneously. It has grown slowly but progressively in size. He describes a constant ache associated with the mass. The mass fluctuates in size and symptoms in direct proportion to activity level.

Surgical findings and comments

Examination of the right posterior thigh reveals a poorly defined, fusiform mass in the posterolateral aspect of the distal thigh. It is significantly tender on palpation. It is fixed to underlying deep tissue.

At surgery, the tumor is noted to be within the biceps musculature with extension into the overlying fascia. A combined marginal and wide excision is performed, with wide margins obtained through expendable areas of muscle and fascia. Because the location of the tumor facilitated surgery under tourniquet control, blood loss is limited to 30cc.

Radiology findings

This case (**Case figs 10.2a** through **10.2e**) demonstrates several characteristic features of vascular lesions. These lesions typically do not have capsules. These tumors are unique in that they typically exert no mass effect and thus do not expand compartments or distort adjacent structures. These tumors also have a characteristic infiltration pattern that seems to gently insinuate into tissues rather than invading or destroying them. The overall appearance is virtually diagnostic of hemangiomas or soft tissue angiomatosis.

Unlike case 10.1 which is entirely intra-muscular, this lesion involves both muscle and subcutaneous tissues and is therefore considered soft tissue angiomatosis. We typically use STIR sequences because they consistently render the lesion high signal providing excellent visualization of these complex tumors as they insinuate into various compartments. On the other hand, T2 fat saturation sequences usually show the lesion has high signal but may be compromised by field inhomogeneity, especially at the large fields of view needed to image these multi-compartment lesions. Field heterogeneity can cause areas of fat saturation to fail, or worse, may cause water saturation to occur which could render the lesion invisible.

Pathology findings

Gross features

The specimen comprises multiple fragments of tan to red soft tissue aggregating to 5.5 × 5 × 2 cm. Cut sections through the fragments reveal yellow to tan glistening surfaces with scattered areas of hemorrhage and interposed strips of skeletal muscle. Representative sections are submitted for processing.

Microscopic features

Low magnification: The lesion comprises numerous, tightly packed, irregular vessel cross sections set in fibrous tissue (**Case fig. 10.2f**).

High magnification: Lesional vessels vary in caliber and thickness (**Case fig. 10.2g**). Cytologic atypia is absent (**Case fig. 10.2h**).

Special studies: Because of characteristic radiologic and histologic features, no special studies are performed.

Pathologic differential or, why isn't it one of the following?

Intramuscular hemangioma: As noted in Case 10.1, angiomatosis and intramuscular hemangioma often are histologically identical. However, angiomatosis involves multiple tissue planes (such as dermis, subcutis, and muscle) or multiple contiguous muscles. This patient's lesion is expansive into subcutis and muscle and thus qualifies as angiomatosis.

Vascular malformation: Angiomatosis most likely represents a vascular malformation. It does not involute, like some pediatric vascular tumors, and it has virtually no risk for malignant transformation. Mixed vessel calibers from capillaries to large veins, irregular shape of single involved vessels, and often poorly developed, partly attenuated vessel walls with no proliferative activity (no mitotic figures and low Ki-67 index) are consistent with a malformation. Lack of, to at most weak nuclear WT-1 expression in lesional endothelial cell nuclei would

Case table 10.2 Summary pathology findings of Case 10.2

Diagnosis	Angiomatosis
Size	5.0 cm (estimated as lesion is submitted in multiple pieces)
Location	Muscle and subcutaneous fat of posterior right thigh
Margin status	Unable to ascertain from pathologic review as lesion is submitted in multiple pieces
Histologic grade (FNCLCC grading system)	Benign (not graded)
Pathologic stage (AJCC TNM classification)	Benign (not staged)

FNCLCC = Fédération Nationale des Centres de Lutte Contre le Cancer (French Federation of Cancer Centers).
AJCC = American Joint Committee on Cancer

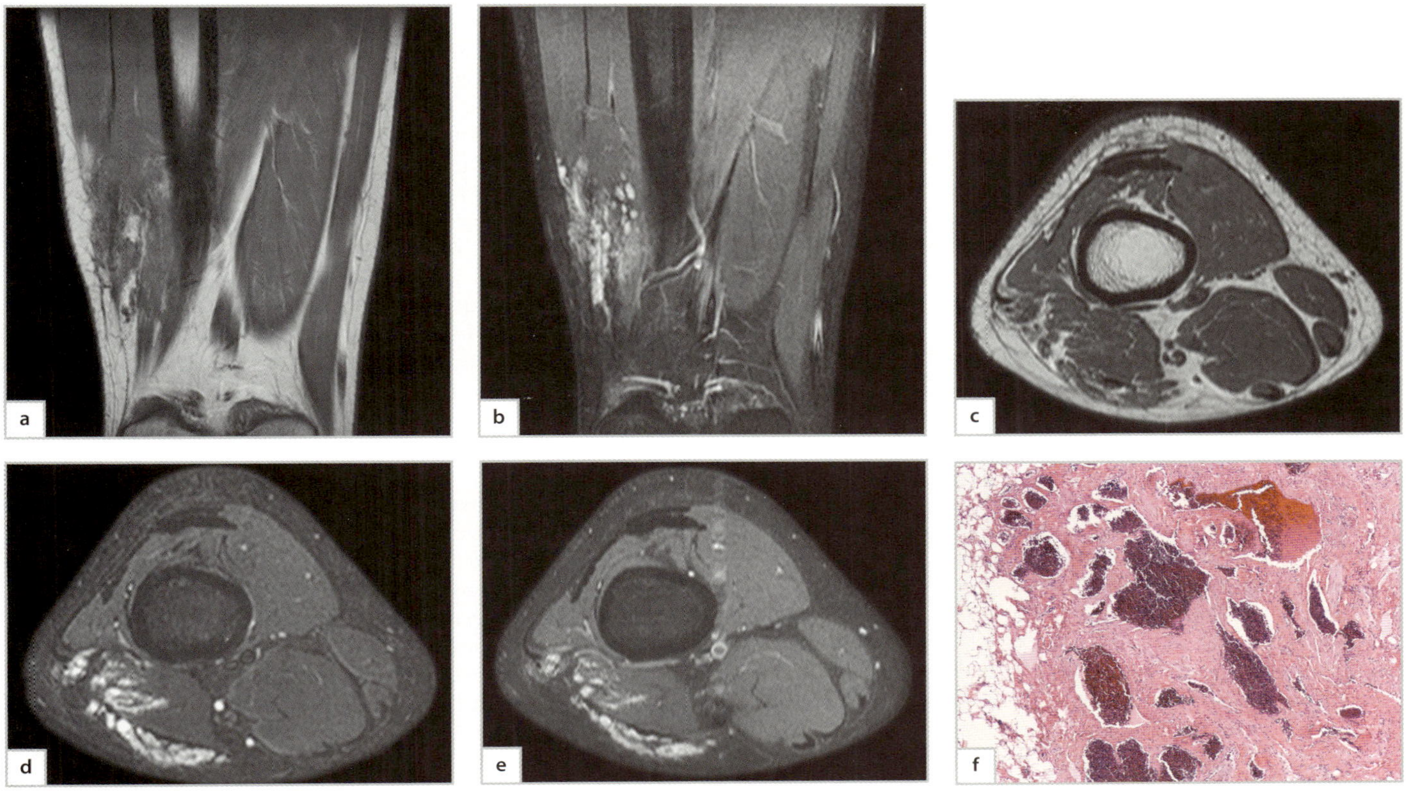

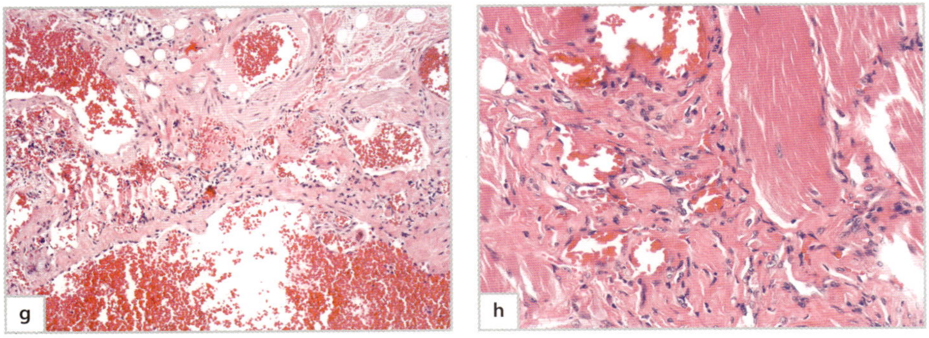

Case figure 10.2 Soft tissue angiomatosis. **10.2a**: Coronal T1 MR image. **10.2b**: Coronal STIR MR image. **10.2c**: Axial T1 MR image. **10.2d**: Axial STIR MR image. **10.2e**: Axial T1 fat saturated post-contrast MR image. The MR images of this 28 year old man show a poorly defined, infiltrative lesion in the subcutaneous tissues and muscles of the distal thigh. Note how the lesion infiltrates into tissues without causing mass effect, best seen on the axial images. **10.2f**: Lower magnification. The lesion comprises tightly packed, malformed, medium sized vessels embedded in adipose tissue. **10.2g**: Higher magnification. Here, smaller vessels arise in the wall of a larger vessel (the lumen of which is facing down in this photomicrograph). This intramural 'cascade' or 'bouquet' of new vessels is reportedly characteristic of angiomatosis though not always present. **10.2h**: High magnification. Small compressed vessels of the lesion spread apart skeletal muscle fibers (right and lower left). Angiomatosis must involve multiple tissue planes or multiple contiguous muscles. In this patient, the lesion extended from the dermis into subcutaneous fat and skeletal muscle.

support vascular malformation etiology (strong diffuse positivity is present in most true vascular neoplasms and normal vessels and negative in malformations, according to three recent studies).

Oncology approach

Medical oncology

This is a benign lesion with no role for medical oncology.

Radiation oncology

There is no definitive role for radiotherapy (RT) in the management of this disease.

Patient outcome

Five years postoperatively, the patient is symptom free with normal function and no clinical evidence of recurrence.

Case 10.3 Lymphangioma

Clinical history and presentation

This is a 6-year-old boy who presents with a three week history of left thigh mass, which was noted spontaneously by the mother. The mass has been persistent. He is asymptomatic.

Physical examination of the left thigh reveals violaceous skin discoloration over a prominent medial distal thigh mass. The mass is soft on palpation. It is deeply situated and fixed to the underlying deep tissue. It is non-tender.

Surgical findings and comments

At surgery, the tumor is noted to be within the subcutaneous tissue. Wide resection is performed, including excision of the underlying fascia. Muscle is uninvolved.

Radiology findings

The images, **Case figs 10.3a** through 10-3e, show a nonspecific mass in the subcutaneous tissues. The mass is largely non-enhancing and likely is cystic. There are fatty septa separating the locules of the mass. Although there is the usual mass effect present, the lesion does not show aggressive invasion of adjacent tissues. The heterogeneous cystic lesion with fat elements could represent a liposarcoma, however, this lesion shows little enhancement and no invasion. A lymphangioma is a likely alternative consideration.

Pathology findings

Gross features

The specimen consists of a 7.5 × 4.5 × 4 cm oblong portion of fatty tissue. Cross sections show a multicystic interior with thin-walled cysts ranging from 0.5 to 1.9 cm dispersed throughout predominantly yellow, lobulated fatty tissue. The fat abnormally bulges above the cut section surface due to fibrous trabeculations (**Case fig. 10.3f**). The cysts contain straw-colored fluid.

Microscopic features

Low magnification: At low magnification, the lesion consists of dilated, thin-walled channels associated with stromal fibrosis and lymphoid aggregates (**Case fig. 10.3g**). Such lymphoid aggregates including lymphoid follicles are common in the stroma of lymphangiomas. The lesion is non-circumscribed. Conservative excision results in a positive margin (**Case fig. 10.3h**). The lymphangioma in this field appears sieve-like because of multiple closely packed, compressed, thin-walled lymphatic channels.

High magnification: The lymphatic channels are dilated and most consist of only a single layer of flattened, uniform endothelial cells (**Case fig. 10.3i**). However, one channel is partially invested with a layer of smooth muscle. An abortive (thin, and/or partial) muscularis is commonly seen in lymphangioma channels, especially in long-standing examples. Some lymphangiomas display myxoid change or fibrosis in the walls or stroma; in this patient, the stroma is fibrotic.

Special studies: No immunohistochemistry or cytogenetic testing is performed because the lesion is classic histologically correlating with the radiologic and clinical impression. However, if performed, IHC for podoplanin (D2-40) would be positive, and expression of CD31 and CD34 would be variable.

Pathologic differential or, why isn't it one of the following?

Vascular malformation: Vascular malformations will often contain blood vessels of varying calibers including veins and well-formed capillaries. These vessels will contain red blood cells instead of lymph fluid. At least some of the veins will demonstrate a well-formed muscularis, which, if present in a lymphangioma, is only focal. In actual cases, some malformations may consist of both veins and lymphatic channels, or normal lymphatic channels may be dilated due to the mass effect of the vascular malformation and may appear to be part of the process. In practical terms, finding a mix of abnormally shaped veins and lymphatic channels in a lesion rather than exclusively one or the other does not alter the treatment approach. This patient, however, has a pure lymphangioma without any venous component.

Oncology approach

Medical oncology

This is a benign lesion with no role for medical oncology. If it recurs, sclerosing therapy could be tried.

Radiation oncology

Surgery is the primary treatment, while more extensive disease can be treated with radiation therapy.

Patient outcome

Fourteen months postoperatively, the patient is symptom free with normal function and no clinical evidence of recurrence.

Case table 10.3 Summary pathology findings of Case 10.3

Diagnosis	Lymphangioma
Size	7.5 cm
Location	Subcutaneous adipose tissue
Margin status	Negative
Histologic grade (FNCLCC Grading System)	Benign (not graded)
Pathologic stage (AJCC TNM classification)	Benign (not staged)

FNCLCC: Fédération Nationale des Centres de Lutte Contre le Cancer (French Federation of Cancer Centers).

AJCC: American Joint Committee on Cancer

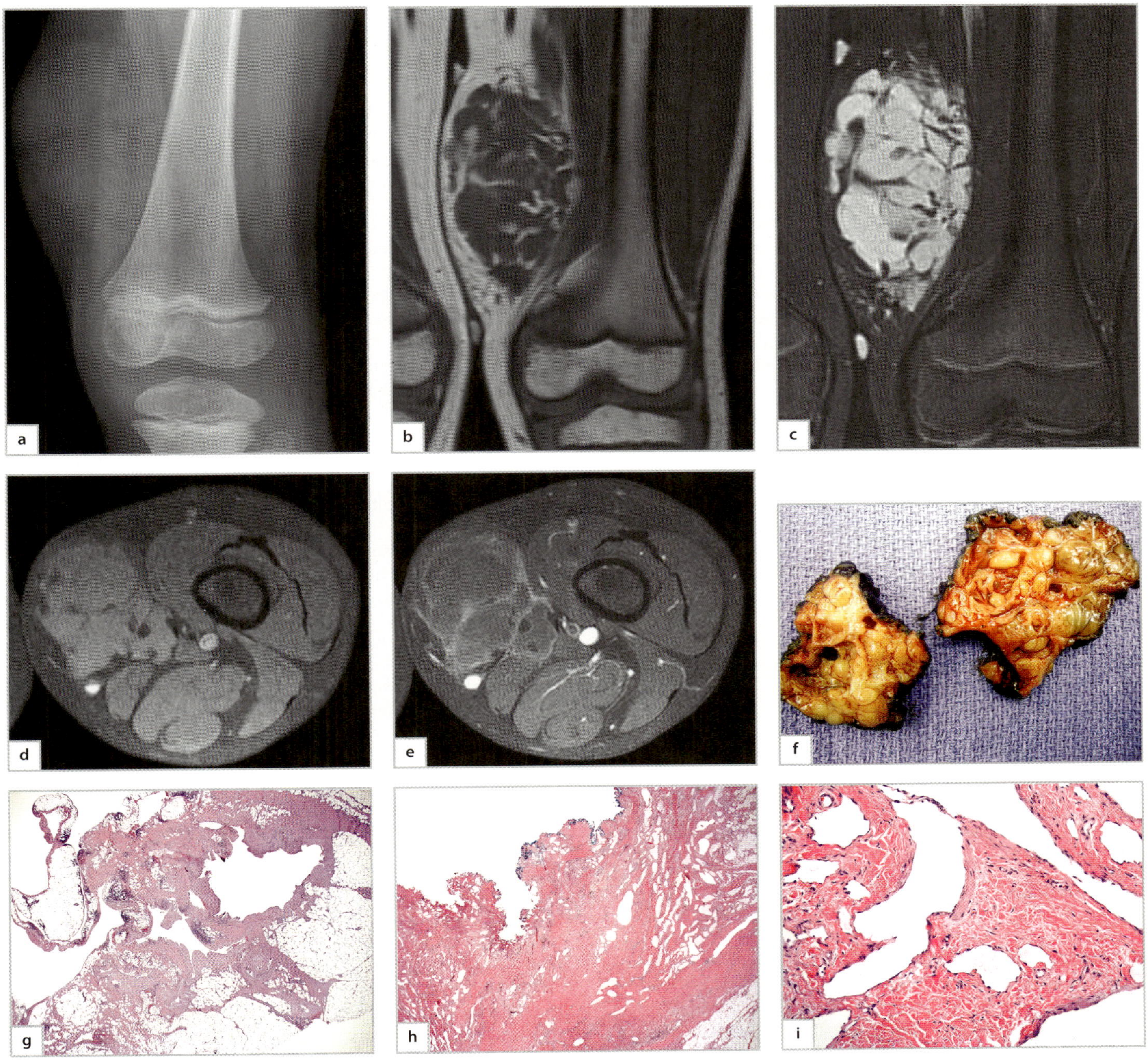

Case figure 10.3 Lymphangioma. Radiographs of this 6 year old boy **10.3a**: AP radiograph: Shows a medial mass of the distal thigh with fat density septations. **10.3b**: Coronal T1 MR image. **10.3c**: Coronal STIR MR image. **10.3d**: Axial T1 fat saturation MR image. **10.3e**: Axial T1 fat saturation post-contrast MR image. The MR images show a T1 low signal, STIR high signal mass measuring 8.3 × 4.7 × 5.0 cm in the deep subcutaneous tissues of the distal thigh. The mass shows modest peripheral rim enhancement indicating much of the mass comprises locules of liquid or non-enhancing matrix. The lobules are separated by fatty tissue septa. Note the expected degree of mass effect is present. **10.3f**: Gross photo of cross section. Cross sections reveal thin walled cysts appearing like empty spaces embedded in lobulated adipose tissue. The surface bulges due to constriction by thin fibrous trabeculations of the lymphangioma. **10.3g**: Low magnification. The lesion is non-circumscribed and consists of variously sized, ectatic channels with stromal fibrosis and lymphoid aggregates. **10.3h**: Low magnification, margin. The lesion extends to inked surgical margins and consists of multiple compressed lymphatic channels imparting a sieve-like appearance. **10.3i**: High magnification. The dilated lymphatic channels appear empty or contain fine flocculent material consistent with lymph fluid. The central channel features a partial, thin muscular wall.

Case 10.4 Epithelioid hemangioendothelioma

Clinical history and presentation

This is a 48 year old man who complains of a slowly enlarging tumor on his right foot. He noticed the tumor approximately two years ago. He said it started as a small lump on the dorsal lateral aspect of the foot. Over the past six months he has noticed it has increased in size, such that it is now extending down to the plantar surface of the foot and has grown in size also on the dorsal part of the foot. He describes no pain. He says it does not fluctuate in size. It is not causing him any discomfort or problems with shoe wear or any other functional problems.

Physical examination reveals a visible soft tissue mass on the dorsal lateral aspect of the foot extending to the plantar surface. The tumor has a lobulated spongy quality on palpation. It is non-tender. It is not pulsatile.

Surgical findings and comments

Open biopsy reveals a subcutaneous tumor intimately involved with the overlying skin.

The patient is placed on a six month course of chemotherapy in an effort to shrink the tumor and decrease the likelihood of metastasis.

Following chemotherapy, there is no gross change in the tumor. Wide resection is performed along with free fasciocutaneous flap coverage.

Radiology findings

This unusual appearing lesion, **Case figs 10.4a** through **10.4d**, has several interesting features. The bulky, exophytic nature is suggestive of a dermatofibrosarcoma. However, there is no ulceration. The lesion shows a focal area of deep invasion without mass effect suggesting a benign vascular entity. There is a lobulated or loculated appearance that suggests vascular pools as can be seen with cavernous hemangiomas. Finally, there is a grossly serpentine morphology. These findings direct the diagnosis to a vascular lesion.

Pathology findings

Gross features

Biopsy: The incisional biopsy comprises irregular, white, rubbery, nodular tumor fragments aggregating to 4 × 2.5 × 1 cm. A small portion of tumor is submitted fresh for cytogenetic analysis, and the remainder is processed for microscopic review.

Resection: The specimen comprises a roughly mushroom shaped portion of skin, subcutaneous adipose tissue and scant skeletal muscle (**Case fig. 10.4e**). Before sectioning, two bosselated nodularities are appreciated under the skin which is otherwise unremarkable. Cross sections reveal a multifocal, multinodular, infiltrating, tan to pale yellow tumor that appears confined to the subcutaneous tissues grossly. Tumor nodules infiltrate an area measuring 7 × 4 × 3 cm and are solid and rubbery to palpation. There is no gross necrosis or hemorrhage (**Case fig. 10.4e**). Margins appear negative for tumor with the closest approximately 0.3 cm from tumor. Tissue is collected fresh for cytogenetics and tumor banking. Nine cassettes of tumor are submitted including representative margins.

Microscopic features

The histologic features of the tumor are identical in the biopsy and the resection. Therefore, only photos from the resection are presented.

Low magnification: The tumor forms multiple adjacent nodules 1 to 3 cm in diameter. These nodules are centered in the dermis and subcutaneous fat. The nodules have discrete borders but are unencapsulated (**Case fig. 10.4f**).

High magnification: At medium magnification, the nodules feature intermixed hypocellular fibrotic areas and myxoid cellular areas in which are suspended small, epithelioid (round cells with round nuclei and discrete cell borders) tumor cells (**Case fig. 10.4g**). Scattered tumor cells contain cytoplasmic vacuoles consistent with 'blister cells' (endothelial tumor cells with early vessel formation) (**Case fig. 10.4h**). Tumor nuclei are uniform, round to ovoid with fine chromatin and generally inconspicuous nucleoli. There is no pleomorphism or necrosis. The mitotic rate is low (0.5 mitoses/10 high power microscopic fields), and there are no atypical mitotic figures. Lymphovascular invasion is not identified. There are no areas of tumor obstructing and emerging from a large vessel (as is seen in some cases of epithelioid hemangioendothelioma).

Special studies: Because the histologic differential is lengthy, a number of antibodies are applied to the tumor. The tumor is diffusely strongly positive for CD34 (**Case fig. 10.4i**) and FLI1 with approximately 15% of cells reactive for mixed D2-40/CD31 antigens. There is no reactivity for S-100 protein, desmin, Melanocytic antigen, mixed keratins (AE1-AE3), Claudin-1 or GLUT1 (all controls are appropriately reactive. INI-1 expression is retained. Approximately 5% of cells express smooth muscle actin, and a similar percentage express epithelial membrane antigen (EMA) (**Case fig. 10.4j**). The patient's karyotype, obtained at the time of biopsy and then at the time of resection, is identical: 46,add(X)(q24),Y,t(3;9)(q21;q;13),add(4)(q31),-6,add(9)(q34),add(13(p13),+mar. Perhaps 10% of EHE do not contain the t(1;3)(p36;q25). Of note, the karyotype contains extra material at 9q34, one of the partners involved in a translocation reported in two cases of epithelioid sarcoma-like hemangioendothelioma (now considered the same tumor as pseudomyogenic hemangioendothelioma).

Pathologic differential or, why isn't it one of the following?

Case table 10.4a lists variant pathology features of epithelioid hemangioendothelioma.

Angiosarcoma: Angiosarcoma often has more vasoformative regions including slit like channels lined by atypical endothelial cells. Mitotic activity is generally higher than in most cases of EHE. Most angiosarcomas lack the distinctive myxochondroid or hyaline matrix of EHE. The 'high grade' or 'malignant' EHE is considered by some experts to be frank angiosarcoma. This anaplastic type of EHE shows increased mitotic activity, nuclear pleomorphism, and sheet-like growth. This patient's tumor lacks these anaplastic features. EHE and angiosarcoma share the same immunohistochemical profile. However, at least 50% of EHE exhibit a thus far specific genetic change: t(1;3)(p36)(q25) that is absent in angiosarcoma. This translocation can be searched for in formalin-fixed, paraffin-embedded sections. This patient's karyotype does not feature the t(1;3), so it is an unusual finding for EHE.

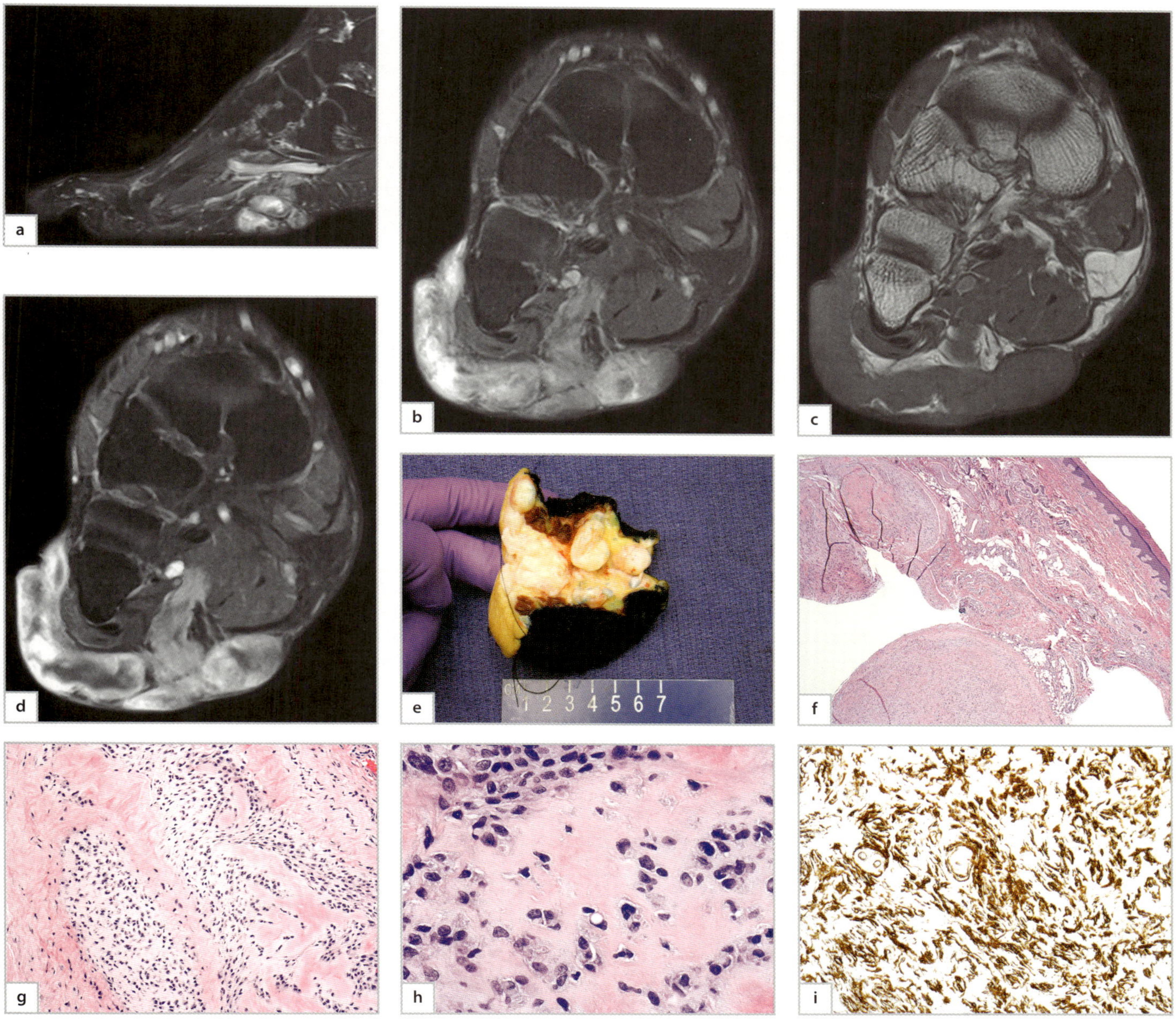

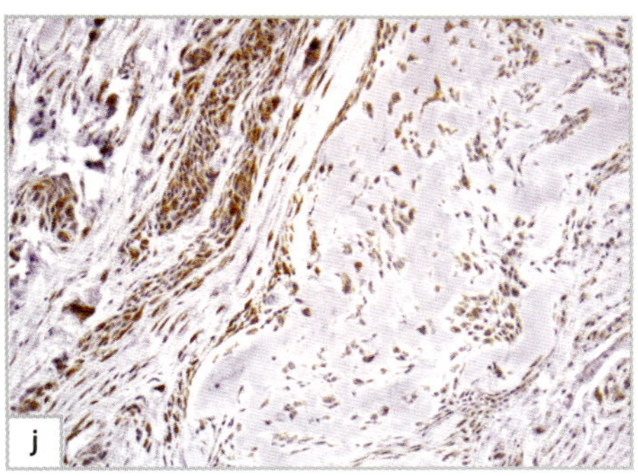

Case figure 10.4 Epithelioid hemangioendothelioma. **10.4a**: Sagittal STIR MR image. **10.4b**: Coronal proton density fat saturated MR image. **10.4c**: Coronal T1 MR image. **10.4d**: Coronal T1 fat saturated post-contrast MR image. The MR images show a subcutaneous lesion of the plantar midfoot with intense heterogeneous enhancement. The mass is bulky and partially exophytic with a serpentine morphology suggesting vessels. There is a small portion of the deep margin which shows insinuating type extension best shown in Figure 10-4d, without mass effect. **10.4e**: Gross photo of cross section of tumor. The tumor is grossly infiltrative into the subcutaneous fat forming multiple white nodules. It is rubbery to palpation and devoid of necrosis and hemorrhage. **10.4f**: Low magnification. The patient's tumor consists of multiple circumscribed but unencapsulated nodules that are predominantly located in the deep dermis and subcutaneous adipose tissue. **10.4g**: Medium magnification. Tumor cells loosely aggregate in pools of myxoid matrix with intervening hyaline matrix. **10.4h**: Higher magnification. Scattered tumor cells feature cytoplasmic vacuoles that represent primitive blood vessel lumina. These cells are known as 'blister cells'. Tumor nuclei are round to ovoid with minimal variation in size and contain fine chromatin with generally inconspicuous nucleoli. **10.4i**: Antibody to CD34. Tumor cells are diffusely and strongly reactive for CD34, a marker of vascular differentiation (but not 100% specific). **10.4j**: Antibody to EMA. Tumor cells are also reactive for epithelial membrane antigen but focally only.

Perineurioma, sclerosing variant: The sclerosing variant of perineurioma is generally smaller than 3 cm. Acral location, however, is the preferred site, although the great majority occurs in the hands rather than feet. It is heavily collagenized with cords, swirls, and clusters of uniform spindle to oval or slightly cuboidal tumor cells that may aggregate around small nerves or blood vessels; this description actually summarizes aspects of this patient's tumor also. Perineurioma tumor cells are commonly reactive for EMA, Claudin-1 and GLUT1, and some soft tissue tumor authors report reactivity for CD34, while others specifically state perineurioma is negative for this marker. Perineuriomas do not express CD31 or Fli1. Cytogenetically, many cases of EHE harbor the t(1;3), while at least some perineuriomas show loss of 22q. This patient's tumor shows overlap in some of its histologic features with perineurioma, but it is CD31 reactive and contains scattered 'blister cells,' vacuolated tumor cells that can look like signet ring cells or lipoblasts but can contain red blood cells and represent earliest vessel formation. Such blister cells are absent in perineurioma. Moreover, myxoid regions are also present, which would not be present in a sclerosing perineurioma except in a very rare variant that combines sclerosing and classic perineurioma features.

Dermatofibrosarcoma protuberans (DFSP): The relatively large size and predominantly superficial location of this tumor would be a good fit for DFSP. One variant of DFSP, myxoid DFSP, can exhibit a matrix that is myxoid, but it is not myxochondroid or hyaline like in this patient's tumor. DFSP is usually diffusely CD34 positive but does not express CD31 or EMA, and it does not contain blister cells, all of which are present in this patient's tumor. DFSP genetically features a t(17;22)(q22;q13) fusing the collagen type I gene with the platelet derived growth factor β gene. Thus, in difficult cases, cytogenetics may be useful, because the two tumors exhibit different translocations.

Extraskeletal myxoid chondrosarcoma (ESMCS): This tumor usually arises in a deep location, but about 25% are subcutaneous. The myxoid matrix is more watery than chondroid and the tumor is often gelatinous and hemorrhagic on gross examination unlike this patient's tumor which is firm to rubbery. Nests and cords of small epithelioid to spindle cells condense at the periphery of tumor lobules which are separated by fibrous septae. This distinctive look is not seen in this patient's tumor. By IHC, extraskeletal myxoid chondrosarcoma is sometimes positive for S-100 protein and EMA, but it is negative for CD34 and CD31. Many cases demonstrate a t(9;22)(q22;q12) or t(9;17)(q22;q11) which can help distinguish it from EHE. FISH can be used to show translocation of the Ewing sarcoma gene in ESMCS that would be absent in EHE.

Epithelioid sarcoma: Epithelioid sarcoma lacks the myxochondroid matrix of EHE. The classic form consists of multiple pseudogranulomatous nodules of tumor cells with central necrosis. While it can be positive for CD34 and EMA, it is negative for CD31 and often shows loss of INI-1 which is retained in EHE. A newly described type of hemangioendothelioma (HE), epithelioid sarcoma-like HE, is a much closer mimic of epithelioid sarcoma than EHE. It shares with EHE a vasculogenic immunohistochemical profile of reactivity for CD31 and FLI-1 but interestingly is negative for CD34.

Sclerosing epithelioid fibrosarcoma (SEFS): This higher grade relative of low grade fibromyxoid sarcoma can occur superficially and is characterized by cords and nests of small epithelioid cells embedded in a dense collagenized matrix. It does not contain blister cells, and it may have areas indistinguishable from adult type fibrosarcoma. Although sometimes EMA positive, SEFS is CD31 and CD34 negative. A translocation t(7;16)(q33;p11), is found in low grade fibromyxoid

Case table 10.4a Variant histologic features of EHE

Feature	Frequency	Comment
'Blister cells': intracytoplasmic vascular lumina that may contain red blood cells	Common	Although common, some tumors may only have widely scattered cells with these vacuoles
Poorly marginated, infiltrative borders	Common	
Intravascular growth	Common	May involve one large vein, multiple small to medium sized veins, or less commonly, small arteries
Dense myxochondroid or myxohyaline stroma	Common	Characteristic of EHE
Central sclerosis and peripheral myxochondroid stroma	Common	Seen in smaller tumors
Multinodularity	Uncommon	
Osseous metaplasia or calcifications	Uncommon	Seen in 10-15% of cases
Multicellular vascular channels formed by tumor	Uncommon	
Metastasis to lymph nodes	Uncommon	
Spindle cells	Uncommon	If present, usually not predominant
Dendritic cells	Uncommon	Polygonal, multipolar cells with elongate cytoplasmic processes; usually not predominant
High nuclear grade, frequent mitotic figures, necrosis, sheet-like growth	Uncommon	Up to one-third of cases have these features; may correlate with more aggressive behavior; referred to as 'malignant' or 'high grade' EHE
Expression of low modular weight keratins	Uncommon	One source states a 25% incidence in EHE of LMW keratin expression. Another source reports 100% reactivity for keratin 18, 25% of keratin 7 and 8, and no reactivity for keratin 19
EMA (epithelial membrane antigen) expression	Uncommon	Variably reported as present in 25% of cases to absent in all cases
D2-40 (podoplanin) expression	Uncommon	~25% of cases. May be cytoplasmic or membranous
Smooth muscle actin expression	Uncommon	~25% of cases. If present, usually focal

sarcoma and SEFS and is absent in EHE. Recently, MUC4 expression has been found in both SEFS and low grade fibromyxoid sarcoma; this may be helpful diagnostically.

Clear cell sarcoma (CCS): Clear cell sarcoma (previously designated 'melanoma of soft parts') is a melanocytic differentiating sarcoma with a predilection for the foot. It is usually cellular and composed of vague nests of round to spindled clear cells some of which may be vacuolated resembling blister cells of EHE. A myxochondroid matrix is absent. Multinucleated tumor cells are common in CCS and unusual to absent in EHE. By immunohistochemistry, CCS expresses S-100 protein and MelanA103 with a few cases reactive for CD34. There is no reactivity for FLI-1 or CD31. Cytogenetically, CCS exhibits t(12;22)(q13;q12) or t(2;22)(q13;q12) and not t(1;3)(q36;q25). FISH can be used to show translocation of the Ewing sarcoma gene in CCS that would be absent in EHE.

Melanoma: While it is true that melanoma is a great histologic imitator of other tumors, it generally does not feature a myxochondroid matrix and would typically have spread beyond the foot by the time it had reached a size of 7 cm. Moreover, almost all melanomas express S-100 protein +/- MelanA103, and melanoma is usually negative for EMA and does not express CD31 or FLI-1.

Case table 10.4b Summary pathology findings of Case 10.4

Diagnosis	Epithelioid hemangioendothelioma
Size	7 × 4 × 3 cm
Location	Predominantly subcutaneous adipose tissue of right foot with focal invasion of fascia and skeletal muscle
Margin status	Negative; one margin is 0.3 cm from tumor; all other margins > 1.0 cm from tumor.
Histologic grade (FNCLCC grading system)	Intermediate grade (grade rendered because of the diagnosis)
Pathologic stage (AJCC TNM classification)	III = T2b/N0/M0 extending into fascia and skeletal muscle

FNCLCC: Fédération Nationale des Centres de Lutte Contre le Cancer (French Federation of Cancer Centers).

AJCCL American Joint Committee on Cancer

Oncology approach

Medical oncology

Usually, there is no role for medical oncology in this tumor. However, in this particular case, the size of the epithelioid hemangioendothelioma are deciding factors in trying a neoadjuvant approach. Unfortunately, the treatment does not help and is thus stopped to allow for surgery.

Radiation oncology

Surgery is the primary treatment, if the disease is localized at initial presentation. Radiation therapy is typically reserved for palliation to relieve bony pain. A common fractionation scheme is 30 Gy in 10 fractions.

Patient outcome

Thirteen months postoperatively, the patient's wound is healed, he is ambulatory, and has no evidence of recurrence or metastasis.

Case 10.5 Angiosarcoma, epithelioid subtype

Clinical history and presentation

The patient is a 58-year-old man with a 15-year history of right-sided neck mass. He states that it has gradually enlarged over the years and has now gotten to be quite large. It has been its current size for approximately six months. He has had no trouble breathing and no changes in his voice.

Physical examination reveals a 6 × 4 cm neck mass on the right with greatest dimension in the vertical plane. It is firm to palpation with a small amount of fluctuance superiorly. There is no overlying erythema or induration. No crepitus is palpated over the neck.

Surgical findings and comments

Fine needle aspiration biopsy is performed yielding a diagnosis of 'high grade malignant neoplasm.'

Following final confirmation of the biopsy result and staging, a right modified radical neck dissection is performed, sparing cranial nerve-11, along with a right thyroid lobectomy. At surgery, a bulky right neck tumor is identified, adherent to the marginal mandibular nerve, as well as the platysma muscle. The tumor is adherent to the internal jugular vein on the right, and this is sacrificed, along with the sternocleidomastoid. The tumor is dissected off of the carotid artery and vagus nerve. The recurrent laryngeal nerve is identified and preserved.

Radiology findings

The bilobed tumor presented, **Case figs 10.5a** through **10.5c**, is deceiving because of its intimate relation to the thyroid. Indeed, **Case fig. 10.5c**, shows the mass appears to originate in the lateral aspect of the gland with a 'claw' sign of thyroid tissue tracking along the margins of the tumor. The organ creating the 'claw' is usually the organ of origin and would lead the radiologist to propose a differential of thyroid cystic tumors. Furthermore, the superior portion of the lesion shows high density areas which could represent calcification or intense enhancement supporting the diagnosis of a thyroid tumor. A precontrast CT would help delineate whether these areas represent calcification or enhancement. However, since the high density areas exactly match the density of adjacent vessels, these areas likely represent highly vascular tissue.

The radiologist might include a vascular tumor in the differential such as hemangioma. However, these rarely show such large cystic portions. Unfortunately, tissue diagnosis proved this to be an angiosarcoma. Interestingly, no calcification was seen at pathology and only superficial focal penetration of the thyroid was found.

Pathology findings

Gross features

The resection consists of a 10 × 8 × 6 cm portion of soft tissue with part of the thyroid gland and a right neck dissection specimen including multiple lymph nodes. Cross sections through the soft tissue and adjoining thyroid gland reveal a 6.5 × 6 × 6 cm markedly necrotic and hemorrhagic tumor that appears well circumscribed (**Case fig. 10.5d**). Twenty sections of the tumor, including inked surgical margins, are

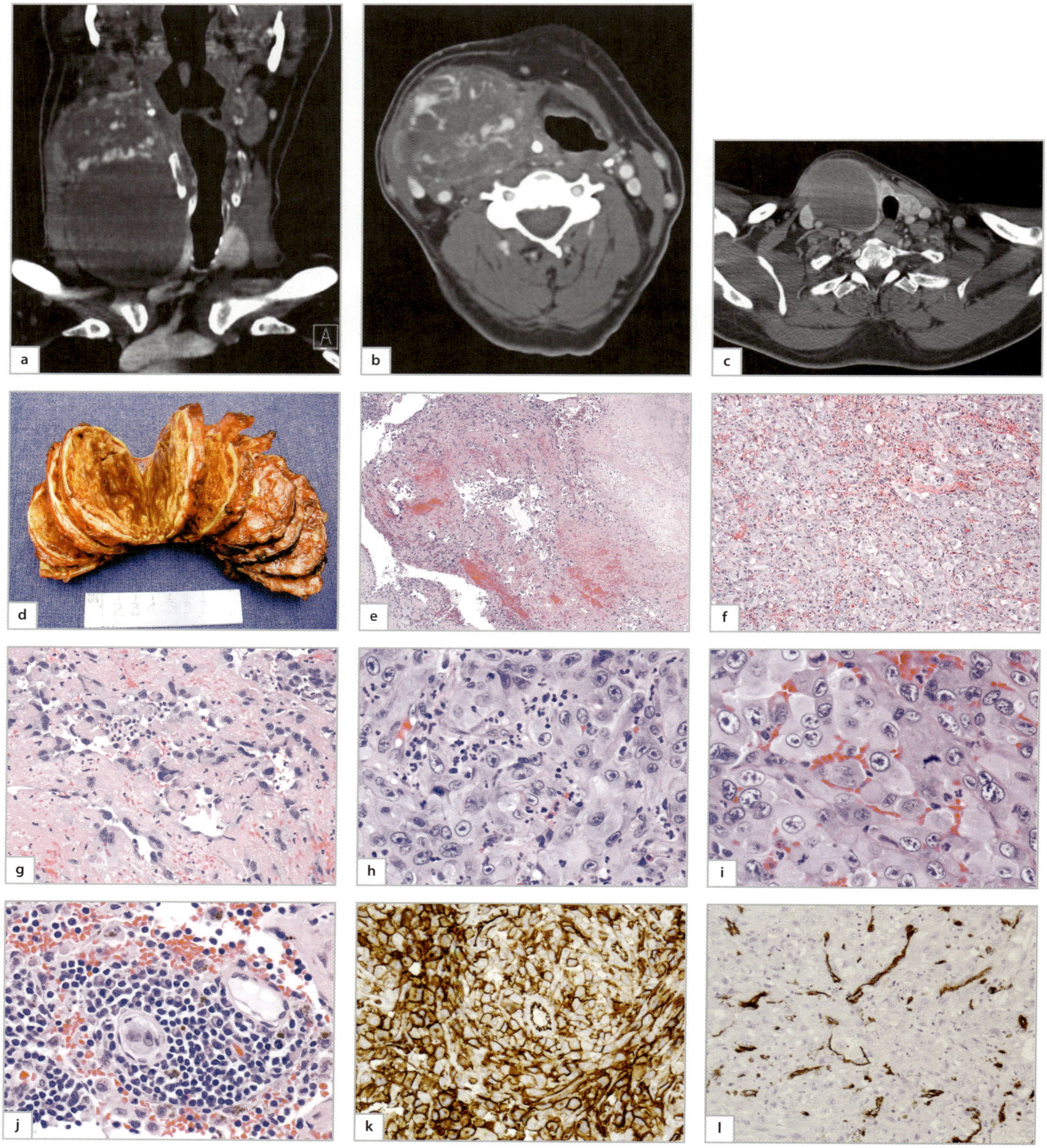

Case figure 10.5 Angiosarcoma. Images from an IV contrast enhanced CT of the neck including: **10.5a**: Coronal reformation, **10.5b**: Axial image through the superior portion. **10.5c**: Axial image from the inferior portion of the mass. This 58 year old man shows a large bilobed mass in the neck with narrowing and displacement of the trachea. The superior portion (Case fig. 10.5b) of the tumor shows heterogeneous areas of high density which exactly match the density of adjacent contrast enhanced vessels (both had Hounsfield density of 230). The inferior portion appears cystic and simple with Hounsfield density of 29. The mass contacts and deforms the thyroid. The appearance suggests a complex tumor with very high vascularity possibly of thyroid etiology. **10.5d**: Gross photograph of representative tumor. Serial cuts through the tumor reveals a hemorrhagic and yellow necrotic parenchyma; commonly seen in high grade angiosarcoma. Unusually, the tumor appears sharply circumscribed and encapsulated.

Case figure 10.5: Continued from page 226

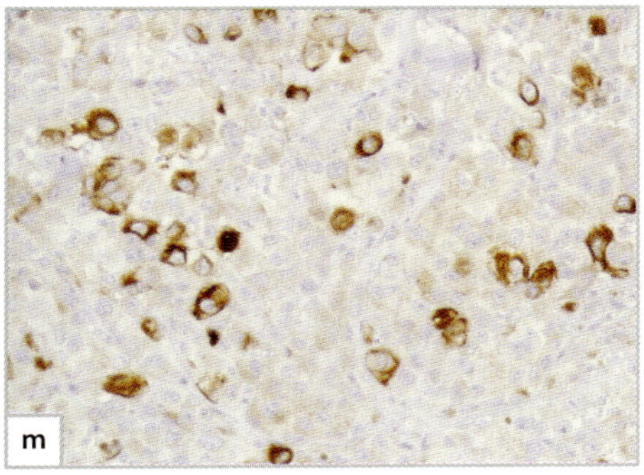

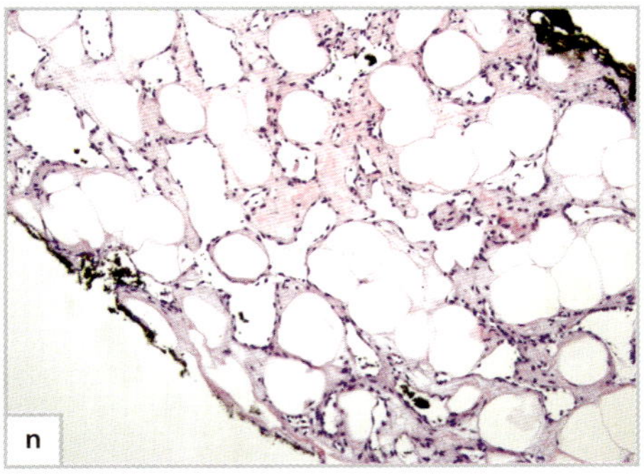

10.5e: Lower magnification. Microscopically, the tumor is approximately 70% necrotic with widespread hemorrhage and fibrin deposition. **10.5f**: Medium magnification. Many fields of viable tumor appear like this with vague nests and columns of epithelioid cells intimately associated with extravasated red blood cells. Even at relatively low magnification, one can appreciate nuclear atypia and scattered cytoplasmic clear spaces suggestive of early vessel lumen formation. **10.5g**: Medium magnification. In this area, jagged spaces are lined by tumor cells that bulge into the clefts. The surrounding stroma is fibrinous. Tumor cells adherent to fibrin and neutrophils float in the spaces. These could represent primitive blood vessels but they are not definitive. Such spaces lined by malignant epithelial cells can be seen in carcinomas, for example, and in that setting have been termed 'pseudovessels' **10.5h**: High magnification. Neutrophils and eosinophils intercalate between epithelioid tumor cells. Epithelioid AS often is inflamed. **10.5i**: High magnification. The tumor is highly mitotically active. In this field, two mitoses are seen. Epithelioid angiosarcoma most often demonstrates marked nuclear pleomorphism as seen here. The nuclei are vesicular (cleared) with irregularly clumped chromatin and prominent, sometimes misshapen and multiple nucleoli. **10.5j**: High magnification of lymph node. A binucleate tumor cell is seen in an intranodal capillary. Notice the intracytoplasmic hemosiderin (brown globular pigment) in macrophages throughout the image. This is consistent with a lymph node draining the hemorrhagic tumor. **10.5k**: CD31 antibody at higher magnification. Diffuse membranous expression of CD31 strongly supports the diagnosis of a vascular tumor. Notice the small non-neoplastic capillary in the center of the field. The normal endothelial cells, much smaller than the tumor endothelial cells, also express CD31 in a membranous pattern. **10.5l**: CD34 antibody at higher magnification. Oddly shaped and of erratic width, these vessels may represent malignant tumor vessels. CD34, while a sensitive marker of vascular differentiation, tends to be expressed in the more vasoformative areas of high grade angiosarcoma. It can commonly be absent in high grade angiosarcoma. **10.5m**: Angiosarcoma, pankeratin antibody at higher magnification. Epithelioid angiosarcomas may be reactive for keratins. Here, scattered tumor cells show cytoplasmic expression for antibody to a broad spectrum of keratins. Notice the reactivity is patchy as is the case in most keratin positive angiosarcomas (carcinomas tend to have diffuse strong expression of keratins). **10.5n**: Angiosarcoma, low grade, higher magnification. For comparison with the patient's high grade epithelioid angiosarcoma, this patient's low grade angiosarcoma is deceptively bland with well-developed blood vessels and small, uniform endothelial cells. However, it permeates or invades the adipose tissue in a telltale, aggressive malignant manner, dissecting between clusters of adipocytes.

submitted to Histology. Multiple lymph nodes are identified and processed for histology. An additional separate 2 cm, partly necrotic tumor nodule is found in the neck dissection soft tissues.

Microscopic features

Low magnification: Corresponding to the gross impression of necrosis and hemorrhage, large areas of the tumor exhibit both (**Case fig. 10.5e**). The tumor infiltrates surrounding tissues although appearing circumscribed on gross examination.

High magnification: Non-necrotic areas of tumor consist entirely of epithelioid tumor cells meaning the cells resemble epithelial cells, as they are round with well-defined cell borders and contain round nuclei with a low to moderate nuclear to cytoplasmic ratio (**Case fig. 10.5f**). These cells form sheets or seem to line jagged channels that represent abortive vessel formation (**Case fig. 10.5g**). A prominent inflammatory infiltrate of neutrophils and eosinophils swirls around tumor cells (**Case fig. 10.5h**). The tumor is replete with intermingled erythrocytes and dotted with hemosiderin and fibrin deposition, features often seen in high grade angiosarcoma. Mitoses are abundant (average of 25/10 high magnification microscopic fields)(**Case fig. 10.5i**) and necrosis involves approximately 70% of tumor parenchyma. Of twenty three lymph nodes, three contain isolated malignant tumor cells, predominantly in intralymphatic blood vessels (**Case fig. 10.5j**). The tumor extends to multiple inked surgical margins. Vascular invasion other than in the lymph nodes is not identified.

Special studies: Because of a wide histologic differential including anaplastic thyroid carcinoma (which can have a pseudovasoformative appearance), melanoma and other types of sarcoma, multiple immunohistochemical stains are performed. All tumor cells show strong membranous reactivity for CD31 (**Case fig. 10.5k**). Normal reactive blood vessels and possibly a few early malignant vessels express CD34 (**Case fig. 10.5l**). About 10% of cells exhibit cytoplasmic reactivity for pankeratin (**Case fig. 10.5m**). All other antibodies show negative expression (S-100 protein and MelanA103 [to help exclude melanoma], keratins 5/p63 [to exclude a high grade squamous carcinoma], calcitonin and CEA [to exclude medullary thyroid carcinoma], thyroglobulin and thyroid transcription factor 1 [to exclude anaplastic thyroid carcinoma] and CD45 [to help exclude high grade lymphoma]. The diffuse membranous reactivity for CD31, focal staining only for pan-keratins and primitive vessel formation enable a diagnosis of epithelioid angiosarcoma.

Pathologic differential or, why isn't it one of the following?

Carcinoma: Radiologically, the tumor was considered to be arising from the thyroid gland. This was also the impression at the time of fine needle aspiration biopsy. However, on histology, the thyroid gland was only focally involved. Anaplastic thyroid carcinoma (ATC) would be in the differential, and some thyroid carcinomas mimic vasoformation by demonstrating elongate clefts lined by tumor cells. However, ATC often has lower grade areas and many cases exhibit focal reactivity for TTF-1 (less commonly thyroglobulin). Moreover, diffuse membranous CD31 reactivity would not be expected. Medullary carcinoma is likewise excluded because of the CD31 expression and lack of CEA and calcitonin expression. This patient's tumor lacks a low grade component. When present, it is very helpful diagnostically.

Case fig. 10.5n is an example of a low grade AS for comparison with this patient's tumor. The vessels in low grade angiosarcoma are well-formed with deceptively bland endothelial cells; the key feature of malignancy is permeative growth into surrounding normal tissue.

Melanoma: Melanoma is notorious for its wide spectrum of cytologic morphologies from epithelioid to spindle cell to small round blue cell. Many examples do not contain melanin pigment. Thus, while unlikely based on the absence of history of melanoma in this patient, it is still reasonable to exclude the possibility given its protean appearances, unpredictable behavior and ability to regress at the primary site, showing up as a metastasis. The tumor is negative for sensitive melanoma markers including S-100 protein and Melan-A. The CD31 reactivity supports the diagnosis of vascular differentiation, because only very rarely does CD31 expression occur in melanoma. The vasoformative areas are also consistent with angiosarcoma.

Proximal type epithelioid sarcoma: By cytologic appearance, this patient's tumor could be consistent with proximal type epithelioid sarcoma. However, that tumor is seldom CD31 positive, although it can express CD34 (in about 50% of cases) and keratins (33-50%). The vasoformative areas in this patient's tumor would not be seen in proximal type epithelioid sarcoma. INI-1 expression is lost in about 50% of epithelioid sarcomas and retained in angiosarcoma.

Oncology approach

Medical oncology

One month postoperatively, the patient is noted to have a local recurrence. He refuses radiation therapy but agrees to chemotherapy. He receives a combination of weekly paclitaxel with bevacizumab and tolerates the treatment well.

Case table 10.5 Summary pathology findings of Case 10.5

Diagnosis	Angiosarcoma, epithelioid subtype
Size	6.5 × 6 × 6 cm
Location	Deep soft tissues of right neck with focal minimal invasion of thyroid gland
Margin status	Positive
Histologic grade (FNCLCC grading system)	High grade (grade 3)
Pathologic stage (AJCC TNM classification)	IV (T2b/N1*/M0) Only rare tumor cells in lymph nodes, predominantly in intranodal vessels.

FNCLCC: Fédération Nationale des Centres de Lutte Contre le Cancer (French Federation of Cancer Centers).
AJCC: American Joint Committee on Cancer

Radiation oncology

Following standard treatment guidelines for high-grade sarcoma, radiation therapy is given usually post-operatively to optimize local regional control. Doses in the post-operative setting are typically 60-66 Gy, depending on margin status. A common type of AS is secondary to prior history of RT, and occurs in the area of prior treatment. Treatment usually consists of surgery. Primary AS can be managed with RT alone, if surgery is not feasible. Definitive doses range from 60-70 Gy.

Patient outcome

Six month postoperatively, the patient remains on chemotherapy with stable recurrent disease.

REFERENCES

Abraham JA, Hornicek FJ, Kaufman AM, et al. Treatment and outcome of 82 patients with angiosarcoma. Ann Surg Oncol 2007;14:1953–1967.

Agulnik M, Okuno S, Von Mehren M. An open-label multicenter phase II study of bevacizumab for the treatment of angiosarcoma. Proc Am Soc Clin Oncol 2009;27:A10522.

Ahmed I, Hamacher KL. Angiosarcoma in a chronically immunosuppressed renal transplant recipient: report of a case and review of the literature. Am J Dermatopathol 2002;24:330–5.

Al Dhaybi R, Powell J, McCuaig C, et al. Differentiation of vascular tumors from vascular malformations by expression of Wilms tumor 1 gene: evaluation of 126 cases. J Am Acad Dermatol 2010;63:1052–1057.

Andersson HC, Parry DM, Mulvihill JJ. Lymphangiosarcoma in late-onset hereditary lymphedema: case report and nosological implications. Am J Med Genet 1995;56:72–5.

Antman K, Chang Y. Kaposi's sarcoma. N Engl J Med 2000;342:1027–38.

Antonescu CR, Yoshida A, Guo T, et al. KDR activating mutations in human angiosarcomas are sensitive to specific kinase inhibitors. Cancer Res 2009;69:7175–9.

Billings SD, Folpe AL, Weiss SW. Epithelioid sarcoma-like hemangioendothelioma. Am J Surg Pathol 2003;27:48–57.

Billings SD, Folpe AL, Weiss SW, et al. Epithelioid sarcoma-like hemangioendothelioma (pseudomyogenic hemangioendothelioma). Letter to editor with comments. Am J Surg Pathol 2011;35:1088–1089.

Bosetti C, La Vecchia C, Lipworth L, et al. Occupational exposure to vinyl chloride and cancer risk: a review of the epidemiologic literature. Eur J Cancer Prev 2003;12:427–30.

Budd GT. Management of angiosarcoma. Curr Oncol Rep 2002;4:515–9.

Burns B, Blakey S, Harris W. Complete response of metastatic angiosarcoma to liposomal doxorubicin and interferon-2a. Proc Am Soc Clin Oncol 2002;A2939.

Canavese F, Soo BC, Chia SK, et al. Surgical outcome in patients treated for hemangioma during infancy, childhood, and adolescence: a retrospective review of 44 consecutive patients. J Pediatr Orthop 2008;28(3):381–6.

Cattamanchi A, Saracino M, Selke S, et al. Treatment with valacyclovir, famciclovir, or antiretrovirals reduces human herpesvirus-8 replication in HIV-1 seropositive men. J Med Virol 2011;83:1696–703.

Cattelan AM, Calabrò ML, De Rossi A, et al. Long-term clinical outcome of AIDS-related Kaposi's sarcoma during highly active antiretroviral therapy. Inter J Oncol 2005;27:779–785.

Chang Y, Cesarman E, Pessin MS, et al. Identification of herpesvirus-like DNA sequences in AIDS-associated Kaposi's sarcoma. Science 1994;266:1865–9.

Connell FC, Ostergaard P, Carver C, et al. Analysis of the coding regions of VEGFR3 and VEGFC in Milroy disease and other primary lymphedemas. Hum Genet 2009;124:625–31.

Coppin C, Kollmannsberger C, Le L, et al. Targeted therapy for advanced renal cell cancer (RCC): a Cochrane systematic review of published randomized trials. BJU Int 2011;108:1556–63.

DeMartelaere SL, Roberts D, Burgess MA, et al. Neoadjuvant chemotherapy-specific and overall treatment outcomes in patients with cutaneous angiosarcoma of the face with periorbital involvement. Head Neck 2008;30:639–46.

Deyrup AT, Tighiouart M, Montag AG, et al. Epithelioid hemangioendothelioma of soft tissue: a proposal for risk stratification based on 49 cases. Am J Surg Pathol 2008;32:924–927.

Dezube BJ. Management of AIDS-related Kaposi's sarcoma: advances in target discovery and treatment. Expert Rev Anticancer Ther 2002;2:193–200.

Dim D, Ravi V, Tan J, et al. The actin-bundling motility protein fascin and vascular endothelial growth factor (VEGF) are universally over-expressed in human angiosarcoma. Proc Am Soc Clin Oncol 2007;25:A10068.

Errani C, Zhang L, Sung YS, et al. A novel WWTR1-CAMTA1 gene fusion is a consistent abnormality in epithelioid hemangioendothelioma of different sites. Genes Chromosomes Cancer 2011;50:655–653.

Evans SR, Krown SE, Testa MA, et al. Phase II evaluation of low-dose oral etoposide for the treatment of relapsed or progressive AIDS-related Kaposi's sarcoma: an AIDS Clinical Trials Group clinical study. J Clin Oncol 2002;20:3236–41.

Fayette J, Martin E, Piperno- Neumann S, et al. Angiosarcomas, a heterogeneous group of sarcomas with specific behavior depending on primary site: a retrospective study of 161 cases. Ann Oncol 2007;18:2030–2036.

Fernandez AP, Sun Y, Tubbs RR, et al. FISH for MYC amplification and anti-MYC immunohistochemistry: useful diagnostic tools in the assessment of secondary angiosarcoma and atypical vascular proliferations. J Cutan Pathol 2012;39:234–42.

Folpe AL, Chand EM, Goldblum JR, et al. Expression of Fli-1, a nuclear transcription factor, distinguishes vascular neoplasms from potential mimics. Am J Surg Pathol 2001;25:1061–1066.

Fury MG, Antonescu CR, Van Zee KJ, et al. A 14-year retrospective review of angiosarcoma: clinical characteristics, prognostic factors, and treatment outcomes with surgery and chemotherapy. Cancer J 2005;11:241–7.

Garcia JM, Gonzalez R, Silva JM, et al. Mutational status of K-ras and TP53 genes in primary sarcomas of the heart. Br J Cancer 2000;82:1183–5.

Garzon MC, Huang JT, Enjolras O, et al. Vascular malformations. Part II: associated syndromes. J Am Acad Dermatol 2007;56:541–64.

George S, Merriam P, Maki RG, et al. Multicenter phase II trial of sunitinib in the treatment of nongastrointestinal stromal tumor sarcomas. J Clin Oncol 2009;27:3154–60.

Gill PS, Tulpule A, Espina BM, et al. Paclitaxel is safe and effective in the treatment of advanced AIDS-related Kaposi's sarcoma. J Clin Oncol 1999;17:1876–83.

Gill PS, Wernz J, Scadden DT, et al. Randomized phase III trial of liposomal daunorubicin versus doxorubicin, bleomycin, and vincristine in AIDS-related Kaposi's sarcoma. J Clin Oncol 1996;14:2353–64.

Gill R, O'Donnell RJ, Horvai A. Utility of immunohistochemistry for endothelial markers in distinguishing epithelioid hemangioendothelioma from carcinoma metastatic to bone. Arch Pathol Lab Med 2009;133:967–972.

Goh SGN, Calonje E. Cutaneous vascular tumors: an update. Histopathol 2008;52:661–673.

Guadagnolo BA, Zagars GK, Araujo D, et al. Outcomes after definitive treatment for cutaneous angiosarcoma of the face and scalp. Head Neck 2011;33(5):661–7.

Hart J, Mandavilli S. Epithelioid angiosarcoma: a brief diagnostic review and differential diagnosis. Arch Pathol Lab Med 2011;135:278–272.

Hauerstock D, Gerstein W, Vuong T. Results of radiation therapy for treatment of classic Kaposi sarcoma. J Cutan Med Surg 2009;13(1):18–21.

Holloway CL, Turner AR, Dundas GS. Cutaneous angiosarcoma of the scalp: a case report of sustained complete response following liposomal Doxorubicin and radiation therapy. Sarcoma 2005;9:29–31.

Hornick JL, Fletcher CDM. Pseudomyogenic hemangioendothelioma: a distinctive, often multicentric tumor with indolent behavior. Am J Surg Pathol 2011;35:190–201.

Huu ARL, Jokinen CH, Ruben BP, et al. Expression of Prox1, lymphatic endothelial nuclear transcription factor, in Kaposiform hemangioendothelioma and tufted angioma. Am J Surg Pathol 2010;34:1563–1573.

Itakura E, Yamamoto H, Oda Y, et al. Detection and characterization of vascular endothelial growth factors and their receptors in a series of angiosarcomas. J Surg Oncol 2008;97:74–81.

Italiano A, Cioffi A, Penel N, et al. Comparison of doxorubicin and weekly paclitaxel efficacy in metastatic angiosarcomas. Cancer 2012;118(13):3330–6.

Jennings TA, Peterson L, Axiotis CA, et al. Angiosarcoma associated with foreign body material. A report of three cases. Cancer 1988;62:2436–44.

Johnson KD, Glinskii OV, Mossine VV, et al. Galectin-3 as a potential therapeutic target in tumors arising from malignant endothelia. Neoplasia 2007;9:662–70.

Kamo R, Ishii M. Histological differentiation, histogenesis and prognosis of cutaneous angiosarcoma. Osaka City Med J 2011;57:31–44.

Kandil A, Rostom AY, Mourad WA, et al. Successful control of extensive thoracic lymphangiomatosis by irradiation. Clin Oncol (R Coll Radiol) 1997;9(6):407–11.

Kolloway CL, Turner AR, Dundas GS. Cutaneous angiosarcoma of the scalp: a case report of sustained complete response following liposomal Doxorubicin and radiation therapy. Sarcoma 2005;9:29–31

Koontz BF, Miles EF, Rubio MA, et al. Preoperative radiotherapy and bevacizumab for angiosarcoma of the head and neck: two case studies. Head Neck 2008;30:262–6.

Krishnamoorthy N, Viswanathan S, Rekhi B, et al. Lymphangiosarcoma arising after 33 years within a background of chronic filariasis: a case report with review of literature. J Cutan Pathol 2012;39:52–5.

Lahat G, Dhuka AR, Hallevi H, et al. Angiosarcoma clinical and molecular insights. Ann Surg 2010;251:1098–1106.

Lau K, Massad M, Pollak C, et al. Clinical patterns and outcome in epithelioid hemangioendothelioma with or without pulmonary involvement: insights from an internet registry in the study of a rare cancer. Chest 2011;140:1312–8.

Laubenstein LJ, Krigel RL, Odajnyk CM, et al. Treatment of epidemic Kaposi's sarcoma with etoposide or a combination of doxorubicin, bleomycin, and vinblastine. J Clin Oncol 1984;2:1115–20.

Lawley LP, Cerimele F, Weiss SW, et al. Expression of Wilms tumor 1 gene distinguishes vascular malformations from proliferative lesions. Arch Dermatol 2005;141:1297–1300.

Lim ST, Tupule A, Espina BM, et al. Weekly docetaxel is safe and effective in the treatment of advanced-stage acquired immunodeficiency syndrome-related Kaposi sarcoma. Cancer 2005;103:417–21.

Limaye N, Wouters V, Uebelhoer M, et al. Somatic mutations in angiopoietin receptor gene *TEK* cause solitary and multiple sporadic venous malformations. Nat Genet 2009;41:118–124.

Maki RG, D'Adamo DR, Keohan ML, et al. Phase II study of sorafenib in patients with metastatic or recurrent sarcomas. J Clin Oncol 2009;27:3133–40.

McMenamin ME, Fletcher CD. Expanding the spectrum of malignant change in schwannomas: epithelioid malignant change, epithelioid malignant peripheral nerve sheath tumor, and epithelioid angiosarcoma: a study of 17 cases. Am J Surg Pathol 2001;25:13–25.

Mendlick MR, Nelson M, Pickering D, et al. Translocation t(1;3)(p36.3;q25) is a nonrandom aberration in epithelioid hemangioendothelioma. Am J Surg Pathol 2001;25:684–687.

Mhawech-Fauceglia P, Herrmann FR, Bshara W, et al. Friend leukemia integration-1 expression in malignant and benign tumors: a multiple tumour tissue microarray analysis using polyclonal antibody. J Clin Pathol 2007;60:694–700.

Miettinen M, Wang ZF. Prox1 transcription factor as a marker for vascular tumors-evaluation of 314 vascular endothelial and 1086 nonvascular tumors. Am J Surg Pathol 2012;36:351–9.

Miettinen M, Sarlomo-Rikala M, Wang Z-F. Claudin-5 as an immunohistochemical marker for angiosarcoma and hemangioendotheliomas. Am J Surg Pathol 2011;35:1848–1856.

Mosam A, Shaik F, Uldrickd TS, et al. A randomized controlled trial of HAART versus HAART and chemotherapy in therapy-naive patients with HIV-associated Kaposi sarcoma in South Africa. J Acquir Immune Defic Syndr 2012;60(2):150–7.

Muramatsu K, Ihara K, Tani Y, et al. Intramuscular hemangioma of the upper extremity in infants and children. J Pediatr Orthop 2008;28(3):387–90.

Nagano T, Yamada Y, Ikeda T, et al. Docetaxel: a therapeutic option in the treatment of cutaneous angiosarcoma: report of 9 patients. Cancer 2007;110:648–51.

Naito S, Shimizu K, Nakashima M, et al. Overexpression of Ets-1 transcription factor in angiosarcoma of the skin. Pathol Res Pract 2000;196:103–9.

Naqvi J, Ordonez NG, Luna MA, et al. Epithelioid hemangioendothelioma of the head and neck: role of podoplanin in the differential diagnosis. Head Neck Pathol 2008;2:25–30.

Nasti G, Errante D, Talamini R, et al. Vinorelbine is an effective and safe drug for AIDS-related Kaposi's sarcoma: results of a phase II study. J Clin Oncol 2000;18:1550–7.

Northfelt DW, Dezube BJ, Thommes JA, et al. Efficacy of pegylated-liposomal doxorubicin in the treatment of AIDS-related Kaposi's sarcoma after failure of standard chemotherapy. J Clin Oncol 1997;15:653–9.

Pansuriya T, van Eijk R, d'Adamo P, et al. Somatic mosaic IDH1 and IDH2 mutations are associated with enchondroma and spindle cell hemangioma in Ollier disease and Maffucci syndrome. Nat Genet 2011;43:1256–1260.

Penel N, Bui BN, Bay JO, et al. Phase II trial of weekly paclitaxel for unresectable angiosarcoma: the ANGIOTAX Study. J Clin Oncol 2008;26:5269–74.

Penel N, Italiano A, Ray-Coquard I, et al. Metastatic angiosarcomas: doxorubicin-based regimens, weekly paclitaxel and metastasectomy significantly improve the outcome. Ann Oncol 2012;23:517–23.

Penn I. Kaposi's sarcoma in organ transplant recipients: report of 20 cases. Transplantation 1979;27:8–11.

Perkins P, Weiss SW. Spindle cell hemangioendothelioma. An analysis of 78 cases with reassessment of its pathogenesis and biologic behavior. Am J Surg Pathol 1996;20:1196–204.
Pritchard DJ. Surgical management of common benign soft-tissue tumors. In: Simon MA, Springfield D, eds. Surgery for Bone and Soft-tissue Tumors. *Philadelphia:* Lippincott-Raven Publisher, 1998:534–537.
Riccardi VM, Wheeler TM, Pickard LR, et al. The pathophysiology of neurofibromatosis. II. Angiosarcoma as a complication. Cancer Genet Cytogenet 1984;12:275–80.
Ron E. Cancer risks from medical radiation. Health Phys 2003;85:47–59.
Rouhani P, Fletcher CD, Devesa SS, et al. Cutaneous soft tissue sarcoma incidence patterns in the U.S. : an analysis of 12,114 cases. Cancer 2008;113:616–27.
Ryan C, von Mehren M. Phase II intergroup study of sorafenib (S) in advanced soft tissue sarcomas (STS): SWOG 0505. Proc Am Soc Clin Oncol 2008;26:A10532.
Scott MT, Portnow LH, Morris CG, et al. Radiation Therapy for Angiosarcoma: The 35-year University of Florida Experience. Am J Clin Oncol 2013;36(2):174–80.
Seinen JM, Styring E, Verstappen V, et al. Radiation-associated angiosarcoma after breast cancer: high recurrence rate and poor aurvival despite surgical treatment with R0 resection. Ann Surg Oncol 2012;19(8):2700–6.
Shon W, Ida CM, Boland-Froemming JM, et al. Cutaneous angiosarcoma arising in massive localized lymphedema of the morbidly obese: a report of five cases and review of the literature. J Cutan Pathol 2011;38(7)560–4.
Skubitz KM, Haddad PA. Paclitaxel and pegylated-liposomal doxorubicin are both active in angiosarcoma. Cancer 2005;104:361–6.
Stewart S, Jablonowski H, Goebel FD, et al. Randomized comparative trial of pegylated liposomal doxorubicin versus bleomycin and vincristine in the treatment of AIDS-related Kaposi's sarcoma. International Pegylated Liposomal Doxorubicin Study Group. J Clin Oncol 1998;16:683–91
Stoler MH, Bonfiglio TA, Steigbigel RT, et al. An atypical subcutaneous infection associated with acquired immune deficiency syndrome. Am J Clin Pathol 1983;80:714–8.
Styring E, Fernebro J, Jonsson PE, et al. Changing clinical presentation of angiosarcomas after breast cancer: from late tumors in edematous arms to earlier tumors on the thoracic wall. Breast Cancer Res Treat 2010;122:883–7.
Tam HK, Zhang ZF, Jacobson LP, et al. Effect of highly active antiretroviral therapy on survival among HIV-infected men with Kaposi sarcoma or non-Hodgkin lymphoma. Int J Cancer 2002;98:916–22.
Tanas MR, Sboner A, Oliveira AM, et al. Identification of a disease-defining gene fusion in epithelioid hemangioendothelioma. Sci Transl Med 2011;3:98ra82.
Trombetta D, Magnusson L, von Steyem FV, et al. Translocation t(7;19) (q22;q13) – a recurrent chromosome aberration in pseudomyogenic hemangioendothelioma? Cancer Genetics 2011;204:211–215.
Tsai J-W, Huang H-Y, Lee J-C, et al. Composite haemangioendothelioma: report of four cases with emphasis on atypical clinical presentation. Pathology 2011;43:176–180.
Trindade F, Tellechea O, Torrelo A, et al. Wilms tumor 1 expression in vascular neoplasms and vascular malformations. Am J Dermatopathol 2011;33: 569–572.
Ueda T, Oji Y, Naka N, et al. Overexpression of the Wilms' tumor gene WT1 in human bone and soft-tissue sarcomas. Cancer Sci 2003;94:271–6.
Verschraegen CF, Arias-Pulido H, Lee SJ, et al. Phase IB study of the combination of docetaxel, gemcitabine, and bevacizumab in patients with advanced or recurrent soft tissue sarcoma: the Axtell regimen. Ann Oncol 2012;23:785–90.
Weihrauch M, Bader M, Lehnert G, et al. Mutation analysis of K-ras-2 in liver angiosarcoma and adjacent nonneoplastic liver tissue from patients occupationally exposed to vinyl chloride. Environ Mol Mutagen 2002;40:36–40.
West JG, Weitzel JN, Tao ML, et al. BRCA mutations and the risk of angiosarcoma after breast cancer treatment. Clin Breast Cancer 2008;8:533–7.
Yildiz F, Atahan IL, Ozyar E, et al. Radiotherapy in congenital vulvar lymphangioma circumscriptum. Int J Gynecol Cancer 2008;18(3):556–9.
Young RJ, Brown NJ, Reed MW, et al. Angiosarcoma. Lancet Oncology 2010;11:983–991.

FURTHER READING

Folpe AL, Inwards CY (eds). Bone and Soft Tissue Pathology. A volume in the series: Foundations in Diagnostic Pathology. Goldblum JR (series ed). Philadelphia: Elsevier Saunders, 2010.
Sarcoma Meta-analysis Collaboration (SMAC). Adjuvant chemotherapy for localized resectable soft tissue sarcoma in adults. Cochrane Database Syst Rev 2000; CD001419.
Fisher C, Mentzel T, Montgomery EA, et al. Diagnostic Pathology Soft Tissue Tumors. Salt Lake City: AMIRSYS, 2011.
Fritz A, Percy C, Jack A (Eds). International Classification of Diseases for Oncology,3rd ed. Geneva, World Health Organization 2000;45.
Miettinen M. Modern Soft Tissue Pathology. Cambridge: Cambridge University Press, 2010.
Fletcher CDM, Krishnan Unni K, Mertens F (Eds). World Health Organization Classification of Tumours. Pathology and Genetics Tumours of Soft Tissue and Bone. Lyon: IARC Press, 2002.

Chapter 11 Chondro-osseous tumors of soft tissues

OVERVIEW

Three unrelated tumors are classified as chondro-osseous by the World Health Organization (WHO): soft tissue chondroma, mesenchymal chondrosarcoma, and extraskeletal (extra-osseous) osteosarcoma. Authors of other soft tissue tumor texts books include additional entities in this category such as synovial chondromatosis, soft tissue chondrosarcoma, phosphaturic mesenchymal tumor, myositis ossificans and fibro-osseous pseudotumor, among others. In this book, these tumors and mesenchymal chondrosarcoma are described in other chapters.

Soft tissue chondroma and extraskeletal osteosarcoma are considerably less common than their correlates in bone, enchondroma and conventional intraosseous osteosarcoma, respectively. Extraskeletal osteosarcoma, for example, comprises only 2-4% of all cases of osteosarcoma (Lee et al. 2010).

CLASSIFICATION

Table 11.1 lists the three entities in this category of chondro-osseous soft tissue tumors (WHO 2013). Mesenchymal chondrosarcoma is described in Chapter 16, Cartilage tumors of bone.

DEMOGRAPHICS

Soft tissue chondroma is uncommon. Males and females are approximately equally affected across a broad age range including children, but most patients are in the 4th to 6th decades.

Soft tissue osteosarcoma is rare. A review of cases registered with the Surveillance, Epidemiology and End Results (SEER) program from 1994-2008 reveals the age-adjusted incidence rate for extraskeletal osteosarcoma is 0.1 per million with a total of 72 cases. For a comparison, the age-adjusted incidence rate for osteosarcoma of bone and joints is 2.0 per million with a total of 1,151 cases; thus, primary osseous osteosarcoma is 16 times more common than its primary soft tissue counterpart. The mean age at diagnosis is 56.6 years (median = 62.5 years), and the range is 10 to 87 years. In the SEER research database, there are more females (N=40, 55.6%) diagnosed with extraskeletal osteosarcoma than males (N=32, 44.4%), although the difference is not statistically significant.

Most primary soft tissue osteosarcomas are located in the connective tissue, subcutaneous tissue and other soft tissues of the lower limb or hip, as shown in **Table 11.2**.

PATHOGENESIS/ETIOLOGY

Table 11.3 lists the genetic findings in soft tissue chondroma and osteosarcoma. Mesenchymal chondrosarcoma is discussed in Chapter 16.

PATHOLOGY

Histologic features of the tumors are listed in **Table 11.4**. Representative photomicrographs included in the table are just that, representative, and do not capture the range of appearances of these tumors. Their intent is to render the verbal depictions of the lesions more comprehensible.

Table 11.1 WHO classification of chondro-osseous tumors of soft tissue (2013)

Tumor	Behavior	Additional comments
Soft tissue chondroma	Benign	Most occur in hands and feet Up to 25% non-aggressive local recurrence rate
Mesenchymal chondrosarcoma	Malignant	Occurs in bone and soft tissue
Primary soft tissue osteosarcoma	Malignant	Rare and aggressive

Benign: does not recur aggressively and does not metastasize. Intermediate: can recur aggressively and/or rarely metastasizes (<5%). Malignant = can recur and commonly metastasizs.

Table 11.2 Extraskeletal osteosarcoma by soft tissue site for cases in 13 SEER registries diagnosed between 1994 and 2008.

Connective, subcutaneous, and other soft tissues								
Head/face/ neck	Upper limb/ shoulder	Lower limb/hip	Thorax	Abdomen	Pelvis	Trunk	Overlap*	NOS
3	6	37	14	4	5	2	0	1

*'A tumor that overlaps the boundaries of two or more subcategories and whose point of origin cannot be determined.' (Fritz et al., 2000). Date from 13 SEER program registries were evaluated for the 15-year period, 1994-2008. All osteosarcoma cases (ICDO-3) = 9180/3) were limited to connective, subcutaneous and other soft tissues (ICD-O topography codes = C49.0 – C49.9)

Table 11.3 Genetics of chondro-osseous tumors of soft tissue

Tumor	Chromosomal abnormality	Genes involved	Percentage of tumors with abnormality
Soft tissue chondroma	12q13-15 rearrangements or amplification seems most common, trisomy 5 reported in 3 cases -6, 11q13 rearrangements, inversion 12 (p12.3q15) reported in single separate cases	HMGA2 (12q15) LPP (3q27) reported in one case translocated to HMGA2	Unknown but majority may have HMGA2 alterations (fusions, amplifications, overexpression)
Extraskeletal osteosarcoma	Complex aneuploid karyotype not different from intraosseous osteosarcoma (only a few cases reported, however) High grade intra-osseous osteosarcoma shows no universal karyotypic changes but the following abnormalities are seen with increased frequency: gain of 1; loss of parts of 6, 9, 10, 13, and 17 with rearrangements of 1p11-13, 1q11-12, 1q21-22, 11p14-15, 14p11-13, 15p1-13, 17p and 19q12-13 Copy number changes occur at 1q21, 3q26, 6p, 8q, 12q12-q13, 14q24-qter, 17p11.2-p12, 19q12-q13	See Chapter 17 for genes involved in syndromes predisposing to osteosarcoma	Unknown (too few cases to be definitive), but it is likely that the majority of the tumors contain a complex aneuploid karyotype
See References for papers pertaining to this table. This static list of genetic abnormalities must be viewed in the context of continuing discovery and refinement of genetic findings.			

Table 11.4 Predominantly adult chondro-osseous tumors of soft tissue grouped by behavior

Tumor	Incidence	Age and sex distribution	Body site (in order of occurrence)	Histopathology description including IHC	
				Medium magnification	High magnification
Benign: does not recur or recurs non-aggressively and does not metastasize					
Soft tissue chondroma	Common	Adults; most in 30s to 60s (case reports in children) M > F	Hands and feet (primarily fingers and toes) >> soft tissues around joints elsewhere	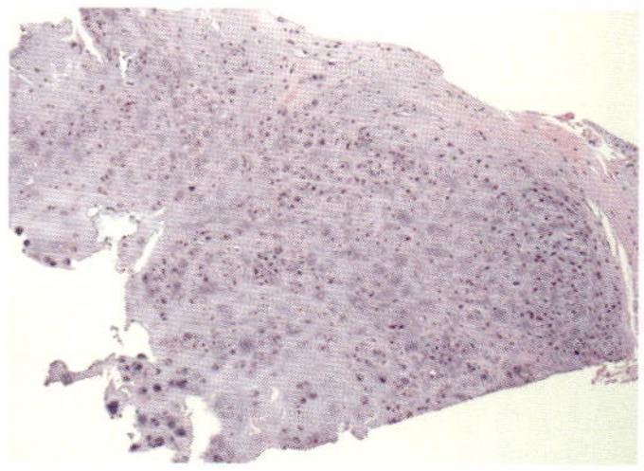	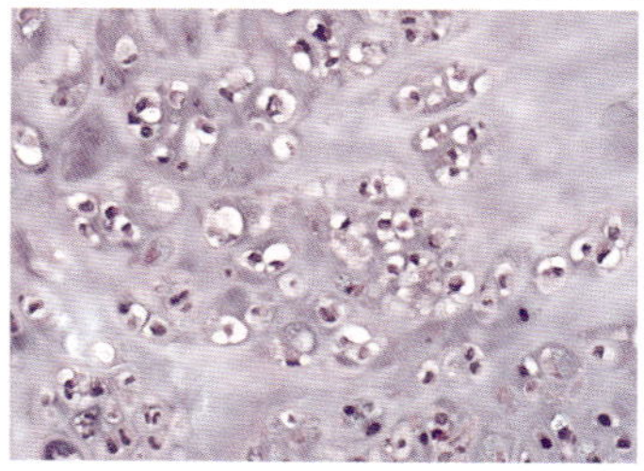
Nodules of hyaline cartilage showing sharp border with surrounding soft tissue. Many are calcified; some with bony ('osteochondroma'), myxoid ('myxochondroma') fibrous ('fibrochondroma'), cystic or peripheral granulomatous change. May be hypercellular with rare but not atypical mitoses. There is also a rare pure, chondroblastoma-like variant, although chondroblastoma-like areas are focally common in the other variants. Tumor cells are S-100 protein positive.					
Malignant: can recur and commonly metastasizes					
Extraskeletal osteosarcoma	Very rare	Adults; most in 50s to 70s M > F	Deep soft tissues of thigh, buttock, shoulder area, trunk. Only 10% are superficial in the dermis or subcutis	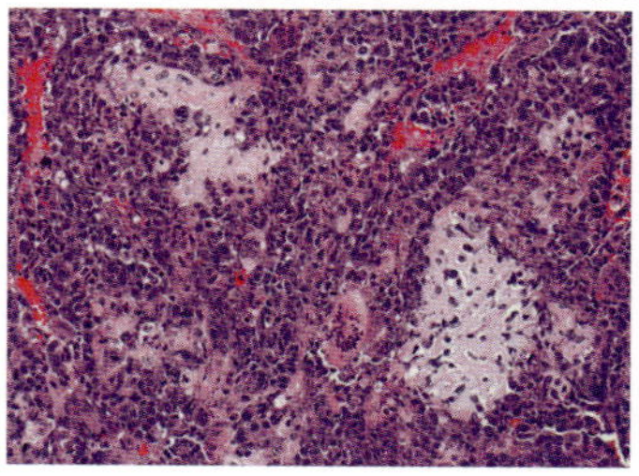	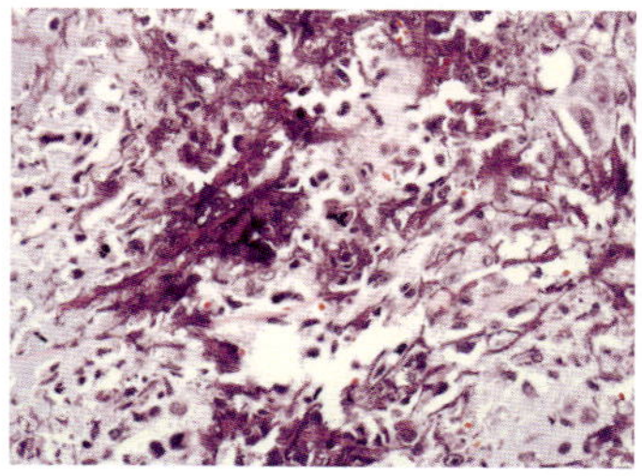
95% are histologically high grade and are identical to the intra-osseous variants of osteosarcoma: osteoblastic, chondroblastic, fibroblastic, telangiectatic, and small cell. Mixed patterns are common. Rare reports of primary low grade extraskeletal osteosarcoma mimicking parosteal osteosarcoma.					
Incidence note: 'Common to very common' indicates that a medium sized practice will treat at least several to dozens of patients with the lesion annually, 'Uncommon to rare' indicates the same practice size will treat one to two patients with the lesion every five years, 'Rare to very rare' indicates the same sized practice will see zero to one patient with the lesion every 20 years.					

Histologic grading

Soft tissue chondroma

This is a benign lesion that is not graded. Although benign, some examples imitate lower grade chondrosarcoma in degree of cellularity, slight nuclear pleomorphism (comprising nuclear enlargement with hypochromic rather than condensed pyknotic chromatin) and sparse mitotic activity. One variant resembles chondroblastoma with a myxoid stroma, chicken wire type calcifications and rounded to spindled tumor cells featuring vacuolated or eosinophilic cytoplasm and grooved or reniform nuclei.

Extraskeletal osteosarcoma

Nearly all cases are high grade. Histologically, they are indistinguishable from high grade intraosseous osteosarcoma subtypes such as osteoblastic, chondroblastic, fibroblastic, telangiectatic, giant cell rich, and small cell. High grade characteristics include marked cellular atypia, necrosis, many mitotic figures, and atypical mitoses. Many cases of extraskeletal osteosarcoma exhibit a mixed morphology with various combinations of osteoblastic osteosarcoma, chondroblastic osteosarcoma, fibroblastic osteosarcoma and/or one of the rarer patterns (Bane et al. 1990).

A small needle core biopsy may not be representative of the lesion and could lead to an erroneous diagnosis of another tumor. The neoplastic osteoid (unmineralized, organic portion of the bone matrix) may be focal, and multiple sections may be required before it is identified.

Low grade extraskeletal osteosarcoma has been reported as individual case reports. It resembles parosteal osteosarcoma.

Behavior

Soft tissue chondroma

Soft tissue chondroma is benign. The local recurrence rate is estimated at 10-25%. Recurrences are successfully managed by conservative re-excision.

Extraskeletal osteosarcoma

This is an aggressive tumor with historically a poor five year survival rate of 30-40% that is much worse than for comparable intraosseous osteosarcoma (Lee et al. 2010; Ahmad et al. 2002). Relatively favorable prognostic factors include size < 5 cm, chondroblastic subtype and low proliferation rate (measured by Ki67 or MIB-1 immunohistochemical staining) (Fisher et al. 2011). Almost all extraskeletal osteosarcomas are histologically high grade; the extremely rare, well-differentiated, primary soft tissue, parosteal osteosarcoma may have a better outcome than other soft tissue osteosarcomas.

Additional laboratory testing

Immunohistochemistry

Soft tissue chondroma is a chondrocytic neoplasm. Thus, the tumor cells express S-100 protein. S-100 protein is not exclusively reactive in cartilaginous tumors. Other antibodies that react with soft tissue chondroma include those detecting SOX9 (nuclear reactivity), neuron specific enolase and CD57, among others (Mietttinen 2010). Nearly all cases can be diagnosed without resorting to immunohistochemistry.

Extraskeletal osteosarcoma shows the same broad range of reactivity seen in intra-osseous versions in that it expresses non-specific antigens such as vimentin and smooth muscle actin. However, reactivity for osteocalcin in malignant osteoblasts, and osteocalcin and osteonectin in osteoid matrix may be relatively specific (Miettinen 2010). SATB2 antibody is also expressed in normal and neoplastic osteoblasts and may also prove diagnostically useful (Conner et at. 2013).

Routine cytogenetics

Soft tissue chondroma karyotypes may be abnormal (see **Table 11.3**). However, there are to date no broadly consistent findings.

Like intra-osseous osteosarcoma, extra-osseous high grade osteosarcoma usually discloses a complex aneuploid karyotype with extensive numerical and structural abnormalities (see **Table 11.3**). While some areas of the genome are more commonly affected, there are no universal changes found in every tumor.

Molecular genetics

A few soft tissue chondromas have been reported to show translocations of, or full-length or truncated transcripts of HMGA2.(Fletcher et al. 2013). This gene is a non-histone chromosomal high mobility group (HMG) gene that may act as a transcription regulator. It is found overexpressed or otherwise altered in a wide variety of benign and malignant tumors (NCBI 2013).

Extraskeletal osteosarcoma shows gene abnormalities similar to those found in intra-osseous osteosarcoma. None thus far are universal in osteosarcomas. See Chapter 17 for more details.

RADIOLOGY

Soft tissue chondroma

Soft tissue chondroma is a benign cartilaginous tumor. These commonly occur in the hands (64%) and feet (20%) and patients tend to present in the 3rd or 4th decade of life (Chung et al. 1978). Calcification is variable. In one series, 5 of 6 cases showed calcification, of which only one showed the characteristics of cartilage matrix. Soft tissue chondroma can be difficult to distinguish from sarcomas with calcification. MR imaging may be helpful to assess for heterogeneity of the lesion and enhancement. Also, soft tissue chondrosarcomas tend to be larger with more irregular calcification (Zlatkin et al. 1985).

Extraskeletal osteosarcoma

Primary soft tissue osteosarcoma or extra-skeletal osteosarcoma is a rare mesenchymal malignancy that shows predominant osteoid components but can have portions with chondroblastic or fibroblastic elements. By definition, there is no attachment to bone or periosteum. Compared to skeletal osteosarcoma, extra-skeletal osteosarcoma tends to occur in older individuals with an average age of 54 years, (Chung 1987). The lower extremity is affected in 46% of cases with the thigh being the single most common location (27%). The tumors presented with are pain or tenderness in 19% of cases. These tumors often are deep seated and fixed to adjacent structures. Radiographically, extra-skeletal osteosarcomas often show spotty or extensive calcifications described as 'cloud like'. This is the typical appearance for osteoid on radiographs. There are scant MR descriptions in the literature. The case has a calcification pattern that suggests both chondroid elements and osteoid production.

SURGERY

Soft tissue chondroma

These are benign tumors with a low rate of local recurrence. Marginal excision is the primary treatment of choice. The rare recurrence has been successfully treated in most cases with repeat resection.

Extraskeletal osteosarcoma

This is a malignant tumor with relatively poor outcome. Wide surgical resection is the operative procedure of choice.

MEDICAL ONCOLOGY

Soft tissue chondroma

This is not a disease that requires medical treatment

Extraskeletal osteosarcoma

Extraskeletal osteosarcoma is treated like intraosseous osteosarcoma (see Chapter 17).

However, these tumors have also been treated like soft tissue sarcoma with a combination of doxorubicin and ifosfamide with some success. The chemotherapy starts the multidisciplinary approach and response is evaluated histologically after complete resection. Adjuvant chemotherapy is then determined according to the percentage of necrosis obtained after neoadjuvant chemotherapy, following the same principles as the intraosseous osteosarcoma paradigm.

With the combination of ifosfamide, mesna, and doxorubicin, a 25% response rate was observed, with 50% progressing despite this ifosfamide-based treatment. When cisplatin and doxorubicin was used, the overall objective response rate was 13%, with 40% of patients progressing. Because of the small numbers of patients, it is not possible to recommend a regimen over the other in this situation; but in case of progression with one regimen, the alternate regimen should be tried (Ahmad 1992).

RADIATION ONCOLOGY

Soft tissue chondroma

Soft-tissue chondromas are benign entities and are best managed with surgical resection. No role for adjuvant radiation therapy has been demonstrated.

Extraskeletal osteosarcoma

Extraskeletal osteosarcoma is a rare entity with a poor prognosis. Data on the best approach for clinical treatment is limited. Most oncologists extrapolate data from osteosarcoma of the bone for treatment recommendations. This would lead one to believe that there is no, or at least, a limited role for adjuvant radiation therapy. Given that the majority of failures appear to be distant (lung), perhaps this is true. However, local recurrence does occur with a frequency of around 20% (Chung 1987). This statistic comes mostly from surgeries that are less than a wide local excision. Better surgery is consistent with local recurrences of around 7% (McCarty 2000). Also, local recurrences can be painful and morbid as this case demonstrated. Consequently, a tentative recommendation would be to offer patients adjuvant radiation therapy in the case of close or positive margins. Upfront radiation is likely to be more effective at preventing recurrence than as palliation after a gross resection.

Of interest, extraosseous osteosarcoma is known to be a radiation-induced histology with approximately 5% of all cases being associated with prior radiation therapy (Chung 1987) and 10% of radiation induced sarcomas are extraosseous osteosarcoma (Wiklund 1991).

CASES

Case 11.1 Soft tissue chondroma

Clinical history and presentation

The patient is a 37 year old man who presents with a mass on the volar aspect of the small finger which was first noted several years prior to presentation and has been steadily increasing in size. Mild pain and tenderness is associated with the mass, but the patient is most concerned about its interference with function.

Physical examination reveals a firm mass located on the volar aspect of the right small finger centered over the proximal interphalangeal joint in the midline. It is minimally tender. The mass limits motion at the associated joint.

Surgical findings and comments

These are benign tumors with a low rate of local recurrence. Marginal excision is the primary treatment of choice. The rare recurrence has been successfully treated in most cases with repeat resection.

Radiology findings

The radiographs in **Case figs 11.1a** and **11.1b** show a soft tissue mass with calcification. The absence of periosteal reaction and erosion suggest a longstanding lesion without aggressive behavior. The calcification density is higher than that typically seen with a tophus. Soft tissue chondromas do not often show characteristic calcified cartilage matrix (arc and rings) rendering this a difficult diagnosis to make. If radiographs show aggressive or heterogeneous features, MR may be helpful to further characterize the lesion for features that might indicate a soft tissue sarcoma such as intense and heterogeneous enhancement and invasive margins.

Pathology findings

Gross features

The specimen consists of a firm, 2.2 cm gray to white nodule that on cross sections is firm and semi-translucent with a 0.5 cm diameter softer red center. Representative sections are submitted for microscopic review.

Microscopic features

Low magnification: The tumor forms a heterogeneous nodule that has a sharp border with surrounding tissue. It is not associated with synovium or bursa. Cross sections show hyaline cartilage that is variably calcified with interspersed fibrosis (**Case fig. 11.1c**).

High magnification: At medium magnification, the hyaline cartilage is hypercellular matching the cellularity of a finger or toe enchondroma or Grade 2 chondrosarcoma of the long bones (**Case fig. 11.1d**). This hypercellularity is of no significance in soft tissue chondroma. Peripheral areas of the tumor mimic a chondroblastoma with chicken wire calcifications, fibrous to chondroid stroma, and round tumor cells (**Case fig. 11.1e**). High magnification of this area also shows stippled matrix calcifications commonly seen in soft tissue chondroma. The tumor cells are large and round with pale nuclei a few of which are reniform similar to chondroblastoma tumor cells. The matrix is chondroid to myxofibrous (**Case fig. 11.1f**). These chondroblastoma-like areas are not uncommon in soft tissue chondroma (Cates et al. 2001).

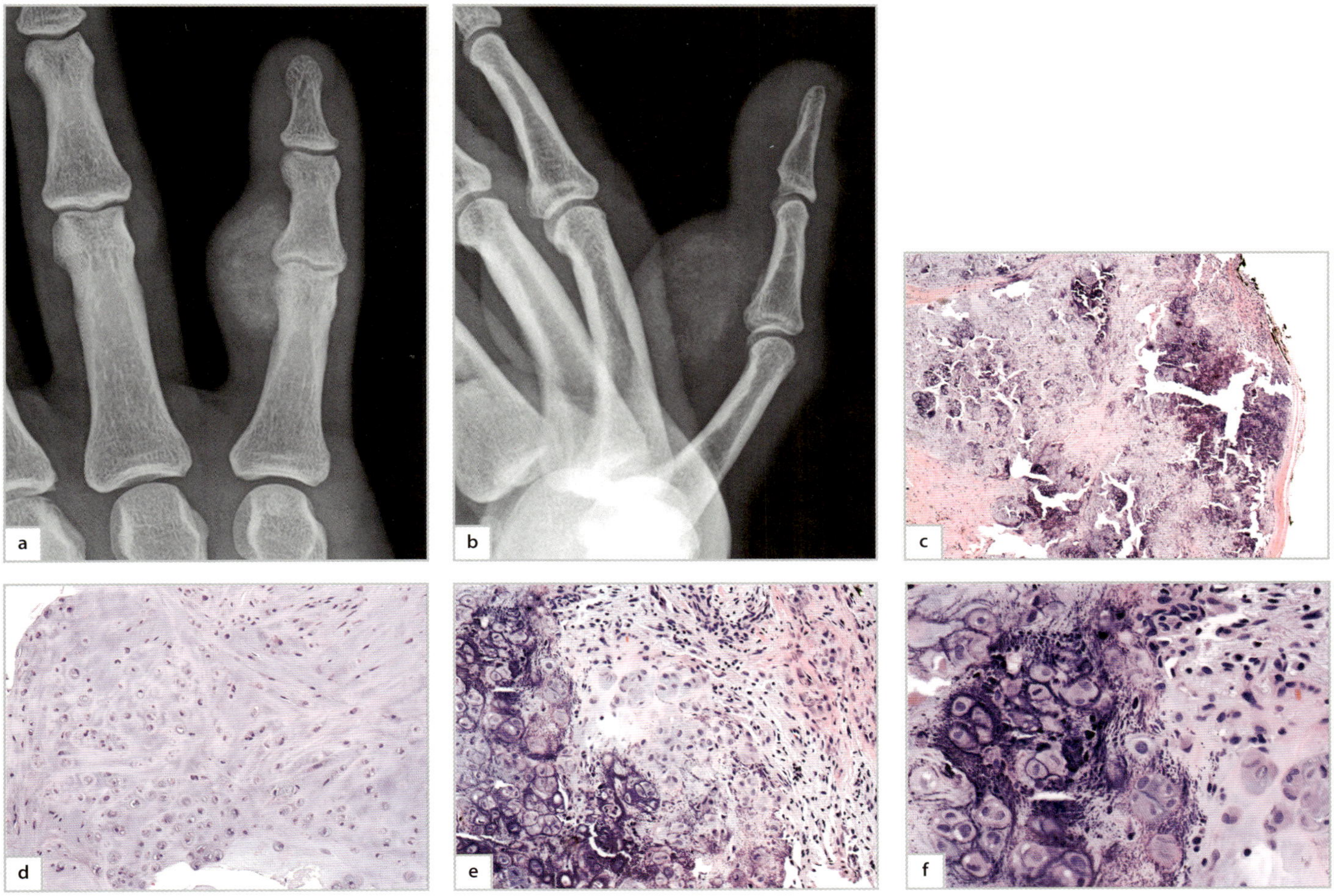

Case figure 11.1 Soft tissue chondroma imaging. **11.1a**: Posteroanterior radiograph. **11.1b**: Lateral radiograph. The radiographs show a 2.2 × 1.6 × 1.5 cm soft tissue mass with fairly homogeneous calcifications of the 5th digit. There is no bone erosion or periosteal reaction. **11.1c**: Low magnification. The tumor is composed primarily of hyaline cartilage that is variably calcified. Fibrous areas are intermixed. Scant normal tissue, partially inked black, is present on the right and reveals a pushing, sharp margin at the interface of tumor and surrounding connective tissue. **11.1d**: Medium magnification. The cellularity rivals that seen in finger or toe enchondroma or even Grade 2 chondrosarcoma of long bones. The nuclei are pale with 'open' chromatin also similar to many cells of Grade 2 chondrosarcoma. **11.1e**: Higher magnification. Here the lesion exhibits a chondroblastoma like appearance with 'chicken wire' calcifications, chondroid to fibrous stroma, and clusters of round cells with pale nuclei. **11.1f**: High magnification. In a chondroblastoma-like area, the calcifications are stippled as well as chicken wire-like. The tumor cells are large and round with pale eosinophilic cytoplasm. Some nuclei are reniform (like tumor cells of chondroblastoma) and all are hypochromatic with inconspicuous nucleoli. The stroma ranges from chondroid to myxofibrous.

Special studies: Because the clinical history, radiologic findings and histology are classic, no special studies such as IHC or cytogenetics are conducted.

Pathologic differential or, why isn't it one of the following?

Synovial chondromatosis: This is usually a diffuse process comprising multiple nodules arising in synovium, bursa or tendon sheath. It is more common around the large joints than in the hands and feet. Generally, the nodules are more lobulated and demonstrate more defined chondrocyte clustering than in soft tissue chondroma. Both soft tissue chondroma and synovial chondromatosis may exhibit increased cellularity and rare mitotic figures, and both can contain metaplastic bone complete with fatty marrow.

Juxtacortical chondroma: This lesion by definition must be adherent to the cortex of a bone.

Synovial chondrosarcoma: This is an extremely rare tumor that can emerge out of synovial chondromatosis. It displays the same features of intraosseous chondrosarcoma including peripheral spindling of malignant chondrocytes, nuclear atypia, and necrosis.

Case table 11.1 Summary pathology findings of Case 11.1

Diagnosis	Soft tissue chondroma
Size	2.2 cm
Location	Soft tissue of right fifth finger
Margin status	Negative
Histologic grade (FNCLCC grading system)	Not graded – lesion is benign
Pathologic stage (AJCC TNM classification)	Not staged – lesion is benign

Oncology approach

Medical oncology

This is a benign lesion with no role for chemotherapy.

Radiation oncology

There is no defined role for radiation therapy in soft tissue chondroma.

Patient outcome

Six months following excision, the patient has regained normal function of the digit and has no evidence of recurrence.

Case 11.2 Extraskeletal osteosarcoma

Clinical history and presentation

The patient is a 46 year old man who presents with a six month history of an enlarging thigh mass. The mass was first noted spontaneously. No history of trauma is noted. He has mild tenderness associated with the mass.

Physical examination reveals a large mass involving the lateral mid thigh. The mass is firm on palpation. It is mildly tender. It is palpable in the subcutaneous tissue but extends deeply and is fixed to surrounding deep structures. A staging CT-scan shows four lung metastases.

Surgical findings and comments

Open biopsy is performed. Gross findings reveal a large firm mass with a gritty consistency.

The patient receives five cycles of neoadjuvant chemotherapy with doxorubicin and ifosfamide and obtains a partial remission of all lesions. Seven months after presentation, he undergoes wide resection of the primary thigh tumor and thoracoscopic resection of four pulmonary metastases.

Radiology findings

This case (**Case figs 11.2a** through **11.2e**) shows a non-specific heterogeneous mass centered in the subcutaneous tissues of this 46 year old man. No gadolinium contrast could be given (due to gadolinium allergy), thus vascularity and viability could not be assessed. However, on PET, the tumor shows high metabolic activity. The CT scan has calcified matrix with a few questionable arcs and areas of cloud like calcification indicating osteoid. The radiologist should identify this as a worrisome aggressive tumor and might reasonably suspect this to be a soft tissue chondrosarcoma or osteosarcoma based on the calcifications.

Pathology findings

Gross features

The initial biopsy comprises fragments of white to tan and hemorrhagic soft tissue aggregating to 2.5 cm.

The wide resection consists of skeletal muscle from the right thigh with adipose tissue and ellipses of skin. One skin ellipse is perforated by necrotic tumor. Cross sections of the 11 × 9 × 6 cm tumor reveal white, firm areas consistent with ossification, gray, semi-translucent areas suggestive of cartilage, fleshy tan areas consistent with sarcoma, NOS, and red, hemorrhagic areas (**Case fig. 11.2f**).

Four pulmonary nodules are excised one month after the wide resection is performed. The nodules range from 0.2 to 2.0 cm. On cross sections, the nodules exhibit a viable, marbled gray and dark red appearance. All margins are grossly negative for metastatic tumor.

Six weeks later, he has a rapidly growing local recurrence which is palliatively excised because of ulceration associated with severe pain. The recurrent tumor comprises nodules up to 6.5 cm in diameter that on cut section range from gray and firm (smaller nodules) to hemorrhagic, soft and necrotic (larger nodules). Further chemotherapy does not help, and the patient is referred to hospice.

Microscopic features

Initial biopsy

Low magnification: The initial biopsy contains an equal mixture of cell rich tumor and less cellular, matrix rich tumor. (Examples of the cellular regions will be shown from the resection.) At low power, the matrix rich areas comprise intermixed nodules of malignant cartilage, osteochondroid, and mineralized osteoid (**Case fig. 11.2g**).

High magnification: Mineralized and un-mineralized osteoid formed by pleomorphic malignant osteoblasts is diagnostic of osteosarcoma (**Case fig. 11.2h**).

Resection (The lung metastases and locally recurrent tumor are histologically identical)

Low magnification: The tumor features cellular areas (**Case fig. 11.2i**) mixed with nodules of malignant cartilage (**Case fig. 11.2j**).

High magnification: Consistent with many extraskeletal osteosarcomas which contain multiple osteosarcomatous patterns, this patient's tumor has areas that resemble giant cell rich osteosarcoma (**Case fig. 11.2k**), chondroblastic osteosarcoma (**Case fig. 11.2l**) and fibroblastic osteosarcoma (**Case fig. 11.2m**). Scattered throughout the tumor are foci of diagnostic, lacelike tumor osteoid (**Case fig. 11.2n**). Necrosis is found in many sections and grossly encompasses 50% of the tumor. Mitotic figures, including atypical forms, consistently number >100 per 10 high magnification microscopic fields. Lymphovascular invasion is present in adjacent normal tissue.

Special studies: Immunohistochemistry is not performed because classic morphologic features easily enable diagnosis on standard sections. In cases with less obvious tumor osteoid, antibody to osteocalcin could be useful, as it is expressed in osteoblasts and osteoid matrix (Miettinen 2010). A new marker of osteoblastic differentiation has just been initially described, SATB2, and it may be more specific and sensitive than osteocalcin (Conner et al 2013).Other antigens that may be seen in osteosarcoma include S-100 protein (in cartilaginous areas), smooth muscle actin, desmin, keratins and EMA, among others.

Three karyotypes are obtained from the initial resection and recurrences. All reveal a markedly abnormal male chromosome complement with extensive numerical and structural abnormalities and 66 to 80 chromosomes. One of the karyotypes is presented

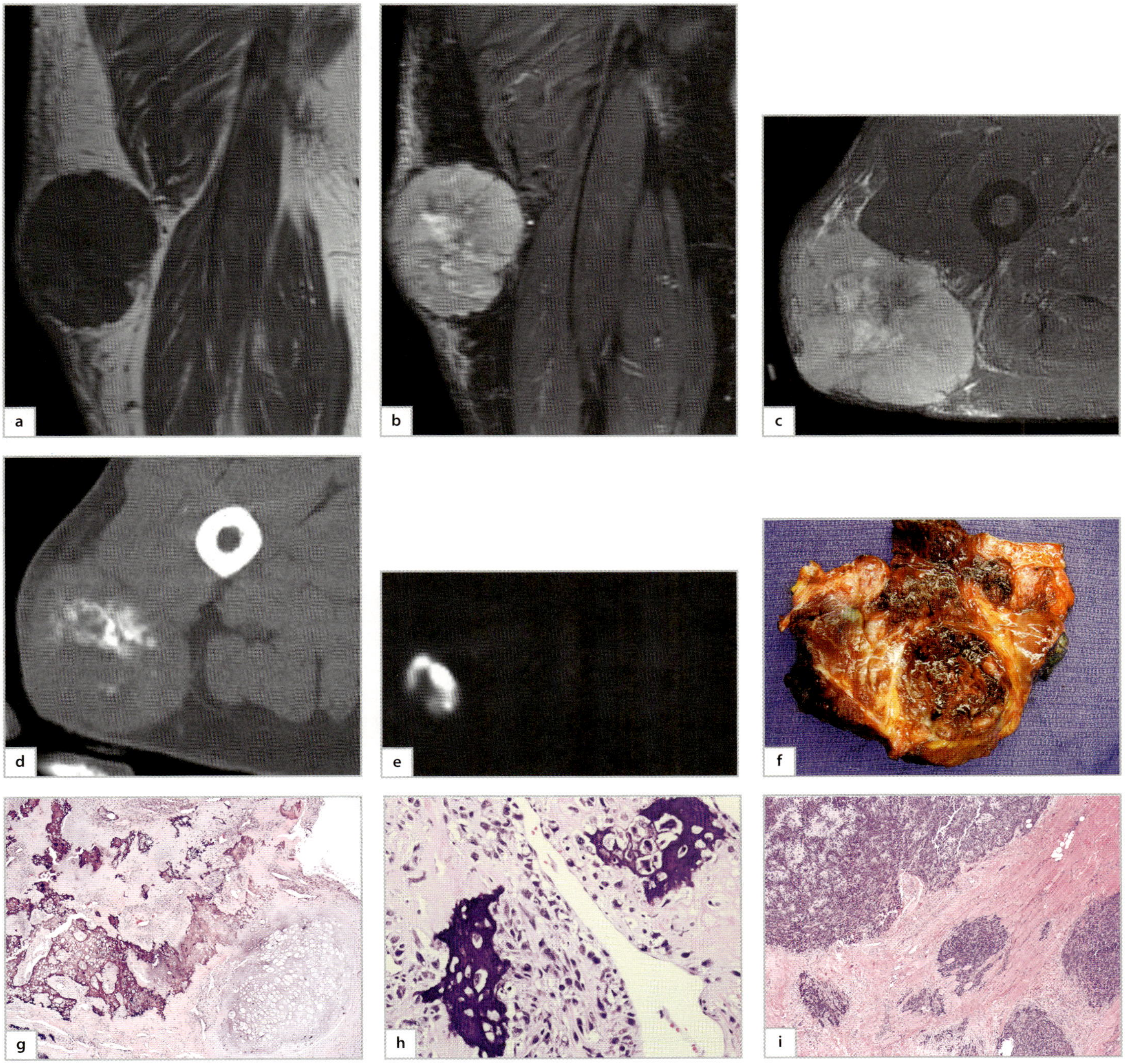

Case figure 11.2 Extraskeletal osteosarcoma imaging. **11.2a**: Coronal T1 MR image. **11.2b**: Coronal STIR MR image. **11.2c**: Axial STIR MR image. **11.2d**: Axial CT scan image without IV contrast. **11.2e**: Axial FDG - PET image. The MR images show a non-specific 8.3 × 9.4 × 9.4 cm heterogeneous T1 low signal, STIR high signal mass in the subcutaneous tissues of the thigh. There is deep stranding along the vastus lateralis muscle. No gadolinium contrast was given due to allergy. The CT image shows a mass with amorphous calcification. PET images show marked FDG uptake in the mass. **11.2f**: Gross photo of tumor resection. The tumor is lobulated and has soft, disrupted hemorrhagic areas and solid white to gray, semi-translucent regions. **11.2g**: Low magnification of initial biopsy. A less cellular, matrix- rich portion of the biopsy contains distinct nodules of malignant cartilage and blended chondroid and osteoid regions. **11.2h**: High magnification of initial biopsy. Diagnostic malignant osteoid is present, both mineralized and non-mineralized. Cytologically atypical osteoblasts are located in the lacunae of the tumor osteoid/bone and in the surrounding matrix.

Case figure 11.2: Continued from page 237

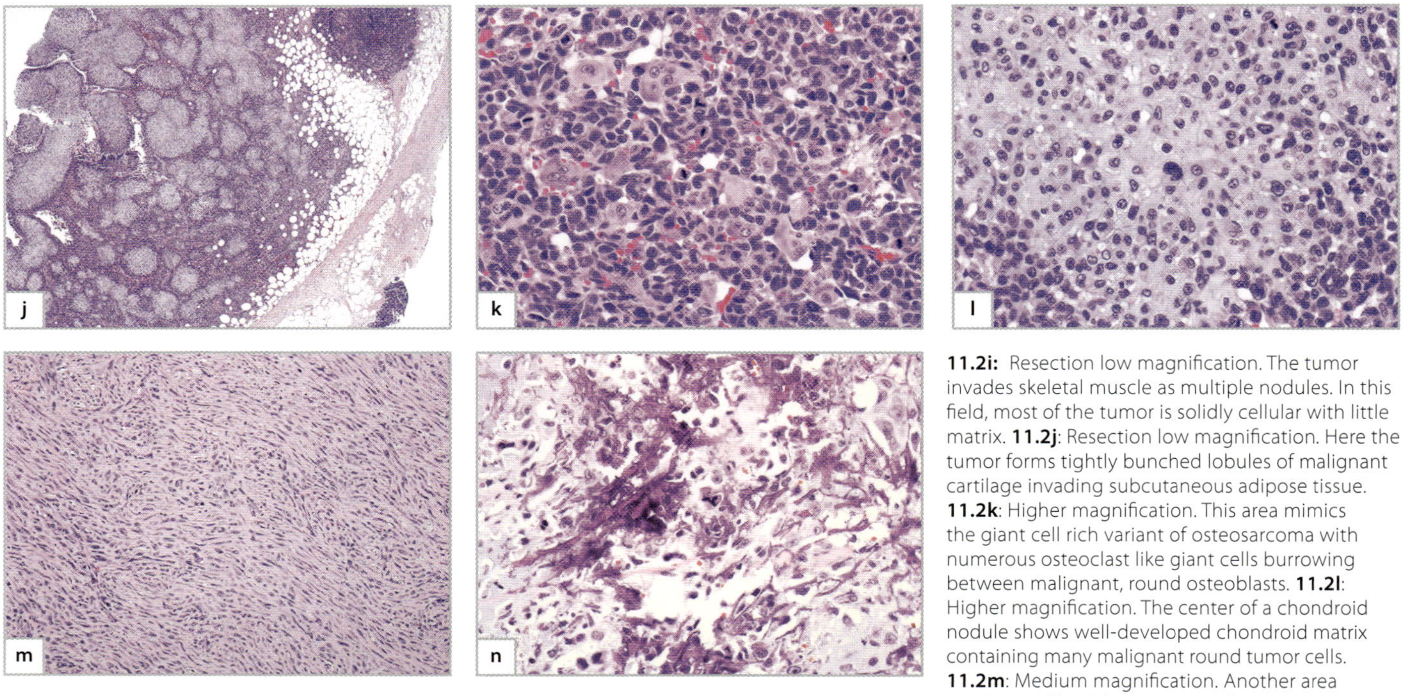

11.2i: Resection low magnification. The tumor invades skeletal muscle as multiple nodules. In this field, most of the tumor is solidly cellular with little matrix. **11.2j**: Resection low magnification. Here the tumor forms tightly bunched lobules of malignant cartilage invading subcutaneous adipose tissue. **11.2k**: Higher magnification. This area mimics the giant cell rich variant of osteosarcoma with numerous osteoclast like giant cells burrowing between malignant, round osteoblasts. **11.2l**: Higher magnification. The center of a chondroid nodule shows well-developed chondroid matrix containing many malignant round tumor cells. **11.2m**: Medium magnification. Another area mimics the fibroblastic variant of osteosarcoma with a pasty collagenous matrix causing the tumor cells to stream in parallel rows. **11.2n**: High magnification. Characteristic 'lace-like' malignant osteoid with atypical mitotic figure.

in more detail: 70-77<3n>,add(X)(p11.3),add(X)(p21),Y, +Y,add(1)(p13),del(1)(p36.1),-2,+add(3)(p24),+add(3)(q13.1),add(4)(q21),-5,-5,-6,add(6)(q12),+7,add(8)(p11.2)x2, -9,+add(10)(p11.2),add(11)(q34),del(11)(q23),add(12)(q21),+add(12)(q22),-13,-13,add(13)(p11.2),add(14)(q24),-15,add(15)(p11.2),+add(16)(q24),-17,+18,add(19)(p13.3),+add(19)(p12),-20,+21,-22,add(22)(q13),+6-13mar[cp9]/46,XY,inv(1)(q22p42)[2]/46,XY[9]

This karyotype shows abnormalities of some of the chromosomes listed in **Table 11.3** that occur with greater frequency in osteosarcoma than would be expected by chance. None of the abnormalities are specific for osteosarcoma, although complex aneuploidy is characteristic.

Pathologic differential or, why isn't it one of the following?

Dedifferentiated liposarcoma (LPS) with osteosarcomatous component: Dedifferentiated liposarcoma with osteosarcoma and/or chondrosarcoma could be histologically indistinguishable from extraskeletal osteosarcoma. However, some dedifferentiated LPS retain areas of lower grade liposarcoma that would be absent in extraskeletal osteosarcoma. Also, dedifferentiated LPS may show IHC nuclear expression of MDM2 and CDK4; such reactivity is absent in high grade osteosarcoma (Dujardin et al. 2011).

Pleomorphic, undifferentiated high grade sarcoma (PUS): PUS does not contain cytologically atypical osteoid. Malignant cartilage would also be uncommon.

Mesenchymal chondrosarcoma: This is a biphasic tumor that combines groups of small round blue cells interrupted by islands of usually low to moderate grade malignant cartilage. The small round blue cells often contain a dilated, branching blood vessels in a hemangiopericytomatous pattern. The cartilaginous areas may undergo endochondral ossification but areas of pure malignant osteoid are absent. In addition, some of the small round cells are reactive for S-100 protein, and all demonstrate expression of SOX9 which would be absent in small cell extraskeletal osteosarcoma, a rare type of extraskeletal OS that could mimic the small round blue cell component of mesenchymal chondrosarcoma (Miettinen 2010).

Malignant peripheral nerve sheath tumor (MPNST) with malignant cartilage and bone: Areas of typical MPNST will be present that consist of long sweeping fascicles of spindle cells with tapered elongate nuclei. The tumor cells in the typical MPNST areas may show spotty S-100 expression +/- GFAP and neurofilament expression. Many patients have NF1 (although osteosarcoma also occurs with increased frequency in patients with NF1).

Other sarcomas with metaplastic bone formation such as synovial sarcoma or solitary fibrous tumor: Most synovial sarcomas and solitary fibrous tumors are not as pleomorphic as this tumor. Malignant cartilage is not found in synovial sarcoma or solitary fibrous tumor. The presence of unequivocal malignant (in other words, cytologically atypical) osteoid confirms the diagnosis of osteosarcoma, as metaplastic (reactive, non-neoplastic) osteoid is not cytologically atypical.

Oncology approach

Medical oncology

After initial biopsy diagnosis, the patient undergoes five cycles of combination doxorubicin and ifosfamide. He shows initial response

Case table 11.2 Summary pathology findings of Case 11.2

Diagnosis	Primary soft tissue osteosarcoma
Size	11 × 9 × 6 cm
Location	Deep soft tissues of thigh
Margin status	Negative
Histologic grade (FNCLCC grading system)	High grade = Grade 3
Pathologic stage (AJCC TNM classification)	Stage IV (T2b/N0/M1) at initial presentation. (Deep high grade tumor >5 cm in size with distant metastases)

to four courses but progression of the primary lesion and the lung metastases during the fifth course. The plan had been for 6 cycles prior to definitive resection.

Six weeks after wide resection of the thigh tumor and resection of pulmonary nodules, the cancer recurs. Chemotherapy is resumed with a combination of irinotecan and temsirolimus on a clinical trial. He continues to demonstrate progressive disease on chemotherapy including new lesions forming around the primary site excision and enlargement of inguinal lymph nodes.

Radiation oncology

No radiation therapy was administered to this patient. In non-metastatic cases with close or positive resection margins, adjuvant radiation therapy should be considered. Radiation therapy may also be quite helpful as palliation.

Patient outcome

Despite wide resection of his primary tumor, resection of pulmonary metastases and multiple courses of chemotherapy, the patient rapidly develops a fulminant local recurrence in the thigh and progressive pulmonary metastases. He succumbs to his disease four months after wide resection.

REFERENCES

Ahmad SA, Patel SR, Ballo MT, et al. Extraosseous osteosarcoma: response to treatment and long-term outcome. J Clin Oncol 2002;20:521–527.

Bane BL, Evans HL, Ro JY, et al. Extraskeletal osteosarcoma. A clinicopathologic review of 26 cases. Cancer 1990;65:2762–70.

Cates JM, Rosenberg AE, O'Connell JX, et al. Chondroblastoma-like chondroma of soft tissue: an under recognized variant and its differential diagnosis. Am J Surg Pathol 2001;25(5):661–666.

Chung EB, Enzinger FM. Chondroma of soft parts. Cancer 1978;41(4):1414–1424.

Chung EB, Enzinger FM. Extraskeletal osteosarcoma. Cancer 1987:60(5):1132–1142.

Conner JR, Hornick JL. SATB2 is a novel marker of osteoblastic differentiation in bone and soft tissue tumors. Mod Pathol 2013;26(sup 2):11A.

Dujardin F, Binh MBN, Bouvier C, et al. MDM2 and CDK4 immunohistochemistry is a valuable tool in the differential diagnosis of low grade osteosarcomas and other primary fibro-osseous lesions of the bone. Mod Pathol 2011;24:624–637.

Fritz, A Percy C Jack A, et al (Eds). International Classification of Diseases for Oncology, 3rd ed. Geneva: World Health Organization, 2000;45.

Goldstein-Jackson SY, Gosheger G, Delling G, et al. Extraskeletal osteosarcoma has a favourable prognosis when treated like conventional osteosarcoma. J Can Res Clin Oncol 2005;131(8):520–526.

Lee S, Lee MR, Lee SJ, et al. Extraosseous osteosarcoma: single institutional experience in Korea. Asia Pac J Clin Oncol 2010;6:126–129.

Surveillance, Epidemiology, and End Results (SEER) Program (www.seer.cancer.gov) SEER*Stat Database: Incidence - SEER 13 Regs Research Data, Nov 2010 Sub (1992-2008) <Katrina/Rita Population Adjustment> - Linked To County Attributes - Total U.S., 1969-2009 Counties, National Cancer Institute, DCCPS, Surveillance Research Program, Cancer Statistics Branch, released April 2011 (updated 10/28/2011), based on the November 2010 submission.

Zlatkin MB, Lander PH, Begin LR, et al. Soft-tissue chondromas. Am J Roengenol 1985;144:1263–1267.

FURTHER READING

Fisher C, Mentzel T, Montgomery EA, et al. Diagnostic Pathology Soft Tissue Tumors. Salt Lake City: AMIRSYS, 2011.

Folpe AL, Inwards CY (eds). Bone and Soft Tissue Pathology. A volume in the series: Foundations in Diagnostic Pathology. Goldblum JR (series ed). Philadelphia: Elsevier Saunders, 2010.

Miettinen M. Modern Soft Tissue Pathology. Cambridge: Cambridge University Press, 2010.

Fletcher CDM, Krishnan Unni K, Mertens F (Eds). World Health Organization Classification of Tumours. Pathology and Genetics of Tumours of Soft Tissue and Bone. Lyon: IARC Press, 2013.

Chapter 12 Myoepithelial tumors of soft tissue (myoepithelioma, mixed tumor, 'parachordoma' and myoepithelial carcinoma)

OVERVIEW

Myoepithelial tumors of soft tissue comprise three types: mixed tumor, myoepithelioma, and myoepithelial carcinoma. Rare malignant versions of mixed tumor and 'parachordoma' also occur (Guedes et al. 2009). A myoepithelioma of specific histology occurring primarily in the tongue is termed ectomesenchymal chondromyxoid tumor (of tongue). Mixed tumor is commonly referred to as chondroid syringoma when it arises in skin. Its rare malignant version comprises a sarcomatous element combined with epithelial and myoepithelial components. The sarcomatous portion may be heterologous and may comprise osteosarcoma or chondrosarcoma, among others.

All three types of soft tissue myoepithelial tumor are composed of cells differentiated along the lines of myoepithelium; namely, a cell that expresses epithelial markers, smooth muscle markers and also often S-100 protein and GFAP. The normal myoepithelial cell provides contractility around the perimeter of exocrine duct structures (such as in salivary gland or breast) imparting a squeezing action to express duct secretions. In addition to containing myoepithelial differentiated cells, mixed tumors of soft tissue also contain recognizable tubules or ducts formed by cells of epithelial differentiation. 'Parachordoma' is a variant of myoepithelioma that histologically resembles chordoma. (True chordomas of soft tissue are exceptionally rare.)

Myoepithelial tumors of soft tissue were only relatively recently described beginning in the 1970s, although similarly appearing salivary gland and breast tumors have been well known for much longer. The relationship of myoepithelial tumors of soft tissue to their salivary gland counterparts is not entirely resolved. Myoepithelial tumor and myoepithelial carcinoma of soft tissue may not be related to the salivary gland versions. However, there are reports of mixed tumors of the salivary gland sharing some genetic findings with mixed tumors of the soft tissues (Bahrami et al. 2012). It is speculated that soft tissue myeopithelial tumors that very closely resemble salivary myoepithelial tumors probably also share similar genetic changes (Fletcher et al. 2013).

Interestingly, some of the myoepithelial tumors are translocation specific and show EWSR1 as a fusion partner with one of several other genes (Antonescu et al. 2010). Thus, at least some myoepithelial tumors join the growing list of mesenchymal tumors with EWSR1 translocations.

Malignant myoepithelial tumors are not treated with a unique chemotherapy regimen. Myoepithelial carcinoma can be misdiagnosed because of a close resemblance to mesenchymal tumors such as extraskeletal myxoid chondrosarcoma and ossifying fibromyxoid tumor (Hornick et al. 2003).

CLASSIFICATION

The World Health Organization (WHO) classification of myoepithelial tumors of soft tissue is provided in **Table 12.1** (Fletcher et al. 2013). Although WHO 2013 lists them as 'Tumors of uncertain differentiation', the myoepithelial tumors of soft tissue are accorded a separate chapter in this text. Analogous to the other chapters of this book, myoepithelial tumors are divided according to behavior: benign tumors do not recur (or recurrences are nonagressive) and do not metastasize, intermediate tumors can recur locally aggressively and/or rarely metastasize, and malignant tumors can both recur and commonly metastasize.

Table 12.1 WHO classification of myoepithelial tumors of soft tissue (2013)*

Tumor	Behavior	Additional comments
Mixed tumor, not otherwise specified	Benign to intermediate	In the skin, this is also termed chondroid syringoma A few cases may recur if incompletely excised
Mixed tumor, malignant, not otherwise specified	Malignant	Malignant epithelial, myoepithelial and sarcomatous components present
Myoepithelioma	Intermediate*	Becoming increasingly recognized; ~20% local recurrence if incompletely excised. *Very rare cases of metastasis reported in cytologically benign tumor
Parachordoma	Intermediate**	This is a type of myoepithelioma that histologically mimics chordoma Low rate of local recurrence **Very rare reported cases of malignant parachordoma
Myoepithelial carcinoma	Malignant	Very rare but may be under recognized currently

*The 2013 WHO classification officially lists myoepithelial tumors as 'Tumors of uncertain differentiation'. However, they have well-defined pathology features and are thus presented in this separate chapter in this text. Benign: does not recur aggressively and does not metastasize. Intermediate: can recur aggressively and/or rarely metastasizes (<5%). Malignant: can recur and commonly metastasizes.

DEMOGRAPHICS

Myoepithelial tumors of soft tissue are relatively rare (an extremely rare case also occurs within bone) (Rekhi et al. 2011). The largest series reviewed 101 patients and found that most tumors occur in adults in the young to middle aged age group affecting equally men and women. In this study, the myoepithelioma was the most common subtype of myoepithelial tumor followed by mixed tumor (tumors with both myoepithelial and ductal differentiation) and no cases of 'parachordoma' were described (Hornick et al, 2003). Myoepithelial carcinoma is the least common subtype of myoepithelial tumor. It usually occurs in middle aged to older individuals, although children to young adults may also be affected.

Myoepithelial tumors in children occur in a broad age range from newborn to seventeen years with a median of nine years and equal distribution among boys and girls (Gleason et al. 2007). The behavior of myoepithelial tumors in children may be particularly aggressive (see below in behavior section) (Hornick et al. 2004; Gleason et al. 2007).

PATHOGENESIS

As with other mesenchymal tumors, the pathogenesis of myoepithelial tumors of soft tissue has not been entirely elucidated. A combination of genetic, possibly epigenetic, and environmental factors are presumed to be causative. Approximately 45% of patients with myoepithelial tumors exhibit an EWSR1 gene fusion (Antonescu et al. 2010). The fusion partners included TOU5F1 (which was more common in patients of pediatric or young adult age), PBX1 and ZNF444. An FUS rather than EWSR1 rearrangement has also been reported (Antonescu et al. 2010).

Other research groups have confirmed the occurrence of the EWSR1-PBX1 fusion and also recently presented a myoepithelial carcinoma of soft tissue bearing an EWSR1-ZNF444 fusion (Brandal et al. 2008, Brandal et al. 2009) and another example with an EWSR1-ATF1 transcript similar to that seen in clear cell sarcoma and angiomatoid fibrous histiocytoma (Flucke et al. 2012). Thus, it appears that myoepithelial tumors of soft tissue, at least some proportion thereof, join the growing list of Ewing sarcoma specific translocation tumors that includes Ewing sarcoma, desmoplastic small round cell tumor, extraskeletal myxoid chondroid sarcoma, myxoid liposarcoma, the aforementioned clear cell sarcoma and angiomatoid fibrous histiocytoma, a few leukemias, and a few epithelial tumors.

Obviously, because of the long list of EWSR1 translocation tumors, some of which show overlap in specific fusion partners, additional factors must weigh in to lead to a specific myoepithelial differentiated tumor rather than, for example, clear cell sarcoma. These additional moderating factors may include differences in degree, duration and timing of cell pathways integral to the specific tumor cells, disparate, localized intercellular environmental factors, and additional, specific modifying genetic and epigenetic changes. All of the EWS gene fusions thus far described for myoepithelial tumors encode for abnormal transcription factors that have also been reported in non-myoepithelial tumors.

Additional genetic findings in myoepithelial tumors include trisomies of various chromosomes such as 11, 15 and 17 and various chromosomal gains and deletions of which none are widely recurrent. Most tumors are hypodiploid to diploid (Hallor et al. 2008). A rare case has been reported with a hypotetraploid karyotype (van der Berg et al. 2004).

Myoepithelial carcinoma, in contrast to benign myoepithelial tumors, may show loss of INI-1 expression (located at chromosome 22q11.2 and known as the SMARCB1 gene) (Hollmann et al. 2011). Loss of INI-1 expression is more common in the pediatric age group at a 40% incidence as opposed to a 10% incidence in adults with myoepithelial carcinoma (Hollmann et al. 2011). Since INI-1 expression is lost only in the malignant variant of myoepithelial tumors, such loss may play a major role in malignant transformation. Loss of INI-1 protein expression is not specific to myoepithelial carcinoma but is frequently seen in malignant rhabdoid tumor (98% of cases), medullary renal cell carcinoma (100%), epithelioid sarcoma (90%), epithelioid malignant peripheral nerve sheath tumor (50%), and extraskeletal myxoid chondrosarcoma (17%) (Hollmann et al. 2011). Of note, most recently, poorly differentiated chordoma and ossifying fibromyxoid tumor of soft tissue have also been reported to lose INI expression (Mobley et al. 2010, Graham et al. 2011).

PATHOLOGY

Table 12.2 lists the incidence, histologic features and immunohistochemical profile of myoepithelial tumors of soft tissue.

Histologic grading of myoepithelial tumors of soft tissue

Benign myoepithelial tumors (benign mixed tumor, myoepithelioma, and 'parachordoma') are not graded. The malignant mixed tumor comprises a malignant ductal component, a malignant myoepithelial

Table 12.2 Incidence and pathologic features of myoepithelial tumors

Tumor	Incidence	Age and sex distribution	Body site (in order of frequency)	Histopathology description including IHC: Medium magnification	High magnification
Benign: does not recur aggressively and does not metastasize					
Mixed tumor, not otherwise specified	Rare	Adults > children M = F	Skin, subcutis and less frequently deep soft tissue of upper extremities, lower extremities, limb girdles, head and neck	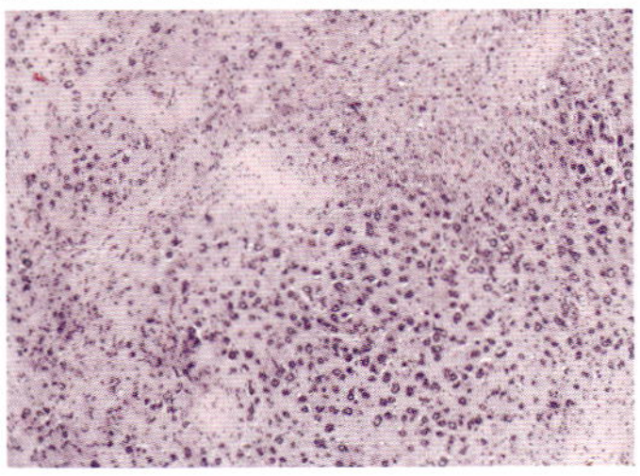	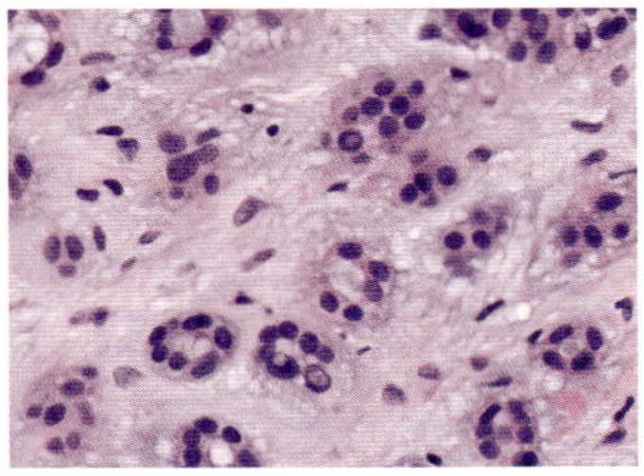
Same description as for myoepithelioma except for the addition of ducts or tubular structures.					

Table 12.2: Continued from page 241

Tumor	Incidence	Age and sex distribution	Body site (in order of frequency)	Histopathology description including IHC Medium magnification	High magnification
Intermediate: can recur aggressively and/or can rarely metastasize (<5%)					
Myoepithelioma	Rare	Older adults > children M = F	Subcutis, skin, deep soft tissue, viscera	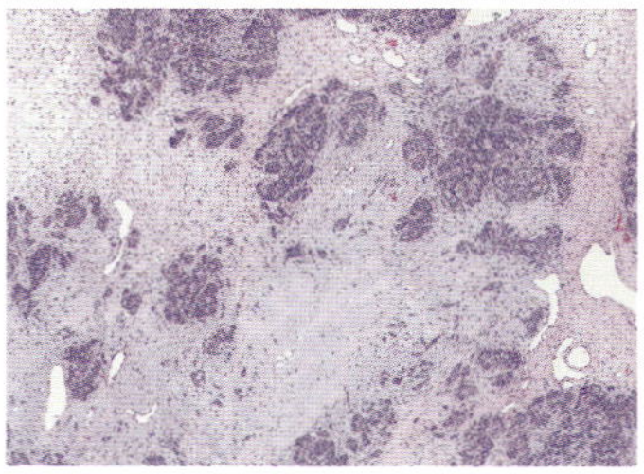	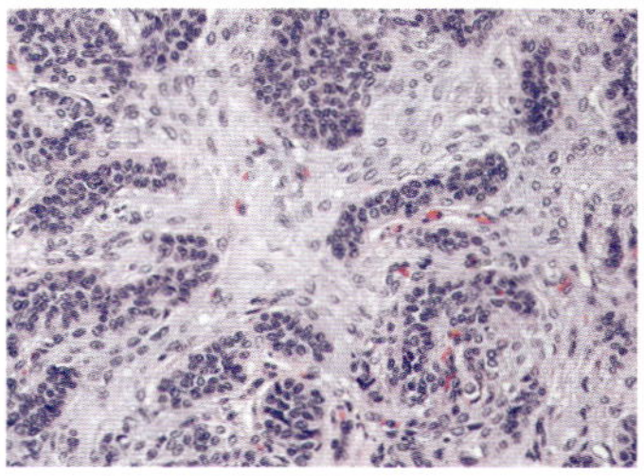
Multinodular or lobulated tumor that is characteristically heterogeneous with epithelioid, clear, histiocytoid, plasmacytoid, and/or spindle cells arranged in cords, nests, trabeculae, reticulae and/or sheets and set in a myxoid, chondromyxoid, chondroid, fibrous, and/or hyaline matrix. Lacks definite ducts or tubules. Minimal nuclear atypia and mitotic rate is usually low (< or = 2/10 hpf). May have infiltrative growth. Rare monomorphic tumors occur that are entirely composed of spindle cells. IHC: Positive for pankeratins, CAM5.2 and/or EMA. 50% + for SMA. Often reactive for S-100 protein (85%). Sometimes positive for: GFAP, p63, calponin, caldesmon. INI-1 intact. Negative for CD34.					
Parachordoma	Very rare	Adults most commonly but broad age range including children. M = F	Deep soft tissue and subcutis most often of arm, then leg; can involve hands and feet; trunk, head and neck far less common	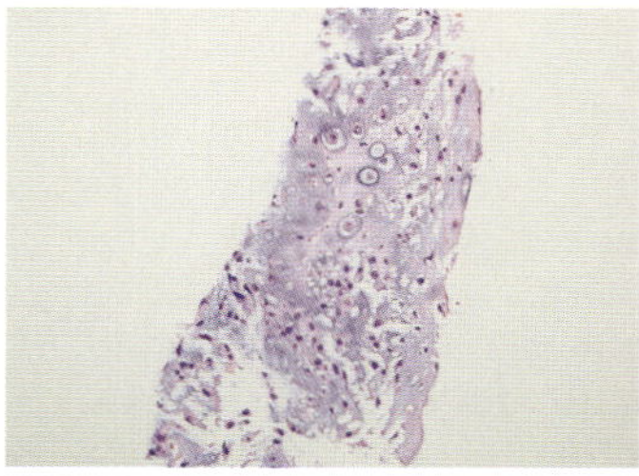	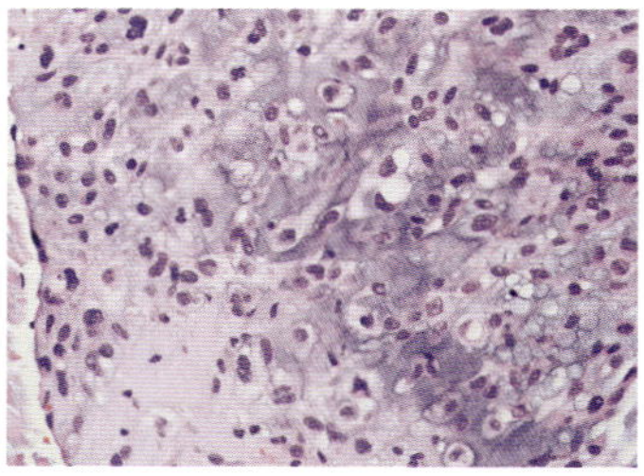
Typical parachordoma: Nests and cords of epithelioid appearing cells set in a myxoid or chondromyxoid matrix. Some cells are multivacuolated and clear suggestive of physaliphorous cells of chordoma. No ducts, no tubules, and no other patterns of myoepithelioma. Low mitotic rate. IHC: PanKeratins CAM5.2 keratin, EMA and S-100 positive. Negative for calponin. Negative for brachyury. Very rare malignant parachordoma: Same epithelioid and clear cells and matrix of benign version but with nuclear atypia, increased mitotic activity and often necrosis. IHC: similar to benign parachordoma.					
Malignant: can recur and commonly metastasizes					
Mixed tumor, malignant, not otherwise specified	Very rare	Adults > children M = F	Soft tissue, subcutis, skin of extremities, limb girdles, head and neck (only a few cases reported)	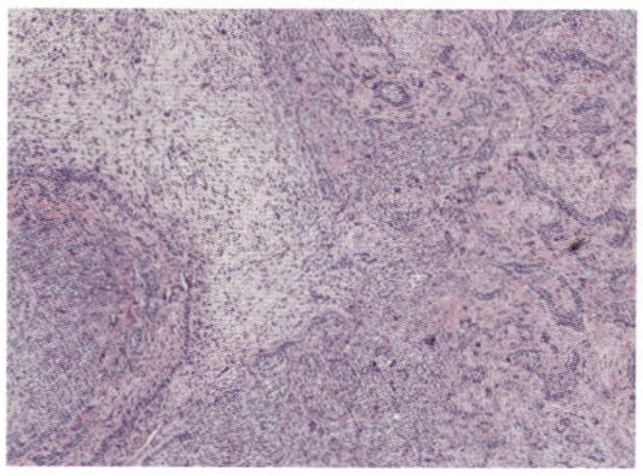	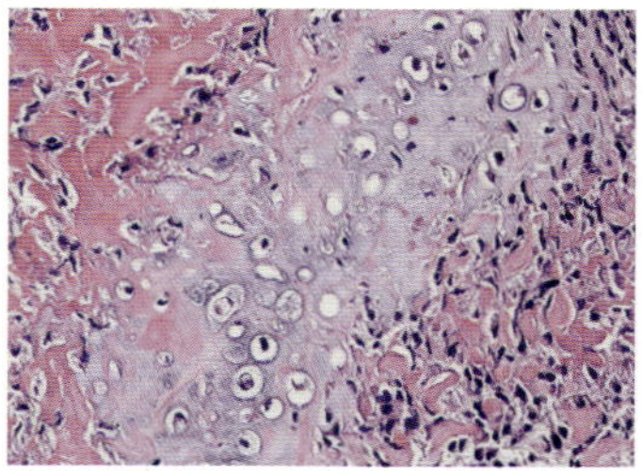 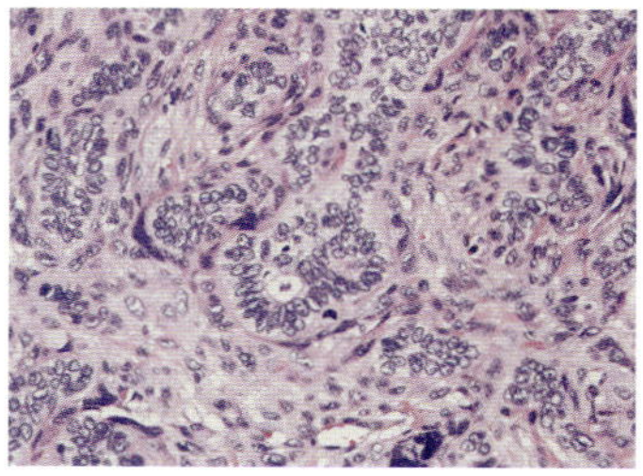
Malignant epithelium, malignant myoepithelium, and sarcoma present with various architectures and matrix as for benign mixed tumor. Histology includes nuclear pleomorphism (prominent nucleoli +/-coarse chromatin +/- variable nuclear shape and size), increased mitotic rate sometimes with atypical mitotic figures and often necrosis.					

Table 12.2: Continued from page 242

Tumor	Incidence	Age and sex distribution	Body site (in order of frequency)	Histopathology description including IHC	
				Medium magnification	High magnification
Myoepithelial carcinoma	Very rare	Adults > Children (4:1) M = F	Deep soft tissue, subcutis and skin of extremities, viscera and rarely bone	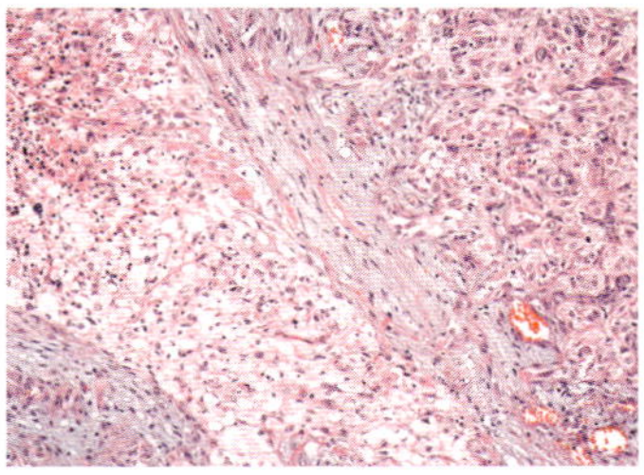	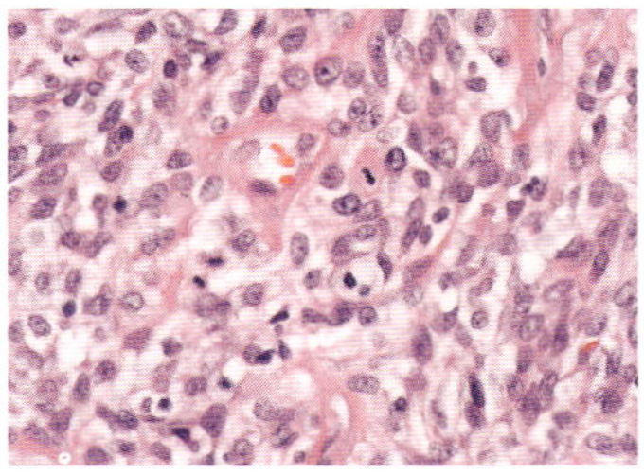
Heterogeneous lobulated or multinodular tumor with cytologically malignant spindle cells, epithelioid cells, clear cells, and/or plasmacytoid cells arranged in cords, trabeculae, reticular pattern, nests, and/or sheets set in myxoid, fibrous, hyaline and or/chondroid matrix. 10-15% have ducts or tubules (but not malignant sarcomatous element as in malignant mixed tumor). Increased mitotic activity and necrosis often present. IHC: Keratin (CAM5.2, panker) and/or EMA positive. S-100 protein and/or GFAP positive. Calponin positive. SMA positive in 50%. CD99 may be patchy membranous and cytoplasmic positive (rarely may show diffuse membranous reactivity mimicking ESFT). INI-1 expression lost in 40% of pediatric and 10% of adult cases. Rare cases positive for p63 chromogranin.					
M: male, F: female. IHC: immunohistochemistry. Ker: keratin, ESFT: Ewing sarcoma family tumors, SMA: smooth muscle actin.					

component and a sarcomatous component which can include chondrosarcoma or osteosarcoma, among others.

Histologic malignant features of myoepithelial carcinoma that separate it from myoepithelioma include nuclear atypia comprising nuclear pleomorphism, coarse chromatin, and macronucleoli, alone or in combination (Hornick et al. 2003). Increased mitotic activity (possibly as little as >5/10 hpf) often accompanies the other histologic indicators of aggressive behavior. Microscopic infiltrative growth does not by itself connote malignancy.

Malignant parachordoma is characterized by malignant histologic features (nuclear atypia, increased mitoses, atypical mitoses, necrosis) superimposed on the epithelioid and physaliphorous appearing myoepithelial cells that are disposed in the typical chondromyxoid and/or chondroid stroma. It lacks the other patterns of myoepithelial carcinoma and malignant mixed tumor.

Myoepithelial carcinoma in children may contain a small round cell population in the tumors (approximately 34% of the cases thus far described) (Gleason et al. 2007, Guedes et al. 2009).

Tumors occurring in the skin and subcutaneous tissue may behave more aggressively if a high mitotic rate is present (Hornick et al. 2004). An elevated mitotic rate (greater than 5/10 hpf) often is accompanied by other ominous features such as nuclear atypia and/or necrosis (Gleason et al. 2007).

Behavior of myoepithelial tumors of soft tissue

Benign myoepithelial tumors may locally recur (up to 20%) but only exceptionally undergo malignant transformation (Hornick et al. 2003). Malignant myoepithelial tumors demonstrate a higher rate of local recurrence (approximately twice that of benign tumors) and in one study, up to one-third of afflicted adults experienced metastasis(es) with a mean follow-up of fifty months (Hornick et al. 2003).

Children with myoepithelial carcinomas may have a particularly aggressive course with a greater then 50% chance of metastasis and a high, often early, mortality rate of 40% (Gleason et al. 2007).

Superficial location does not preclude malignant behavior, as a small subset of dermal and subcutis myoepithelial tumors comprise malignant mixed tumors or myoepithelial carcinoma (Mentzel et al. 2003, Hornick et al. 2004).

Special stains or tests used to diagnose myoepithelial tumors of soft tissue

Immunohistochemistry

By definition, myoepithelial tumors of soft tissue differentiate along a myoepithelial cell phenotype. This means that the tumors cells are reactive by IHC for a combination of the following, the exact mix varying per individual tumor: epithelial markers (pan-keratin, EMA, p63), myoid markers (calponin, smooth muscle actin), and additional markers of myoepithelium (S100 protein, GFAP). Superficial tumors may more prominently express EMA rather than keratins (80% vs 60% in a review of fourteen cases) (Hornick et al. 2004). About 50% of myoepitheliomas and myoepithelial carcinomas express p63 (Jo et al. 2011).

Myoepithelial carcinomas, in contrast to the benign myoepithelial tumors, may far less frequently express smooth muscle actin. Also dissimilar to myoepithelioma, myoepithelial carcinoma exhibits a 40% pediatric and 10% adult rate of loss of INI-1 protein expression (Hollmann et al. 2011).

The variant of myoepithelial soft tissue tumor known as parachordoma (nests of variably vacuolated cells set in a myxochondroid matrix mimicking chordoma) are negative for brachyury in comparison to true chordoma which in almost all cases strongly expresses brachyury (Tirabasco et al. 2008).

Genetic testing

Genetic testing may be used in an ancillary manner to confirm the diagnosis of myoepithelial tumor and exclude histologic mimics. As approximately 50% of myoepithelial tumors demonstrate an EWSR1 fusion, FISH using a break apart probe set for the EWSR1 chromosome site (22q12) may be helpful. Of course, a negative result does not exclude the diagnosis. A positive result has its own caveat, because entities in the differential include tumors with EWSR1 translocations such as Ewing sarcoma and extraskeletal myxoid chondrosarcoma. Fortunately, the most challenging entity to distinguish from myoepithelioma/myoepithelial carcinoma , extraskeletal myxoid chondrosarcoma, exhibits translocations only with NR4A3, whereas thus far, no myoepithelial carcinoma has been reported with this fusion of EWSR1 to NR4A3 (Antonescu et al. 2010, Flucke et al. 2012).

RADIOLOGY

On MR imaging, myoepitheliomas show T1 homogeneous isointensity, T2 hyperintensity and have homogeneous enhancement (Hiwatashi et al. 2000). The overall appearance is non-specific.

Myoepithelial carcinoma is a very rare tumor. There is little published regarding its imaging appearance. Harada et al. 2005 presented a case report showing an ill-defined T2 high signal mass with infiltrative margins centered in the muscles.. Unfortunately, we do not have a case with imaging to present.

SURGERY

Benign mixed tumor

Marginal excision of these tumors is generally curative. Incompletely excised tumors can result in a local recurrence rate approximating 20%.

Myoepithelial carcinoma

Because this tumor represents a malignancy with aggressive potential, wide surgical resection is advocated.

MEDICAL ONCOLOGY

Myoepithelial carcinomas are a rare group of neoplasms with myoepithelial differentiation which usually affect salivary glands (Savera, et al. 2000), but have also been diagnosed in soft tissues (Harada, et al. 2005), lungs (Miura, et al. 2000) or breasts. Whether these tumors have a similar pathophysiology or are different depending on their anatomical site of origin is not clear (Pattari, et al. 2008). These cancers usually affect middle aged adults but 20% are seen in children (Gleason, et al. 2007). Usual tumor sizes range from 2 to 5 cm, and pain is the most common presentation. When occurring in the salivary glands, swelling and facial weakness from cranial nerve VII compression are also observed. Despite sometimes low grade features, about half of the patients will develop metastases with a poor prognosis (Tanahashi, et al. 2007). A fine needle aspiration might not be sufficient to make a final diagnosis (Khademi, et al. 2010).

Because this cancer is so rare and even more so when occurring in skin and soft tissues, there is no standard medical treatment. A localized tumor should be excised. Medical oncology intervention is indicated in cases of unresectable or metastatic disease. Case reports describe the use of intra-arterial cisplatin with radiation therapy (Takayama, et al. 2006) or with systemic platinum-based chemotherapy (Noronha, et al. 2006, Pierard, et al. 2006). No biological agents have been tried, but epidermal growth factor receptors (EGFR) are expressed in salivary glands and could offer a new target for therapy, at least in salivary gland based tumors (Yamada, et al. 1989). Whether soft tissue and skin myoepithelial carcinoma would benefit from anti-EGFR therapy is currently unknown.

RADIATION ONCOLOGY

Myoepithelial tumors range from low grade to high grade lesions. Benign mixed tumors contrast with myoepithelial carcinoma which is often aggressive. Due to the rare incidence of this disease, treatment guidelines are not established. In general, complete resection is the treatment of choice. Experience on the use of adjuvant radiation therapy is limited to small case series and case reports.

Even though most reports in the literature show good local control with the use of adjuvant radiation therapy for locally advanced malignant disease, the benefit is still uncertain. Reports on the use of radiation therapy for unresected myoepithelial carcinoma are even scarcer. Case reports show mixed results in terms of tumor control from radiation therapy for gross disease.

Incidence note: 'Common to very common' indicates that a medium sized practice will treat at least several to dozens of patients with the lesion annually, 'Uncommon to rare' indicates the same practice size will treat one to two patients with the lesion every five years, 'Rare to very rare' indicates the same sized practice will see zero to one patient with the lesion every 20 years.

CASES

Case 12.1 Myoepithelioma of soft tissue

Clinical history and presentation

The patient is a 49 year old man who presents with a 15 year history of a right lower extremity mass. He relates that it grew slowly up until two years ago. Two years ago it stopped growing and has been stable in size. The patient states it is nontender and does not bother him except that he knocks it against furniture. He also states that he had a similar mass on his right arm, which was removed by a dermatologist and was found to be an angiolipoma.

Physical examination reveals a 4.5 cm soft mobile mass on the anterior aspect of the right leg near his knee. It is nontender to palpation.

Surgical findings and comments

Findings at surgery reveal an encapsulated soft tissue tumor which is completely excised.

Radiology findings

The lesion, **Case figs 12.1a** through **12.1e**, is a relatively simple solid tumor in the skin. There is no MR evidence for calcification or fat tissue. The intermediate signal on T2 suggests this may be a fibrous lesion. There is no association with nerves or vessels, and the adjacent bone appears unaffected. No aggressive features of infiltration or destruction are seen. Even though the tumor appears non-aggressive, it is an indeterminant solid lesion and ultimately, tissue diagnosis is needed.

Pathology findings

Gross features

The tumor is marginally resected in one excision, and two other specimens are submitted as additional margins. After differential inking, cross sectioning reveals a 5 × 4.5 × 3 cm solid, pink to tan-white,

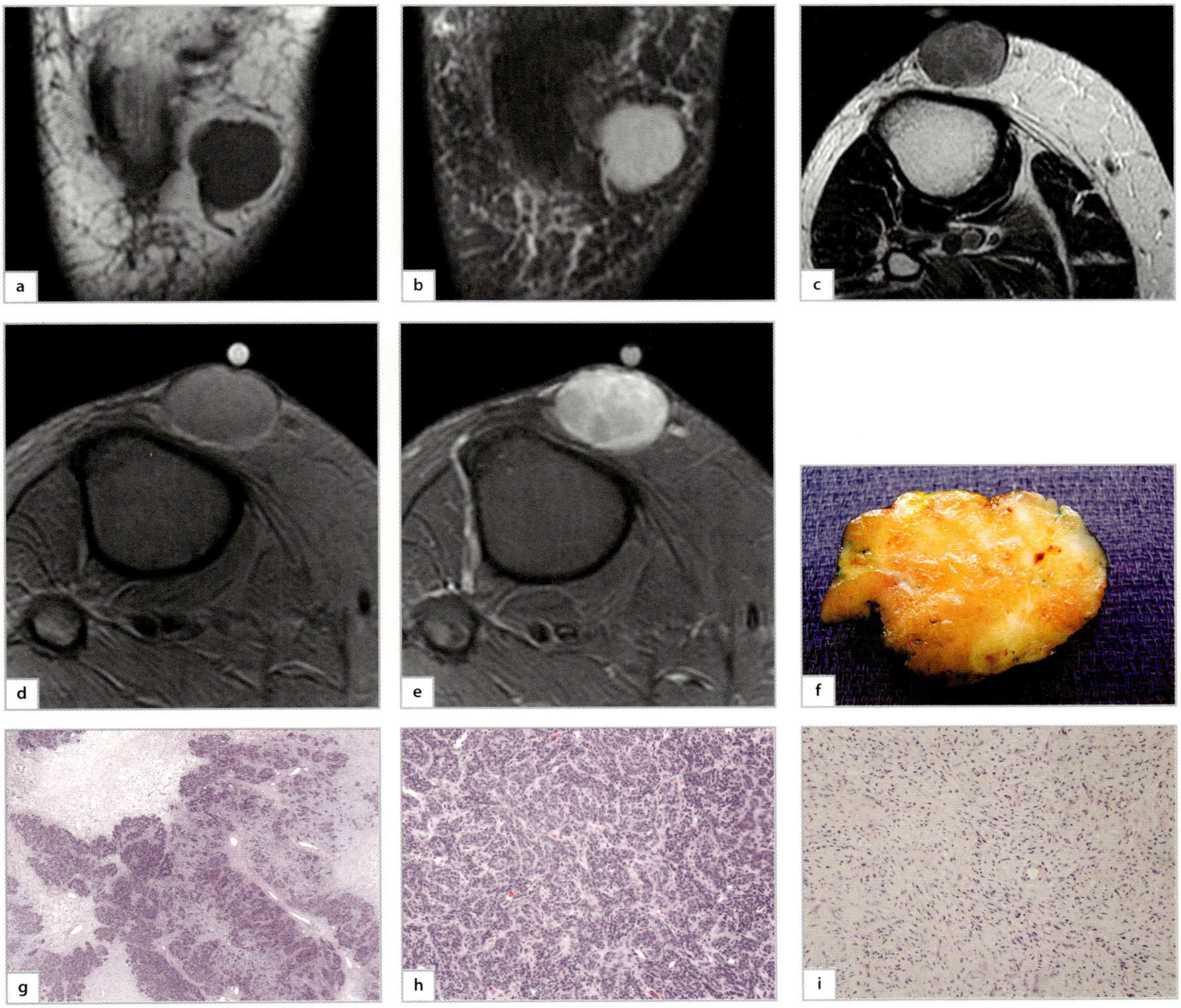

Case figure 12.1 Myoepithelioma imaging. MR imaging including. **12.1a:** Coronal T1, **12.1b**: Coronal STIR, **12.1c:** Axial T2, **12.1d**: Axial T1 fat saturation pre-contrast and **12.1e**: Axial T1 fat saturation post-contrast. There is a 3.4 × 3.3 × 2.6 cm mass in the subcutaneous tissues anterior to the proximal tibia. The lesion shows homogeneous T1 isointensity and T2 intermediate signal with fairly uniform intense enhancement. This is an overall non-specific appearance. **12.1f**: Myoepithelioma, gross photograph of cross section of tumor. The tumor is not necrotic and appears vaguely lobulated with pale pink and white to tan areas. **12.1g**: Low magnification. A typical region of this patient's tumor includes nests and cords of blue cells juxtaposed to myxoid and chondroid areas. This marked architectural heterogeneity is classic for myoepithelioma, although a few cases may show just one pattern. **12.1h**: Medium magnification, more epithelial appearing area. A braided, cordlike pattern of tightly cohesive tumor cells may be attempting but does not quite form ducts or tubules. **12.1i**: Medium magnification, pure spindle cell area. About 30% of the patient's tumor comprises a spindle cell proliferation that ranges from low to moderate cellularity.

Case figure 12.1: Continued from page 245

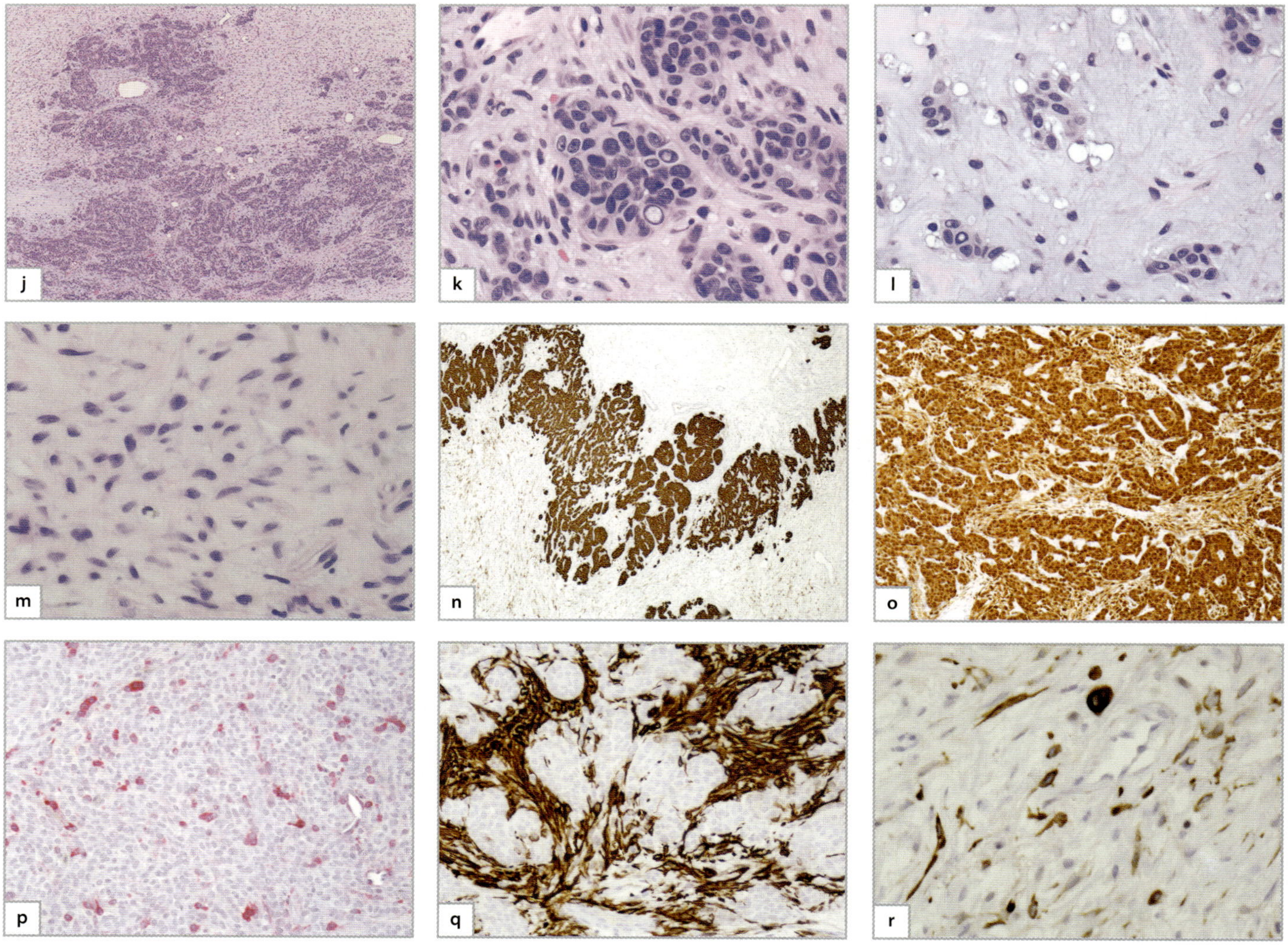

12.1j: Medium magnification, mixed spindle and corded/nested area. Many of the cords and nests of tumor cells are centered around ectatic blood vessels as is seen here. The spindle cell component flows around the nests and cords of smaller rounded cells. **12.1k**: High magnification, tumor cell nests. Cells forming the nests and cords exhibit scant cytoplasm (thus conferring a small round blue cell appearance at low and medium magnification) and small, oval nuclei with scattered nuclear pseudo-inclusions and grooves. **12.1l**: High magnification, chondroid matrix. This patient's tumor features a minority component of chondroid matrix in which are disposed clusters of epithelioid appearing tumor cells with microcyst formation. **12.1m**: High magnification, pure spindle cell area. Although there is slight variation in nuclear shape, the tapered to round ended nuclei feature fine, evenly dispersed chromatin and inconspicuous nucleoli consistent with a benign or low grade tumor. **12.1n**: Low magnification, pan-keratins IHC stain. The corded nested areas are diffusely strongly reactive for pan-keratins. Closer inspection reveals some reactivity in the spindle cell component as well. **12.1o**: Medium magnification, S-100 protein IHC stain. Consistent with myoepithelial cells, the corded areas (which on histology might otherwise resemble epithelium) exhibit diffuse strong reactivity for S-100 protein. **12.1p**: Medium magnification, calponin IHC stain. Even the epithelioid appearing areas contain scattered cells reactive for calponin (red Chromagen) consistent with myoepithelial differentiation. **12.1q**: Medium magnification, GFAP IHC stain. Many of the spindled tumor cells enveloping nests of tumor express GFAP, another marker fairly commonly seen in myoepithelial cells. Interestingly, despite the common myoepithelial differentiation of all cells in this patient's tumor, cell subsets differ in range and intensity of expression of the various myoepithelial antigens. **12.1r**: High magnification, pan-keratins IHC stain in spindle cell area. Weak to strong cytoplasmic expression of keratins is notable even in the pure spindle cell areas. This is an expected reactivity given the myoepithelial nature of the tumor cells.

glistening tumor (**Case fig. 12.1f**). Multiple cassettes are submitted after samples are collected fresh for cytogenetics and tumor banking. The additional margins comprise slips of skin and scant subjacent soft tissue. Tumor is not grossly identified in the additional margin excisions. All additional marginal tissue is submitted for microscopic evaluation.

Microscopic features

Low magnification: The most remarkable feature of this tumor is its histologic heterogeneity. Hypocellular myxoid spindle cell areas abut and extend beyond cellular, epithelial like nests and cords, and foci of blue-gray chondroid matrix are scattered throughout (**Case fig. 12.1g**). This diversity is highly characteristic of myoepithelioma, although rare cases may just comprise spindle cells. Necrosis is absent. The tumor exhibits a slightly infiltrative perimeter.

High magnification: Medium magnification of some of the cellular areas reveals interweaving cords of cells with scant cytoplasm (**Case fig. 12.1h**) and pure spindle cell areas (**Case fig. 12.1i**). Spindle cells also course among nests of tumor cells (**Case fig. 12.1j**). At highest magnification, the more cohesive tumor cells forming nests and cords feature scant cytoplasm and oval nuclei with scattered nuclear pseudoinclusions and grooves (**Case fig. 12.1k**). A chondroid like matrix is the least prevalent pattern (**Case fig. 12.1l**). Pure spindle cell areas exhibit a myxoid to fibrotic matrix, and the nuclei are not atypical with fine, evenly dispersed chromatin and inconspicuous nucleoli (**Case fig. 12.1m**). Mitoses are few and range up to 2 per 10 high magnification microscopic fields. Abnormal mitotic figures are absent. Lymphovascular invasion is not identified. The additional tissue submitted as new margins are positive in the deep aspect for tumor.

Special studies: The nests and cords of tumor cells are diffusely and strongly reactive for pan-keratins (**Case fig. 12.1n**) and S-100 protein (**Case fig. 12.1o**). A few cells also express calponin (**Case fig. 12.1p**) and GFAP (**Case fig. 12.1q**) (all controls are appropriately reactive). This staining profile is typical of tumors with myoepithelial differentiation. Scattered expression of keratins, SMA, and S-100 protein is notable in the pure spindle cell areas (**Case fig. 12.1r**).

The tumor karyotype reveals two related and evolving cell lines with an interstitial deletion of the short arm of chromosome 12 (12p-) in both cell lines and translocation t(1;7) in the side line: 46,XY,del(12)(p11.2p12)[18]/46,idem,t(1;7)(q21;p15)[2]. This karyotype is not specific for myoepithelioma but does not exclude the diagnosis. Most myoepitheliomas are diploid to hypodiploid, as is this patient's tumor and some but not all display trisomies and/or demonstrate 22q12 rearrangement.

There is no evidence for EWSR1 gene rearrangement by FISH using a Vysis, Inc. dual color break apart probe set (controls were appropriately reactive). About 50% of myoepitheliomas are negative for EWSR1 translocations, so this result does not exclude the diagnosis.

Pathologic differential or, why isn't it one of the following?

Benign mixed tumor of soft tissue: This closely related entity to myoepithelioma differs only in having ducts or tubules with true epithelial cell differentiation in addition to a myoepithelial component. This patient's tumor was extensively sampled, and no tubules or ducts were found.

Parachordoma: Parachordoma is considered by most soft tissue pathologists to represent a myoepithelioma that is composed exclusively of round to spindled myoepithelial cells embedded in a chondromyxoid matrix. It was initially called parachordoma because at one time it was thought to represent chordoma of soft tissue. However, immunohistochemical results clearly show it is myoepithelial rather than notochordal in differentiation. This patient's tumor certainly contains foci resembling 'parachordoma,' but the predominant pattern is sheets of spindled myoepithelial cells. Thus, it is best termed myoepithelioma.

Ossifying fibromyxoid tumor of soft tissue (OFMT): This rare tumor may have myxoid, fibrotic and cellular zones, bland appearing oval to spindle cells, and a peripheral (less often random) arrangement of metaplastic bone. Tumor cells are most often reactive for S-100 protein but can also express keratins, smooth muscle actin, desmin, CD57, NSE, and/or GFAP in a minority of cases. INI-1 expression may be partially lost resulting in a mosaic pattern on IHC in ~70% of cases (Graham et al. 2011). Thus, immunohistochemically, there is some overlap with myoepithelial tumors. The characteristic peripheral rim of bone, lack of chondroid stroma, even spacing of tumor cells, and lack of EWSR1 translocation help distinguish it from myoepithelioma with metaplastic bone.

Skin adnexal tumor: Various skin adnexal tumors enter the diagnosis of myoepithelioma, and especially mixed tumor of soft tissue can be confused with eccrine tumors. The IHC profile of myoepithelioma, with multi-marker expression of both myoid and epithelial proteins, is not seen in primary skin adnexal tumors.

Myoepithelial carcinoma: This is a rare tumor that differs from its benign counterpart in showing histologic features consistent with malignancy including increased nuclear pleomorphism, higher mitotic activity, infiltrative growth, and necrosis. Forty percent of pediatric and 10% of adult cases demonstrate loss of INI-1 expression by IHC. Nuclear INI-1 expression is retained in myoepithelioma, 'parachordoma' and benign mixed tumor.

Case table 12.1a lists the variant histologic features that may be seen in myoepithelioma of soft tissue and skin.

Case table 12.1a Variant histologic features of myoepithelial tumors of skin and soft tissue

Histologic feature	Frequency	Comment
Mixed architecture: includes tight nests and cords of small myoepithelial cells, myxoid, hyalinized or fibrotic spindle cell regions, chondroid areas, and reticular areas.	Most common	Not all patterns are present in every tumor. Most tumors have at least two patterns, however
Pure cellular spindle cell tumor	Uncommon	May mimic leiomyoma or a myofibroblastic tumor
Mixed cell population including: small condensed cells with scant cytoplasm, plasmacytoid cells, polygonal histiocytoid cells, clear cells, spindle cells.	Common	These different cell types usually are associated with multiple architectural patterns, and all types may not be present in one tumor
Metaplastic cartilage or bone	Uncommon	May be found in up to 15% of cases
Metaplastic adipocytic component	Uncommon	
'Parachordoma' appearance	Uncommon	Vacuolated clear cells and round myoepithelial cells set in a chondromyxoid matrix superficially resembling chordoma
Small round blue cell morphology mimicking Ewing sarcoma family of tumors	Uncommon	Found in some aggressive malignant pediatric cases (perhaps up to one third). Does not form the entire tumor; other areas histologically consistent with myoepithelial differentiation are present
Pure plasmacytoid cell tumor	Rare	Tumor cells are round with discrete cell borders, eosinophilic cytoplasm and eccentrically placed round nuclei
Malignant myoepithelioma (myoepithelial carcinoma)	Very rare	Nuclear pleomorphism including coarse chromatin and prominent nucleoli, increased mitotic activity including atypical mitotic figures, and necrosis are all usually present. Skin tumors may behave badly only with increased mitotic activity. Some tumors may contain ducts or tubules; such cases differ from malignant mixed tumor in lacking a sarcomatous component. Some cases show loss of INI-1 nuclear expression by IHC.
Histologically benign tumor mixed with myoepithelial carcinoma	Very rare	Suggests a rare benign tumor may undergo malignant transformation

Case table 12.1b Summary pathology findings of Case 12.1

Diagnosis	Myoepithelioma
Size	5 × 4.5 × 3 cm.
Location	Superficial
Margin status	Positive (deep margin only)
Histologic grade (FNCLCC grading system)	This is a benign lesion and therefore is not graded.
Pathologic stage (AJCC TNM classification)	This is a benign lesion and therefore is not staged.

FNCLCC: Fédération Nationale des Centres de Lutte Contre le Cancer (French Federation of Cancer Centers).

AJCC: American Joint Committee on Cancer

Oncology approach

Medical oncology

This patient has a benign tumor. There is no medical oncology intervention.

Radiation oncology

The patient undergoes excision with positive margins. The patient has the option of undergoing further excision in order to obtain negative margins. No radiation therapy is indicated, since surgery alone should control this benign tumor.

Patient outcome

Three years postoperatively the patient has no evidence of recurrence.

REFERENCES

Antonescu CR, Zhang L, Chang NE, et al. EWSR1-POU5F1 fusion in soft tissue myoepithelial tumors. A molecular analysis of sixty-six cases, including soft tissue, bone, and visceral lesions, showing common involvement of the EWSR1 gene. Genes Chromosomes Cancer 2010;49(12):1114–24.

Bahrami A, Dalton JD, Krane JF, et al. A subset of cutaneous and soft tissue mixed tumors are genetically linked to their salivary gland counterpart. Genes Chromosomes Cancer 2012;51:140–148.

Balogh Z, Deak L, Sapi Z. Malignant myoepithelioma of soft tissue: A case report with cytogenetic findings. Cancer Genetics Cytogenetics 2008;183(2):121-4.

Barnes L, Appel BN, Perez H, et al. Myoepithelioma of the head and neck: case report and review. J Surg Oncol 1985;28(1):21–8.

Behzatoglu K, Canberk S, Bahadir B, et al. Parachordoma or myoepithelioma? A case report of a rare soft tissue tumor. Pathol Inter 2007;57:167–170.

Brandal P, Panagopoulos I, Bjerkehagen B, et al. Detection of a t(1;22)(q23;q12) translocation leading to an EWSR1-PBX1 fusion gene in a myoepithelioma. Genes Chomosomes Cancer 2008;47(7):558–64.

Brandal P, Panagopoulos, Bjerkehagen B, et al. t(19:22)(q13;q12) Translocation leading to the novel fusion gene EWSRI-ZHF444 in soft tissue myoepithelial carcinoma. Genes Chromosomes Cancer 2009;48(12):1051–6.

El-Kabany M, Al-Abdulghani R, Ali AE, et al. Soft tissue high grade myoepithelial carcinoma with round cell morphology: report of a newly described entity with EWSR1 gene rearrangement. Gulf J Oncolog 2011;1(9):73–7.

Fletcher CDM, Unni KK, Mertens F. World Health Organization Classification of Tumours: Pathology and Genetics of Tumours of Soft Tissue and Bone. Lyon: IARC Press 2002.

Flucke U, Mentzel T, Verdijk MA, et al. EWSR1-ATF1 chimeric transcript in a myoepithelial tumor of soft tissue: a case report. Hum Pathol 2012;43(5):764–8.

Flucke U, Tops BBJ, Verdijk MAJ, et al. NR4A3 rearrangement reliably distinguishes between the clinicopathologically overlapping entities myoepithelial carcinoma of soft tissue and cellular extraskeletal myxoid chondrosarcoma. Virchows Arch 2012;460(6):621–8.

Gleason BC, Fletcher CDM. Myoepithelial carcinoma of soft tissue in children: an aggressive neoplasm analyzed in a series of 29 cases. Am J Surg Pathol 2007;31:1813–1824.

Graham RP, Dry S, Li S, et al. Ossifying fibromyxoid tumor of soft parts: a clinicopathologic, proteomic and genomic study. Am J Surg Pathol 2011;35:1615–25.

Guedes A, Barreto BF, Barreto LGS, et al. Metastatic parachordoma. J Cutan Pathol 2009;36(2):270–3.

Hallor KH, Teixeira MR, Fletcher CDM, et al. Heterogeneous genetic profiles in soft tissue myoepitheliomas. Mod Pathol 2008;21(11):1311–9.

Harada O, Ota H, Nakayama J. Malignant myoepithelioma (myoepithelial carcinoma) of soft tissue. Pathol Int 2005;55:510–3.

Hiwatashi A, Matsumoto S, Kamoi I, et al. Imaging features of myoepithelioma arising from the hard palate. A case report. Acta Radiol 2000;41(5):417–9.

Hollmann TJ, Hornick JL. INI1-Deficient tumors: Diagnostic features and molecular genetics. Am J Surg Pathol 2011;35(10):e47–63.

Hornick JL, Fletcher CSM. Cutaneous myoepithelioma: A clinicopathologic and immunohistochemical study of 14 cases. Hum Pathol 2004;35(1):14–24.

Hornick JL, Fletcher CDM. Myoepithelial tumors of soft tissue. A clinicopathologic and immunohistochemical study of 101 cases with evaluation of prognostic parameters. Am J Surg Pathol 2003;27(9):1183–1196.

Jo VY, Fletcher CDM, et al. p63 Immunohistochemical staining is limited in soft tissue tumors. Am J Clin Pathol 2011;136(5):762–6.

Khademi B, Kazemi T, Bayat A, et al. Salivary gland myoepithelial neoplasms: a clinical and cytopathologic study of 15 cases and review of the literature. Acta Cytol 2010;54:1111–7.

Mentzel T, Requena L, Kaddu S, et al. Cutaneous myoepithelial neoplasms: clinicopathologic and immunohistochemical study of 20 cases suggesting a continuous spectrum ranging from benign mixed tumor of the skin to cutaneous myoepithelioma and myoepithelial carcinoma. J Cutan Pathol 2003;30(5):294–302.

Miura K, Harada H, Aiba S, et al. Myoepithelial carcinoma of the lung arising from bronchial submucosa. Am J Surg Pathol 2000;24:1300–4.

Mobley BC, McKenney JK, Bands CD, et al. Loss of SMARCB1/INI1 expression in poorly differentiated chordomas. Acta Neuropathologica 2010;120: 745–753.

Noronha V, Cooper DL, Higgins SA, et al. Metastatic myoepithelial carcinoma of the vulva treated with carboplatin and paclitaxel. Lancet Oncol 2006;7:270–1.

Pattari SK, Dey P, Gupta SK, et al. Myoepithelial cells: any role in aspiration cytology smears of breast tumors? Cytojournal 2008;5:9.

Pierard S, Gregoire V, Weynand B, et al. Epithelial-myoepithelial carcinoma of the submandibular gland with symptomatic lung metastases treated with chemotherapy. Eur Arch Otorhinolaryngol 2006;263:1158–60.

Rekhi B, Amare P, Gulia A, et al. Primary intraosseous myoepithelioma arising in the iliac bone and displaying trisomies of 11, 15, 17 with del (16q) and del (22q11) – A rare case report with review of literature. Pathol Res Pract 2011;207(12):780–5.

Savera AT, Sloman A, Huvos AG, et al. Myoepithelial carcinoma of the salivary glands: a clinicopathologic study of 25 patients. Am J Surg Pathol 2000;24:761–74.

Takayama O, Yokoyama J, Ito S. Therapeutic experience of recurrent myoepithelial carcinoma by superselective intra-arterial chemotherapy infused high-dose CDDP. Auris Nasus Larynx 2006;33:235–8.

Tanahashi J, Kashima K, Daa T, et al. A case of cutaneous myoepithelial carcinoma. J Cutan Pathol 2007;34:648–53.

Tirabosco R, Mangham DC, Rosenberg AE, et al. Brachyury expression in extra-axial skeletal and soft tissue chordomas: A marker that distinguishes chordoma from mixed tumor/myoepithelioma/parachordoma in soft tissue. Am J Surg Pathol 2008;32(4):572–80.

van den Berg E, Zorqdrager H, Hoekstra HJ, et al. Cytogenetics of a soft tissue malignant myoepithelioma. Cancer Genetics Cytogenetics 2004;151(1):87–9.

Yamada K, Iwai K, Okada Y, et al. Immunohistochemical expression of epidermal growth factor receptor in salivary gland tumours. Virchows Arch A Pathol Anat Histopathol 1989;415:523–31.

Chapter 13 Neural and perineural tumors of soft tissues

OVERVIEW

Neural tumors of soft tissue include nerve sheath differentiated neoplasms such as schwannoma, neurofibroma and perineurioma, paragangliomas and rare ectopic CNS type tumors: meningioma, hemangioblastoma, and ependymoma. Behavior ranges from benign to aggressively malignant (malignant peripheral nerve sheath tumor (MPNST)).

Diagnosis and treatment strategies continue to evolve as the exploration of these tumors at the molecular genetic level proceeds.

CLASSIFICATION

Table 13.1 lists the neural and perineural tumors of soft tissue. Neuroblastoma and pure dermal tumors are excluded. This table includes the 2013 WHO classified nerve sheath tumors and is also partly based on another suggested classification (Rodriguez et al. 2012).

DEMOGRAPHICS

Neuromas and benign nerve sheath tumors are common. Most occur in adults as single sporadic lesions. Sporadic schwannomas and sporadic neurofibromas occur with approximately equal frequency on a per patient basis, but NF1 patients may have multiple neurofibromas resected per individual. **Figure 13.1** indicates the surgical incidence of these lesions compared with malignant peripheral nerve sheath tumors resected from 2000 to 2010 at the University of New Mexico Health Sciences Center (UNM HSC), a medium sized, academic hospital system. At all ages, benign tumors far outnumber malignant tumors, and overall, resected benign tumors are 16 times more common than malignant peripheral nerve sheath tumors (n = 280).

Perineurioma has a predilection for differing ages and gender according to subtype. The sclerosing variant of soft tissue perineurioma, the most common type of perineurioma found in soft tissue unassociated with a nerve, occurs most commonly in the fingers and hands of young adults (M > F by 2:1). A rare reticular variant of soft tissue perineurioma also affects young adults (F > M by ~2:1). Typical soft tissue perineurioma is found in a broad age range from childhood to older adults and may or may not slightly favor females (Hornick et al. 2005; Pina-Oviedo et al. 2008). Intraneural perineurioma is very rare and occurs in children and young adults with a slight female predominance.

Nerve sheath myxoma can affect patients at any age, but young adults are favored and males slightly more than females.

Head and neck paragangliomas occur most often in middle-aged patients with an equal sex distribution in carotid body tumors and 2:1, F:M predominance in vagal body tumors. In accord with several larger series, of 26 patients recently treated at UNM HSC, approximately 25% of patients were aged 21-40 years, 50% were aged 40-60 years, and no children were affected.

Ependymomas of soft tissue are rare and generally occur in young adults. Ectopic meningiomas are also rare with the more common site comprising the subcutis of the scalp in older adults and the less common site comprising the paraspinous soft tissue of children. Soft tissue hemangioblastoma is another very rare tumor that can occur outside the CNS in the soft tissue. From the few cases reported, it occurs in adults.

Regarding malignant neural and perineural tumors, Surveillance, Epidemiology, and End Results (SEER) data were evaluated from 13 registries during a 15 year period (USA, 1994-2008). All tumors presented in this section arose in the connective tissue. The average annual incidence rates for neural/perineural tumors, along with their respective ICDO-3 codes, are presented in **Table 13.2**. There are no statistically significant differences in the incidence rates between males and females. Although MPNST is not a particularly uncommon sarcoma, as it accounts for up to 10% of all soft tissue sarcomas, in absolute terms, it is indeed rare. Malignant perineurioma, malignant granular cell tumor, and malignant paraganglioma are truly exotic entities. The actual number of cases reported in the 13 SEER registries illustrates the paucity of these tumors (**Figure 13.2**).

Patients with malignant peripheral nerve sheath tumors are diagnosed at a wide range of ages. Within this group, patients with rhabdomyoblastic differentiation are diagnosed at a younger age (mean = 28.0 years) compared to the other tumor types. The age distribution for selected neural/perineural tumors is shown in **Figure 13.3**.

PATHOGENESIS/ETIOLOGY

Traumatic and Morton's neuromas are reactive lesions that consist of a haphazard proliferation of axons following tissue injury.

Schwannomas occur much more commonly sporadically than in the setting of neurofibromatosis type 2 or schwannomatosis (sometimes also called neurilemmomatosis or neurofibromatosis type 3). Somatic mutations or allelic loss of the chromosome 22 merlin (schwannomin) gene account for many of the sporadic cases (see **Table 13.3**). The hallmark of neurofibromatosis type 2 is bilateral vestibular (acoustic) schwannomas, but other associated tumors include schwannomas at other soft tissue and skin sites, meningiomas and glial neoplasms. Schwannomatosis is distinguished from NF2 by the lack of vestibular schwannomas and presence of commonly painful cutaneous and spinal root tumors. Patients with Carney complex type 1 also can develop multiple schwannomas of a particular variant: psammomatous melanotic schwannoma (Carroll 2012).

Granular cell tumors (GCT) consist of a variant of a Schwann cell neoplasm in which the tumor cells contain abundant lysosomes imparting a granular eosinophilic appearance to the cytoplasm. Most patients are adults, but any age may be affected. Up to 25% of patients may have multiple lesions, but these individuals do not have schwannomatosis or NF2. The tumors occur more frequently in women. The rare malignant granular cell tumor most commonly afflicts older patients (> 60 years) and does not arise from a benign GCT (Folpe et al. 2010).

Solitary neurofibromas are more common in men, and the prevalent age is young adulthood. However, patients with NF1 often develop neurofibromas at an earlier age in childhood or adolescence. NF1 is an autosomal dominant condition affecting 1 in 2500 to 1 in

Table 13.1 Neural and perineural tumors and lesions of soft tissue

Tumor or lesion	Behavior	Additional comments
Neuromuscular hamartoma (benign Triton tumor)	Benign	Not a true monoclonal neoplasm
Neuromas Morton Traumatic	Benign	These are reactive proliferations
Granular cell tumor	Benign	There is a rare malignant version
Schwannoma Conventional Cellular Plexiform Melanotic Microcystic/reticular Others	Benign	Sporadic or associated with NF2 or schwannomatosis (also known as NF3)
Neurofibroma Circumscribed Diffuse and massive soft tissue Plexiform Others	Benign	Sporadic or associated with NF1
Perineurioma Intraneural Soft tissue Sclerosing Reticular	Benign	There is a very rare malignant version
Hybrid peripheral nerve sheath tumors	Benign	Combinations include schwannoma and perineuroma, schwannoma and neurofibroma, and some cannot be specifically defined (these are termed 'hybrid benign nerve sheath tumor NOS')
Nerve sheath myxoma	Intermediate	Usually limited to the dermis
Malignant peripheral nerve sheath tumor (MPNST) Low grade High grade Epithelioid MPNST with divergent differentiation MPNST ex schwannoma Malignant melanotic schwannoma Perineurial MPNST	Malignant	Sporadic or associated with NF1
Synovial sarcoma of nerve	Malignant	Rare intraneural variant of synovial sarcoma
Paraganglioma of head and neck	Benign to malignant	Most carotid body tumors (~90%) behave in a benign fashion
Ependymoma of soft tissue	Intermediate to malignant	Rare; occurs as a soft tissue mass at tip of coccyx
Ectopic meningioma	Benign	Rare; scalp and distal paraspinal soft tissue
Hemangioblastoma of soft tissue	Benign?	Too few cases in soft tissue to confirm behavior

Benign: does not recur or recurs non-aggressively and does not metastasize. Intermediate: can recur aggressively and/or rarely metastasizes . Malignant: can recur and commonly metastasizes.

3500 newborns. Half of patients experience a new mutation, so there will be no family history in these individuals. The NF1 gene, located on chromosome 17, is large, and a broad spectrum of mutations may cause the disease which is completely penetrant but of variable expression. The NF1 gene codes for neurofibromin, a protein that is involved in inhibiting the RAS pathway, among other functions. It acts as a tumor suppressor. NF1 patients are at risk for other tumors including malignant peripheral nerve sheath tumor (MPNST), optic gliomas, glioblastomas, pheochromocytoma, rhabdomyosarcoma, gastrointestinal stromal tumor, and juvenile chronic myelogenous leukemia (Carroll 2012). Sporadic and NF1 related neurofibromas exhibit biallelic inactivation of the NF1 gene. Plexiform neurofibroma is almost exclusive to NF1 patients, while diffuse neurofibroma has an approximately 10-20% association with NF1.

Perineuriomas are associated with mutations or allelic losses of the NF2 gene, and a single case of t(2;10)(p23;q24) has been reported (Brock et al. 2005; Mietttinen et al. 2010). However, only a few cases to date have been examined genetically.

Malignant peripheral nerve sheath tumor affects 3--20% of patients with NF1 and usually arises in a deep plexiform neurofibroma in these cases. It contains additional mutations beyond biallelic inactivated neurofibromin genes (see **Table 13.3**). For both the NF1 associated tumors and the sporadic tumors, females are slightly more frequently affected. MPNST in NF1 accounts for approximately 50-60% of all MPNST, and it occurs at an earlier age (most commonly adolescence to young adulthood) than sporadic MPNST (middle aged and older adults), although any age can be affected in either situation.

Paragangliomas of the head and neck may be associated with a defined genetic syndrome (see **Table 13.3**) but are more commonly sporadic. These are neural autonomic nervous system tumors that show differentiation toward paraganglionic cells. They are discussed in this chapter, because orthopaedic surgeons may resect those occurring in the head and neck. Chronic hypoxia (such as living at high altitude or due to pulmonary disease) can predispose to head and neck paraganglioma.

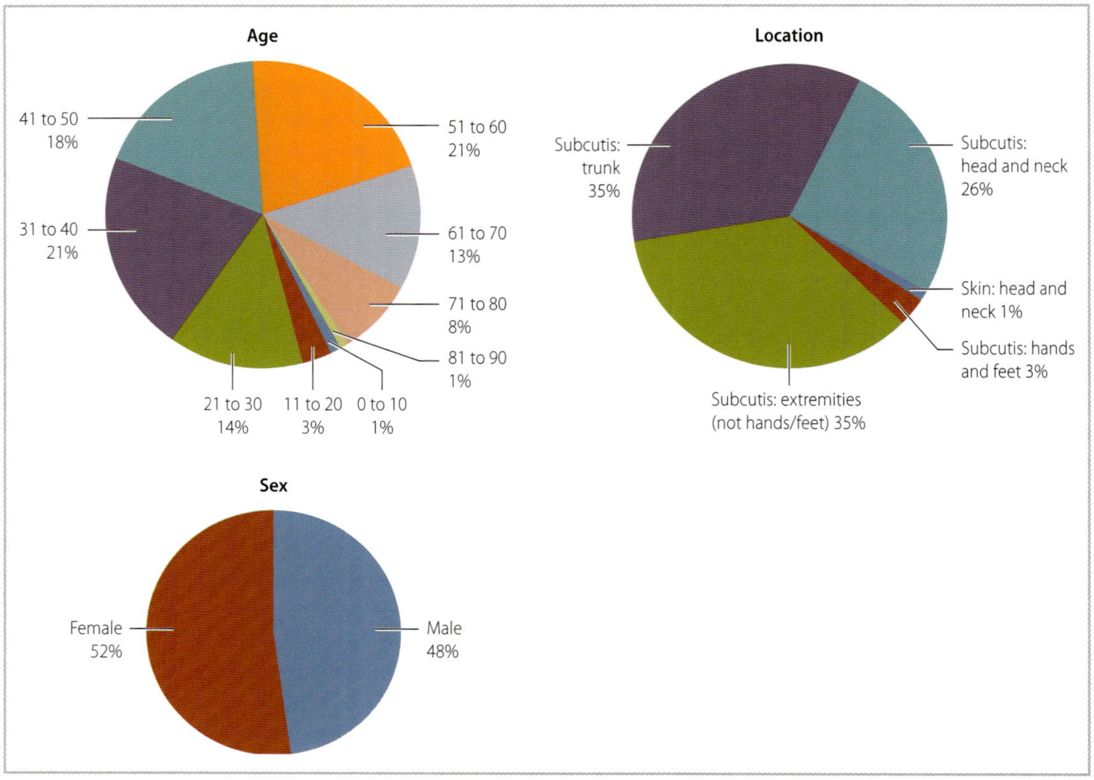

Figure 13.1 Schwannomas resected at University of New Mexico Health Sciences Center 2000-2010 (n=92).

Table 13.2 Average annual incidence rates of neural/perineural tumors of the soft tissue in 13 SEER registries between the years 1994 and 2008.

Neural/perineural tumor type	ICDO-3 Code	Incidence rate per million
Malignant peripheral nerve sheath tumors (MPNST)		
Malignant peripheral nerve sheath tumor*	9540 and 9560	0.5
MPNST with rhabdomyoblastic differentiation	9561	0.0
Malignant perineurioma	9571	0.0
Malignant granular cell tumor	9580	0.0
Malignant paragangliomas		
Malignant extra-adrenal paraganglioma	8693	0.0
Malignant paraganglioma	8680	0.0
* Malignant neurilemmoma tumors (ICDO-3 = 9560) were combined with MPNST		

PATHOLOGY

Table 13.4 briefly describes the soft tissue neural/perineural tumors by incidence, body site, and pathologic features. SEER data compiled from 13 registries (1994-2008) indicate the most common body locations for the malignant peripheral nerve sheath tumors and malignant paragangliomas (**Figure 13.4**).

Histologic grading

Benign neural and perineural tumors

Benign neural and perineural tumors are not graded. However, it should be noted that some benign tumors may exhibit degenerative nuclear atypia ('ancient' change in schwannoma, neurofibroma, hybrid peripheral nerve sheath tumors, and perineurioma). Degenerative atypia includes cells with nuclear enlargement, irregular contours, sometimes multinucleation and dark, smudgy chromatin. Importantly, coarse chromatin, irregularly distributed chromatin and increased mitotic activity are absent.

Paragangliomas of the head and neck may contain scattered pleomorphic tumor cells with hyperchromasia and multinucleation. These cells do not forecast malignant behavior (see below).

Malignant neural and perineural tumors

Malignant peripheral nerve sheath tumors may be graded by the FNCLCC system which is collapsed to low and high grade by the American Joint Committee on Cancer (7th ed; FNCLCC grade 2 is considered high grade by the AJCC). In practice, most MPNST are high grade tumors (~85%). Possibly, grading of MPNST may have prognostic significance, but a commonly accepted, prognostically proven system is not in place at this time (Rodriguez et al. 2012).

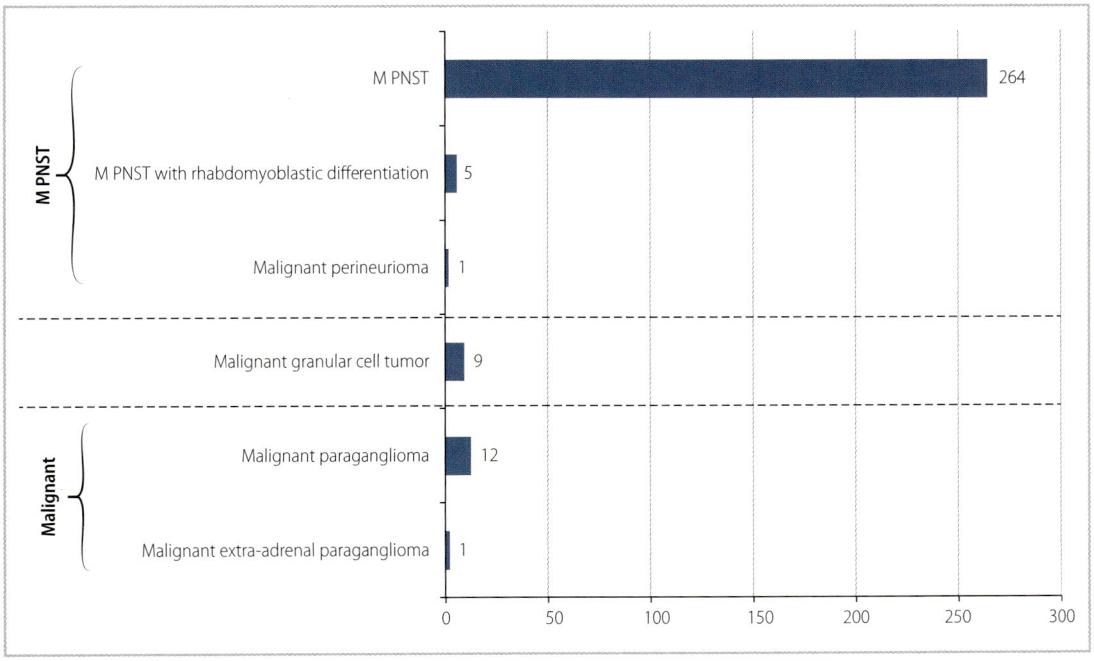

Figure 13.2 Frequency of neural/perineural tumors of the soft tissue in 13 seer registries between the years 1994 and 2008.

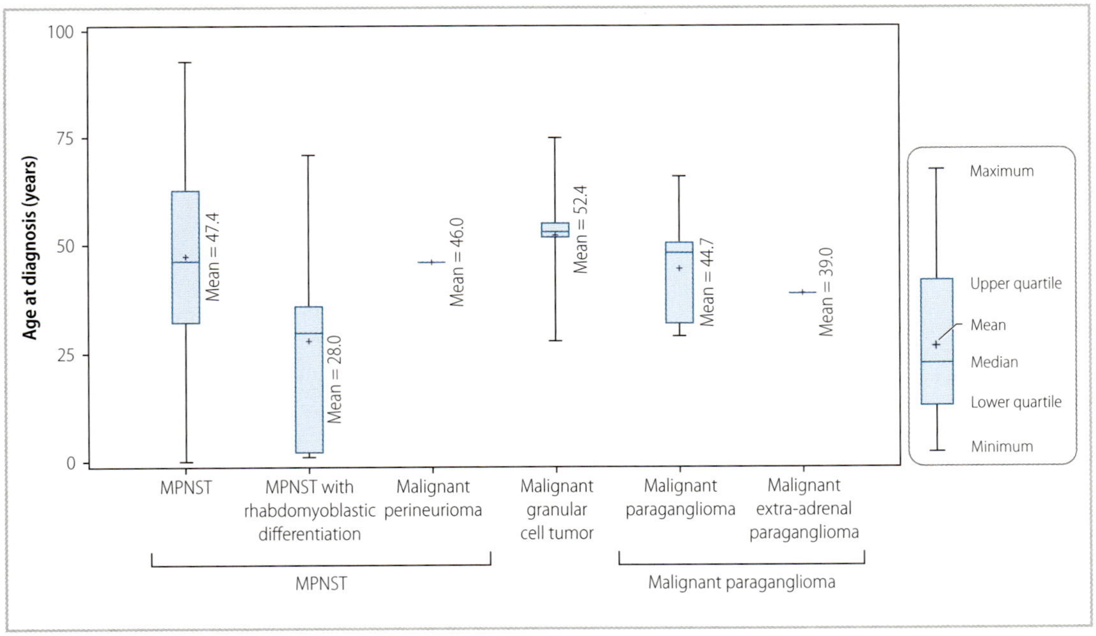

Figure 13.3 Age distribution of neural/perineural tumors of the soft tissue among cases in 13 SEER registries during the time period 1994-2008 (n=292).

Behavior

Benign neural and perineural tumors

Traumatic neuromas, despite a reactive nature, do not spontaneously regress. Solitary, non-plexiform, non-diffuse neurofibromas very rarely transform to malignant peripheral nerve sheath tumor. Even a solitary neurofibroma may be associated with NF1, and therefore excision may be recommended for molecular genetic confirmation of the diagnosis.

Diffuse neurofibromas may locally recur but do not have a high risk for transformation to MPNST. By contrast, plexiform neurofibromas, especially those in the deep soft tissue (associated with a large peripheral nerve), are the origin of NF1 related MPNST. Focal early transformation to MPNST in a portion of a plexiform neurofibroma can be considered behaviorally analogous to a low grade sarcoma (Folpe et al. 2010).

Schwannomas are benign. Very rarely, an otherwise typical schwannoma may transform to the epithelioid variant of MPNST or angiosarcoma.

Benign granular cell tumors far outnumber the malignant variant. Although benign, they habitually demonstrate infiltrative margins

Table 13.3 Genetics of neural and perineural tumors of soft tissue

Tumor	Chromosomal abnormality (karyotyping methodology)	Genes involved (molecular methodology)	Percentage of tumors with abnormality
Granular cell tumor	Benign GCT: diploid or hyperdiploid Malignant GCT: aneuploid, hyperdiploid, t(5;15)(p14;q25) +X, abnormalities of 5, 15	Unknown	Most benign tumors are diploid Very few karyotypes of malignant GCT reported. No consistent chromosomal findings (n= 10 cases)
Schwannoma sporadic	22, 7, X, Y alterations most common. Many tumors are diploid without chromosomal abnormalities. Cellular schwannoma may have trisomy 17 among other non-recurring changes leading to diploidy, tetraploidy, or aneuploidy (66% diploid)	Biallelic inactivation of merlin (schwannomin) gene (22q12.2), both somatic	Majority have biallelic inactivation of merlin
Schwannoma in NF2	Unknown whether karyotype is significantly different than in sporadic schwannoma	Biallelic inactivation of merlin (schwannomin) gene (22q12.2). One inactivation is germline; other is somatic	100% have biallelic inactivation of merlin
Schwannoma in schwannomatosis	Unknown whether karyotype is significantly different than in sporadic schwannoma	Inactivating mutation of merlin (schwannomin/NF2 gene) (22q12.2) as a somatic event combined with inactivating mutation of SMARCB1/INI1 gene (22q11.2) in the germline	Majority have merlin gene alteration (somatic but not germline) ~30% have SMARCB1/INI1 gene alteration
Schwannoma in carney complex type 1 (carney syndrome)	Unknown whether karyotype is significantly different than in sporadic schwannoma	Carney complex type 1 (Carney syndrome) gene: PRKAR1A (17q) gene alterations, one germline	Most have PRKAR1A gene alterations
Neurofibroma, sporadic	9p21-22 rearrangements. Many cutaneous and diffuse neurofibromas have diploid karyotype	Somatic alterations of NF1 gene	Majority have NF1 gene alterations
Neurofibroma in nf1	9p21-22 rearrangements	*NF1* alterations of both alleles: one germline and the second somatic	5% of patients have complete loss of NF1 gene in germline; remainder of NF1 patients has nonsense, missense, frameshift and mutations affecting RNA splicing of NF1 gene as germline change. Patients with whole gene loss usually have increased risk for plexiform neurofibroma, MPNST, cognitive impairment and many dermal neurofibromas
Perineurioma, intraneural	Monosomy 22	*NF2* gene alterations	Too few cases to determine frequency of *NF2* alterations
Perineurioma, soft tissue	22q11.2-12 rearrangements or Monosomy 22	*NF2* gene alterations	Too few cases to determine frequency of *NF2* alterations
Perineurioma, sclerosing	Monosomy 22 Monosomy 10 t(2;10)(p23;q24)	*NF2* gene alterations	Too few cases to determine frequency of *NF2* and chromosome 10 alterations
Hybrid peripheral nerve sheath tumor	Unknown	*NF2* alterations *NF1* alterations *SMARCB1/INI1* alterations	Majority may have *NF2* gene alterations Minority may have *NF1* or *SMARCB1/INI1* alterations
Malignant peripheral nerve sheath tumor in NF1	Complex aneuploid karyotype affecting nearly all chromosome regions. Recurrent changes include: Losses: 1p, 9p, 11, 12p, 14q, 17q, 22q, x or Y Gains: 2,7, 8, 9p or all of 9	Both *NF1* gene (neurofibromin) (17q11) alleles inactivated by mutation and/or loss *EGF* and *EGFR* and other growth factors and receptors may be mutated, amplified, or overexpressed. Gains: *PDCD1* (2p25.3), *SOX5* (12p12.1) *FOXM1* (12p13.33), *NOL1* (12p13.31), *CDK4* (12q14.1). Losses: *CDKN2A/p16* (9p21), *PSIP/p75* (9p22/3), *PTPRD* (9p23 to 9p24.1), *PTEN* (10q23.31); *RB* (13q14); *p53* (17q13). Mutations of *CDKN2A/p16* Some recurrent sites harbor unknown genes.	Most tumors exhibit complex aneuploidy. Some may show triploid karyotype. Gain: *PDCD1*, (~45%); *SOX5*, (~30%); *FOXM1*, (~30%); *NOL1*, (~30%); *CDK4*, (~15%). Loss: *p53* (50-75%); *PSIP/p75* (~50%); *PTPRD*, (50%); *PTEN*, (~30%); *RB* (~25%). Mutations: *CDKN2A/p16* (~50%)
Malignant peripheral nerve sheath tumor, sporadic	Complex aneuploid karyotype Recurrent changes include: Loss: 1p, 9p, 11, 12p, 14q, 17q, 22q, Xor Y Gain: 2,7, 9p or all of 9	NF1 gene also often affected but not in 100% of cases. Remaining findings similar to MPNST arising in NF1	Most tumors exhibit complex aneuploidy. Some may show triploid karyotype (which may confer a worse prognosis) NF1 gene alterations not identified in all cases. Other gene gain and loss frequencies as for NF1-associated MPNST

Table 13.3: Continued from page 254

Tumor	Chromosomal abnormality (karyotyping methodology)	Genes involved (molecular methodology)	Percentage of tumors with abnormality
Paraganglioma of head and neck	PGL1 syndrome: 11q23 PGL2 syndrome: 11q13.1 PGL3 syndrome: 1q23.3 PGL4 syndrome: 1p36.1-p35 MEN2a and MEN2b: 10g11.2 Von Hippel Lindau: 3p26-p25 Carney triad:	PGL1: SDHD/SDH4 PGL2: Unknown gene PGL3: SDHC/SDH3 PGL4: SDHB/SDH1 RET gene VHL gene	Majority of tumors are sporadic unassociated with a syndrome. However, the PGL1-3 syndromes may account for ~25% of seemingly sporadic head and neck paragangliomas PGL1-3 mostly head and neck paragangliomas; PGL4 various sites Rare patients with MEN2a and MEN2b develop head and neck paragangliomas Rare patients with Von Hippel-Lindau develop head and neck paragangliomas Some patients with Carney triad have head and neck paragangliomas

Amp: amplification. O-e: over-expressed, loh: loss of heterozygosity,

See references for papers and texts pertaining to this table. This static list of genetic abnormalities must be viewed in the context of continuing discovery and refinement of genetic findings.

Table 13.4 Neural and perineural tumors of soft tissue grouped by behavior

Tumor	Incidence	Age and sex	Body site (in order of occurrence)	Histopathology description including IHC	
				Medium magnification	High magnification
Benign: does not recur or recurs non-aggressively and does not metastasize					
Neuromuscular hamartoma and benign triton tumor	Very rare	Infants > young children >> young adults	Head and neck, upper trunk major nerve or nerve plexus May be associated with a desmoid tumor	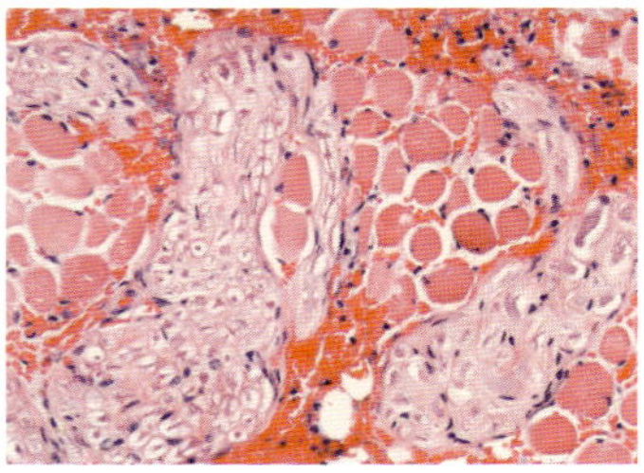	
Neuromuscular hamartoma: Enlarged nerves that contain clusters of mature skeletal muscle cells. **Benign Triton tumor**: A neurofibroma that contains mature skeletal muscle cells. IHC is usually not necessary to make diagnosis, but skeletal muscle cells are positive for desmin and myogenin.					
Neuromas Morton traumatic	Very common	All ages for traumatic (post injury including surgery) Morton: adult woman	traumatic: digits and extremities Morton: interdigital nerve between 3rd and 4th metatarsal heads	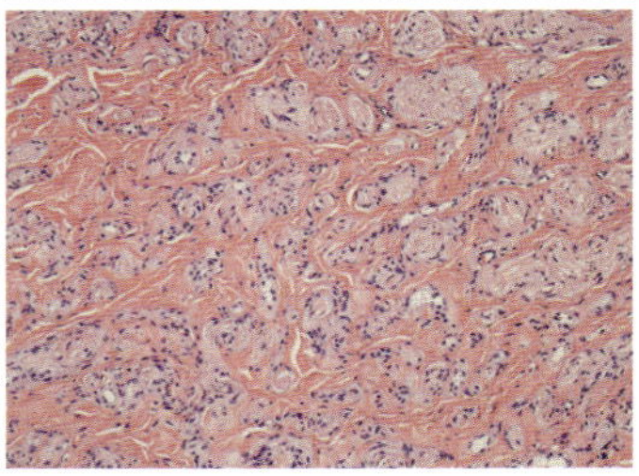	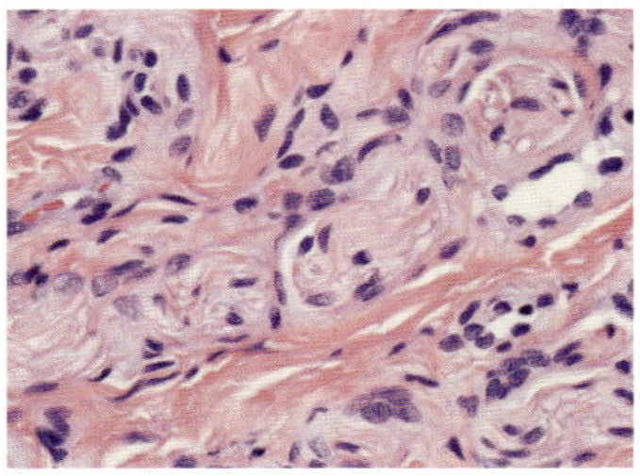
Traumatic: Unencapsulated, haphazard proliferation of small nerve twigs (Schwann cells, axons, and perineurial cells) encased in fibrous stroma (scar tissue). **Morton neuroma**: Variant of traumatic neuroma with thickening +/- thrombosis of intraneural vessels, intraneural and extraneural fibrosis with loss of axons, and increased Schwann cells and fibroblasts.					
Granular cell tumor	Common	Broad age range but adults (20s-50s) most common. F slightly > M	Trunk, upper extremity, head, lower extremity. Most commonly superficial but can occur in muscle	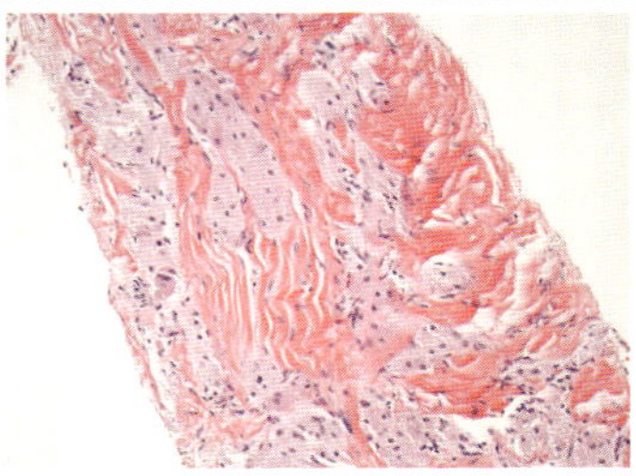	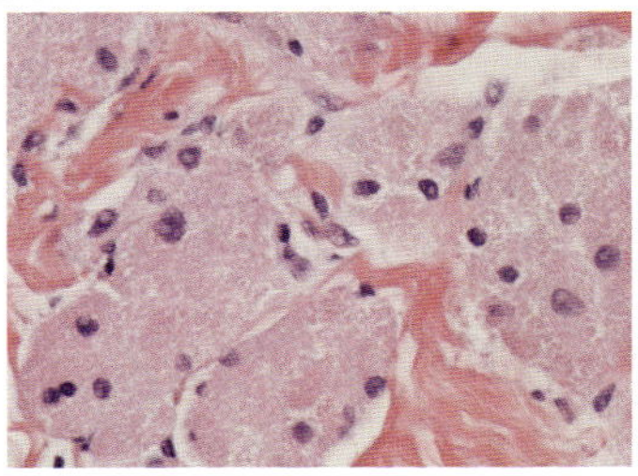
Benign GCT: Solid sheets or clusters of polygonal to epithelioid cells. Infiltrative edges. Tumor cells have granular, eosinophilic cytoplasm (due to lysosomes) with round to ovoid nuclei that are hyperchromatic or vesicular with nucleoli. The cytoplasm may also clump. Mitoses rare. Focal nuclear atypia and spindling of cells can be present. **Malignant GCT**: Usually larger than benign tumors. Increased nuclear atypia, necrosis, extensive cell spindling and higher mitotic activity than benign GCT. Borderline tumors may also occur. IHC: S-100 and CD68 positive in both benign and malignant GCT.					

Table 13.4: Continued from page 255

<table>
<tr><th rowspan="2">Tumor</th><th rowspan="2">Incidence</th><th rowspan="2">Age and sex</th><th rowspan="2">Body site (in order of occurrence)</th><th colspan="2">Histopathology description including IHC</th></tr>
<tr><th>Medium magnification</th><th>High magnification</th></tr>
<tr><td>Schwannoma
Conventional
Cellular
Plexiform
Melanotic
Microcystic/reticular
Others</td><td>Very common</td><td>Broad age range, but most common in middle age. Rare in children except cellular plexiform schwannoma</td><td>Head and neck, distal extremities, superficial tissue. Also: vestibular and retroperitoneal locations</td><td>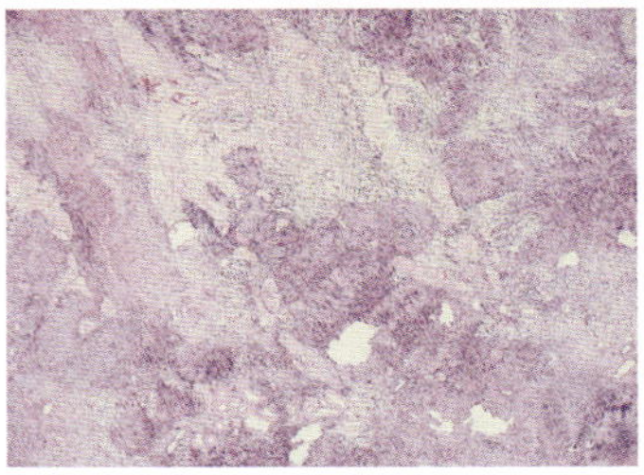</td><td>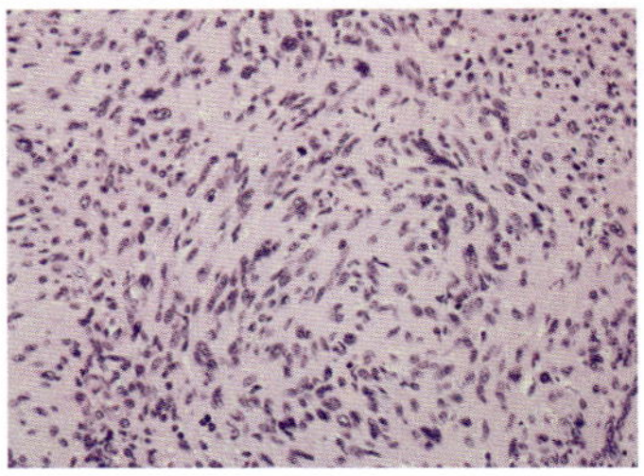</td></tr>
<tr><td colspan="6">Conventional: Encapsulated tumor of Schwann cells arranged in cellular (Antoni A) and hypocellular (Antoni B) areas. Nuclei may line up (Verocay body). Vessels may be hyalinized. Light sprinkling of chronic inflammatory cells common. Schwann cells- elongate spindle cells with spindled, pointy-ended nuclei that may also be wavy or show a 'shepherd's crook' bend. Mitoses absent to rare.
Cellular: Only Antoni A areas present. Cells may be more ovoid rather than slender and spindled.
Plexiform: Multiple nodules present.
Plexiform cellular: Multiple nodules all cellular.
Others: see Cases Table of Schwannoma variants.
IHC: Schwann cells S-100 positive. EMA positive at edge of tumor nodules.</td></tr>
<tr><td>Neurofibroma
Circumscribed
Diffuse and massive soft tissue
Plexiform
Others</td><td>Common</td><td>Broad age range but most common in young adults; NF1 patients may present in childhood</td><td>Trunk = head, upper extremity, lower extremity, neck</td><td>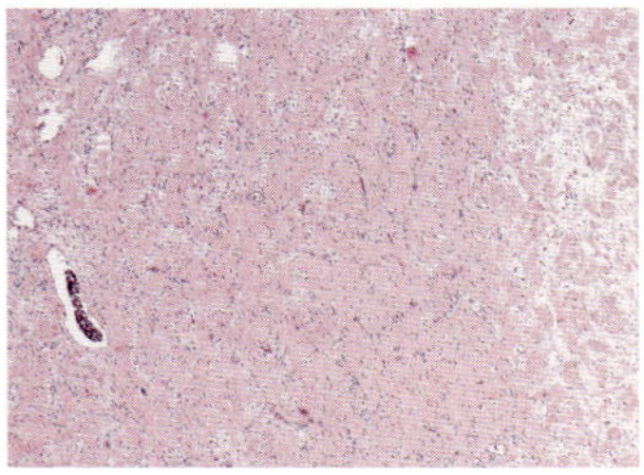</td><td>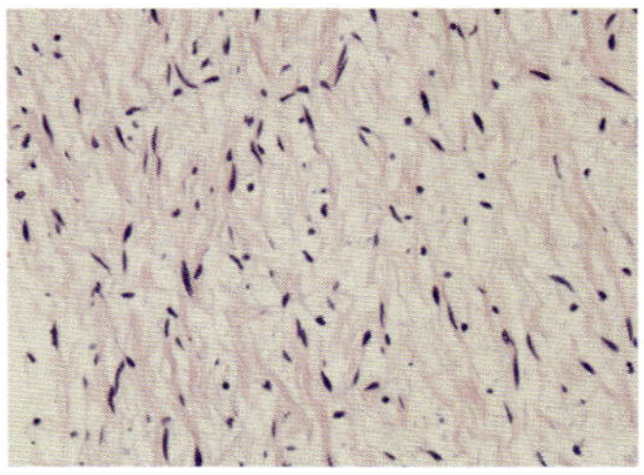</td></tr>
<tr><td colspan="6">Circumscribed: Random or subtly palisading assortment of Schwann cells, fibroblasts, axons, and collagen fibers often with scattered mast cells. Mitoses absent to very rare.
Diffuse: Same features as above but diffusely infiltrating (usually subcutis).
Plexiform: Multiple intraneural (encapsulated by perineurium) tumors with or without diffuse component.
Others: Pigmented, epithelioid, 'ancient', myxoid, cellular, intraneural (encapsulated), dendritic cutaneous.
IHC: Schwann cells S-100 positive, fibroblasts CD34 positive, axons neurofilament positive.</td></tr>
<tr><td>Perineurioma
Intraneural
Soft tissue
Sclerosing
Reticular
Others</td><td>Rare</td><td>Intraneural: children to young adults.
Soft tissue: Broad age but middle aged adults most common
Sclerosing: young adults
M > F</td><td>Intraneural: major extremity nerves.

Soft tissue: Extremities, trunk, head and neck, 2:1 superficial: deep

Sclerosing: Fingers, hands >> elsewhere</td><td>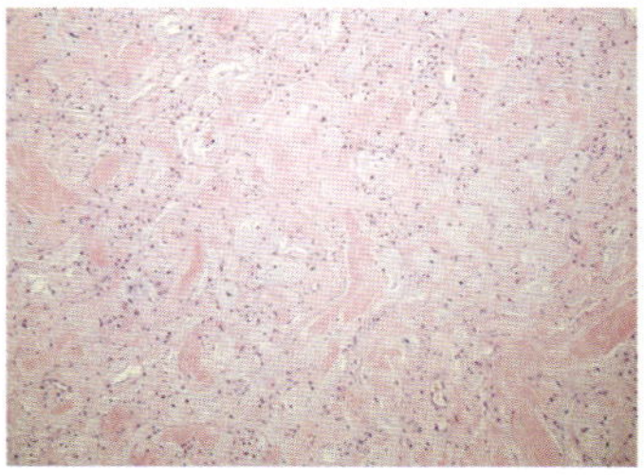</td><td>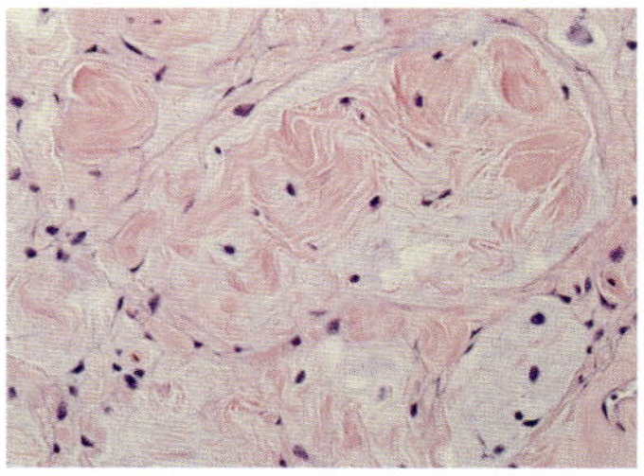</td></tr>
<tr><td colspan="6">Intraneural: Affected nerve contains tight balls of increased perineurial cells with central residual axons and Schwann cells set in a fibrous endoneurial background.
Soft tissue: Circumscribed, unencapsulated nodule of slender, very elongate spindled perineurial cells that can storiform, form fascicles or lamellae and often swirl around thin-walled vessels. Background can be fibrous, myxoid or both. Can be hypocellular, hypercellular or both. Mitotic rate generally low. May have cytologic atypia (does not affect behavior).
Sclerosing: Circumscribed unencapsulated nodule that is densely fibrous with cords, clusters and perivascular and/or perineural arrangements of cuboidal or epithelioid uniform cells (+/- spindled perineurial cells).
Reticular/Myxoid: Hypocellular due to extensive myxoid stroma sometimes with tumor cells forming fishnet like patterns.
IHC: perineurial cells are EMA positive (but may be focal) GLUT1, collagen IV and laminin positive. Claudin-1 and SMA may be positive. CD34 may be positive in soft tissue variant.</td></tr>
<tr><td>Hybrid peripheral nerve sheath tumors</td><td>Rare</td><td>Adults mostly.
M = F.
May be sporadic or associated with NF1, NF2 or NF3 (schwannomatosis)</td><td>Primarily subcutaneous or dermal/subcutis of extremities, head and neck, trunk</td><td>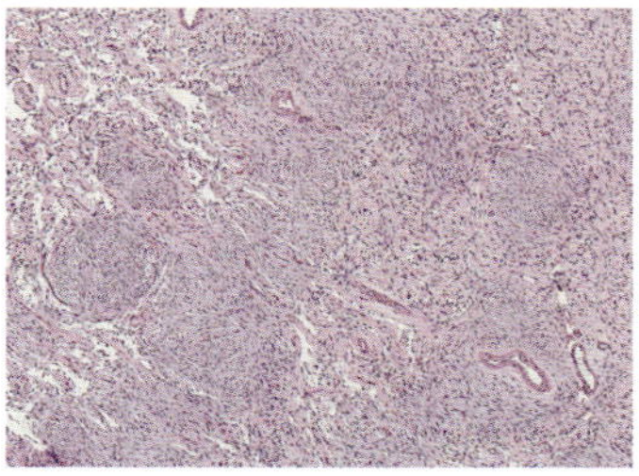</td><td></td></tr>
<tr><td colspan="6">Benign peripheral nerve sheath differentiation in combinations of neurofibroma/schwannoma, schwannoma/perineurioma, neurofibroma/perineurioma and others. May have degenerative nuclear atypia ('ancient change') and low mitotic rate. May show plexiform architecture.
IHC: S-100 positive in schwannoma part; S-100, CD34 and neurofilaments in neurofibroma part; EMA and GLUT1 in perineurioma part.</td></tr>
</table>

Table 13.4: Continued from page 256

Tumor	Incidence	Age and sex	Body site (in order of occurrence)	Histopathology description including IHC Medium magnification	High magnification
Paraganglioma of head and neck	Common	Middle age M = F for carotid body and F > M for vagal body lesions	Neck or any site along the vagus nerve	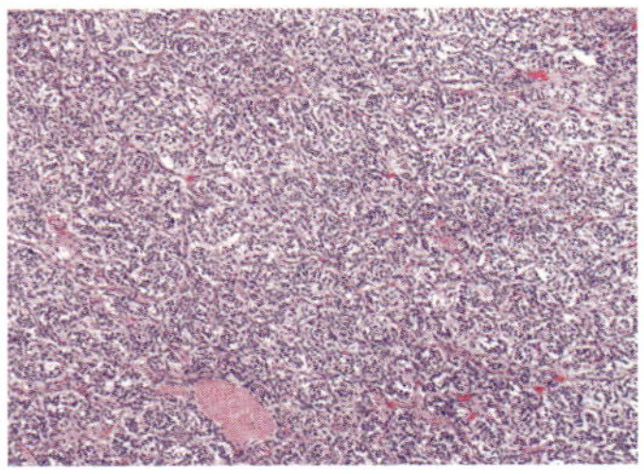	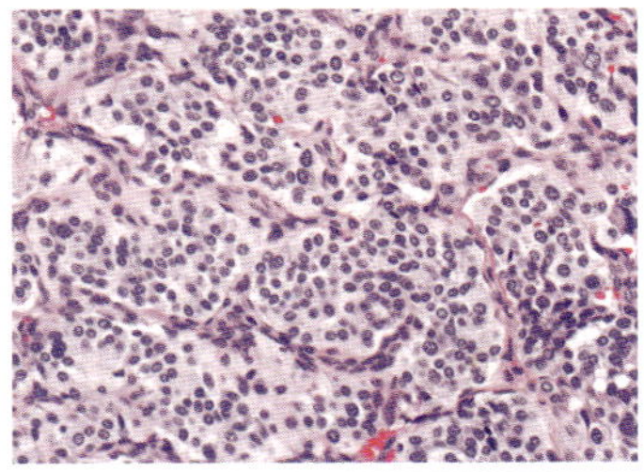
Clusters or balls of cells separated by fibrous bands (Zellballen). Tumor cells are usually round with a moderate N/C ratio and clear to basophilic to eosinophilic cytoplasm. Nuclei are usually uniform, but scattered large nuclei and multilobulated nuclei may be present. Mitotic rate is usually low. Prominent vessels often with hemorrhage and hemosiderin deposition. IHC: tumor cells positive for NSE, chromogranin and synaptophysin; sustentacular cells positive for S-100 protein. Some cases have necrosis and increased mitoses.					
Ectopic meningioma	Rare	Children to young adults, most commonly. May be congenital	Superficial scalp, and soft tissue/ subcutis/dermis over spine	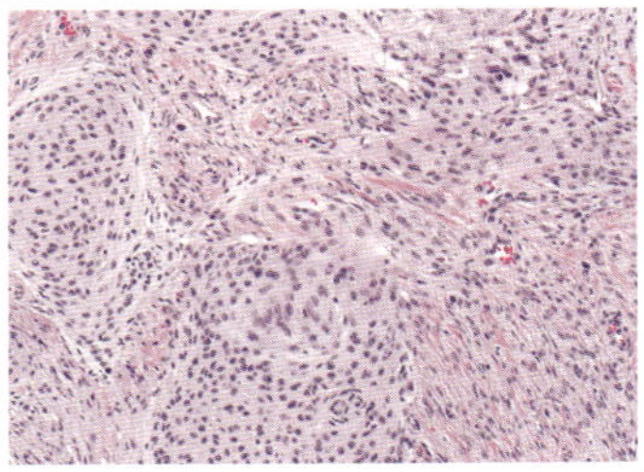	
Most commonly of meningothelial type with syncytial nodules of uniform meningothelial cells with scattered nuclear pseudoinclusions. Some tumors consist of less obvious strands and nests set in fibrous stroma. May have psammoma bodies. IHC: Positive for EMA and negative for S-100 protein like perineurioma.					
Hemangioblastoma of soft tissue	Very rare	Older adults. F > M	Extremities; may be associated with a peripheral nerve	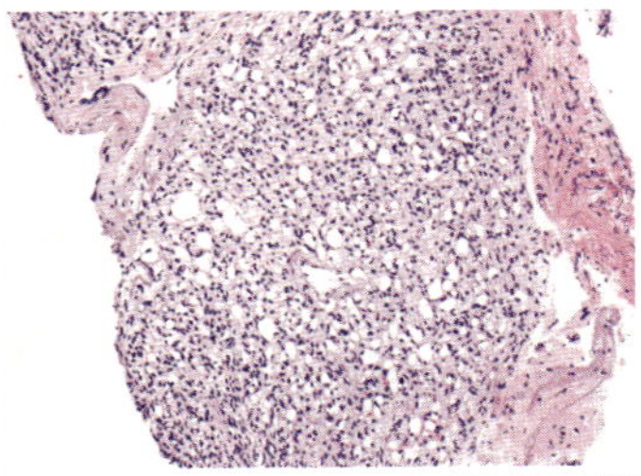	
Cellular neoplasm of multivacuolated, clear cells and plump spindle cells enmeshed in a prominent capillary network. May have nuclear atypia but mitotic rate is low. No necrosis. IHC tumor cells strongly express S-100 protein and α-inhibin and other SMA. Negative for keratins, CD10 and RCC antigen expression.					
Nerve sheath myxoma	Rare	Broad age range but young to middle aged adults most common M slightly > F	Usually confined to dermis Hand most common, arm, leg, foot, head and neck, trunk	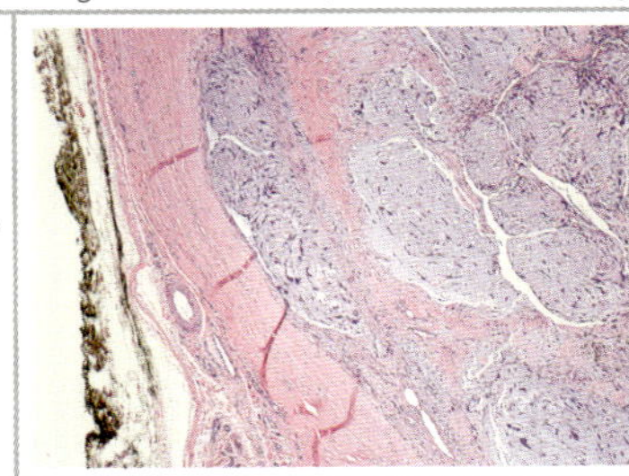	
Multilobulated myxoid tumor mostly of dermis with pushing border. Lobules often divided by thick fibrous bands. Hypocellular with bland spindle or epithelioid cells sometimes clustering together, forming a meshwork, or rings. Tumor cells include mostly Schwann cells (S-100 +), but also fibroblasts (CD34 +) and perineurial cells (EMA+).					
Intermediate: can recur aggressively and/or rarely metastasizes					
Ependymoma of soft tissue	Rare	Children to young adults but broad age range	Exclusive to subcutaneous tissue of coccygeal region	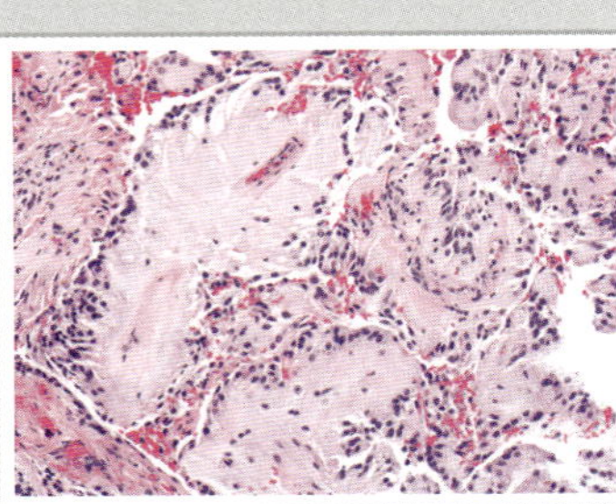	
Cellular, minimally atypical, glial to epithelial appearing tumor with true and, more commonly, pseudo-rosettes (perivascular). Myxopapillary variant has pseudopapillae and abundant myxoid matrix. GFAP strongly diffusely positive; S-100 protein usually positive. May also express EMA and keratins.					

Table 13.4: Continued from page 257

Tumor	Incidence	Age and sex	Body site (in order of occurrence)	Histopathology description including IHC: Medium magnification	High magnification
Malignant: can recur and commonly metastasizes					
Malignant peripheral nerve sheath tumor (MPNST) Low grade High grade Epithelioid MPNST with divergent differentiation MPNST ex schwannoma Malignant melanotic schwannoma Perineurial MPNST	Common	Adults most commonly (20-50 years). NF1 patients tend to be younger M = F Up to 50% of patients have NF1 Up to 10% have history of radiation	Usually subfascial. Extremities, head and neck, trunk	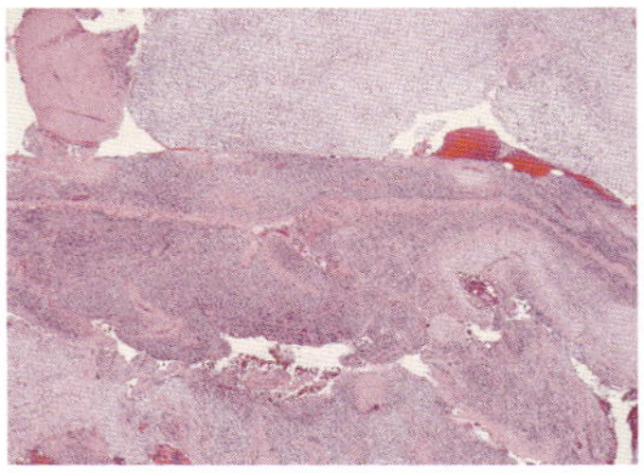	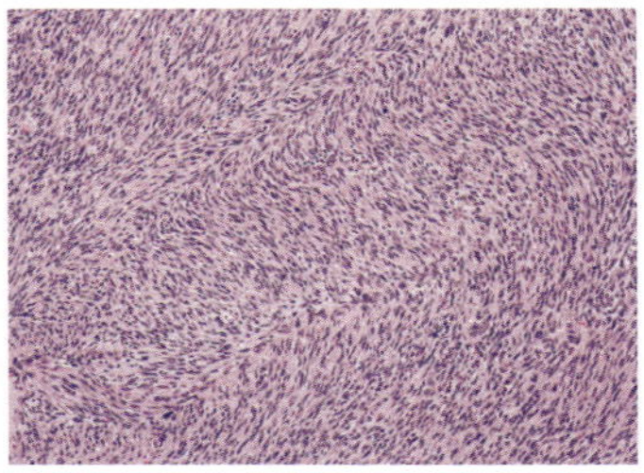
Notoriously variable in appearance but most (80%) are fascicular spindle cell tumors, and most of these are hypercellular with necrosis, numerous mitotic figures and malignant nuclear features. Intratumoral heterogeneity is also prominent (with varying cellularity, myxoid change, and fibrosis). 15% Have heterologous elements including rhabdomyosarcoma (also called malignant Triton tumor), osteosarcoma, angiosarcoma, chondrosarcoma or benign glandular/ epithelial elements. 5% are epithelioid and these are commonly diffusely S-100 protein positive, whereas spindle fascicular MPNST usually shows only patchy positivity. GFAP and neurofilaments sometimes positive; rarely EMA positive. Heterologous elements express antigens appropriate to differentiation.					
Synovial sarcoma of nerve	Rare	Adults, young to middle-aged, but also children M = F	Usually affects a larger peripheral nerve of extremities or trunk	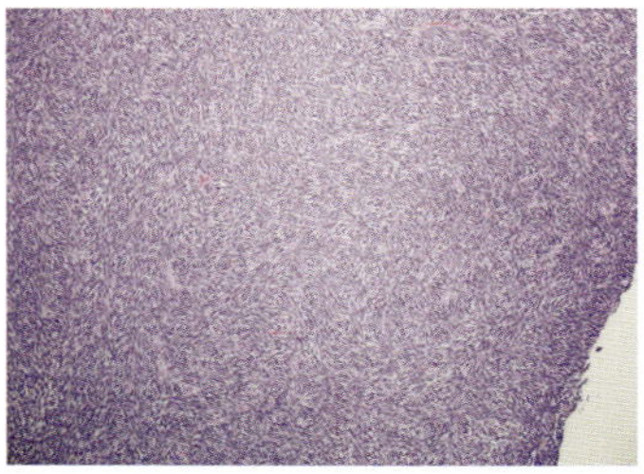	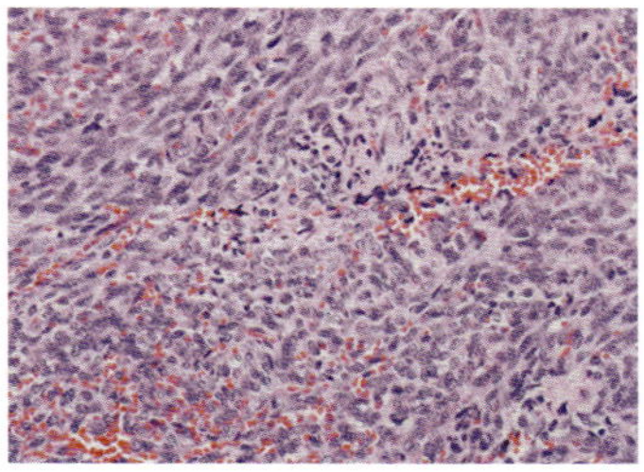
Usually consists of the monophasic spindle cell type of SS when occurring intraneurally, but biphasic examples also occur. Does not usually appear plexiform. **Monophasic**: Cellular fascicular growth of spindle cells, often with only mild to moderate atypia but relatively high N/C ratio. **IHC**: Usually EMA +, usually simple keratin +, majority strongly TLE-1 positive; can be focally S-100 protein positive. Requires genetic confirmation showing t(X;18) (or rarely t(X;20)).					
Incidence note: 'Common to very common' indicates that a medium sized practice will treat at least several to dozens of patients with the lesion annually, 'Uncommon to rare' indicates the same practice size will treat one to two patients with the lesion every five years, 'Rare to very rare' indicates the same sized practice will see zero to one patient with the lesion every 20 years.					

Connective, subcutaneous, and other soft tissues

		Head/ face/ neck	Upper limb/ shoulder	Lower limb/ hip	Thorax	Abdomen	Pelvis	Trunk	Overlap*	NOS
MPNST	MPNST	33	44	81	26	14	42	19	4	1
MPNST	MPNST with rhabdomyoblastic differentiation	0	0	3	0	1	1	0	0	0
MPNST	Malignant perineurioma	0	0	1	0	0	0	0	0	0
	Malignant granular cell tumor	0	1	2	2	1	2	1	0	0
Malignant paraganglioma	Malignant extra-adnenal paraganglioma	0	0	0	0	0	1	0	0	0
Malignant paraganglioma	Malignant paraganglioma	1	0	1	1	4	4	0	0	1
	Total	34	45	88	29	20	50	20	4	2

* "A tumor that overlaps the boundaries of two or more subcategories and whose point of origin cannot be determined." (Fritz et al., 2000)

Figure 13.4 Neural/perineural tumors of the soft tissue by site for cases in 13 SEER registries diagnosed between 1994 and 2008.

which can result in incomplete initial excision and a risk for local recurrence.

Nerve sheath myxomas are benign but exhibit a local recurrence rate of up to 50%.

Perineuriomas are benign with a very low rate of local recurrence (Hornick et al. 2005).

Paragangliomas of the head and neck behave in a benign fashion in approximately 90% of cases. However, metastases may occur in up to 10% of cases; those with only lymph node involvement have a 75% five year survival, whereas the five year survival diminishes to 10-15% in patients with distant metastases (Lee et al. 2002).

Regarding peripherally occurring rare CNS tumors: ectopic meningiomas are benign, soft tissue ependymomas can metastasize in up to 20% of cases, sometimes decades after initial diagnosis, and soft tissue hemangioblastoma appears to behave in a benign fashion (fewer than 20 cases reported).

Malignant neural and perineural tumors

Historically, malignant peripheral nerve sheath tumor was associated with a grim prognosis with five year survival rates hovering around 15% (in NF1 patients) and 50% (in sporadic cases). However, more recent series report five year disease specific survival rates ranging up to 85% for patients with and without NF1 (Folpe et al. 2010, Stucky et al. 2012). A Mayo Clinic review of 175 patients treated from 1985 to 2010 reported the following features auguring a poor outcome: size >/= 5 cm, local recurrence, high tumor grade (using a Mayo Clinic specific method), and trunk location (Stucky et al. 2012). Recent better outcomes may be related to improved local control by surgery and radiation as well as earlier detection.

Whether histologic grade predicts behavior is controversial with most experts noting that 'low grade' MPNST does not portend an improved survival. However, a specific grading scheme tailored just to MPNST may have predictive value; such a system has yet to be disseminated and accepted (Rodriguez et al. 2012). As with many other malignancies, molecular genetic findings are being assessed for prognostic value. A sampling of recently reported negative prognostic features includes: CDK4 gene gain or amplification, increased FOXM1 protein expression (Yu et al. 2011), phosphorylation of the MET protein (Torres et al. 2011), inactivation of p14 and p16 (Endo et al. 2011). Additional studies will determine the prognostic value of these and other molecular markers.

Malignant granular cell tumors (~1% of all granular cell tumors) behave as high grade sarcomas. Features associated with metastases include marked nuclear atypia with high nuclear to cytoplasmic ratio and prominent nucleoli, cell spindling, tumor necrosis, mitotic rate >2/10 hpf and Ki67 index > 10%; with three or more of these features, there is a 50% incidence of metastasis (Fanburg-Smith et al. 1998).

It is difficult to predict behavior of head and neck paragangliomas. However, vascular invasion, increased mitotic rate, and necrosis have been reported to be significantly associated with metastasis.

Additional laboratory testing

Immunohistochemistry

Table 13.4 includes the immunohistochemical profile of neural/perineural tumors. As with nearly all other soft tissue tumors, no single antibody is 100% specific for a single tumor. Antibody reactivity is contextual and augments rather than supercedes histologic features.

Routine cytogenetics

Karyotyping may be of value in the diagnosis of perineurioma (chromosome 22 and sometimes chromosome 10 abnormalities in sclerosing variant) and malignant peripheral nerve sheath tumor (complex aneuploidy in most cases). Perineurioma may resemble low grade fibromyxoid sarcoma (LGFMS) histologically and to some extent shares immunohistochemical results, as both may be reactive for EMA and Claudin-1. However, LGFMS commonly exhibits one of two specific translocations: (t(7;16)(q33;p11) or t(11;16)(p11;p11). Synovial sarcoma, the major sarcoma in the differential of MPNST, also demonstrates translocations that may be identified by karyotyping or FISH: t(X;18)(p11;q11) or t(X;20)(p11;q13). Fluorescence in situ hybridization may be performed on formalin-fixed, paraffin embedded tissues or touch prints and may be the only option in cases where karyotyping fails or fresh tissue is not obtained.

Molecular genetics

PCR is an alternative method that can find the specific translocations described above in the differential diagnosis of perineurioma and synovial sarcoma.

Although laborious, sequencing of the NF1 or NF2 genes in patients with NF1 and NF2 can provide limited prognostic information that may be clinically useful. For example, patients with deletion of the entire gene develop a severe form of NF1 with increased risk for MPNST, while those with a specific 3 base pair deletion in exon 17 of the gene have a mild expression of the disease with no risk for MPNST (Jouhilahti et al. 2010). NF2 patients with truncating nonsense mutations or frameshift mutations have a more severe form of the disease than those patients with large deletions, in-frame indels and missense mutations (Carroll 2012). At least some patients with schwannomatosis have alterations of the SMARCB1 tumor suppressor gene; however, not as much work has occurred in determining genotype:phenotype correlations in this disease.

Molecular markers may predict behavior in MPNST. These include overexpressed activated MET (Torres et al. 2011), overexpressed lysine-specific demethylase 1 (Schildhaus et al. 2011), inactivation of p14, p15, and p16 (Endo et al. 2011), and CDK4 and FOXM1 alterations (Yu et al. 2011) among others. These are early basic research results, but delineating these and other genetic level (or epigenetic level) changes could lead to targeted, more effective therapy for MPNST.

RADIOLOGY

A peripheral nerve sheath tumor (PNST) usually appears as a several centimeter, discrete, fusiform shaped mass originating from a peripheral nerve and represents either a schwannoma or a neurofibroma. On CT imaging, these may show decreased density due to the myelin sheath fat content. MRI typically shows tapering ends of the tumor with longitudinal axis oriented with the nerve. MR may show a T2 target sign or an enhancement target sign where the peripheral aspect of the tumor shows a rim with respectively brighter T2 signal or brighter enhancement. Occasionally, fatty muscle atrophy can be shown on T1 images in the distribution associated with the nerve. The split fat sign can be seen as a beak or triangle of fat tissue that tapers away from each pole of the fusiform mass. The fascicular sign has multiple low signal foci on T2 or PD images correlating with numerous nerve fascicles seen end-on when imaged in cross-section (Chee, 2011).

If in fact the nerve of origin is identifiable, then gross features may be helpful to differentiate between neuromas and schwannomas. Beaman, 2004 suggests in schwannomas, the nerve is eccentric to the mass. On the other hand, the neurofibroma should lie central to the nerve and may obliterate visualization of the nerve. However, (Jee, 2004) in a series of 52 patients showed no statistically significant difference for central versus peripheral orientation of the affected nerve in distinguishing schwannoma from neuroma. Likewise, no significant difference was shown between the two tumors for cystic areas and peripheral enhancement or contrast target sign. The series from Jee, 2004 did show statistical significance for T2 target sign (58% neurofibroma, 15% schwannoma), central enhancement (75% neurofibroma, 8% schwannoma), fascicular appearance on T2 images (25% neurofibroma, 63% schwannoma), and thin hyperintense rim on T2 images (8% neurofibroma, 58% schwannoma). In our experience, the fascicular appearance is not as common as a smudged or dirty appearance to the tumor on T2 images. The fascicular sign is related to enlargement of the underlying nerve fascicules which appear as dots when viewed on transverse images. Perhaps the 'dirty' appearance results when enlargement causes distortion and discrete fascicles can no longer be discerned.

There is clearly overlap in the appearance of the two benign PNST tumors. Finding a split fat sign and a nerve of origin will at least help the radiologist determine the lesion is a PNST. The ability to distinguish between schwannoma and neurofibroma is an interesting exercise and may be clinically important to the surgeon for preoperative planning and to prepare the patient for surgery. The schwannoma can usually be surgically removed while sparing the nerve of origin whereas a neurofibroma is inseparable from the nerve and requires the nerve to be sacrificed.

In addition to distinguishing between the two benign peripheral nerve sheath tumors, the radiologist must also assess if the tumor has malignant features worrisome for a peripheral malignant nerve sheath tumor (PMNST). In the setting of neurofibromatosis type 1, the patient may have multiple neurofibromas and these patients are at higher risk to have a neurofibroma malignancy (Ducatman 1986). Chee, 2011 estimated approximately 50% of MPNST occur in the setting of neurofibromatosis; however, only about 5% of patients with neurofibromatosis develop a MPNST. In a series by Wasa, 2010, features that favored a PMNST include large size, on average 14.5 cm; whereas benign neurofibromas averaged 6 cm. Unfortunately, there was significant overlap in size between PNST and PMNST. Heterogeneous appearance on T1 images, perilesion edema, intra-tumor cystic change and peripheral enhancement also favor PMNST. Features which were not statistically significant for distinguishing PMNST from neurofibroma include margin definition and T2 heterogeneity (Wasa, 2010). We present a case of epithelioid MPNST, (see Case 13.7). There is scant literature describing the imaging appearance of epithelioid MPNST.

Despite the significant overlap in appearance between neuroma, schwannoma and PMNST, the radiologist hopefully can at least determine whether a given tumor is neurogenic and then render an opinion regarding possible malignant features.

Neurofibromas are divided into three categories including: local (90%), plexiform and diffuse. The plexiform neurofibromas are essentially pathognomonic of Neurofibromatosis type 1. The diffuse subtype is quite rare. Diffuse neurofibroma tends to be a poorly defined, infiltrative lesion that spreads along connective tissue septa. It typically involves the skin and hence is evaluated clinically.

In a series of 339 patients published by Hassell in 2008, only 10 had advanced imaging. 50% of diffuse neurofibromas showed a plaque like growth pattern and 30% had an infiltrative pattern with the remaining lesions showing a mixed or mass like pattern. 90% of diffuse neurofibroma involved the skin and subcutaneous tissues, with 20% infiltrating into deep muscle structures. The lesion showed intense enhancement and most were either mildly or markedly hyperintense on T2 images. In the entire series, gender distribution was about equal and the mean age was 35 years. Overall, 34% of diffuse neurofibromatosis involved the extremities, 35% the trunk, and 28% the head and neck regions. 3% of the patient's had an underlying malignancy of which approximately half were malignant peripheral nerve sheath tumors.

Plexiform neurofibromas are the hallmark lesion of neurofibromatosis type 1. They typically show diffuse nerve thickening and nodularity with involvement of nerve branches. The appearance has been likened to a 'bag of worm'. The lesions are typically T1 low signal or isointense to muscle and high signal on fluid sensitive sequences. Enhancement is variable. STIR sequences are ideally suited for imaging these extensive lesions because the fat suppression is homogeneous over the large field of views commonly needed; and, the neurofibromas are consistently very conspicuous with high signal on STIR sequences.

Perineurioma is a rare benign peripheral nerve sheath tumor. There are two types of lesions seen: intra-neural perineurioma and extra-neural perineurioma also called soft tissue perineurioma. Of the soft tissue variant, approximately half occur in the subcutaneous tissues (Hornick 2005) and the sexes are almost equally affected. 44% occur in the lower extremity and 23% occur in the upper extremity. The intraneural subtype causes symmetric tubular enlargement without affecting side branches, thus distinguishing it from plexiform neurofibroma. The intraneural perineuriomas have T2 high signal and enhancement with rope-like enlargement of a long segment of a nerve (Kransdorf 2006).

Granular cell tumor is typically a benign superficial tumor that arises from nerve tissue. These are not usually imaged because of their superficial location and indeed, we do not have imaging of a case. Adequate surgery is usually curative of these benign lesions; however, there are rare malignant granular cell tumors. Granular cell tumors are common in the head and neck region and particularly involve the tongue. In a small series of granular cell tumors of the extremity, Blacksin 2005, found the tumors had T1 iso or hyperintensity to muscle and T2 high signal peripherally low T2 signal centrally. They found malignant lesions tended to be larger than 4 cm, showed invasive margins and had association with major nerve trunks.

SURGERY

Schwannoma

Marginal excision of these tumors results in a very low rate of recurrence. Extreme care must be taken to avoid injury to the involved nerve during dissection to separate the tumor from the nerve.

Granular cell tumor

Recurrence is rare following marginal excision of these tumors.

Plexiform neurofibroma

These tumors can be quite challenging to manage. Occurring exclusively in patients with neurofibromatosis, they are typically large, infiltrative, and multiple. Attempts at surgical resection can be associated with substantial blood loss and relatively high rates of recurrence. Most are asymptomatic, or mildly symptomatic, and therefore can be managed conservatively. Occasionally, surgery will be indicated if a tumor becomes particularly disabling or is impinging on vital structures.

GRAY AREA

Although malignant degeneration can occur in these tumors (typically in deeply situated tumors of long standing) with relatively high frequency (2-29%), prophylactic excision is rarely possible due to the extensive and multiple nature of these tumors. Rapid growth of a solid area in these otherwise typically soft and spongy tumors should raise concern of malignant degeneration.

GRAY AREA

Symptomatic patients with painful tumors that involve the skin can achieve significant relief with staged partial resection of the tumor, allowing interval healing, until enough of the tumor has been removed to improve symptoms. However, continued growth of the residual tumor will often occur in the intermediate term, resulting in recurrence of symptoms.

PERINEURIOMA

Marginal excision of these tumors results in a low recurrence rate. However, excision of an intraneural perineurioma can result in significant associated nerve damage. Since malignant degeneration has not been reported in these tumors, any decision to remove them must be weighed against the likelihood and consequences of possible associated nerve damage.

Malignant peripheral nerve sheath tumor

Malignant peripheral nerve sheath tumors (MPNSTs) are high-grade malignancies and should be treated with wide resection. Surgery of these tumors can prove particularly challenging, even in relation to sarcoma surgery in general, particularly when they occur in a plexiform neurofibroma in patients with neurofibromatosis.

MEDICAL ONCOLOGY OF NEURAL AND PERINEURAL TUMORS OF SOFT TISSUES

Malignant peripheral nerve sheath tumor

MPNST is slightly more preponderant in women than in men with a median age at diagnosis of 30 to 35 years of age. Most MPNST occur in patients with a genetic anomaly of the neurofibromatosis (NF) 1 gene, which causes neurofibromatosis type 1. The prevalence of MPNST in this genetically autosomal dominant disease is about 5%. In the general population, MPNST incidence is much lower (0.001%) (Ducatman et al. 1986). There is no specific chemotherapy treatment to this type of sarcoma. Tumors smaller than 5 to 10 cm are treated by surgical resection (Zou et al. 2009). The bigger the tumor, the worse the prognosis. Any tumor greater than 5 cm should be evaluated for multidisciplinary chemotherapy therapy, including neoadjuvant of adjuvant chemotherapy (Kroep, et al. 2011). The general medical oncology principles apply to this sarcoma subtype (See Chapter X). In patients with NF, lifelong awareness of MPNST is indicated (Anghileri, et al. 2006).

Neurofibromatosis type I

NF1 gene is on chromosome 17 (Kalamarides et al 2011, Upadhyaya 2011). The product of the NF1 gene is a large and complex protein called neurofibromin, which is primarily active in neural cells as a regulator of cell division. NF1 is the most common type of the neurofibromatoses. By age 10, patients have already some of the characteristics signs of neurofibromatosis, which include light brown spots on the skin ('café-au-lait' spots), two or more hamartomas on the iris of the eye, tumor on the optic nerve, a larger than normal head circumference, and abnormal development of the spine, the skull, and bones such as the tibia, and multiple neuromas. NF1 also increases the risk of tumor development, particularly, meningiomas, gliomas, pheochromocytomas, and more rarely, leukemia.

Neurofibromatosis type II

The NF2 gene product is a tumor-suppressor protein called merlin, a cytoskeletal protein. The merlin gene is located on chromosome 22q. NF2 gene mutation is less common and causes slow-growing tumors on the eighth cranial nerves. Symptoms include deafness, cataracts at an early age or retinal changes that may affect vision, and other nervous system tumors. NF type 2 also increases the risk of meningiomas and ependymomas.

Schwannomatosis

Schwannomatosis is the development of multiple schwannomas everywhere in the body except on the vestibular branch of the 8th cranial nerve. Major symptoms include motor or sensory changes by compression of nerves or adjacent tissue. The gene alteration responsible for schwannomatosis is not established.

Neurofibromatosis type I pathogenesis and potential therapies

Ras is a small GTPase, which is related in structure to the Gα subunit of heterotrimeric G proteins (large GTPases). GTPases hydrolyze a bound guanosine triphosphate (GTP) molecule into guanosine diphosphate (GDP). Ras GTPase activity is rather inefficient and requires additional controls (Spyk et al. 2011).

In many cancers, mutations of Ras cause this G-protein to be in a permanent activated state, with bound GT. However, in NF, the dysregulation of Ras occurs at the control level for Ras. A Ras GTPase activating protein (GAP) binds to and stabilizes the GTPase catalytic machinery of Ras by forcing the catalyzation of GTP to GDP, causing Ras to be deactivated. Guanine nucleotide exchange factors (GEFs) catalyzes the release of GDP from Ras. Thus GEFs facilitates Ras activation. The balance between GEF and GAP activity determines the guanine nucleotide status of Ras, thereby regulating Ras activity. The binding and unbinding of GTP causes conformational changes into activated and inactivated states, respectively. Hence, activation and deactivation of Ras and other small G proteins are controlled by cycling between the active GTP-bound and inactive GDP-bound forms (Reuter et al. 2000). Neurofibromin is a regulator of GTPase activating proteins (GAPs) and functions as a tumor suppressor gene (Klose et al. 1998). In NF1, where neurofibromin activity is decreased or lacking, Ras remains activated because the absence of a fully functioning neurofibromin prevents normal inactivation of Ras through GAP. The loss of inhibitory control on the ras oncoprotein induces cellular proliferation, resulting in tumor development. Ras also attaches to plasma membranes and Golgi apparatus for optimal cellular functions. This attachment adjacent to the C-terminal CaaX box of Ras depends on prenylation and/or palmitoylation of one or two Cys residues, respectively, which are mediated by farnesyltransferase and geranylgeranyltransferase (Berndt et al. 2011). Thus Ras inhibition could happen at various molecular levels.

Inhibition of farnesylation interferes with the membrane binding and has been tested in cancers with mutated Ras. Farnesyl transferase inhibitors include salirasib, tipifarnib, and lonafarnib and others. These drugs exhibit profound anti-oncogenic effects in many cancer cell lines. Other non-specific inhibitors of GTPase include the botulic toxin and fusidic acid, an antibiotic agent. Reovirus target Ras activation and is being studied in clinical trials as an oncolytic viral therapy (Thurukkumaran, et al. 2009). None of these agents have been studied for MPNST.

RADIATION ONCOLOGY

Schwannoma

Neural/perineural tumors are composed of a histologic variety of tumors originating from peripheral nerves. The most common location of intracranial schwannomas is the vestibulocochlear nerve. Standard treatments of these tumors have transitioned from surgery to radiation therapy over many years. Morbidity of surgery is relatively high compared to radiation therapy. For example, facial nerve function is preserved in only 60% of patients who undergo surgery while 98% of patients who undergo radiation therapy preserve facial nerve function. A big difference also exists for hearing preservation in favor of radiation therapy. Tumor control rates with radiation therapy are similar to the excellent control rates seen with surgery. Radiation therapy for acoustic schwannomas is commonly delivered using radiosurgical technique in which one treatment consisting of a single dose of between 12 to 13 Gray is used.

Granular cell tumor

Radiation therapy for granular cell tumor is generally not recommended. Surgery alone is usually highly effective for benign granular cell tumor so no radiation therapy is needed. Malignant granular cell tumor does not respond well to radiation therapy, and there is no proven benefit for the use of radiation therapy for these tumors.

Plexiform neurofibroma

Plexiform neurofibroma is usually treated with surgery. When surgery is contraindicated, case reports have demonstrated successful use of radiation therapy for local control and palliative benefit (Robertson et al. 2004).

Malignant peripheral nerve sheath tumors (MPNST)

Malignant peripheral nerve sheath tumors are aggressive tumors usually treated with a multimodality approach. Surgery with negative margins should be attempted. Adjuvant radiation therapy clearly improves local control and possibly survival. The Mayo Clinic reviewed 134 patients treated at their institution. 54% underwent radiation therapy as part of the initial treatment. Surgical margin status was statistically significant for survival. Both surgical margin status and the use of radiation therapy were statistically significant for local control. In particular, radiation dose of at least 60 Gray improved local control (Wong et al. 1998).

Perineurioma

There is no known role for the use of radiation therapy for perineurioma.

CASES

Case 13.1 Schwannoma

Clinical history and presentation

The patient is a 75-year-old man who notes a mass in the posterior aspect of the left knee which has been present for the past 3 years. He reports this mass has not grown in the last couple of years, but that it has become slightly more painful. He relates pain in the knee with ambulation and with prolonged standing.

The patient has a palpable nodular mass in the left popliteal fossa. He has exquisite tenderness with palpation of this mass, which radiates down to the mid-calf level.

Surgical findings and comments

Findings at surgery reveal a tumor within the substance of the posterior tibial nerve. The tumor is removed without damaging the associated nerve.

Radiology findings

This patient's lesion, **Case figs 13.1a** through **13.1g**, is a fusiform, soft tissue density mass visible on radiographs due to the adjacent fat tissues outlining the mass. The MR images show the tumor originates from the sciatic nerve and has the classic fusiform shape oriented with the nerve of origin. There is also the 'split fat sign' shown at the ends of the lesion by a triangle of fat. The tumor has intense enhancement. Traditionally, schwannomas were thought to have an eccentric relationship to the nerve of origin; however sequential axial images showed this schwannoma to align centrally with the sciatic nerve. This underscores the unreliable nature of some of these imaging signs. Careful review of the axial T2 images did not show fascicles (no fascicular sign), instead, there is overall high signal with a 'dirty' or smudged appearance. Given the morphology and relationship to a nerve, a peripheral nerve tumor can be diagnosed with confidence. The absence of destruction, necrosis or infiltration is reassuring that there is no malignancy.

Also included is an additional case of schwannoma (**Case figs 13.1h** through **13.1l**) involving the tibial nerve. This case also shows the fusiform morphology aligning with the nerve of origin and the split fat sign. The lesion is somewhat unusual for being bilobed. The patient did not have Neurofibromatosis Type 1. Note the 'dirty' or smudged appearance on T2 imaging.

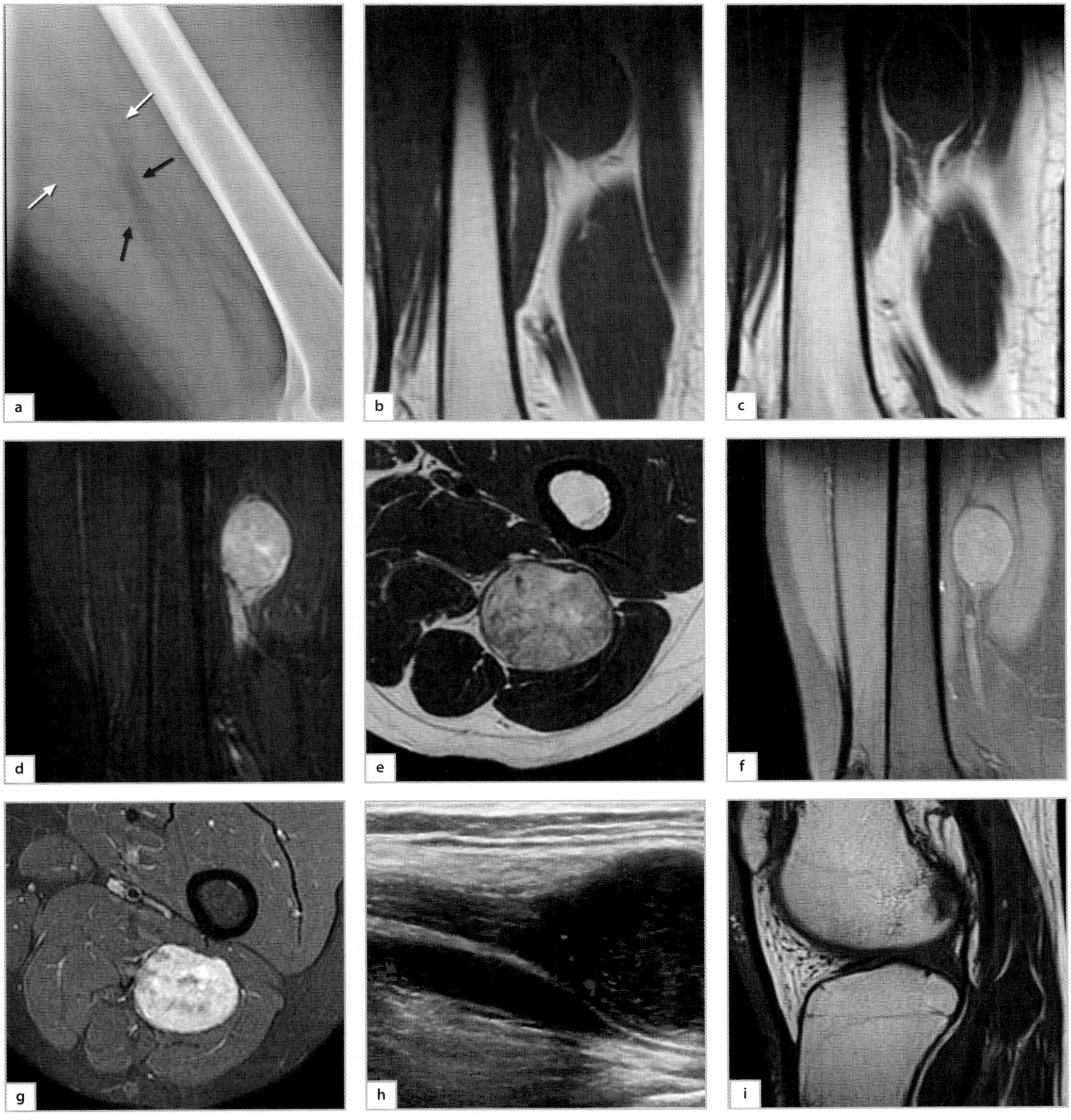

Case figure 13.1 Schwannoma imaging: **13.1a**. Is a lateral radiograph showing a subtle soft tissue mass in the posterior compartment of the thigh, white arrows. The black arrows show the fat beak distal to the mass. MR images. **13.1b** through **13-1c**: Are adjacent sagittal T1 images, **13.1d**: Sagittal STIR, **13.1e**: Axial T2, **13.1f**: Sagittal T1 fat saturated, **13.1g**: Axial T1 fat saturated post-contrast. The MR images show a T1 low signal, T2 high signal fusiform mass with tapering ends. The tumor did not show a distinct fascicular sign but does have the smudged or 'dirty' appearance on T2 images. The mass enhances intensely and uniformly. The sagittal image Figure 13-1c and sequential axial images (not included) show the mass blending with the sciatic nerve. Schwannoma – additional case. **13.1h**: Color doppler sagittal ultrasound image posterior to the knee in a 75 year old man shows a mildly heterogeneous fusiform solid mass with minimal vascularity that blends into the tibial nerve. **13.1i**: Is a sagittal T1 MR image, **13.1j**: Sagittal STIR MR image, **13.1k**: Axial T2 fat saturated MR image, and **13.1l**: Axial T1 fat saturated post-contrast MR image. The MR images show a bilobed fusiform T1 low signal, T2 and STIR high signal mass which blends with the tibial nerve. The nerve of origin was best demonstrated on sequential axial images which are not included. There is no fascicular sign but the mass did have a smudged or 'dirty' appearance on T2 images, Figure 13.1k, sometimes evident in schwannomas. The mass demonstrates intense, uniform enhancement.

Case figure 13.1: Continued from page 263

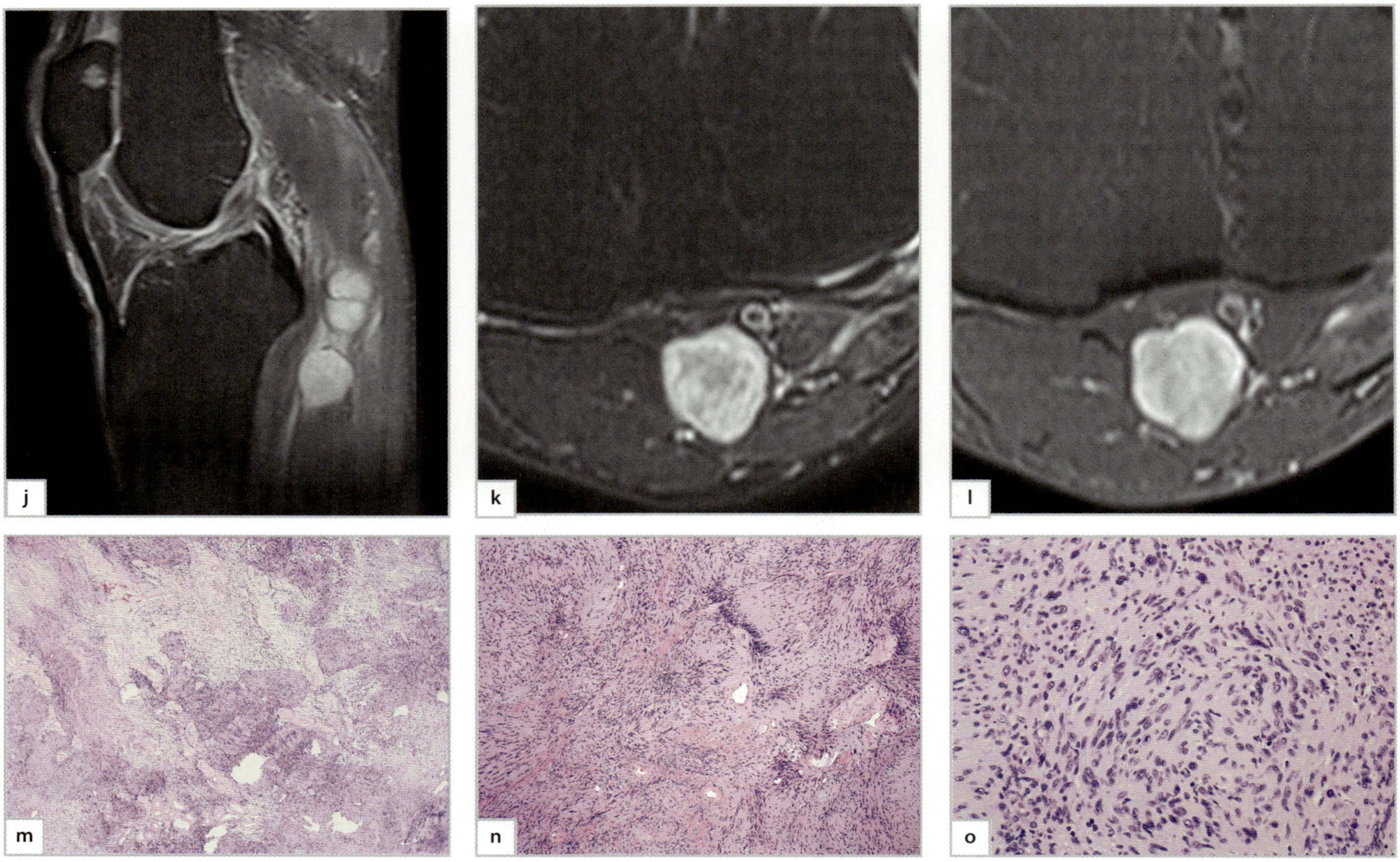

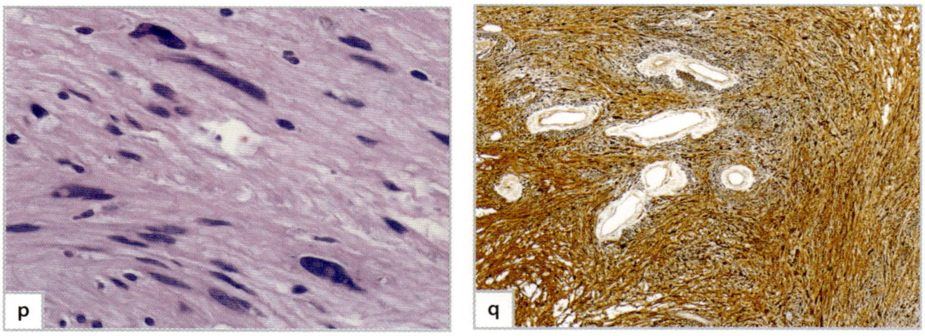

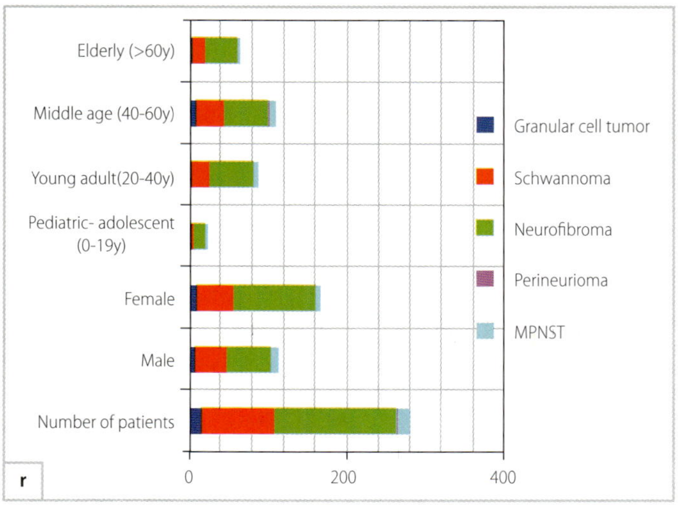

13.1m: Low magnification. Characteristic of schwannoma, the tumor displays hypercellular (Antoni A) areas and hypocellular (Antoni B) areas irregularly intermixed. Blood vessels with thick hyalinized walls are also apparent (these are common in long-standing tumors such as schwannoma). **13.1n**: Medium magnification. A Verocay body is seen in the upper portion of the field. It consists of a linear alignment of tumor nuclei forming a palisade with cytoplasm flowing away on either side of the nuclear lineup. This is a characteristic feature of schwannoma, but smooth muscle tumors may also rarely form these from neoplastic smooth muscle cells. **13.1o**: Higher magnification. A cellular area of the tumor consists of swirls of Schwann cells. The nuclei appear to float in a sea of pink cytoplasm because of indistinct cell borders. There is moderate variation in nuclear size and shape, a fairly unusual feature of a benign mesenchymal tumor but common in schwannomas. A single mitotic figure is present. Rare normal mitotic figures are acceptable in schwannoma. Lymphocytes are also present as scattered, small, dark round nuclei; sprinkles of lymphocytes are common in schwannoma. **13.1p**: High magnification. Often, schwannomas contain cells with degenerative atypia such as in this field. The nuclei are large, may be unusually shaped, and appear hyperchromatic. However, these features are considered innocuous when seen in conjunction with smudged or smearly chromatin rather than well-defined chromatin granularity. Nuclear vacuoles and breaks in the nuclear rim (chromatinic rim) are also degenerative changes. Care must be taken not to mistake these changes for malignant cells. **13.1q**: S-100 protein antibody at low magnification. Expression of S100 protein is diffuse and strong (notice the lack of staining of the thick-walled vessels). Although difficult to appreciate at this magnification, expression is both nuclear and cytoplasmic. **13.1r**: Nerve sheath tumors at UNM Health Sciences Center 2000-2010.

Pathology findings

Gross features

The specimen consists of a 2.7 × 1.8 × 1.6 cm portion of soft tissue covered by yellow adipose tissue. Cross sections reveal a circumscribed, tan to yellow nodule with a gritty texture. The nodule grossly abuts margins. A portion is collected fresh for cytogenetics, and a small amount is saved for tissue banking.

Microscopic features

Low magnification: The tumor is heterogeneous at low magnification with hypocellular (Antoni B areas) and hypercellular regions (Antoni A areas) (**Case fig. 13.1m**). Even at low power, hyalinized blood vessels are obvious. The tumor is sharply circumscribed. At slightly higher magnification, a well-formed palisade of tumor nuclei is apparent (Verocay body)(**Case fig. 13.1n**). There is no necrosis.

High magnification: Higher magnification reveals swirling and jumbled spindle cells. The cells exhibit indistinct cell borders so that the nuclei appear to float in a sea of pale pink cytoplasm. Scattered nuclei are larger and irregularly shaped but not hyperchromatic (**Case fig. 13.1o**). A rare mitotic figure is identified (less than 1 per 20 high power microscopic fields in this tumor)(**Case fig. 13.1o**). At highest magnification, some tumor cells contain enlarged, hyperchromatic nuclei with nuclear inclusions (**Case fig. 13.1p**). The chromatin in these cells is smudgy (not sharply granulated as in well preserved cells) consistent with degenerative cellular atypia. At 400x magnification, the cell cytoplasm appears wiry and the some of the nuclei display pointy ends with a curved shape (**Case fig. 13.1p**).

Special studies: The tumor shows diffuse strong expression of S-100 protein in both the cytoplasm and nuclei of tumor cells (**Case fig. 13.1q**). Non-staining cells in the tumor are lymphocytes and the endothelial nuclei of blood vessels.

Karyotyping is successful and reveals the following: 46,XY,-22,+mar in 19 cells with one non-clonal aberration (46,XY,t(1;2)(p33;q10)-22,+mar. Loss of chromosome 22q material or loss of the entire chromosome is a recurrent finding in schwannomas.

Pathologic differential or, why isn't it one of the following?

Neurofibroma, circumscribed type: Neurofibroma is also a peripheral nerve sheath tumor that is relatively common as a sporadic neoplasm. Like schwannoma, it contains Schwann cells (these are usually slender spindle cells with bipolar, elongate, sometimes wavy nuclei and wiry pale eosinophilic cytoplasm). However, neurofibroma also contains other cells including axons, CD34 expressing fibroblasts, and perineurial cells (all in varying intermixed proportions per individual tumor). Until recently, it was almost dogma that a schwannoma would not contain axons (identified by reactivity for neurofilaments). However, it has recently been recognized that schwannomas may contain scattered axons and otherwise still meet the definition of the tumor; namely, 99% plus of all the cells are benign Schwann cells.

Neurofibroma, by virtue of its varying cells, generally does not form Verocay bodies and often contains short broad swatches of collagen (courtesy of the fibroblast element of the tumor). Such distinctive collagen deposition is not seen in schwannoma. Cellularity is generally more uniform in neurofibroma than schwannoma with its abrupt Antoni A and Antoni B regions. Neurofibromas tend to feature a more mucoid matrix than schwannoma. Mast cells are more common in neurofibroma than in schwannoma. Both schwannoma and conventional, sporadic neurofibroma are circumscribed; schwannomas feature a perineurial capsule (highlighted by EMA reactivity). Both tumors may also show chromosome 22 loss or 22q loss, but these losses are more frequently seen in schwannoma.

Combined schwannoma/neurofibroma: This recently described hybrid tumor may be more common in syndromes such as NF1 and NF2 than in sporadic tumors. Both components would need to be identified histologically and could be confirmed by uniform S-100 expression in the schwannoma areas and erratic or patchy expression in the neurofibroma areas.

Leiomyoma or leiomyosarcoma: Smooth muscle tumors often consist of spindle cells. In most such cases, the cells are brightly eosinophilic (more so than in peripheral nerve sheath tumors) and feature cigar shaped, blunt-ended, or train car shaped nuclei. However, a few tumors may contain nuclei more akin to Schwann cells in shape: wavy and pointy ended. Nuclear inclusions common in Schwann cells are distinctly uncommon in smooth muscle tumor nuclei. Uncommonly, nuclear palisading simulating Verocay bodies may occur in smooth muscle tumors. Immunohistochemistry can resolve any diagnostic doubt, as smooth muscle tumors must express desmin, and/or actin, and/or caldesmon. While they can occasionally show reactivity for S-100 protein, this is usually focal and the muscle markers will enable a definitive diagnosis. It is of course, important to recognize that any soft tissue tumor, including a schwannoma, may contain reactive, actin-positive myofibroblasts; these should not be mistaken for actual tumor cells.

Malignant peripheral nerve sheath tumor (MPNST): MPNST is composed most commonly of malignant Schwann cells. It does occur as various histologic grades; however, the low grade form is almost always confined to a pre-existing plexiform neurofibroma. Unlike a schwannoma, most MPNST display permeative tumor borders. Nuclear atypia can be subtle but is not degenerative. Mitotic activity is often higher than a rare division figure, and atypical mitoses may be found. The non-epithelioid MPNST is only focally S-100 protein positive in contrast to schwannoma which is diffusely reactive for antibody to S-100.

Although conventional schwannoma is the principal type of schwannoma, a number of subtypes and unusual histologic findings have been described. **Case table 13.1a** lists the main histologic variants and variant features.

Case fig. 13.1r provides gender, age and body location data for 92 schwannomas resected at the University of New Mexico Health Sciences Center 2000-2010, a moderately sized academic institution. Only four percent are children or adolescents, there is an equal gender distribution, and subcutaneous tissue of extremities (not hands/feet), trunk and head and neck are approximately equally affected.

Oncology approach

Medical oncology

This is a benign lesion with no role for medical oncology.

Radiation oncology

The tumor is removed surgically, and the patient is disease free years later. No radiation therapy is recommended.

Patient outcome

Two years postoperatively the patient has no symptoms, normal neurologic function, and no evidence of recurrence.

Case table 13.1a Variants and variant histologic features of schwannoma

Feature or variant	Frequency	Comment
Degenerative or 'ancient' change	Very common	Surmised to occur from mechanical trauma in long-standing lesions. Changes include cyst formation, fresh and old hemorrhage, histiocyte influxes, hyalinized, thick-walled, sometimes thrombosed vessels, calcifications, and nuclear enlargement and variable nuclear shape with hyperchromaticity and inclusions, but smudgy (poorly preserved) chromatin. Degenerative changes may be so extensive (with massive cyst formation) that multiple sections may be needed to find diagnostic Schwann cells. No clinical significance
Cellular schwannoma	Uncommon	Occurs mostly around spine in soft tissues. Composed of fascicles of spindled Schwann cells without significant atypia. There are no Antoni B areas, and Verocay bodies are absent. It is encapsulated, often with subcapsular lymphoid aggregates. It may be mitotically active, but the rate is low and there are no atypical mitoses. Necrosis is rare but if present is focal. Can recur but does not metastasize
Plexiform schwannoma	Uncommon	Plexiform growth of multiple nodules with Antoni A and Antoni B areas and Verocay bodies. Most common in skin. Not associated strongly with any syndromes (unlike plexiform neurofibroma with NF1)
Plexiform cellular schwannoma	Uncommon	Most plexiform schwannomas disclose a cellular schwannoma morphology (cellular fascicles of elongate Schwann cells) in encapsulated, adjacent nodules. Two reports describe trisomy 17 in plexiform cellular schwannoma (Joste et al. 2004, Tassano et al. 2010). More common in soft tissue of young children. May have mitotic rate up to 18/10hpf
Melanotic (pigmented or psammomatous melanotic schwannoma)	Rare	50% of patients have Carney syndrome (cardiac myxoma, dermal spotty pigmentation, endocrine overactivity and adrenal and pituitary neoplasia). Most common in adults around spinal nerves or autonomic nerves, but can occur in soft tissue and viscera. Exhibits both Schwannian and melanocytic differentiation with spindle and epithelioid cells, prominent melanin pigment deposition, and reactivity for melanocytic markers as well as S-100 protein. Psammoma bodies are common. May contain mature adipose tissue. May be multiple in 20%. May metastasize, especially those with atypia and/or increased mitotic activity
Schwannoma with lipoblasts	Rare	Conventional schwannoma that contains scattered signet-ring type lipoblasts. No clinical significance
Schwannoma with metaplastic cartilage or bone	Rare	Conventional morphology with metaplastic, non-atypical cartilage or bone. No clinical significance
Hybrid peripheral nerve sheath tumor	May be Uncommon rather than Rare	Combination of schwannoma and neurofibroma or schwannoma and perineuroma. Histology resembles both components. Immunohistochemistry may be required to confirm multiple constituents (diffuse S-100 reactivity in schwannoma, patchy S-100 with more CD34 and neurofilaments in neurofibroma, and EMA, GLUT1 or claudin-1 in perineuroma areas without S-100 reactivity). May be associated with NF1 and NF2
Epithelioid schwannoma	Rare	Circumscribed, encapsulated tumor composed of epithelioid Schwann cells with a solid, fibrous and/or myxoid background. May have small component of conventional schwannoma. Rare mitoses and no necrosis or significant nuclear atypia. Diffusely strongly S-100 reactive with no reactivity for keratins or EMA. Usually occurs in adults; females > males. No clinical significance
Schwannoma with true epithelial elements	Rare	This may actually consist of cutaneous schwannomas with entrapped adnexal structures such as eccrine glands or ducts rather than true glandular metaplasia. Glands or ducts express keratins and not S-100 protein. No clinical significance
Pseudoglandular schwannoma	Rare	Schwannoma with degenerative cysts lined by round or columnar Schwann cells mimicking cystic glands. Lining cells are S-100 protein positive and keratin negative. No clinical significance
Neuroblastoma-like schwannoma	Rare	Schwann cells are predominantly small and round (cytologically similar to neuroblasts) with a background of spindle and/or epithelioid Schwann cells. Tumor cells may aggregate around nodules of collagen 'giant rosettes' somewhat simulating true rosettes of neuroblastoma. Usually forms a small subcutaneous nodule. Diffusely S-100 protein positive. Negative for MUC4. No clinical significance
Microcystic/reticular schwannoma	Rare	Elongate interconnecting strands of elongate Schwann cells in a background that is myxoid, fibrillary, or collagenous. May strongly resemble myxoma or perineuroma. Diffusely S-100 protein reactive and negative for EMA. More common in viscera. No clinical significance
Malignant transformation to malignant peripheral nerve sheath tumor or angiosarcoma	Extremely rare	Conventional schwannoma converts to MPNST or angiosarcoma. MPNST is usually epithelioid variant and high grade. Most angiosarcomas arising in schwannoma occur in head and neck in older men. Prognosis is generally poor

Case table 13.1b Summary pathology findings of Case 13.1

Diagnosis	Schwannoma
Size	2.7 cm maximal diameter
Location	Soft tissue of left posterior knee, subcutis
Margin status	Positive
Histologic grade (FNCLCC grading system)	Benign (not graded)
Pathologic stage (AJCC TNM classification)	Benign (not staged)

FNCLCC: Fédération Nationale des Centres de Lutte contre le cancer (French Federation of Cancer Centers). AJCC: American Joint Committee on Cancer

Case 13.2 Epithelioid schwannoma

Clinical history and presentation

This is a 44-year-old woman who presents with a three year history of a left arm mass. The mass has been stable in size but increasingly symptomatic. She relates severe tenderness associated with the mass as well as pain which radiates up and down her arm and occasionally to her chest. She denies numbness, tingling, or weakness.

Examination of the arm shows a palpable 1 × 1 cm mass of the medial arm just proximal to the elbow that is very tender to palpation. She exhibits a strongly positive Tinel sign with radiation of symptoms into her ulnar nerve distribution of her hand. She is hypersensitive in her hand and ulnar nerve distribution as well. She has pain in the area of the mass with range of motion of the elbow, wrist, and digits.

Surgical findings and comments

At surgery, the tumor is noted to be within the ulnar nerve. Marginal excision is performed without damage to the nerve.

Radiology findings

The MR images (**Case figs 13.2a** through **13.2e**) show a mass originating in the ulnar nerve, perhaps best demonstrated with the sequential axial images. This in conjunction with a split fat sign indicates a PNST. The subtle eccentricity relative to the nerve is suggestive of schwannoma as opposed to neurofibroma; however there is limited specificity for this sign. Fortunately, no aggressive features such as heterogeneity on T1, perilesion edema, intra-tumor cystic change or peripheral pattern of enhancement were found.

Pathology findings

Gross features

The 2.4 × 1.7 × 1.3 cm nodular tumor appears grossly encapsulated with a gray to tan external surface. Cross sections reveal a slightly compressible, yellow to tan interior with areas of acute hemorrhage. The specimen is entirely submitted for microscopic review in three cassettes.

Microscopic features

Low magnification: Low magnification reveals a circumscribed, variably fibrotic and myxoid, cellular tumor (**Case fig. 13.2f**). Necrosis is absent.

High magnification: Medium magnification reveals that 95% of the cells have an epithelioid appearance; that is, the cells are round with discrete cell borders and a moderate nuclear to cytoplasmic ratio. The collagenized or solid areas contain vague, back to back clumps of pale eosinophilic cells with or without fibrosis (**Case fig. 13.2g**) while the myxoid regions demonstrate similar epithelioid cells in tight clusters suspended in a gray myxoid matrix (**Case fig. 13.2h**). Tumor nuclei are relatively uniform, ovoid and hypochromatic with scattered nuclear pseudoinclusions. Mitotic figures are identified but number less than 1/10 high magnification fields and are not atypical. One edge of the tumor consists of typical schwannoma with elongate, spindled Schwann cells exhibiting scattered degenerative nuclear atypia (**Case fig. 13.2i**).

Special studies: Tumor cells are diffusely positive for S-100 protein which highlights the encapsulated nature of the tumor (**Case fig. 13.2j**). As would be expected for Schwann cells, the reactivity is both nuclear and cytoplasmic (**Case fig. 13.2k**). Collagen IV is expressed in a latticework fashion around clumps of tumor cells and around individual tumor cells consistent with abundant basement membrane material. Tumor cells do not express smooth muscle actin.

Pathologic differential or, why isn't it one of the following?

Epithelioid neurofibroma: Epithelioid neurofibroma is even rarer than epithelioid schwannoma. It comprises strands and clusters of epithelioid Schwann cells intermixed with usual neurofibroma elements. The typical patient has NF1.

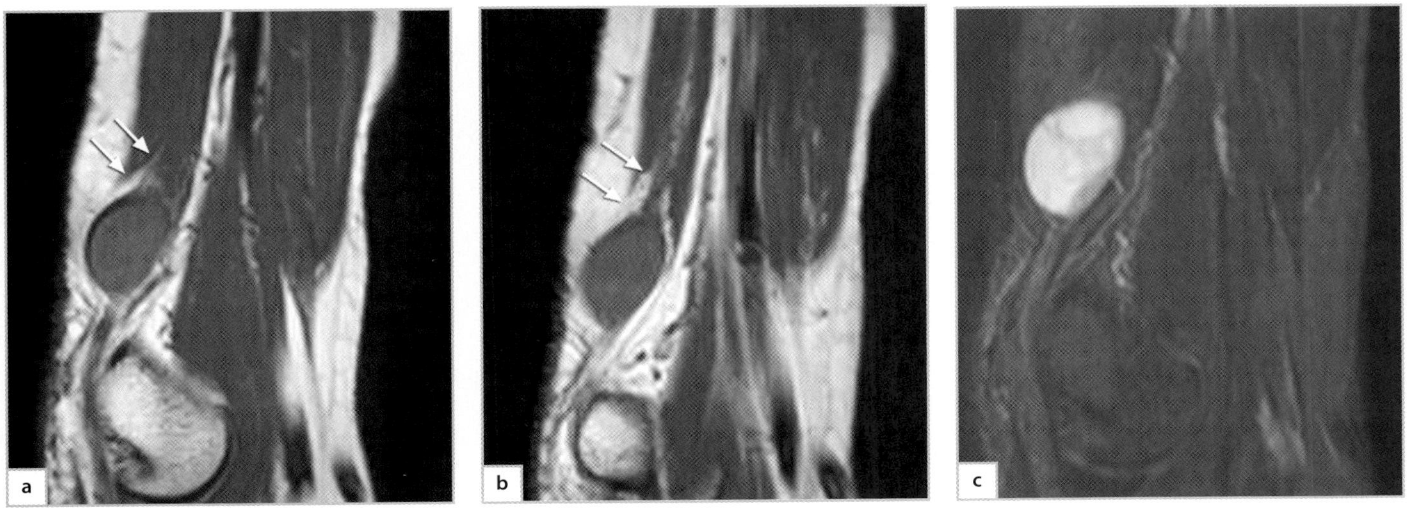

Case figure 13.2 Epithelioid schwannoma imaging. **13.2a** and **13.2b**: Two adjacent sagittal T1 MR images. **13.2c:** Sagittal STIR MR image.

Case figure 13.2: Continued from page 267

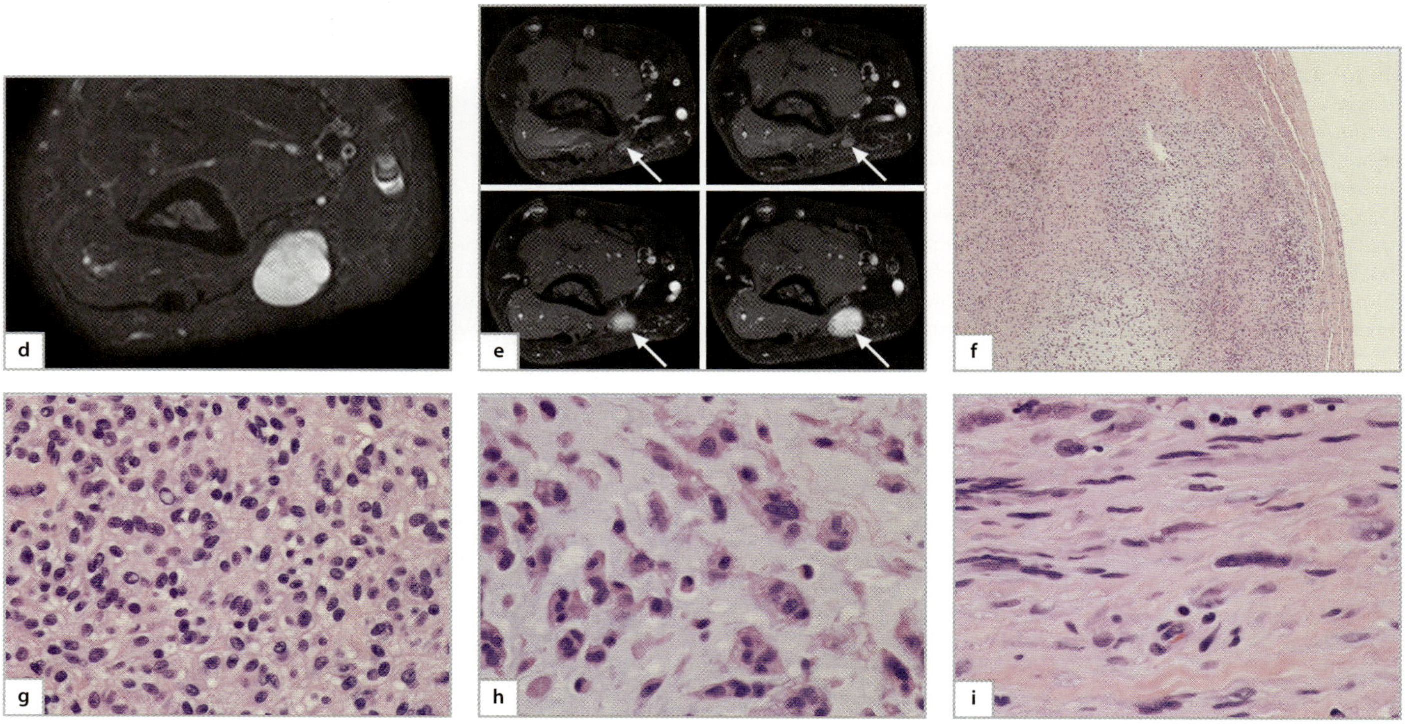

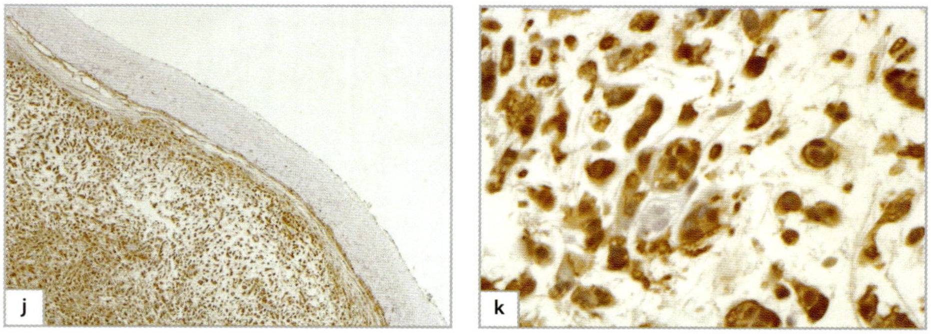

13.2d: Axial STIR MR image. **13.2e**: Four contiguous axial T1 fat saturation post-contrast MR images. The MR images show a fusiform shaped sharply circumscribed mass adjacent to the media margin of the distal triceps muscle and expanding into the subcutaneous tissues. The mass measures 18 × 13 × 21 mm and has T1 isointensity and STIR high signal with uniform intense enhancement. The four contiguous axial images show the mass originates from the ulnar nerve, arrows in Case fig. 13.2e. There is a slight eccentricity of the mass relative to the nerve. There is a fat tissue layer forming a partially visualized triangle (arrows in Case figs 13.2a and b) proximal to the mass. This has been described as that split fat sign. **13.2f**: Low magnification. The tumor is cellular with a pushing rather than invasive border. Areas appear myxoid or solid with variable fibrosis. A small cyst is present in the myxoid area. **13.2g**: Medium magnification. There is a suggestion of clumping or nesting in this field. Tumor cells are epithelioid and relatively uniform with pale round to ovoid nuclei and scattered nuclear inclusions. Cell borders are well defined. **13.2h**: Medium magnification. A myxoid field shows small clusters of epithelioid cells suspended in a blue-gray mucoid matrix. **13.2i**: High magnification. About 5% of this patient's tumor exhibits features of typical or conventional schwannoma: elongate, wavy spindle cells with equally wavy, elongate nuclei, wiry cytoplasm, pink basement membrane collagen deposition and mild degenerative nuclear atypia. **13.2j**: S-100 protein antibody, low magnification. Tumor cells are diffusely positive for S-100 protein, and the stain highlights the tumor's reassuring pushing border and capsule (the latter shows no S-100 IHC reactivity). **13.2k**: S-11 protein antibody, high magnification. Consistent with both conventional schwannoma and the epithelioid variant of MPNST, tumor cells diffusely strongly express S-100 protein in the nucleus and cytoplasm.

Myoepithelioma: Myoepithelioma may have a similar histologic appearance to this tumor. However, it sometimes will also contain epithelial tubular structures, chondroid or cartilaginous matrix, and will exhibit reactivity for myoepithelial markers including calponin, smooth muscle actin, and keratins as well as showing some (usually not diffuse) expression of S-100 protein and GFAP.

Epithelioid malignant peripheral nerve sheath tumor (epithelioid MPNST): Epithelioid MPNST demonstrates more cytologic atypia including cells with macronucleoli, and coarse, irregularly distributed chromatin, and the mitotic rate is higher (well above 5/50 hpf). Necrosis may also be present. MPNST usually exhibits at least focally permeative invasion. Both epithelioid schwannoma and epithelioid MPNST diffusely express S-100 protein, so this does not discriminate between the two entities. Epithelioid MPNST are usually larger than 2.4 cm. Very few cases of epithelioid schwannoma have been reported, so genetic information is sparse. However, like conventional schwannoma, loss of heterozygosity (LOH) of the NF2 gene on chromosome 22 or deletions of 22q and, interestingly, LOH of the NF1 gene (17q) have been reported (Laskin et al. 2005). MPNST usually demonstrate complex aneuploidy on karyotyping which may include losses of chromosome 22 and 17 (entirely or in part).

Intraneural synovial sarcoma, predominantly epithelioid: Rarely, synovial sarcoma may arise within a nerve. Thus far, only the monophasic spindle cell type has been found intraneurally. This patient's tumor could resemble the biphasic synovial sarcoma. Immunohistochemistry would be discriminatory, as synovial sarcoma is rarely diffusely S-100 protein reactive, and would also show keratin and/or EMA expression in 95% of cases. Genetic testing would be definitive as synovial sarcoma exhibits t(X;18) and rarely others which are not seen in epithelioid schwannoma.

Melanoma: Melanoma is a mimicker of many tumors and certainly can appear epithelioid. It would be rare to first be detected associated with the ulnar nerve. Immunohistochemically, it would very likely (~90%) express additional markers of melanocytes such as HMB45, and Melanocyte antigen A as well as S-100 protein. It would most likely show increased nuclear atypia and mitotic activity compared with this patient's tumor.

Leiomyosarcoma, epithelioid variant: Epithelioid leiomyosarcoma is rare in the soft tissues. It will demonstrate increased nuclear atypia and mitotic activity compared with this patient's tumor. Leiomyosarcoma is rarely diffusely S-100 protein reactive, although 15% of smooth muscle tumors may express S-100 protein focally. Muscle markers such as desmin, smooth muscle actin, muscle specific actin, and caldesmon (at least one) will be positive in contrast to this patient's tumor.

Case table 13.2 Summary pathology findings of Case 13.2

Diagnosis	Schwannoma, epithelioid variant
Size	2.4 cm maximal diameter
Location	Ulnar nerve
Margin status	Positive
Histologic grade (FNCLCC Grading System)	Benign (not graded)
Pathologic stage (AJCC TNM classification)	Benign (not staged)

FNCLCC: Fédération Nationale des Centres de Lutte Contre le Cancer (French Federation of Cancer Centers). AJCC: American Joint Committee on Cancer

Oncology approach

Medical oncology

This is a benign lesion with no role for medical oncology.

Radiation oncology

A marginal excision is performed, and the patient has no evidence of recurrence years later.

Patient outcome

Four years postoperatively the patient has no symptoms, normal neurologic function, and no evidence of recurrence.

Case 13.3 Diffuse neurofibroma

Clinical history and presentation

The patient is a 22-year-old man with a history of neurofibromatosis, Type I, who presents with an enlarging tumor of the left hip. He relates significant pain associated with the mass. Symptoms are constant and poorly related to activity.

Physical examination of the left hip reveals a large mass over the left iliac crest. It is intimately associated with overlying skin. It has a soft and spongy consistency on palpation. It is moderately tender.

The tumor is too extensive to warrant complete resection given moderate symptoms. Options are presented to the patient and he elects to proceed with partial excision.

Surgical findings and comments

At surgery, the central 50% of the tumor is removed along with associated skin. The wound is closed primarily. Blood loss is 350 cc.

Radiology findings

This case (**Case figs 13.3a** through **13.3d**) shows an extensive infiltrating lesion of the skin and subcutaneous tissues. There is overall thickening and marked enhancement of the lesion. **Case fig. 13.3d** shows a small area with deep muscle invasion. Note the absence of mass effect. There is no focalization or plaque like raised portion. This lesion primarily demonstrates the infiltrative pattern of growth as seen in approximately 30% of cases. There is no serpentine pattern or 'bag of worms' appearance that can be seen with plexiform neurofibromas. Likewise, no surface ulceration is seen as in dermatofibrosarcoma protuberans which can also present as expansive or plaque like skin lesions.

Pathology findings

Gross features

The specimen consists of an 18 × 4.5 × 4.5 cm strip of skin and underlying subcutaneous tissue. The skin surface is without abnormalities. Cross sections reveal a diffuse amber to mustard colored, glistening edematous process with interspersed yellow fat lobules. The process or lesion extends to deep and peripheral margins. Representative sections including margins are submitted in six cassettes, and fresh tissue is collected for cytogenetic analysis and tissue banking.

Microscopic features

Low magnification: This large lesion diffusely infiltrates dermis and subcutaneous fat. It is unencapsulated (**Case fig. 13.3e**). It envelops and stunts rather than effaces eccrine ducts of the skin (**Case fig. 13.3f**).

Case figure 13.3: Continued from page 269

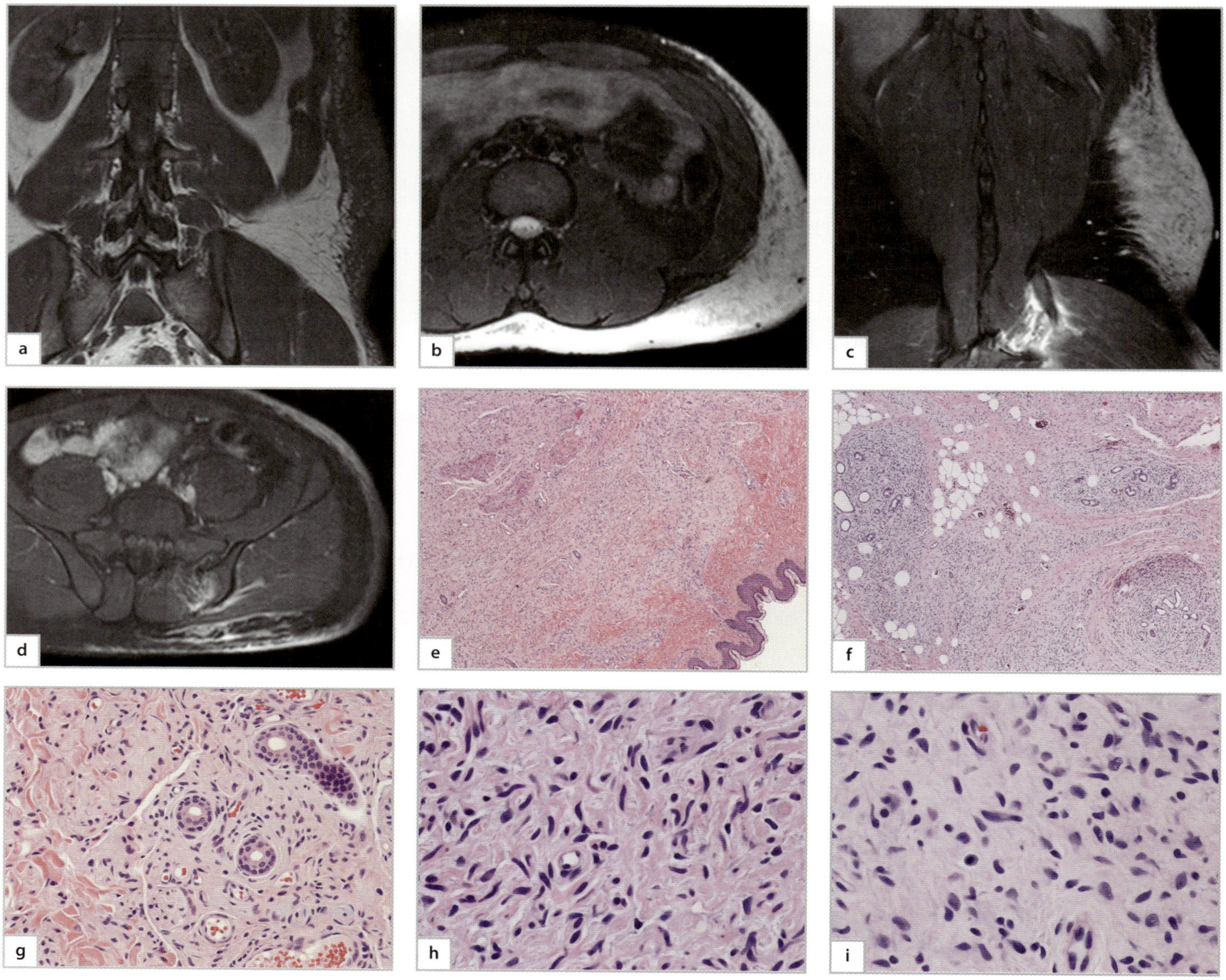
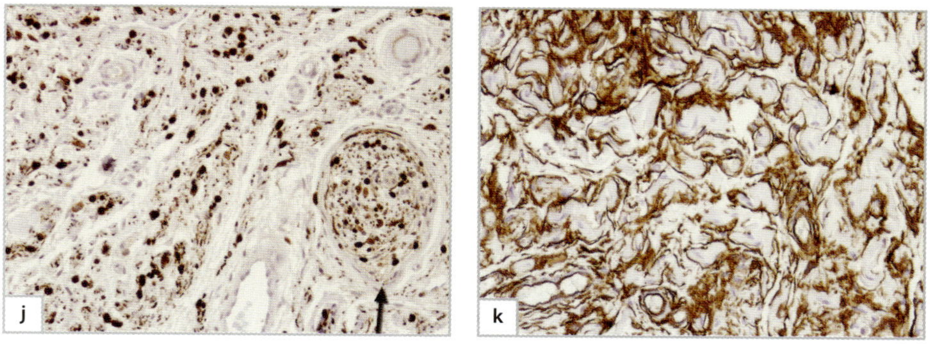

Case figure 13.3 Diffuse neurofibroma imaging. **13.3a**: Coronal T1 MR image. **13.3b**: Axial STIR MR image. **13.3c**: Coronal T1 fat saturated post-contrast MR image. **13.3d**: Axial T1 fat saturated post-contrast MR image. The MR images show an extensive infiltrative lesion involving the skin and subcutaneous tissues over much of the left flank. There is intense uniform enhancement without matrix or necrosis seen. The lesion surface is smooth without ulceration or raised plaque. Note on 13-3d the lesion has infiltrated into the left gluteal muscles and the left paraspinal muscles. **13.3e**: Low magnification. The tumor is unencapsulated and irregularly infiltrates dermis. **13.3f**: Medium magnification. Rather than destroying adnexal structures, the tumor spreads around them causing atrophy of the eccrine glands and ducts. The tumor is slightly more cellular than the normal dermis. **13.3g**: Higher magnification. In this field, several eccrine ducts are surrounded by vague nodular aggregates of tumor cells resembling Wagner-Meissner type corpuscles. These Meissner-like structures are reportedly characteristic of diffuse neurofibroma. Note the similarity of appearance of small peripheral nerve cross section to the tumor cells. **13.3h**: Higher magnification. Tumor cells in this field are consistent with Schwann cells: wavy or buckled, bipolar spindle nuclei with indistinct cell borders. No mitotic activity is identified. **13.3i**: High magnification. Mast cells accompany the tumor. Mast cells are often present in neurofibroma but are nonspecific. Slightly variable in shape, the tumor cells exhibit fine, evenly distributed chromatin and inconspicuous nucleoli. Nuclear inclusions are also present (common in peripheral nerve sheath tumors but not specific).

Case figure 13.3: Continued from page 270

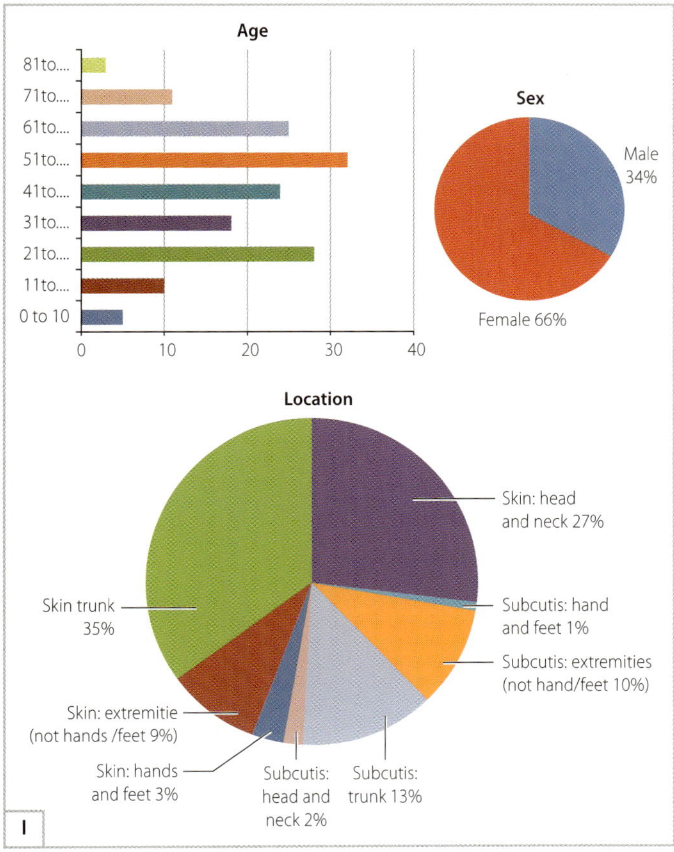

13.3j: Neurofibroma, diffuse type, S-100 protein antibody. Many of the tumor cells express S-100 protein in both the cytoplasm and nucleus. The intensity and type of staining matches that of a peripheral nerve (arrow). **13.3k**: Neurofibroma, diffuse type, CD34 antibody. The tumor also contains many CD34- expressing fibroblasts consistent with neurofibroma. **13.3l**: Neurofibromas resected at UNM Health Sciences Center 2000-2010 (n=156)

High magnification: Medium magnification demonstrates vague rounded clusters of tumor cells resembling Wagner-Meissner-like bodies or tactile differentiation (**Case fig. 13.3g**). In some areas, the tumor consists of buckled or wavy spindle Schwann cells curling through fibrous and myxoid stroma (**Case fig. 13.3h**). Highest magnification of a typical area discloses Schwann cells with non-atypical nuclei, wiry cytoplasm, and scattered mast cells (**Case fig. 13.3i**). Mitotic figures are not identified.

Special studies: Because of classic histologic features, the sample retained for possibly cytogenetic analysis is not processed. However, immunohistochemical staining is performed and reveals a mix of S-100 positive Schwann cells (**Case fig. 13.3j**) and CD34-expressing fibroblasts (**Case fig. 13.3k**) as would be expected for neurofibroma.

Pathologic differential or, why isn't it one of the following?

Malignant peripheral nerve sheath tumor (MPNST): Most malignant peripheral nerve sheath tumors are deep to the fascia, and this patient's tumor is located in the dermis and subcutaneous fat. Most MPNST are high grade with frequent mitoses, marked nuclear pleomorphism, and regional necrosis. S-100 protein expression is usually focal rather than diffuse, and most MPNST do not express CD34. Some experts report frequent focal positivity for keratins 8 and 18 and nestin in MPNST. A diffuse neurofibroma very rarely transforms to MPNST, whereas deep plexiform neurofibromas pose a much greater risk for malignant change. Most MPNST display a complex aneuploid karyotype. At the molecular level, it often shows loss of the NF1 gene at 17q11 and commonly loss of the p53 gene at 17q13.

Dermatofibrosarcoma protuberans (DFSP): Radiologically, as noted above, DFSP could appear similar. However, the characteristic pattern of growth is storiforming of short, plump spindle cells spreading around adnexal structures in the dermis and sandwiching layers of subcutaneous fat between bands of tumor. Conceivably, the myxoid variant of DFSP might present a greater diagnostic challenge. However, although both this patient's tumor and DFSP are CD34 expressing, DFSP does not express S-100 protein. Genetically, DFSP carries a specific translocation: t(17;22)(q21;q13) which fuses the collagen type 1 α1 gene to platelet derived growth factor β chain.

Case table 13.3a lists the histologic variants and variant histologic features of neurofibroma. As with schwannoma, there are quite a few.

Case fig. 13.3l provides gender, age and body location data for 156 neurofibromas resected at the University of New Mexico Health Sciences Center 2000-2010, a moderately sized academic institution. Similar to schwannoma, most patients are adults (15% children to adolescents), but in contrast to schwannoma, females outnumber males, and ~75% occur in the skin compared with only 1% of schwannomas.

Oncology approach

Medical oncology

This is a benign lesion with no role for medical oncology.

Case table 13.3a Variants and variant histologic features of neurofibroma

Feature or variant	Frequency	Comments
Localized cutaneous neurofibroma	Common	90% are sporadic, those occurring in NF1 patients may have overlying café-au-lait spot
Diffuse type neurofibroma	Uncommon	Usually large, usually in children, 10% occur in NF1 patients
Plexiform neurofibroma	Uncommon	Nearly always associated with NF1. May undergo malignant change. A diffuse component may coexist with the wormlike involved nerve branches
Localized intraneural neurofibroma	Uncommon	Segmental fusiform enlargement of one nerve. May be superficial or deep. Usually sporadic. May be associated with NF1, especially if multiple
Pseudo-Meissnerian corpuscles ('tactile differentiation')	Uncommon	Reported to be commonly seen in diffuse neurofibroma. Comprises balls of Schwann cells with peripheralized nuclei
Hybrid neurofibroma/schwannoma	Uncommon?	May be more often associated with NF1 and NF2 patients than sporadic. True frequency not yet known. Schwannian component (diffusely expressing S-100 protein) may appear as small nodules embedded in neurofibroma
'Ancient neurofibroma' or 'atypical neurofibroma'	Uncommon	Neurofibroma with scattered cells showing degenerative nuclear atypia including smudgy chromatin and nuclear inclusions. No clinical significance
'Cellular neurofibroma'	Uncommon	Neurofibroma with increased cellularity with or without low level of normal mitotic activity. Must exclude low grade MPNST arising in plexiform neurofibroma (extensive sampling may be required)
Pigmented neurofibroma	Rare	Scattered melanin containing cells present in otherwise typical neurofibroma, usually superficial diffuse type. 50% occur in NF1 patients
Massive soft tissue neurofibroma	Rare	Gigantism of limb due to diffuse and often plexiform components. Occurs only in NF1 patients. Low risk for malignant change
Dendritic cell neurofibroma with pseudorosettes	Rare	Cutaneous neurofibroma containing pseudorosettes of small cells surrounding, larger pale cells. EMA expressing perineurial cells form the rims of the structures
Epithelioid neurofibroma	Rare	Neurofibroma with clusters and cords of epithelioid Schwann cells. Most patients have NF1. No clinical significance
Granular cell neurofibroma	Rare	Many tumor cells contain abundant, PAS positive, granular, eosinophilic cytoplasm
Neurofibroma with metaplastic epithelium	Rare	Neurofibroma that contains true glands or tubules. No clinical significance
Lipoblastic neurofibroma	Rare	Neurofibroma that contains signet ring lipoblast-like cells. No clinical significance
Neurofibroma with metaplastic bone	Rare	No clinical significance

Radiation oncology

The neurofibroma is partially excised. It continues to grow slowly but is not symptomatic. If the lesion becomes symptomatic again, further surgery should be considered. Alternatively, radiation therapy may be used if surgery is not a good option.

Patient outcome

Three years postoperatively, the patient has had slow growth of the tumor but has had very minimal symptoms since surgery.

Case table 13.3b Summary pathology findings of Case 13.3

Diagnosis	Diffuse neurofibroma
Size	At least 18 cm in maximal dimension
Location	Dermis and subcutis of left hip
Margin status	Positive
Histologic grade (FNCLCC grading system)	Benign (not graded)
Pathologic stage (AJCC TNM classification)	Benign (not staged)

FNCLCC: Fédération Nationale des Centres de Lutte Contre le Cancer (French Federation of Cancer Centers). AJCC: American Joint Committee on Cancer

Case 13.4 Plexiform neurofibroma

Clinical history and presentation

The patient is a 21-year-old female with a history of neurofibromatosis type 1 who presents with recurrence of a mass in the hypothenar aspect of the left palm. The mass was initially excised 10 years ago with benign pathology, but has slowly recurred. She has pain associated with the mass, but no neurologic complaints.

Physical examination of the left palm reveals a soft tissue mass arising from the hypothenar eminence. It is intimately associated with overlying skin. It has a soft and spongy consistency on palpation. It is moderately tender.

Surgical findings and comments

Complete surgical excision of the tumor during a single operation would necessitate flap coverage and would likely compromise function of the ulnar aspect of the hand substantially. Options are presented to the patient and she opts for a staged surgical excision of the most symptomatic portion of the tumor.

During the initial surgical procedure, the central 50% of the tumor is removed and the wound closed primarily. Eight weeks later, after an appropriate interval of wound healing, the patient is returned to surgery for excision of approximately 90% of the residual tumor.

Radiology findings

Neurofibroma - plexiform. This is a more subtle case of plexiform neurofibroma (**Case figs 13.4a** through **13.4d**) without the classic 'bag of worms' sign and less extensive disease than often seen. There is a somewhat serpentine appearance seen on the coronal STIR image (**Case fig. 13.4b**). There is an infiltrative pattern of growth extending from subcutaneous tissues, through fascia, into the thenar eminence muscles. The insinuating pattern of spread involving skin and muscle with modest mass effect might suggest a soft tissue angiomatosis. However, the skin surface expansion and distortion caused by the lesion in conjunction with the clinical setting with presumed stigmata of neurofibromatosis 1 would help render the correct diagnosis.

We also present MR images from two additional patients with plexiform neurofibroma. The first patient, **Case fig. 13.4e** through **13-4i** shows the classic extensive disease involving multiple nerves. There is confluent bilateral disease of the brachial and sacral plexus with extension into nerve branches. The second patient, **Case figs 13.4j** through **13.4m**, shows a very large infiltrative lesion with the classic 'bag of worms' sign. Note also the bilateral involvement of the sacral plexus and the scattered cutaneous lesions.

Pathology findings

Gross features

Both the initial specimen and the later excision consist of boggy subcutaneous tissue containing multiple, circumscribed nodules which on cross section are slightly myxoid and gray.

Microscopic features

Low magnification: The tumor comprises numerous enlarged peripheral nerves (**Case fig. 13.4n**). Compared with a normal peripheral nerve, the involved nerves are less cellular and more myxoid (**Case fig. 13.4o**). Consistent with the radiologic impression of a diffuse mass, there is a diffuse neurofibroma component to the lesion (**Case fig. 13.4p**). This extraneural extension is common with plexiform neurofibroma.

High magnification: Medium magnification reveals swatches and bands of collagen (which may be intermixed with a few Schwann cells). This appearance has been likened to 'chopped carrots' or 'shredded carrots' and is a notable feature of cutaneous and plexiform neurofibroma (**Case fig. 13.4q**). Other areas of the tumor are much more myxoid and contain neoplastic cells (some with inspissated mucin) and residual nerve fibers (**Case fig. 13.4r**). Highest magnification reveals some nuclear atypia including multilobate nuclei with well-preserved chromatin, and nuclei with nucleoli and nuclear pseudo-inclusions (**Case fig. 13.4s**). Atypical cells are not uncommon in plexiform neurofibroma (see below for differential diagnosis with malignant peripheral nerve sheath tumor).

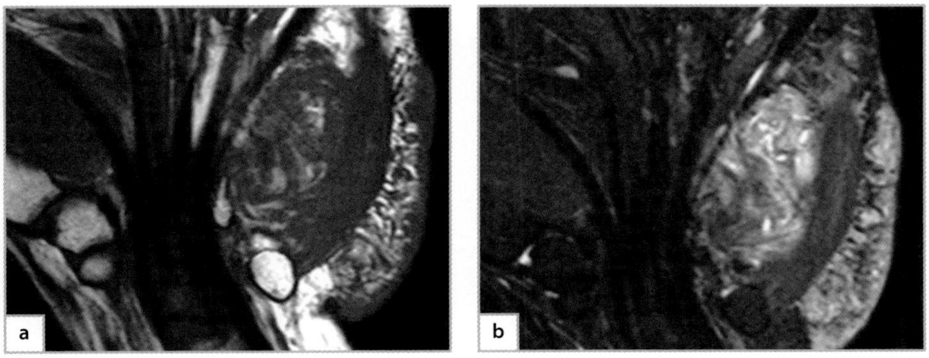

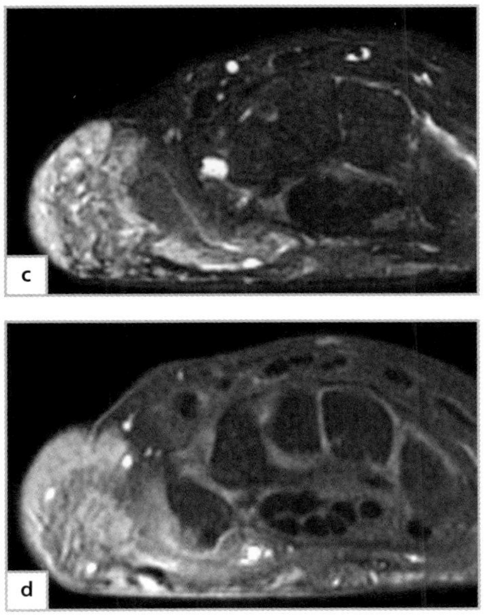

Case figure 13.4 Neurofibroma – plexiform. **13.4a**. Coronal T1 MR image. **13.4b**: Coronal STIR MR image. **13.4c**: Axial STIR MR image, **13.4d**: Axial T1 fat saturated post-contrast MR image. The MR images of this 21 year old woman show a heterogeneous mass with moderate irregular enhancement involving the skin and infiltrating into the muscles of the thenar eminence. The mass measures 6.4 × 4.5 × 2.5 cm. The coronal images show a serpentine appearance, although no classic 'bag of worms' sign is present, probably due to the small size of the lesion. No clear nerve of origin is seen.

Case figure 13.4: Continued from page 273

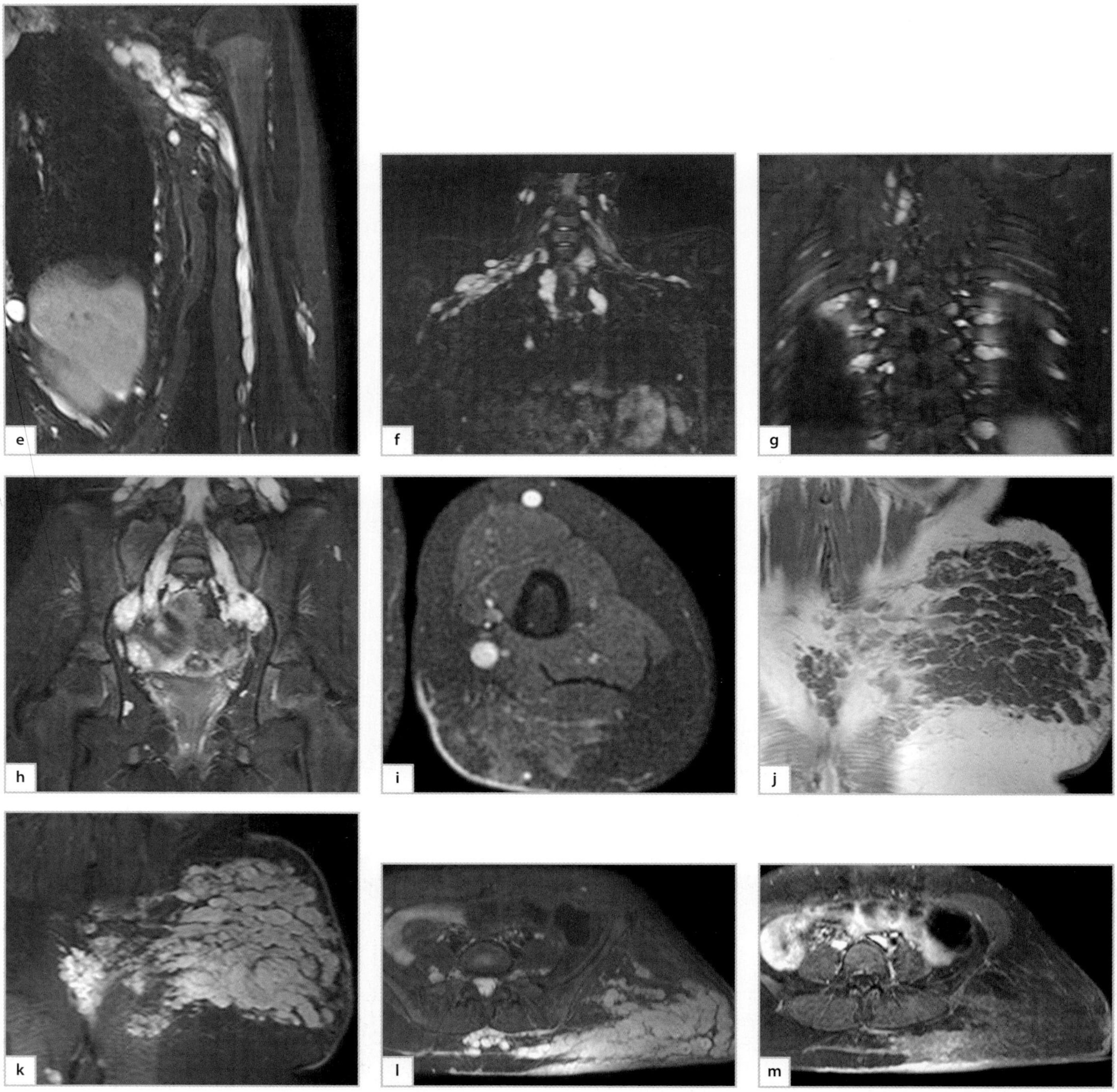

13.4e: Additional patient with plexiform neurofibroma. Coronal STIR MR image of the arm. **13.4f**: coronal STIR MR image of the chest. **13.4g**: Coronal STIR MR image of the posterior ribs. **13.4h**: Coronal STIR MR image of the pelvis. **13.4i**: Axial T1 fat saturated post-contrast MR image of the arm. This second case of plexiform neurofibroma in an 11 year old female shows the extensive disease burden with bilateral involvement of the brachial plexus, numerous intercostal nerves and the sacral plexus. There is involvement of nerve branches. Interestingly, the extensive arm lesion shows little enhancement, Figure 13-4i. Additional patient with Plexiform Neurofibroma. **13.4j**: Coronal T1 MR image. **13.4k**: Coronal STIR MR image. **13.4l**: Axial STIR MR image. **13.4m**: axial T1 fat saturated post-contrast MR image. These images of a 17 year old female show the classic 'bag of worms' appearance of a plexiform neurofibroma. Note there are also multiple other lesions seen involving the skin and sacral plexus. This lesion shows moderate heterogeneous enhancement. **13.4n**: Low magnification. The tumor consists of serpentine enlarged peripheral nerves filled with tumor. **13.4o**: Low magnification. A normal peripheral nerve in the center is contrasted with the larger, tumorous nerves. The involved nerves contain intermixed fibrotic and myxoid areas.

Case figure 13.4: Continued from page 274

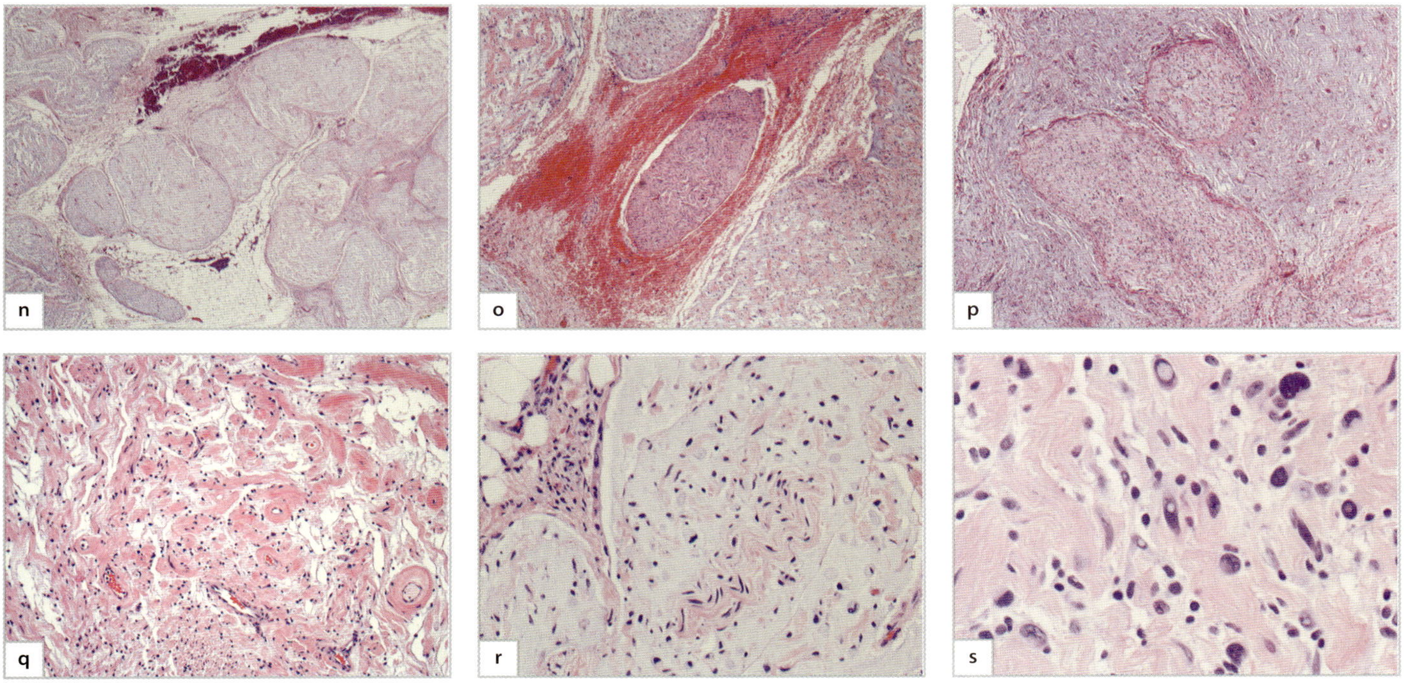

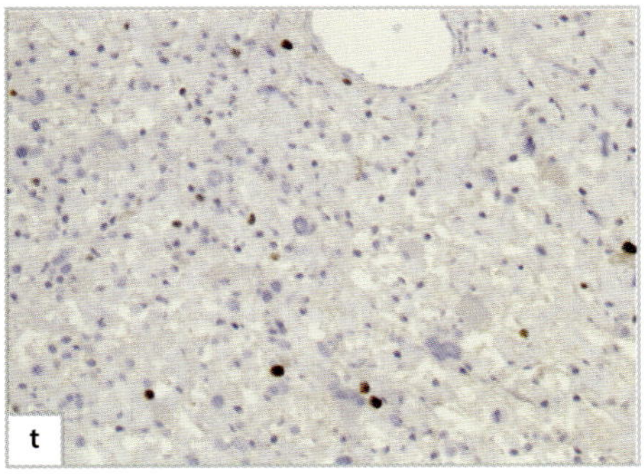

13.4p: Low magnification. Commonly, a diffuse component coincides with the plexiform tumor as is notable here. **13.4q**: Medium magnification, cross section of involved nerve. The pink bands and swatches in this field have been likened to chopped or shredded carrots. They predominantly consist of collagen, although a few Schwann cells may be coursing alongside. Notice the intraneural blood vessels are sheathed in hyalinized collagen, also. **13.4r**: High magnification. The tumor here is particularly myxoid with bundles of wiry Schwann cells floating in a gray gelatinous matrix. The rounded cells with absorbed myxoid material most likely consist of Schwann cells and histiocytes.**13.4s**: High magnification. Nuclear atypia is not unusual in plexiform neurofibroma. Notice the variation in size and shape of the tumor cells and scattered nuclear inclusions. The chromatin is generally well preserved rather than smudgy and degenerated. The border between low grade MPNST and atypical neurofibroma is not well-defined. Hypercellularity, more than a rare mitotic figure, and coarse chromatin and chromatin clearing are all features that would suggest malignant transformation has occurred. **13.4t**: Ki67 immunohistochemical stain. Notice the large atypical cells do not express Ki67 indicating that these cells are not proliferating. The overall Ki67 percentage positivity is low consistent with a plexiform neurofibroma.

Special studies: A Ki67 immunohistochemical stain is performed and shows a low rate of proliferative activity of about 2%, even in areas with atypical cells (**Case fig. 13.4t**).

Pathologic differential or, why isn't it one of the following?

Plexiform schwannoma: The typical plexiform schwannoma is more homogeneous in terms of cell constituents. It may consist entirely of Antoni A areas. Expression of S-100 protein is diffuse rather than focal as in plexiform neurofibroma. A 'chopped or shredded' carrot look of collagen deposition is absent. Myxoid change, frequent in plexiform neurofibroma, is unusual in plexiform schwannoma.

Cellular neurothekeoma: This tumor is usually dermal but can extend into the subcutaneous tissue. It may mimic a plexiform tumor because it is composed of closely packed nodules (sometimes with focal sheet like growth) with interposed collagen strands. The tumor cells are usually round but may be spindled. The cytoplasm is eosinophilic, and tumor nuclei are usually round and hypochromatic but atypia and atypical mitoses may also be seen in ~15-20%. Multinucleated osteoclast-like giant cells and myxoid change are relatively common. The tumor may be related to plexiform fibrohistiocytic tumor, as both tumors express NKI-C3 and MiTF (microphthalmia-associated transcription factor), and both do not express S-100 protein or melan-A or HMB-45.

Case table 13.4 Summary pathology findings of Case 13.4

Diagnosis	Plexiform neurofibroma
Size	~6 × 4 × 4 cm of involved tissue
Location	Subcutaneous tissue of hand
Margin status	Focally positive
Histologic grade (FNCLCC grading system)	Benign (not graded)
Pathologic stage (AJCC TNM classification)	Benign (not staged)

FNCLCC: Fédération Nationale des Centres de Lutte Contre le Cancer (French Federation of Cancer Centers). AJCC: American Joint Committee on Cancer

Oncology approach

Medical oncology

This is a benign lesion with no role for medical oncology, as the pathologist finds no evidence of transformation to malignant peripheral nerve sheath tumor. However, the patient should be closely followed, as she is at risk for development of MPNST from any other deep plexiform neurofibromas she may have.

Radiation oncology

The patient undergoes partial excision and is minimally symptomatic years later. If she becomes symptomatic again, further surgery should be considered. Radiation therapy can be used in case surgery is not a good option.

Patient outcome

Two years postoperatively, the patient has a small area of residual tumor which has not increased appreciably in size since surgery and is associated with very mild tenderness. She has normal function of the hand.

Case 13.5 Perineurioma, sclerosing variant

Clinical history and presentation

The patient is a 51-year-old woman who has a history of a right groin mass which she describes as a fatty-type mass which was excised three and one-half years ago. The patient noted return of the mass several months following surgery which has since remained unchanged. She relates mild tenderness associated with the mass.

Physical examination reveals a firm deep mass in the right groin. It is mobile within the deep tissue. It is mildly tender on palpation. Neurologic examination of the extremity is normal.

Surgical findings and comments

Marginal excision is performed.

Radiology findings

The case (**Case figs 13.5a** through **13.5c**) shows an ovoid homogeneous mass in the deep tissues of the groin. There is no linear extension or clear nerve involvement. The tumor is separate from adjacent bone, joint and vessels. There is no fusiform shape or clear connection to a nerve and no split fat sign is seen. None of the usual signs of neurogenic lesion is seen. The lack of infiltration, heterogeneity or necrosis indicates a non-aggressive lesion. The radiologist can be helpful with groin lesions in confirming they are not due to hernia or aneurysm. Unfortunately, there are otherwise no specific features evident.

Pathology findings

Gross features

The specimen is received fresh and consists of a 9 × 5 × 3.5 cm tan mass that on cross sectioning is glistening, tan and solid with ill-defined nodularity. It extends to inked surgical margins. One portion of tumor is sent to Cytogenetics and another is rapidly frozen for tumor banking. Representative sections are submitted in seven cassettes for routine processing.

Microscopic features

Low magnification: The tumor is remarkable for evenly mixed bands of sclerosis and myxoid stroma throughout all sections (**Case fig. 13.5d**). Cellularity is low, and there is no acute hemorrhage or necrosis. In some fields, the tumor cells interconnect forming delicate cobwebs that frame bands of hyalinized collagen (**Case fig. 13.5e**). Thin walled vessels are also encircled by cuffs of dense collagen.

High magnification: The tumor cells are uniform with pale ovoid nuclei, pale eosinophilic cytoplasm and indistinct cell borders on routine hematoxylin and eosin staining (**Case fig. 13.5f**). Nuclear atypia is absent. Mitotic figures are rare (less than 1 per 50 high power microscopic fields) and without atypical forms.

Special studies: Consistent with the diagnosis, the tumor cells are reactive for EMA which highlights the elongate spindled cytoplasm of many of the cells (**Case fig. 13.5g**). In addition, Collagen IV is also prominently present, consistent with basement membrane production (**Case fig. 13.5h**). The tumor cells do not express CD34, S-100 protein, or keratins (as a few sclerosing perineuriomas have been described to do). Approximately 5% of cells weakly express smooth muscle actin (reactivity for SMA has been reported in sclerosing perineurioma). Although not performed in this case, GLUT1 would be likely to expressed and also possibly Claudin-1. Staining for both of these antibodies can be diagnostically very helpful but may be focal (GLUT1) or absent (Claudin-1).

Karyotyping is successful and reveals the following: 45-46,XX,add(2)(q37),del(6)(q21),t(10;14)(q22;q24),add(10)(q26),add(22)(q13)[cp2]/46XX[17] with two non-clonal aberrations: 46,XXdel(16)(q10)[1] and 46,XX,add(22)(q13)[1].

This karyotype is consistent with the few genetic findings reported for sclerosing perineurioma which includes abnormalities of chromosome 22q13 and rearrangements or deletions of chromosome 10q (Brock et al. 2005).

Pathologic differential or, why isn't it one of the following?

Soft tissue perineurioma: This patient's tumor is located in an unusual site and is large for the sclerosing variant of perineurioma, which usually presents as a small nodule in the dermis of the hands. So, size and site would fit more harmoniously with the soft tissue variant of perineurioma. However, the extensive sclerosis and genetic finding of abnormalities of chromosome 10q support the diagnosis of sclerosing variant of perineurioma. Soft tissue perineurioma is reminiscent of meningioma histologically (not surprising, since meningothelial cells and perineurial cells are most likely related) with usually moderate to high cellularity, sometimes prominent whorls of cells, and additional architectural patterns that include storiform, lamellar and/or fascicular. Hyalinization of collagen can be present but is unusual and typically focal when occurring in soft tissue perineurioma.

Malignant peripheral nerve sheath tumor, malignant perineurioma variant: This variant of malignant peripheral nerve sheath tumor demonstrates permeative borders, nuclear atypia, necrosis, and increased

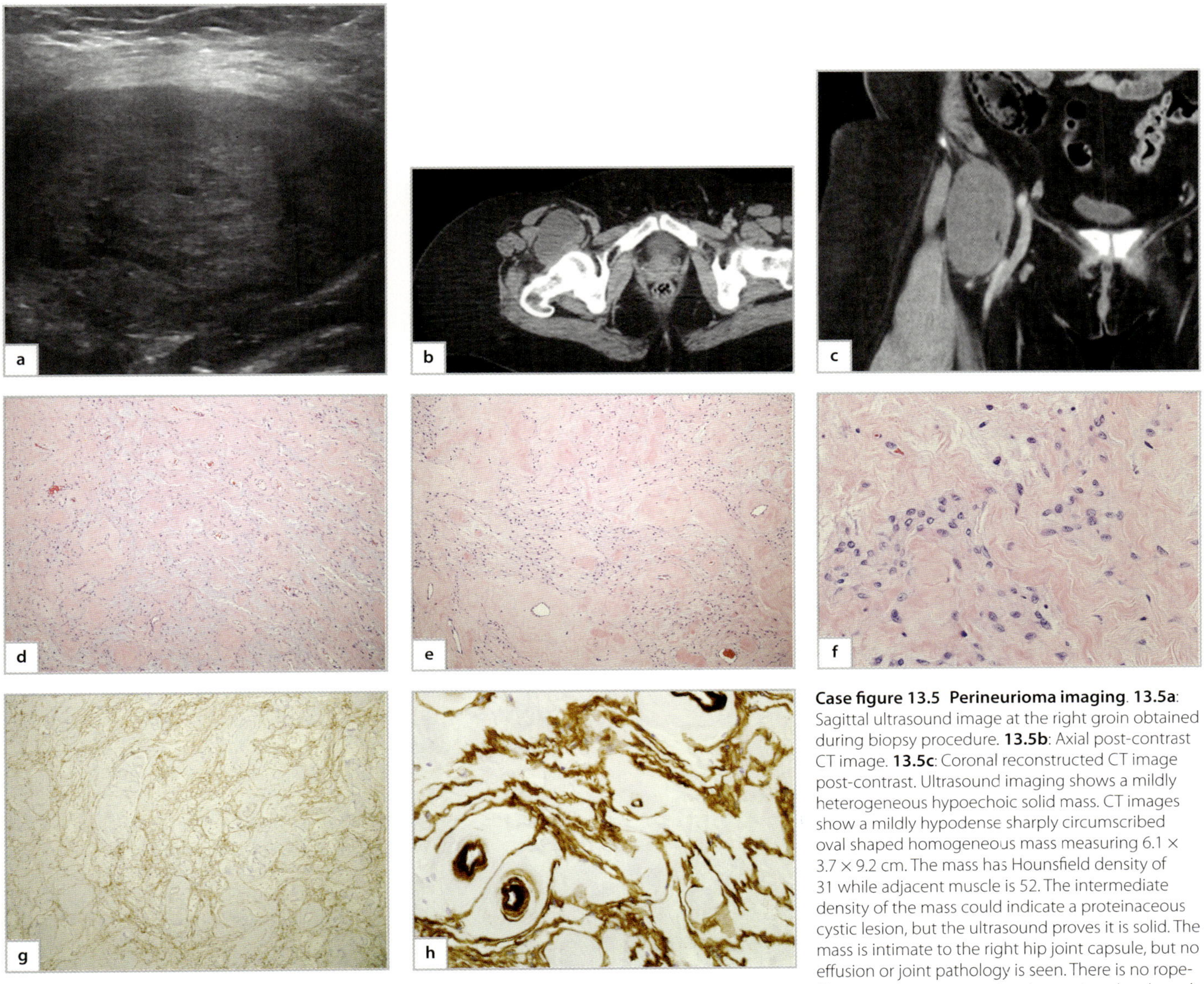

Case figure 13.5 Perineurioma imaging. 13.5a: Sagittal ultrasound image at the right groin obtained during biopsy procedure. **13.5b**: Axial post-contrast CT image. **13.5c**: Coronal reconstructed CT image post-contrast. Ultrasound imaging shows a mildly heterogeneous hypoechoic solid mass. CT images show a mildly hypodense sharply circumscribed oval shaped homogeneous mass measuring 6.1 × 3.7 × 9.2 cm. The mass has Hounsfield density of 31 while adjacent muscle is 52. The intermediate density of the mass could indicate a proteinaceous cystic lesion, but the ultrasound proves it is solid. The mass is intimate to the right hip joint capsule, but no effusion or joint pathology is seen. There is no rope-like or contiguous nerve involvement and no branch disease is seen. There is no gross fat tissue and no calcifications are evident. **13.5d**: Lower magnification. The hypocellular tumor consists of alternating bands of collagen and myxoid stroma. **13.5e**: Lower magnification. Elongate spindle tumor cells form a characteristic delicate mesh that entraps collagen. Thin walled vessels are cuffed by hyalinized collagen. **13.5f**: High magnification. Tumor cells are ovoid to spindled with pale, uniform nuclei. The collagen matrix is wiry to matte in this field. Cell borders are inconspicuous. There is no nuclear atypia and no mitotic activity. **13.5g**: EMA (epithelial membrane antigen) antibody. The long delicate tumor cell cytoplasmic extensions course around hyalinized vessels and enmesh collagen. **13.5h**: Collagen IV antibody. Perineurial cells are modified fibroblasts and as such produce basement membrane components such as Collagen IV and laminin (chromogen is brown color).

mitotic activity. It is very rare. Although benign perineuriomas may exhibit cytologic atypia, the tumors are circumscribed with pushing borders, and necrosis and increased mitotic activity are absent. Based on the history, this patient may have shown an ability to recur which is unusual. However, the original tumor resection was not available for review and may have consisted of a lipoma.

Low grade fibromyxoid sarcoma (LGFMS): LGFMS is generally a subfascial sarcoma that consists of spindle cells, a mixed myxoid and collagenous stroma, and arcing blood vessels. It may show focal expression of EMA and Claudin-1 (reactivity similar to perineurioma). The spindle cells may also resemble those of perineurioma. However, the tumor cells express MUC4, and most cases demonstrate a t(7;16)(q34;p11) translocation.

Epithelioid hemangioendothelioma (EHE): Some cases of EHE show extensive sclerosis and minimal cytologic atypia similar to sclerosing perineurioma. The stroma can appear chondroid which is dissimilar to sclerosing perineurioma. Immunohistochemically, the tumor cells are seldom EMA reactive, usually CD31, FLI-1, ERG, and CD34 reactive, and some will exhibit cytoplasmic vacuoles consistent with early blood vessel formation. Most cases of EHE also bear a specific translocation: t(1;3)(p36.3;q25).

Case table 13.5a lists the variants and variant histologic features of perineurioma. Like other peripheral nerve sheath tumors, perineuriomas are histologically diverse, but all contain cells with a specific line of differentiation (as in Schwann cells for schwannoma, Schwann cells, axonal cells and fibroblasts for neurofibroma, and perineurial cells for perineurioma).

Case table 13.5a Variants and variant histologic features of perineurioma

Variant or feature	Frequency	Comment
Sclerosing perineurioma	Rare but may be most common variant of perineuroma	Usually located in hands and forms a small dermal nodule in young adults, M>F
Soft Tissue perineurioma	Rare	Occurs most commonly in subcutaneous adipose tissue. Rare cases reported in the mandible
Intraneural perineurioma	Very rare	Onion bulb like whorls of neoplastic perineurial cells encircling residual nerve fibers
Plexiform perineurioma	Very rare	Typical plexiform architecture of serpentine nodules of tumor
Reticular perineurioma	Very rare	Delicate lacelike pattern of elongate spindle tumor cells in a myxoid or edematous stroma Degenerative cytologic atypia and microcysts may be present
Epithelioid perineurioma	Very rare, case report	Predominant component is epithelioid perineurial cells with minor typical component
Combined sclerosing and soft tissue perineurioma	Rare	
Hybrid perineurioma and schwannoma or perineurioma and neurofibroma	Rare	Components are discrete in acral examples and intermixed at other sites. Most are dermal or subcutaneous. Degenerative nuclear atypia may be present. The largest series (n = 42) reported no association with neurofibromatosis
Sclerosing pacinian-like perineurioma	Very rare, case reports only	Dermal location
Perineurioma with adipocytes	Very rare, case reports only	May occur with soft tissue or sclerosing variants
Perineurioma with granular cells or hybrid perineuroma and granular cell tumor	Very rare, case reports only	Cell may mimic granular cells of granular cell tumor. Single case report of acral plexiform combined perineuroma and granular cell tumor
Perineurioma with metaplastic bone	Very rare, case reports only	A rare case has also been reported with psammomatous calcifications
'Atypical cellular perineurioma'	Very rare, case reports only	Uniformly hypercellular with nuclear atypia. Possibly may have increased risk for local recurrence
Malignant perineurioma (perineuroma variant of MPNST)	Very rare	Infiltrative with necrosis, increased mitotic activity and nuclear atypia

Case table 13.5b Summary pathology findings of Case 13.5

Diagnosis	Perineurioma, sclerosing variant
Size	9 × 5 × 3.5 cm
Location	Subcutaneous tissue of right groin
Margin status	Positive
Histologic grade (FNCLCC grading system)	Benign lesion so not graded
Pathologic stage (AJCC TNM classification)	Benign lesion so not staged

FNCLCC: Fédération Nationale des Centres de Lutte Contre le Cancer (French Federation of Cancer Centers). AJCC: American Joint Committee on Cancer

Oncology approach

Medical oncology

This is a benign lesion with no role for medical oncology.

Radiation oncology

Radiation therapy has no known role in perineurioma.

Patient outcome

Two years postoperatively, the patient has had no evidence of recurrence.

Case 13.6 Malignant peripheral nerve sheath tumor

Clinical history and presentation

The patient is a 28-year-old woman who complains of an approximately 5 week history of insidious onset of mass in the left buttock region. She notes that the mass is painful when she is seated.

Physical examination reveals a somewhat soft mass in the left buttock area on deep palpation.

Surgical findings and comments

Open biopsy is performed, confirming the diagnosis.

Following pre-operative chemotherapy, the patient is returned to surgery for wide resection of the tumor. The tumor is contained within the central portion of the gluteus maximus muscle. The central two thirds of the muscle is removed along with the tumor, providing a satisfactory wide margin. The sciatic nerve is preserved.

Radiology findings

In this case (**Case figs 13.6a** through **13.6f**), shows an overall nonspecific aggressive appearing tumor in the gluteal muscles. The nerve of origin is not identifiable as is often the case with MPNST. Therefore, the radiologist cannot ascertain that this is a neurogenic tumor, but can only diagnose an aggressive tumor such as a sarcoma.

Pathology findings

Gross features

The incisional biopsy consists of a 3 × 2.2 × 0.4 cm aggregate of solid to soft gelatinous lobulated soft tissue. A small portion is submitted to Cytogenetics. The remainder is embedded for standard histology.

The resection specimen consists of an 18 × 14.5 × 11 cm roughly ovoid mass with an attached ellipse of skin. The specimen is received

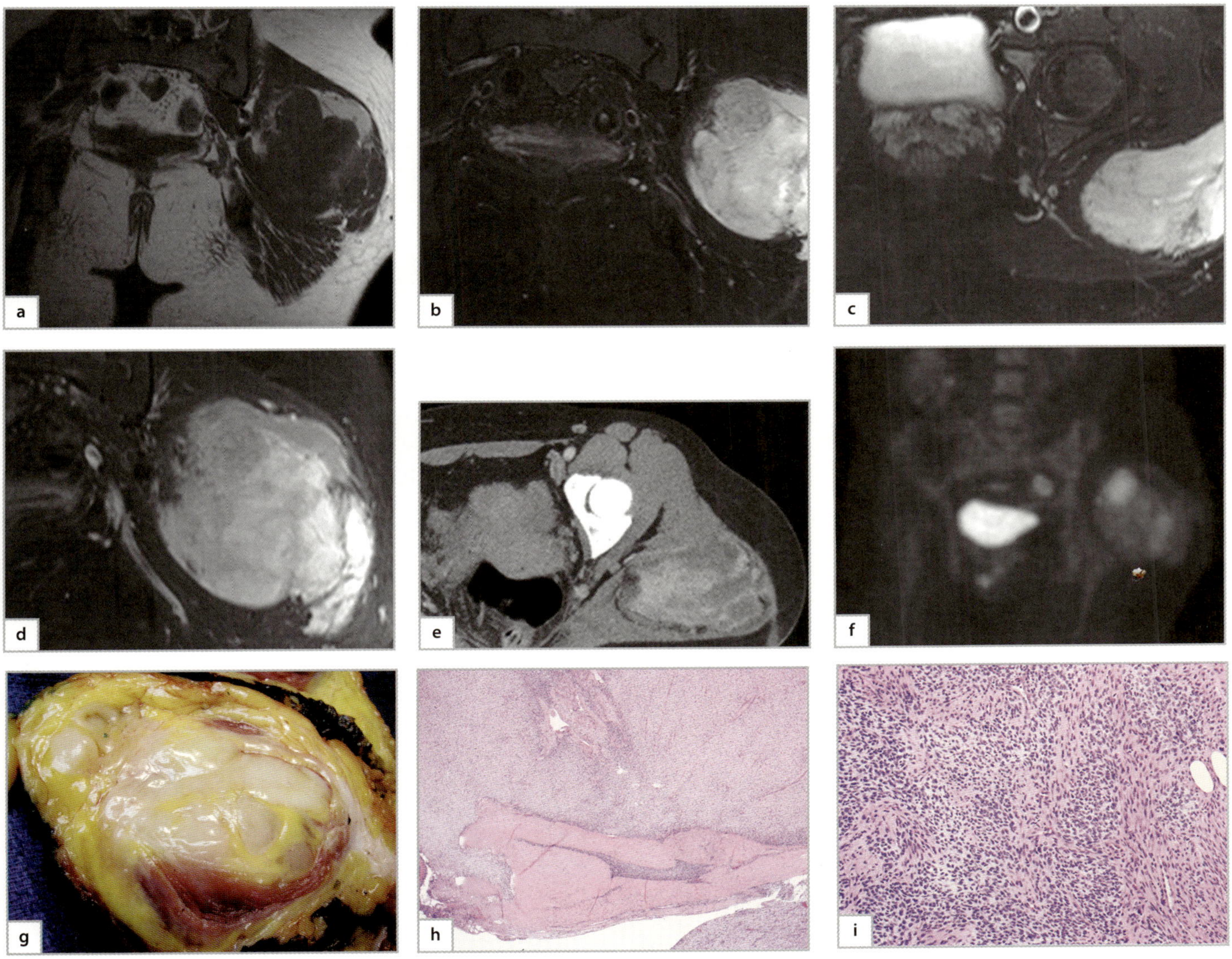

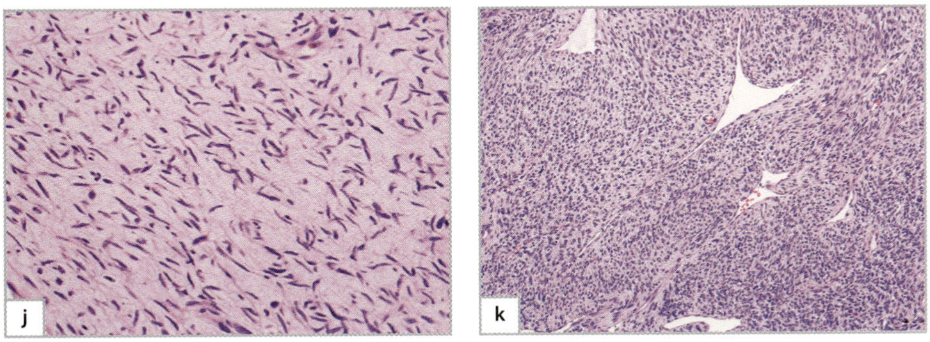

Case figure 13.6 Malignant peripheral nerve sheath tumor (MPNST) imaging. **13.6a**: Coronal T1 MR image. **13.6b**: Coronal STIR MR image. **13.6c**: Axial T2 fat saturated MR image. 13.6d: Coronal T1 fat saturated post-contrast image. **13.6e**: Axial CT image post IV contrast. **13.6f**: PET image. There is a heterogeneous 13.2 × 9.9 × 5.7 cm, T1 low signal, T2 and STIR high signal mass in the gluteal muscles. The mass shows intense, somewhat heterogeneous enhancement. The mass has heterogeneous density and enhancement on CT images. The PET shows heterogeneous increased metabolic activity. A nerve of origin is not found, the mass is separate from the sciatic nerve which passes about 1.5 cm inferomedial to the mass as seen on the coronal images. The overall appearance is non-specific but is worrisome for malignancy or sarcoma. **13.6g**: Gross photo of tumor resection. This cross section of tumor reveals coalescing, glistening tan to white nodules that infiltrate adipose tissue and impinge on skeletal muscle. Other cross sections of tumor are more gelatinous, focally cystic, and soft yellow consistent with necrosis. **13.6h**: Low magnification. Typical of a sarcoma, the tumor infiltrates surrounding normal tissue which in this field consists of fascia or tendon. **13.6i**: Medium magnification. This field features two distinct cell populations: eosinophilic spindle cells and clusters of small round cells with scant cytoplasm. This area resembles biphasic synovial sarcoma. However, immunohistochemistry reveals no reactivity for keratins or EMA. S-100 protein expression is present and limited to the small round cell population. **13.6j**: Medium magnification. In this area, the tumor appears low grade or even benign with uniform elongate spindle cells loosely dispersed in a myxoid or edematous matrix. **13.6k**: Medium magnification. Some of the vessels assume a hemangiopericytomatous appearance with tumor cells bulging into and irregularly compressing the veins.

Case figure 13.6: Continued from page 279

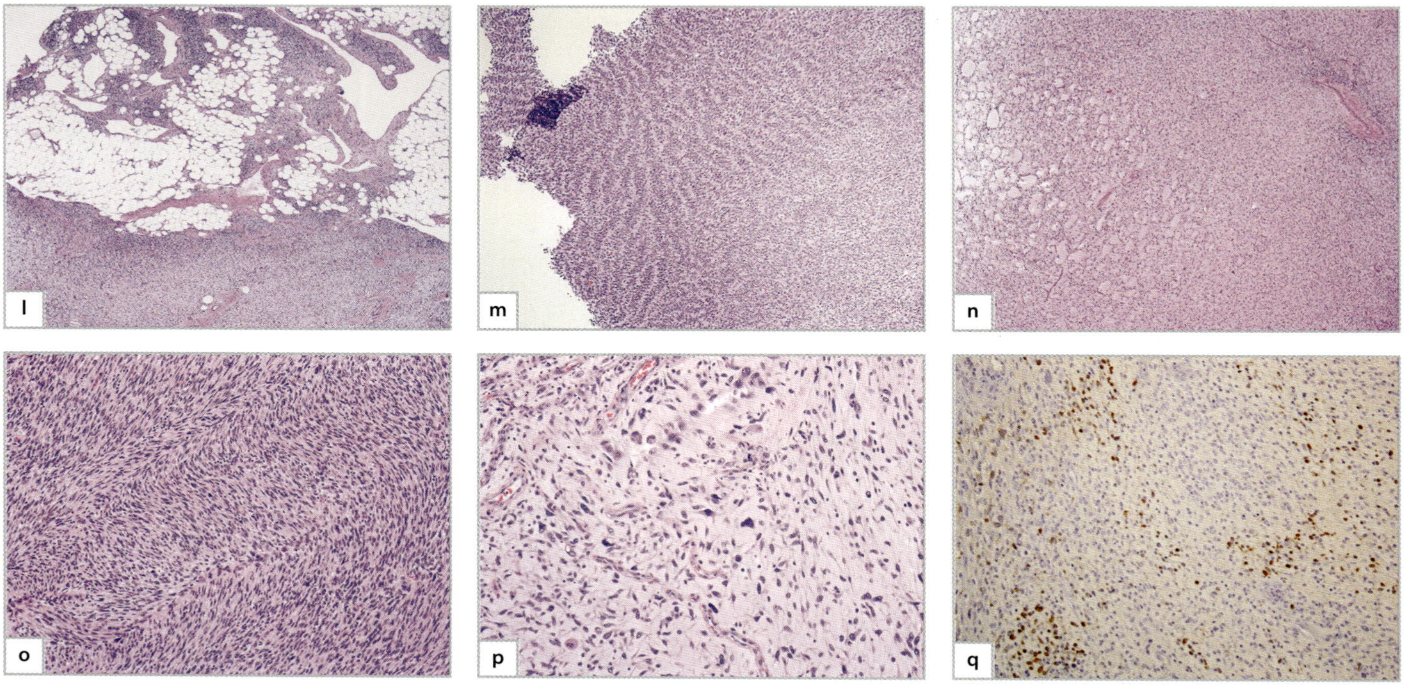

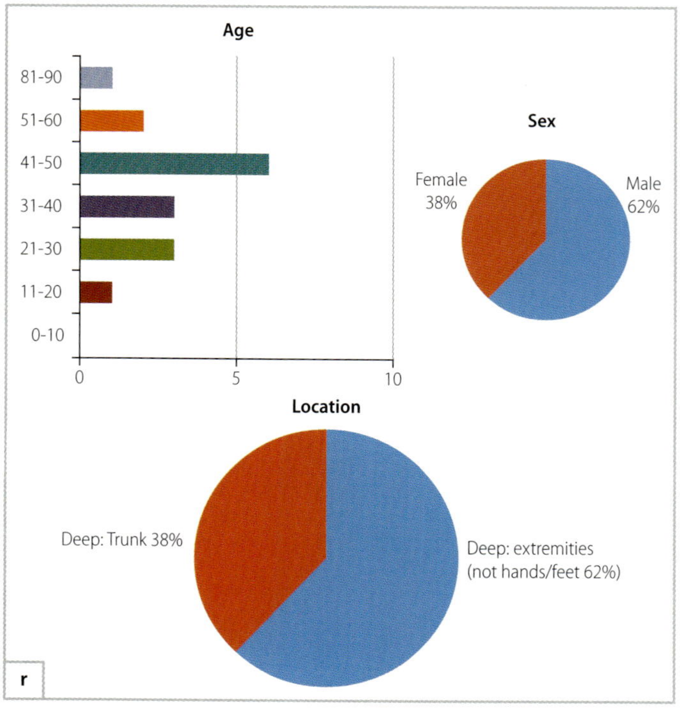

13.6l: Malignant peripheral nerve sheath tumor, resection, low magnification. The tumor infiltrates adipose tissue in this field following a perivascular route. **13.6m**: Low magnification. Marbled or tigroid appearance imparted by alternating hypocellular and hypercellular stripes of tumor. This example simulates Verocay bodies of schwannoma. **13.6n**: Medium magnification. In this area, the tumor focally is microcystic. **13.6o**: Medium magnification. Another zone comprises spindle tumor cells arranged in a herringbone or fascicular pattern. **13.6p**: Higher magnification. A cellular myxoid area comprises cells of various shapes (from spindled to epithelioid) and nuclear features (from wavy or buckled to polygonal to rounded, mono-lobated to multilobated with some multinucleation). The degree of nuclear atypia is moderate. **13.6q**: Medium magnification. Clusters of tumor cells express S-100 protein primarily in the nuclei. These positive cells compose about 10% of the entire tumor cell population. **13.6r**: MPNSTs resected at University of New Mexico Health Sciences Center 2000-2010 (n=16)

oriented and inked accordingly. Serial sections reveal an intramuscular 14.7 × 11.2 × 11 cm tumor with a heterogeneous cut surface. Thirty percent is yellow and soft consistent with necrosis, 40% is multicystic and gelatinous (possibly also necrotic) and 30% is tan to white, more firm solid tissue (**Case fig. 13.6g**). All margins are grossly negative for tumor.

Microscopic features

Low and high magnification, incisional biopsy: The incisional biopsy includes large enough fragments to assess the margin of the tumor. It is permeative which is more consistent with a sarcoma than benign mesenchymal tumor (**Case fig. 13.6h**). At medium magnification, in accord with many examples of MPNST, the tumor is heterogeneous with varying cellularity and architecture. Some areas feature spindled eosinophilic cells flowing around smaller cells with scant cytoplasm and round nuclei (**Case fig. 13.6i**). In other areas, the tumor appears low grade and comprises uniform elongate spindle cells floating in a pale eosinophilic myxoid matrix (**Case fig. 13.6j**). A hemangiopericytomatous vascular pattern is fairly common in MPNST and is present in this patient's tumor (**Case fig. 13.6k**).

Low and high magnification, resection: Low magnification confirms the gross impression of invasion into adipose tissue (**Case fig. 13.6l**). Back to back, hypocellular and hypercellular bands cause a tigroid or marbled appearance (**Case fig. 13.6m**). It is frequent finding in MPNST (in this example it mimics Verocay bodies of schwannoma). Other patterns in this patient's tumor include microcystic or reticular (**Case fig. 13.6n**) and fascicular or herringbone (**Case fig. 13.6o**). Higher magnification of a cellular myxoid area reveals epithelioid to spindled tumor cells with moderate nuclear pleomorphism (**Case fig. 13.6p**).

Special studies: Immunohistochemical staining is performed and reveals scattered clusters of cells reactive for S-100 protein (**Case fig. 13.6q**). Tumor cells do not express keratins, EMA, TLE-1, glial fibrillary acidic protein (GFAP), actin or desmin.

The tumor's karyotype is complex aneuploid: 46,XX,add(2)(p13),+5,t(7;12)(p10;p10),-8,-9,add(9)(p13),-19,-22,+3mar [5]. 47~51,XX,add(2)(p13),+add(2)(p13),t(7;12)(p10,p10),-8,-9,-9,add(9)(p13),+12,+14,+16,-19,add(19)(q13.4),-22,+3~5mar[cp13]. 46,XX[1].

Malignant peripheral nerve sheath tumors often display complex aneuploidy. Loss of chromosome 22, while not specific, is in line with chromosome 22 deletions seen in other peripheral nerve sheath tumors.

Pathologic differential or, why isn't it one of the following?

Synovial sarcoma: The most difficult entity in the pathologic differential of MPNST is synovial sarcoma. Both tumors can show protean patterns even within one example, and the most common architecture is shared: long fascicles of spindle cells that have scant cytoplasm. Both may have epithelioid areas and keratin expression, although these are more common in synovial sarcoma. Fifteen percent of synovial sarcomas may focally express S-100 protein. MPNST does not express TLE-1 in contrast with ~90% of synovial sarcomas. Nearly all cases of synovial sarcoma show a specific translocation: t(X;18)(p11;q11) which fuses the SS18 (SYT) gene to one of five subtypes of the SSX gene (most commonly SSX1 or SSX2). This translocation can be identified by FISH or PCR and is highly useful diagnostically.

High grade sarcoma, NOS: A significant percentage of high grade sarcomas currently are not specifically classifiable (~20%). However, in this case, the characteristic marbling pattern, architectural and cytologic heterogeneity but with some cells featuring buckled or wavy slender spindled nuclei, and focal S-100 protein expression enable a specific diagnosis of MPNST.

Case fig. 13.6r provides gender, age and body location data for 16 MPNST resected at the University of New Mexico Health Sciences Center 2000-2010, a moderately sized academic institution. Although the number of patients is small, 44% of patients are under the age of 40 years. Most of these younger patients have NF1.

Oncology approach

Medical oncology

This patient presents with a large tumor of the thigh. She is offered participation in a clinical trial of neoadjuvant chemotherapy with a combination of gemcitabine, docetaxel and bevacizumab (Verschraegen, et al. 2012). She receives the planned four courses. Her tumor remains stable by PET-scan or MRI, but the patient's pain decreases considerably with chemotherapy. She is then referred to surgery.

Radiation oncology

Despite wide margins, adjuvant radiation therapy is indicated in order improve local control. Fortunately, the patient is disease free years later.

Patient outcome

Three years postoperatively, the patient has normal function and no evidence of local recurrence or metastatic disease.

Case table 13.6 Summary pathology findings of Case 13.6

Diagnosis	MPNST
Size	14.7 × 11.2 × 11 cm
Location	Intramuscular, buttock
Margin status	Negative
Histologic grade (FNCLCC grading system)	High grade
Pathologic stage (AJCC TNM classification)	Stage III = T2b/N0/M0

FNCLCC: Fédération Nationale des Centres de Lutte Contre le Cancer (French Federation of Cancer Centers). AJCC: American Joint Committee on Cancer

Case 13.7 Epithelioid malignant peripheral nerve sheath tumor

Clinical history and presentation

A 36 year old man presents with a one-month history of right hip pain and swelling which began after a work-out and has been slowly progressive, to the point where he now has a large mass associated with paresthesias in the posterior aspect of the right leg. On further questioning, he does relate a history of intermittent right sided sciatica over the past three to four years. The pain is increased with activity and at night and decreased with rest.

Physical examination of the right hip reveals a large ill-defined deeply seated soft tissue mass involving the right buttock and lateral hip.

Surgical findings and comments

Open biopsy is performed. Final pathologic findings are consistent with a benign nerve sheath tumor. The patient is returned to surgery two weeks following the biopsy where marginal excision of the tumor is performed.

On pathologic examination of the entire removed specimen, malignancy is identified.

Amputative hemipelvectomy is recommended to the patient. Under the realization that there is a high risk of metastatic disease, the patient opts for a course of radiation and chemotherapy rather than further surgery on the extremity, pending the possibility of local recurrence.

Radiology findings

The MR images of this case (**Case figs 13.7a** through **13.7d**), shows a very large multicompartment tumor of the gluteal region with extension into the pelvis and invasion of the ischial tuberosity. The mass is very heterogeneous with areas of intense enhancement and other cystic appearing areas. The sciatic nerve is surrounded by the tumor, and lies anterior to the cystic portion as seen on **Case fig. 13.7c**. The sciatic nerve may be invaded by the tumor, but does not appear to be the nerve of origin. Overall, the appearance is not specific, however; clearly this is an aggressive tumor likely a sarcoma.

Pathology findings

Gross features

The incisional biopsy consists of several portions of pale yellow, semi-translucent soft tissue ranging up to 2.3 cm in maximum diameter. A small amount is sent to Cytogenetics, and the remainder is submitted in three cassettes for histology processing.

The resection consists of multiple fragments of tan pink lobulated tumor ranging in diameter from 1 to 10.5 cm and aggregating to 23 × 20 × 5cm. Cross sections reveal a solid, grossly heterogeneous interior with opaque to semi-translucent solid to gelatinous tumor and brown areas of ragged soft parenchyma consistent with necrosis (**Case fig. 13.7e**). The tumor multifocally extends to inked surgical margins. Some tumor is collected fresh for Cytogenetics and for tissue banking, and 20 cassettes are submitted for histology processing.

Microscopic features

Incisional biopsy low and high magnification*:* Unfortunately, this tumor appears deceptively low grade on the incisional biopsy. In many areas, tumor cellularity is low, and it exhibits a pushing margin with normal tissue (**Case fig. 13.7f**). A few areas are more cellular and composed of storiforming, uniform cells with indistinct cell borders (**Case fig. 13.7g**). These areas mimic perineuroma or schwannoma. Some of the more cellular areas reveal epithelioid tumor cells cordoned off by bands of vascularized fibrous tissue (**Case fig. 13.7h**). No melanin pigment or psammomatous calcifications are found. High magnification of a more cellular region reveals epithelioid tumor cells with variable nuclei in terms of shape and size (**Case fig. 13.7i**). However, coarse chromatin, irregularly distributed chromatin, macronucleoli, and hyperchromasia (nuclear features typical of malignant cells) are absent. An intensive search for mitotic activity fails to find any mitoses. Spindled tumor cells are also present and also show no overtly malignant nuclear features.

Special studies performed on incisional biopsy: All epithelioid tumor cells and intermixed spindled tumor cells strongly express S-100 protein by immunohistochemistry (**Case fig. 13.7j**). Intercolated bands of fibrovascular tissue are negative for S-100 protein and instead show strong expression of smooth muscle actin consistent with reactive myofibroblasts. Scattered cells are reactive for neurofilaments (**Case fig. 13.7k**). Similar to what has been described in epithelioid schwannomas, foci of CD-34 expressing fibroblasts form a mesh around epithelioid tumor cells (**Case fig. 13.7l**) (Laskin et al. 2005). The number of proliferating cells is low and estimated at less than 1% by Ki67 IHC (**Case fig. 13.7m**).

The karyotype of the tumor is reported as 46,XY[19] with one non-clonal cell showing the following: 45,XY,t(1;17)(q32;p11.2),-15,add(18)(q21.1)-19,+mar[1]. This represented one cell of 20 metaphases analyzed. There are no identifiable abnormalities of chromosome 17q (site of NF1 gene) or chromosome 22 (site of NF2 gene). Of course, the non-clonal abnormal cell may represent an artifact of tissue culture.

The tumor is signed out by the surgical pathologist as a peripheral nerve sheath tumor most suggestive of epithelioid schwannoma. However, because the tumor is large and aggressive appearing on radiology, the surgical pathology report also states that this is a relatively small sample and may not be representative of the entire tumor. Additionally, the report notes that schwannomas may undergo malignant transformation, albeit rarely, and caution is advised in assuming with 100% confidence that the tumor is benign.

Resection (debulking) specimen low and high magnification: In contrast to the pushing border noted on the incisional biopsy, many areas of the resection specimen reveal permeative growth into skeletal muscle and adipose tissue (**Case fig. 13.7n**). Approximately 25% of tissue sections are necrotic and hemorrhagic. Ten percent consists of high grade tumor with increased cellularity, individual cell necrosis, and mitotic activity (**Case fig. 13.7o**). The maximum mitotic rate in the high grade areas is 3/10 hpf. In the high grade foci, tumor cells are round to polygonal with scant cytoplasm and hyperchromatic nuclei without nuclear inclusions. In the low grade areas, the cells are predominantly epithelioid, 10% exhibit nuclear inclusions, and mitotic activity and necrosis are absent.

Special studies performed on resection: Diffuse S-100 reactivity is retained in the high grade areas consistent with the epithelioid variant of MPNST (**Case fig. 13.7p**). Higher grade regions also show nuclear reactivity for MDM2 (**Case fig. 13.7q**). The proliferation marker, Ki67, has increased expression in high grade areas of tumor (30-50% of cells reactive). All tumor cells express INI-1 in the nuclei.

Repeat karyotyping of the patient's resection specimen reveals a single clonal abnormality distinct from the first non-clonal abnormal karyotype: 46,XY,inv(6)(p12p23)[7]/46,XY[12]. Although clonal, the finding is not specific for a particular tumor and is unusually simple for MPNST which typically demonstrates complex aneuploidy with multiple numerical and structural chromosome changes.

Pathologic differential or, why isn't it one of the following?

Epithelioid schwannoma: Areas of this patient's tumor are consistent with epithelioid schwannoma: the regions of low to moderate cellularity composed of epithelioid tumor cells without overt malignant nuclear features and no mitotic activity. In fact, benign epithelioid nerve sheath tumors may actually be highly cellular, but most are well circumscribed, many are suprafascial, and average size is small 1.5 cm (range of 0.3 to 6.8 cm)(Laskin et al. 2005).

Most epithelioid MPNST are larger and often hypercellular with or without a myxoid background matrix. The tumors are usually composed of relatively uniform epithelioid cells with amphophilic or eosinophilic cytoplasm and large, vesicular nuclei with prominent eosinophilic nucleoli (Fisher et al. 2011, Miettinen et al. 2010). Tumor cells may be arranged as nodules, cords, or solid sheets. Rhabdoid and clear cells may be present, and a more typical MPNST spindle cell fascicular component is common. Necrosis and mitotic activity are usually conspicuous.

This patient's tumor is atypical for epithelioid MPNST in its lack of the characteristic vesicular nuclei with prominent nucleoli. However, infiltrative growth, foci of geographic necrosis, large size, high grade areas with prominent mitotic activity, and some nuclear atypia comprising hyperchromatic nuclei with coarse chromatin enable a diagnosis of malignant sarcoma. Furthermore, diffuse S-100 reactivity is in keeping with epithelioid MPNST. The lack of reactivity for melanoma markers and focal reactivity for neurofilaments and GFAP also support the diagnosis of epithelioid MPNST. The majority of MPNST display a complex aneuploid karyotype; this patient's tumor karyotyping yielded a normal karyotype with one non-clonal abnormal cell. It is possible that the cells karyotyped may have represented overgrowth of normal cells. The single abnormal cell may not accurately depict the genetic state of the tumor.

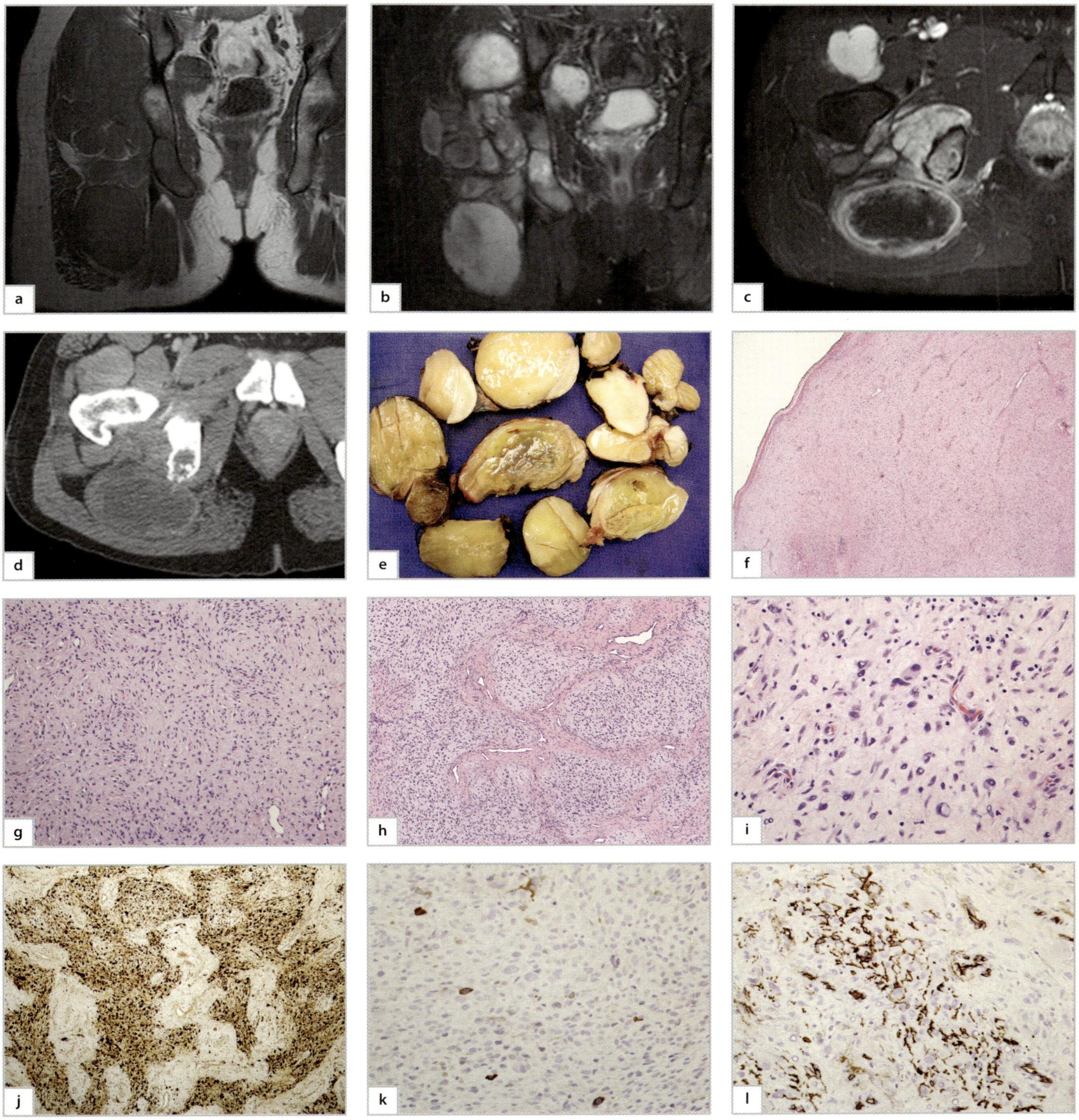

Case figure 13.7 Epithelioid malignant peripheral nerve sheath tumor (MPNST) imaging. **13.7a**: Coronal T1 MR image. **13.7b**: Coronal STIR MR image. **3.7c**: Axial T1 fat saturated post-contrast MR image. The MR images in this 35 year old man show a 23.6 × 12.7 × 16cm multilobulated mass of the buttock extending into the pelvis and displacing the bladder. The mass surrounds the sciatic nerve. The mass shows heterogeneity with cystic areas and areas of intense enhancement. The CT image. **13.7d**: Axial post IV contrast CT scan with bone window shows bone destruction. The overall appearance is non-specific, but indicates an aggressive lesion consistent with a sarcoma. **13.7e**: Gross photograph of tumor cross sections. The tumor is almost entirely solid but varies in consistency from semi-firm to soft and mucoid in color from opaque tan to brownish-green and mucoid. The tumor extends to inked surgical margins. Green and gelatinous areas may be necrotic. **13.7f**: Low magnification. Much of the biopsy consists of a low cellularity tumor with a pushing rather than infiltrative border. Necrosis and hemorrhage are absent. **13.7g**: Medium magnification. Storiforming, slightly more cellular areas form the minority of the biopsy. The cells are uniform and on H&E stain suggest Schwann cells or possibly perineural cells. **13.7h**: Medium magnification. Moderately cellular are of nodules of epithelioid tumor cells encased by bands of vascular fibrous tissue. Even at this magnification, tumor cell variability is appreciable.

Case figure 13.7: Continued from page 283

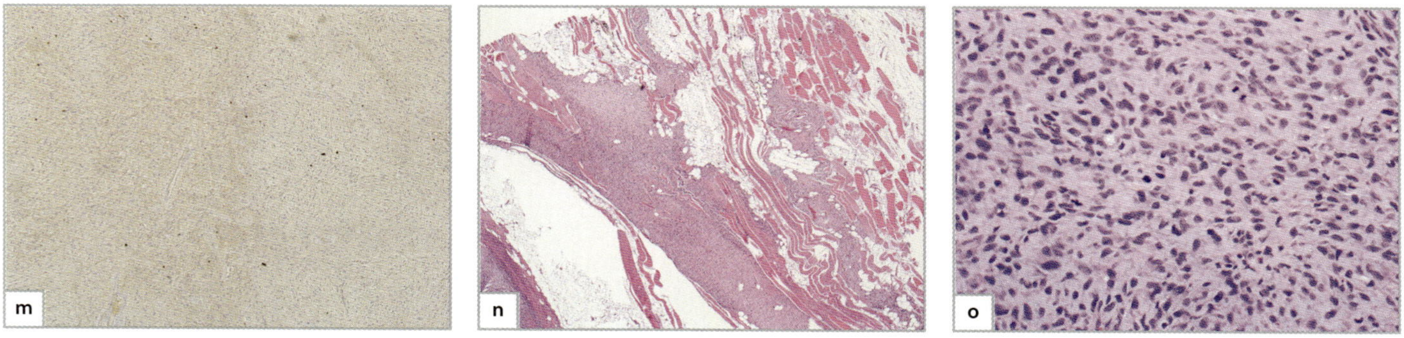

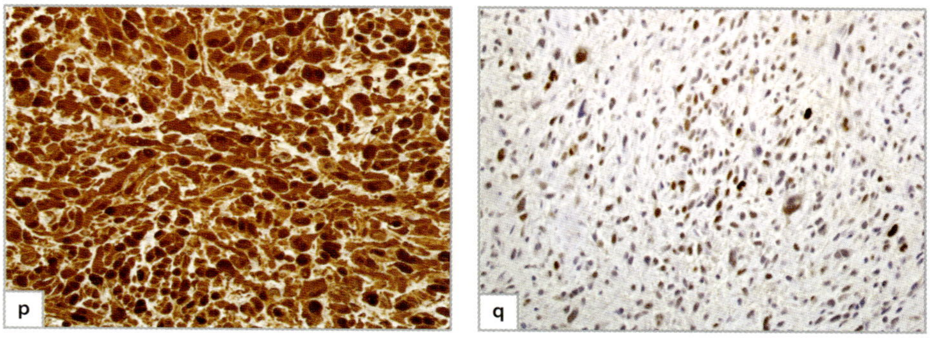

13.7i: High magnification. Many of the tumor cells are epithelioid (rounded with discrete cell borders). Some cells display nuclear inclusions. Although variable in nuclear size and shape, coarse, irregularly distributed chromatin, hyperchromaticity, and macronucleoli, aspects often notable in malignant nuclei, are absent in these nuclei. Mitotic figures are not identified. **13.7j**: S-100 IHC stain. All epithelioid and intermixed spindled tumor cells strongly express S-100 protein. The interwoven bands of fibrovascular tissue show reactivity for smooth muscle actin (not demonstrated on this slide which instead reveals lack of reactivity for S-100 in these bands). **13.7k**: Neurofilaments IHC stain. Scattered tumor cells are reactive for neurofilaments. Such axonally differentiated cells occur in half of conventional schwannomas. **13.7l**: CD34 stain IHC stain. Similar to what is seen in some epithelioid schwannomas; CD34-expressing fibroblasts form a mesh around epithelioid tumor cells. These meshes are spottily distributed throughout the epithelioid areas of the biopsy. **13.7m**: Ki67 IHC stain. The proliferation rate is low (less than 1%) in the biopsy material. **13.7n**: Low magnification. The resection specimen clearly shows area of aggressive permeation by tumor into adjacent normal tissue. **13.7o**: High magnification. Three mitotic figures are present in this field of high grade tumor. **13.7p**: S-100 protein IHC stain. The epithelioid high grade tumor cells diffusely express S-100 protein in both the nuclei and cytoplasm. **13.7q**: Resection specimen, MDM2 IHC stain. Numerous cells in higher grade areas show nuclear reactivity for MDM2 protein.

Proximal type epithelioid sarcoma (PT-ES): Proximal type epithelioid sarcoma could mimic the typical epithelioid MPNST histologically because it consists of sheets of epithelioid cells with vesicular nuclei and prominent nucleoli. However, it should express epithelial markers (keratins 8, 14 and 19 and EMA most commonly), while it will not express S-100 protein. Many cases show loss of INI-1 nuclear expression, but about 50% of epithelioid MPNST also show loss of reactivity.

Sarcoma, high grade with epithelioid cells, not otherwise specified: Some sarcomas cannot be specifically diagnosed. A few are epithelioid in morphology. This patient's tumor does not fall into the category of sarcoma with epithelioid morphology, NOS, because of IHC results indicating peripheral nerve sheath differentiation.

Case table 13.7a lists the histologic variants and variant features reported for malignant peripheral nerve sheath tumors. Just as with benign peripheral nerve sheath tumors, MPNST exhibits diverse appearances.

Oncology approach

Medical oncology

After resection of the primary tumor, the patient is found to have positive margins. He receives four courses of adjuvant chemotherapy with docetaxel, gemcitabine, and bevacizumab. The multidisciplinary treatment is completed with a course of adjuvant radiotherapy to the bed of the tumor.

Six months later the patient presents with multiple bony and pulmonary metastases with involvement of the base of the skull and cord compression, requiring emergent radiotherapy. The radiation treatment is followed by one course of doxorubicin and ifosfamide, but the patient develops a neutropenic septicemia, requiring intensive care monitoring. He does not respond to the treatment and is transferred to palliative care.

Radiation oncology

An amputative hemipelvectomy is needed in order to remove the tumor completely, but the patient decides to undergo definitive radiation therapy instead in light of the overall poor prognosis. He later develops metastatic disease.

Patient outcome

Despite aggressive treatment, the patient develops pulmonary metastases nine months post-operatively. One year postoperatively he is alive with progressive disease.

Case table 13.7a Histologic variants or variant features of MPNST

Variant or feature	Frequency	Comment
MPNST arising in plexiform neurofibroma	Common	20-50% of all MPNST arise in NF1 patients, mostly in deep plexiform neurofibromas Overall lifetime risk for NF1 patient to develop MPNST: 8-13%
Spindle cells arranged in fascicles	Common	Resembles synovial sarcoma
Spindle cells arranged in herringbone files	Common	Resembles synovial sarcoma
Alternating hypocellular and hypercellular bands	Common	This is a diagnostic clue to but is not specific for MPNST
Perivascular accentuated hypercellularity	Common	Tumor cells may also invade vessel walls; this is also a diagnostic clue but not specific to MPNST
Necrosis- geographic palisading or diffuse	Common	Geographic palisading = edges of tumor nodules exhibit a rim of necrotic cells Diffuse = broad areas are necrotic with residual viable cells cuffing vessels
Patchy hyalinization (dense collagen deposition with few cells)	Common	Contributes to the heterogeneous microscopic appearance
Spindle cells with wavy or buckled, pointy ended, spindled nuclei; often nuclei are lanceolate (shaped like an arrowhead)	Common	Most common appearance of MPNST nuclei Lanceolate nucleus: one end is pointed and the other blunt. Nuclei of synovial sarcoma tend to be ovoid and appear overlapping
Relatively bland, uniform nuclei in a tumor that otherwise has features of high grade MPNST	Uncommon	Other features of high grade MPNST include many mitoses =/- atypical mitoses, permeative growth, and necrosis
Small round cell appearance	Uncommon	Mimics other small round cell tumors including small round cell or poorly differentiated variant of synovial sarcoma
Verocay bodies	Uncommon	Palisading tumor nuclei
Hemangiopericytomatous vessels	Uncommon	Thin walled, ectatic sharply angulated vessels 'staghorn' like
Marked nuclear pleomorphism	Uncommon	Marked variability in nuclear size and shape with multi-lobulation and scattered tumor giant cells
Numerous tumor giant cells	Uncommon	
Divergent mesenchymal differentiation	Uncommon	Seen in 15% of MPNST. Usually takes form of a sarcoma, most commonly rhabdomyosarcoma (malignant Triton tumor) but also includes osteosarcoma, chondrosarcoma, and angiosarcoma. Malignant Triton tumors may have a worse prognosis
Divergent epithelial differentiation	Rare	Differential includes biphasic synovial sarcoma Epithelium is most commonly mucin producing glands but columnar, flat or squamous epithelium also occurs. In most cases, epithelium is cytologically benign. Neuroendocrine cells frequently mixed in with glandular cells (this is absent in synovial sarcoma). Glandular cell often CK20 +/CK7- (opposite pattern in synovial sarcoma). Most patients have NF1
Epithelioid MPNST	Rare	May arise from pre-existing schwannoma. No increased association with NF1. Diffusely S-100 protein positive in contrast to typical MPNST which usually exhibits patchy positivity
MPNST with perineurial differentiation ('malignant perineuroma')	Rare	Tumor cells express perineurial type markers (EMA, Claudin-1, GLUT1) but show increased mitotic activity, necrosis and atypia
MPNST arising from schwannoma	Extremely rare	Most such MPNST are of the epithelioid variant
MPNST arising from ganglioneuroma	Extremely rare	May be associated with history of radiation to benign tumor

Case table 13.7b Summary pathology findings of Case 13.7

Diagnosis	Epithelioid MPNST
Size	23 cm (approximately)
Location	Gluteal muscle with invasion into pelvis
Margin status	Positive (resection is intended as a debulking)
Histologic grade (FNCLCC grading system)	High grade (some areas of resection show increased cellularity, individual cell necrosis, and mitotic rate of 8/10 hpf)
Pathologic stage (AJCC TNM classification)	III = T2b/N0/M0 (deep high grade tumor > 5cm; no lymph node or distant metastases at presentation)

FNCLCC: Fédération Nationale des Centres de Lutte Contre le Cancer (French Federation of Cancer Centers). AJCC: American Joint Committee on Cancer

REFERENCES

Anghileri M, Miceli R, Fiore M, et al. Malignant peripheral nerve sheath tumors: prognostic factors and survival in a series of patients treated at a single institution. Cancer 2006;107:1065–74.

Antonescu CR. The role of genetic testing in soft tissue sarcoma. Histopathol 2006;48(1);13–21.

Beaman FD, Kransdorf MJ, Menke DM. Schwannoma: radiologic-pathologic correlation. Radiographics 2004;24:1477–1481.

Berndt N, Hamilton AD, Sebti SM. Targeting protein prenylation for cancer therapy. Nat Rev Cancer 2011;11:775–91.

Blacksin MF, White LM, Hameed M, et al. Granular cell tumor of the extremity: magnetic resonance imaging characteristics with pathologic correlation. Skeletal Radiol 2005;34(10):625–31.

Brock JE, Perez-Atayde AR, Kozakewich PW, et al. Cytogenetic aberrations in perineurioma, variation with subtype. Am J Surg Pathol 2004;29(9):1164–9.

Carter JM, O'Hara C, Dundas G, et al. Epithelioid malignant peripheral nerve sheath tumor arising in a schwannoma, in a patient with 'neuroblastoma-like' schwannomatosis and a novel germline SMARCB1 mutation. Am J Surg Pathol 2012;36:154–160.

Chee, DWY, Peh WCG, Shek TWH. Pictorial essay: imaging of peripheral nerve sheath tumours. Can Assoc Radiol J 2011;62:176–182.

Chetty R. Reticular and microcystic schwannoma: a distinctive tumor of the gastrointestinal tract. Ann Diag Pathol 2011;15(3):198–201.

Ducatman BS, Scheithauer BW, Piepgras DG, et al. Malignant peripheral nerve sheath tumors. A clinicopathologic study of 120 cases. Cancer 15;57(10):2006–2021.

Endo M, Kobayashi C, Setsu N, et al. Prognostic significance of p14ARF, p15INK4b and p16INK4a inactivation in malignant peripheral nerve sheath tumors. Clin Can Res 2011;17:3771–3782.

Feldman DS, Jordan C, Fonseca L. Orthopaedic manifestations of neurofibromatosis type 1. J Am Acad Orthop Surg 2010;18(6):346–57.

Frank D, Gunawan B, Holtrup M, et al. Cytogenetic characterization of three malignant peripheral nerve sheath tumors. Cancer Genetics Cytogenet 2001;144(1):18–22

Guillou L, Aurias A. Soft tissue sarcomas with complex genomic profiles. Virchows Arch 2010;456(2):201–17.

Gupta G, Mammis A, Maniker A. Malignant peripheral nerve sheath tumors. Neurosurg Clin N Am 2008;19(4):533–543.

Harder A, Wesemann M, Hagel C, et al. Hybrid neurofibroma/schwannoma is overrepresented among schwannomatosis and neurofibromatosis patients. Am J Surg Pathol 2012;36(5):702–9.

Hassell DS, Bancroft LW, Kransdorf MJ, et al. Imaging appearance of diffuse neurofibroma. AJR 2008;190(3):582–588.

Hornick JL, Bundock EA, Fletcher CDM. Hybrid schwannoma/perineurioma: clinicopathologic analysis of 42 distinctive benign nerve sheath tumors. Am J Surg Pathol 2009;33(10):1554–61.

Hornick JL, Fletcher CD. Soft tissue perineurioma: clinicopathologic analysis of 81 cases including those with atypical histologic features. Am J Surg Pathol 2005;29:845–858.

Ingham S, Huson SM, Moran A, et al. Malignant peripheral nerve sheath tumours in NF1: Improved survival in women and in recent years. Eur J Cancer 2011;47(18):2723–8.

Jee WH, Oh SN, McCauley T, Ryu KN, et al. Extraaxial neurofibromas versus neurilemomas: discrimination with MRI. AJR Am J Roentgenol 2004;183(3):629–633.

Joste NE, Racz MI, Montgomery KD, et al. Clonal chromosome abnormalities in a plexiform cellular schwannoma. Cancer Genetics Cytogenet 2004;150(1):73–7.

Jouhilahti E-M, Peltonen S, Heape AM, et al. The pathoetiology of Neurofibromatosis 1. Am J Path 2011;178:1932–1939.

Kalamarides M, Acosta MT, Babovic-Vuksanovic D, et al. Neurofibromatosis 2011: a report of the Children's Tumor Foundation Annual Meeting. Acta Neuropathol 2012;123(3):369–80.

Klose A, Ahmadian MR, Schuelke M, et al. Selective disactivation of neurofibromin GAP activity in neurofibromatosis type 1. Hum Mol Genet 1998;7:1261–8.

Kransdorf MJ, Murphey MD. Imaging of Soft Tissue Tumors, 2nd ed. Baltimore: Lippincott Williams and Wilkins, 2006:349–351.

Kroep JR, Ouali M, Gelderblom H, et al. First-line chemotherapy for malignant peripheral nerve sheath tumor (MPNST) versus other histological soft tissue sarcoma subtypes and as a prognostic factor for MPNST: an EORTC soft tissue and bone sarcoma group study. Ann Oncol 2011;22:207–14.

Laskin WB, Fetsch JF, Lasota J, et al. Benign epithelioid peripheral nerve sheath tumors of the soft tissues: clinicopathologic spectrum of 33 cases. Am J Surg Pathol 2005;29(1):39–51.

Macarenco RS, Ellinger F, Oliveira AM. A distinctive and underrecognized peripheral nerve sheath neoplasm. Arch Pathol Lab Med 2006;131(4):625–36.

McMenamin ME, Fletcher CDM. Expanding the spectrum of malignant change in schwannomas. Am J Surg Path 2001;25(1):13–25.

Mentzel T, Kutzner H. Reticular and plexiform perineurioma: clinicopathological and immunohistochemical analysis of two cases and review of perineurial neoplasms of skin and soft tissues. Virchows Archives 2005;447(4):677–82.

Mertens F, Dal Cin P, De Wever I, et al. Cytogenetic characterization of peripheral nerve sheath tumours: a report of the CHAMP study group. J Pathol 2000;190:31–38.

Nasser H, Danforth Jr RD, Sunbuli M, et al. Malignant granular cell tumor: case report with a novel karyotype and review of the literature. Ann Diag Pathol 2010;14(4):273–8.

Papachristou DJ, Palekar A, Surti U, et al. Malignant granular cell tumor of the ulnar nerve with novel cytogenetic and modular genetic findings. Cancer Genetics Cytogenet 2009;191(1):46–50.

Patton KT, Satcher RL, Laskin WB. Capillary hemangioblastoma of soft tissue: report of a case and review of the literature. Hum Pathol 2005;36:1135–1139.

Reuter CW, Morgan MA, Bergmann L. Targeting the Ras signaling pathway: a rational, mechanism-based treatment for hematologic malignancies? Blood 2000;96:1655–69.

Robertson TC, Buck DA, Schmidt-Ullrich R, et al. Isolated plexiform neurofibroma: treatment with three-dimensional conformal radiotherapy. Laryngoscope 2004;114(7):1139–42.

Rodriguez FJ, Folpe AL, Giannini C, et al. Pathology of peripheral nerve sheath tumors: diagnostic overview and update on selected diagnostic problems. Acta Neuropathol 2012;123(3):295–319.

Rodriguez FJ, Stratakis CA, Evans DG. Genetic predisposition to peripheral nerve neoplasia: diagnostic criteria and pathogenesis of neurofibromatoses, Carney complex, and related syndromes. Acta Neuropathol 2012;123(3):349–367.

Scheithaueer BW, Amrami KK, Folpe AL, et al. Synovial sarcoma of nerve. Hum Pathol 2011;42(4);568–77.

Schildhaus H-U, Riegal R, Hartmann W, et al. Lysine-specific demethylase 1 is highly expressed in solitary fibrous tumors, synovial sarcomas, rhabdomyosarcomas, desmoplastic small round cell tumors, and malignant peripheral nerve sheath tumors. Hum Pathol 2011;42:1667–1675.

Spyk SL, Thomas N, Cooper DN, et al. Neurofibromatosis type 1-associated tumours: Their somatic mutational spectrum and pathogenesis. Hum Genomics 2011;5:623–90.

Stucky C-C, Johnson KN, Gray RJ, et al. Malignant peripheral nerve sheath tumors (MPNST): The Mayo Clinic Experience. Ann Surg Oncol 2012;19(3):878–885.

Tassano E, Sementa AR, Tavella E, et al. Trisomy 17 in congenital plexiform (multinodular) cellular schwannoma. Cancer Genetics Cytogenet 2010;203(2):313–5.

Thirukkumaran C, Morris DG. Oncolytic viral therapy using reovirus. Methods Mol Biol 2009;542:607–34.

Tommaso LD, Magrini E, Consales A, et al. Malignant granular cell tumor of the lateral femoral cutaneous nerve: report of a case with cytogenetic analysis. Hum Pathol 2002;33(12):1237–40.

Upadhyaya M. Genetic basis of tumorigenesis in NF1 malignant peripheral nerve sheath tumors. Front Biosci 2011;16:937–51.

Wasa J, Nishida Y, Tsukushi S, et al. MRI features in the differentiation of malignant peripheral nerve sheath tumors and neurofibromas. AJR Am J Roentgenol 2010;194(6):1568–1574.

Wong WW, Hirose T, Scheithauer BW, et al. Malignant peripheral nerve sheath tumor: analysis of treatment outcome. Int J Radiat Oncol Biol Phys 1998;42(2):351.

Yu J, Deshmukh H, Payton JE, et al. Array-based comparative genomic hybridization identifies CDK4 and FOMX1 alterations as independent predictors of survival in malignant peripheral nerve sheath tumor. Clin Can Res 2011;17(7):1924–34.

Zou C, Smith KD, Liu J, et al. Clinical, pathological, and molecular variables predictive of malignant peripheral nerve sheath tumor outcome. Ann Surg 2009:1014–22.

FURTHER READING

Fisher C, Mentzel T, Montgomery EA, et al. Diagnostic Pathology Soft Tissue Tumors. Salt Lake City: AMIRSYS, 2011.
Folpe AL, Inwards CY (eds). Bone and Soft Tissue Pathology. A volume in the series: Foundations in Diagnostic Pathology. Goldblum JR (series ed). Philadelphia: Elsevier Saunders, 2010.
Miettinen M. Modern Soft Tissue Pathology. Cambridge: Cambridge University Press, 2010.
Fletcher CDM, Krishnan Unni K, Mertens F (Eds). World Health Organization Classification of Tumours. Pathology and Genetics of Tumours of Soft Tissue and Bone. Lyon: IARC Press, 2013.
Scheithauer BW, Woodruff JM, Erlandson RA (Eds). Atlas of Tumor Pathology Tumors of the Peripheral Nervous System. Washington DC: Armed Forces Institute of Pathology 1999.
Hornick JL (Ed). Practical Soft Tissue Pathology: A Diagnostic Approach. Philadelphia: Elsevier Saunders, 2013.

Chapter 14 Miscellaneous soft tissue tumors of uncertain differentiation

OVERVIEW

These tumors are grouped together because each one is enigmatic in the same manner: each neoplasm can be well characterized morphologically, immunohistochemically and to some degree genetically, yet the cell of differentiation is unknown. In fact, some of these tumors may not possess a normal cell analog; this could be the case for epithelioid sarcoma and alveolar soft part sarcoma, for example. Most other soft tissue tumors differentiate along a specific cellular phenotype. Examples include the liposarcomas, rhabdomyosarcomas, and vascular tumors. Others most likely represent neoplastic counterparts of primitive neuroectodermal blastic cells such as with the Ewing sarcoma family of tumors. Finally, some sarcomas are poorly differentiated and have lost any resemblance to a normal cell type. By comparison, this chapter's group differs from these undifferentiated and poorly differentiated tumors by being highly distinctive yet untethered to a cell type, which is an unusual combination.

While undefined regarding origin and phenotype, nonetheless, these tumors are fairly well defined regarding behavior, prognosis, and treatment approaches. So, from a practical standpoint, when one of these tumors is diagnosed, the patient can be appropriately counseled and treated. Much work continues to discover the relationship of these tumors to other tumors and normal cells, uncover each entity's pathogenesis, elaborate specific molecular genetic features, and, perhaps most importantly, identify key molecular targets to enable refined, more effective therapy. As with many sarcomas, research is hampered by the paucity of these tumors. Therefore, when possible, it is highly desirable to collect fresh tumor for banking, as each case is of immense value for investigators and hence for future patients.

CLASSIFICATION

The World Health Organization (WHO) 2013 classification of these tumors is provided in **Table 14.1**. Note that none of these tumors are closely related to one another. They represent odds and ends in the spectrum of soft tissue tumors: those that remain once all the others have been binned into 1) specific lines of differentiation (schwannoma or leiomyosarcoma, for example); 2) classified as undifferentiated (primitive or blastic; Ewing sarcoma family of tumors, for example); or 3) classified as poorly differentiated or dedifferentiated (undifferentiated high grade pleomorphic sarcoma, or dedifferentiated liposarcoma, for example). Although the WHO considers myoepithelial tumors neoplasms of uncertain differentiation, these tumors are discussed in Chapter 12. Giant cell tumor of soft tissue is considered in this chapter and in Chapter 7.

DEMOGRAPHICS

Surveillance Epidemiology and End Results (SEER) data were evaluated to provide incidence and body site location of seven malignant tumors described in this chapter. SEER sites do not track benign tumors or the rare malignant PEComa, malignant OFMT and malignant behaving AFH, so no population based data are available for the incidence of these sarcomas. SEER data were evaluated from 13 registries during a 15 year period (1994-2008). All tumors presented in this section arise in the connective, subcutaneous and 'other' tissues. The average annual incidence rates of miscellaneous soft tissue tumors of uncertain differentiation, along with their respective ICDO-3 code, are presented in **Table 14.2**. Compared to females, males have statistically higher rates of epithelioid sarcoma (0.5 versus 0.3 per million), extraskeletal myxoid chondrosarcoma (0.3 versus 0.2 per million), and desmoplastic small round cell tumors (0.2 versus 0.0 per million). The number of cases reported in 13 SEER registries is shown in **Figure 14.1**.

Although there is overlap between the ages at diagnosis for the different tumor types, the youngest mean ages at diagnosis are found in patients with alveolar soft part sarcoma, desmoplastic small round cell tumor and extrarenal rhabdoid tumor, and the oldest mean age at diagnosis is seen in the extraskeletal myxoid chondrosarcoma group (**Fig. 14.2**).

The majority of these tumors are diagnosed in the lower long limb and hip (**Fig. 14.3**).

Ten year survival rates for these seven tumors abstracted from SEER data are present in **Table 14.3**. Ten-year relative survival (or relative to the general population of corresponding sex and age) for miscellaneous soft tissue tumors of uncertain differentiation range from 9.7 to 67.4%, with desmoplastic small round cell tumor patients having the worst prognosis, and biphasic synovial sarcoma patients the best.

PATHOGENESIS

The pathogenesis of these tumors is not known. Some arise more commonly in childhood and thus may be related in part to defective differentiation or maturation. Some occur more commonly in young adults, and these may develop under the influence of high levels of circulating hormones, certain proteins, inflammatory mediators, and others. The remaining members of the set tend to occur more commonly in older individuals, and the usual etiologic suspects can be invoked: diminished immune response, accumulating mutations, lengthened exposure time to oncogenic agents, etc.

Table 14.4 lists the genetic findings of these tumors.

PATHOLOGY

Table 14.5 provides demographic and pathologic features of these neoplasms with representative photomicrographs. See the Cases portion of the chapter for a more detailed discussion of selected tumors with additional pathology images.

Table 14.6 lists recently published local recurrence, metastatic and survival rates and adverse prognostic features of these tumors.

Table 14.1 WHO classification of soft tissue tumors of uncertain differentiation (2013)*

Tumor	Behavior	Possible cell of differentiation	Additional comments
Acral fibromyxoma	Benign	Fibroblast, possibly specialized	Usually periungual. Dermal based lesion so it is not discussed further in this text
Intramuscular myxoma **Juxta-articular myxoma**	Benign*	Fibroblast, possibly specialized	Common soft tissue tumor. May be associated with fibrous dysplasia (Mazabraud syndrome). Only rarely locally recurs. Does not metastasize and does not appear to dedifferentiate. *Juxta-articular myxoma is a related tumor with a risk for local recurrence
Deep 'aggressive' angiomyxoma	Benign	Myofiboblastic, possibly specialized	Occurs almost exclusively in adult women. Pelvic/perineal region tumor so it is not discussed further in this text
Ectopic hamartomatous thymoma	Benign	Branchial cleft cells	NOT a thymoma. Almost exclusive to the neck
Atypical fibroxanthoma	Benign	Myofibroblastic or mixed fibroblastic/myofibroblastic	This is a dermal tumor so it is not discussed further in this text
Pleomorphic hyalinizing angiectatic tumor (PHAT)	Intermediate*	Fibroblast, possibly specialized	Rare cases may transform to myxofibrosarcoma
Hemosiderotic fibrolipomatous tumor (HsFIT)	Intermediate	Fibroblast, possibly specialized	May be related to myxoinflammatory fibroblastic sarcoma (MIFS) and possibly to pleomorphic hyalinizing angiectatic tumor (PHAT)
Angiomatoid fibrous histiocytoma (AFH)	Intermediate*	Fibroblastic reticulum cell of lymph node versus other fibroblastic-myoid cell	* Rare cases may metastasize A translocation specific sarcoma
Ossifying fibromyxoid tumor (OFMT)	Intermediate*	Mixed neuronal, Schwannian, and cartilaginous differentiation; unlikely myoepithelial	* Up to 30% local recurrence rate Rare cases metastasize: these comprise both histologically bland and histologically atypical tumors
Synovial sarcoma (SS)	Malignant	Unknown	One of the most common sarcomas occurring in young adults. No relationship to synovium. A translocation specific sarcoma
Epithelioid sarcoma (ES)	Malignant	Unknown	Despite its name, spindle cells often are present and may predominate
Alveolar soft part sarcoma (ASPS)	Malignant	Unknown	A translocation specific sarcoma
Clear cell sarcoma of soft tissue (CCS)	Malignant	Unknown but exhibits some melanocytic features	A translocation specific sarcoma
Extraskeletal myxoid chondrosarcoma (ESMCS)	Malignant	Unknown but often expresses S-100 protein and neuroendocrine markers	A translocation specific sarcoma
Desmoplastic small round cell tumor (DSRCT)	Malignant	Unknown	A translocation specific sarcoma
Perivascular epithelioid cell tumor (PECOMA)	Benign*	Perivascular epithelioid cell with some melanocytic and myoid features	*Tumors with atypical histologic features are able to metastasize
Extrarenal rhabdoid tumor (ERRT)	Malignant	Unknown	This is a diagnosis of exclusion as many other tumors can contain rhabdoid cells (cells with an appearance mimicking small round rhabdomyoblasts)
Intimal sarcoma	Malignant	Smooth muscle or fibroblastic cells of large vessel	Very rare tumor that occurs in large pulmonary vessels or aorta. Not discussed further in this text

* Myoepithelial tumors are considered 'Tumors of uncertain differentiation' and are covered in Chapter 12 of this publication. Giant cell tumor of soft tissue is presented in Chapter 7 and in tables and figures in this chapter. It is currently considered a 'fibrohistiocytic tumor' but is most likely a fibroblastic/myofibroblastic tumor.

RADIOLOGY

As noted, this chapter includes a menagerie of unrelated tumors.

Intramuscular myxoma

The intramuscular myxoma is a common tumor encountered in a sarcoma practice. This is a benign tumor that usually appears homogeneously T1 iso- or low signal intensity to muscle and has T2 and STIR high signal. Myxomas have variable and heterogeneous enhancement. The margins of the tumors are sharply defined without infiltration or invasion evident. The appearance is nonspecific but the absence of aggressive features is reassuring. A thin rim of fat can be seen surrounding intramuscular myxomas. This is usually more prominent adjacent to the proximal and distal poles of the mass. The fat rim may represent focal fatty atrophy of the muscle. Kransdorf and Murphey, 2006, state they 'believe the MR appearance of an intramuscular mass with low signal intensity on T1 weighting, high signal intensity on T2 weighting, and a peripheral rim of fat and surrounding edema is nearly pathognomonic of myxoma.' However, not all intramuscular myxomas demonstrate the peripheral rim of fat. A differential for a sharply circumscribed, homogeneous, T1 low signal, T2 high signal intramuscular mass might include nodular fasciitis or peripheral nerve sheath tumor. Nodular fasciitis has a predilection for the subcutaneous tissues and is most common on the volar aspect of the forearm. The fat rim sign is not described with nodular fasciitis. Peripheral nerve sheath tumors (PNST) may have the split fat sign, showing a triangle or beak of fat tissue adjacent to the proximal or distal poles of the tumor. Also, PNST may show the nerve of origin extending into the mass indicating the neurogenic etiology.

Table 14.2 Average annual incidence rates of miscellaneous soft tissue tumors of uncertain differentiation in 13 SEER registries between the 1994 and 2008

Tumor type	ICDO-3 code	Incidence rate per million
Alveolar soft part sarcoma	9581/3	0.1
Clear cell sarcoma	9044/3	0.2
Desmoplastic small round cell tumor	8806/3	0.1
Epithelioid sarcoma	8804/3	0.4
Extrarenal rhabdoid tumor	8963/3	0.1
Extraskeletal myxoid chondrosarcoma	9231/3	0.2
Synovial sarcoma		
Biphasic	9043/3	0.3
Epithelioid cell	9042/3	0.0
Spindle cell	9041/3	0.4
NOS	9040/3	0.6

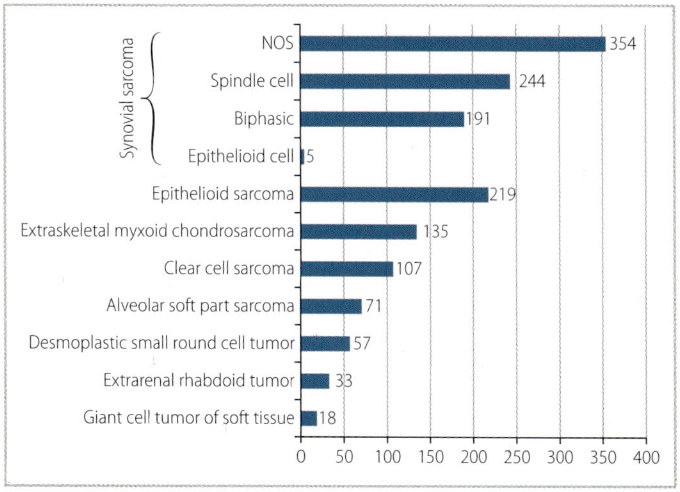

Figure 14.1 Frequency of miscellaneous soft tissue tumors of uncertain differentiation in 13 SEER registries between the years 1994 and 2008.

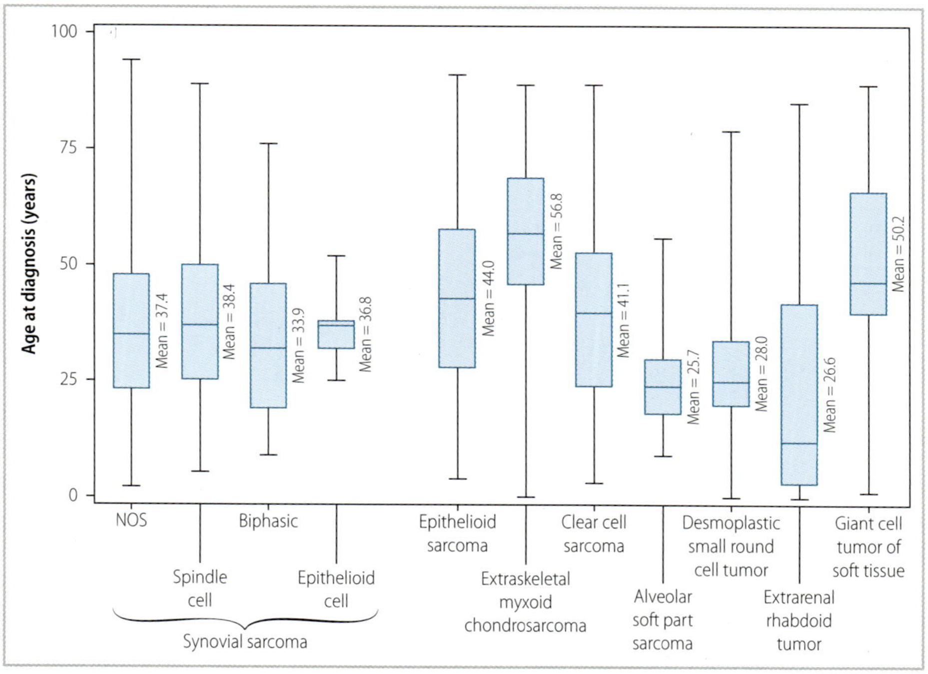

Figure 14.2 Age distribution of miscellaneous soft tissue tumors of uncertain differentiation among cases in 13 SEER registries during the time period 1994-2008 (N=1,434).

There is a rare syndrome of associating myxomas and fibrous dysplasia called Mazabraud syndrome. This is more common with polyostotic fibrous dysplasia, and there is a propensity for the myxomas to occur near the bone lesions. The myxomas are usually multiple in Mazabraud syndromes (Dundaram et al. 1989).

Pleomorphic hyalinizing angiectatic tumor and hemosiderotic fibrolipomatous tumor

These two tumors tend to involve the subcutaneous tissues and have a predilection for the lower extremity, particularly the foot and ankle. Little is published on the imaging appearance. The histologic variation and complexity of these lesions will likely result in significant heterogeneity of imaging appearance.

Angiomatoid fibrous histiocytoma

Angiomatoid fibrous histiocytoma (AFH) is usually superficial in location and involves the extremities. Approximately half of tumors will have pseudovascular blood filled spaces which will show fluid-fluid levels on imaging. A differential for a large aggressive mass comprised predominantly by cystic spaces with fluid-fluid levels might include; angiosarcoma, cavernous hemangioma, and angiomatosis. These lesions are not definitively characterizable on imaging and tissue diagnosis is required.

Ossifying fibromyxoid tumor

The lower extremity is most often affected, followed by upper extremity, trunk, and the head and neck regions. Presentation is usually with a slow growing painless mass, (Miettinen et al. 2008).

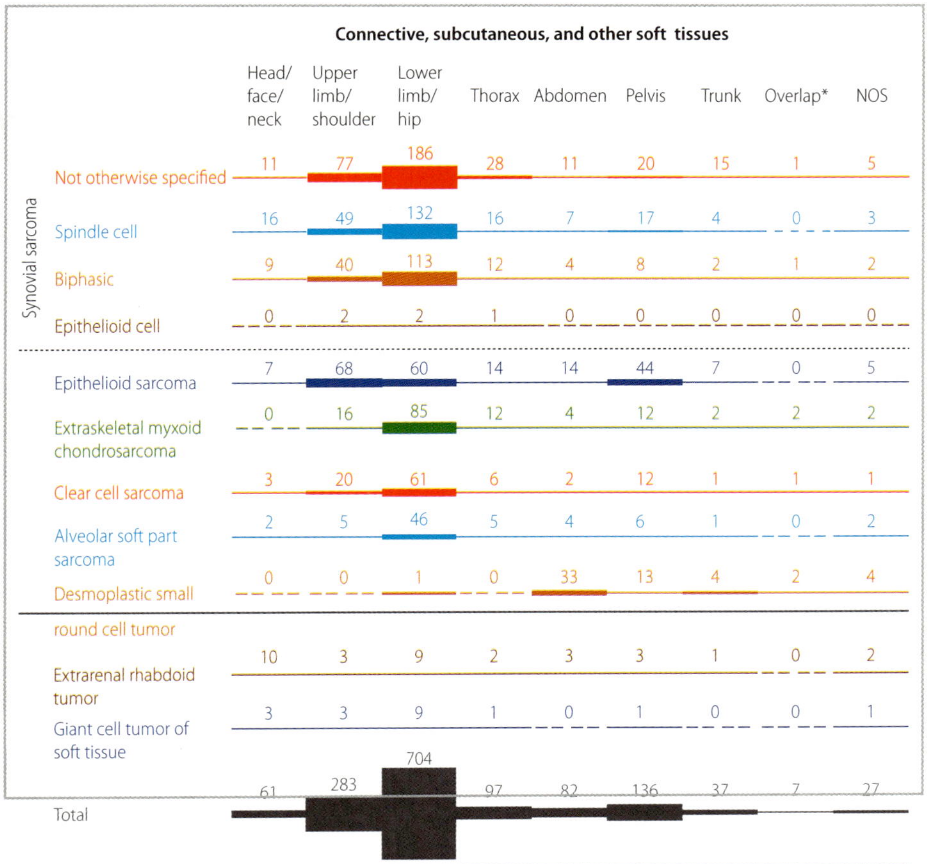

*"A tumor that overlaps the boundaries of two or more subcategories and whose point of origin cannot be determined." (Fritz et al., 2000)

Ten-year relative survival (or relative to the general population of corresponding sex and age) for miscellaneous soft tissue tumors of uncertain differentiation range from 9.7% to 67.8%, with desmoplastic small round cell tumor cases having the worst prognosis, and giant cell tumor of soft tissue cases the best.

Figure 14.3 Miscellaneous soft tissue tumors of uncertain differentiation by site for cases in 13 SEER registries diagnosed between 1994 and 2008.

Table 14.3 Ten-year relative survival rate in 13 SEER registries for years 1994 and 2008, percent survival (SE=standard error)

Tumor type	Percent survival (SE)
Synovial sarcoma	
NOS	62.3% (3.4%)
Spindle cell	51.1% (5.0%)
Biphasic	67.4% (4.4%)
Epithelioid cell	*
Epithelioid sarcoma	50.7% (4.8%)
Extraskeletal myxoid chondrosarcoma	64.1% (8.0%)
Clear cell sarcoma	46.9% (6.2%)
Alveolar soft part sarcoma	42.9% (8.1%)
Desmoplastic small round cell tumor	9.7% (5.6%)
Extrarenal rhabdoid tumor	39.3% (9.8%)

*Due to a small number of cases, 10 year survival could not be calculated.

Schaffler et al. 1997, presented a case with irregular calcifications in an intramuscular mass with significant enhancement seen on CT. The literature describes variable radiographic and MR appearance depending on the amount of mineralization and ossification. Eighty-one percent have an incomplete shell of mature bone in the capsular region of the tumor (Enzinger et al. 1989). Unfortunately, we do not have imaging of a case to present.

Synovial sarcoma

Synovial sarcoma has an equal sex distribution with74% in the extremities, particularly the lower extremity. Eighty-five percent occur in the extremities if the hip and shoulder are included, 20% occur in the foot and ankle and 8% occur in the hand and wrist (Kransdorf et al.1995). Imaging features have prognostic significance.

On CT scan, calcifications are seen in 10% of low grade and 17% of high grade synovial sarcomas. A poorer prognosis is predicted by: tumor >10 cm, absence of calcification, tumor cysts, presence of hemorrhage, proximal location (Tateishi et al. 2004). Patients usually present with a slow growing painful mass. Synovial sarcomas will have punctate calcifications in up to one-third, usually with a peripheral pattern. The slow tumor growth may result in pressure erosions of adjacent bone, frank bone invasion is unusual. MR imaging shows a nonspecific heterogeneous mass with T1 iso or low signal and T2 high signal. Approximately 40% will show evidence of hemorrhage and about 18% will have predominant cystic areas with fluid-fluid levels. The 'triple signal intensity' sign has been described in 35% of cases showing hypo-, iso- and hyper-intensity of the tumor relative to fat on T2 images (Jones et al. 1993). This is apparently due to a combination of cystic and solid

Table 14.4 Genetics of soft tissue tumors of uncertain differentiation

Tumor	Chromosomal abnormality	Genes involved	Percentage of tumors with abnormality
Intramuscular myxoma (IM-M) **Juxta-articular myxoma (JA-M)**	Usually diploid karyotype If abnormal, no specific consistent karyotypic findings. One case of JA-M with inv(2), +7, t(8;22)(q11-12;q12-13)	*GNAS1* gene mutations except in juxta-articular myxoma	50-60% of IM-M feature *GNAS1* activating mutations. JA-M lack *GNAS1* mutations
Giant cell tumor (GCT) of soft tissue	No consistent abnormalities. One case report of telomeric associations (same as in GCT of bone)	Unknown	Unknown
Pleomorphic hyalinizing angiectatic tumor (PHAT) **Hemosiderotic fibrolipomatous tumor (HsFIT)** **Myxoinflammatory fibroblastic sarcoma (MIFS)**	t(1;10)(p22-31;q24-25) and abnormalities of chromosome 3p	t(1;10) = *TGFBR3* (1p22) fused to *MGEA5* (10q24) or a nearby gene causing upregulation of *FGF8* Amplification of *VGLL3* (3p11-12)	Unknown but likely to be a majority of cases of PHAT, HsFIT and MIFS
Angiomatoid fibrous histiocytoma (AFH)	t(2;22)(q33;q12) t(12;16)(q13;p11) t(12;22)(q13;q12) Some cases may also be polysomic	*EWSR1-CREB1* *FUS-ATF1* *EWSR1-ATF1*	~100% (Almost all cases have one of the three translocations.)
Ossifying fibromyxoid tumor (OFMT)	22q deletions in many cases 6p21 rearranged in some cases Few cases studied show variable abnormalities including: t(10;18)(q26;q11), t(6;12)(p21;?), t(3;11)(p21;p15), t(5;13)(q13;q34) t(11;19)(q11;q13) unbalanced translocation involving 14q and various deletions (8p21, 9p22, 12q13) and additions	*PHF1* is abnormal (rearranged) in most cases (located on chromosome 6p21) *INI-1* gene is deleted which parallels mosaic pattern of nuclear expression by IHC (loss of normal INI-1 expression in some cells)	~70% show *INI-1* gene deletions Most cases show *PHF1* gene rearrangements
Synovial sarcoma (SS)	t(X;18)(p11.2;q11.2) t(X;20)(p11.2;q13.3)	*SS18 (SYT)-SSX1, SSX2, SSX3*, or *SSX4* *SS18L1-SSX1*	100% (Most cases have SS18-SSX1 or SS18-SSX2 translocations)
Epithelioid sarcoma (ES)	-22, del or t(22)(q11.2) t(8;22)(q22;q11) in a few classic ES t(10;22) in two cases of proximal ES.	*INI-1* gene loss or translocation	Majority of ES, conventional and proximal types
Alveolar soft part sarcoma	der(17)t(X;17)(p11;q25)	*ASPL-TFE3*	~100%
Clear cell sarcoma of soft tissue	t(12;22)(q13;q12) t(2;22)(q33;q13) Secondary numerical and structural abnormalities may be present involving chromosomes 1,2,3,6,7,8,9,11-17, 21, 22	*EWSR1-ATF1* *EWSR1-CREB1*	~100% (These are the same translocations as in AFH)
Extraskeletal myxoid chondrosarcoma	t(9;22)(q22;q12) t(9;17)(q22;q11) t(9;15)(q22;q21) t(3;9)(q12;q22) May have additional changes including del(22)(q12-13) and trisomies of 1q, 7, 8, 12, 19	*EWSR1-NR4A3* *TAF15-NR4A3* *TCF12-NR4A3* *TFG-NR4A3*	~100% (t(9;22) is most common). All cases to date involve *NR4A3* gene as a fusion partner
Desmoplastic small round cell tumor	t(11;22)(p13;q12)	*WT1-EWSR1*	100%
Perivascular epithelioid cell tumor	16p13 LOH 9q34 LOH	*TSC2* *TSC1* (These are the tuberous sclerosis genes)	Majority may have *TSC2* LOH; rare cases have both *TSC2* and *TSC1* LOH
Extrarenal rhabdoid tumor	Deletion of 22q11.2 or specific gene mutation at 22q11.2	*hSNF5/SMARCB1* (INI-1) gene deleted on 22q11.2. - Some are germline mutations. p53 mutations common Keratin 8 gene mutations common	~100% (INI-1 gene abnormalities seen in almost all cases and may become definitional)

Amp = amplification. O-E = over-expressed, LOH = loss of heterozygosity, t = translocation, CR = case report

See References for papers and texts pertaining to this table. This static list of genetic abnormalities must be viewed in the context of continuing discovery and refinement of genetic findings.

Table 14.5 Soft tissue tumors of uncertain differentiation grouped by behavior

<table>
<tr><th rowspan="2">Tumor</th><th rowspan="2">Incidence</th><th rowspan="2">Age and sex</th><th rowspan="2">Body site (in descending order of involvement)</th><th colspan="2">Histopathology description including IHC</th></tr>
<tr><th>Medium magnification</th><th>High magnification</th></tr>
<tr><td colspan="6">Benign: does not recur or does not aggressively recur and does not metastasize</td></tr>
<tr><td>Intramuscular myxoma (IM-M)
Juxta-articular myxoma (JA-M)</td><td>Common</td><td>Middle aged adults most commonly.
F > M
JA-M is M > F</td><td>Deep soft tissue of thigh, buttock, shoulder, proximal arm.
Juxta-articular myxoma is most often around knee; superficial and deep soft tissue involvement</td><td>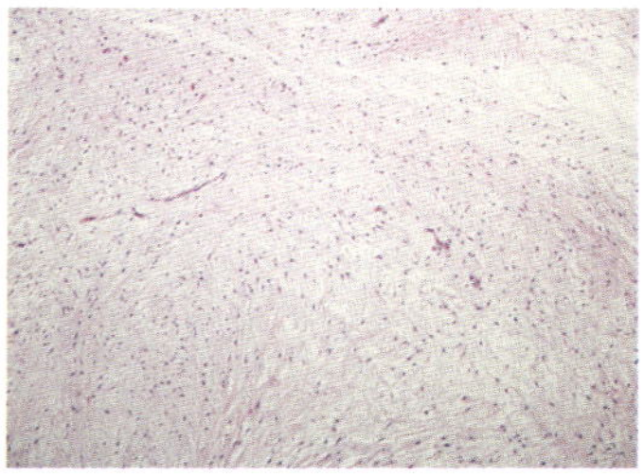</td><td>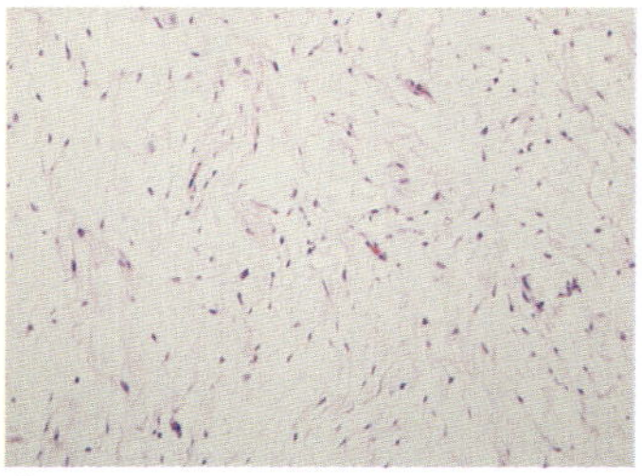</td></tr>
<tr><td colspan="6">Uniform, bland spindle or polygonal cells set in a myxoid matrix. Extremely to mildly hypocellular in most cases except JA myxoma which is more cellular and rare cellular IM myxoma. Vessels are few, small, and short (more vascularity in JA-M). Tumor often invades skeletal muscle permeating between muscle fibers.
Fibrosis, cyst formation, hemorrhage, and mild inflammation may be present. Necrosis, atypia absent. Mitoses absent to rare.
IHC: No specific findings. May be CD34 and/or weakly SMA positive. Negative: S-100, desmin, keratins</td></tr>
<tr><td>Ectopic hamartomatous thymoma</td><td>Very rare</td><td>Adults
M >> F</td><td>Superficial or deep ST of lower neck</td><td>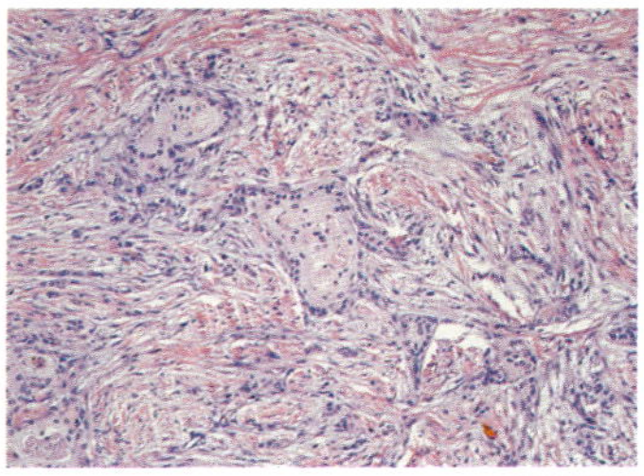</td><td>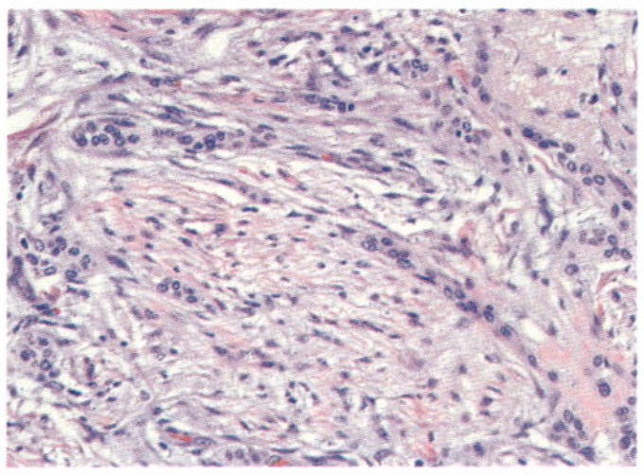</td></tr>
<tr><td colspan="6">Mixture of fat, spindle cells, squamous cell nests and/or glands. Rare cases are cytologically atypical.
Does not contain thymic tissue. Recapitulates branchial tissues; may be a type of myoepithelial tumor</td></tr>
<tr><td colspan="6">Intermediate: can recur aggressively and/or rarely metastasizes (<5%)</td></tr>
<tr><td>Pleomorphic hyalinizing angiectatic tumor (PHAT)</td><td>Rare</td><td>Middle aged adults, older adults; rarely children.
F slightly > M</td><td>Superficial tissue of ankle, leg, arm, chest wall, uncommon in deep soft tissues</td><td>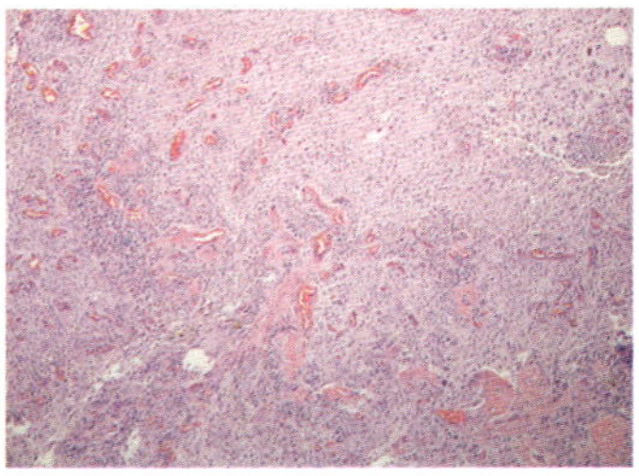</td><td>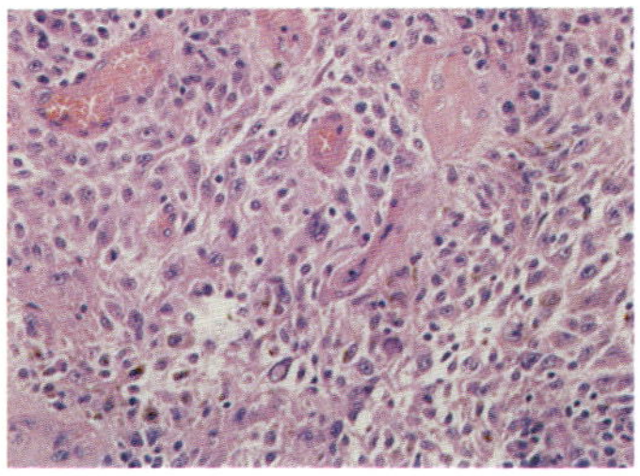</td></tr>
<tr><td colspan="6">Circumscribed moderately cellular tumor with prominent dilated (angiectatic) medium to large vessels, often clustered. The vessels look damaged with fibrin and hyaline deposits. Tumor cells are spindled to polygonal with nuclear size and shape variability. Nuclear pseudoinclusions prominent. Secondary myxoid change and hemosiderin deposits common. Necrosis, marked mitotic activity, and coarse nuclear chromatin with irregular chromatin clearing are absent. Rare cases may recur as myxofibrosarcoma.
IHC: CD34 usually positive. Other markers negative.</td></tr>
<tr><td>Hemosiderotic fibrolipomatous tumor (HsFIT)</td><td>Rare</td><td>Middle aged adults
F > M</td><td>Superficial tissue at acral sites, foot > hand >>> proximal extremities or head and neck</td><td>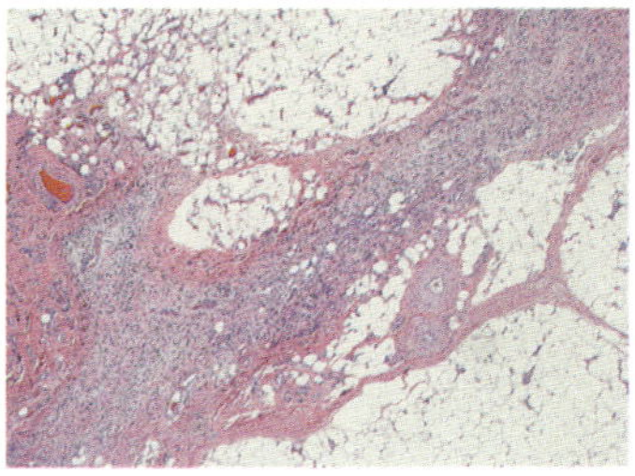</td><td>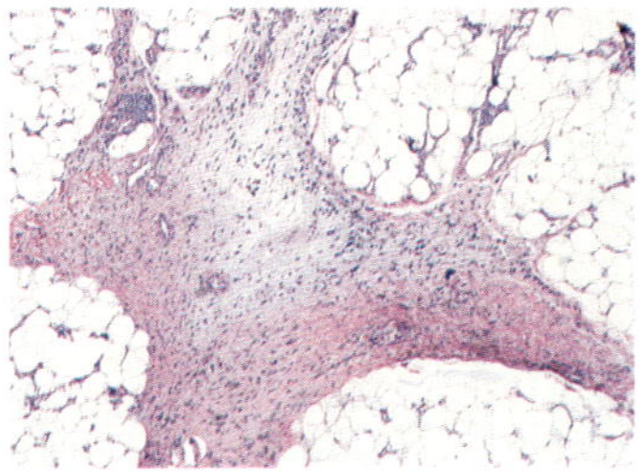</td></tr>
<tr><td colspan="6">Lobulated lipomatous tumor with prominent foci of spindled fibroblasts some of which contain hemosiderin pigment, siderophages, and osteoclastic giant cells.
Some cases overlap histologically with PHAT or MIFS. IHC: CD34 and calponin positive. Negative for desmin, S-100 protein, keratins, and caldesmon.</td></tr>
</table>

Table 14.5: Continued from page 293

Tumor	Incidence	Age and sex	Body site (in descending order of involvement)	Histopathology description including IHC Medium magnification	 High magnification
Angiomatoid fibrous histiocytoma (AFH) **Rare cases metastasize to local lymph nodes or to lungs**	Rare	Children to young adults. Rarely in older adults. F slightly > M	Extremities, trunk, head and neck. Most are superficial	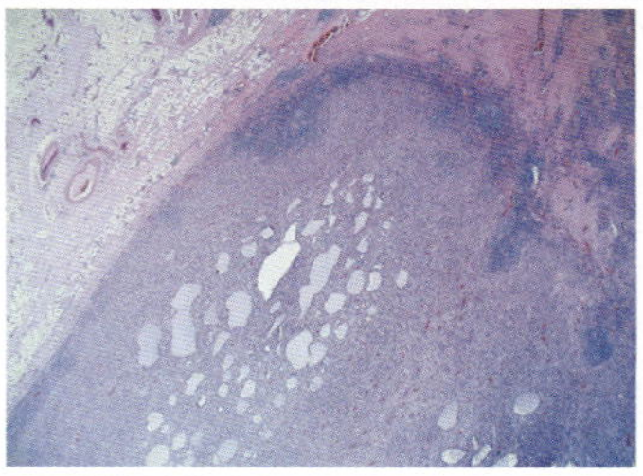	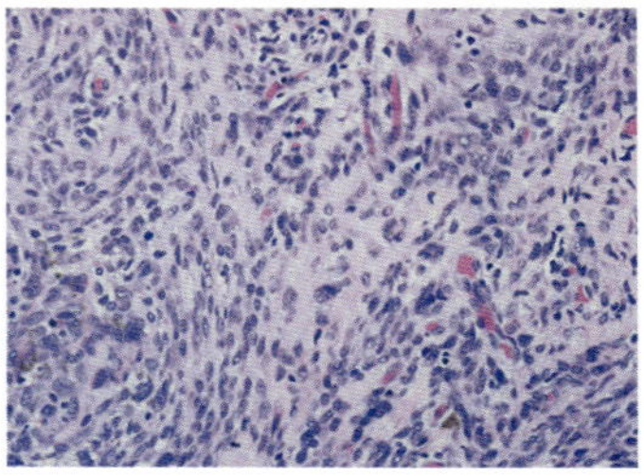
Nodules of histiocytoid ovoid to spindled cells cuffed by a lymph node-like band of lymphocytes and plasma cells. Hemorrhage, hemosiderin, cystic pseudovascular spaces also typical. Rare cases show nuclear pleomorphism. IHC: CD68, CD99 (sometimes membranous) positive; often desmin, SMA, ALK-1, and EMA positive. Negative for CD34, S-100 protein, keratins.					
Ossifying fibromyxoid tumor (OFMT) **Rare cases metastasize**	Rare to very rare	Middle aged adults (often of years' duration), but older children to old age also affected. M slightly > F	Subcutaneous but often connected to tendons, fascia or skeletal muscle. Proximal and distal extremities, H&N, trunk	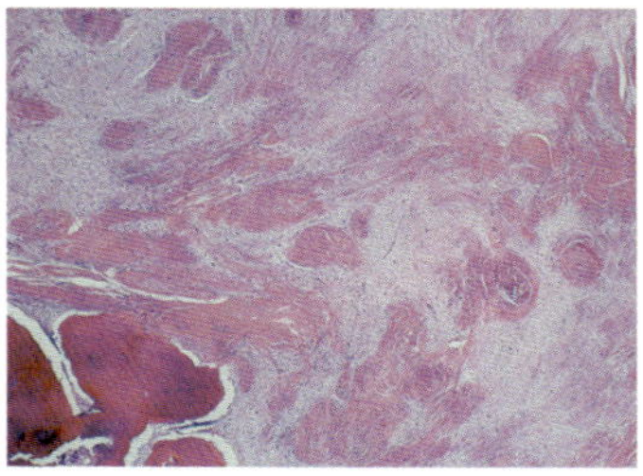	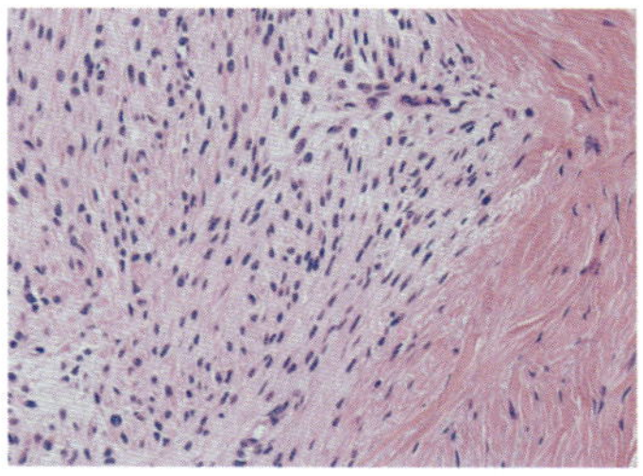
Uni– to multinodular encapsulated tumor of round to focally spindled clear to eosinophilic cells. Nodules may be septated. Most show peripheral osteoid in capsule which may extend centrally. Tumor nuclei are pale, often with small nucleoli; +/- nuclear pseudoinclusions. Low mitotic rate. *Malignant variant is more pleomorphic with necrosis and increased mitotic activity.* 'Atypical' OFMT falls between benign and malignant. IHC: S-100 protein positive, INI-1 mosaic pattern (30-60%). Some positive for desmin, GFAP, SMA, EMA, keratins.					
Perivascular epithelioid cell tumor (PEComa) **Rare cases metastasize**	Very rare	Middle aged adults but broad age range F >> M	Rare in deep soft tissues, more common sites include: kidney, uterus, intestinal wall, falciform ligament (special variant)	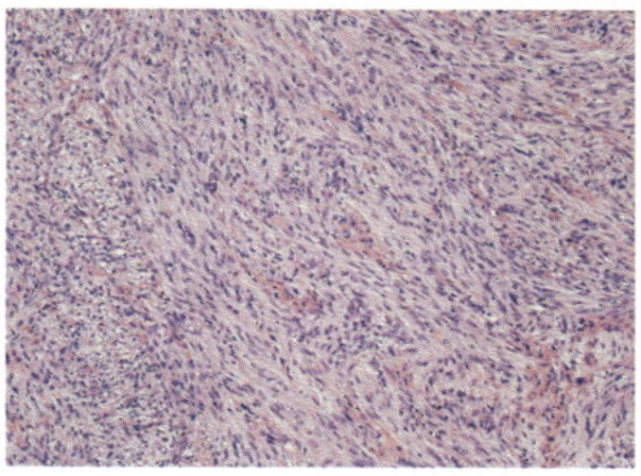	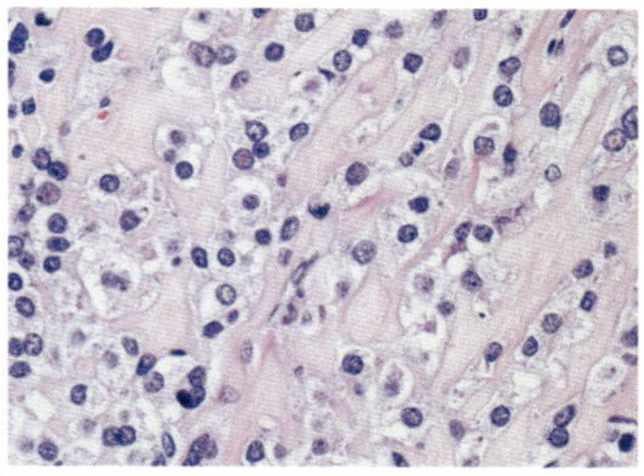
Nests of clear cells radiating away from blood vessels often also with eosinophilic round to spindle cells and clear spindle cells. May resemble clear cell renal cell carcinoma with nests girded by blood vessels. *Malignant version exhibits increased nuclear atypia, necrosis, high mitotic rate and/or atypical mitoses.* IHC: mixed myoid and melanocytic markers positive including SMA, caldesmon, calponin, HMB-45, Mart-1. Negative markers: keratins; desmin and S-100 usually negative.					
Giant cell tumor of soft tissue (GCT-ST) or Giant cell tumor of low malignant potential. **Very rare cases metastasize**	Very rare	Young to middle aged adults but broad age range including children. M = F	Arm, thigh, calf but can also occur in head and neck, trunk, hands and feet. 67% superficial 33% deep	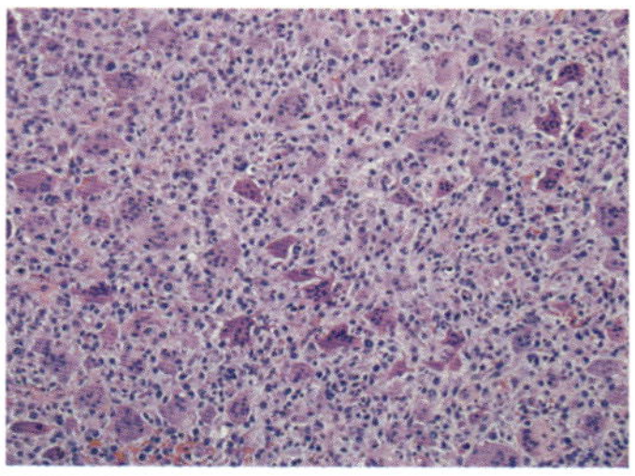	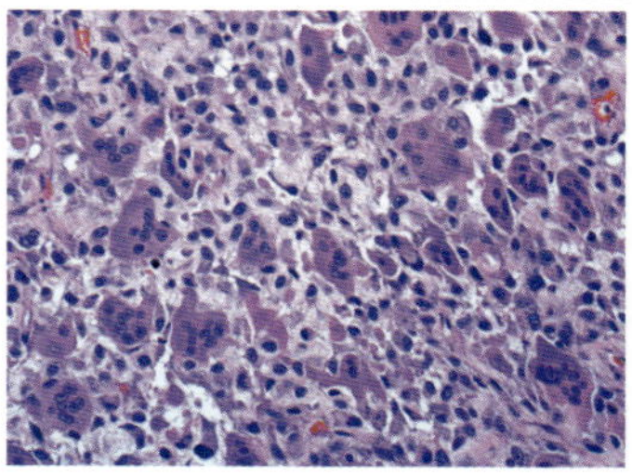
Nodules of tumor that remarkably resemble giant cell tumor of bone with mononuclear stromal cells the nuclei of which are identical to those of evenly distributed osteoclast like giant cells. Peripheral rim of new bone common. Central hemorrhage, fibrosis, and ABC like changes common. Vascular invasion in 33%. No cytologic atypia. Mitoses usually low with no atypical mitoses. IHC: CD68 +, p63 +/-, SMA +/-.					

Table 14.5: Continued from page 294

Tumor	Incidence	Age and sex	Body site (in descending order of involvement)	Histopathology description including IHC: Medium magnification	Histopathology description including IHC: High magnification
Malignant: can recur and commonly metastasizes					
Synovial sarcoma (SS)	Common	Young to middle aged adults. Rare in children < 5 years and patients > 70 years. M > F	70% occur in extremities (lower > upper) then trunk (abdominal wall, inguinal area most common), head and neck (neck, larynx/pharynx, intra-oral most common), then other sites such as pleura, bone. Hands/feet not uncommonly affected. Very rarely involves synovium. Almost all cases are deep (subfacial)	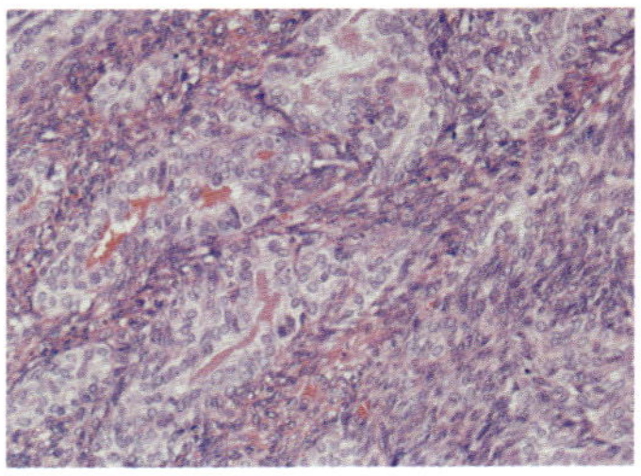	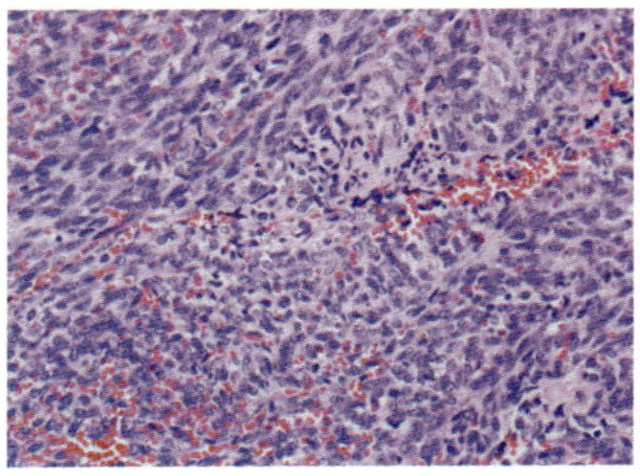
Monophasic type: Hypercellular fascicles of plump spindle cells with mildly atypical ovoid nuclei and moderate mitotic rate. Commonly have calcifications. *Biphasic type:* Spindle cells as above mixed with solid nests or glands of epithelial cells. *Poorly differentiated type:* Hypercellular small round blue cell tumor mimicking Ewing sarcoma family of tumors, Rarely pleomorphic fascicular or large epithelioid. IHC: EMA, pan-keratins, TLE1 positive in most. S-100 and CD99 focal in ~50%; latter may be membranous. FLI1 in 25%. CD34 rarely positive (5%).					
Epithelioid sarcoma (ES)	Rare	Young adults most commonly but also occurs in children and elderly. M > F	Classic or conventional ES: distal upper extremity, lower extremity (knee, lower leg, ankle feet). Often superficial and may form granuloma annulare like, non-healing, cutaneous ulcers. May also be deep running along tendons or fascia. Proximal type ES: Usually deep at limb girdles. However, some examples are superficial and in distal extremities	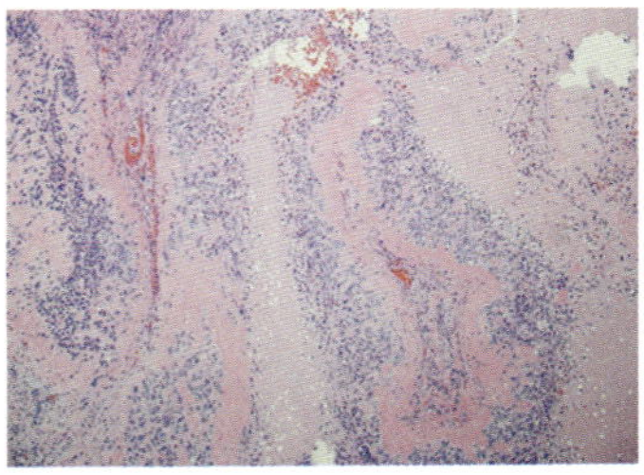	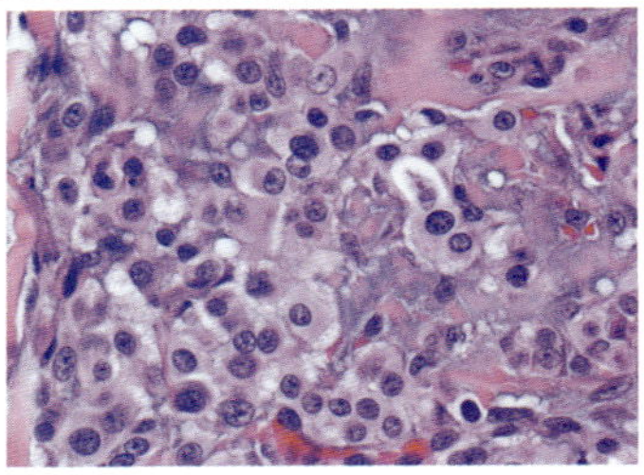
Classic variant: Centrally necrotic nodules surrounded by a cuff of viable tumor cells resembling necrotizing granulomas at low magnification. Tumor cells rounded in center and more spindled at periphery of nodule. Tumor cells are mildly atypical with eosinophilic cytoplasm. Subvariants include: fibroma-like, angiomatoid, spindle cell, and myxoid. *Proximal variant:* Necrotic nodules with more pleomorphic tumor cells including rhabdoid cells. IHC: Pankeratin and EMA positive. FLI1 often positive. CD34 positive (50%). INI1 lost in ~90%. SMA may be positive; desmin usually negative. CD31 negative.					
Alveolar soft part sarcoma (ASPS)	Very rare	Adolescents and young adults but any age may be affected. F slightly > M under age 30y	Extremities (thigh or buttock most commonly), head and neck (orbit or tongue). Rarely arises in bone, stomach, other visceral sites	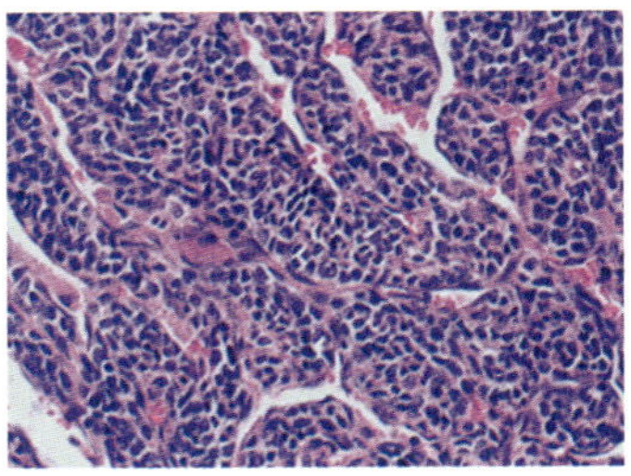	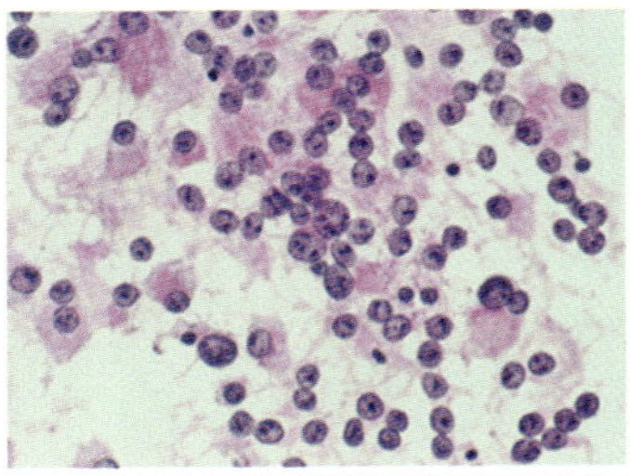
Nests of granular polygonal cells that show central sloughing resembling lung alveoli. Solid pattern also occurs. Tumor cells have eosinophilic cytoplasm, granules or crystals on PAS/D staining, and generally uniform round nuclei with prominent nucleoli. Mitotic rate usually low. IHC: TFE3 positive. Desmin focal. Negative for vimentin, melanocytic markers, keratins, CD34, S-100 protein.					

Table 14.5: Continued from page 295

Tumor	Incidence	Age and sex	Body site (in descending order of involvement)	Histopathology description including immunhistochemistry Medium magnification	 High magnification
Clear cell sarcoma of soft tissue (CCS)	Rare	Young adults but children to old age may be affected. F may be slightly > M	Extremities (foot/ankle, hand, thigh most commonly), trunk Special variant occurs in gastrointestinal tract Most are perifascial infiltrating tendons but some are purely superficial	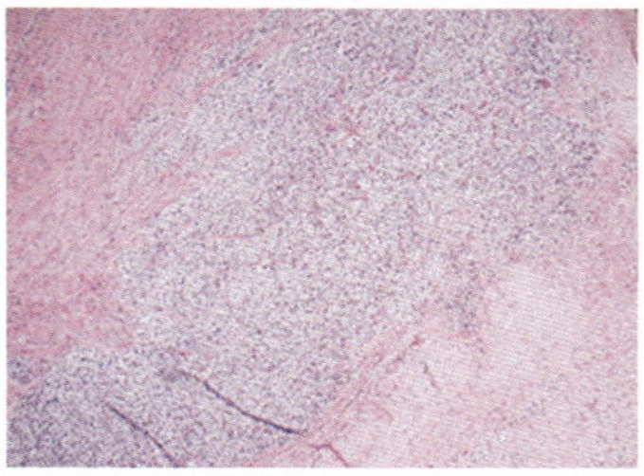	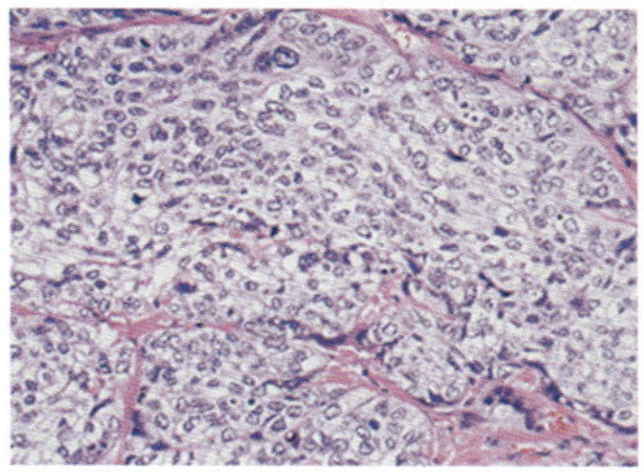
Sheets or nests of clear to eosinophilic round to spindle cells usually infiltrating tendon sheath. PAS stain usually shows glycogen. Nuclei vesicular with nucleoli. Scattered 'wreath-like' MN tumor cells. Atypia usually minimal. Necrosis usually absent. Mitotic rate usually low. May have melanin pigment. IHC: S-100 protein in almost all cases, HMB-45, MelA103 in majority. May also express EMA, keratins, CD34, synaptophysin. 50% show variable loss of INI-1 expression..					
Extraskeletal myxoid chondrosarcoma (ESMCS)	Rare	Middle aged to older adults Rare cases only in children and adolescents M > F	Deep soft tissues of proximal extremities (thigh most common), limb girdles, trunk, foot, H&N Rare cases reported elsewhere such as pleura	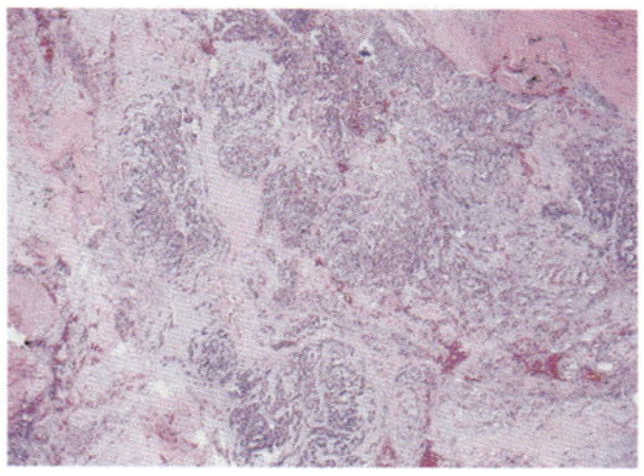	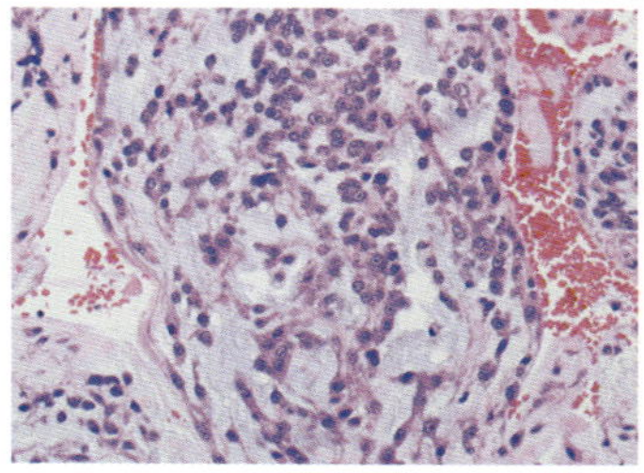
Classic type: Multiple lobules of myxoid material containing cords, webs, and clusters of uniform small eosinophilic cells with round to spindled nuclei. Hemorrhage and necrosis common. Hyaline cartilage absent. *Poorly differentiated type:* Scant to absent myxoid matrix. Tumor cells more pleomorphic including rhabdoid forms. May have spindle cell, high grade areas. More mitoses. IHC: S-100 focal to diffuse in most cases. Some also express NSE and synaptophysin. 50% show variable loss of INI-1 expression.					
Desmoplastic small round cell tumor (DSRCT)	Rare	Children to young adults. Rare in older adults M > F	Abdominal cavity, paratesticular, thoracic cavity, head and neck (rarely other visceral locations)	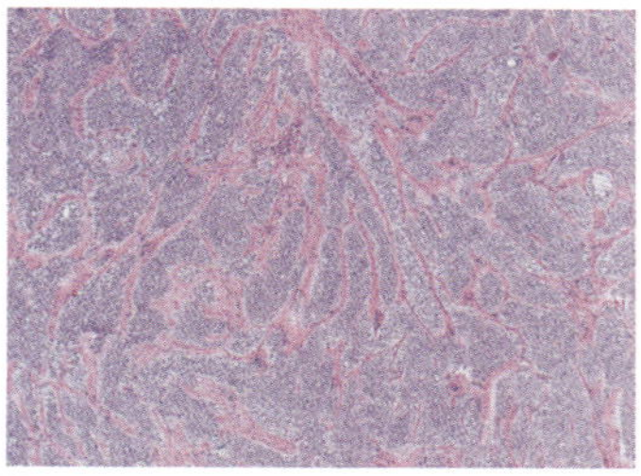	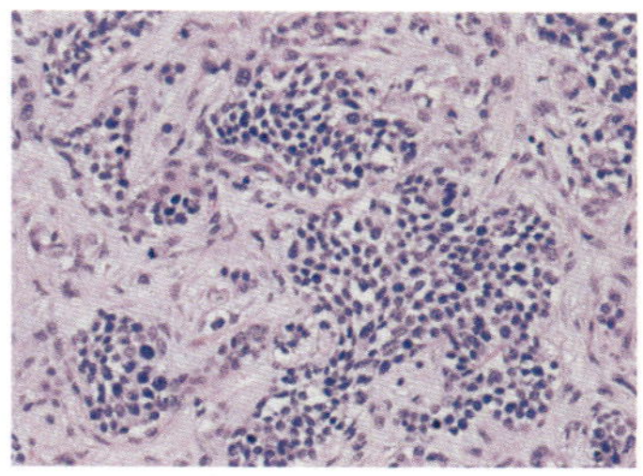
Nests of small round to slightly spindled blue cells embedded in dense sclerotic or desmoplastic stroma. Some cells have more cytoplasm than usually seen in SRBCT. May have overt squamous differentiation and/or rosette formation. High mitotic rate. Necrosis common, often in centers of nests. IHC: 'polyphenotypic' : desmin, keratins, NSE, EMA, WT1, S-100 protein, CD56, chromogranin, synaptophysin always to often positive. Dot like reactivity for desmin and vimentin is typical.					
Extrarenal rhabdoid tumor (ERRT)	Very rare	Infants and children; rare in young to middle aged adults Rare cases are congenital Rare cases are familial	Usually deep neck or paraspinous tissues Rarely may be cutaneous or visceral	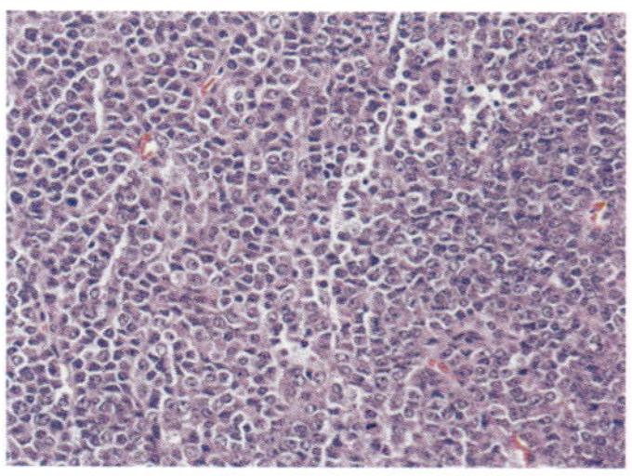	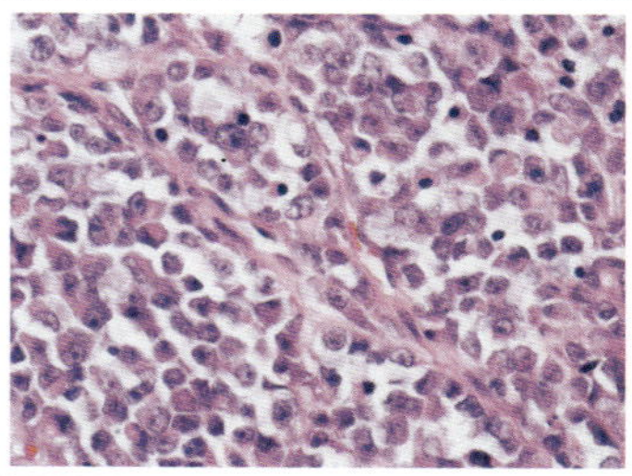
Sheets, trabeculae +/- discohesive alveolar pattern of round to polygonal, uniform cells with round to bean shaped nuclei, nucleoli, and glassy, eosinophilic, globoid cytoplasmic inclusions. Necrosis and high mitotic rate common. IHC: Loss of INI-1 is almost definitional. Most are vimentin, EMA, and keratins positive, the last in the inclusions (which are composed of intermediate filaments).					

M: male, F: female. IHC: immunohistochemistry, UMP: uncertain malignant potential. MN: multinucleate.

Incidence note: 'Common to very common' indicates that a medium sized practice will treat at least several to dozens of patients with the lesion annually, 'uncommon to rare' indicates the same practice size will treat one to two patients with the lesion every five years, 'rare to very rare' indicates the same sized practice will see zero to one patient with the lesion every 20 years.

Photomicrographs are representative only and do not capture all the variant histologic features that may be seen in these tumors (see cases section for more details).

Table 14.6 Local recurrence, metastasis, survival rates and adverse prognostic factors of soft tissue tumors of uncertain differentiation

Tumor	Local recurrence rate by 5 years	Metastasis rate	5 year survival/10 year survival	Adverse prognostic factors
Intramuscular myxoma	<1%	0%	~100%	None
Juxtaarticular myxoma	33%	0%	~100%	Recurrence may be related to incomplete conservative excision
Ectopic hamartomatous thymoma	5-10%	0%	~100%	Rare cases are histologically consistent with carcinoma, but there is little date on behavior of such cases Recurrence may be related to incomplete conservative excision
Hemosiderotic fibrolipomatous tumor	~50%	0%	~100%	Recurrence may be related to incomplete conservative excision
Pleomorphic hyalinizing angiectatic tumor	33%	0%	No data Presumed ~100%	Rare cases reported to recur as myxofibrosarcoma, but there is little data on behavior of these cases
Angiomatoid fibrous histiocytoma	12%	1-5%	~100%/~95%	Large size (>5 cm) and deep location may be associated with increased risk for LR and metastasis
Ossifying fibromyxoid tumor (OFMT), classic type	22-27%	<5%	No data Presumed ~95%	Malignant OFMT is more aggressive with higher metastasis and mortality rates
Synovial sarcoma	50%	40%	36-76%/20-63%	Large size (>5 cm)
Epithelioid sarcoma - Classic variant - Proximal variant	80% (classic) 65% (proximal)	45% (classic) 75% (proximal)	50%-80% range (classic) 35% range (proximal)	Large size (>5 cm) Positive regional lymph nodes at presentation Vascular or perineural invasion
Alveolar soft part sarcoma	<10%	>80%	60%/38%	Older patient age, mets at presentation, large tumor size
Clear cell sarcoma of soft tissue	22%	60-65%	47-59%/36-41%	Large size (> 5 cm)
Extraskeletal myxoid chondrosarcoma	48%	46%	90%/70%	Large size (>5 cm), older patient age, location in proximal extremity or limb girdle High nuclear grade (+/- rhabdoid cells) have shortened survival
Desmoplastic small round cell tumor	60-80%%	30-40%	30%/5%	Patients usually expire of uncontrollable massive LR (most are located in abdominal cavity)
Perivascular epithelioid cell tumor	<10% cutaneous Low for completely excised classic PEComa	0% for classic PEComa >50% for malignant PEComa	~100% for classic PEComa <50% 10 year survival for malignant PEComa	Most PEComas of soft tissue are histologically and clinically benign Malignant PEComas have 2 or more of the following: size >5 cm, infiltrative, high nuclear grade and cellularity, mitoses >/= 1/50 HPF, necrosis, vascular invasion
Giant cell tumor of soft tissue or giant cell tumor of low malignant potential	12%	<5%	98%/98%	Incomplete surgical excision increases risk for LR
Extrarenal rhabdoid tumor	30%	85%	15%/Unknown	Nearly 100% fatality rate at 5 years

elements with hemorrhage and fibrous tissue. The authors of the triple signal intensity note it is not specific to synovial sarcoma.

The appearance of synovial sarcoma is too variable for a classic description. However, when an aggressive soft tissue mass of the extremity is encountered, the radiologist should look for extensive cystic change and the presence of punctate calcifications which would favor the diagnosis of synovial sarcoma.

Epithelioid sarcoma

Epithelioid sarcoma (ES) is a rare high grade tumor with a propensity for local recurrence, regional lymph node involvement and distant metastasis. It is the most common primary soft tissue sarcoma of the hand. Epithelioid sarcoma often presents innocuously as a skin nodule and primarily affects young men. There is described a 'proximal-type' of ES which has a predilection for the pelvis and perineum and may be a more aggressive tumor. We present two cases, a conventional ES of the axilla and proximal type ES involving the perineum. The proximal-type is described as having multilobulated contours in 88% (Tateishi et al. 2002). Nodal involvement is seen in 63%, which is much more frequent than most sarcomas. MR appearance is not specific with iso- to hyperintense appearance on both T1 and T2 images, perhaps related to hemorrhage products.

Alveolar soft part sarcoma

Alveolar soft part sarcoma (ASPS) occurs in the extremities (60%) and in the trunk in 20% with a particular predilection for the buttock and thigh. ASPS is known for its poor prognosis with late metastasis which are most common to lung, brain and bone (Folpe et al. 2006). Brain metastasis was noted in 19% of patients with Stage IV disease, all of whom had metastatic disease elsewhere (Portera et al. 2001). MR imaging shows a T1 iso to slightly hyperintense, T2 mildly hyperintense mass with intense enhancement and flow voids related to vessels in the tumor (Kim et al. 2005). Other than the presence of vascular flow voids, the appearance is not specific. If the tissue diagnosis is known, brain imaging should probably be included in metastatic surveillance. Our case of ASPS was originally treated at an outside facility three years prior and then presented to our institution with metastatic disease of the adrenal glands and lungs. We do not have imaging of the primary tumor which involved the abdominal wall.

Clear cell sarcoma

Clear cell sarcoma (CCS) occurs in the extremities in 92% of cases with the lower extremity being most common location; particularly, the foot and ankle are involved (Kransdorf et al. 1995). Clear cell sarcoma tends to involve tendon, aponeurosis or fascial structures. Melanin is detected in 72% of tumors at pathology (Chung et al. 1983). The quantity of melanin is microscopic and probably does not contribute to T1 high signal on MRI.

Metastases can occur to lymph nodes in up to 50% which is much more common than most sarcomas. We present a case involving the knee which originates from the patellar tendon.

Extraskeletal myxoid chondrosarcoma

Extraskeletal myxoid chondrosarcoma (ESMC) is common in the proximal extremities and limb girdles and occurs in adulthood with an average age of 53 years. The MR appearance is usually T1 isointense and T2 heterogeneously high signal, and there is usually mild to moderate heterogeneous enhancement. Cystic change was seen in 21% and hemorrhage was seen in 5% (Tateishi et al. 2006). The overall appearance is nonspecific. The cotyledonous appearance with lobulated substance and surface of the tumor is at least suggestive of a cartilage tumor.

Desmoplastic small round cell tumor

Desmoplastic small round cell tumor (DSRCT) occurs in young adults with a male preponderance and the tumor tends to occur in the peritoneal cavity of the pelvis. Specifically, the tumor usually arises in the retrovesical space. Cross sectional imaging may show single or multiple intraperitoneal soft tissue masses. The tumor can have calcifications.

DSRCT spreads via peritoneal seeding and can metastasize to lymph nodes, liver and bone. Pleural involvement is common, occurring in approximately 63%. Seeding of the tumor tract has been reported (Kis et al. 2012).

Although we do not have pathologic findings, we present an imaging case of DSRCT, (**Figs 14.4a** and **14.4b**).

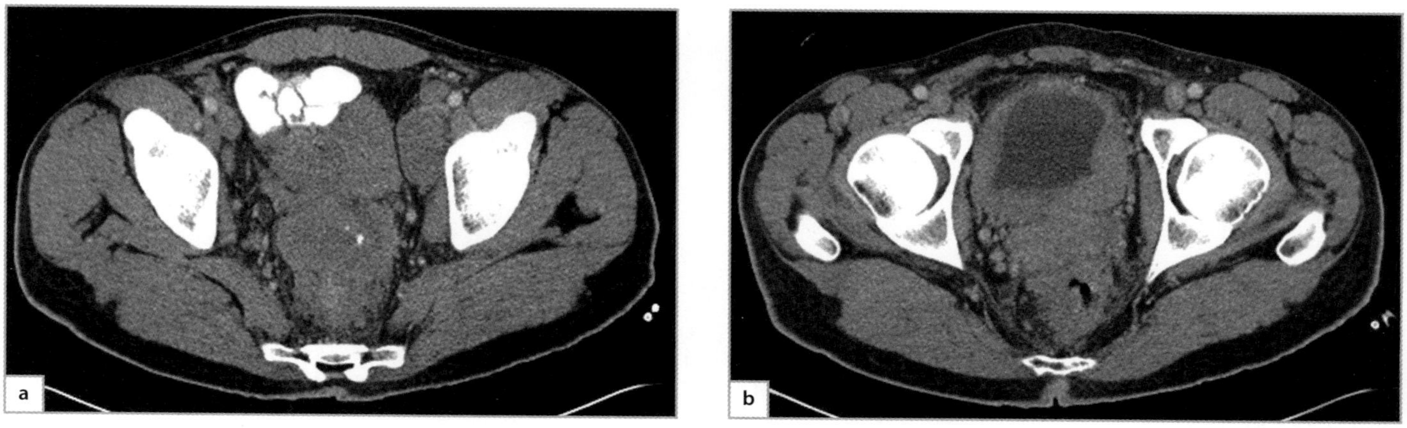

Figures 14.4a and **14.4b** Shows a desmoplastic small round cell tumor. (a) is an axial CT images post IV contrast, showing a 6.9 × 4.9 × 7.2 cm isodense mass in the retrovesticular space. The mass shows minimal enhancement without low density areas or necrosis. There are several small calcifications and there is a left pelvic adenopathy. There is no ascites yet present. (b) is an axial scan showing urinary bladder wall thickening indicating tumor invasion.

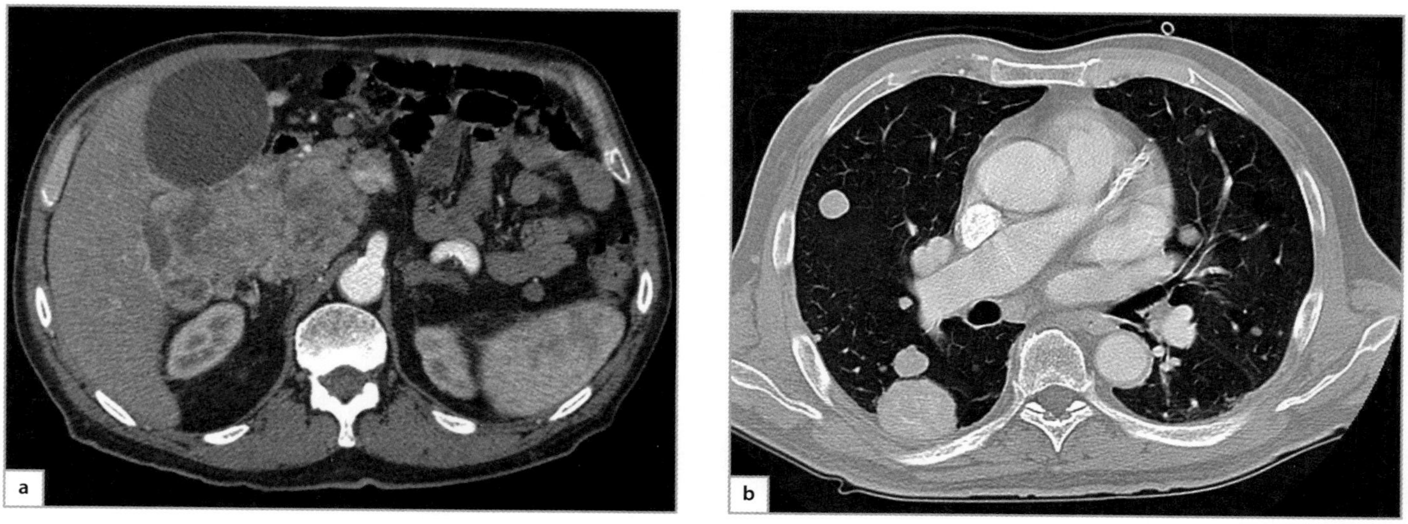

Figures 14.5a and **14.5b** Show a perivascular epithelioid cell tumor. (a) is an axial CT image post IV contrast through the upper abdomen and (b) is through the lung bases of a 78-year old man showing a 6 × 11 cm heterogeneously enhancing mass of the porta hepatis region. There is no ascites or adenopathy. The lungs show multiple masses undoubtedly from metastasis.

Perivascular epithelioid cell tumor

Perivascular epithelioid cell tumor (PEComa) is a family of mesenchymal neoplasms including angiomyolipoma, lymphangiomyomatosis and clear cell sugar tumors. Some patients may have tuberous sclerosis complex. These tumors can occur throughout the body and may involve visceral organs, peritoneum and retroperitoneum.

Radiologically, tumors may appear heterogeneous on CT with heterogeneous enhancement. With MR imaging, these tumors show T1 low signal and T2 high signal intensity with heterogeneous enhancement and increased vascularity (Akitake et al. 2009) (**Figs 14.5 a** and **14.5b**). The differential for a renal mass in a patient with tuberous sclerosis includes AML or PEComa. The presence of visible fat tissue or signal dropout on out-of-phase gradient echo MR imaging favors the diagnosis of AML.

Giant cell tumor of soft tissue

These are usually superficial lesions of the extremities and imaging is not typically obtained. We do not have imaging to present.

Extrarenal rhabdoid tumor

Extrarenal rhabdoid tumors can occur throughout the body. These are described as having T1 predominant isointensity with some hyperintense areas, and T2 heterogeneous hyperintensity with avid contrast enhancement (Dobbs et al. 2011). The appearance is not specific but suggests an aggressive vascular lesion.

SURGERY

Intramuscular myxoma

Marginal excision of these tumors results in a very low rate of recurrence.

Pleomorphic hyalinizing angiectatic tumor and hemosiderotic fibrolipomatous tumor

Marginal excision of these tumors may result in a recurrence rate as high as 50%. Multiple and aggressive recurrences have been reported, although metastasis has not been observed. Due to the aggressive local nature of this tumor, wide surgical resection is recommended.

Angiomatoid fibrous histiocytoma

These tumors behave in a fashion similar to low grade sarcoma. Recurrences are common after incomplete excision. Nodal and pulmonary metastases, although rare, have been reported. Wide surgical excision is therefore recommended.

Ossifying fibromyxoid tumor

Aggressive local behavior has been reported with these tumors, including histologic progression to malignancy and associated metastasis. Wide surgical excision is recommended.

Synovial sarcoma

This tumor represents an aggressive high grade malignancy. Wide surgical excision is the procedure of choice.

Epithelioid sarcoma

This tumor represents a high grade malignancy. Wide surgical excision is recommended.

Alveolar soft part sarcoma

This tumor represents an aggressive high grade malignancy. Wide surgical excision is the procedure of choice.

Clear cell sarcoma of soft tissue

This tumor represents a high grade malignancy. Wide surgical excision is indicated.

Extraskeletal myxoid chondrosarcoma

Wide surgical resection is the procedure of choice with this malignant neoplasm. Late recurrence and metastasis are common.

MEDICAL ONCOLOGY

Pazopanib, an oral angiogenesis inhibitor that targets vascular endothelial growth factor receptor and platelet-derived growth factor receptor, was studied in 142 patients with advanced soft tissue sarcoma (STS). Adipocytic STS were not very sensitive to this antiangiogenic kinase inhibitor. However, patients with leiomyosarcoma, synovial sarcomas, and other STS types had prolonged progression-free and overall survivals, compared to historical controls treated with chemotherapy. The most frequent drug-related adverse events include hypertension, fatigue, hypopigmentation, nausea, liver enzyme elevations, weight loss, myelosuppression, and proteinuria (Sleijfer et al. 2009). Thus, a randomized phase 3 study was performed in patients with angiogenesis inhibitor-naive, metastatic soft-tissue sarcoma, progressing despite previous standard chemotherapy, the PALETTE trial. Patients were randomized in a 2:1 ratio to receive either pazopanib 800 mg once daily or placebo, with no subsequent cross-over. Of 369 patients randomized, 246 received pazopanib and 123, placebo. Median progression-free survival was 4.6 months for pazopanib compared with 1.6 months (hazard ratio = 0·31; p<0·0001). A trend for improved overall survival was seen with pazopanib (van der Graaf et al. 2012). The FDA has approved pazopanib for treatment of refractory sarcoma in 2012 (url). http://www.fda.gov/Drugs/InformationOnDrugs/ApprovedDrugs/ucm302090.htm.

Intramuscular myxoma

No medical oncology is needed.

Pleomorphic hyalinizing angiectatic tumor and hemosiderotic fibrolipomatous tumor

No medical oncology is needed.

Angiomatoid fibrous histiocytoma

No medical oncology is needed, unless the tumor metastasizes.

Ossifying fibromyxoid tumor

No medical oncology is needed in the benign cases.

Synovial sarcoma

Synovial sarcoma contains a characteristic reciprocal translocation t(X;18)(p11.2;q11.2), representing the fusion of SYT on chromosome 18 with either SSX1, SSX2, or rarely SSX4 (all on chromosome X) (Clark et al. 1994, Kawai et al. 1998).The resulting gene fusions appear to be mutually exclusive and concordant in primary and metastatic tumors.

The resulting fusion protein of synovial sarcoma brings together the transcriptional activating domain of SS18 (SYT) and a transcriptional repressor domain of SSX (Ito et al. 2004, Thaete et al. 1999). The transcription factor, SYT, is activated after fusion to the repressor domain, SSX, which can no longer interact properly with its other nuclear protein partners, causing constitutive activation and division of the mesenchymal cell of origin. There is an association between the SS18-SSX1 or SS18-SSX2 fusion type and both tumor morphology and five-year survival (Ladanyi et al. 2002).

However, the most accepted prognostic factor is the size of the primary (Sultan et al. 2009), which correlates with the development of metastases (Deshmukh et al. 2004, Ferrari et al. 2004, Guillou et al. 2004, Okcu et al. 2003). Other good prognostic factors are younger age, negative surgical margins, lower histologic grade, histologic subtype, and the SYT-SSX fusion type which might influence biological markers such as p53 overexpression, Ki-67 proliferative index (Prxybyl et al. 2012, Saito et al. 2004).

Patients with synovial sarcoma may present with a history of a small nodule that rapidly increases in size (Thompson et al. 2000). The mass becomes painful and is usually located deeply (Chotel et al. 2008).

The standard treatment of primary tumor is the wide surgical removal of the lesion with or without addition of radiotherapy.

Whether there is a role for medical oncology for treatment of the primary tumor is not firmly established. For big tumors, neoadjuvant or adjuvant chemotherapy could be administered (Chen et al. 2012). There is also a debate regarding the best combination of chemotherapy for these patients (Canter et al. 2008). In the metastatic setting, a high response rate to ifosfamide-based therapy has been reported (40%-70%) (Rosen et al. 1994), thus, this agent is recommended if chemotherapy is administered as part of multidisciplinary treatment of the primary, usually with doxorubicin (Eilber et al. 2007).

For patients with recurrent disease, there is no standard recommended treatment. If patients are ifosfamide naïve, the combination of doxorubicin and ifosfamide is indicated (Rosen et al. 1994). The role of gemcitabine and docetaxel is not yet defined (Mora et al. 2009). The first choice is to offer participation in a clinical trial.

Targeted inhibitors of the fusion protein are the future of therapy for synovial sarcoma. An innovative approach has been tested in 16 patients (Kawaguchi et al. 2005), where a 9-mer peptide spanning the SYT-SSX fusion region was used to vaccinate patients. Another approach is a monoclonal antibody raised against the frizzled homologue called FZD10, a cell-surface receptor present on the synovial sarcoma cells and absent in the normal organs, which is in preclinical stage (Fukukawa et al. 2008).

Epithelioid sarcoma

Epithelioid sarcoma presents as a firm-to-hard palpable mass. Superficial lesions might ulcerate and deep tumors might be mistaken for ganglion cysts or giant cell tumors of tendon sheath. Pain or tenderness is uncommon. This tumor is slow growing with an average duration of symptoms before surgical resection of 29 months (Chase et al. 1985).

The prognosis depends on the presentation (Jawad et al. 2009, Nunes et al. 2010). A more central location is worse than a distal extremity presentation. Patients with an isolated primary have a 70% chance of survival at 10 years, while patients with lymph node involvement have only a 30% chance of being alive after 10 years. Thus the surgical intervention not only has a therapeutic intent, but also a staging intent. Primary amputation offers no survival benefit to patients presenting with regional metastases. Wide local excision with negative margins is indicated and sentinel lymph node biopsy should be considered given that 25-35% of patients will have positive nodes. The benefit of adjuvant therapy is not established, but most patients with positive margins, metastatic lymph nodes, or local recurrence are treated with a multidisciplinary approach including radiotherapy and chemotherapy (Ross et al. 1997, Whitworth et al. 1991). Local recurrence is common, but should be treated locally and aggressively, as many patients will survive free of disease.

Despite its benign appearance and the multidisciplinary approach, this tumor tends to rapidly metastasize to lymph nodes (Daigeler et al. 2009, Loya et al. 2007), lungs, bones, and soft tissues (Matsushita et al. 2002) in about 30 to 50% of patients. In the setting of metastatic disease, the role of chemotherapy is not well defined. Standard soft tissue sarcoma chemotherapies are used, and about 30% of patients will demonstrate a response. The best data are registry data (Jones et al. 2011). In a small series, it is suggested that regimens with doxorubicin might be better than those without (Galanis et al. 1997).

Alveolar soft part sarcoma

These tumors are extremely vascular, and might present as a pulsatile mass associated with a bruit (Torres et al. 2010). The mass is usually painless, slow-growing, and rarely causes functional impairment. Thus it might take months to make the diagnosis.

Because of the relative lack of symptoms, many patients present with metastases to the lung or other sites as the first disease manifestation (Cordier et al. 1985). The most common metastatic sites are lung, bone, central nervous system, and liver (Reichardt et al. 2003). Metastases might occur 15 years after initial resection of the tumor. Metastases often affect the lungs in a miliary fashion, while the patient retains a quasi normal respiratory function. In a series of 70 patients brain metastases were almost always detected in conjunction with metastases to other sites (Portera et al. 2001). Thus an MRI of the brain should be part of the work-up of these patients. In another series of 15 patients with alveolar soft part sarcoma, 9 presented with metastatic disease and one developed early metastases (Anderson et al. 2005).

Despite poor response to treatment of metastatic disease, overall survival was 75% at 5 years and 40% at 10 years with a mean survival of 6.5 years (Pappo et al. 1996).

Radical resection is the therapy of choice for localized disease (Kayton et al. 2006). Complete microscopic R0 resection is critical to prevent recurrence of localized alveolar soft part sarcoma. Modern surgical treatment results in good local control of primary tumors. Local recurrence rates range from 11- 50% (Portera et al. 2001).

Despite the occurrence of metastases in about 70% of patients, 5-year overall survival rates range from 45 to 88% (Salvati et al. 2010). There is no evidence that conventional chemotherapy, radiation or excision increase the survival of patients who have metastases at diagnosis (Portera et al. 2001). In case of oligometastases, resection of the metastases might help prolong survival (218 months versus 63.5 months) (Salvati et al. 2010).

Antiangiogenesis

This tumor is resistant to chemotherapy and medical treatment was unsuccessful until the discovery of VEGFR tyrosine kinase inhibitors, which have changed the course of this disease. Expression of proangiogenic genes in oligo microarrays identified eighteen up-regulated angiogenesis-related genes in ASPS (Lazar et al. 2007). Pazopanib has received fast track approval from the FDA (van der Graaf et al. 2012). Sunitinib and cediranib have shown activity in alveolar part sarcoma. Sunitinib showed 5 partial responses in 9 ASPS patients (Stacchiotti et al. 2011). Cediranib showed single-agent efficacy in a study of 36 patients with ASPS, causing a >40% response rate and a disease control rate of 78% (Kummar et al. 2011). These preliminary data are promising and suggest effectiveness of tyrosine kinase inhibitors of the VEGF signaling pathway in ASPS.

Other signaling pathway targets

The search for potential targets in ASPS has been studied by testing tissue microarray (Taylor et al. 2011). The c-Met receptor and its downstream effectors (e.g. AKT and ERK) are activated in ASPS. The gene that encodes for c-Met receptor (MET) is an ASPL–TFE3 transcriptional target (Tsuda et al 2007). A Phase II clinical trial evaluated the use of tivantinib, a novel c-Met inhibitor, for the treatment of 27 ASPS patients. Stable disease for durations up to 29+ weeks were observed (Wagner et al. 2012).

In conclusions, antiangiogenic tyrosine kinase inhibitors have shown promising results in the treatment of ASPS and could become a first line of therapy in patients with metastatic disease. The recommendation is to enroll patients on a clinical trial whenever possible.

Clear cell sarcoma of soft tissue

This tumor often arises in tendons and aponeuroses, usually in the lower extremities. The mass grows to be painful and might metastasize to lymph nodes. When it continues to spread, the lungs are usually involved. This tumor is usually slow growing (Goldberg et al. 2005). If the primary tumor is completely surgically resected at diagnosis, the median overall survival is about 50% at 5 year (Kuiper et al. 2003). If the disease is metastatic, the survival drops to 33% (Deenik et al. 1999) despite appropriate therapy.

Surgical resection is the treatment of a localized clear cell sarcoma (CCS). A sentinel lymph node biopsy is recommended, since CCS has a tendency to spread through the lymphatic system first. Radiation may have a role in palliation of local disease when CCS cannot be fully resected (Spunt et al. 1999). There currently is no role for chemotherapy at this stage.

Treatment of metastatic disease

CCS seems more resistant to the standard sarcoma chemotherapy (Scurr 2011). Because of the resemblance to melanoma, chemotherapy treatment recommended for melanoma (dacarbazine, cisplatin, carmustine and taxanes) might be considered, but these drugs do not cure patients. Thus, participation in a clinical trial should be offered. What could practically be offered is a non tumor specific Phase I clinical trial, since this disease is so rare. For example, increased activity of the tyrosine kinase, ERBB3, has been shown on a microarray analysis of CSS (Schaefer et al. 2004). New ERBB3 monoclonal antibodies are currently in clinical trials (Schoeberl et al. 2010).

Immunotherapy has also been reported in a few cases of CCS with intralesional interferon inducing prolonged remission in a few cases (Lauro et al. 1999, Steger et al. 1991). Expression profiling for CCS reveals many activated genes in common with melanoma (Segal et al. 2003). Since the EWS-ATF1 translocation of CCS possibly stimulates the immune system (Worley et al. 2001), it might be appropriate to use the new immunotherapies approved for melanoma such as ipilimumab to treat CCS (Verschraegen 2012).

Desmoplastic small round cell tumor

Desmoplastic small round (blue) cell tumor (DSRCT) is an aggressive and rare tumor that primarily occurs as masses in the abdomen including lymph nodes, the lining of the abdomen, diaphragm, spleen, liver, chest wall, skull, spinal cord, large intestine, small intestine, bladder, brain, lungs, testicles, ovaries, and the pelvis. It metastasizes rapidly to liver, lungs, lymph nodes, brain, skull, and bones (Gerald et al. 1991). It is a childhood cancer that predominantly affects boys and young adults. In females, it is often mistaken for ovarian cancer.

DSRCT is associated with a unique chromosomal translocation (t11;22)(p13:q12)[3] resulting in a EWS/WT1 transcript[4] which codes for a protein that acts as a transcriptional activator. The EWS/WT1 translocation product targets ENT4,[5] a pH-dependent adenosine transporter (Gerald et al. 1998, Li et al. 2008).

Like ovarian cancer, DSRCT can grow to huge size before being noticed by the patient. The tumors are hard, round masses felt by palpation of the abdomen. Patients may present with abdominal distention, abdominal or back pain, gastrointestinal obstruction, lack of appetite, ascites, anemia, and/or cachexia. Despite intense treatments, the prognosis is poor. Five year survival rate of DRSCT is only approximately 15%.

Treatment

A multi-modality approach of high dose chemotherapy, aggressive surgical resection, radiation, and stem cell rescue improves survival for selected patients (Philippe-Chomette et al. 2012). Patients initially respond to first line chemotherapy but relapse is common. Best approach is to offer participation in a clinical trial. High dose chemotherapy similar to Ewing protocols should be offered, within the context of a multidisciplinary approach that includes debulking surgery and radiation therapy (Kushner et al. 1996). Other treatment options include: stem cell transplantation, intensity-modulated radiation therapy, radiofrequency ablation, stereotactic body radiation therapy, intraperitoneal hyperthermic chemoperfusion. In relapsed patients, metronomic low dose chemotherapy offers a good palliation (Aguilera et al. 2008).

Extraskeletal myxoid chondrosarcoma

Extraskeletal myxoid chondrosarcoma (ESMCS) are predominantly located in the deep soft tissues of the lower extremity (60%) and buttock (20%), with a mean tumor size around 10 to 15 cm at diagnosis, and spread distantly more often than their skeletal counterpart. Approximately 13% of patients presented with metastases. In a series of 87 patients (Drilon et al. 2008), the median age of the patients at the time of diagnosis was 49 years, with a male-to-female ratio of 2:1. The 5-year, 10-year, and 15-year overall survival rates were 82%, 65%, and 58%, respectively. For patients presenting without metastases, 37% developed local recurrence (median time of 3.3 years) and 26% developed distal recurrence (median time of 3.2 years).

Three cases of extraskeletal myxoid chondrosarcoma have been associated with Hu antibodies (Hoosien et al. 2011, Verschraegen 2009, Verschuuren et al. 1994). The specific neurologic syndrome caused by Hu antibodies is called paraneoplastic encephalomyelitis/sensory neuronopathy (PEM/SN) (Dalmau et al. 1992). However, most patients with Hu antibodies do not have neurologic symptoms. Hu antibodies are IgGs directed against the Hu antigens, a family of proteins found in all neurons of the central and peripheral nervous system, and a few extraneuronal cells. The function of Hu antigens has not been completely elucidated, but they appear to play a role in early neuronal embryogenesis by interfering with mRNA to promote differentiation and maintenance of the neuronal phenotype. For a comprehensive review of antineuronal antibody, see Senties-Madrid and Vega-Boada (Senties-Madrid et al. 2001). Thus, for patients presenting with a neurological symptomatology associated with a new soft tissue tumor, ESMCS should be in the differential diagnosis.

Unfortunately, this sarcoma is chemotherapy resistant with a short median time to disease progression while receiving chemotherapy of 5.2 months, with more than 70% of patients progressing within 6 months of therapy. Aggressive control of localized disease and prevention of recurrence is the primary approach to management, because patients with systemic disease do not respond to chemotherapy (Ogura et al. 2012, Patel et al. 1995). Again, these patients should be offered participation in a clinical trial.

Extrarenal rhabdoid tumor

Malignant rhabdoid tumor (MRT) is one of the most aggressive and lethal malignancies in pediatric oncology. MRT usually occurs in the kidney. The second most frequent site is the central nervous system (CNS) and the tumor is then called Atypical Teratoid/Rhabdoid Tumor (AT/RT) (Hilden et al. 2004). Non-CNS tumors are all called non CNS MRT or extrarenal rhabdoid tumor (ERT). The ERT is the rarest (less than 10% of MRTs) and could originate anywhere.

MRT is characterized by the early onset of local and distant metastases and resistance to chemotherapy. Overall survival rate is only 20-25%. Younger patient have a worse prognosis compared to toddlers older than 2 years. Girls have a slightly higher survival rate. Synchronous or metachronous brain tumors with MRT are found in 10-15% of patients. Paraneoplastic hypercalcemia is seen in 25% of patients (Reinhard et al. 2008, Weeks et al. 1989).

Most MRTs and AT/RTs contain deletions at chromosome locus 22q11.1 where in lies the (*SMARCB1*) gene which acts as a classic tumor suppressor (Roberts et al. 2009). *SMARCB1* encodes a member of the human *SWI/SNF* complex, also known as the integrase interactor 1 (*INI1*). The *SWI/SNF* complex acts in an adenosine triphosphate (ATP)-dependent manner to remodel chromatin, which regulates gene transcription and DNA repair. Malignant rhabdoid tumor lacks *INI1* immunohistochemical staining, whereas most other tumors have detectable INI1 protein. This genetic anomaly is used to help making a differential diagnosis Hoot et al. 2004).

Genetic counseling is highly recommended for all malignant rhabdoid tumor affected families. Germline mosaicism is suggested because usually neither parent has a mutation in their own peripheral blood.

Treatment of extra-renal MRT is the same as the renal MRT and should be multidisciplinary (Puri et al. 2008), however in most children the disease will recur (Bourdeaut et al. 2008). The treatment for disseminated MRT remains investigational. Thus, enrollment of patients on clinical trials is encouraged. Most chemotherapy regimens combine ifosfamide, platinum, etoposide, vincristine, doxorubicin, and cyclophosphamide with granulocyte colony-stimulating factor.

Perivascular epithelioid cell tumor

PEComas form a panel of tumors that span from an uncertain malignant potential to a very aggressive malignant disease (Bleeker et al. 2012, Nese et al. 2011). The most common PEComas are renal angiomyolipoma and pulmonary lymphangioleiomyomatosis, both of which are associated with tuberous sclerosis complex (Kenerson et al. 2007, Martignoni et al. 2008). More recently, PEComas harboring TFE3 gene fusions have also been isolated (Argani et al. 2010)

PEComas are rare and can have various features; thus, they are often mistaken for other tumoral proliferation such as carcinomas, smooth muscle tumors, adipocytic tumours, clear cell sarcomas, melanomas and gastrointestinal stromal tumors.

Most malignant PEComas are resistant to chemotherapy. However interference of the tuberous sclerosis complex with the mTOR pathway offers a potential new therapy with drugs such as temsirolimus or everolimus (Italiano et al. 2010, Wagner et al. 2010).

Giant cell tumor of soft tissue

Giant cell tumor of soft tissue, giant cell tumor of low malignant potential, the counterpart of the giant cell tumor of bone (Chapter 22), tumor of low malignant potential, formed of a proliferation of osteoclasts.

They rarely metastasize, and therefore medical treatment is not necessary.

RADIATION ONCOLOGY

Miscellaneous tumors of uncertain differentiation are a group of unrelated histologic entities with diverse clinical behaviors ranging from purely benign to highly aggressive and lethal. Intramuscular myxoma lies within the purely benign spectrum of clinical behavior. Marginal excision is usually sufficient for excellent local control. Reports in the literature do not recommend the use of radiation therapy for intramuscular myxoma. On the other hand, several other histologic entities such as pleomorphic hyalinizing angiectatic tumor, angiomatoid fibrous histiocytoma, and ossifying fibromyxoid tumor are inadequately treated with only a marginal excision due to the high risk of local recurrence with this treatment. Therefore, adjuvant radiation therapy has been used in this circumstance even though the true impact of radiation therapy is not known due to small numbers of cases. If wide local excision is achieved for these types of tumors, no adjuvant therapy is needed due to low rates of local recurrence.

Synovial sarcoma, epithelioid sarcoma, alveolar soft part sarcoma, and clear cell sarcoma of soft tissue usually have a high risk of local recurrence despite wide local excision. A randomized trial has established the routine use of adjuvant radiation therapy as standard of care unless the estimated risk of local recurrence is low (Yang et al. 1998). Another group of tumors including desmoplastic small round cell tumor, extraskeletal myxoid chondrosarcoma, and extrarenal rhabdoid tumor are on the highly aggressive spectrum of clinical behavior. Multimodality therapy is usually required in order to maximize control of these tumors. Due to the lack of success from surgery alone in obtaining local control, radiation therapy is usually added to the treatment regimen. Nonetheless, the optimal treatment is not known in part due to the rarity of these diseases.

Perivascular epithelioid cell tumor also known as PEComa, can vary significantly in terms of the aggressiveness of histologic and clinical features. Those in the more aggressive category may benefit from radiation therapy. On the other hand, many are indolent and do not benefit from radiation therapy. Thus, clinical judgement is necessary in making a treatment decision for PEComa. Finally, treatment for giant cell tumor of soft tissue is based on the much more common giant cell tumor of bone. Surgery is the treatment of choice. For those cases in which surgery is not possible, radiation therapy is effective therapy for giant cell tumor of soft tissue.

CASES

Case 14.1 Intramuscular myxoma

Clinical history and presentation

The patient is a 59 year old man who notes a mass in the lateral aspect of the mid-thigh which has been present for the past 2-3 years. It was first noted after a fall. He reports this mass has not changed appreciably in size. He has no symptoms.

On exam, a palpable firm mass deep in the lateral aspect of the mid-thigh is appreciated. It is non-tender.

Surgical findings and comments

Findings at surgery reveal a solid myxoid tumor within the substance of the vastus lateralis. It is removed intact.

Radiology findings

Case figs 14.1a through **14.1f**, show a typical appearance for this common benign tumor. The lesion is bland isointense to low signal on T1 image and is also homogeneously high signal on T2 and STIR sequences with variable enhancement. This appearance is not specific but has a non-aggressive appearance without obvious invasion or destruction of adjacent tissues. Our main case has only a subtle beak sign of fat adjacent to the inferior pole of the tumor.

The bonus case, **Case figs 14.1g** and **14.1h**, shows a more obvious example of the fatty beak that can be seen with some non-aggressive tumors in muscle. The two additional cases presented (**Case figs 14.1i** through **14.1l**) are remarkably similar showing an oblong intramuscular mass with homogeneous low T1 and high signal on T2 and STIR imaging with modest heterogeneous enhancement. None of these cases have invasive or destructive appearing margins. Some of the intramuscular myxomas have the fat beak sign; this is not reliable in our experience and may simply indicate an indolent intramuscular mass with resulting displacement or atrophy of adjacent muscle.

Pathology findings

Gross features

The specimen consists of a 4 × 3 × 2.6 cm ovoid soft tissue mass that on cut sectioning is uniformly gray, myxoid, and glistening (**Case fig. 14.1m**).

Microscopic features

Low magnification: Although the tumor appeared well circumscribed grossly, it superficially infiltrates nearby skeletal muscle (**Case fig. 14.1n**). Intramuscular myxoma insinuates between slips of skeletal muscle rather than completely effacing muscle fibers. This is one of the uncommon examples of a benign tumor with irregular permeation into nearby normal tissue.

High magnification: Medium magnification reveals a typical hypocellular myxoid example. Spindled tumor cells are suspended in a myxoid matrix that also supports long, fine coursing strands of collagen (**Case fig. 14.1o**). Most cases of intramuscular myxoma contain only a few vessels which are primarily capillary sized and widely dispersed. At high magnification, muciphages (histiocytes ingesting the myxoid matrix) can be prominent or may intermingle with the tumor cells (**Case fig. 14.1p**). The tumor nuclei are small, pyknotic (very dark) and uniform. Mitotic activity is absent. Some deep myxomas, and especially the juxta-articular type, have regions of increased fibrosis (**Case fig. 14.1q**), hemosiderin deposition, mildly increased cellularity, more prominent vasculature, or secondary cystic degeneration.

Special studies: An alcian blue stain highlights the myxoid matrix (**Case fig. 14.1r**). Alcian blue is a histochemical stain that marks neutral and acidic carbohydrate components such as hyaluronic acid. Tumor cells express CD34 by immunohistochemistry and are nonreactive for S-100 protein (**Case fig. 14.1s**). Alcian blue and CD34 reactivity are consistent with the diagnosis but not specific or required. A few myxomas may express smooth muscle actin (SMA) in a 'tram track' pattern of reactivity consistent with myofibroblastic differentiation. This patient's tumor is nonreactive for SMA.

Pathologic differential or, why isn't it one of the following?

Myxoid peripheral nerve sheath tumor: Schwannoma and neurofibromas may be predominantly myxoid. However tumor

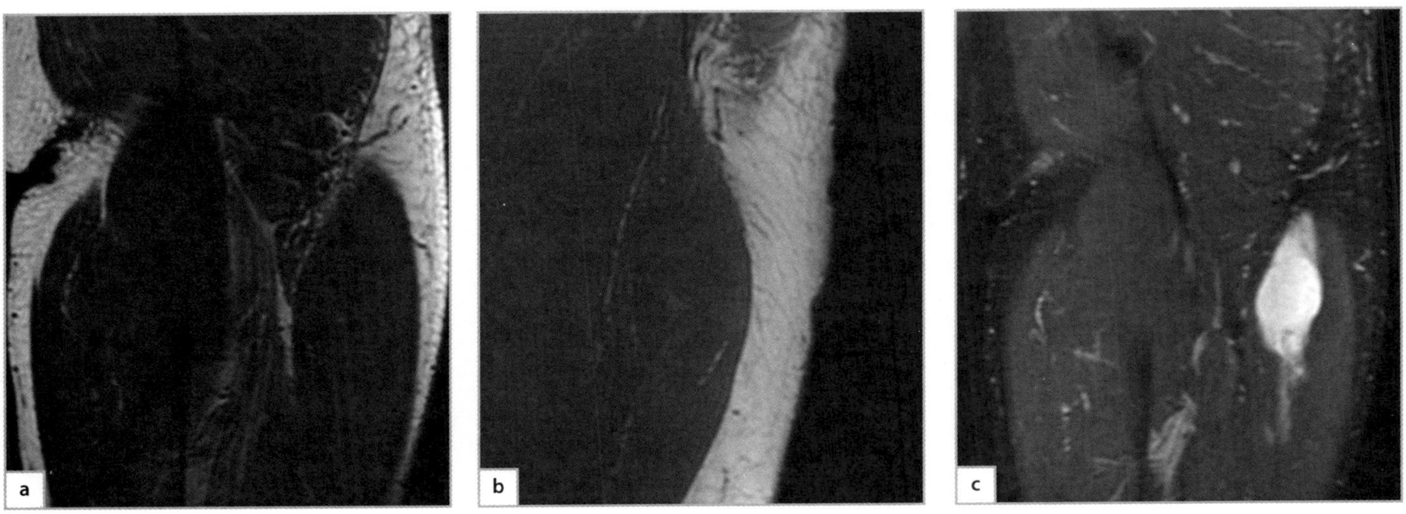

Case figure 14.1 Intramuscular myxoma. MR images including **14.1a**: Coronal T1, **14.1b**: Sagittal T1, **14.1c**: Coronal STIR.

Case figure 14.1: Continued from page 303

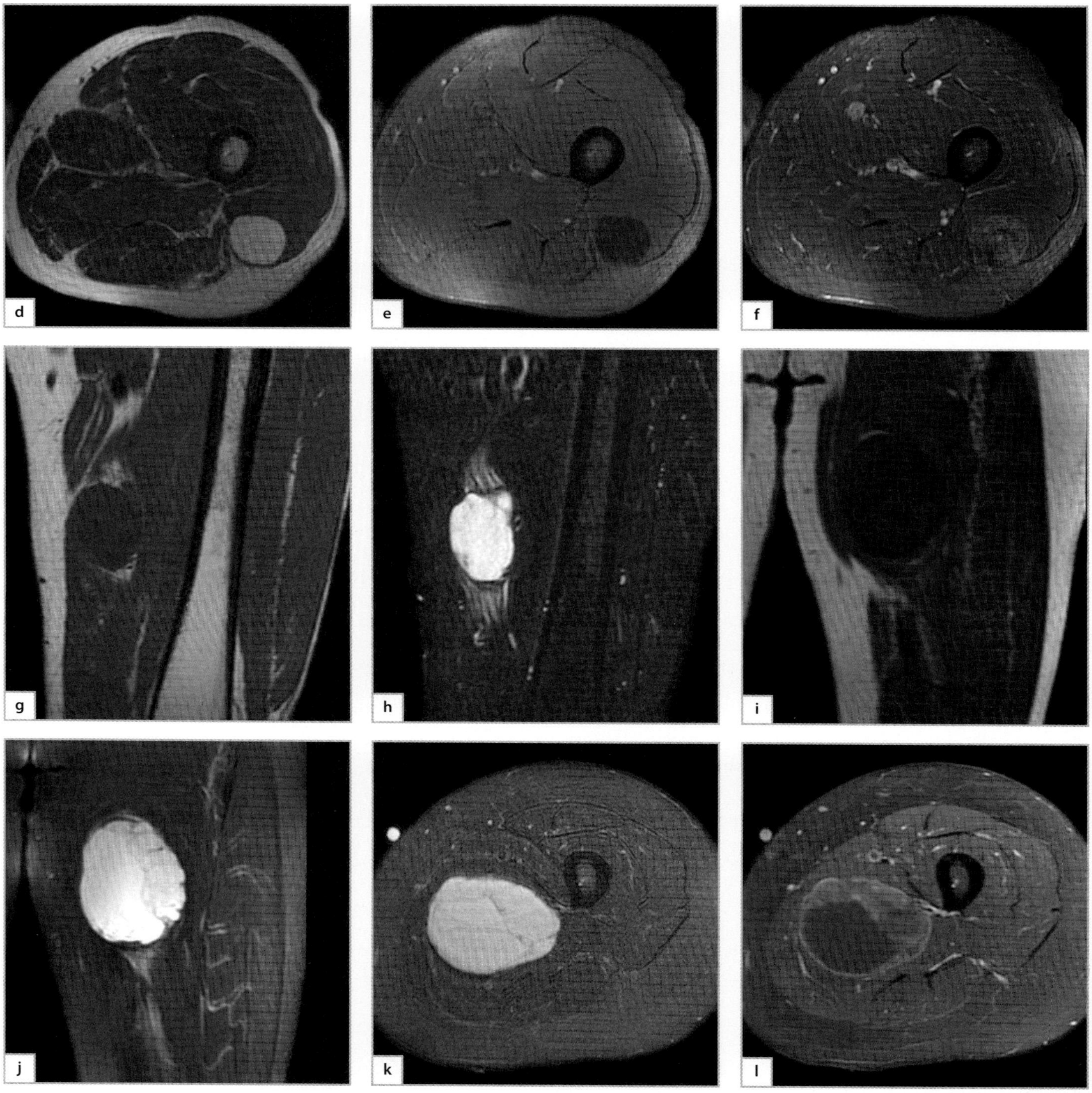

14.1d: Axial T2, **14.1e**: Axial T1 fat saturated and **14.1f**: Axial T1 fat saturated post-contrast. The MR images show a 2.7 × 3.1 × 3.5 cm sharply circumscribed mass, short arrows in Case fig. 14.1a, in the vastus laterlalis muscle of this 59 year old man. The mass show homogeneous T1 isointensity to muscle with T2 and STIR high signal intensity. There is a suggestion of a fat signal beak or triangle adjacent to the inferior pole of the mass, long arrow, 14.1a and 14.1b. There is modest heterogeneous enhancement, and the STIR sequence shows mild edema adjacent to the proximal and distal poles of the mass. We present two additional cases of intramuscular myxoma. **14.1g**: Coronal T1 and **14.1h**: Coronal STIR shows a 4.7 × 3.1 × 3.6 cm mass in the adductor compartment of this 72 year old man. The fat beak adjacent to the proximal and distal poles of the mass is well demonstrated. The second additional case is of a 58 year old woman with a 5.1 × 8.6 × 6.9 cm mass in her adductor magnus muscle. MR images including **14.1i** Coronal T1, **14.1j** Coronal STIR, **14.1k** Axial T2 fat saturation and **14.1l** Axial T1 fat saturation post-contrast. The mass in both of these cases is oblong shaped with homogeneous T1 iso-low signal intensity with T2 and STIR high signal intensity and modest heterogeneous enhancement. The second additional case shows moderate septation on fluid sensitive sequences, Case figs 14.1j–14.1k.

Case figure 14.1: Continued from page 304

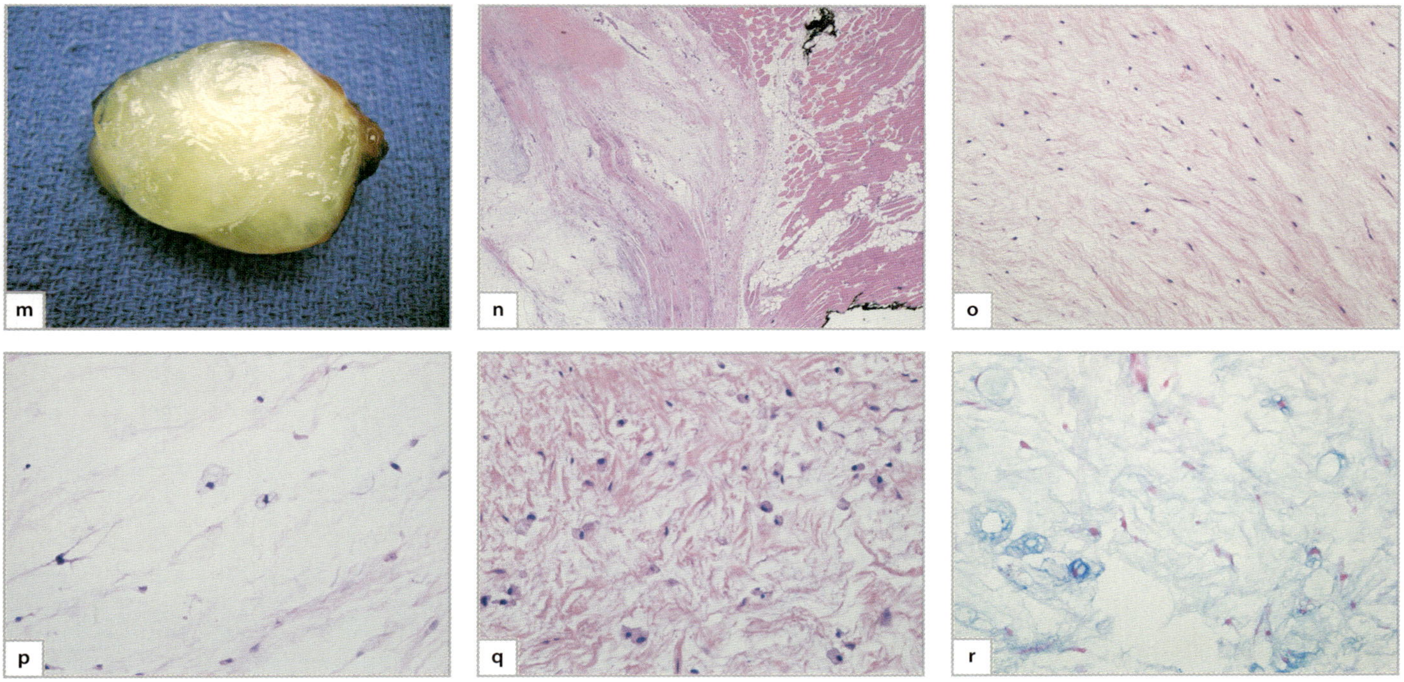

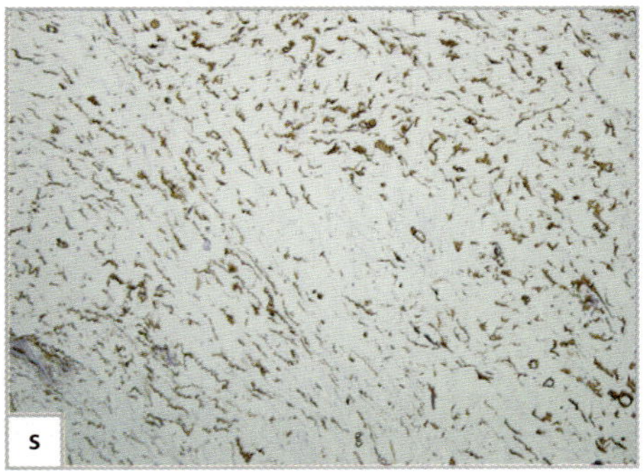

14.1m: Gross photo, cut section of tumor. Cut sections reveal a glistening, soft, semitranslucent tumor without hemorrhage or necrosis. **14.1n**: Low magnification. The tumor is hypocellular with some peripheral layers of collagen fibers. Characteristically, it focally extends into skeletal muscle, separating the muscle fibers but not destroying them. Secondary edema and fat deposition are present in the muscle and are commonly associated with intramuscular myxoma. **14.1o**: Medium magnification. The tumor contains dispersed nuclei along with thin streaming collagen fibers. The background consists of a gray myxoid matrix. There is no necrosis and no blood vessels. **14.1p**: High magnification. Tumor cells may be spindled or polygonal in myxomas: in this case, they are elongate spindled with some branching processes. Tumor nuclei are small, pyknotic, and uniform. The two rounded cells in the center are histiocytes that have engulfed myxoid matrix (muciphages). **14.1q**: High magnification, fibrotic area. In this field, cellularity remains low, but collagen is increased. Most of the cells present are muciphages. Scattered areas of increased fibrosis are common in intramuscular myxoma and characteristic of juxta-articular myxoma. **14.1r**: Alcian blue stain. This histochemical stain highlights hyaluronic acid by turning it a light blue. Note the muciphages are also positive. Lipid is alcian blue negative. **14.1s**: Medium magnification, CD34 immunohistochemical stain. CD34 reveals the slender, undulating and branching shapes of the tumor cells.

cells exhibit wavy or buckled nuclei, nuclear palisading may occur (in schwannoma), and tumor cells express S-100 protein (all in schwannomas and most in neurofibromas). CD34 and alcian blue may be positive in myxoid peripheral nerve sheath tumors which may also contain muciphages.

Myxoid variant of extraabdominal or deep fibromatosis (desmoid tumor): Cellularity is higher in myxoid desmoid tumors, vessels are more numerous, and areas of conventional desmoid tumor are usually present. Some desmoids may express CD34 and/or SMA, but nuclear β catenin, present in about 75% of desmoids, is absent in myxomas.

Low grade myxofibrosarcoma: Low grade myxofibrosarcoma may look deceptively bland at low magnification mimicking a myxoma. However, unequivocal nuclear atypia is present, and the blood vessels are more well developed forming long, slightly curving shapes. Both tumors may express CD34 and focal SMA. Alcian blue reactive myxoid matrix is also present in both tumors.

Low grade fibromyxoid sarcoma (LGFMS): This tumor enters the differential of myxomas that exhibit regions of increased fibrosis and cellularity. LGFMS contains arcades of blood vessels, a whorling,

Case table 14.1 Summary pathology findings of Case 14.1

Diagnosis	Intramuscular myxoma
Size	4 cm
Location	Deep (intramuscular)
Margin status	Negative
Histologic grade (FNCLCC grading system)	Not graded: benign soft tissue tumor.
Pathologic stage (AJCC TNM classification)	Not staged: benign soft tissue tumor.

FNCLCC: Fédération Nationale des Centres de Lutte Contre le Cancer (French Federation of Cancer Centers).

AJCC: American Joint Committee on Cancer

thumbprint like arrangement of collagen fibers, and the transition from myxoid to fibrous areas is usually abrupt. Although a few LGFMS may express CD34, none have been reported to express SMA (as is the case with a few myxomas). Reactivity for MUC4 antibody has been proposed as a relatively specific marker of LGFMS. Finally, LGFMS exhibits one of two specific translocations: t(7;16)(q32-34;p11) = *FUS-CREB3L2* or t(11;16)(p11;p11) = *FUS-CREB3L1*.

Oncology approach

Medical oncology

This is a surgical disease. There is no role of medical oncology.

Radiation oncology

The patient undergoes excision of a left thigh intramuscular myxoma. The risk of future recurrence is low and no radiation therapy is indicated.

Patient outcome

Thirty months postoperatively the patient has no symptoms, normal function, and no evidence of recurrence.

Case 14.2 Pleomorphic hyalinizing angiectatic tumor

Clinical history and presentation

This is a 55 year old woman who presents with a left ankle mass present for many years. Five years ago the patient underwent an MRI but was told the mass was nothing to be concerned about.

Surgical findings and comments

Marginal excision was performed by a podiatrist and the patient referred for further management. Examination reveals a healed incision over the medial ankle. Wide resection of the surgical bed is performed.

Radiology findings

Case figs 14.2a through **14.2e** shows an ill-defined complex mass of the subcutaneous tissues. The lesion has heterogeneous signal but most of the tissue appears to follow fat tissue signal (T1 and T2 high signal) and has minimal enhancement. There is a small central nodule that has T1 low signal and T2 high signal suggesting this is more cellular or more edematous area and also has moderate enhancement. Overall, the lesion is not specific but does not show invasive or destructive features. Tissue diagnosis is needed.

Pathology findings

Gross features

The original resection specimen (removed by a podiatrist at a private clinic) is not available for review. The re-excision consists of 4.5 × 4 × 2 cm portion of skin and underlying soft tissue. Cross sections reveal a blood filled cavity consistent with recent surgery. The cavity has a periphery of firm tissue with interspersed areas of adipose tissue. No discrete tumor is identified. However, a small portion of the firm cavity wall is submitted fresh for karyotyping.

Microscopic features

Low magnification: Despite the lack of discrete tumor grossly, the patient has multiple residual tumor foci surrounding the biopsy cavity. These are recognizable at low magnification as clusters of ectatic hyalinized blood vessels embedded in a cellular to fibrotic background (**Case fig. 14.2f**).

High magnification: Medium magnification reveals the clustered blood vessels have a battered or injured appearance with fibrin deposition and recanalization (**Case fig. 14.2g**). However, many intratumoral vessels are normal in appearance (**Case fig. 14.2h**). Hemosiderin is nearly always found in pleomorphic hyalinizing angiectatic tumor (PHAT); in this patient's tumor, it is readily identifiable (**Case fig. 14.2h**). The vessels that show damage with fibrin deposition range in size, and small vessels may be affected as well as large veins (**Case fig. 14.2i**). Another area of tumor discloses the large range of nuclear size and shape. Several nuclei contain pseudo-inclusions, a characteristic finding in PHATs (**Case fig. 14.2j**). Areas also resemble myxoinflammatory fibroblastic sarcoma (MIFS)(**Case fig. 14.2k**). There is no necrosis, and mitotic figures are rare (up to 1/20hpf).

Special studies: Tumor cells are diffusely strongly reactive for CD34 (**Case fig. 14.2l**). They do not express S-100 protein. Smooth muscle actin is not expressed by tumor cells. However, it does bring into sharp relief the increased number, various calibers, and odd, distorted shapes of tumor vessels (**Case fig. 14.2m**).

The karyotype is reported as 46,XX[19] with one cell showing non-clonal changes: 47,XX,+8,t(16;18)(p11.2;p11.2)[1]. This non-clonal change cannot be considered representative of the tumor.

Pathologic differential or, why isn't it one of the following?

Entities in the pathologic differential include those tumors that occur in the superficial tissue of the extremities, contain scattered pleomorphic or atypical cells, and show myxoid or hyalinized areas and hyalinized blood vessels. These include benign lesions such as 'ancient' schwannoma, ischemic fasciitis, hemosiderotic fibrolipomatous tumor, and malignant tumors including myxofibrosarcoma, and myxoinflammatory fibroblastic sarcoma (acral myxoinflammatory fibroblastic sarcoma). **Case table 14.1a** sorts these tumors with key diagnostic features.

In reality, a considerable overlap has been noticed among PHAT, 'early PHAT,' hemosiderotic fibrolipomatous tumor (HSFLT), myxofibrosarcoma (**Case fig. 14.2n**), and myxoinflammatory fibroblastic sarcoma (MIFS) (**Case fig. 14.2o**). Close age ranges, same body sites, shared microscopic features, similar IHC staining profiles, and lately, hints of genetic concordance suggest a close relationship among these entities. Some cases of PHAT reveal a remarkable resemblance to HSFLT especially in the leading edge of the tumor (Folpe et al. 2004, Luzar et al. 2006). Some PHATs appear to recur

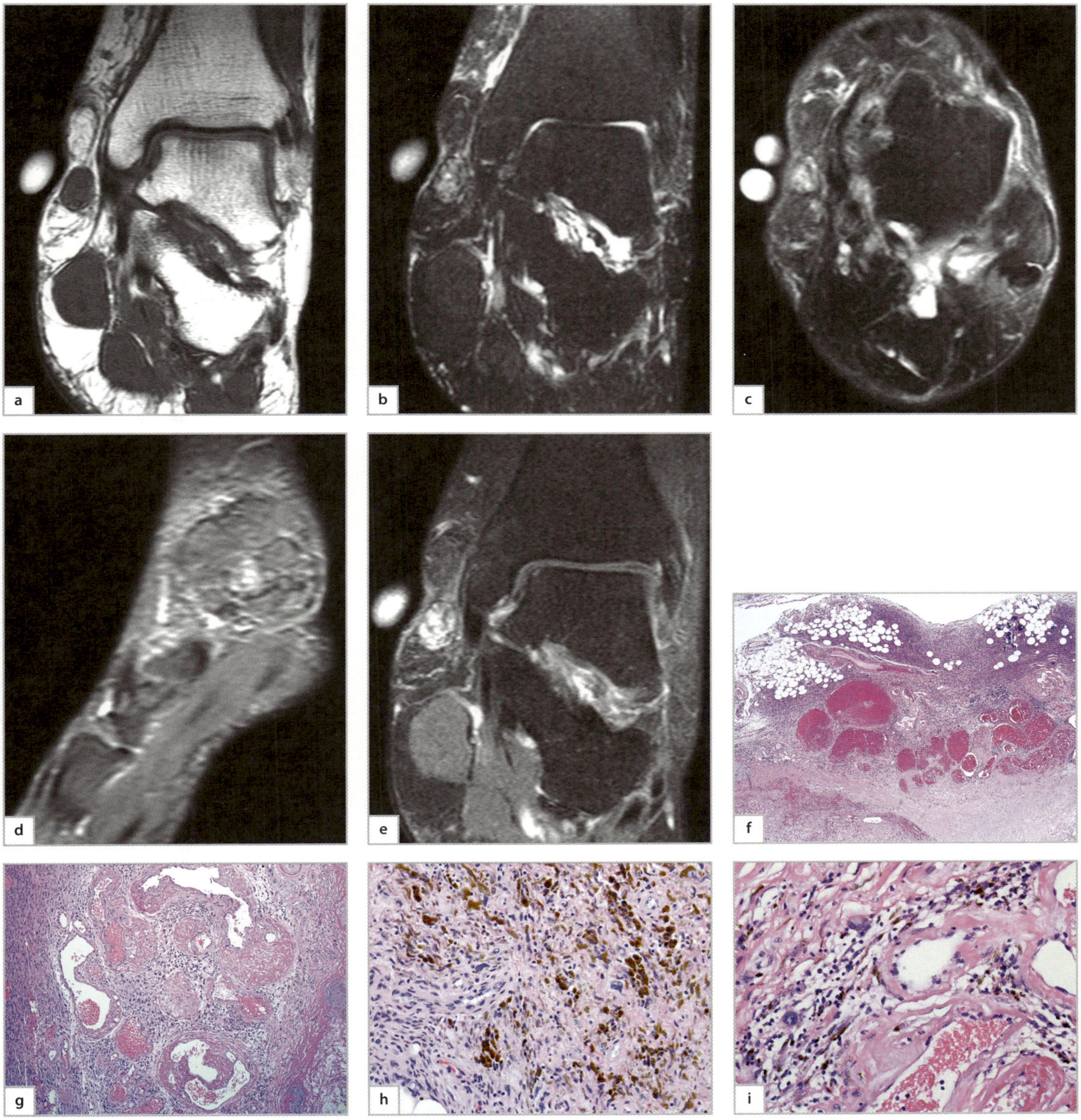

Case figure 14.2 Pleomorphic hyalinizing angiectatic tumor. MR images including. **14.2a**: Coronal T1, **14.2b**: Coronal T2 fat saturated, **14.2c**: Axial proton density fat saturated, **14.2d**: Sagittal STIR, **14.2e** Coronal T1 fat saturated post-contrast are presented. There is an ill-defined mass of the medial subcutaneous tissues measuring approximately 1.6 × 4.6 × 4.8 cm in this 53 year old woman. The mass is heterogeneous and is predominately T1 high signal with corresponding low signal on T2 fat saturated and STIR sequences. The mass has a small central nodule of T1 low signal with heterogeneous high signal on T2 fat saturated and STIR sequences. There is overall no enhancement except for the small central nidus. **14.2f**: Low magnification. The tumor consists of clustered, ectatic blood vessels embedded in a cellular spindle cell proliferation. Tumor invades fat in a honeycomb pattern. **14.2g**: Medium magnification. Typical blood vessels of PHAT appear traumatized with fibrin deposition, distorted lumens, and recanalization. The vessel at top shows fibrin extending beyond the adventitia. Surrounding tumor is cellular with myxoid and fibrotic foci. **14.2h**: Higher magnification. Not all intratumoral vessels are damaged: several small vessels appear normal in this field. Striking hemosiderin deposition is present. Nearly all PHATs contain hemosiderin, although an iron stain may be necessary to find more subtle deposits. The hemosiderin in primarily intracytoplasmic in histiocytes and a few tumor cells. **14.2i**: High magnification. Small vessels also may exhibit mural fibrin deposition. Notice the hemosiderin, sprinkles of lymphocytes, and scattered large multinucleated or mononuclear atypical tumor cells.

Case figure 14.2: Continued from page 307

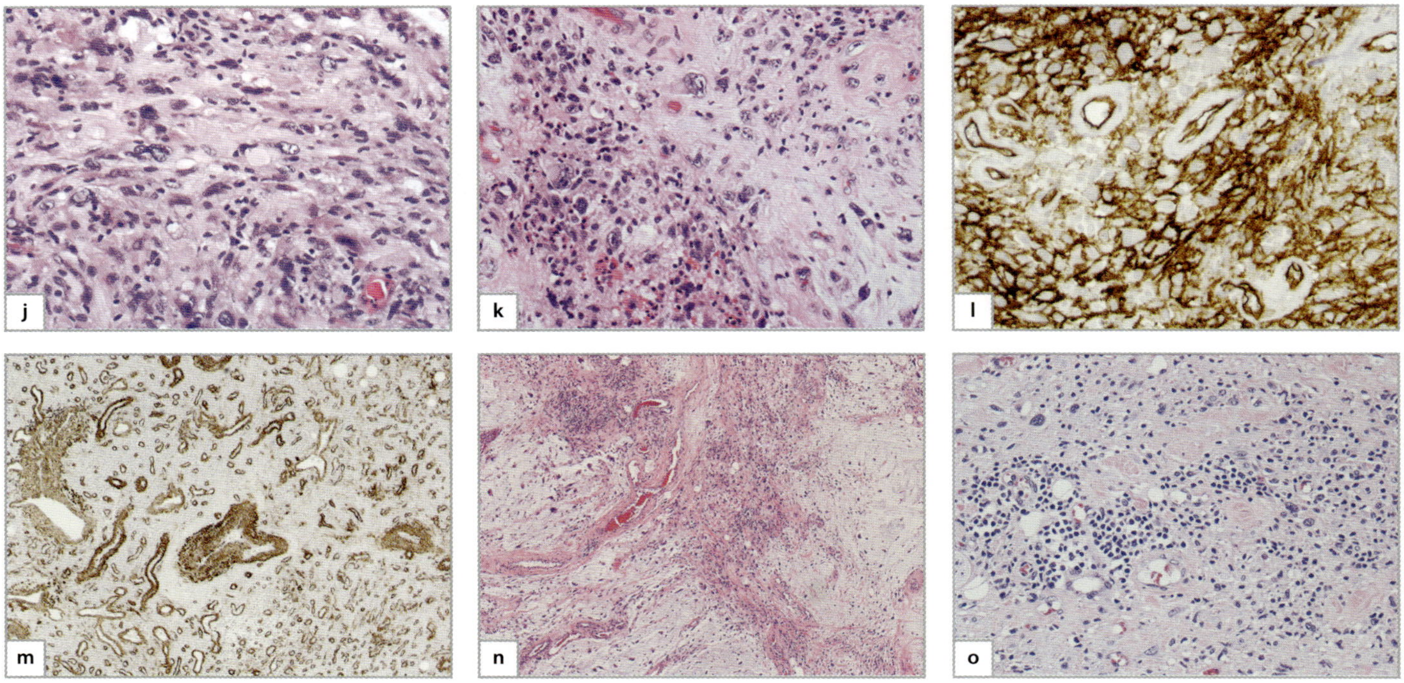

14.2j: High magnification. Tumor cells in the central portion of the tumor nodules exhibit a range of nuclear size and shape. Cell borders are ill defined. Three nuclei contain pseudo-inclusions, a typical feature in PHATs. **14.2k**: High magnification. Aside from the hyalinized small vessel, this field resembles myxoinflammatory fibroblastic sarcoma (MIFS). Genetic, morphologic, and IHC results indicate a close relationship between MIFS and PHAT. **14.2l**: CD34 IHC stain, medium magnification. Nearly all tumor cells express CD34. The endothelial cells in the hyalinized vessels are also reactive and serve as a positive internal control. **14.2m**: Smooth muscle actin IHC stain, lower magnification. SMA highlights the muscular layer of blood vessels. Here it reveals the increased numbers, various sizes, and peculiar, distorted shapes of intratumoral vessels. **14.2n**: Myxofibrosarcoma (MFS) medium magnification. Myxofibrosarcoma may be related to PHAT, HSFLT, and MIFS. This area of intermediate grade MFS could easily be mistaken for PHAT or MIFS. Not all MFS show this morphology, however. **14.2o**: Myxoinflammatory fibroblastic sarcoma (MIFS) medium magnification. This tumor infiltrating the dermis could be mistaken for a region in a myxofibrosarcoma or PHAT. MIFS contains Reed-Sternberg like cells (large tumor cells with cleared nuclei and macronucleoli), lacks conspicuous hyalinzed vessels, and usually does not contain much hemosiderin.

as a tumor indistinguishable from myxofibrosarcoma (Mitsuhashi et al. 2005; Kazakov et al. 2007, Illueca et al. 2011; authors' personal experience in one recent case). Finally, two specific, consistent genetic alterations have been reported in both myxoinflammatory fibroblastic sarcoma and hemosiderotic fibrolipomatous tumor (Hallor et al. 2009, Antonescu et al. 2011; see **Case table 14.2a**).

It is likely that PHAT, HSFLT, and MIFS will merge into one entity based on the aforementioned accumulating evidence. These most likely represent morphologic variants or perhaps distinct phases of progression of one tumor type (Antonescu et al. 2011). Here is an area of soft tissue pathology that may simplify: lumping rather than splitting diagnostic categories. Simplification is occurring due to enough cases accrued to enable adequate clinical, radiologic, morphologic, immunohistochemical, and genetic evaluation.

Oncology approach

Medical oncology

This is a surgical disease. There is no role of medical oncology despite the small risk of transformation to a higher grade.

Radiation oncology

The patient continues to have positive margins after two resections for pleomorphic hyalinizing angiectatic tumor of the left ankle. Even though radiation therapy is an option for the positive margins, it is decided to observe the patient for recurrence.

Patient outcome

Two years postoperatively the patient has no symptoms, normal function, and no evidence of recurrence.

Case table 14.2a Histologic differential diagnosis of pleomorphic superficial soft tissue tumors/lesions (all lesions occur in adults)

Tumor or lesion	Most common body site location	Main histologic features	Variant histologic features or significant absent features	IHC profile	Genetics	Behavior
'Early pleomorphic hyalinizing angiectatic tumor (PHAT)'	Sup. ST of distal extremities	Fascicles of small spindle cells with wavy nuclei infiltrating fat in the manner of DFSP. Myxoid matrix, inflammation and intracytoplasmic hemosiderin common	Rare pleomorphic cells with intranuclear pseudo-inclusions. Abnormally congregated small vessels +/- ectasia and fibrin. Typical PHAT present simultaneously May recur as PHAT	CD34 usually positive	Unknown	Recurs
PHAT	As above, rarely deep or other sites such as axilla	Cellular tumor of aggregated ectatic vessels with fibrinized walls surrounded by spindled and pleomorphic cells set in hyalinized to myxoid stroma. Tumor cells with pseudo-inclusions but rare mitoses. Intracytoplasmic hemosiderin	May have periphery of 'Early PHAT.' Rare cases have increased mitotic activity. Rare cases have punctate necrosis. Exceptional cases have myxofibrosarcoma like areas or recur with myxofibrosarcoma histology	CD34 usually positive	One case of two unbalanced translocations: der(1)t(1;3)(p31;q12),-3, der(10) t(1;10)(p31;q25)	Recurs. Rare cases transform to myxofibrosarcoma
Ischemic fasciitis	Soft tissue over bony prominences: extremities, limb girdles, buttock	Cellular lesion of fibroblasts and myofibroblasts with zones of fibrinoid necrosis surrounded by a cuff of new vessels, damaged vessels and degenerative nuclear atypia of some cells	Intracytoplasmic hemosiderin is not reported. Abnormal clusters of ectatic vessels not reported	CD34 often positive SMA +/-	Unknown. Presumed diploid because the lesion is not currently considered a neoplasm but rather a reactive process	Recurs if inciting event continues
'Ancient' schwannoma	Any body site. Primarily superficial when occurring in extremities.	Variably cellular to myxoid or fibrotic tumor with damaged, hyalinized often ectatic vessels. Tumor cells have buckled or wavy nuclei, may show degenerative nuclear atypia, may have nuclear palisading (verocay bodies)	No virocyte like cells (large tumor cells with vesicular nuclei with prominent macronucleoli)	S-100 protein positive GFAP often positive CD34 usually negative or only focally positive	Schwannomin (22q) +/- Neurofibromin (17q) gene abnormalities	Does not recur or metastasize
Hemosiderotic fibrolipomatous tumor (HSFLT)	Sup. ST of distal extremities	Nodules, fascicles or percolations (reminiscent of DFSP) of bland, uniform spindle cells in fat Prominent hemosiderin (in macrophages or extracellular). Virtually identical to 'Early PHAT'	Myxoid foci. Calcifications. Aggregates of osteoclastic giant cells. Metaplastic ossification. Floret type multinucleate cells. Mural hyalinization of small vessels	CD34 positive in most cases	t(1;10)(p22;q24) = TGFBR3-MGEA5 in most cases (n=~25). Amplification of 3p11-12 in most cases = VGLL3 gene amplified (n =~25)	Recurs
Myxoinflammatory fibroblastic sarcoma (MIFS)	Distal extremities of arm, leg; less commonly proximal extremities. Sup ST, also may involve dermis and tendons fascia	Cellular tumor of alternating fibrous and myxoid zones. Three types of tumor cells: spindled, pleomorphic ('virocyte like') and pseudolipoblastic Inflammation commonly heavy, acute and chronic	Fibrous or myxoid zones may form the large majority of the tumor. Pseudolipoblastic cells may be absent. Necrosis may be present. Rare cases show progression to high grade sarcoma. One case of hybrid tumor with foci consistent with HSFLT	CD34 positive in most cases SMA +/- Keratins focally positive in a few cases	t(1;10)(p22;q24) = TGFBR3-MGEA5 in most cases (n=~20). Amplification of 3p11-12 in most cases = VGLL3 gene amplified (n = ~20)	Recurs; rarely metastasizes. Very rare high grade cases of uncertain behavior – may be more aggressive
Myxofibrosarcoma	Sup. ST of extremities, proximal and distal, lower > upper. Rarely hands/feet, trunk, H&N	Mixed fibrous and myxoid tumor with marked nuclear pleomorphism but not virocyte like cells. Vessels are 'curvilinear' but not hyalinized. Inflammation usually minimal. Pseudolipoblasts may be present	Low grade tumors mimic myxoma and would not be in the differential of the other tumors in this table. High grade tumors often have low grade regions, however. Epithelioid variant	CD34 positive in some cases SMA focal +/-	Complex karyotype common with no specific recurrent findings but often triploid or tetraploid with ring chromosomes	Recurs. Metastatic potential present and lower with superficial tumors, lower grade tumors

DFSP: dermatofibrosarcoma protruberans,
SMA: smooth muscle actin, Sup: superficial, ST: soft tissue, H&N: head and neck

Case table 14.2b Summary pathology findings of Case 14.2

Diagnosis	PHAT
Size	4 cm originally; resection comprises microscopic foci of tumor up to 0.5 cm
Location	Superficial (subcutaneous adipose tissue of ankle)
Margin status	Focally positive at the deep aspect
Histologic grade (FNCLCC grading system)	This is a benign tumor (although with a risk for recurrence and possible dedifferentiation to myxofibrosarcoma). It is not graded.
Pathologic stage (AJCC TNM classification)	This is currently considered a benign tumor and is not staged.

FNCLCC: Fédération Nationale des centres de Lutte Contre le Cancer (French Federation of Cancer Centers). AJCC: American Joint Committee on Cancer

Case 14.3 Angiomatoid fibrous histiocytoma

Clinical history and presentation

The patient is a 25 year old man who presents with a one year history of a thigh mass. The mass was first noted after a fall from a ladder during which the patient believes he sustained a blow to the thigh. Work-up was felt to be consistent with a hematoma. Over the ensuing year, the patient underwent multiple needle aspirations and operative evacuations of the presumed hematoma. Due to the refractory nature of the 'hematoma,' pathologic specimen was finally submitted and the patient referred for further management.

Surgical findings and comments

Physical examination reveals a large mass in the anterior aspect of the proximal thigh. Multiple, haphazardly placed surgical scars are noted. The mass is soft on palpation and tender. Multiple enlarged groin nodes are palpable. Wide resection of the tumor is performed with lymph node dissection of the groin.

Radiology findings

Our case, **Case figs 14.3a** through **14.3e**, shows a large mass of the thigh with the most remarkable feature being the extensive multiloculated cysts showing fluid-fluid levels. This is not a specific feature and can be seen with angiosarcoma and synovial sarcoma. The tumor shows heterogeneous enhancement of the lateral aspect. Clearly, this is an aggressive tumor and tissue diagnosis is needed.

Pathology findings

Gross features

The patient's tumor is originally interpreted at an outlying center as a hematoma and is surgically evacuated three times over a period of one year. Tissue or fluid that is removed is not evaluated in pathology until the fourth attempt at surgical cure of the 'hematoma.' A gross description of this fourth procedure biopsy is not available, although histology is available (see below).

The main resection specimen consists of a large wedge of skin, subcutaneous tissue and skeletal muscle. The skin contains three linear surgical scars. After inking the margins, sectioning reveals a 19 × 15.8 × 8.1 cm multiloculated, smooth-surfaced cavity filled with sanguinous fluid. Surrounding the cavity are ill-defined, gray, firm foci that push into surrounding muscle (**Case fig. 14.3f**). Tissue is collected fresh for cytogenetics and tumor banking. Additional tissue is also submitted as 'deep distal lateral margin' and groin lymph nodes are also separately removed. The latter range from 0.4 to 2.6 cm maximally; the largest contains soft, white to gray areas that bulge above the cut surface highly suspicious for nodal metastasis.

The locally recurrent tumor removed approximately eight months later consists of a 2.5 cm in maximum diameter, similarly cavitated tumor with a thickened rim of dense, fibrous white tissue. Margins are grossly positive.

Microscopic features

Biopsy: The biopsy comprises sheets of cells with central cyst formation. Medium magnification (**Case fig. 14.3g**) reveals ovoid cells with indistinct cell borders and pale eosinophilic cytoplasm. Tumor nuclei are pale and only slightly pleomorphic with inconspicuous nucleoli. Hemosiderin is present.

Resection low magnification: The microscopic appearance matches the gross impression of raised cords or tumor jutting into a large blood filled space (**Case fig. 14.3h**).

Resection high magnification: Medium magnification of the edge of the tumor shows a prominent lymphocytic response (**Case fig. 14.3i**). Higher magnification discloses a fairly well defined border between tumor cells and reactive inflammation (which also includes plasma cells)(**Case fig. 14.3j**). Much of the tumor appears similar to the biopsy regarding individual cell morphology (**Case fig. 14.3k**). However, some areas comprise cells with more atypia including an increased nuclear to cytoplasmic ratio, nuclear hyperchromasia, and increased mitotic activity (**Case fig. 14.3l**). Mitoses in these areas number up to 30/10 high power microscopic fields. Necrosis and vascular invasion are absent. Margins are negative (closest is 0.2 cm).

Sections of the lymph node grossly suspicious for metastasis confirm involvement (**Case fig. 14.3m**) in two of 15 nodes.

Special studies: Immunohistochemical staining reveals 30% of tumor cells express desmin (**Case fig. 14.3n**), 10% express EMA , and there is no reactivity for antibodies to: CD34, smooth muscle actin, mixed keratins, or S-100 protein. INI-1 expression is preserved.

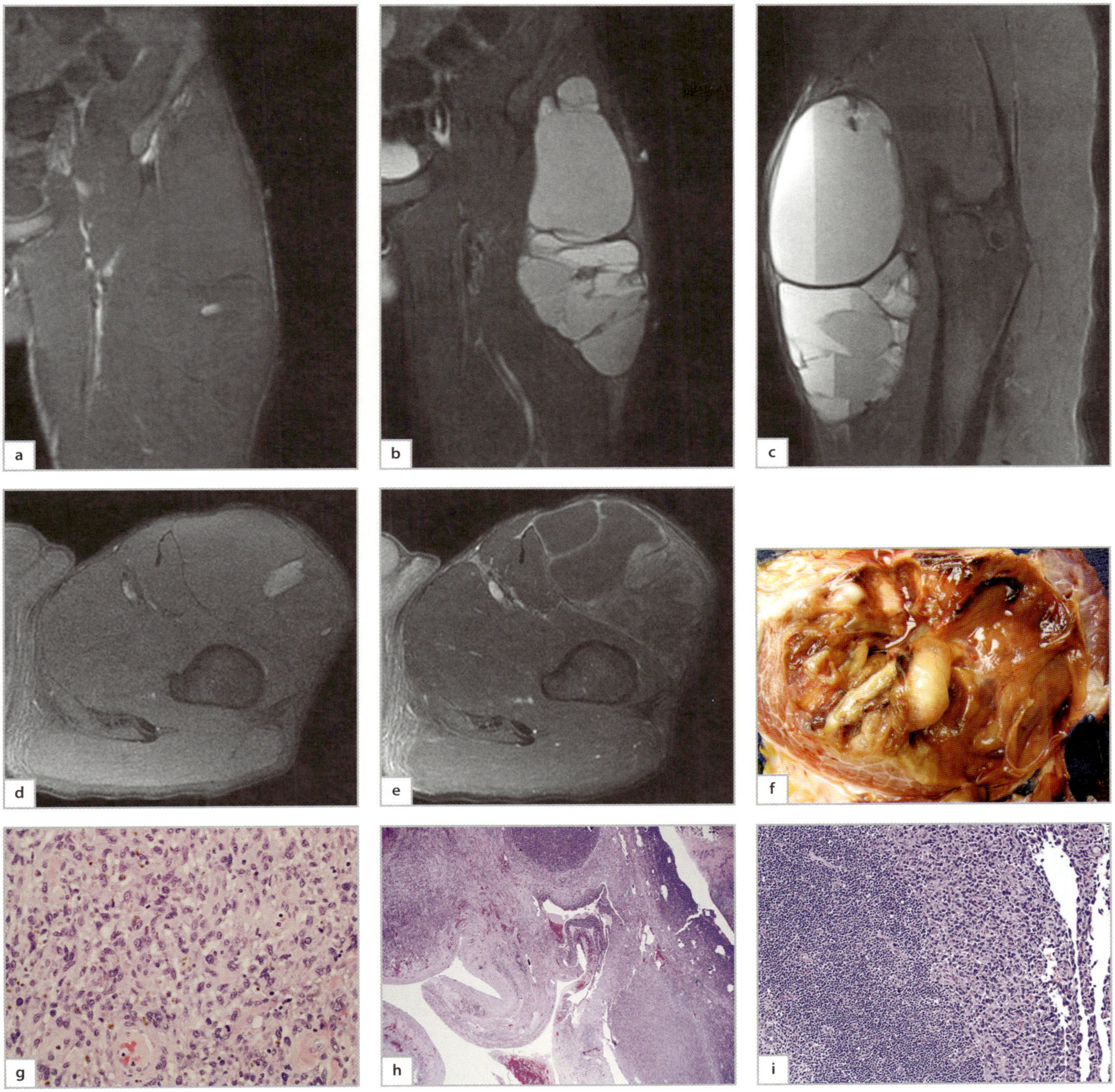

Case figure 14.3 Angiomatoid fibrous histiocytoma. MR images including **14.3a**: Coronal T1, **14.3b**: Coronal STIR, **14.3c**: Sagittal proton density fat saturated, **14.3d**: Axial T1 fat saturated and **14.3e**: Axial T1 fat saturated post-contrast. There is a very large, cystic and solid mass of the proximal quadriceps muscle measuring 7.8 × 20.1 × 8.9 cm in this 24 year old man. The mass shows extensive, large cystic areas with fluid-fluid levels as seen on Figure 14-3c. The mass has a small focus of T1 high signal tissue that does not decrease in signal with fat saturation indicating this is likely blood breakdown products such as met-hemoglobin. There is heterogeneous enhancement of the anterolateral portion of the mass with smooth, thin septa that enhance. **14.3f**: Gross cross section of main tumor resection. The tumor is striking for massive cavitary change. Color ranges from golden to reddish brown and blood clot adheres focally to the smooth inner surface. Raised cords and a central cylinder form the cellular bulk of the tumor. The striated skeletal muscle curving around the edge of the tumor is pale and directly abuts the neoplasm. **14.3g**: Medium magnification, initial biopsy. On the fourth evacuation, the lesion is biopsied and reveals a proliferation of ovoid cells with pale nuclei and indistinct cell borders. Hemosiderin is focally prominent and present in this field. **14.3h**: Low magnification, resection. Corresponding to the gross impression, the tumor forms cords extending into a blood filled cavity. **14.3i**: Medium magnification, resection. The outer edge of the tumor is cuffed by a chronic inflammatory cell infiltrate. This lymphocytic reactive band is characteristic of AFH and a clue to the diagnosis.

Case figure 14.3: Continued from page 311

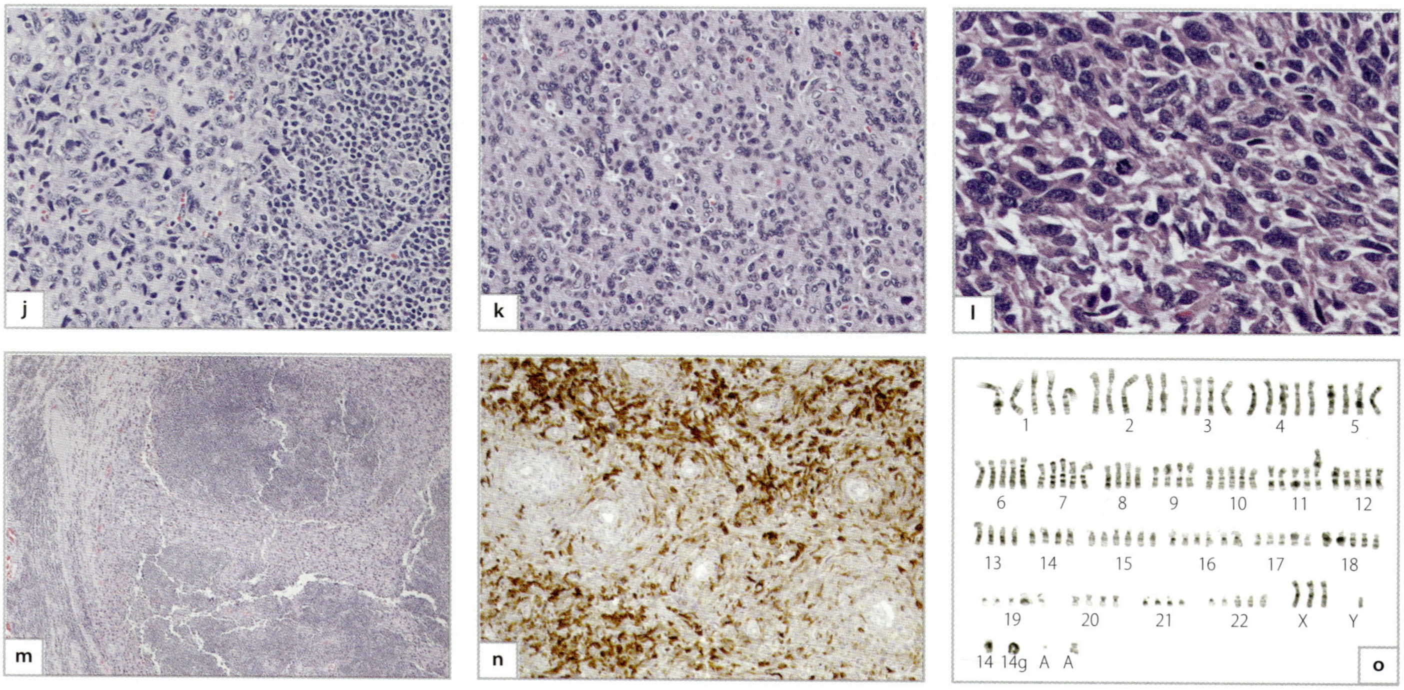

14.3j: Higher magnification, resection. The interface between tumor cells at left and reactive inflammatory cells is fairly sharp. The inflammatory cells include lymphocytes and plasma cells. Notice the relative size of the tumor cells compared to the lymphocytes. **14.3k**: Higher magnification, resection. The morphology in much of the tumor matches the biopsy findings. **14.3l**: High magnification, resection. In some areas, the neoplastic cells are more atypical with an increased N/C ratio, hyperchromasia, and increased mitotic activity. **14.3m**: Medium magnification, largest inguinal lymph node. Tumor is present. **14.3n**: Medium magnification, desmin IHC stain. About 50% of AFH contain cells expressing desmin. This patient's tumor shows strong desmin expression in 30% of tumor cells (brown chromagen). **14.3o**: Karyotype. The karyotype is complex and includes duplications of some chromosomal material and unidentifiable ring and marker chromosomes. The positive lymph node is also karyotyped and yields identical findings.

The tumor karyotype discloses a near pentaploid chromosome complement (**Case fig. 14.3o**): 112-112<5n>XXX,Y,-Y,add(2)(q31),-3,-5,-8,-9,add(11)(p11.2),-13,-14,+15,+16,-20,del(21)(q11.2),add(22)(q11.2)x3,+r,+3mar[cp2]. A karyotype is also performed of the positive lymph node and is identical. Two recent reports of a cytologically pleomorphic AFH noted multiplication of the genome as seen in this patient (but also an EWSR1-CREB1 fusion (Rossi et al. 2007,Tornoczky et al. 2012).

FISH using an EWS break apart probe set is equivocal for translocation (attempted twice on paraffin embedded, formalin-fixed tissue). PCR is not performed.

Pathologic differential or, why isn't it one of the following?

This is an exceptionally large example of an angiomatoid fibrous histiocytoma. One other large deep AFH (23 cm) with early metastases has been reported (Matsumura et al. 2010). Multiple prior surgical interventions may have played a stimulatory role in the growth of this patient's tumor. Its morphology, expression of desmin and EMA, body site location (at a conclave of lymph nodes in the groin region), and young adult age of the patient support the diagnosis. It does behave uncharacteristically aggressively, but infiltrative margins and deep location (both features of this patient's tumor) have been reported to increase the risk for metastasis.

Epithelioid sarcoma: Epithelioid sarcoma does not usually appear angiomatoid, although tumors with prominent hemorrhage ('angiomatoid variant') have been described. The classic version comprises centrally necrotic nodules surrounded by a band of relatively uniform epithelioid cells. Necrosis is usually absent in AFH. ES does not elicit a lymphoid cuff or a fibrous capsule present in ~80% of AFH. Most ES are non-reactive for desmin (positive in ~50% of AFH), and at least 90% show loss of nuclear expression of INI-1 (preserved in AFH). Both tumors occur commonly in young adults, but classic ES is usually superficial and <5 cm. The proximal ES can be larger and deep, but histologically is more atypical than most cases of pleomorphic AFH including this example. Genetically, ES may demonstrate abnormalities of 22q (INI-1 gene), while the great majority of AFH disclose one of three specific translocations, t(12;22), t(12;16) or t(2;22).

Undifferentiated high grade pleomorphic sarcoma: This sarcoma differs from AFH in usually occurring in middle aged to older adults. It does not typically contain blood filled spaces, and a fibrotic capsule with a lymphoid cuff has not been described. By definition, it does not show a specific pattern of IHC reactivity such as this patient's tumor. The karyotype is usually nonspecifically complex.

Leiomyosarcoma: Leiomyosarcoma would be rare in a young adult. Desmin reactivity might suggest the diagnosis, and LMS would have to be the diagnosis rather than leiomyoma because of the high mitotic activity and deep location. However, LMS will not form a fibrous capsule or lymphoid cuff, and other muscle markers are also usually expressed including smooth muscle actin and caldesmon. LMS lacks the specific translocations of AFH.

Synovial sarcoma (SS): The age of the patient, site, and size would be consistent with synovial sarcoma. Some SS can cavitate like the patient's tumor. However, SS does not form a lymphoid cuff or fibrous capsule. Some cases are distinctly biphasic with glandular, ductal or squamous components in addition to a fascicular growth of plump spindle cells. Most cases are negative for desmin. SS and AFH commonly express EMA (SS > AFH). Genetically, both are distinguished by specific separate translocations: t(X;18) or t(X;20) for SS and t(12;22), t(12;16) or t(2;22) in AFH.

Most AFH are small (<3 cm), superficial, and contain nodules of uniform small cells with un-alarming nuclei. The differential diagnosis for these more morphologically innocuous tumors includes a different set of entities than for this patient's large, deep, cytologically atypical tumor. For the small, cytologically bland AFH the histologic differential includes spindle cell hemangioma (true endothelial spaces; positive for CD34 and CD31), aneurysmal fibrous histiocytoma (balled collagen at edges, mixed inflammatory cells, desmin negative), giant cell tumor of tendon sheath (mixed cell population including foamy macrophages), Kaposi sarcoma (true endothelial spaces, HHF8 and CD34 positive) and epithelioid sarcoma (necrosis prominent, negative for desmin, most cases INI-1 negative) (Thway 2009, Fanburg-Smith et al. 1999, Weinreb et al. 2008).

Angiomatoid fibrous histiocytoma may exhibit some variety in morphology and immunostaining profile. **Case table 14.3a** lists these variant features.

Oncology approach

Medical oncology

The malignant counterpart can cause metastases in less than 5% of cases and most can be cured by surgical resection (Costa, et al. 1990). Widespread disease is so rare that the role for medical oncology is not defined. However, because this patient presents with positive lymph nodes and evidence of pulmonary metastases, he is treated with combination chemotherapy including doxorubicin and ifosfamide × 5 courses but progresses. He is then placed on an institutional trial combination of irinotecan and temsirolimus which stabilizes his disease for approximately one year. His regularly scheduled follow-up CT scan then reveals slight enlargement of some of his cavitary lung lesions and a new 1.5 cm right lower lobe nodule.

Although AFH harbors the same translocations as somatic clear cell sarcoma (CCS), the latter is an aggressive tumor that exhibits melanocytic marker expression and a distinctly different gene expression profile including increased transcription of melanocytic genes, *MET* and SOX10 while AFH overexpressed *TFE3* (Antonescu et al. 2007). However, rare cases of AFH, such as occurring in this patient, behave more aggressively and may possibly benefit from chemotherapy regimens developed for CCS.

Radiation oncology

The patient is diagnosed with metastatic angiomatoid fibrous histiocytoma of the left thigh. Treatment consists of resection of

Case table 14.3a Variant pathology features of AFH

Feature	Frequency	Comments
Complete circumferential cuff of lymphocytes and plasma cells	Common	This reactive pattern is rarely seen in other mesenchymal tumors and is a strong clue to the diagnosis May include reactive lymphoid follicles with germinal centers and be florid enough to mimic tumor metastatic to a lymph node low magnification
Partial circumferential cuff of lymphocytes and plasma cells	Common	Several sections may be required to find the characteristic lymphoid cuff (+/- lymphoid follicles)
Absent cuff of lymphocytes and plasma cells.	Rare	May occur de novo or may be lost with recurrent tumor
Angiomatoid pattern of spaces filled with red blood cells and not lined by endothelium	Common	These spaces may be macroscopic or microscopic or both
Multinodular growth without angiomatoid spaces	Rare	Nearly all cases of AFH are multinodular. Most are multinodular and angiomatoid. Rare cases are multinodular and not angiomatoid
Fibrous pseudocapsule	Common	Reactive lymphoid cuff may occur in the capsule or just outside it
Hemosiderin deposition	Common	
Myxoid stroma	Uncommon	Usually focal but may be diffusely present
Reticulated macrocystic or microcystic pattern	Rare	Requires diffuse myxoid change
Sclerotic stroma	Common	Usually focal but may be diffusely present
Storiform architecture	Common	Usually mixed with short fascicular pattern
Short fascicular architecture	Common	Usually mixed with storiform pattern
Cannonball like architecture	Uncommon	Focal and consists of round swirls of tumor cells surrounded by fibrous, myxoid or lymphoid tissue
Short spindly or oval tumor cells often with indistinct cell borders and minimal nuclear atypia (oval to round vesicular nuclei)	Common	These are the characteristic tumor cells of AFH
Scattered cells with large hyperchromatic nuclei	Common	These are dispersed among the typical, uniform smaller tumor cells
Clusters of pleomorphic tumor cells with multinucleation and hyperlobated nuclei with prominent single or multiple nucleoli	Uncommon	Focal areas of pleomorphism do not seem to affect prognosis

Case table 14.3a: Continued from page 313

Feature	Frequency	Comments
Diffuse pleomorphism as described above. May also have mummified tumor cells (individual necrotic cells with smudgy chromatin and condensed cytoplasm) and hyperchromatic nuclei with coarse chromatin	Rare	It is unclear whether diffuse pleomorphism portends aggressive behavior
Tumor cells with nuclear pseudoinclusions	Uncommon	When present, occurs in scattered cells
Tumor cells with nuclear grooves	Uncommon	When present, occurs in scattered cells
High mitotic rate	Uncommon	
Calcifications	Uncommon	May rarely be prominent possibly more often when primary to bone
Small round blue cells	Rare	Form small aggregates that may mimic Ewing sarcoma family of tumors
Clear cells	Rare	May be prominent and comprise round cells with oval uniform nuclei and clear cytoplasm
Multinucleated osteoclast like giant cells	Rare	These reactive cells are dispersed among the neoplastic cells. May be responding to hemosiderin
Serpentine growth of tumor separated by desmoplastic stroma	Rare	May mimic metastatic carcinoma at low magnification
Small irregular clefts some containing RBC mimicking EHE	Rare	Tumor cells are negative for CD31 and CD34 unlike hemangioendothelioma
Less common IHC expression of: SMA, MSA, calponin, caldesmon, CD68, CD99, CD21, mixed keratins	Uncommon to Rare	AFH tumor cells do NOT react for CD31, CD34, S-100 protein Most characteristic IHC expression is for desmin (50%) and EMA (40-60%). INI-1 expression is retained.
Deep soft tissue location (subfascial)	Uncommon	May be associated with more aggressive course
Other body site locations: bone, omentum, lungs, brain, mediastinum, vulva, ovary, retroperitoneum	Rare	Single case reports supported in most cases by FISH evidence of characteristic translocations
Cases without fusion of: EWSR1-CREB1 (75%+ of cases), EWSR1-ATF1 and FUS-ATF1	Rare	Cases occurring outside of soft tissue may more frequently involve ATF1 than CREB1. Rare cases otherwise classic for AFH may not contain these translocations. This could be due to breakpoints not detectable in probe sets or due to as yet uncharacterized genetic changes

IHC: immunohistochemistry, SMA: smooth muscle actin, MSA: muscle specific actin, EMA: epithelial membrane antigen, EHE: epithelioid hemangioendothelioma.

Case table 14.3b Summary pathology findings of Case 14.3

Diagnosis	AFH
Size	19 × 15.8 × 8.1 cm
Location	Deep (subfascial)
Margin status	Positive
Histologic grade (FNCLCC grading system)	This is an intermediate category tumor and is not graded using the FNCLCC system. However, it does meet tumor specific criteria for the pleomorphic variant of AFH
Pathologic stage (AJCC TNM classification)	T2b/N1/M1(two lung nodules) = Stage IV at presentation. (The lung nodules were not sampled but radiologically and clinically are consistent with metastases.)

FNCLCC: Fédération Nationale Des Centres de Lutte Contre le Cancer (French Federation of Cancer Centers). AJCC: American Joint Committee on Cancer

the primary tumor followed by chemotherapy. During the course of treatment, the patient develops local recurrence treated with reexcision followed by postoperative radiation therapy. He has good local control and continues on chemotherapy.

Patient outcome

Three years postoperatively, the patient is alive with asymptomatic, bilateral, recently slowly growing pulmonary metastatic disease. He continues to experience pain at the site of his original tumor which on imaging shows heterotopic ossification but no recurrent disease. He is currently undergoing chemotherapy (third regimen of gemcitabine and docetaxel).

Case 14.4 Ossifying fibromyxoid tumor

Clinical history and presentation

The patient is a 67 year old man who presents with a left medial arm mass which has been present for four years. The mass has enlarged slowly but progressively over the past two years. The mass is painless, but he relates intermittent episodes of radiating numbness to the medial elbow. These episodes occur particularly at night.

Surgical findings and comments

Physical examination reveals a firm, three centimeter diameter, superficial mass over the medial aspect of the arm. It is mobile and separable from underlying muscle. It is non-tender. Marginal excision is performed. Due to concern regarding the pathologic diagnosis, the patient is referred to musculoskeletal oncology for further management. The patient is returned to surgery for wide surgical resection.

Radiology findings

No radiology is available. The initial clinical impression was lipoma; therefore, the general surgeon did not request imaging studies.

Pathology findings

Gross features

The resection specimen consists of the ovoid tumor itself measuring 3.5 × 3.5 × 2.7 cm with an overlying ellipse of skin and no additional non-neoplastic tissue. Cross sections reveal a mixed fibrous to calcified, tan to tan white tumor with a whorled cut surface. More than 80% of the tumor is submitted for routine histology, and three blocks require decalcification. Since the specimen is received in formalin, tissue is not available for karyotyping and banking.

The re-excision specimen comprises an ellipse of skin and underlying centrally firm soft tissue measuring 4.4 × 1 × 1.9 cm. Cross sections reveal areas of fat necrosis and firm fibrous regions. No discrete tumor mass is identified.

Microscopic features

Low magnification: At low magnification, the tumor is solid, unencapsulated with a pushing border. It is striking for alternating pale myxoid and dense pink, hypocellular fibrous areas (**Case fig. 14.4a**). Primarily at the periphery, nodules of well-formed mature bone arise suddenly in the tumor (**Case fig. 14.4b**).

High magnification: Medium magnification of bone interface reveals collagen bands attached to one edge of bone, well formed lines of calcification and lack of osteoblastic rimming (**Case fig. 14.4c**). The two main components of the tumor are 1) mildly cellular myxoid regions that swirl around: 2) hypocellular collagenous areas (**Case fig. 14.4d**). However, in one area, the tumor causes a reactive hyperplasia of eccrine glands (**Case fig. 14.4e** and **Case fig. 14.4f**). This phenomenon has been reported in OFMT (Folpe et al. 2003, Min et al. 2005). Dense

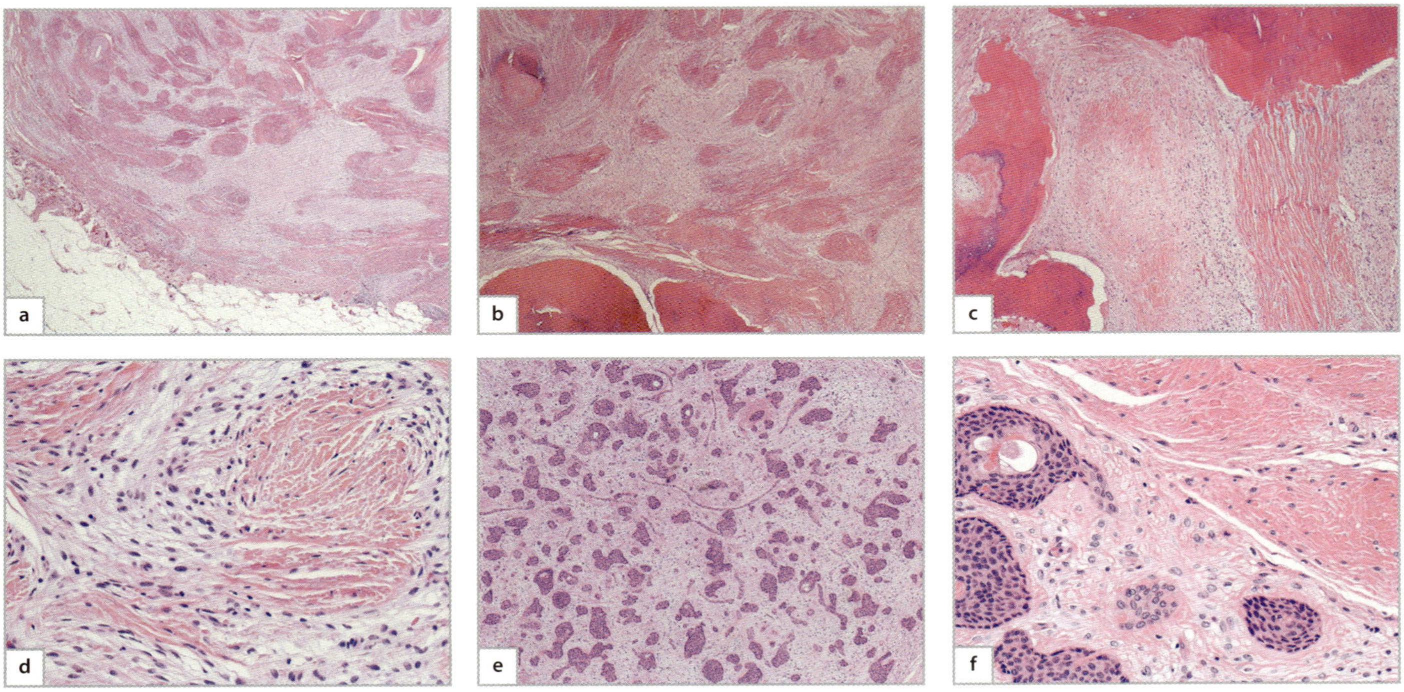

Case figure 14.4 Ossifying fibromyxoid tumor. **14.4a**: Low magnification. The tumor pushes into the subcutaneous fat without a pseudocapsule. It consists of alternating dense fibrous zones and myxoid regions. **14.4b**: Low magnification. In this field, two nodules of well-formed bone arise suddenly (meaning adjacent tumor is histologically no different than distant tumor) at the periphery. **14.4c**: Medium magnification. Tassels of collagen emanate off one of the bone spicules. Notice the lack of osteoblastic rimming, and the well-formed lines of calcification in the neoplastic bone. **14.4d**: Medium magnification. Most of the tumor consists of myxoid cellular regions that swirl around dense, collagenous, fibrous areas. **14.4e**: Lower magnification. Entrapped eccrine ducts and glands exhibit reactive hyperplasia, a phenomenon previously described in OFMT. **14.4f**: Medium magnification, entrapped proliferated eccrine ducts. Notice the tumor edges right up to the proliferated ducts with no fibrosis, inflammation, or edema.

Case figure 14.4 Continued from page 315

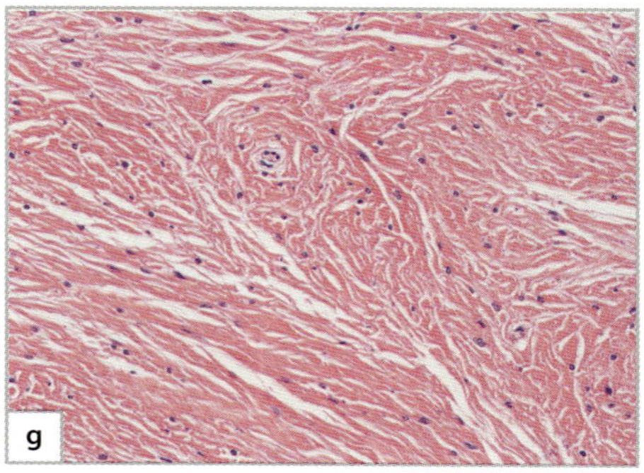

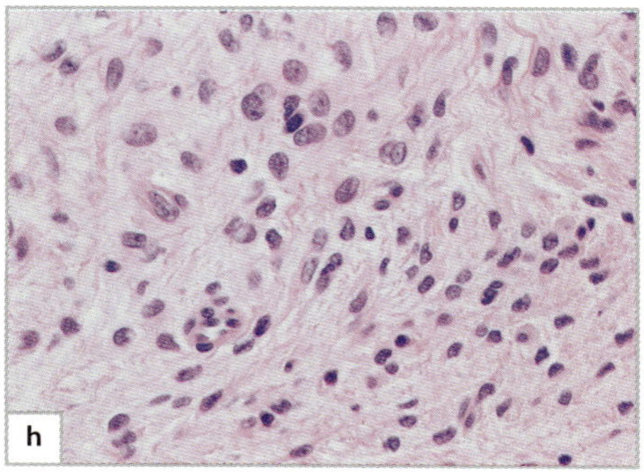

14.4g: Higher magnification, dense area. The dense regions of the tumor show artifactual clefting or cracking. Tumor cells are widely dispersed without clear cell borders. **14.4h**: High magnification, myxoid area. The lesional cells are uniform with indistinct cell borders and hypochromatic oval nuclei with absent to single small nucleoli. Mitoses are not identified. Necrosis is absent.

areas of tumor comprise bands of collagen that crack during sectioning (**Case fig. 14.4g**). High magnification of the myxoid areas reveals ovoid uniform pale nuclei with inconspicuous to single small nucleoli. Cytoplasm is eosinophilic, and cell borders are not distinguishable (**Case fig. 14.4h**). There is no mitotic activity, no necrosis, and no nuclear atypia (the last is typified by greater variation in nuclear size and shape, hyperchromasia, macronucleoli, multilobation, and often coarse, unevenly distributed chromatin).

Special studies: By IHC, about 20% of tumor cells weakly express S-100 protein. Tumor cells do not express keratins, p63, smooth muscle actin, calponin, or EMA .

Pathologic differential or, why isn't it one of the following?

Soft tissue myoepithelioma (myoepithelial tumor of soft tissue): Myoepithelioma of soft tissue often contains spindled cells and myxoid areas. However, ducts or tubules are commonly present as is chondromyxoid matrix rather than bone (although the latter can occur uncommonly). This patient's tumor has entrapped hyperplastic but recognizable eccrine ducts that should not be mistaken for true tubule/duct formation by the tumor.

By immunohistochemistry, myoepithelioma and OFMT commonly express S-100 protein, but myoepithelioma shows a broader repertoire of reactivity which includes p63 (~60% of cases), mixed keratins, GFAP, calponin, and smooth muscle actin (consistent with the dual epithelial-smooth muscle differentiation of the constituent cells). However, rare OFMT may express keratins, GFAP and SMA, but p63 is not expressed (Min et al. 2005, Miettinen et al. 2008, Jo et al. 2011). A few myoepitheliomas, mainly some pediatric myoepithelial carcinomas, show loss of INI-1 expression (Hollman et al. 2011). INI-1 expression is mosaic (patchy loss of expression in 30-60% of tumor cells) in up to 75% of OFMT (Graham et al. 2011). Thus, there can be overlap in IHC reactivity patterns in a given case of OFMT and myoepithelioma; at such a juncture, classic morphologic features including a peripheral rim of lamellar bone, absence of epithelioid myoepithelial cells, and lack of tubules/ducts supports OFMT.

At the genetic level, many cases of OFMT exhibit rearrangement of the *PHF1* gene on chromosome 6p21 which can be detected on interphase FISH or PCR testing (Gebre-Medhin et al. 2012). By contrast, at least 50% of soft tissue myoepithelial tumors and a smaller proportion of cutaneous examples contain fusions of the *EWSR1* gene with other partners including *POU5F1* (younger patients with clear cell morphology), *PBX1, ZNF444, FUS*, and *ATF-1* (Flucke et al. 2011, Antonescu et al. 2010, Flucke et al. 2012). EWSR1 negative tumors tend to be superficial, benign and feature ducts or tubules facilitating discrimination from OFMT (Antonescu et al. 2010).

Soft tissue perineurioma (STP): STP is relatively rare, is composed of slender uniform spindled cells and can feature alternating areas of myxoid and collagenized stroma. Occasional cases ossify. Perineuriomas do not express S-100 protein, can exhibit a distinctive meningothelial like whirling of cells, and express EMA, GLUT1, Claudin-1 and CD34 (the last in about 67%). Genetically, soft tissue perineuriomas disclose abnormalities of the *NF2* gene on chromosome 22 and/or 10q changes.

Low grade fibromyxoid sarcoma (LGFMS): LGFMS is characterized by alternating myxoid and collagenous zones like OFMT. Rare cases may ossify and further mimic OFMT. The spindled neoplastic fibroblasts are generally uniform with minimal atypia (in most cases; recurrences may also exhibit more pleomorphism) similar to OFMT. Subtle differences include arcades of blood vessels and thumbprint-like whorls of tumor cells in LGFMS. By IHC, only rare cases react for S-100 protein which is expressed in 75-95% of OFMT. MUC4 has been proposed as specific and sensitive for LGFMS (Doyle et al. 2011) but a few OFMT may also express this antigen (Graham et al. 2011). The lesions are very distinct genetically, as LGFMS contains one of two balanced translocations: t(7;16)(q32-34;p11) = *FUS-CREB3L2* or t(11;16)(p11;p11) = *FUS-CREB3L1*. These translocations have not been reported in OFMT.

Extraskeletal myxoid chondrosarcoma (ESMCS): Based on histologic features, ESMCS is seldom in the differential of OFMT.

Malignant ossifying fibromyxoid tumor (malignant OFMT): This type of OFMT exhibits high nuclear grade or high cellularity and mitotic activity of >2 figures/50 high power microscopic fields (Folpe et al. 2003). This patient's tumor is low nuclear grade, moderately cellular, and mitotic figures are not identified in 50 fields. (High cellularity is indicated by nuclear crowding with loss of intervening matrix encompassing at least one 4x microscopic field)(Graham et al. 2011). Importantly, although malignant OFMT by these criteria exhibit a higher rate of recurrence and metastasis, rare histologically bland tumors may also metastasize. Malignant OFMT may contain areas of typical OFMT, and thus extensive sampling is strongly urged (Graham et al. 2011).

Case table 14.4a lists variant pathologic features reported for OFMT.

Oncology approach

Medical oncology

Malignant variants occur in about 10 to 20% of cases. Usually, the disease has a low malignant potential and the treatment remains surgical, even in the metastatic setting (Enzinger, et al. 1989,

Case table 14.4a Variant pathology features of OFMT

Feature	Frequency	Comments
Peripheral shell of tumor osteoid	Common (60-80%)	Usually the osteoid is hypocellular lamellar bone that arises abruptly from surrounding tumor. In a few cases, the bone may extend into the center of the tumor or comprise the bulk (>50%) of the tumor. Centrally situated bone may be more common in malignant OFMT. A few cases may show disintegration of the bone with a multinucleated osteoclastic giant cell reaction
Fibrous pseudocapsule	Common (80%-90%)	Infiltrative margin may be associated with increased local recurrence
Evenly spaced round to plump spindled cells arranged in nests and cords in vague lobules	Common (80%)	Tumor cells may have indistinct cell borders Cytoplasm is pale eosinophilic
Uniform round to oval nuclei with absent to small nucleoli with mitotic rate <2/50hpf	Common (80%)	Nuclear clefts, grooves, and pseudo-inclusions may be seen
Fibrous (collagenous) or myxofibrous matrix	Common (>90%)	Fibrous and myxoid aras often abut sharply
Hyalinized blood vessels	Common	Resemble those seen in ancient schwannoma
S-100 protein reactivity by IHC	Common (65-95%)	Reactivity may be weak and is seldom diffuse
Mosaic INI-1 reactivity by IHC	Common (30-60%)	FISH tests may not show deletion of 22q
Calcifications or cartilage	Uncommon	
Necrosis	Uncommon	Not a predictor of recurrence or metastasis
Satellite nodules	Uncommon	Not a predictor of recurrence or metastasis
Malignant OFMT: high nuclear grade or high cellularity and >2 mitoses/50 hpf	Uncommon	Tumors with high nuclear grade also often have high cellularity, increased mitoses and necrosis Tumor lobulation may be accentuated in malignant OFMT Some malignant OFMT have areas of typical OFMT
Atypical OFMT: may have increased mitotic rate but not high cellularity and vice versa	Rare	Behavior of these tumors is much closer to typical OFMT than malignant OFMT
Additional IHC Reactivity **Keratins, EMA, GFAP, SMA, desmin, MUC4**	Uncommon to rare	Profile of immunohistochemical reactivity can overlap with myoepithelial tumors OFMT commonly express CD10 but this is of low diagnostic value

Case table 14.4b Summary pathology findings of Case 14.4

Diagnosis	OFMT
Size	3.5 × 3.5 × 2.7 cm
Location	Subcutaneous tissue of arm.
Margin status	Initial margins widely positive. No residual tumor on re-excision.
Histologic grade (FNCLCC grading system)	This is considered a benign tumor by the WHO, as most cases behave in a benign fashion. This tumor does not show histologic features of 'malignant' OFMT.
Pathologic stage (AJCC TNM classification)	Since this patient's tumor is a benign OFMT, it is not staged. However, rare histologically benign OFMT may metastasize, so the patient must be followed long term.

FNCLCC: Fédération Nationale des Centres de Lutte Contre le Cancer (French Federation of Cancer Centers). AJCC: American Joint Committee on Cancer

Folpe, et al. 2003). In patients with multiple metastases or rapidly recurrent metastatic disease, there is no consensus for medical therapy. Chemotherapy regimens for soft tissue sarcoma or for osteosarcoma have been used in rapidly progressive cases, usually unsuccessfully. Interestingly, a genomic analysis of these tumors shows a disappearance of IN1 expression, similar to the one observed in malignant rhabdoid tumors (Graham, et al. 2011).

Radiation oncology

The patient undergoes two surgeries including wide resection for ossifying fibromyxoid tumor of the left arm. No radiation therapy is indicated after wide resection.

Patient outcome

Five years postoperatively the patient is asymptomatic and has no evidence of recurrence.

Case 14.5 Synovial sarcoma

Clinical history and presentation

This 22 year old physically active man presents with a right shoulder mass discovered incidentally on an MRI performed for unrelated shoulder pain. He had a right clavicle closed fracture sustained after a mountain biking accident five years previously that was treated non-operatively. One year previous to presentation, he had removal of a bony prominence at the site of the right clavicle fracture.

The patient complains of shoulder discomfort with overhead activities, mild dull aching pain, and limitations in range of motion.

The incidentally discovered mass is most consistent on imaging with a benign lesion such as complicated perilabial cyst, joint bodies, or myositis ossificans, but a sarcoma cannot be entirely excluded. The recommendation is to follow the lesion with careful serial imaging.

Surgical findings and comments

Physical examination reveals no obvious masses or other pathology regarding the shoulder.

Due to the persistence of the mass along with inability to definitively rule out malignancy without a tissue sample, marginal excision is performed. Following confirmation of malignancy, the patient is returned to surgery for wide resection of the tumor bed along with reconstruction of the anterior shoulder soft tissue with a pectoralis tendon transfer.

Radiology findings

Synovial sarcoma, monophasic variant. We present a difficult case, **Case figs 14.5a** through **14.5i**, of a young man presenting with calcifications found on radiographs, at first thought to be joint bodies. His initial imaging workup includes a bone scan which shows no uptake, **Case fig. 14.5e**. MR arthrography is performed (**Case figs 14.5b** through **14.5d**) to determine if the calcifications are in fact intra-articular and to hopefully also identify the presumed intra-articular process causing them. Instead, a well-defined encapsulated appearing mass is found associated with the inferior glenohumeral ligament (IGHL). Given the tumor has little T2 or proton density high signal (**Case figs 14.5b** and **14.5c**) and has an apparent capsule, it is thought to be a fibrous process perhaps related to exuberant healing response from previous or repeated shoulder injury of the IGHL ligament. This correlates with the patient's active outdoor lifestyle that includes rock climbing and mountain biking.

After considerable discussion with the patient, he elects for close interval follow up. Unfortunately, his tumor grows during the five month interval (**Case figs 14.5f** through **14.5h**) prompting the pursuit of tissue diagnosis. Interestingly, the tumor has only moderate enhancement and only modest interval growth. This underscores the highly variable appearance and course for synovial sarcoma.

We present two additional cases of synovial sarcoma (**Case figs 14.5i** through **14.5p**) which happen to also involve the right shoulder area. These two additional cases show more aggressive features such as larger size, absence of calcification, proximal location and cystic component. The second case has T1 high signal areas that could represent hemorrhage.

Pathology findings

Gross features

The initial excision consists of a 4.5 × 3 × 1.9 cm ovoid portion of soft tissue that is partially disrupted. Cut sections reveal a gray, fibrous, spottily calcified mass that occupies the entire specimen (**Case fig. 14.5q**). Small portions are collected fresh for cytogenetics and tissue banking, and five cassettes are submitted for routine histology.

The re-excision consists of two parts: skin and superficial soft tissue (4.5 × 4 × 2 cm) and deep soft tissue of the right shoulder (three fragments, largest 8 cm). The first portion contains a healing skin scar and no discrete lesions. The second portion contains yellow necrotic areas but no discrete lesions. Both portions are extensively sampled for histology review.

Microscopic features

Low magnification Initial Specimen: Consistent with the gross impression, the tumor contains scattered calcifications and is variably fibrotic (**Case fig. 14.5r**).

High magnification initial specimen: At medium magnification, some of the calcifications are small and round and dispersed evenly in collagen rich areas (**Case fig. 14.5s**). Most of the tumor consists of short, hypercellular fascicles of plump spindle cells. The nuclei are minimally pleomorphic and normochromatic without prominent nucleoli, cell borders are indistinct, and mitoses are few (**Case fig. 14.5t**). This hypercellularity imparts a blue color at low magnification and is characteristic of most synovial sarcomas, at least focally. Only one other tumor consistently shows a similar blue fascicular pattern at low magnification: malignant peripheral nerve sheath tumor.

Re-excision: The re-excision contains foci of tumor identical to the original excision (**Case fig. 14.5u**). Tumor extends to cauterized inked tissue edges but because the specimen is received in pieces, it is not possible to determine margin status microscopically.

Special studies initial specimen: On IHC staining, about 15% of tumor cells express keratins AE1/AE3 and EMA (**Case fig. 14.5v**). Tumor nuclei are diffusely intensely reactive for TLE1 (**Case fig. 14.5w**), a sensitive and fairly specific marker of synovial sarcoma (positive predictive value of 92% in one review; Jagdis et al. 2009). TLE1 expression correlates with finding t(X;18) genetically (Knosel et al. 2010: review of 259 cases of SS with 96% of cases expressing TLE1). However, TLE1 is expressed in other tumors that may enter the differential diagnosis such as malignant peripheral nerve sheath tumor (up to 30% of cases), mesothelioma (strongly positive in 70%) and rarely other sarcomas such as solitary fibrous tumor (Kosemehmetoglu et al. 2009, Matsuyama et al. 2010, Terry et al. 2007).

Karyotyping reveals a normal chromosome complement of 46,XY. This is interpreted as not representative of tumor and most likely consists of overgrowth of normal fibroblasts. FISH is not performed, because of the characteristic clinical, morphologic, and IHC findings.

Additional case: Although the monophasic spindle cell variant of synovial sarcoma outnumbers the biphasic variant by an estimated 3-4:1, an example of biphasic SS is provided. In this example (**Case fig. 14.5x**), the epithelial cells are pale, round, some form tubules and are surrounded by spindled tumor cells identical to those seen in spindle cell monophasic SS. Some biphasic SS are dominated by glands or tubules, and a few cases contain foci of squamous metaplasia (Fisher et al. 2011).

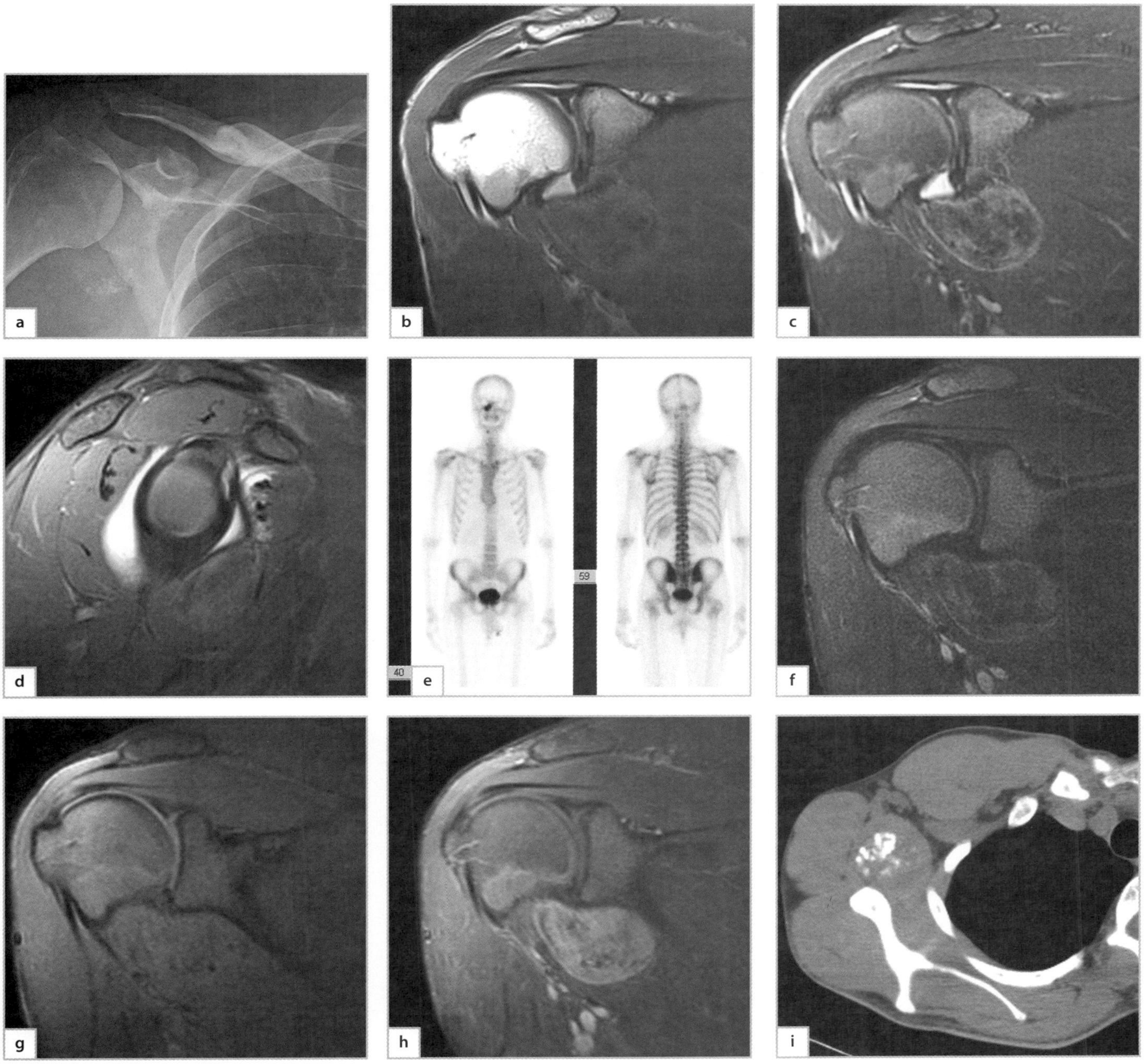

Case figure 14.5 Synovial sarcoma, monophasic. Anteroposterior radiograph, **14.5a**: Shows a cluster of irregular calcifications in the inferior aspect of the right shoulder in this 22 year old athletically active man. There is an old healed clavicle fracture related to remote prior mountain biking accident. The orientation of the calcification is suggestive of intra-articular joint bodies although there are no signs of osteoarthritis. An MR arthrogram was performed to ascertain if these calcifications might be related to intra-articular pathology. The MR arthrogram images including **14.5b**: Coronal proton density, **14.5c**: Coronal T2 fat saturated and **14.5d**: Sagittal proton density fat saturated show an extra-articular encapsulated appearing mass measuring 4.2 × 3.0 × 2.8 cm. The tumor shows stippled low signal areas corresponding to the calcifications seen on radiographs. The tumor has mild heterogeneous T2 high signal and appears adherent to or originates from the inferior glenohumeral ligament. Nuclear medicine bone scan at the time of presentation. **14.5e**: Shows no significant uptake by the lesion, there is right maxillary sinus disease incidentally noted. The patient elected to have short interval follow-up and returned 5 months later for repeat MR exam with IV contrast including; **14.5f**: Coronal STIR, **14.5g**: Coronal T1 fat saturated and **14.5h**: Coronal T1 fat saturated post-contrast images. These images show the mass is homogeneously T1 isointense to muscle, except for the stippled calcification. The mass has minimal STIR high signal and shows moderated enhancement. The mass had increased modestly in size now measuring 4.8 × 3.2 × 3.1 cm. CT imaging at the time. **14.5i**: Showed the stippled calcification of the mass and no lung lesions. We present two additional cases of synovial sarcoma also involving the shoulder. figures 14.5j through 14.5m are from a 19 year old man with shoulder girdle mass. MR images include.

Case figure 14.5: Continued from page 319

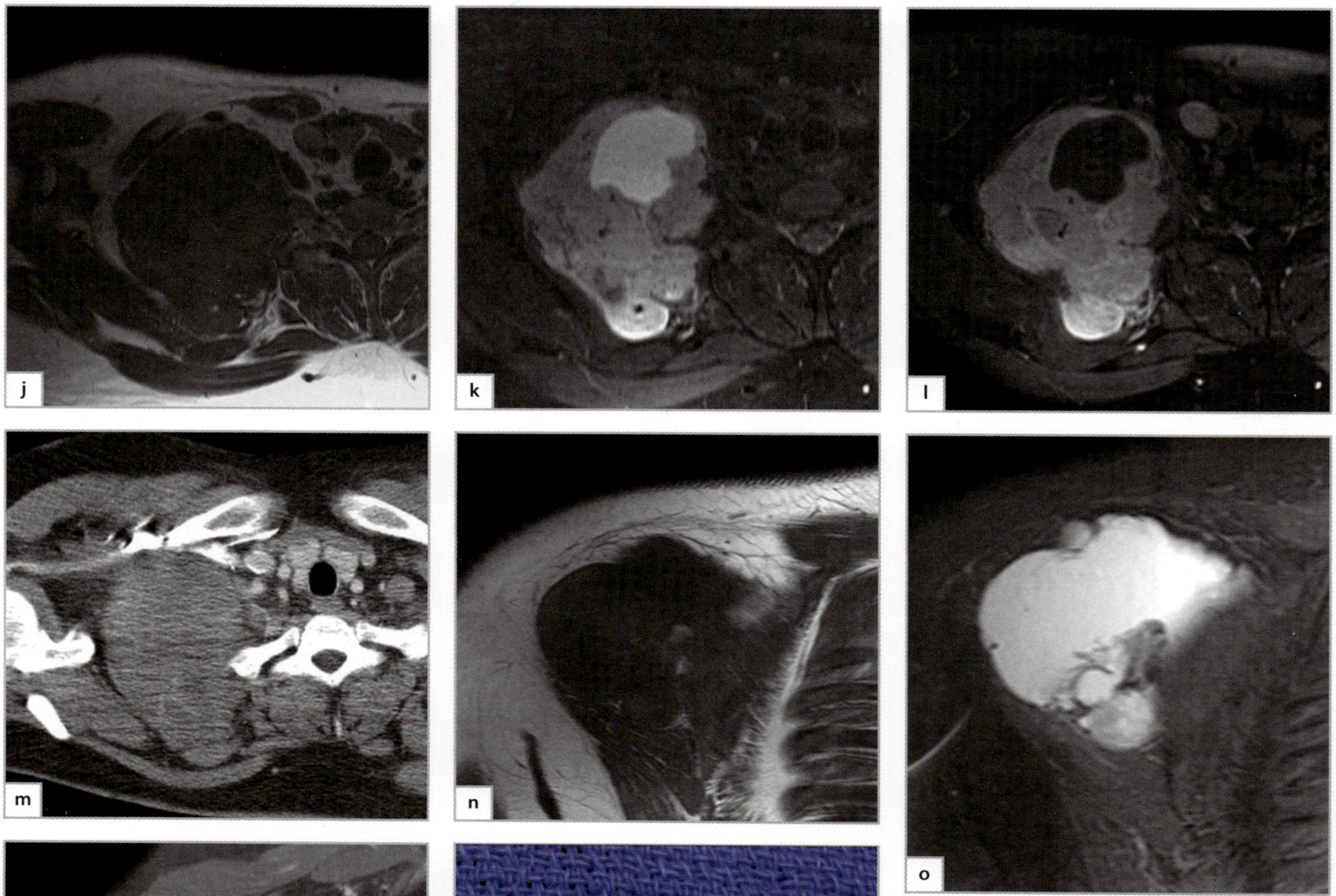

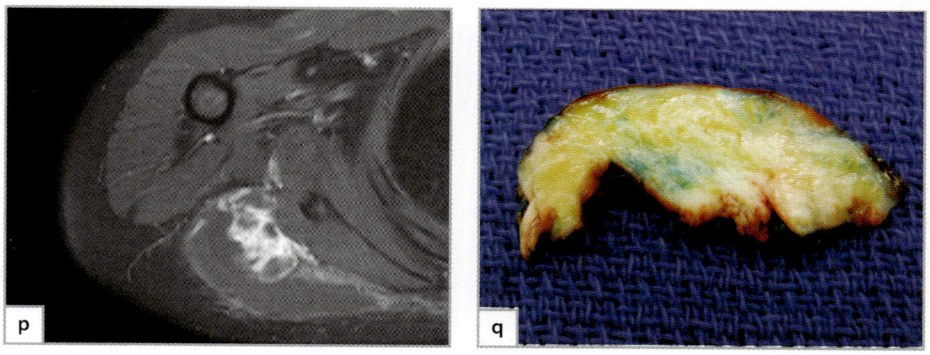

14.5j: Axial T1, **14.5k**: Axial STIR, **14.5l**: Axial T1 fat saturated post-contrast . There is an 11 × 12.1 × 8.6 cm mass with T1 isointensity to muscle and STIR heterogeneous high signal. There is intense enhancement with a large cystic or necrotic portion. There are low signal intensity thin branching structures likely from feeding vessels. CT scan axial image, **14.5m**: Ahows mild heterogeneous density without calcifications. The second additional case of synovial sarcoma is presented on images figues 14.5n through 14.5p involving the shoulder in this 18 year old woman. MR images include; **14.5n**: Coronal T1, **14.5o**: Coronal STIR, **14.5p**: Axial T1 fat saturated post-contrast. There is a 8.9 × 10.2 × 10.6 cm mass with T1 heterogeneous isointensity and STIR high signal. Post-contrast images show much of the tumor is cystic or necrotic with a nodular solid portion along the inferior aspect. The nodular portion shows some T1 high signal pre-contrast which could be from hemorrhage or proteinaceous material. **14.5q**: Synovial sarcoma (SS) 350 gross photo of cross section of tumor. The tumor is firm, pale yellow, with fibrous striations. It is gritty on sectioning consistent with small calcifications. Although not specific, the features of a large, deep firm, gritty tumor are suggestive of synovial sarcoma which commonly is calcified.

Case figure 14.5: Continued from page 320

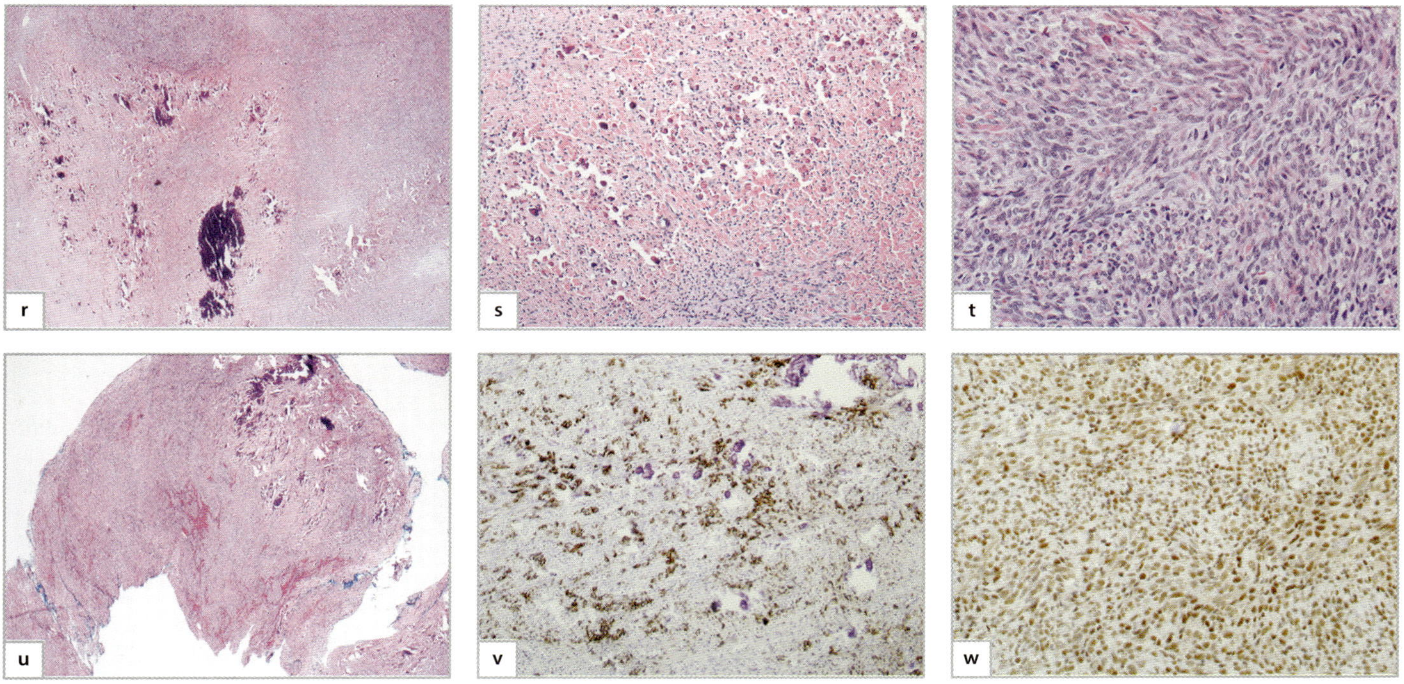

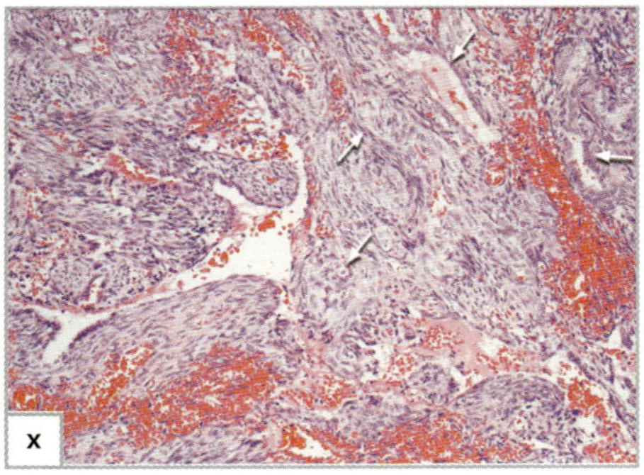

14.5r: Low magnification. The tumor contains scattered calcifications and is variably fibrotic consistent with the gross impression. **14.5s**: Medium magnification. The range of calcifications includes small round, evenly dispersed nodules resembling cementum bodies. In this patient's tumor, they are particularly prominent in collagenized areas. **14.5t**: High magnification. The most typical histology of synovial sarcoma comprises short fascicles of crowded, plump, uniform spindle cells with indistinct cell borders as seen in this field. Mitotic figures are uncommon. **14.5u**: Re-excision specimen low magnification. Residual tumor is present histologically identical to the original marginal excision. It is present in small amounts in the deep portion of the re-excision. **14.5v**: Medium magnification, keratins AE1/AE3 IHC stain. Although no overt epithelial differentiation is present on standard staining, 15% of tumor cells express these keratins (brown chromagen). **14.5w**: Higher magnification, TLE1 IHC stain. Nearly all tumor nuclei strongly express this antigen which is highly sensitive and fairly specific for synovial sarcoma. **14.5x**: Another case: biphasic synovial sarcoma, medium magnification. Arrows point to the epithelial component which forms nests and tubules. Intraluminal mucin is present (which can be highlighted with mucicarmine, Alcian blue or PAS/D stains). The other component consists of crowded, uniform plump spindle cells that flow around the epithelial foci.

Pathologic differential or, why isn't it one of the following?

Malignant peripheral nerve sheath tumor (MPNST): In many aspects, MPNST may closely resemble synovial sarcoma. Both may consist of cellular blue fascicles of plump spindle cells with a relatively low mitotic rate and uniform nuclear features. Both may also be biphasic (although this is more common in SS) with glands or tubules strewn amidst fascicles of plump spindle cells. Calcifications are more common in SS. MPNST may exhibit a striped appearance at low magnification, with alternating hypocellular and hypercellular bands. It may also demonstrate hypercellularity around vessels and undermining of vessel walls by tumor cells.

Similarities continues at the level of immunohistochemistry. Both tumors may express S-100 protein in a patchy manner (up to ~35% of SS and 50% of MPNST). Rare SS express GFAP or neurofilaments, and so does MPNST. A few MPNST express TLE1 in a nuclear pattern as ~95% of SS do. Keratins may be expressed in both tumors, although SS can express keratins 7 and 19 which MPNST does not. However, MPNST does not express EMA which is present in ~95% of monophasic, biphasic and poorly differentiated variants of SS. The majority of SS diffusely express Bcl-2 while only 30% of MPNST express it and usually in a patchy distribution (Fisher et al. 2011).

Genetic testing is diagnostically very useful. More than 90% of SS contain the translocation t(X;18) which is absent in MPNST.

Adult type fibrosarcoma (FS): This is a diagnosis of exclusion. It consists of long fascicles and herringbone arrangements of more elongate spindle cells than are seen in typical SS. It does not express keratins, EMA, or TLE1.

FS does not have a characteristic genetic signature, but it lacks t(X;18).

Fibrosarcomatous transformation of dermatofibrosarcoma protuberans (FS-DFSP): Lower grade areas of tumor may also be present. It lacks an epithelial component. It is often patchily positive for CD34, and does not express keratins, EMA, or TLE1. Genetically, it features a t(17;22)(q21;q13) = COL1A1-PDGFB translocation rather than the t(X;18) of SS (rare SS contain an alternate t(X;20)).

Synovial sarcoma, poorly differentiated variant (PDSS): This variant contains more mitoses and necrosis than classic monophasic or biphasic SS. It may consist entirely of small round blue cells and thus mimic Ewing sarcoma family of tumors. Uncommonly, PDSS consists of highly mitotically active spindle cells or large round epithelioid cells. Genetic testing is highly recommended to detect the t(X;18).

Leiomyosarcoma (LMS): LMS does not usually enter the differential of SS, because the tumor cells are more eosinophilic with blunt ended or cigar shaped nuclei. Furthermore, LMS cells express muscle markers including SMA, MSA, desmin, and caldesmon (less than 10% of SS express SMA or desmin).

Solitary fibrous tumor (SFT): SFT may have calcifications, may have areas of fascicular spindle cell architecture, and often exhibits an hemangiopericytomatous pattern of vasculature (ectatic angulated vessels resembling antler or stag horns). SFT often expresses bcl2 and CD99 as does SS. However, keratins, EMA, and TLE1 are rarely expressed in SFT, and the jumbled mix of hypocellular and cellular areas typical of SFT are less common in SS. Most SFT express CD34 which is rarely seen in SS. Finding t(X;18) excludes SFT and confirms SS.

Ectopic hamartomatous thymoma (enters the differential of biphasic SS): This is a rare benign tumor confined to the base of the neck in adult men. It consists of epithelial and spindle cells. Keratins and EMA are expressed as in SS, but also SMA and CD34 (only rarely in SS). TLE1 has not been reported to be expressed in this tumor. Genetic testing is highly recommended in difficult cases.

Sarcomatoid carcinoma (enters the differential of biphasic SS): This tumor is more common than biphasic SS when the patient is older and the location is the head and neck. Both tumors can contain fascicles of spindled cells and epithelial nests and tubules. Sarcomatoid carcinoma usually exhibits a higher mitotic rate, more pleomorphism, and necrosis. Both tumors express keratins and EMA. However, TLE1 is rare in sarcomatoid carcinoma. Genetic testing is highly recommended in difficult cases.

Sarcomatoid mesothelioma or biphasic mesothelioma: These enter the differential when SS occurs in the pleura or peritoneum. The tumors may appear similar histologically. Both tumors express keratins and EMA. TLE1 may also be expressed in both. Calretinin IHC is not discriminatory. Genetic testing may be required.

Case table 14.5a Variant pathology features of SS

Feature	Frequency	Comments
Hypercellular fascicles of plump spindle cells that look blue at low magnification due to cell crowding and scant cytoplasm	Common	This is the most common histologic pattern of synovial sarcoma. It is often present at least focally
Monophasic spindle cell synovial sarcoma	Common	Outnumbers biphasic SS by at least 3-4 to 1. Lacks widespread nuclear atypia, high mitotic rate, or prominent necrosis
Biphasic synovial sarcoma	Uncommon	Consists of typical short, plump spindle cells arranged in fascicles plus nests and tubules or glands of epithelial cells. Intraluminal secretions often present and positive on PAS/D, mucicarmine, and Alcian blue stains. Reticulin stain surrounds small nests of cells unlike in many sarcomas Rarely may have squamous metaplasia, papillary architecture, or intracytoplasmic mucin vacuoles in epithelial cells
Poorly differentiated synovial sarcoma (PDSS)	Uncommon	Must comprise the bulk of the tumor to be considered PDSS. Characterized by increased mitotic activity and necrosis Three cellular variants: most common is small round blue cell PDSS which looks like Ewing sarcoma family of tumors, large epithelioid cell type which can resemble metastatic carcinoma, and elongate spindle cell type which can be mistaken for adult type fibrosarcoma. Associated with worse prognosis in multiple studies May have a distinctive gene expression profile compared with typical synovial sarcoma. Rare additional features include myxoid stroma, nodules of tumor set in desmoplastic stroma like desmoplastic small round cell tumor, and strands of small epithelioid cells in a myxoid matrix mimicking extraskeletal myxoid chondrosarcoma
Hemangiopericytomatous vessels	Common	Sharply angulated, ectatic, antler-horn like medium sized vessels
Tigroid striping at low magnification due to nuclear palisading of tumor cells	Uncommon	This striped pattern may be seen most commonly in benign and malignant peripheral nerve sheath tumor but also occurs in benign and malignant smooth muscle tumors
Microcalcifications	Common	Present in ~35% of SS May be extensive ('calcifying variant'), cementum-like, or dystrophic
Ossification	Uncommon	Rarely, ossification may be massive: these tumors may have a better prognosis than typical SS Ossification comprises osteoid or woven (immature) bone
Myxoid stroma	Uncommon	May be reticulated or microcystic and mimic a myoepithelial tumor Myxoid stroma may be very extensive, but usually there are foci of typical spindle cell SS also present
Heavily hyalinized or collagenized stroma	Uncommon	Fibrotic stroma is fairly common as a focal finding Diffuse sclerosis can mimic sclerosing epithelioid fibrosarcoma
Tumor cells with eosinophilic granular cytoplasm	Uncommon	Rarely, these cells may predominate May show reactivity for α-inhibin and synaptophysin

Case table 14.5: Continued from page 322

Feature	Frequency	Comments
Markedly pleomorphic tumor cells with hyperlobation or multiple nuclei, hyperchromasia, and macronucleoli	Rare	Focal only
Epithelioid cells only: 'monophasic epithelioid SS'	Extremely rare	May not exist
Rhabdoid cells	Extremely rare	Focal only
Immunohistochemical reactivity: EMA (90%), keratins (90%), TLE1 (95%), Bcl-2 (95%)	Common	Other proposed commonly expressed antibodies include CD56 (80%) and NY-ESO-1 (75%). Percent reactivity may vary slightly across institutions due to differing fixation and staining conditions
Immunohistochemical reactivity: S-100 protein (40%), calretinin (40%), β-catenin (40%, nuclear), FLI-1 (20%)	Uncommon	May introduce other entities in the differential such as MPNST, Ewing sarcoma family of tumors, sarcomatoid carcinoma, mesothelioma
Immunohistochemical reactivity: CD34 (5%)	Rare	CD34, if present, is usually focal. Positivity for CD34 should prompt consideration of another diagnosis such as solitary fibrous tumor, epithelioid sarcoma, GIST
t(X;18)(p11;q11) = *SS18 (SYT)*-SSX translocation	Common	These translocations of *SSX1*, *SSX2*, or rarely *SSX4* and *SS18* are found in >90% of SS and are tumor specific. May be considered definitional of SS *SSX2* gene is rarely rearranged in biphasic SS
t(X;20)(p11;q13) = *SS18L1-SSX1*	Rare	This is a rare variant translocation reported only in SS

Case table 14.5b Summary pathology findings of Case 14.5

Diagnosis	Synovial sarcoma, monophasic spindle cell type
Size	4.5 × 3.9 × 1.9 cm
Location	Deep soft tissue of shoulder
Margin status	Most likely focally positive after re-excision
Histologic grade (FNCLCC grading system)	High grade = 3
Pathologic stage (AJCC TNM classification)	T1b/N0/M0 = Stage IIA (high grade, deep tumor <5cm)

FNCLCC: Fédération Nationale des Centres de Lutte Contre le Cancer (French Federation of Cancer Centers). AJCC: American Joint Committee on Cancer

Case table 14.5a lists variant pathology features reported for synovial sarcoma.

Oncology approach

Medical oncology

The patient is seen in medical oncology consultation, where the risk of metastatic disease is estimated below 15%. Therefore chemotherapy, which has not been shown to impact survival, is not indicated. Because the margin is positive, a wide resection with postoperative radiation is recommended to decrease the risk of local recurrence. Eighteen months later, the patient has no evidence of local recurrence or metastatic disease.

For patients with localized disease, local control with surgery and radiotherapy is excellent (Guadagnolo, et al. 2007). Primary tumor size, margin of resection, and mean mitotic activity are the main prognostic factors for survival (Brennan, et al. 2010, Guillou, et al. 2004, Lewis, et al. 2000, Palmerini, et al. 2009, Shi, et al. 2012, Spurrell, et al. 2005). Favorable prognosis is seen in tumors smaller than 5cm, with negative margins, low grade, and mean mitotic rate below 10 mitoses per 10 hpf. In patients with unfavorable factors, neoadjuvant chemotherapy yields a high objective response rate, but its effect on survival is not clear (Canter, et al. 2008, Italiano, et al. 2009, Singer, et al. 1996). Randomized studies to clarify the role of chemotherapy are lacking.

Radiation oncology

The patient eventually undergoes wide resection for high grade synovial sarcoma. Post operative radiation therapy is indicated despite negative margins due to the high risk of local recurrence. The patient tolerates radiation therapy well.

Patient outcome

Two years postoperatively, the patient has no evidence of local recurrence or metastatic disease. He has near normal shoulder function. In addition to the favorable prognostic factors of small tumor size and low stage at presentation, the tumor is diffusely calcified. Such synovial sarcomas may behave less aggressively than non-calcified examples.

Case 14.6 Epithelioid sarcoma, proximal type

Clinical history and presentation

The patient is a 35 year old man who presents with a tender mass in the left groin/hip area. Five years previously, he sustained a hamstring muscle pull while engaged in Tai Kwan Do. His symptoms resolved spontaneously but three years ago, he noticed a mass in the same area as his injury. The mass has grown. It is tender to palpation and painful with activity.

Surgical findings and comments

Physical examination reveals a large, firm, deeply situated mass in the medial aspect of the left hip/groin area that is firmly fixed to underlying deep tissue. It is mildly tender. He has full and painless range of motion of the hip.

Open biopsy is performed, and abundant viable tumor is submitted fresh for Pathology evaluation. Upon diagnosis of epithelioid sarcoma, the patient undergoes two rounds of neoadjuvant chemotherapy. Thereafter, wide resection of the subcutaneous tumor is performed widely ellipsing the previous biopsy tract.

Radiology findings

Case figs 14.6a through **14.6d** shows a nonspecific, aggressive appearing mass of the subcutaneous tissues of the inner thigh, perineal region. Epithelioid sarcomas of this location are considered a proximal subtype and may have a worse prognosis. Regional adenopathy is seen in 63% of cases, but only a single borderline lymph node is present in the left inguinal region of this patient. Multilobulated morphology is described in 88% which is demonstrated best on coronal STIR images, **Case fig. 14.6b**, however, this is not specific to epithelioid sarcoma and is seen in many aggressive tumors.

Case figs 14.6e through **14.6i** is a case of conventional subtype epithelioid sarcoma, showing a nonspecific aggressive tumor of the axilla in a 58 year old woman. The tumor surrounds the subclavian artery and displaces the subclavian vein posteriorly. Although the brachial plexus nerves are not specifically identified with this exam, (due to motion and the large field of view employed) the location of the tumor splaying the subclavian vessels indicates high likelihood of nerve involvement. Indeed, clinically the patient had progressive

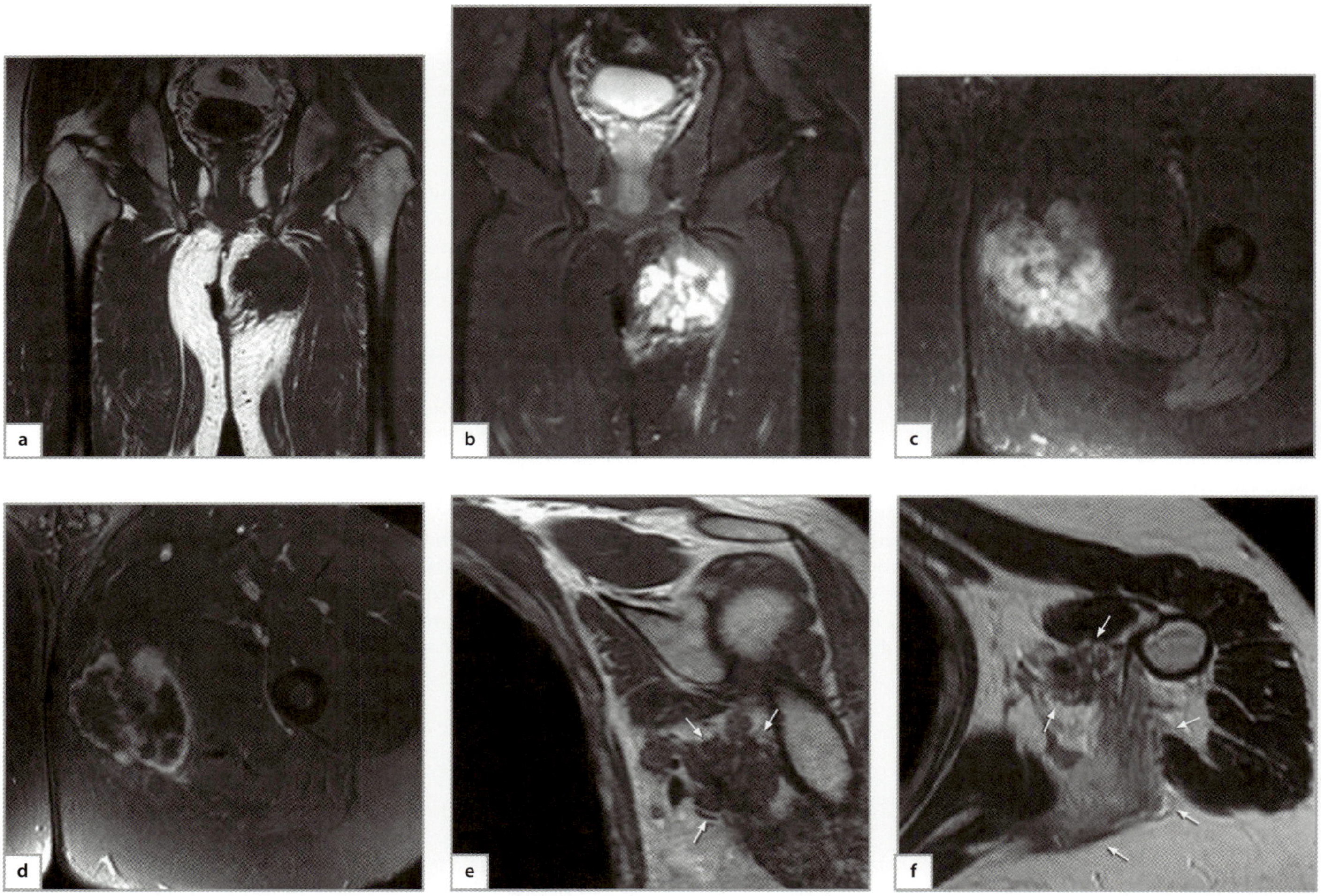

Case figure 14.6 Epithelioid sarcoma. MR images. **14.6a**: Coronal T1, **14.6b**: Coronal STIR, **14.6c**: Axial STIR and **14.6d**: Axial T1 fat saturated post-contrast of this 35 year old man. The subcutaneous perineal mass measures 6.7 × 6.3 × 6.7 cm and is predominantly T1 iso-intense to muscle and shows heterogeneous STIR high signal. The mass has intense irregular rim enhancement. The margins appear shaggy and infiltrative. The appearance is nonspecific but indicates an aggressive lesion warranting tissue diagnosis. This location is considered a proximal subtype Epithelioid Sarcoma. There was a single borderline enlarged left inguinal lymph node (images not included). MR images of this conventional type epithelioid sarcoma include. **14.6e**: Coronal T1, **14.6f**: Axial T2.

Case figure 14.6: Continued from page 324

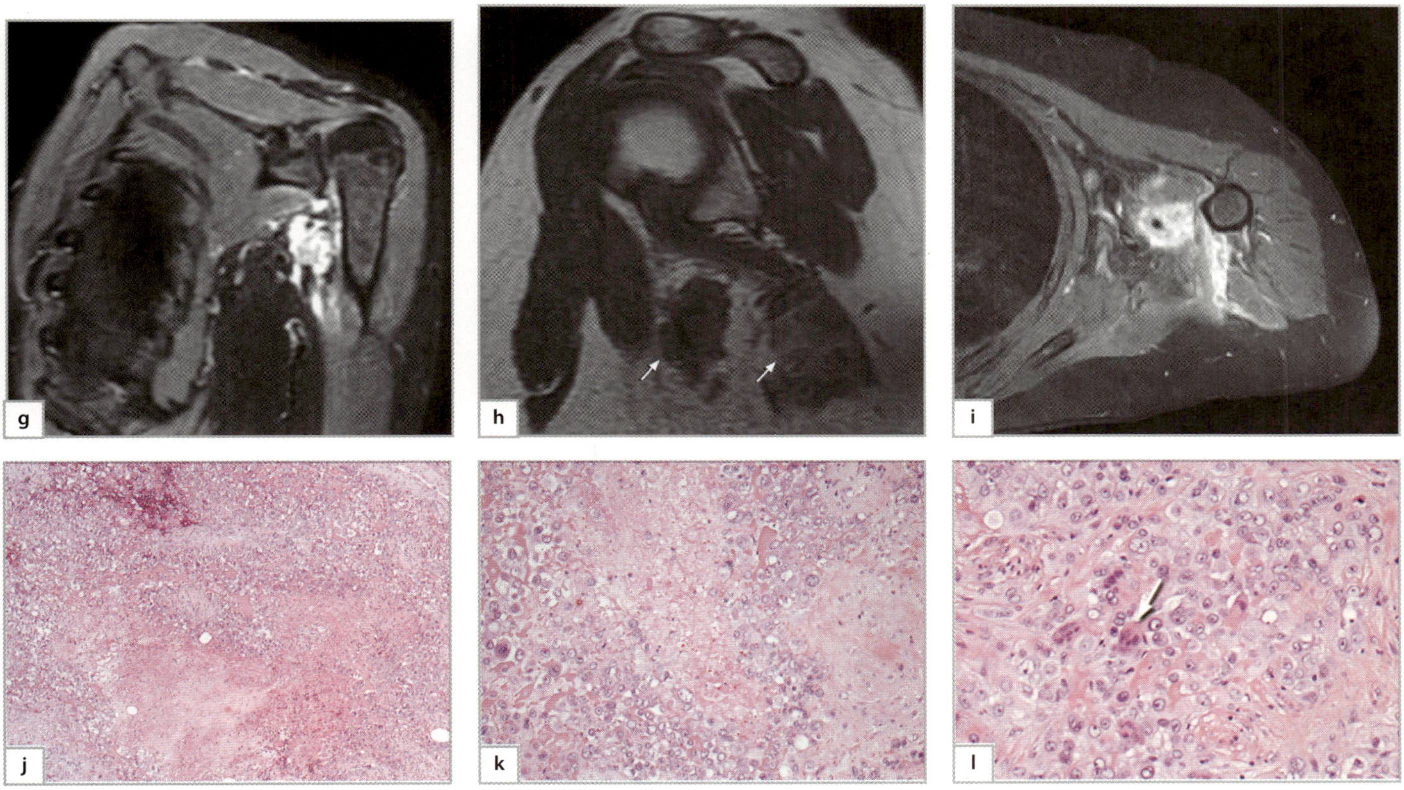

14.6g: Coronal STIR, **14.6h**: Sagittal T1 and **14.6i** axial T1 fat saturated post-contrast. There is a 3.7 × 2.9 × 2.5 cm irregular mass of the left axilla in this 58 year old woman, small arrows in 14.6e, 14.6f and 14.6h. The tumor is T1 isosignal and T2 mildly hyperintense with high signal on STIR and intense enhancement. There is fatty atrophy of the teres major muscle, large arrows in 14.6f and 14.6h. The tumor surrounds the subclavian artery without causing appreciable vessel narrowing. The subclavian vein is displaced posteriorly by the tumor. **14.6j**: Low magnification. The tumor consists of multiple centrally necrotic nodules, one of which is presented in this field. **14.6k**: Medium magnification. The central necrotic foci are abruptly delimited by pale epithelioid tumor cells. The background matrix in viable areas is fibrotic or cast-like hyaline material. **14.6l**: Medium magnification. A minority of tumor cells exhibit a spindled shape. Multinucleate, osteoclast-like giant cells (arrow) are interspersed among the tumor cells. Blood vessels are relatively inconspicuous and vary in caliber.

neurologic deficit and there is fatty atrophy of the teres major muscle shown on the MR exam. The intimate circumferential tumor contact of the subclavian artery lends high suspicion that the vessel is involved with tumor. The patient also had enlarged axillary lymph nodes on the MR exam, images not included.

Pathology findings

Gross features

The biopsy comprises multiple portions of gray to pale yellow rubbery soft tissue aggregating to 3 × 2.5 × 0.6 cm. A portion is submitted fresh to Cytogenetics.

The resection consists of a 13.5 cm × 9.5 × 8.5 cm ovoid portion of soft tissue with attached ellipse of skin. It is received oriented and is differentially inked. Serial sectioning reveals a 13.5 × 9 × 8 cm heterogeneous pink to tan tumor with areas of hemorrhage and a mucoid central area consistent with prior biopsy site. Multiple sections are taken for margin assessment and tumor histology. Additional material is submitted fresh for karyotyping.

Microscopic features

Low magnification: The tumor is multinodular with most nodules featuring large, central areas of geographic necrosis (**Case fig. 14.6j**).

High magnification: Medium magnification reveals abrupt tumor necrosis and pale eosinophilic, round tumor cells embedded in a hyalinized or fibrous matrix (**Case fig. 14.6k**). A few tumor cells are spindled (less than 10%), and some areas contain scattered multinucleated osteoclast-like giant cells (**Case fig. 14.6l**). There is moderate variation in nuclear size and shape, and a pasty matrix is focally prominent (**Case fig. 14.6m**). Characteristically, tumor nuclei are pale or vesicular with moderately sized nucleoli (**Case fig. 14.6n**). The mitotic rate averages 12 mitoses/10hpf with atypical forms. Rhabdoid cells, often a hallmark of proximal type ES, are absent. Margins are negative with the closest at 0.8 cm (posterior).

Special studies: Tumor cells express the following antigens: EMA, low molecular weight keratin (both diffusely positive)(**Case figs 14.6o** and 14-6p), vimentin, CD99, and CD56 (diffusely positive) with a few cells reactive for bcl-2, S-100 protein, MelanA103 antigen, inhibin, and NSE. Tumor cells do not express smooth muscle actin, desmin, myogenin, CD34, CD31, or HMB45 (all controls are appropriately reactive). INI-1 nuclear expression is lost in tumor cells. This immunoprofile is overall consistent with epithelioid sarcoma with characteristic vimentin, EMA and keratin reactivity and loss of INI-1 nuclear expression. CD34 is absent in ~50% of cases. Some proximal type ES express desmin, and

Case figure 14.6: Continued from page 325

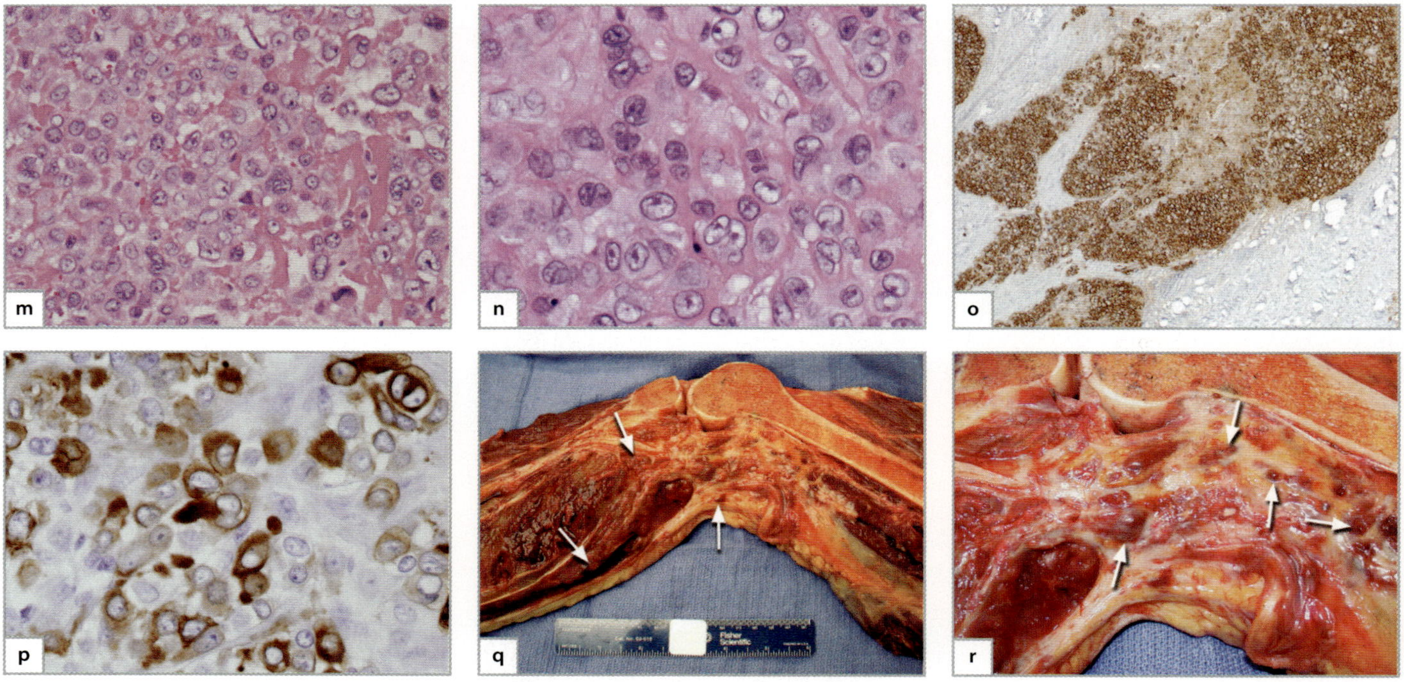

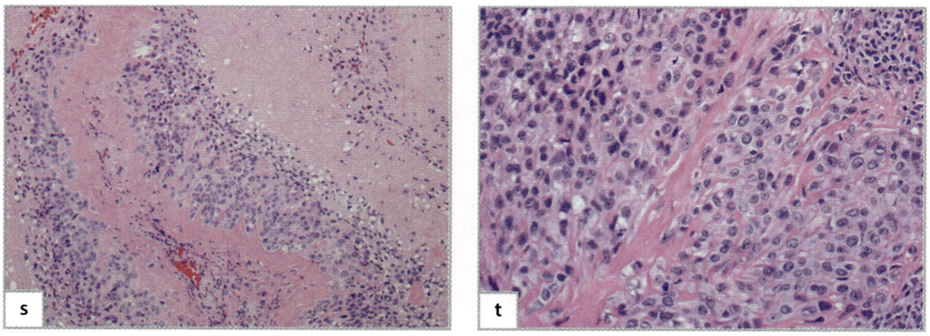

14.6m: Epithelioid sarcoma, proximal type, medium magnification. Moderate nuclear pleomorphism is evident with a 3x range in size, with multilobation and odd shapes. The background matrix is pasty and focally prominent. **14.6n**: High magnification. For a high grade tumor, the nuclei are remarkably pale or vesicular. Some cells have moderately enlarged single nucleoli. **14.6o**: Low magnification, EMA IHC stain. Tumor cells are strongly reactive for epithelial membrane antigen (the central necrotic cells less so; brown chromagen). About 95% of ES diffusely express EMA. **14.6p**: High magnification, keratins AE1/AE3 IHC stain. Tumor cells express mixed keratins with varying intensity. Most ES express keratins (~95%). **14.6q**: Gross photo of tumor. This patient's tumor shows the in transit pattern of tumor growth that occurs in some cases of classic ES. Multiple nodules advance proximally from the patient's initial distal posterior calf primary tumor (arrows point to several of these nodules). **14.6r**: Closer view of tumor nodules. The nodules are raised, numerous and appear dark red (arrows point to several). **14.6s**: Medium magnification. Tumor cells comprising classic or conventional ES form nests with central necrosis that can mimic granulomas on low magnification. **14.6t**: High magnification. The tumor cells are more uniform with less mitotic activity than in proximal type ES. Both tumors may contain spindled tumor cells, especially at the edges of nodules. (Spindled tumor cells are not present in this field).

SMA may be present in ~15% of cases, especially in spindled tumor cells. The reactivity for A103, S-100 protein, and inhibin is unusual, but reactivity is focal.

The biopsy karyotype is insufficient, as less than 20 cells are cultured. The resection karyotype is as follows: 46,XY,t(10;22)(p12;q13)[4]/46,XY[13]. Three non-clonal translocations comprise: t(2;6)(q32;p21)[1], t(7;11)(p22;q21)[1] and t(6;21;10;12)(q11;q13;q22;q22)[1]. Proximal type ES may show -22, deletion or translocation of 22q11.2 (*INI-1* gene). This patient's clonal translocation may encompass the 22q11.2 region. Proximal type ES has been reported to show t(10;22) in two cases (Lualdi et al. 2004).

Reverse transcriptase PCR results are negative for the fusion transcript characteristic of synovial sarcoma.

Conventional (classic) epithelioid sarcoma: For comparison, a classic type ES is also presented. Classic type ES may show 'in transit' metastases similar to some melanomas, in that the tumor creeps proximally as multiple nodules before spreading to lymph nodes or more distant sites. This proximal spread often occurs along tendons or aponeuroses and may be found on initial presentation, as some patients are undiagnosed for years. This patient, a young adult man, presented with both in transit metastases and inguinal adenopathy after suffering for four years with a non-healing distal leg ulcer (the primary tumor) (**Case figs 14.6q** and **14.6r**).

Microscopic review of the primary site tumor reveals nodules with central necrosis mimicking necrobiotic granulomas at low magnification (**Case fig. 14.6s**). High magnification reveals cells with more uniform nuclei than seen in proximal type ES (**Case fig. 14.6t**).

Pathologic differential or, why isn't it one of the following?

Synovial sarcoma: The only SS that could resemble this patient's tumor is the rare, poorly differentiated SS with large epithelioid cells and prominent necrosis (PDSS). Patient age and location of the tumor would fit well with PDSS, and the immunoreactivity for vimentin, keratin, and EMA would be consistent with the diagnosis, also. However, PDSS features diffuse rather than focal Bcl-2 reactivity, and genetically would contain the diagnostic translocation t(X;18) (or, more rarely, t(X;20)).

Classic epithelioid sarcoma: The patient's tumor contains larger, more pleomorphic tumor cells than are seen in classic ES. Both proximal type ES and classic ES may occur at limb girdles, so the site does not automatically clinch the diagnosis of proximal rather than classic type. Many classic ES are superficial rather than deep, however. The immunohistochemical profile is the same for proximal and classic ES. A translocation of chromosomes 22 and 10 has only been described thus far in proximal type ES.

Other sarcomas with epithelioid morphology: Quite a few sarcomas may have epithelioid variants including malignant peripheral nerve sheath tumor (which may show loss of INI1 expression but is usually only focally EMA or keratins reactive and usually CD34 negative), leiomyosarcoma (which expresses muscle markers and retains INI-1), myxofibrosarcoma (older patient population, retains INI1, lacks EMA and keratin reactivity), and liposarcoma (retains INI-1, MDM2 and CDK4 positive in most cases, ring and marker chromosomes on karyotyping).

Myoepithelial carcinoma (MEC): This tumor is rarer than proximal type ES. In contrast to proximal type ES, MEC is usually histologically heterogeneous with reticulated, solid, fibrotic, and chondromyxoid areas. It may contain ductal structures and metaplastic bone or cartilage. Tumor cells may be spindled, epithelioid, plasmacytoid, small round blue cell shaped or a mixture of these. The range of nuclear pleomorphism is usually more pronounced than in proximal ES. Tumor cells also express markers of myoepithelial differentiation such as S-100 protein, GFAP, calponin, and SMA all of which are rare to uncommon in proximal ES. Rare myoepithelial carcinomas exhibit loss of INI-1 expression (10% of adult cases and 40% of pediatric cases; Hollmann et al. 2011). In contrast to ES, at least 40% of MEC disclose one of several specific translocations most of which involve the *EWSR1* gene.

Metastatic melanoma: Since melanoma may assume many different morphologies, including a pure epithelioid cell morphology, it enters the differential of proximal type ES. Melanin pigment has not been described in ES and may be found in ~30% of metastatic melanomas. Some epithelioid melanomas feature cells with macronucleoli ('cherry red nucleoli') and prominent multinucleate tumor giant cells. By IHC, only rare melanomas express keratins and EMA. A majority will express S-100 protein, HMB45, or MelanA103, although a distressing minority lacks any melanocytic antigenicity. These last non-expressing tumors, however, do not lose INI1 expression (lost in 95% of ES). Genetically, many melanomas exhibit BRAF or c-kit mutations.

Case table 14.6a lists variant pathology features reported for epithelioid sarcoma.

Oncology approach

Medical oncology

This patient was treated with 2 cycles of doxorubicin and ifosfamide prior to be referred to surgery. It might have been prudent to perform a sentinel lymph node dissection to rule out lymph node invasion given the MRI findings. The value of sentinel lymph node dissection

Case table 14.6a Variant pathology features of ES

Feature	Frequency	Comments
Nodules comprising central necrosis rimmed by viable epithelioid tumor cells mimicking necrobiotic granulomas at low magnification	Common	This is the typical appearance of classic ES Proximal ES, however, may grow in sheets with more haphazard necrosis Similarity to non-neoplastic granulomas also occurs clinically, as the tumors may present as non-healing, targetoid skin ulcers with raised, 'sealing wax' margins suggestive of granuloma annulare
Spindled tumor cells located primarily at the edges of tumor nodules	Common	Although in classic and proximal ES, the predominant component is epithelioid tumor cells, spindled tumor cells are also present (less commonly in proximal ES). The spindled cells can express SMA (~20% of ES cases have SMA expression)
Proximal type ES: Increased cell size with pleomorphic nuclei and increased mitotic figures	Uncommon	Proximal type ES usually is deep and occurs at limb girdles, but it can also occur in the head and neck and in the distal extremities Rhabdoid tumor cells are common (small round cells with glassy eosinophilic cytoplasmic inclusions that push the nucleus to the side)
Mixed classic and proximal type ES	Uncommon	Consists of areas of lower grade classic ES and high grade proximal ES
Fibroma-like variant of ES	Rare	Sclerotic stroma in which spindled tumor cells form storiform patterns Minimal cytologic atypia Recurrences of classic ES may take on this appearance
Angiomatoid or angiosarcoma-like variant of ES	Rare	Tumor cell line anastomosing spaces that simulate blood vessels. Hemorrhage and intraluminal red blood cells are also present. Some tumor cells may contain cytoplasmic vacuoles like the true endothelial tumor cells of epithelioid hemangioendothelioma. Tumor cells are mixed epithelioid and spindled
Extensive myxoid stroma	Rare	May lack necrsosis and instead feature central areas of fibrosis May contain foci of classic ES
Osteoid or calcifications	Uncommon	Can occur in classic ES and fibroma-like variant of ES Osteoid, woven bone or woven bone with focal lamellar maturation may occur
Multinucleated osteoclast-like giant cells	Uncommon	Can occur in classic and proximal type ES
Tumor cells with cytoplasmic vacuoles	Rare	May be seen in classic ES or angiomatoid ES Vacuoles may be due to lipid May mimic mucinous carcinoma or epithelioid hemangioendoethelioma tumor cells

Case table 14.6a: Continued from page 327

Feature	Frequency	Comments
Plasmacytoid tumor cells	Rare	May mimic plasmacytoid cells of myoepithelial carcinoma or myoepithelioma
Intra-articular or intra-osseous location	Rare	Intra-articular cases (n = 2) consisted of mixed classic and proximal type ES Fibroma-like variant may be most likely type to arise in bone
IHC: Vimentin (100%), pan keratins (95%), EMA (95%), keratin 8 (90%), keratin 14 (50%), CD34 (50%), Cyclin D1 (95%), INI1 loss of expression (95%)	Common	This is the typical IHC profile of ES including all variants
IHC: Keratins 5/6 (20%), SMA (20%), keratin 7 (20%)	Uncommon	Expression is usually focal (restricted primarily to spindled tumor cells for SMA)
IHC: CD31 (1%), HMB45 or A103 (1%?), S-100 protein (?3%) desmin (5%?)	Rare	Expression of these antigens is focal
Genetics: 22q deletions or translocations	Common	Involves INI1 (SMARCB1, hSNF5) gene

Case table 14.6b Summary pathology findings of Case 14.6

Diagnosis	ES, proximal type
Size	13.5 × 9 × 8 cm
Location	Deep soft tissue of proximal thigh/hip
Margin status	Negative (closest is posterior margin at 0.8 cm from tumor edge)
Histologic grade (FNCLCC grading system)	High grade
Pathologic stage (AJCC TNM classification)	T2b/N0/M0 = Stage III (high grade deep tumor > 5 cm)

FNCLCC: Fédération Nationale des Centres de Lutte Contre le Cancer (French Federation of Cancer Centers). AJCC: American Joint Committee on Cancer

is not proven for epithelioid sarcoma. If a node had been invaded, consideration of adjuvant chemotherapy would have been discussed more aggressively. Because the tumor did not shrink with neoadjuvant chemotherapy, additional adjuvant chemotherapy was not administered. Instead the patient was referred to radiation oncology.

Radiation oncology

The patient receives neoadjuvant chemotherapy followed by wide resection for epithelioid sarcoma of the left thigh. Postoperative radiation therapy is recommended due to the high risk of local recurrence. The patient tolerates a full course of radiation therapy well.

Patient outcome

Thirty months postoperatively, the patient has normal function and no evidence of local recurrence or metastatic disease.

Case 14.7 Alveolar soft part sarcoma

Clinical history and presentation

A 17 year old teenaged boy presents to an outside facility with an abdominal wall mass of at least one year's duration. It is asymptomatic but slowly growing. The patient initially considered the tumor to be a bruise sustained in football.

Surgical findings and comments

Physical examination reveals a four centimeter in diameter firm mass in the rectus abdominis. Marginal excision is initially performed, followed one month later by a wide resection with negative margins.

A staging work-up is negative. The patient is diagnosed with a Stage II alveolar soft part sarcoma and chooses to resume a normal life, without surveillance. Three years later the patient returns for a follow-up and a new staging work-up is done, revealing metastatic disease in the lungs ad adrenals. The patient is asymptomatic. A biopsy of one of the adrenal masses confirms the recurrence.

Radiology findings

Our case, **Case figs 14.7a** and **14.7b** show the metastatic disease involving the adrenal gland and lungs in the patient, now 21 years old. In general, lung metastases are very common with sarcomas, however, the adrenal disease is quite unusual with sarcoma and might errantly lead a radiologist to search for a different primary. Given that 19% of patients with Stage IV ASPS have brain metastases, one might reasonably include brain imaging in the patient's imaging surveillance program. Unfortunately, no brain imaging is performed.

Pathology findings

Gross features

The resected abdominal wall tumor consists of a 4 × 3 × 2.5 cm solid but soft, pale yellow to gray mass. It grossly closely approaches resection margins. The patient's small tumor (<5 cm) is in keeping with his lack of discernable metastases at presentation. A recent Japanese review of 26 patients noted a significant correlation of tumor size with metastases at presentation (< or = 5 cm: 30% mets at presentation versus >5 cm: 80% mets at presentation)(Ogura et al. 2012).

The adrenal mass biopsy comprises multiple white needle cores that are submitted in one cassette for routine processing. Touch preps are first made, however, because the pathologist is present in Interventional Radiology to ensure adequate specimen is obtained.

Microscopic features

Low magnification: The tumor forms back to back nests of eosinophilic granular cells with sprinkles of lymphocytes (**Case fig. 14.7c**).

High magnification: Medium magnification reveals solid balls of tumor cells separated by thin fibrous septations (**Case fig. 14.7d**). Blood vessels run in the septations, and consequently the tumor is richly vascularized (a feature that may be apparent at the time of surgical resection with increased bleeding). A touch prep (cytology smear) of the tumor using a modified Papanicolaou stain reveals only mild nuclear variation with many nuclei demonstrating single prominent nucleoli (**Case fig. 14.7e**). The mitotic rate is relatively high for ASPS at 4/10 hpf, and a few nests show central necrosis. These last two features are atypical and may be associated with a more accelerated aggressive behavior. Multiple foci of vascular invasion are present (this is characteristic of ASPS).

Margins of resection are negative for tumor by at least 0.5 cm. This patient presented at age 17 years with at least a one year history of a mass. Therefore, his tumor appears more like the pediatric cases of ASPS that feature solid nests rather than nests with central dropout and dyscohesion (the classic pseudoalveolar pattern).

Special studies: A PAS/D (periodic acid-schiff with diastase) stain highlights granular cytoplasmic crystals (**Case fig. 14.7f**). These crystals are also notable on trichrome and Alcian blue stains. Immunohistochemistry is performed and reveals strong diffuse nuclear reactivity for TFE3 (**Case fig. 14.7g**). This is a highly sensitive and fairly highly specific marker for ASPS. A few cells express desmin (~10%). There is no expression of S-100 protein, smooth muscle actin, keratins, HMB45, myogenin, or keratins. Desmin and SMA may be expressed in up to 50% of ASPS, usually focally (Folpe et al. 2006).

A karyotype cannot be performed, because the original resection and biopsy specimens are submitted to Pathology in formalin. In histologically non-classic cases, genetic testing can be very helpful diagnostically by demonstrating the characteristic der(17)t(X;17)(p11;q25) = *ASPL-TFE3* translocation.

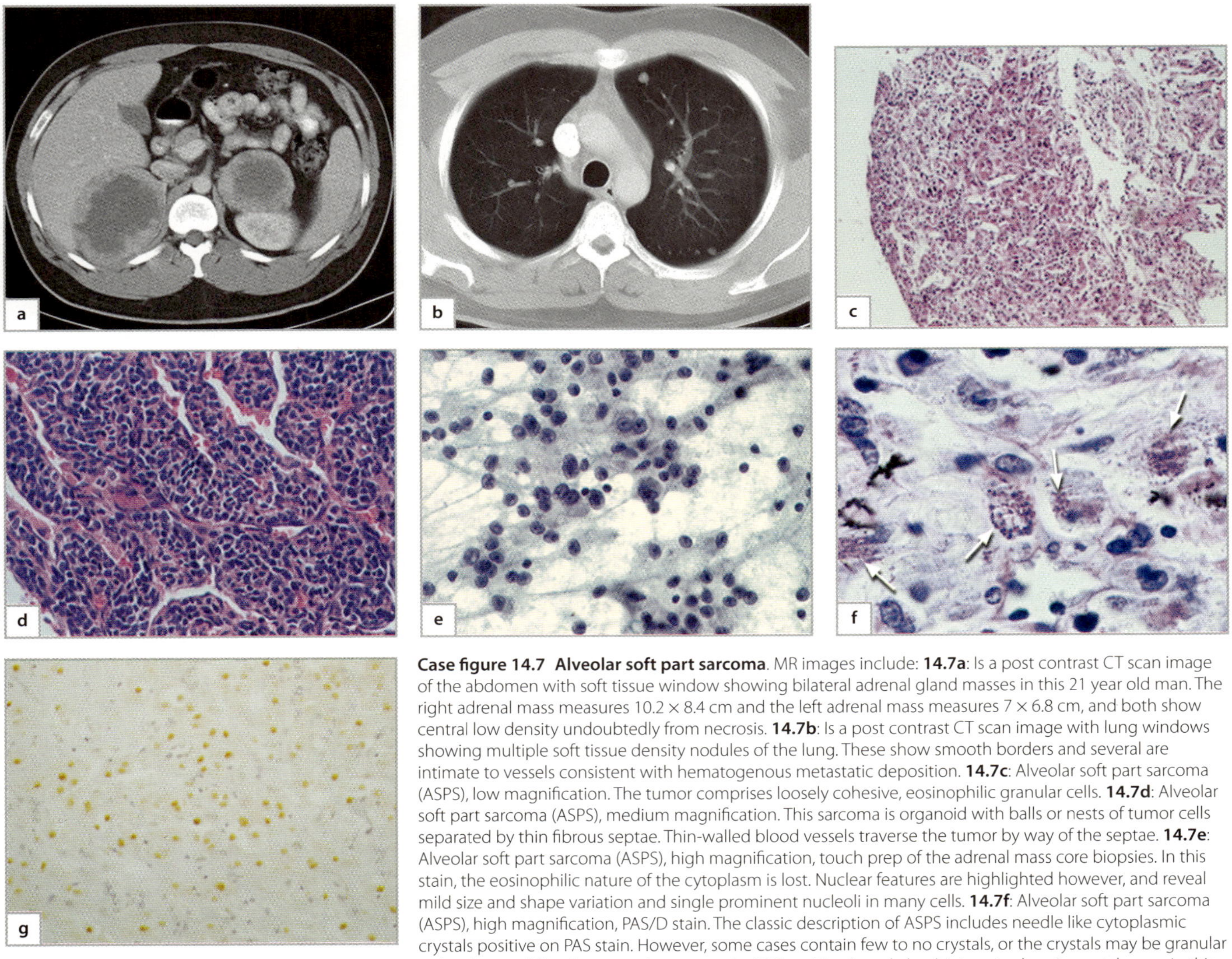

Case figure 14.7 Alveolar soft part sarcoma. MR images include: **14.7a**: Is a post contrast CT scan image of the abdomen with soft tissue window showing bilateral adrenal gland masses in this 21 year old man. The right adrenal mass measures 10.2 × 8.4 cm and the left adrenal mass measures 7 × 6.8 cm, and both show central low density undoubtedly from necrosis. **14.7b**: Is a post contrast CT scan image with lung windows showing multiple soft tissue density nodules of the lung. These show smooth borders and several are intimate to vessels consistent with hematogenous metastatic deposition. **14.7c**: Alveolar soft part sarcoma (ASPS), low magnification. The tumor comprises loosely cohesive, eosinophilic granular cells. **14.7d**: Alveolar soft part sarcoma (ASPS), medium magnification. This sarcoma is organoid with balls or nests of tumor cells separated by thin fibrous septae. Thin-walled blood vessels traverse the tumor by way of the septae. **14.7e**: Alveolar soft part sarcoma (ASPS), high magnification, touch prep of the adrenal mass core biopsies. In this stain, the eosinophilic nature of the cytoplasm is lost. Nuclear features are highlighted however, and reveal mild size and shape variation and single prominent nucleoli in many cells. **14.7f**: Alveolar soft part sarcoma (ASPS), high magnification, PAS/D stain. The classic description of ASPS includes needle like cytoplasmic crystals positive on PAS stain. However, some cases contain few to no crystals, or the crystals may be granular rather than rod-like. Arrows point to granular PAS positive (purple hue) intracytoplasmic crystals seen in this patient's tumor. **14.7g**: Alveolar soft part sarcoma (ASPS), medium magnification, TFE3 IHC stain. Tumor nuclei are diffusely positive for TFE3, an antibody that stains few other tumors and is highly sensitive for ASPS.

Pathologic differential or, why isn't it one of the following?

Paraganglioma (PG): Paraganglioma is perhaps the closest histologic mimic to ASPS especially those with solid nests, as both tumors can be described as showing a zellballen architecture. Despite the benign nature of most PG, there is usually more nuclear pleomorphism than is seen in most ASPS. Most patients are middle aged adults. Common locations including the carotid body can also be involved by ASPS. Cytoplasmic crystals are absent. By IHC, paragangliomas are chromogranin reactive and negative for TFE3, while the opposite obtains for ASPS. Paragangliomas lack the t(X;17) of ASPS.

Metastatic carcinoma such as renal cell carcinoma or hepatocellular carcinoma: The patient is young, and therefore metastatic carcinoma would be unlikely. However, a subtype of renal cell carcinoma, Xp11 translocation renal cell carcinoma, does preferentially affect children to young adults and also exhibits strong diffuse nuclear TFE3 expression. It may show a papillary pattern unlike ASPS or a nested pattern with cells containing abundant clear or eosinophilic cytoplasm similar to ASPS. Prominent nucleoli are common as with ASPS. Unlike ASPS, the tumor cells consistently express RCC antigen, CAM5.2 keratins and sometimes EMA. Genetically, Xp11 RCC may demonstrate the translocation *ASPL-TFE3* but other translocation partners include *PRCC* (1q21), *PSF* (1p34), and *NonP* (X). A renal primary tumor noted on imaging or biopsy would be diagnostically helpful, although rare ASPS may arise in visceral locations including potentially the kidney.

Granular cell tumor (GCT): GCT usually grows as round to polygonal cells in clusters, sheaves or sheets without a distinctive organoid pattern. Malignant GCT is rare and features solid growth of pleomorphic round to spindled tumor cells with necrosis and increased mitotic activity. A solid variant of ASPS could overlap histologically with malignant GCT. Unfortunately, a few GCT express nuclear TFE3. However, granular cell tumors are diffusely reactive for S-100 protein dissimilar to ASPS and do not express desmin or SMA (seen in up to 50% of ASPS).

Neuroendocrine carcinoma (NEC): Few neuroendocrine tumors exhibit the marked granular eosinophilic cytoplasm of ASPS. An organoid pattern of growth, however, is common in NEC, but pseudoalveolar central cell sloughing is not. NEC is characteristically

Case table 14.7a Variant pathology features of ASPS

Feature	Frequency	Comments
Nests of round or polygonal epithelioid cells separated by thin fibrous septae that contain thin-walled blood vessels. Nests show central sloughing of cells and dyscohesion = pseudoalveolar pattern.	Common	This is the most typical appearance of alveolar soft part sarcoma
Solid nests of cells without central sloughing.	Uncommon	The solid nests may be smaller and may be seen more often in children
Solid sheets of cells without nests.	Uncommon	This pattern may be more common in children in the head and neck
Myxoid change	Rare	
Cystic change	Rare	
Prominent hemorrhage	Rare	
Necrosis	Uncommon	May be more common in children and with solid pattern
Hemangiopericytomatous vascular pattern	Uncommon	Sharply angulated, ectatic stag-horn shaped blood vessels
Prominent lymphocytic inflammatory cell infiltrate	Rare	
Infiltrates of xanthomatous histiocytes	Very rare	
Clear cell change	Common	This can occasionally be extensive and mimic metastatic renal cell carcinoma
Multinucleate tumor cells	Common	These are dispersed among the typical tumor cells and do not exhibit increased nuclear pleomorphism
Tumor cells with cytoplasmic vacuoles	Uncommon	May be a degenerative change and usually patchy
Marked cellular pleomorphism	Rare	Marked variation in nuclear size and shape. This is usually patchy Rhabdoid cells may also be present
Spindled tumor cells	Very Rare	May require genetic confirmation of the diagnosis
Frequent mitotic figures	Rare	May coincide with cellular pleomorphism and necrosis.
Cytoplasmic crystals	Common	Highlighted on PAS/D, Alcian blue or trichrome stains Usually consists of rod shaped but may be coarse granules Absent or rare in 30% of cases
IHC: TFE3 (92%), desmin (50%), SMA (50%)	Common	Nuclear TFE3 is sensitive and relatively specific for ASPS. Other tumors reported to show nuclear TFE3 include Xp11 translocation renal cell carcinoma, some granular cell tumors, rare PEComas, chordoma, adrenal cortical carcinoma, urothelial or bile duct carcinoma, MPNST, and high grade myxofibrosarcoma (some of these are in single case reports)
IHC: NSE (30%), vimentin (30-50%)	Uncommon	This sarcoma is unusual in that vimentin may be entirely absent
Genetics: unbalanced translocation t(X;17) (p11;q25)	Common	This translocation is highly sensitive and found in ~100% of cases. It is not entirely specific for ASPS, however and has been reported in Xp11 translocation renal cell carcinoma and rare PEComas

reactive for synaptophysin and chromogranin and does not express nuclear TFE3, a profile opposite that of ASPS. NEC lacks the t(X;17) of ASPS.

Perivascular epithelioid cell tumor (PEComa): PEComas more commonly occur in the abdominal cavity and uterus than in soft tissue. Females are more commonly affected than males, even at soft tissue sites. Tumor cells may be epithelioid, or spindled, and some cases feature a prominent sclerotic stroma. Consistent with the name, the vasculature of PEComa is often prominent and may include large, thick walled vessels that are absent in ASPS. However, tumors composed of nested clear to eosinophilic epithelioid cells can overlap histologically with ASPS. TFE3 may uncommonly be expressed in PEComas (Mitton et al. 2012, Tsuji et al. 2012). Additionally, the *ASPL-TFE3* translocation has also been reported in a few examples of PEComa (Mitton et al. 2012). However, unlike ASPS, PEComas display a myomelanocytic phenotype characterized by IHC expression of HMB45, desmin, and sometimes A103, S-100 protein and SMA. Some PEComas show loss of heterozygosity of the *TSC2* gene (16p13) which has not been reported in alveolar soft part sarcoma.

Case table 14.7a lists variant pathology features reported for alveolar soft part sarcoma. Most ASPS do not vary from the typical morphology.

Case table 14.7b Summary pathology findings of Case 14.7

Diagnosis	ASPS
Size	4 × 3 × 2.5 cm
Location	Deep abdominal wall soft tissue (in rectus abdominis muscle)
Margin Status	Negative
Histologic Grade (FNCLCC Grading System)	High grade
Pathologic Stage (AJCC TNM Classification)	T1b/N0/M0 = Stage IIA (high grade deep tumor <5 cm)

FNCLCC: Fédération Nationale des Centres de Lutte Contre le Cancer (French Federation of Cancer Centers). AJCC: American Joint Committee on Cancer

Oncology approach

Medical oncology

After the patient develops metastases three years after his resection of his primary tumor, he is treated with a combination of ifosfamide and doxorubicin without response. He is then enrolled in a clinical trial of gefitinib, which he takes for 6 months and the lesions stabilize for 17 months. Upon progression, he receives a combination of low-dose docetaxel and gemcitabine on a weekly basis with bevacizumab. He progresses after 4 months and develops a brain metastasis treated with resection followed by γ knife. One month later, he develops hemoptysis caused from invasion of an enlarging soft tissue density in the right mainstem bronchus. A stent is placed and the patient is referred to hospice.

Alveolar soft part sarcomas are slow growing but resistant to chemotherapy as illustrated in this case. Interestingly, they now seem to be more responsive to the new tyrosine kinase inhibitors, in particular cediranib. In this case, the patient had an excellent and durable response to gefitinib, a tyrosine kinase inhibitor targeting EGFR. It might have been informative to sequence the exons to understand whether the EGFR was constitutively activated by phosphorylation. However, it is possible that the target of gefitinib is a different tyrosine kinase receptor, since this cancer harbor a specific *TFE3- ASPSCR1* translocation. This sarcoma also has a tendency to metastasize to the brain as illustrated in this case.

Radiation oncology

This patient is diagnosed with alveolar soft part sarcoma of the rectus muscle which is eventually excised with negative margins. Unfortunately, the patient is lost to follow up, and no adjuvant radiation therapy is prescribed. Three years later, the patient develops metastatic disease. He undergoes palliative chemotherapy and radiosurgery for brain metastases.

Patient outcome

Three years postoperatively the patient develops metastatic tumors in the lungs and adrenal glands and is treated with chemotherapy. Three years following, he develops brain metastases and is treated with further chemotherapy and γ knife irradiation. Two months later, and one month after entering hospice, the patient succumbs to widespread metastatic disease.

Case 14.8 Clear cell sarcoma of soft tissue

Clinical history and presentation

The patient is an 11 year old girl who presents with a one-year history of a painful soft tissue mass in the left small toe. Marginal excision has been performed at an outside facility.

Surgical findings and comments

Physical examination reveals a healing surgical incision over the plantar aspect of the foot involving the proximal aspect of the small toe and extending into the web space between the fourth and fifth toes. The pathology is reviewed, and a clear cell sarcoma is diagnosed, with positive margins. A staging work-up includes an MRI of the left foot and a CT scan of the chest, abdomen, and pelvis. There are no metastases.

Wide surgical resection of the tumor bed is performed one month after initial biopsy.

Radiology findings

We do not have imaging of the 11 year old girl with a CCS of the toe. For comparison, **Case figs 14.8a** through **14.8e** shows an aggressive mass of the right knee in a 19 year old woman. The radiographs show an anterior mass obscuring the patellar tendon. This is not the typical appearance for prepatellar bursitis where the tendon contour is usually visible and the swelling is clearly anterior to the patellar tendon. Indeed, the MR images show the mass appears to originate in the tendon and destroys the lateral portion of the patellar tendon. There is regional lymphadenopathy which occurs more commonly with CCS than other sarcomas (**Case fig. 14.8e**). There are no calcifications which would have suggested a synovial sarcoma. There are no fluid-fluid levels as might be seen in a vascular lesion such as angiosarcoma or hemangioma/angiomatosis. There are no fat tissue elements to guide us toward a lipomatous tumor differential. The lesion abuts the tibia but does not affect the tibia and does not appear to originate from bone. The STIR sequence shows a smudged or 'dirty' appearance which can be seen with schwannoma, however no nerve of origin is demonstrated. The most striking feature of this tumor is its origin from the tendon which directs us to the diagnosis of CCS. Given the aggressive features, tissue diagnosis and removal are warranted.

Pathology findings

Gross features

The initial marginal excision contains a 2.3 × 2.0 × 2.0 cm vaguely lobulated tan mass attached to scant fascia-like tissue. It extends to excision margins.

The re-excision consists of an oriented, ellipse of skin and scant underlying soft tissue measuring 2.8 cm in maximum dimensions. It is differentially inked, and cross sections reveal pale yellow to tan surfaces without a discrete residual mass. The specimen is entirely submitted for microscopic review in five cassettes.

Microscopic features

Low magnification: The patient's tumor forms uniform solid nodules infiltrating deep dermis and tendon (**Case fig. 14.8f**).

High magnification: Medium magnification reveals nests packed tightly together (**Case fig. 14.8g**). Most of the tumor feature round, pale eosinophilic cells with round, only mildly pleomorphic nuclei. Some fields contain clear cells with discrete cell borders (**Case fig. 14.8h**). Melanin pigment is absent, and there is no inflammatory cell infiltrate. Multinucleated tumor giant cells are present but rare. Mitotic activity is sparse (1-2/10hpf). Individual necrotic cells are present but generally inconspicuous. The re-excision specimen contains a 0.2 cm residual nodule of sarcoma. All margins are negative by at least 0.5 cm.

Special studies: Tumor cells show patchy weak to moderate reactivity for S-100 protein. A103 melanocytic antigen is diffusely strongly positive (**Case fig. 14.8i**). The initial biopsy is reviewed by a national expert in soft tissue pathology who performs a chromosome 22q12

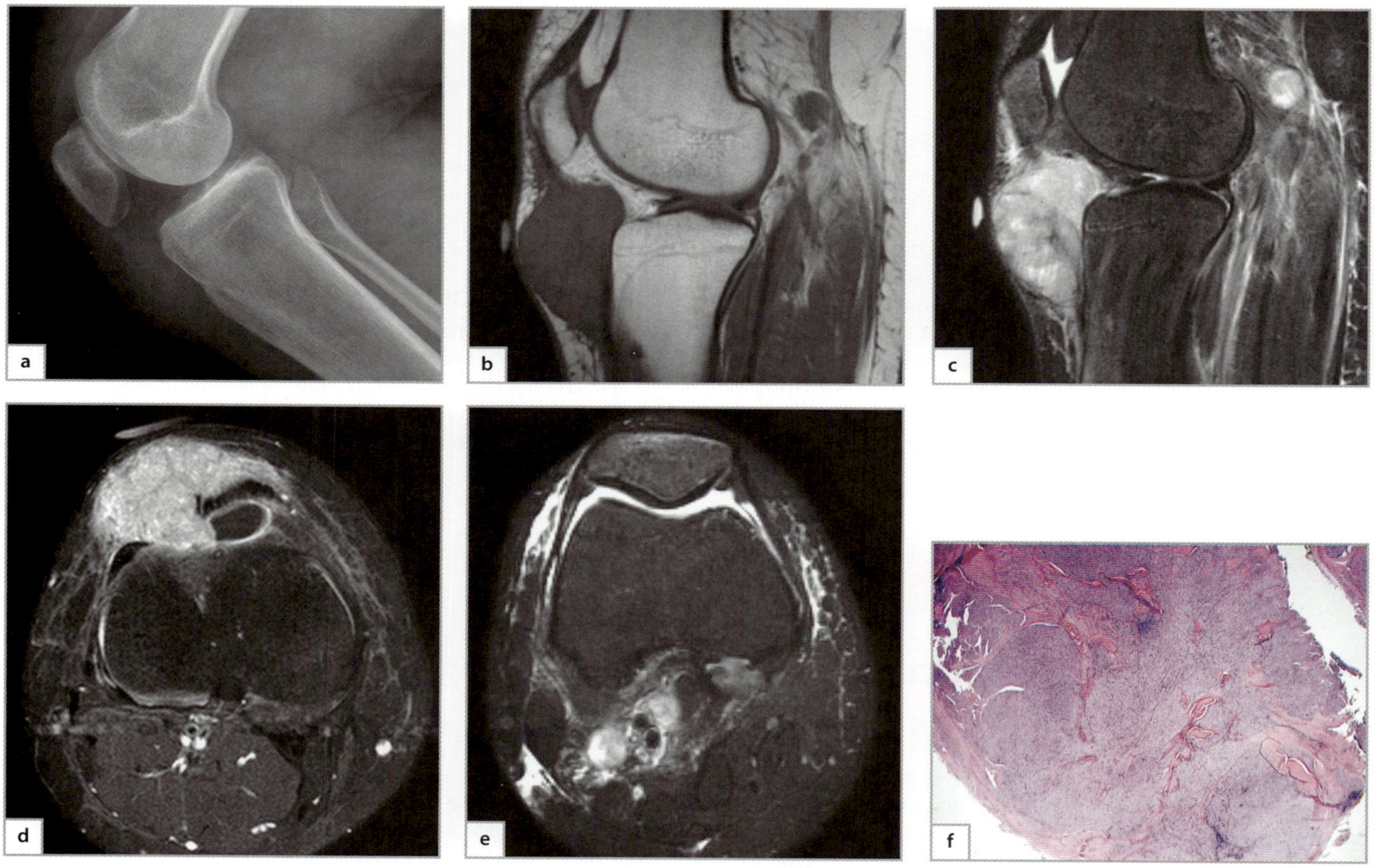

Case figure 14.8 Clear cell sarcoma MR images include: Case figs 14.8a through 14.8f. We do not have imaging of the 11 year old girl with a CCS of the toe. Instead, imaging of a 19 year old woman who presented with a knee mass is provided. **14.8a**: Lateral radiograph shows an ovoid soft tissue mass obscuring the patellar tendon contour. There is no calcification or periosteal reaction. MR imaging of the tumor including. **14.8b**: Sagittal T1, **14.8c**: Sagittal STIR, and **14.8d**: Axial T1 fat saturated post-contrast show a 3 × 5.2 × 5.5 cm mass originating from and destroying the lateral aspect of the right patellar tendon. The tumor is T1 isosignal, STIR high signal and shows intense diffuse enhancement. There is a small knee effusion. The mass is intimate to the anterior surface of the tibia but shows no cortical destruction, periosteal reaction or marrow changes. **14.8e**: Axial STIR image shows several enlarged popliteal lymph nodes with adjacent edema signal suggesting infiltration or inflammatory reaction. There were also enlarged, necrotic lymph nodes of the right inguinal and iliac regions not included. **14.8f**: Low magnification. The tumor forms coalescing solid nodules in the dermis and underlying tendon (this view is of involved tendon). Necrosis and heterogeneous regions (such as fibrosis, hemorrhage or myxoid stroma) are absent.

Case figure 14.8: Continued from page 332

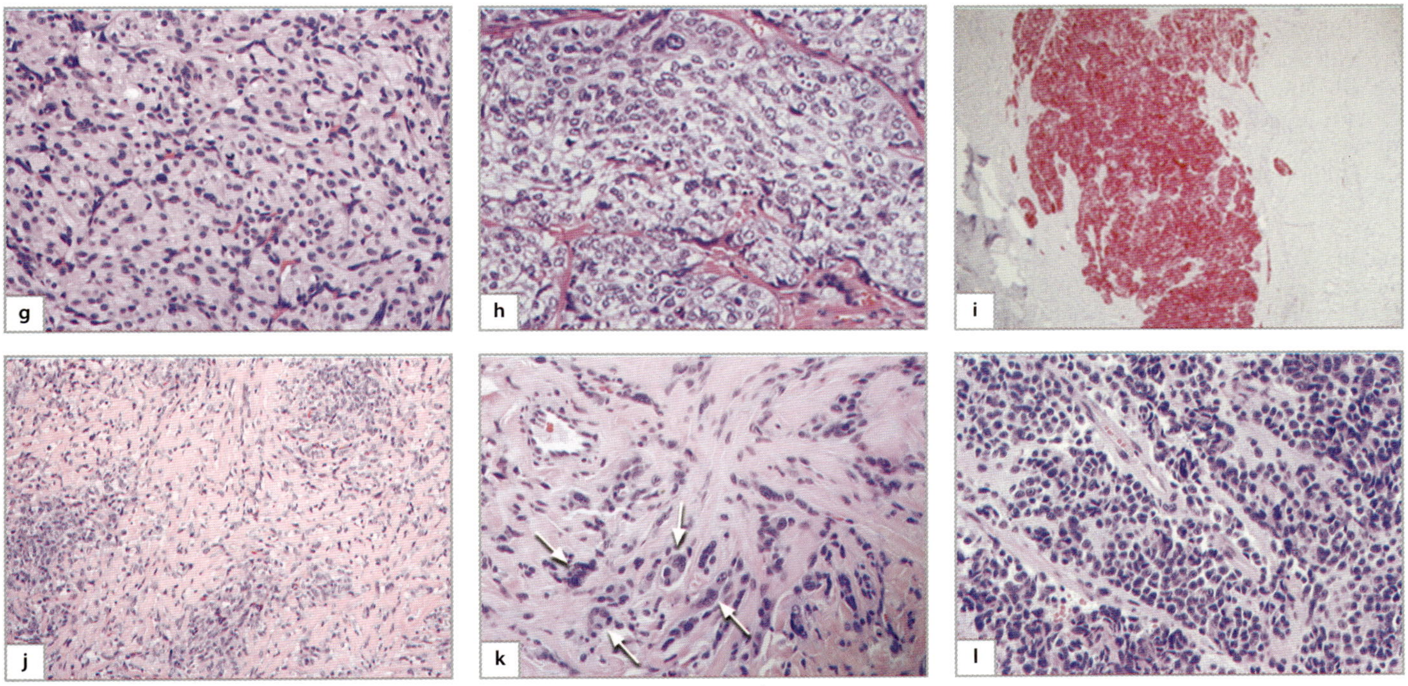

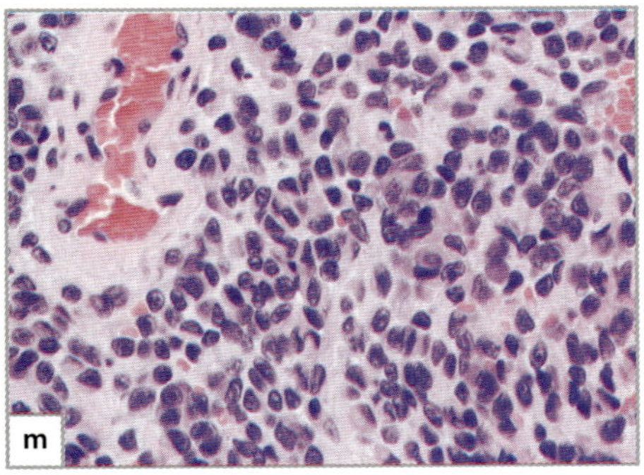

14.8g: Medium magnification. Some clear cell sarcomas consist predominantly of pale eosinophilic cells as in this patient's case. The cells are packed in adjoining nests and there is minimal nuclear pleomorphism. A single mitotic figure is present in the center. **14.8h**: High magnification. Clear cells are focally present and exhibit distinct cell borders. Scattered cell debris consistent with apoptotic bodies are present. Tumor nuclei are vesicular with small to absent nucleoli. **14.8i**: Low magnification A103 melanocyte antigen IHC stain (red chromagen). Consistent with the diagnosis of CCS, tumor cells are diffusely intensely reactive for this melanocytic marker. **14.8j**: Comparison patient with sclerosing variant, low magnification. This patient's tumor is markedly fibrotic and appears histologically similar to sclerosing epithelioid fibrosarcoma. Fortunately, immunohistochemistry and genetic findings enable differentiation. **14.8k** Comparison patient with sclerosing variant, high magnification. Tumor cells are round to spindled with amphophilic cytoplasm. Tumor giant cells, one with a wreath-like arrangement of nuclei, are notable (arrows point to several). These tumor giant cells are often present in CCS. **14.8l**: Comparison patient with small round, dyscohesive cells mimicking seminoma cells, medium magnification. In this patient, the tumor cells form loosely cohesive nests separated by fibrous septae. A few CCS can strongly resemble metastatic seminoma even to the extent of containing internodular infiltrates of plasma cells and lymphocytes. **14.8m**: Comparison patient with small round, dyscohesive cells mimicking seminoma cells, high magnification. The tumor cells are small with a relatively high N/C ratio. Many cells contain single prominent macronucleoli. Clear cells and multinucleate tumor giant cells were not found in this patient's tumor. IHC and FISH studies corroborated the diagnosis.

FISH break apart assay that confirms translocation of the *EWSR1* gene consistent with (though not specific for) clear cell sarcoma.

Two additional comparison cases of clear cell sarcoma: For comparison, two additional cases of CCS are presented. The first is from the thumb of a 54 year old man and represents the sclerosing variant of clear cell sarcoma (**Case fig. 14.8j**). Higher magnification reveals round and spindled cells with pale amphophilic (lavendar) cytoplasm and scattered tumor giant cells (**Case fig. 14.8k**). These multinucleate tumor giant cells, often with nuclei arranged in a wreath-like array, are common in CCS. This tumor was confirmed as CCS sclerosing variant by melanocytic marker expression and the finding of the translocation, t(12;22), on karyotyping.

The second comparison patient is a 19 year old woman with a 9 cm deep soft tissue knee mass. This patient's tumor consists of cells that are small with defined cell borders and which contain single prominent nucleoli (**Case fig. 14.8l**). These cells resemble seminoma cells (**Case fig. 14.8m**) and, in fact, a rare CCS may remarkably mimic metastatic seminoma complete with nodules of this type of tumor cell separated by fibrous strands enriched with plasma cells and lymphocytes. This patient presented with Stage IV disease including metastases to matted regional lymph nodes and lungs.

Pathologic differential or, why isn't it one of the following?

Melanoma: Melanoma is rare in this age group. It often displays more cytologic atypia than the usual CCS. Melanin pigment does not discriminate between the two tumors nor does immunohistochemical staining. At the genetic level, CCS demonstrates one of two translocations: t(12;22)(q13;q12) = *EWSR1-ATF1* or t(2;22)(q34;q12) = *EWSR1-CREB1*. In contrast, melanoma often contains BRAF or c-kit mutations and exhibits a complex aneuploid karyotype. Rare CCS (<5%) may contain a BRAF mutation in addition to a usual translocation (Hocar et al. 2012).

Epithelioid sarcoma: Classic epithelioid sarcoma can occur in the foot and in this age group. However, it does not show such a nested pattern, rather, it more commonly features centrally necrotic nodules that resemble necrobiotic granulomas at low magnification. Melanin pigment is absent (present in ~35-66% of CCS). By IHC, ES expresses keratins and EMA, CD34 in 50% of cases, and loss of INI1 expression; epithelial markers are uncommon and of present focal in CCS, and INI1 expression is preserved. ES does not contain the translocations of CCS.

PEComa: This tumor often assumes a nested pattern composed of round clear or eosinophilic granular cells. It may occur in children and in subcutaneous fat. A sclerotic variant has been described that could mimic sclerotic CCS. IHC separates PEComa from CCS; the former shows a myomelanocytic phenotype (including SMA, muscle specific actin and desmin reactivity as well as HMB45, Melanocyte antigen, or S-100 protein) while CCS lacks the muscle markers and only expresses melanocytic antigens. Genetically, PEComas lack the translocations of CCS.

Myoepithelioma or myoepithelial carcinoma of soft tissue (ME-T): Myoepitheliomas do not have a nested architecture. However, not all CCS are nested, either. Some myoepithelial tumors contain ducts or tubules (~40% or more). Chondromyxoid matrix is often present in ME-tumors and usually absent in CCS. Many ME-T exhibit a more heterogeneous appearance than CCS with mixes of stroma and cell shapes. By IHC, ME-T express myoid markers such as SMA, caldesmon and calponin and epithelial markers including keratins, EMA and p63. In addition, S-100 protein and GFAP are also often expressed. Melanocytic markers are absent to rare. Genetically, both tumors show rearrangements of the *EWSR1* gene.

Extraskeletal myxoid chondrosarcoma (ESMCS): Most patients with ESMCS are adults. However, this entity enters the differential in

Case table 14.8a Variant pathology features of CCS

Feature	Frequency	Comments
Tightly packed nests of predominantly ovoid cells with thin to thick intervening septae. Tumor is attached to or invading tendon or fascia.	Common	This is the characteristic appearance of most clear cell sarcomas ~15% are confined to the dermis; most are subcutaneous with extension into tendon/fascia
Fascicles or compact nests of short spindled cells	Common	Usually focal Pure fascicular growth of spindled cells is rare in CCS Reticulin stains can highlight the nested architecture found in many CCS
Solid sheets of rounded epithelioid cells	Uncommon	Reported as a focal or prominent finding in ~50% of cases in one series*
Seminoma or dysgerminoma-like pattern of dis-cohesive, round epithelioid cells with prominent nucleoli separated by bands of lymphocytes and plasma cells	Rare	Distinguished from metastatic seminoma/dysgerminoma by immunohistochemistry (melanocytic markers expressed in CCS; PLAP in seminoma)
Alveolar like architecture with central sloughing of tumor cells in nests with viable cells clinging to fibrous walls mimicking lung alveoli	Rare	May mimic alveolar rhabdomyosarcoma or alveolar soft part sarcoma
Myxoid stroma or microcystic pattern	Rare	May resemble extraskeletal myxoid chondrosarcoma
Sclerotic variant with marked fibrosis and often hypocellularity	Rare	This may be more common when CCS involves the dermis
Clear cells with central, uniform round nuclei with single nucleoli	Common	Most tumors do not consist of 100% clear cells
Pale eosinophilic or amphophilic cells with the above nuclear features	Common	Most tumors contain some of these cells Some tumors lack clear cells entirely
Multinucleated tumor cells with clumped or wreath-like arrangement of uniform round nuclei with single nucleoli	Common	These cells provide a clue to the diagnosis
Marked cellular pleomorphism	Rare	Usually focal if present
High mitotic rate (>10 mitotes/10 hpf)	Rare	Atypical mitotic figures are absent
Melanin pigment	Common	May be seen in up to 66% of cases Usually focal and not grossly appreciable
Intracellular glycogen	Common	Abundant and accounts for the clear or granular appearance of tumor cells Identified on PAS stains with (no granules) and without diastase (purple granules)
Necrosis	Common	Usually focal Extensive (>50%) necrosis may be associated with a more rapid course
Rhabdoid tumor cells	Rare	Usually focal if present
IHC: S-100 protein (90%), HMB45 (80-90%), A103 (70%), MITF (80-100%)	Common	Indicates the melanocytic differentiation of the tumor MITF is positive in cases of negative other melanocytic markers (less specific)
IHC: c-kit (15%), synaptophysin (40%), EMA (10-25%), keratins AE1/AE3 (10-25%)	Uncommon to Rare	
Genetics: t(12;22)(q13;q12) = EWSR1-ATF1 fusion t(2;22) (q33;q12) = EWSR1-CREB1 fusion	Common	Present in 85-90% of cases (FISH or rtPCR); most are EWSR1-ATF1 fusions. Rare variant translocations may be reported in the future as has occurred for synovial sarcoma, Ewing sarcoma family of tumors and many other translocation specific sarcomas.

*Hisaoka et al. 2008

cases of CCS in older patients with myxoid stroma and lack of nesting or in cases of ESMCS with scant myxoid stroma. In such cases, IHC is very helpful, as CCS expresses melanocytic markers including HMB45, A103, and MITF as well as S-100 protein, while ESMCS only expresses S-100 protein. Genetically, most cases of CCS and ESMCS demonstrate rearrangement of the *EWSR1* gene but the translocation partners are different.

Paraganglioma-like dermal melanocytic tumor (PGDMT): This is a very rare, not yet fully characterized tumor that occurs in the dermis of young adults and may be located in distal extremities. Tumor cells are arranged in zellballen, are clear with minimal nuclear atypia, and exhibit a low mitotic rate. Fine melanin pigment may be present. Both this tumor and CCS express melanocytic markers, so IHC is not discriminatory. However, EWSR1 gene translocation is absent in PGDMT.

Dermal clear cell mesenchymal neoplasm (DCCMN): Another very rare dermal tumor composed of vague lobules of large clear cells that can form a cutaneous nodule and thus far occurs only in adults. Nuclear atypia and mitotic activity is usually minimal but can occasionally be prominent. IHC is helpful in that DCCMN lacks expression of melanocytic markers (including MITF and tyrosinase), and expresses p63 and variably CD68. Genetic findings are awaited.

Metastatic carcinoma such as clear cell renal cell carcinoma (RCC) or adrenal cortical carcinoma (ACC): These tumors occur rarely in children or young adults. However, both these tumors can simulate CCS in a nested organization of clear to eosinophilic round cells. However, by IHC, RCC and ACC can be distinguished in that RCC expresses keratins, EMA, RCC antigen and lacks A103 or HMB45 reactivity, while ACC is inhibin and A103 expressing but lacks HMB45 or S-100 expression in most cases. Genetic testing does not reveal the translocations of CCS

Case table 14.8a lists variant pathology features reported for clear cell sarcoma.

Case table 14.8b Summary pathology findings of Case 14.8

Diagnosis	CCS of soft tissue
Size	2.3 × 2.0 × 2.0 cm
Location	Superficial, primarily subcutaneous adipose but attached to tendon
Margin status	Negative (on re-excision; closest margin is 0.5 cm)
Histologic grade (FNCLCC grading system)	High grade (considered high grade for management purposes although nuclear atypia and mitotic rate is low with no necrosis)
Pathologic stage (AJCC TNM classification)	T1a/N0/M0 = Stage IIA (high grade superficial tumor <5 cm)

FNCLCC: Fédération Nationale des Centres de Lutte Contre le Cancer (French Federation of Cancer Centers). AJCC: American Joint Committee on Cancer

Oncology approach

Medical oncology

In this case, no further treatment is administered, because the surgical procedure is most likely curative. It may have been useful to perform a sentinel lymph node dissection to rule out lymph node invasion, but the tumor is small and the staging work-up negative. The value of sentinel lymph node dissection is not proven for clear cell sarcoma. If a node had been invaded, consideration of adjuvant chemotherapy would have been discussed. However, this tumor is usually resistant to the standard sarcoma therapies and behaves more similarly to melanoma.

Radiation oncology

The patient undergoes wide resection of a clear cell sarcoma located on a toe of the left foot. Even though post-operative radiation therapy is an option to decrease local recurrence, the surgeon does not refer the patient for radiation therapy likely due to the patient's young age.

Patient outcome

Two years postoperatively, the patient has normal function and no evidence of local recurrence or metastatic disease. Because of her small tumor size, she is at lower risk for distant spread. However, she will need to be followed carefully for at least 30 years due to the propensity for late metastases in clear cell sarcoma (the longest latency period for metastasis to develop in CCS is 29 years; Hocar et al. 2012).

Case 14.9 Extraskeletal myxoid chondrosarcoma

Clinical history and presentation

The patient is a 59-year-old man who presents with a one-year history of a painless soft tissue mass in the anterolateral aspect of the right hip. The mass was noted spontaneously and has grown slowly but progressively in size.

Surgical findings and comments

Physical examination reveals a large, deep soft tissue mass over the anterolateral aspect of the right hip. It is firm, fixed, and non-tender. Incisional biopsy is performed. Following confirmation of the pathologic diagnosis, a staging work-up is performed and does not reveal metastases.

The patient is returned to surgery for wide surgical resection of the tumor.

Radiology findings

Our case, **Case figs 14.9a** through **14.9e** show an aggressive lesion in this 59 year old man. The tumor follows the signal characteristics of water with T1 isointensity and T2 high signal. This signal pattern is common to many aggressive, inflammatory or edematous tumors but is also seen with cartilage matrix. The lobulated substance and surface of the lesion gives a cotyledonous pattern and can be seen with cartilage matrix. Unfortunately, there is no calcification of the matrix on radiographs to confirm this appearance. The cystic portion along the anterior aspect of the tumor is T1 high signal and may contain proteinaceous fluid or hemorrhage degradation products. This is clearly an aggressive lesion and tissue diagnosis is needed.

Pathology findings

Gross features

The incisional biopsy consists of grossly myxomatous (gelatinous semitranslucent) tumor tissue aggregating to 4 × 3 × 1 cm. Portions are collected fresh for karyotyping and tissue banking. The remainder is entirely submitted in 3 cassettes for routine processing.

The resection comprises a 15 × 12 × 11.5 oriented portion of adipose tissue and skeletal muscle partially surfaced by an 6 × 2 cm ellipse of skin. The specimen is differentially inked and cross sections reveal a moderately well-circumscribed, 12.1 × 10.2 × 7.1 cm, tan, lobulated, myxoid mass with a single large cyst containing yellow friable material (**Case fig. 14.9f**).

Microscopic features

The incisional biopsy and viable resected tumor are histologically identical, so only the resection slides are described.

Low magnification: Tumor cells aggregate in pools of gray-blue mucin and are separated by varying amounts of pale pink fibrotic stroma (**Case fig. 14.9g**). In these aggregates, tumor cells form lattices and interconnecting strands (**Case fig. 14.9h**). In some areas, the tumor cords are thin and delicately branching (**Case fig. 14.9i**).

High magnification: The tumor cells are round to spindled with pale eosinophilic cytoplasm and variably well-defined cell borders. Nuclei are monotonous, small and round, and many contain single nucleoli (**Case fig. 14.9j**). Mitoses average 1/10 hpf, and marked cellular pleomorphism, cartilage, and apoptotic bodies are absent. Vascular invasion is not identified. All margins are negative with the closest at 0.5 cm from tumor.

Special studies: By IHC, tumor cells strongly express synaptophysin (**Case fig. 14.9k**), chromogranin (**Case fig. 14.9l**) and CD99 (**Case fig. 14.9m**). Interestingly, tumor cells do not express S-100 protein, and there is no reactivity for pan-keratins (all controls are appropriately reactive).

Genetic testing includes FISH for EWSR1 rearrangement which is negative for evidence of translocation at 22q12. The karyotype is reported as follows: 46,XY,der(9)inv(9)(q22q34)t(9;16)

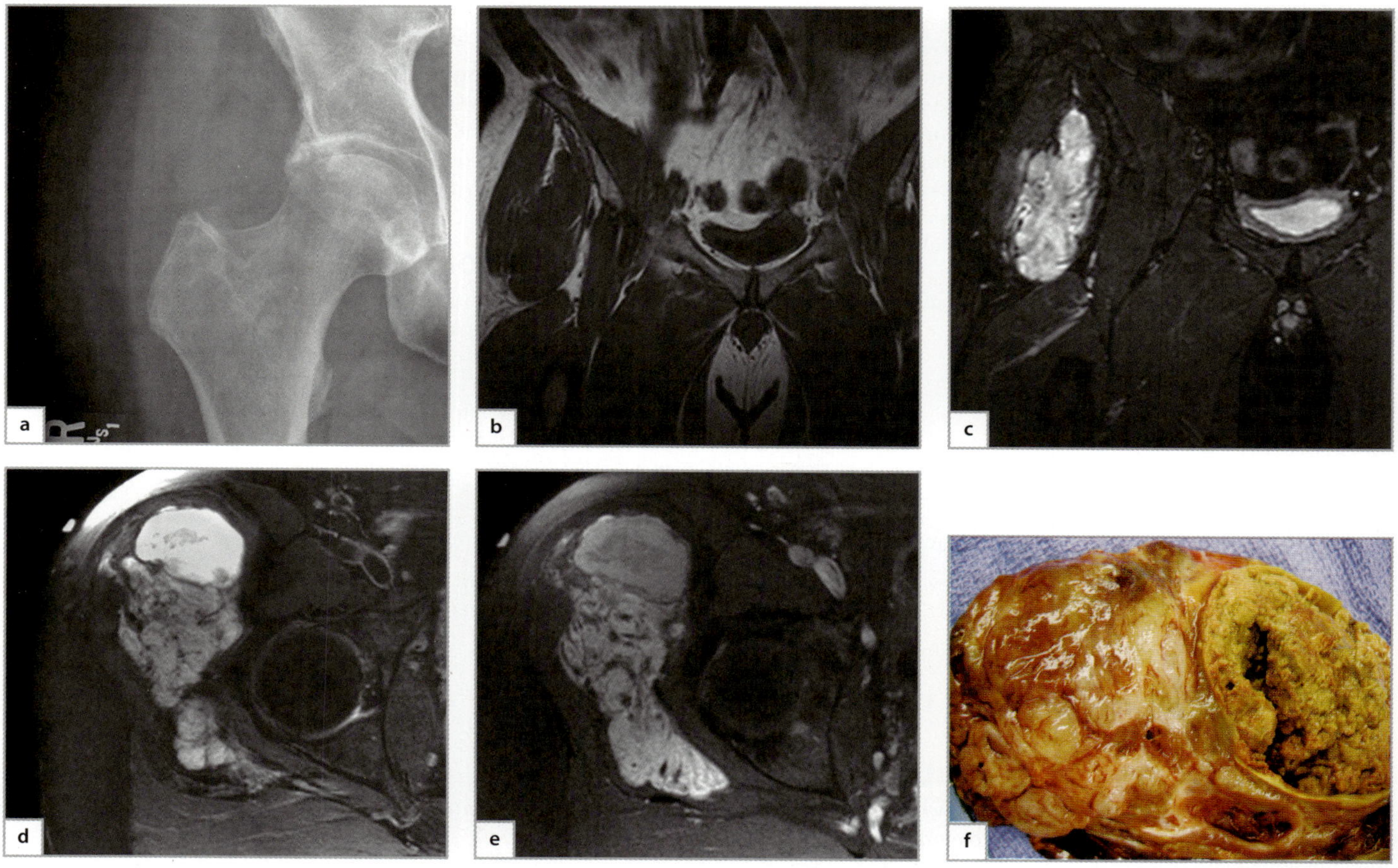

Case figure 14.9 Extraskeletal myxoid chondrosarcoma. **14.9a**: Is an anteroposterior radiograph of the right hip showing a bulging contour to the right gluteus medius muscle. There is no soft tissue calcification or bone findings. MR images include. **14.9b**: Coronal T1, **14.9c**: Coronal STIR, **14.9d**: Axial T2 fat saturation and **14.9e**: Axial T1 fat saturated post-contrast show a 11 × 13 × 5.9 cm heterogeneous mass in the right gluteus medius and minimus muscles of this 59 year old man. The mass is T1 isointense with T2 and STIR high signal and has a lobulated appearance of the tumor substance. There is intense enhancement with invasion into the overlying gluteus medius muscle laterally. There is a cystic portion anteriorly with T1 high signal, not included, likely from hemorrhage or proteinaceous material. **14.9f**: Cross section of 12 cm tumor. The cystic cavity containing yellow friable necrotic tissue is presumed secondary to previous incisional biopsy. The main portion of the tumor comprises non-necrotic lobules of compressible, semi-translucent, glistening gelatinous tumor. The surface is undulating with irregular depressions. Vascularity is web-like and easily appreciated in the near transparent tumor.

Case figure 14.9: Continued from page 336

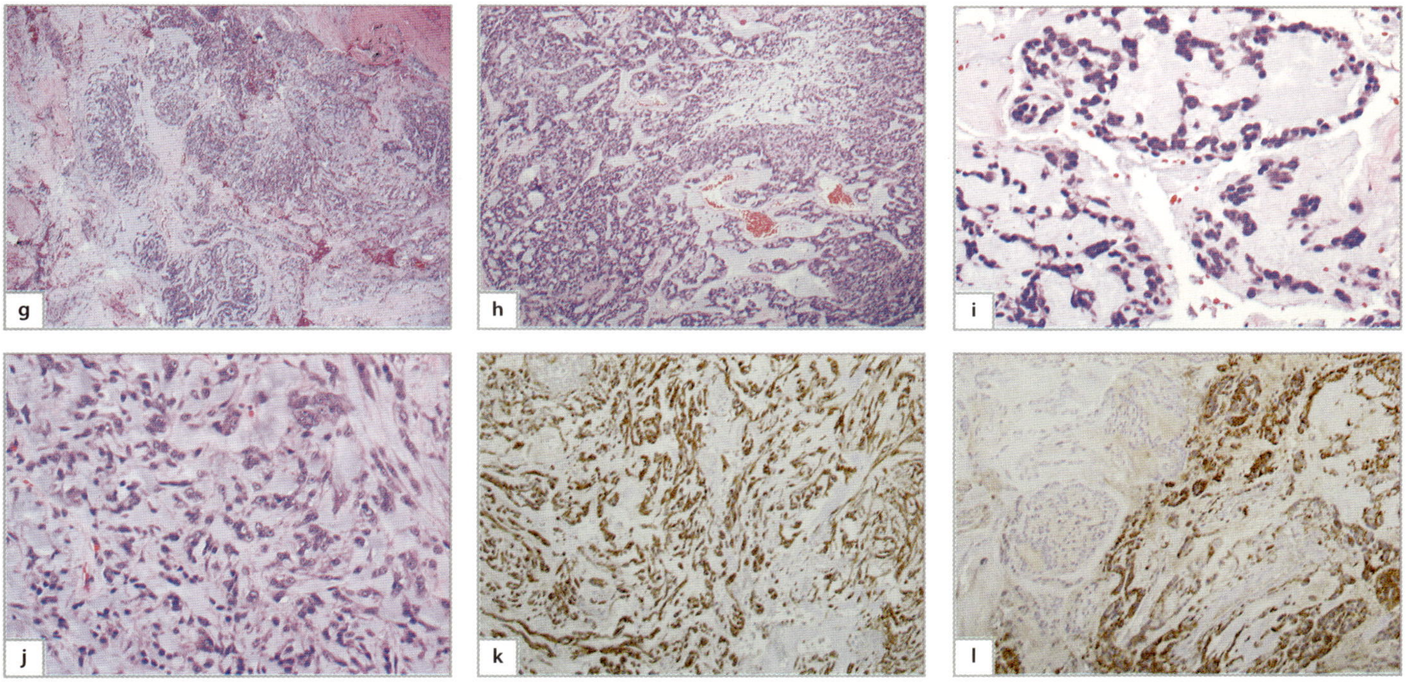

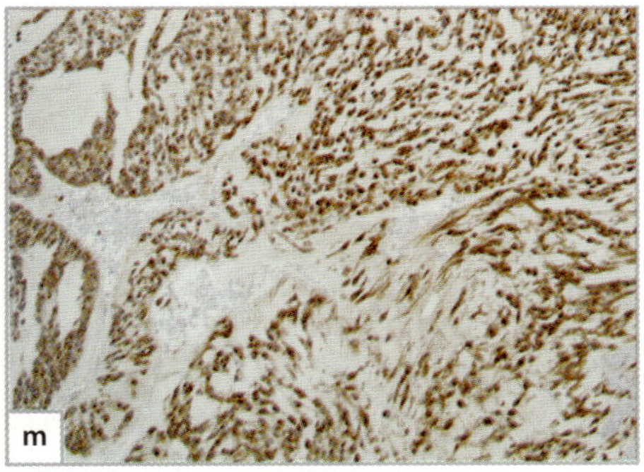

14.9g: Low magnification. The lobularity grossly apparent is recapitulated at the microscopic level. Aggregates of tumor cells reside in pools of gray mucin separated by varying amounts of pink fibrotic stroma. Acute hemorrhage is present, a feature commonly found in ESMCS. **14.9h**: Low magnification. The nodules are formed by lattices and strands of cells floating in gray-blue mucinous material. **14.9i**: Medium magnification. The delicate interconnecting weblike network of tumor cells can be one to just a few cells thick. **14.9j**: High magnification. Lesional cells are round to spindled with monotonous small round nuclei many of which contain single prominent nucleoli. A few cells are multinucleated. Mitotic activity is low throughout the tumor, and individual cell necrosis is absent. **14.9k**: Medium magnification, synaptophysin IHC stain. Tumor cells are diffusely positive for synaptophysin (brown chromagen). This is uncommon in ESMCS. **14.9l**: Medium magnification, chromogranin IHC stain. Tumor cells exhibit variable expression of chromogranin (brown chromagen). This is distinctly unusual but not unreported in ESMCS. **14.9m**: Medium magnification, CD99 IHC stain. Tumor cells exhibit cytoplasmic reactivity for CD99. This is a common and nonspecific finding in ESMCS.

(q22,p11.2),add(11)(q23)[20]. Abnormalities involving the 9q22 region (*NR4A3* gene) are recurrent in extraskeletal myxoid chondrosarcoma (Flucke el al. 2012). The *NR4A3* gene is involved in nearly all ESMCS with various partner genes, the most common of which is *EWSR1* (22q12). However, other partners include *TAF15* (17q11), *TCF12* (15q21) and *TFG* (3q11-12)(Hisaoka et al. 2005, Yasuda et al. 2011, Kohashi et al. 2008). This patient's 9q22 partner at 16p11.2 suggests another novel partner gene.

Pathologic differential or, why isn't it one of the following?

Myoepithelial carcinoma (MEC): Probably the most similar entity in the differential diagnosis is MEC. Both tumors overlap in demonstrating myxoid regions and may both feature uniform small round to spindled cells. Many MEC express S-100 protein which is also expressed in up to 40% of ESMCS. MEC also expresses (in most cases) additional markers of myoepithelial differentiation including keratins, p63, EMA, smooth muscle actin, calponin and h-caldesmon. Only rarely do ESMCS express keratins, SMA, or calponin, although they can show reactivity (~10-20%) for EMA (Hisaoka et al. 2005). Both MEC and up to 20% of ESMCS lose expression of INI1 (Kohashi et al. 2008). Both MEC and ESMCS can show translocations of the EWSR1 gene, but thus far, the fusion partners reported are distinct (Flucke et al. 2012, Vergara-Lluri et al. 2012). In challenging cases, rtPCR or FISH for the fusion partners may be diagnostically confirmatory.

Metastatic neuroendocrine carcinoma (NEC): The large size of the tumor makes occult metastasis an unlikely possibility. Metastatic NEC does not exhibit the festoons and lace like pattern of ESMCS. Myxoid matrix would be unusual. NEC is usually more atypical cytologically. Both tumors can express synaptophysin and chromogranin (more common in NEC than ESMCS especially for chromogranin). S-100 protein reactivity favors ESMCS (absent in this patient, however). Most NEC express keratins (~85%). Translocations involving *NR4A3* are absent in NEC.

Myxoid variant of clear cell sarcoma (CCS-MV): Some ESMCS contain scant myxoid matrix and are hypercellular; these can resemble CCS. ESMCS occurs most commonly in middle aged and older adults, while CCS affects children to young adults. Location in distal extremities (as is common in CCS) is unusual for ESMCS which prefers the thigh or limb girdles. Both tumors may express S-100 protein (~90% of CCS and up to 40% of ESMCS), but additional melanocytic markers are usually seen in CCS and absent in ESMCS. Both sarcomas feature translocations of *EWSR1* but again, as with myoepithelial carcinoma, the fusion partners are different (*ATF1* and *CREB1* in CCS and *NR4A3* in ESMCS).

Case table 14.9a lists variant pathology features reported for extraskeletal myxoid chondrosarcoma.

Oncology approach

Medical oncology

Because the tumor is fully resected, and the patient has no metastasis, he is not offered adjuvant chemotherapy. Regardless, extraskeletal myxoid chondrosarcomas are notoriously resistant to chemotherapy.

Radiation oncology

The patient undergoes wide resection for extraskeletal myxoid chondrosarcoma, and margins are negative on Pathology review. It is decided that the patient does not receive postoperative radiation therapy.

Patient outcome

Two years postoperatively, the patient has normal function and no evidence of local recurrence or metastatic disease. Despite the negative margins, he is at risk for local recurrence and distant relapse. A recent review of 86 patients treated at Memorial Sloan-Kettering Cancer Center and the Royal Marsden Hospital reported a 49% disease recurrence with the median time to any recurrence of 4.7 years (Drilon et al. 2008). Larger tumor size (>10 cm) has been suggested a significant negative prognostic feature and is present in this patient (Ogura et al. 2012).

Case table 14.9a Variant pathology features of ESMCS

Feature	Frequency	Comments
Nodules of tumor cells with peripheral hypercellularity and latticework, filigree, or stranding arrangement embedded in an abundant myxoid matrix	Common	This is the characteristic architecture of ESMCS
Cellular variant with scant myxoid matrix	Uncommon	May be a focal finding in otherwise classic ESMCS. Recurrences may show this morphology of hypercellularity and scant matrix
Small round to plump spindle or polygonal cells with pale eosinophilic cytoplasm, +/- cytoplasmic vacuoles and uniform round nuclei with single small nucleoli. Low mitotic rate: 0-2 mitoses/10 hpf	Common	These are the typical cells in ESMCS
High grade variant: large epithelioid cells, +/- spindle cells, +/- rhabdoid cells with increased nuclear pleomorphism, increased mitotic rate, +/- large areas of necrosis	Uncommon	This variant often contains only sparse myxoid matrix. It is controversial whether this variant is associated with a more aggressive course. High grade areas, if comprising the entire tumor, can mimic synovial sarcoma, epithelioid sarcoma, clear cell sarcoma, extra-renal rhabdoid tumor, metastatic melanoma, and MPNST. High grade areas may be seen focally in otherwise typical tumors. High grade areas may be the predominant pattern with classic areas representing a minority of the tumor
Acute hemorrhage	Common	Hemosiderin may also be present
Dual differentiation with translocation proven synovial sarcoma and ESMCS	Extremely rare	More cases of combination tumors may be described in the future. This case combined classic ESMCS and SS both with their specific translocations
IHC: S-100 protein (~30-40%), NSE (50%), synaptophysin (~20-60%)	Common	The reactivity pattern is not specific or consistent
IHC: chromogranin (2-5%), EMA (~15%), smooth muscle actin (6%), loss of INI1 expression (~15%)	Uncommon to rare	No specific line of differentiation can be confirmed with this reactivity pattern
Genetics: rearrangement of *NR4A3* (9q22) with other partners including *EWSR1* **(22q12)(60% of cases),** ***TAF15*** **(17q11)(18% of cases) and rarely others including** ***TCF12 (15q21)*** **and** ***TFG (3q12)***	Common	To date, no other tumor but ESMCS shows fusion transcripts containing NR4A3. Thus, the finding of a translocation involving this gene can confirm the diagnosis of ESMCS

Case table 14.9b Summary pathology findings of Case 14.9

Diagnosis	ESMCS
Size	12.1 × 10.2 × 7.1 cm
Location	Deep intermuscular tissue of hip/buttock
Margin status	Negative; closest margin is 0.5 cm
Histologic grade (FNCLCC grading system)	ESMCS is not usually graded: FNCLCC system not used
Pathologic stage (AJCC TNM classification)	T2b/N0/M0 = Stage IIB vs Stage III if one considers ESMCS high grade

FNCLCC: Fédération Nationale des Centres de Lutte Contre le Cancer (French Federation of Cancer Centers). AJCC: American Joint Committee on Cancer

REFERENCES

Aguilera D, Hayes-Jordan A, Anderson P, et al. Outpatient and home chemotherapy with novel local control strategies in desmoplastic small round cell tumor. Sarcoma 2008;2008:261589.

Akitake R, Kimura H, Sekoguchi S, et al. Perivascular epithelioid cell tumor (PEComa) of the liver diagnosed by contrast-enhanced ultrasonography. Intern Med 2009;48(24):2083–6.

Anderson ME, Hornicek FJ, Gebhardt MC, et al. Alveolar soft part sarcoma: a rare and enigmatic entity. Clin Orthop Relat Res 2005;438:144–8.

Antonescu CR, Argani P, Erlandson RA, et al. Skeletal and extraskeletal myxoid chondrosarcoma: a comparative clinicopathologic, ultrastructural, and molecular study. Cancer 1998;83:1504–21.

Antonescu CR, Dal Cin T, Nafa K, et al. EWSR1–CREB1 is the predominant gene fusion in angiomatoid fibrous histiocytoma. Genes Chromosomes Cancer 2007;46(12):1051–1060.

Argani P, Aulmann S, Illei PB, et al. A distinctive subset of PEComas harbors TFE3 gene fusions. Am J Surg Pathol 2010;34:1395–406.

Armah HB, Parwani AV. Epithelioid sarcoma. Arch Pathol Lab Med 2009;133(5):814–819.

Baratti D, Pennacchioli E, Casali PG, et al. Epithelioid sarcoma: prognostic factors and survival in a series of patients treated at a single institution. Ann Surg Oncol 2007;14:3542–3551.

Bleeker JS, Quevedo JR, Folpe AL. 'Malignant' perivascular epithelioid cell neoplasm: risk stratification and treatment strategies. Sarcoma 2012;2012:541626.

Bourdeaut F, Freneaux P, Thuille B, et al. Extra-renal non-cerebral rhabdoid tumours. Pediatr Blood Cancer 2008;51:363–8.

Brassesco MS, Valera ET, Castro-Gamero AM, et al. Cytogenetic findings in an epithelioid sarcoma with angiomatoid features: a case report. Genet Mol Res 2009;8:1211–1217.

Brennan B, Stevens M, Kelsey A, et al. Synovial sarcoma in childhood and adolescence: a retrospective series of 77 patients registered by the Children's Cancer and Leukaemia Group between 1991 and 2006. Pediatr Blood Can 2010;55:85–90

Brennan M, Singer S, Maki R, et al. Soft tissue sarcoma. Cancer Principles and Practice of Oncology 2008;1741–1794.

Bu X, Bernstein L, Brynes RK. Reduced risk of synovial sarcoma in females: X-chromosome inactivation? Br J Cancer 2002;87:28–30.

Canter RJ, Qin LX, Maki RG, et al. A synovial sarcoma-specific preoperative nomogram supports a survival benefit to ifosfamide-based chemotherapy and improves risk stratification for patients. Clin Cancer Res 2008;14:8191–7.

Casanova M, Ferrari A, Collini P, et al. Epithelioid sarcoma in children and adolescents: a report from the Italian Soft Tissue Sarcoma Committee. Cancer 2006;106:708–17.

Chase DR, Enzinger FM. Epithelioid sarcoma. Diagnosis, prognostic indicators, and treatments. Am J Surg Pathol 1985;9:241–63.

Chaturvedi M, Khare MS. Epithelioid sarcoma with angiomatous pattern: A diagnostic dilemma. Indian J Pathol Microbiol 2010;53(1):170–171.

Chen G, Folpe AL, Colby TV, et al. Angiomatoid fibrous histiocytoma: Unusual sites and unusual morphology. Group from China. Mayo Clinic, Rochester and Scottsdale, Hospital in France. Mod Pathol 2011;24:1560–1570.

Chen Y, Yang Y, Wang C, et al. Adjuvant chemotherapy decreases and postpones distant metastasis in extremity stage IIB/III synovial sarcoma patients. J Surg Oncol 2012;106(2):162–8.

Chotel F, Unnithan A, Chadrasekar CR, et al. Variability in the presentation of synovial sarcoma in children: a plea for greater awareness. J Bone Joint Surg Br 2008;90:1090–6.

Christopherson WM, Foote FW Jr., Stewart FW. Alveolar soft-part sarcomas: structurally characteristic tumors of uncertain histogenesis. Cancer 1952;5:100–11.

Chung EB, Enzinger FM. Malignant melanoma of soft parts. A reassessment of clear cell sarcoma. Am J Surg Pathol 1983;7(5):405–13.

Clark J, Benjamin H, Gill S, et al. Fusion of the EWS gene to CHN, a member of the steroid/thyroid receptor gene superfamily, in a human myxoid chondrosarcoma. Oncogene 1996;12:229–35.

Clark J, Rocques PJ, Crew AJ, et al. Identification of novel genes, SYT and SSX, involved in the t(X;18)(p11.2;q11.2) translocation found in human synovial sarcoma. Nat Genet 1994;7:502–8.

Cordier JF, Bailly C, Tabone E, et al. Alveolar soft part sarcoma presenting as asymptomatic pulmonary nodules: report of a case with ultrastructural diagnosis. Thorax 1985;40:203–4.

Costa MJ, Weiss SW. Angiomatoid malignant fibrous histiocytoma. A follow-up study of 108 cases with evaluation of possible histologic predictors of outcome. Am J Surg Pathol 1990;14:1126–32.

Daigeler A, Kuhnen C, Hauser J, et al. Alveolar soft part sarcoma: Clinicopathologic findings in a series of 11 cases. World Journal of Surgical Oncology 2008;6:71–77.

Daigeler A, Kuhnen C, Moritz R, et al. Lymph node metastases in soft tissue sarcomas: a single center analysis of 1,597 patients. Langenbecks Arch Surg 2009;394:321–9.

Dalmau J, Craus F, Rosenblum MK, et al. Anti-Hu-associated paraneoplastic encephalomyelitis/sensory neuronopathy. A clinical study of 71 patients. Medicine (Baltimore) 1992;71:59–72.

Deenik W, Mooi WJ, Rutgers EJ, et al. Clear cell sarcoma (malignant melanoma) of soft parts: A clinicopathologic study of 30 cases. Cancer 1999;86:969–75.

Deskmukh R, Mankin HJ, Singer S. Synovial sarcoma: the importance of size and location for survival. Clin Orthop Relat Res 2004;155–61.

Dobbs MD, Correa H, Schwartz HS, et al. Extrarenal rhabdoid tumor mimicking a sacral peripheral nerve sheath tumor. Skeletal Radiol 2011;40(10):1363–8.

Drilon AD, Popat S, Bhuchar G, et al. Extraskeletal myxoid chondrosarcoma: A retrospective review from 2 referral centers emphasizing long-term outcomes with surgery and chemotherapy. Cancer 2008;113(12):3364–3371.

Drilon AD, Popat S, Bhuchar G, et al. Extraskeletal myxoid chondrosarcoma: a retrospective review from 2 referral centers emphasizing long-term outcomes with surgery and chemotherapy. Cancer 2008;113:3364–71.

Edmonson JH, Ryan LM, Blum RH, et al. Randomized comparison of doxorubicin alone versus ifosfamide plus doxorubicin or mitomycin, doxorubicin, and cisplatin against advanced soft tissue sarcomas. J Clin Oncol 1993;11:1269–75.

Eiber FC, Dry SM. Diagnosis and management of synovial sarcoma. J Surg Oncol 2008;97(4):314–320.

Eilber FC, Brennan MF, Eilber FR, et al. Chemotherapy is associated with improved survival in adult patients with primary extremity synovial sarcoma. Ann Surg 2007;246:105–13.

Enzinger FM. Epitheloid sarcoma. A sarcoma simulating a granuloma or a carcinoma. Cancer 1970;26:1029–41.

Enzinger FM, Weiss SW, Liang CY. Ossifying fibromyxoid tumor of soft parts. A clinicopathological analysis of 59 cases. Am J Surg Pathol 1989;13(10): 817–27.

Enzinger FM. Epithelioid sarcoma. A sarcoma simulating a granuloma or a carcinoma. Cancer 1970;26:1029–41.

Fadare O. Myxoid epithelioid sarcoma: Clinicopathologic analysis of two cases. Int J Surg Pathol 2009;17:147–152.

Fanberg-Smith JC, Miettinen M. Angiomatoid 'malignant' fibrous histiocytoma: A clinicopathologic study of 158 cases and further exploration of the myoid phenotype. Hum Pathol 1999;30(11):1336–1343.

Ferrari A, Gronchi A, Casanova M, et al. Synovial sarcoma: a retrospective analysis of 271 patients of all ages treated at a single institution. Cancer 2004;101:627–34.

Fisher C. Epithelioid sarcoma of Enzinger. Adv Anat Pathol 2006;13(3):114–121.

Flucke U, Hulsebos TJ, van Krieken JH, et al. Myxoid epithelioid sarcoma: a diagnostic challenge: A report on six cases. Histopathol 2010;57(5):753–759.

Flucke U, Tops BBJ, Verdijk MAJ, et al. NR4A3 rearrangement reliably distinguishes between the clinicopathologically overlapping entities myoepithelial carcinoma of soft tissue and cellular extraskeletal myxoid chondrosarcoma. Virchows Arch 2012;460:621–628.

Folpe AL, Deyrup AT. Alveolar soft part sarcoma: a review and update. J Clin Pathol 2006;59(11):1127–1132.

Folpe AL, Mentzel T, Lehr HA, et al. Perivascular epithelioid cell neoplasms of soft tissue and gynecologic origin: a clinicopathologic study of 26 cases and review of the literature. Am J Surg Pathol 2005;29:1558–75.

Folpe AL, Morris RJ, Weiss SW. Soft tissue giant cell tumor of low malignant potential: a proposal for the reclassification of malignant giant cell tumor of soft parts. Mod Pathol 1999;12:894–902.

Folpe AL, Weiss SW. Pleomorphic hyalinizing angiectatic tumor: analysis of 41 cases supporting evolution from a distinctive precursor lesion. Am J Surg Pathol 2004;28(11):1417–25.

Folpe AL, Weiss SW. Ossifying fibromyxoid tumor of soft parts: a clinicopathologic study of 70 cases with emphasis on atypical and malignant variants. Am J Surg Pathol 2003;27:421–31.

Fritz A, Percy C, Jack A, et al. (Eds). International Classification of Diseases for Oncology, 3rd ed. Geneva: World Health Organization 2000;45.

Fujimura Y, Ohno T, Siddique H, et al. The EWS-ATF-1 gene involved in malignant melanoma of soft parts with t(12;22) chromosome translocation, encodes a constitutive transcriptional activator. Oncogene 1996;12:159–67.

Fukukawa C, Hanaoka H, Nagayama S, et al. Radioimmunotherapy of human synovial sarcoma using a monoclonal antibody against FZD10. Cancer Sci 2008;99:432–40.

Galanis E, Edmonson JH, Papagelopoulos PJ, et al. Chemotherapy for advanced epithelioid sarcoma. J Clin Oncol 1997:A1817.

Gerald WL, Ladanyi M, de Alava E, et al. Clinical, pathologic, and molecular spectrum of tumors associated with t(11;22)(p13;q12): desmoplastic small round-cell tumor and its variants. J Clin Oncol 1998;16:3028–36.

Gerald WL, Miller HK, Battifora H, et al. Intra-abdominal desmoplastic small round-cell tumor. Report of 19 cases of a distinctive type of high-grade polyphenotypic malignancy affecting young individuals. Am J Surg Pathol 1991;15:499–513.

Goldberg JM, Albritton K. Clear cell sarcoma and alveolar soft part sarcoma. ESUN Article 2005 2:

Graham RP, Dry S, Li X, et al. Ossifying fibromyxoid tumor of soft parts: A clinicopathologic, proteomic and genomic study. Am J Surg Pathol 2011;35(11):1615–1625.

Gross E, Rao BN, Pappo A, et al. Epithelioid sarcoma in children. J Pediatr Surg 1996;31:1663–5.

Guadagnolo BA, Zagars GK, Ballo MT, et al. Long-term outcomes for synovial sarcoma treated with conservation surgery and radiotherapy. Int J Radiat Oncol Bio Phys 2006;69:1173–80.

Guillou L, Benhattar J, Bonichon F, et al. Histologic grade, but not SYT-SSX fusion type, is an important prognostic factor in patients with synovial sarcoma: a multicenter, retrospective analysis. J Clin Oncol 2004;22:4040–50.

Guillou L, Wadden C, Coindre JM, et al. 'Proximal-type' epithelioid sarcoma, a distinctive aggressive neoplasm showing rhabdoid features: clinicopathology, immunohistochemical, and ultrastructural studies of a series. Am J Surg Pathol 1997;21(2):130–146.

Hallor KH, Micci F, Meis-Kindblom JM, et al. Fusion genes in angiomatoid fibrous histiocytoma. Cancer Lett 2007;251:158–163.

Herzog CE. Overview of sarcomas in the adolescent and young adult population. J Pediatr Hematol Oncol 2005;26:215–8.

Hilden JM, Meerbaum S, Burger P, et al. Central nervous system atypical teratoid/rhabdoid tumor: results of therapy in children enrolled in a registry. J Clin Oncol 2004;22:2877–84.

Hisaoka M, Hashimoto H. Extraskeletal myxoid chondrosarcoma: Updated clinicopathological and molecular genetic characteristics. Pathol Interl 2005;55(8):453–463.

Hisaoka M, Ishida T, Kuo TT, et al. Clear cell sarcoma of soft tissue: a clinicopathologic, immunohistochemical, and molecular analysis of 33 cases. Am J Surg Pathol 2008;32(3):452–460.

Hocar O, Le Cesne A, Berissi S, et al. Clear cell sarcoma (malignant melanoma) of soft parts: A clinicopathologic study of 52 cases. Dermatol Res Prace 2012;2012:984096.

Hoosin M, Vredenburgh J, Lanfronco J, et al. A myxoid chondrosarcoma associated with an anti-Hu-positive paraneoplastic encephalomyelitis. J Neurooncol 2011;101:135–9.

Hoot AC, Russo P, Judkins AR, et al. Immunohistochemical analysis of hSNF5/INI1 distinguishes renal and extra-renal malignant rhabdoid tumors from other pediatric soft tissue tumors. Am J Surg Pathol 2004;28:1485–91.

Hornick JL, Cal Cin P, Fletcher CDM. Loss of INI1 expression is characteristic of both conventional and proximal type epithelioid sarcoma. Am J Surg Pathol 2009;33(4):542–50.

Hoshino M, Ogose A, Kawaskima H, et al. Molecular analyses of cell origin and detection of circulating tumor cells in the peripheral blood and alveolar soft part sarcoma. Cancer Genet Cytogenet 2009;190:75–80.

Hosseinzadeh P, Cheung F. Epithelioid sarcoma. Electronic Sarcoma Update Newsletter 2009;6.

Italiano A, Delcambre C, Hostein I, et al. Treatment with the mTOR inhibitor temsirolimus in patients with malignant PEComa. Ann Oncol 2010;21:1135–7.

Italiano A, Penel N, Robin YM, et al. Neo/adjuvant chemotherapy does not improve outcome in resected primary synovial sarcoma: a study of the French Sarcoma Group. Ann Oncol 2009;20:425–30.

Ito T, Ouchida M, Ito S, et al. SYT, a partner of SYT-SSX oncoprotein in synovial sarcomas, interacts with mSin3A, a component of histone deacetylase complex. Lab Invest 2004;84:1484–90.

Jalali GR, Vorstman JA, Errami A, et al. Detailed analysis of 22q11.2 with a high density MLPA probe set. Hum Mutat 2008;29(3):433–440.

Jawad MU, Extein J, Min ES, et al. Prognostic factors for survival in patients with epithelioid sarcoma: 441 cases from the SEER database. Clin Orthop Relat Res 2009;467:2939–48.

Jones BC, Sundaram M, Kransdorf MJ. Synovial Sarcoma: MR imaging findings in 34 patients. AJR 1993;161:827–830.

Jones RL, Constantinidou A, Olmos D, et al. Role of Palliative Chemotherapy in Advanced Epithelioid Sarcoma. Am J Clin Oncol 2013;35(4):351–7.

Judkins AR. Immunohistochemistry of INI1 expression: a new tool for old challenges in CNS and soft tissue pathology. Adv Anat Pathol 2007;14:335–339.

Kato H, Hatori M, Kokubun S, et al. CA125 expression in epithelioid sarcoma. Jpn J Clin Oncol 2004;34(3):149–54.

Kawaguchi S, Wada T, Ida K, et al. Phase I vaccination trial of SYT-SSX junction peptide in patients with disseminated synovial sarcoma. J Transl Med 2005;3:1.

Kawai A, Hosono A, Nakayama R, et al. Clear cell sarcoma of tendons and aponeuroses: A study of 75 patients. Cancer 2007;109(1):109–16.

Kawai A, Woodruff J, Healey JH, et al. SYT-SSX gene fusion as a determinant of morphology and prognosis in synovial sarcoma. N Engl J Med 1998;338:153–60.

Kawashima H, Ogose A, Umezu H, et al. Ossifying fibromyxoid tumor of soft parts with clonal chromosomal aberrations. Cancer Genet Cytogenet 2007;176:156–160.

Kayton ML, Meyers P, Wexler LH, et al. Clinical presentation, treatment, and outcome of alveolar soft part sarcoma in children, adolescents, and young adults. J Pediatr Surg 2006;41:187–93.

Kenerson H, Folpe AL, Takayama TK, et al. Activation of the mTOR pathway in sporadic angiomyolipomas and other perivascular epithelioid cell neoplasms. Hum Pathol 2007;38:1361–71.

Kim HS, Lee HK, Weon YC, et al. Alveolar soft-part sarcoma of the head and neck: clinical and imaging features in five cases. AJNR 2005;26(6):1331–5.

Kis B, O'Regan KN, Agoston A, et al. Imaging of desmoplastic small round cell tumour in adults. Br J Radiol 2012; 85(1010):187–92.

Kohaski K, Oda y, Yamamoto H, et al. SMARCB1/INI1 protein expression in round cell soft yissue sarcomas associated with chromosomal translocations involving EWS: A special reference to SMARB1/INI1 negative variant Extraskeletal Myxoid Chondrosarcoma. Am J Surg Pathol 2008;32:1168–1174.

Koplin SA, Nielsen GP, Hornicek FJ. Epithelioid sarcoma with heterotopic bone: a morphologic review of four cases. Inter J Surg Pathol 2010;18(3):207–212.

Kosemehmetoglu K, Kaygusuz G, Bahrami A, et al. Intra-articular epithelioid sarcoma showing mixed classic and proximal type features: report of two cases, with immunohistochemical and molecular cytogenetic INI1 study. Am J Surg Pathol 2011;35:891–897.

Kransdorf MJ, Murphey MD. Imaging of Soft Tissue Tumors, 2nd ed. Baltimore: Lippincott Williams and Wilkins, 2006: 486.

Kransdorf MJ. Malignant soft-tissue tumors in a large referral population: distribution of diagnoses by age, sex, and location. Am J Roentgenol 1995;164(1):129–34.

Kuiper DR, Hoekstra HJ, Veth RP, et al. The management of clear cell sarcoma. Eur J Surg Oncol 2003;29:568–70.

Kummar S, Strassberger A, Monks A, et al. An evaluation of cediranib as a new agent for alveolar soft part sarcoma (ASPS). J Clin Oncol 2011;29:A10001.

Kushner BH, LaQuaglia MP, Wollner N, et al. Desmoplastic small round-cell tumor: prolonged progression-free survival with aggressive multimodality therapy. J Clin Oncol 1996;14:1526–31.

Ladanyi M, Antonescu CR, Leung DH, et al. Impact of SYT-SSX fusion type on the clinical behavior of synovial sarcoma: a multi-institutional retrospective study of 243 patients. Cancer Res 2002;62:135–40.

Ladanyi M, Lui MY, Antonescu CR, et al. The der(17)t(X;17)(p11;q25) of human alveolar soft part sarcoma fuses the TFE3 transcription factor gene to ASPL, a novel gene at 17q25. Oncogene 2001;20:48–57.

Laskowski J. Sarcoma aponeuroticum. Nowotory 1961;11:61–67.

Lauro S, Bordin F, Trasatti L, et al. Concurrent chemoimmunotherapy in metastatic clear cell sarcoma: a case report. Tumori 1999;85:512–4.

Lazar AJ, Das P, Tuvin D, et al. Angiogenesis-promoting gene patterns in alveolar soft part sarcoma. Clin Cancer Res 2007;13:7314–21.

Le Cesne A, Blay JY, Judson I, et al. Phase II study of ET-743 in advanced soft tissue sarcomas: a European Organization for the Research and Treatment of Cancer (EORTC) soft tissue and Bone sarcoma group trial. J Clin Oncol 2005;23:576–84.

Lewis JJ, Antonescu CR, Leung DH, et al. Synovial sarcoma: a multivariate analysis of prognostic factors in 112 patients with primary localized tumors of the extremity. J Clin Oncol 2000;18:2087–94.
Li H, Smolen GA, Beers LF, et al. Adenosine transporter ENT4 is a direct target of EWS/WT1 translocation product and is highly expressed in desmoplastic small round cell tumor. PLoS One 2008;3:e2353.
Lieberman PH, Brennan MF, Kimmel M, et al. Alveolar soft-part sarcoma. A clinico-pathologic study of half a century. Cancer 1989;63:1–13.
Loya AC, Prayaga AK, Arora A, et al. Lymph node metastasis of soft tissue tumors: a cytomorphologic study. Acta Cytol 2007;51:153–60.
Martignoni G, Pea M, Reghellin D, et al. PEComas: the past, the present and the future. Virchows Arch 2008;452:119–32.
Masson P. Tumeurs Humaines: Histologie, Diagnostics et Techniques, Paris: Maloine, 1956
Matsumura T, Yamaguchi T, Tochigi N, et al. Angiomatoid fibrous histiocytoma including cases with pleomorphic features analyzed by fluorescence in-situ hybridization. J Clin Pathol 2010;63:124–128.
Matsushita Y, Ahmed AR, Kawaguchi N, et al. Epithelioid sarcoma of the extremities: a dismal long-term outcome. J Orthop Sci 2002;7:462–6.
Meis-Kindblom JM, Bergh P, Gunterberg B, et al. Extraskeletal Myxoid Chondrosarcoma: A reappraisal of its morphologic spectrum and prognostic factors based on 117 cases. Am J Surg Pathol 1999;23(6):636–650.
Meis-Kindblom JM. Clear cell sarcoma of tendons and aponeuroses: A historical perspective and tribute to the man behind the entity. Adv Anat Pathol 2006;13(6):286–292.
Miettinen M, Fanburg-Smith JC, Virolainen M, et al. Epithelioid sarcoma: an immunohistochemical analysis of 112 classical and variant cases and a discussion of the differential diagnosis. Hum Pathol 1999;30:934–42.
Miettinen M, Finnell V, Fetsch JF. Ossifying fibromyxoid tumor of soft parts--a clinicopathologic and immunohistochemical study of 104 cases with long-term follow-up and a critical review of the literature. Am J Surg Pathol 2008;32(7):996–1005
Min KW, Seo IS, Pitha J. Ossifying fibromyxoid tumor: Modified myoepithelial cell tumor? Report of 3 cases with immunohistochemical and electron microscopic studies. Ultrastruct Pathol 2005;29:535–548,
Mitton B, Federman N. Alveolar soft part sarcomas: Molecular pathogenesis and implications for novel targeted therapies. Sarcoma 2012;2012:428789.
Mora J, Cruz CO, Parareda A, et al. Treatment of relapsed/refractory pediatric sarcomas with gemcitabine and docetaxel. J Pediatr Hematol Oncol 2009;31:723–9.
Naka N, Takenaka S, Araki N, et al. Synovial sarcoma is a stem cell malignancy. Stem Cells 2010;28:1119–31.
Nese N, Martignoni G, Fletcher CD, et al. Pure epithelioid PEComas (so-called epithelioid angiomyolipoma) of the kidney: A clinicopathologic study of 41 cases: detailed assessment of morphology and risk stratification. Am J Surg Pathol 2011;35:161–76.
Nishimura Y, Yamaguchi Y, Tomita Y, et al. Epithelioid sarcoma on the foot, masquerading as an intractable wound for greater then 18 years. Clin Exp Dermatol 2009;35:263–268.
Nunes LF, Fiod NJ, Vasconcelos RA, et al. [Epithelioid sarcoma: clinical behavior, prognostic factors and survival]. Rev Col Bras Cir 2010;37:251–5.
Oda Y, Tsuneyoshi M. Extrarenal rhabdoid tumors of soft tissue: clinicopathological and molecular genetic review and distinction from other soft tissue sarcomas with rhabdoid features. Pathol Inter 2006;56(6):287–295.
Ogura K, Beppu Y, Chuman H, et al. Alveolar soft part sarcoma: A single centered 26 patient case series and review of the literature. Sarcoma 2012;epub article ID:907179.
Ogura K, Fujiwara, Beppu Y, et al. Extraskeletal myxoid chondrosarcoma: a review of 23 patients treated at a single referral center with long-term follow-up. Arch Orthop Trauma Surg 2012;132(10):1379–86.
Okcu MF, Munsell M, Treuner J, et al. Synovial sarcoma of childhood and adolescence: a multicenter, multivariate analysis of outcome. J Clin Oncol 2003;21:1602–11.
Ordonez NG. Alveolar soft part sarcoma: a review and update. Adv Anat Pathol 1999;6:125–39.
Orrock JM, Abbott JJ, Gibson LE, et al. INI1 and glut-1 expression in epithelioid sarcoma and its cutaneous neoplastic and non-neoplastic mimics. Am J Dermatopathol 2009;31(2):152–156.
Palmerini E, Staals EL, Alberghini M, et al. Synovial sarcoma: retrospective analysis of 250 patients treated at a single institution. Cancer 2009;115:2988–98.
Pappo AS, Parham DM, Cain A, et al. Alveolar soft part sarcoma in children and adolescents: clinical features and outcome of 11 patients. Med Pediatr Oncol 1996;26:81–4.
Patel SR, Burgess MA, Papadopoulos NE, et al. Extraskeletal myxoid chondrosarcoma. Long-term experience with chemotherapy. Am J Clin Oncol 1995;18:161–3.
Pennacchioli E, Fiore M, Collini P, et al. Alveolar soft part sarcoma: Clinical presentation, treatment and outcome in a series of 33 patients at a single institution. Ann Surg Oncol 2010;17(12):3229–33.
Philippe-Chomette P, Kabbara N, Andre N, et al. Desmoplastic small round cell tumors with EWS-WT1 fusion transcript in children and young adults. Pediatr Blood Cancer 2012;58:891–7.
Portera CA Jr, Ho V, Patel SR, et al. Alveolar soft part sarcoma: clinical course and patterns of metastasis in 70 patients treated at a single institution. Cancer 2001;91(3):585–91.
Przybyl J, Jurkowska M, Rutkowski P, et al. Downstream and intermediate interactions of synovial sarcoma-associated fusion oncoproteins and their implication for targeted therapy. Sarcoma 2012;2012:249219.
Puri DR, Meyers PA, Kraus DH, et al. Radiotherapy in the multimodal treatment of extrarenal extracranial malignant rhabdoid tumors. Pediatr Blood Cancer 2008;50:167–9.
Quezado MM, Middleton LP, Bryant B, et al. Allelic loss on chromosome 22q in epithelioid sarcomas. Hum Pathol 1998;29:604–8.
Raoux D, Peoch M, Pedeutour F, et al. Primary epithelioid sarcoma of bone: report of a unique case with immunohistochemical and fluorescent in-situ hybridization confirmation of INI deletion. Am J Surg Pathol 2009;33(6):954–8.
Reichardt P, Lindner T, Pink D, et al. Chemotherapy in alveolar soft part sarcomas. What do we know? Eur J Cancer 2003;39:1511–6.
Reinhard H, Reinert J, Beier R, et al. Rhabdoid tumors in children: prognostic factors in 70 patients diagnosed in Germany. Oncol Rep 2008;19:819–23.
Rekhi B, Ingle A, Agarwal M, et al. Alveolar soft part sarcoma 'revisited': Clinicopathologic review of 47 cases from a tertiary cancer referral center, including immunohistochemical expression of TFE3 in 22 cases and 21 other tumors. Pathology 2012;44(1):11–17.
Roberts CW, Biegel JA. The role of SMARCB1/INI1 in development of rhabdoid tumor. Cancer Biol Ther 2009;8:412–6.
Rosen G, Forscher C, Lowenbraun S, et al. Synovial sarcoma. Uniform response of metastases to high dose ifosfamide. Cancer 1994;73:2506–11.
Ross HM, Lewis JJ, Woodruff JM, et al. Epithelioid sarcoma: clinical behavior and prognostic factors of survival. Ann Surg Oncol 1997;4:491–5.
Saito T, Oda Y, Kawaguchi K, et al. PTEN and other tumor suppressor gene mutations as secondary genetic alterations in synovial sarcoma. Oncol Rep 2004;11:1011–5.
Salvati M, D'Elia A, Frati A, et al. Sarcoma metastatic to the brain: a series of 35 cases and considerations from 27 years of experience. J Neurooncol 2010;98:373–7.
Schaefer KL, Brachwitz K, Wai DH, et al. Expression profiling of t(12;22) positive clear cell sarcoma of soft tissue cell lines reveals characteristic up-regulation of potential new marker genes including ERBB3. Cancer Res 2004;64:3395–405.
Schaffler G, Raith J, Ranner G, et al. Radiographic appearance of an ossifying fibromyxoid tumor of soft parts. Skeletal Radiol 1997;26(10):615–8.
Schoeberl B, Faber AC, Li D, et al. An ErbB3 antibody, MM-121, is active in cancers with ligand-dependent activation. Cancer Res 2010;70:2485–94.
Schoffski P, Dumez H, Wolter P, et al. Clinical impact of trabectedin (ecteinascidin-743) in advanced/metastatic soft tissue sarcoma. Expert Opin Pharmacother 2008;9:1609–18.
Scurr M. Histology-driven chemotherapy in soft tissue sarcomas. Curr Treat Options Oncol 2011;12:32–45.
Segal NH, Pavlidis P, Noble WS, et al. Classification of clear-cell sarcoma as a subtype of melanoma by genomic profiling. J Clin Oncol 2003;21:1775–81.
Senties-Madrid H, Vega-Boada F. Paraneoplastic syndromes associated with anti-Hu antibodies. Isr Med Assoc J 2001;3:94–103.
Shi W, Indelicato DJ, Morris CG, et al. Long-term Treatment Outcomes for Patients With Synovial Sarcoma: A 40-year Experience at the University of Florida. Am J Clin Oncol 2013;36(1):83–8.
Singer S, Baldini EH, Demetri GD, et al. Synovial sarcoma: prognostic significance of tumor size, margin of resection, and mitotic activity for survival. J Clin Oncol 1996;14:1201–8.
Sjogren H, Meis-Kindblom JM, Orndal C, et al. Studies on the Molecular Pathogenesis of Extraskeletal Myxoid Chondrosarcoma-Cytogenetic, Molecular Genetic, and cDNA Microarray Analyses. Am J Pathol 2003;162(3):781–792.

Sleijfer S, Ray-Coquard I, Papai Z, et al. Pazopanib, a multikinase angiogenesis inhibitor, in patients with relapsed or refractory advanced soft tissue sarcoma: a phase II study from the European organisation for research and treatment of cancer-soft tissue and bone sarcoma group (EORTC study 62043). J Clin Oncol 2009;27:3126–32.
Sobanko JF, Meijer L, Nigra TP. Epithelioid Sarcoma: A Review and Update. J Clin Aesthet Dermatol. 2009;2(5):49–54.
Spunt SL, Poquette CA, Hurt YS, et al. Prognostic factors for children and adolescents with surgically resected nonrhabdomyosarcoma soft tissue sarcoma: an analysis of 121 patients treated at St Jude Children's Research Hospital. J Clin Oncol 1999;17:3697–705.
Spurrell EL, Fisher C, Thomas JM, et al. Prognostic factors in advanced synovial sarcoma: an analysis of 104 patients treated at the Royal Marsden Hospital. Ann Oncol 2005;16:437–44.
Stacchiotti S, Negri T, Zaffaroni N, et al. Sunitinib in advanced alveolar soft part sarcoma: evidence of a direct antitumor effect. Ann Oncol 2011;22:1682–90.
Steger GG, Wrba F, Mader R, et al. Complete remission of metastasised clear cell sarcoma of tendons and aponeuroses. Eur J Cancer 1991;27:254–6.
Stockwin LH, Vistica DT, Kenney S, et al. Gene expression profiling of alveolar soft part sarcoma (ASPS). BMC Cancer 2009;9:22–33
Sultan I, Rodriguez-Galindo C, Saab R, et al. Comparing children and adults with synovial sarcoma in the Surveillance, Epidemiology, and End Results program, 1983 to 2005: an analysis of 1268 patients. Cancer 2009;115:3537–47.
Sundaram M, McDonald DJ, Merenda G. Intramuscular Myxoma: A Rare but Important Association with Fibrous Dysplasia of Bone. AJR 1989;153:107–108.
Tanas MR, Rubin BT, Montgomery EA, et al. Utility of FISH in the diagnosis of angiomatoid fibrous histiocytoma: A series of 18-cases. Mod Pathol 2010;23(1):93–97.
Tateishi U, Hasegawa T, Beppu Y, et al. Synovial sarcoma of the soft tissues: prognostic significance of imaging features. J Comput Assist Tomogr 2004;28(1):140–8.
Tateishi U, Hasegawa T, Kusumoto M, et al. Radiologic manifestations of proximal-type epithelioid sarcoma of the soft tissues. AJR 2002;179(4):973–7.
Tateishi U, Hasegawa T, Nojima T, et al. MRI features of extraskeletal myxoid chondrosarcoma. Skeletal Radiol 2006;35(1):27–33.
Taylor BS, Barretina J, Maki RG, et al. Advances in sarcoma genomics and new therapeutic targets. Nat Rev Cancer 2011;11:541–57.
Thaete C, Brett D, Monaghan P, et al. Functional domains of the SYT and SYT-SSX synovial sarcoma translocation proteins and co-localization with the SNF protein BRM in the nucleus. Hum Mol Genet 1999;8:585–91.
Thompson RC, Jr., Garg A, Goswitz J, et al. Synovial sarcoma. Large size predicts poor outcome. Clin Orthop Relat Res 2000;(373):18–24.
Thway K, Fisher C. Tumors with EWSR1-CREB1 and EWSR1-ATF1 Fusions: The Current Status. Am J Surg Pathol 2012;36(7):e1-e11.
Tornoczky T, Bogner B, Krausz T, et al. Angiomatoid fibrous histiocytoma: Pleomorphic variant associated with multiplication of EWSR1-CREB1 fusion gene. Pathology Oncology Research 2012;18(2):545–548.
Torres KE, Pollock RE. Alveolar Soft Part Sarcoma (ASPS). ESUN Article 2010 7.
Tsuda M, Davis IJ, Argani P, et al. TFE3 fusions active met signaling by transcriptional up-regulation, defining another class of tumors as candidates for therapeutic MET inhibition. Cancer Research 2007;67(3):919–929.
Tsuji K, Ishikawa Y, Imamura T. Technique for differentiating alveolar soft part sarcoma from other tumors in paraffin embedded tissue: Comparison of immunohistochemistry for TFE3 and CD147 and of reverse transcription polymerase chain reaction for ASPSCR1-TFE3 fusion transcript. Hum Pathol 2012;43(3):456–363.
van der Graaf WT, Blay JY, Chawla SP, et al. Pazopanib for metastatic soft-tissue sarcoma (PALETTE): a randomised, double-blind, placebo-controlled phase 3 trial. Lancet 2012;379:1879–86.
Vergara-Lluri ME, Stohr BA, Puligandla B, et al. A Novel Sarcoma with Dual Differentiation: Clinicopathologic and molecular characterization of a combined synovial sarcoma and extraskeletal myxoid chondrosarcoma. Am J Surg Pathol 2012;36(7):1093–1098.
Verschraegen C. The monoclonal antibody to cytotoxic T lymphocyte antigen 4, ipilimumab, in the treatment of melanoma. Cancer Manag Res 2012;4:1–8.
Verschraegen C. Unraveling the mystery of a supraclavicular mass. Oncology (Williston Park) 2009;23:721–3.
Verschraegen CF, Glover K. ET-743 (PharmMar/NCI/Ortho Biotech). Curr Opin Investig Drugs 2001;2:1631–8.
Verschuuren J, Twijnstra A, De Baets M, et al. Hu antigens and anti-Hu antibodies in a patient with myxoid chondrosarcoma. Neurology 1994;44:1551–2.
Wagner AJ, Goldberg JM, Dubois SG, et al. Tivantinib (ARQ 197), a selective inhibitor of MET, in patients with microphthalmia transcription factor-associated tumors: Results of a multicenter phase 2 trial. Cancer 2012;118(23):5894–902.
Wagner AJ, Malinowska-Kolodziej I, Morgan JA, et al. Clinical activity of mTOR inhibition with sirolimus in malignant perivascular epithelioid cell tumors: targeting the pathogenic activation of mTORC1 in tumors. J Clin Oncol 2010;28:835–40.
Watabe A, Okuyama R, Hashimoto A, et al. Epithelioid sarcoma-like hemangioendothelioma: a case report. Acta Dermato Venereol 2009;89(2):208–209.
Weeks DA, Beckwith JB, Mierau GW, et al. Rhabdoid tumor of kidney. A report of 111 cases from the National Wilms' Tumor Study Pathology Center. Am J Surg Pathol 1989;13:439–58.
Weinreb I, Rubin BP, Goldblum JR. Pleomorphic angiomatoid fibrous histiocytoma: A case confirmed by fluorescence in-situ hybridization analysis for EWSR1 rearrangement. Cutan Pathol 2008;35(9):855–860.
Weiss SW. Alveolar soft part sarcoma: are we at the end or just the beginning of our quest? Am J Pathol 2002;160:1197–9.
Whitworth PW, Pollock RE, Mansfield PF, et al. Extremity epithelioid sarcoma. Amputation vs local resection. Arch Surg 1991;126:1485–9.
Wick MR, Manivel JC. Epithelioid sarcoma and epithelioid hemangioendothelioma: an immunocytochemical and lectin-histochemical comparison. Virchows Arch A Pathol Anat Histopathol 1987;410:309–16.
Willems SM, Schrage YM, Baelde JJ, et al. Myxoid tumours of soft tissue: the so-called myxoid extracellular matrix is heterogeneous in composition. Histopathol 2008;52(4):465–474.
Williams A, Bartle G, Sumathi VP, et al. Detection of ASPL/TFE3 fusion transcripts and the TFE3 antigen in formalin fixed paraffin embedded tissue in a series of 18 cases of alveolar soft part sarcoma: Useful diagnostic tools and cases with unusual histological features. Virchows Arch 2011;458(3):291–300.
Wolf PS, Flum DR, Tanas MR, et al. Epithelioid sarcoma. The University of Washington Experience. Am J Surg 2008;196(3):407–412.
Worley BS, van den Broeke LT, Goletz TJ, et al. Antigenicity of fusion proteins from sarcoma-associated chromosomal translocations. Cancer Res 2001;61:6868–75.
Yamato M, Nichimura G, Yamaguchi T, et al. Epithelioid sarcoma with unusual radiological findings. Skeletal Radiol 1997;26(10):606–10.
Yang JC, Chang AE, Baker AR, et al. Randomized prospective study of the benefit of adjuvant radiation therapy in the treatment of soft tissue sarcomas of the extremity. J Clin Oncol 1998;16(1):197–203.
Yang L, Chen Y, Chui T, et al. Identification of biomarkers to distinguish clear cell sarcoma from malignant melanoma. Hum Pathol 2012;43(9):1463–70.
Yasuda T, Hori T, Suzuki K, et al. Extraskeletal myxoid chondrosarcoma of the thigh with a t(9;17) translocation. Oncol Lett 2012;3(3):621–624.
Zhong M, De Angelo P, Osborne L, et al. Dual color break-apart FISH assay on paraffin embedded tissues as an adjunct to diagnosis of XP11 translocation renal cell carcinoma and alveolar soft part sarcoma. Am J Surg Path 2010;34(6):757–766.

FURTHER READING

Fisher C, Montgomery EA, Thway K. Biopsy Interpretation Series: Biopsy Interpretation of Soft Tissue Tumors. Philadelphia: Walters Kluwer/Lippincott Williams and Wilkins, 2011.
Fisher C. Epithelioid sarcoma. In: Fisher C, Mentzel T, Montgomery EA, et al (Eds). Diagnostic Pathology Soft Tissue Tumors. Manitoba: AMIRSYS, 2011.

Chapter 15 Metastatic tumors of soft tissue and bone

OVERVIEW

Clinically consequential but microscopically middling describes the tumors in this chapter because the majority are histologically routine but behaviorally ominous carcinomas and melanoma.

Bar none, metastatic carcinoma is the most common skeletal malignancy encountered by orthopedic oncologists. Care of these patients involves radiation oncologists and medical oncologists to treat the metastases or attempt to prevent them.

Data accrued from animal models, clinical studies, and basic research using human samples have yielded numerous texts and thousands of peer-reviewed articles on the subject of bone metastases. Much less has been investigated regarding the far less common event of soft tissue metastasis. As is described in pathology textbooks familiar to all medical students, the path to successful establishment of a tumor distant to the primary site is intricate and multistep, and mapping this path proceeds in ever increasing detail.

The seed and fertile soil hypothesis first proposed over a century ago by the English surgeon Stephen Paget is being championed with new gusto in light of current molecular genetic and biochemical studies exposing the interplay between the metastatic tumor cell and the stroma to which it finds a suitable site for proliferation. It is recognized that not all 'seeds' from even a single tumor are the same: perhaps only a few tumor cells (possibly cancer stem cells) have the capacity to metastasize. Systemic roles of immune surveillance, marrow competence, and immediate stressors of primary tumor resection also modulate metastatic implantation.

This text will not describe the proposed mechanisms of metastasis, as it is a practical volume dealing with how metastases are diagnosed and treated. Fortunately, new oncology approaches are offering improvements in care of patients with bone metastases. Unfortunately, in most patients with soft tissue metastases, the prognosis remains poor, as colonization of this site is usually a late, high stage event.

TUMORS

Bone metastases

Tumors that metastasize to bone are primarily carcinomas followed by melanoma and then, far less frequently, by sarcoma. Eighty percent of the responsible tumors consist of carcinomas of breast, prostate, lung, and kidney. In adult men in the US, prostate cancer accounts for 60% of metastases and lung for 25%. For women, 70% of metastases to the skeleton derive from breast carcinoma with the remainder divided primarily among thyroid, kidney and uterine/cervical carcinomas (Greenspan et al. 2007).

Carcinomas that seldom spread to the skeleton include those from the stomach, anus, pancreas, salivary glands, and colon/rectum (Rekhtman et al. 2011). On the other hand, although itself rare, pheochromocytoma is prone to bone metastasis.

Lymphoma and leukemia also may spread to the skeleton and can form a single or multiple discreet nodules that may mimic metastatic carcinoma.

Soft tissue metastases

A summary of 121 cases of soft tissue metastases noted that primary tumors of the lung, kidney, and colon were the most common originators (Damron et al. 2000). A review of a similar number of cases collected over 30 years from the Ohio State University Medical Center found that the most common sites were from the skin (melanoma) followed equally by lung and breast carcinoma, with kidney and colorectal carcinoma accounting for many of the remaining cases (Plaza et al.2008). In 27% of patients, the soft tissue metastasis was the initial disease-presenting manifestation (Plaza et al. 2008).

DEMOGRAPHICS

Most patients with metastases to the bone or soft tissue are over the age of 50 years, as this is the population with the highest rates of the carcinomas most likely to metastasize. However, younger individuals are not exempt and are at risk for metastasis from a different set of tumors.

Bone metastases

A classic autopsy study published in 1950 reviewing 1000 consecutive patients who died of cancer reported a 27% rate of bone metastasis (Abrams et al. 1950). This is recognizably an underestimate given the technical limitations of the time, and most current estimates consider the overall rate of metastasis to bone is approximately 50% (Kelly et al. 2012). For example, in Canada, with approximately 140,000 annual new cases of cancer, up to 70,000 individuals may develop bone metastases. Viewed from another angle, approximately 70% of patients dying of carcinoma have bone metastases, although most are asymptomatic (Dorfman et al. 1998). Unquestionably, metastatic cancer to bone is a major health problem.

After lungs and liver, the skeleton is the third most common site of metastasis. In most patients, a primary site is found (approximately 85-90%); however, some patients (10-15%) will not have a primary site uncovered, and these patients are considered to have 'CUP' or 'carcinoma of unknown primary'.

Soft tissue metastases

Soft tissue metastases are several orders of magnitude less common than metastases to the skeleton. Most patients are adults. The majority of patients presenting with a soft tissue metastasis have high stage disease and a poor prognosis (Damron et al. 2000). Relatively few series of soft tissue metastases have been reported.

These metastases may be mistaken for abscess, hematoma, hemangioma or varicosities, a degenerative process such as a Baker's cyst, myositis ossificans, or intermittent claudication. In comparison with many sarcomas, a higher proportion of metastatic lesions in the soft tissue are painful, and the possibility of metastasis should be entertained in such a setting (Damron et al. 2000).

PATHOGENESIS

Theories abound regarding why the skeleton suffers from a high proportion of metastases. In mechanical terms, it is a significant site of the body's vasculature. The vertebral plexus of veins lacks valves, and retrograde venous pressure may often be increased in abdominal and chest regions leading to retrograde flow of blood bypassing the caval system to reach the vertebrae (Dorfman et al. 1998). Tumors may metastasize to the bone via direct extension as well as by lymphatic channels and blood vessels. In pathophysiological terms, the hematopoietic bone marrow provides a rich growth medium for many types of tumors.

The incidence of particular carcinoma metastases does not necessarily synchronize with the overall incidence of these tumors. For example, thyroid carcinoma, a relatively uncommon tumor, is one of the top metastasizing carcinomas in women, while kidney carcinoma, likewise relatively uncommon, accounts for a outsized number of skeletal metastases (Nakashima 2010).

In adults, most metastases are located in the axial skeleton, and other common sites include the proximal femur, humerus and tibia (Greenspan et al. 2007). The bone site may provide a clue to source of the metastasis, as metastases located distal to the elbows and knees often derive from breast, lung or kidney carcinoma. Additionally, not only is lung carcinoma the most frequent solitary or acral bone metastasis source; it is also the most frequent subperiosteal or intracortical metastasis (Dorfman et al. 1998).

PATHOLOGY

Metastases to bone

A recent Canadian review of 257 patients presenting with impending or actual pathologic fracture from metastatic malignancy found the most common, fracture-prone sites as follows: femur (70%), humerus (22%), tibia (4%), radius (3%), and ulna (1%) (Kelly et al. 2012). However, in adults, in overall numbers, the axial skeleton is more commonly affected by metastases than the appendicular skeleton. Most skeletal metastases occur as multiple lesions. Skeletal metastases may be associated with a better prognosis than other distant metastases (such as to the lungs) depending on the tumor type (breast carcinoma is an example).

Metastases may be lytic, blastic, or mixed lytic and blastic. Seventy five percent of bone metastases are pure osteolytic, 15% are osteoblastic, and the remainder are mixed. Tumors that are more commonly osteolytic include lung, kidney, breast, thyroid, stomach, and colon. The osteoblastic tumors include breast, prostate, ovary, cervix, carcinoid tumor, bladder carcinoma, and osteosarcoma (Greenspan et al. 2007). Tumors with a mixed pattern are usually breast or lung carcinoma.

Although carcinoma of the stomach is a more frequent metastasizer to the skeleton then colorectal carcinoma, colon carcinoma is the most frequent gastrointestinal carcinoma to present with a solitary skeletal metastasis as the initial clinical event (Dorfman et al. 1998). Pancreatic carcinomas are more likely to metastasize to the bone if they are located in the body or tail.

Thyroid carcinoma, especially follicular subtype, shows a particular propensity for skeletal metastasis, and bone is the most common implantation site after cervical lymph nodes (Dorfman et al. 1998).

In children, sarcomas are more likely to metastasize to the bone than in adults. The most common metastasizing tumors in children include the Ewing sarcoma family of tumors, osteosarcoma, rhabdomyosarcoma, neuroblastoma, and clear cell sarcoma of kidney (Nakashima 2010).

In contrast to a predilection for the axial skeleton for bone metastases in adults, more metastases are appendicular in children and most are osteolytic. Neuroblastoma shows a unique predisposition for metastasizing to bones of the orbit, the jaws and metaphyses of long bones (Dorfman et al. 1998).

Metastases to soft tissue

The most frequent sites of soft tissue metastases in adults are: trunk, thigh muscles, arm muscles, iliopsoas, and paraspinous muscles, but any site may be involved including not only the deep but the subcutaneous tissues. However, deep soft tissue metastases are more likely to be biopsied or resected by an orthopedic oncologist.

Sarcomas themselves may metastasize to the soft tissues, albeit this is estimated to develop in no more than 1.2 to 6.6% of all patients, and it usually occurs as a late event in the setting of widespread disease (Cann et al. 2002). Sarcoma patients with soft tissue metastases are more likely to have a larger tumor (equal to or greater than 10 cm) and high grade histology (Cann et al. 2002). Many sarcomas have been reported to metastasize to the soft tissues including osteosarcoma, high grade pleomorphic spindle cell sarcoma NOS, leiomyosarcoma, synovial sarcoma, chondrosarcoma, and angiosarcoma among others (Damron et al. 2000, Cann et al. 2002, Plaza et al. 2008).

Table 15.1 compares and contrasts tumors metastatic to the skeleton and soft tissue in adults and children.

Radiology

Detection and surveillance for metastatic disease is a routine, if laborious task for the radiologist. In general oncologic imaging, PET/CT is becoming the standard of care for surveillance. However, FDG uptake

Table 15.1 Metastatic tumors to bone and soft tissue in adults and children (US data)

Age and gender	Most common metastatic tumors to bone	Most common metastatic tumors to soft tissue	Most common bone sites	Most common soft tissue sites
Adult males	Prostate, lung	Lung, melanoma, kidney, colon	Axial skeleton, proximal femur, humerus, tibia	Trunk, thigh muscles, arm muscles, iliopsoas, paraspinous muscles
Adult females	Breast, thyroid, kidney, uterus/cervix	Melanoma, breast, lung, kidney, colon		
Children (M&F)	Ewing sarcoma family of tumors, osteosarcoma, rhabdomyosarcoma, neuroblastoma, clear cell sarcoma of kidney	No data	Appendicular skeleton	No data

Note that lymphomas may also present as discrete solitary or multiple bone and soft tissue 'metastases'. Orthopaedic surgeons may also resect soft tissue masses that are found subsequently in Pathology to consist of enlarged lymph nodes involved by metastatic tumor.

is unreliable with sarcomas, and thus, standard CT without PET is the systemic imaging exam of choice for sarcoma patients. The primary sarcoma site is usually imaged using MRI with contrast. The lungs are a common location for sarcoma metastasis and chest CT with IV contrast is the usual exam performed for metastatic surveillance. The liver is the second most common site of metastasis for leiomyosarcoma and hence, abdominal CT imaging should be added for surveillance in these patients.

A given individual metastasis usually does not have a specific imaging appearance. The exception is a metastasis which shows discernible matrix of the primary tumor such as osteoid from osteosarcoma or chondroid matrix from a chondrosarcoma.

Generally, it is the multiplicity of tumors in the setting of known primary tumor that allows the diagnosis of metastatic disease.

Metastases to bone have a variable appearance and may show permeative destruction or may have a punched out lytic appearance with sharply defined smooth margins. Bone metastasis can be blastic as is typically seen with prostate or breast cancer. Bone metastasis can also become blastic with healing response after successful chemotherapy.

Lung metastases are typically spherical and will be associated with pulmonary arteries reflecting their hematogenous route of deposition.

Liver metastases are usually spherical and will have a low density halo or indistinct margins and are commonly described as having a cannon ball appearance.

Metastases to soft tissues are somewhat unusual and may be underreported. The most common tumors to metastasize to soft tissues are lung carcinoma (31%), renal carcinoma (12%) and colon carcinoma (7%). The most common sites of soft tissue metastatic involvement in descending order of frequency is; thigh, psoas, gluteal, and lumbar paraspinal muscles (Damron, et al. 2000). Metastasis to muscle is usually painful leading to clinical presentation. The typical muscle metastasis on MR is T1 low signal with T2 high signal and may have adjacent edema. On the other hand, melanoma metastasis can have T1 high signal related to the presence of hemorrhage or melanin production.

Carcinoma metastasis and lymphoma involving the soft tissues may show extensive inflammatory reaction that may mimic the appearance of infection or phlegmon.

SURGERY OF METASTATIC TUMORS

Tumors metastatic to bone

The role of surgery in the treatment of metastatic bone disease is almost always palliative in nature. Curative surgery is rarely entertained. Cancers metastatic to bone can cause severe pain and disability in terminal patients, and successful palliative surgery can make a substantial contribution to their quality of life. The technical considerations, indications for surgery, and risk of peri-operative complications warrant a voluminous discussion itself and, indeed, several textbooks are devoted to these considerations. In brief, surgical treatment is warranted for prophylactic fixation of impending pathologic fractures, for repair of existing pathologic fractures, for treatment of painful bony lesions refractory to treatment with chemotherapy and/or radiation therapy, for spinal tumors with risk of neurologic compromise, and bony lesions that might otherwise compromise function.

Surgery is almost always performed in close conjunction with systemic treatment and radiation therapy. Polymethylmethacrylate ('bone cement') is often utilized during surgery to augment any defect created by the tumor.

Melanoma

Historically, surgery in stage IV melanoma has been largely reserved for palliation.

CLINICAL PEARL

Prognosis in stage IV melanoma is dismal, even in the presence of aggressive systemic therapy. Prolongation of survival is dependent upon complete response, a situation which is rarely possible with systemic therapy alone. Recent data suggests that long-term survival can be achieved with surgical intervention in carefully selected cases. Surgery with the intent of providing long-term survival should only be considered when all sites of disease are amenable to resection. Incomplete resection does not increase survival. Tumor characteristics favoring slower growth such as low burden of disease, a solitary site of metastasis, and prolonged disease-free interval are associated with better outcome. Patients with M1a disease (isolated skin, soft tissue, or distant nodal metastases) have the most favorable prognosis in stage IV melanoma, and therefore represent better candidates to surgical resection than patients with M1b (pulmonary metastases) or M1c (brain or visceral metastases).

Carcinoma

Surgery plays a minimal role in the treatment of metastatic carcinoma to the soft tissues. Occasionally, a patient will achieve symptomatic benefit from a palliative resection of a soft tissue metastasis. Rarely, amputation will provide palliative relief with extensive metastatic involvement of an extremity.

Lymphoma

Surgery rarely plays a role in the treatment of lymphoma involving the soft tissues.

MEDICAL ONCOLOGY

Bone metastases

Bone metastases are exceedingly common and treatment is specific to the primary histology. However, there are a few issues surrounding bone metastases that should be discussed globally.

- The localized painful bone metastasis: The lesion should be assessed for fracture and the orthopedic surgeon should be consulted. Radiation therapy is very useful for pain control and should also be considered.
- Hypercalcemia of malignancy, or malignancy-associated hypercalcemia (MAH), is commonly paraneoplastic (80% of cases). However, it is also seen in patients with extensive osteolytic lesions (20% of cases). The distinction between humoral and osteolytic hypercalcemia is of diagnostic but not of therapeutic relevance. Often, both mechanisms are involved in the same patient. Metastatic disease activates the RANKL pathway, the production of parathyroid hormone-related protein (PTH-r), and sometimes ectopic production of $1,25(OH)_2D_3$. Bone invasion by cancer causes massive bone reabsorption through release of proteolytic and osteolytic enzymes with paracrine activity on adjacent bone and stromal cells. Patients who develop hypercalcemia present with confusion, constipation, nausea, headache, dehydration, and rarely seizures. However, when calcium levels rise slowly, symptoms are indolent or absent. When patients are symptomatic, MAH is a clinical emergency. Patients with a serum calcium concentration >14 mg/dL (3.5 mmol/L) require treatment, regardless of

symptoms. The widespread use of bisphosphonates for the prevention of skeletal events has decreased the prevalence of MAH. Multiple treatments are available, but by far the two most active ones, besides hydration which should be immediately started, are the use of bisphosphonates or of rank ligand inhibitors. **Table 15.2** describes available treatments for hypercalcemia.

- In patients with widespread bone metastases, skeletal events should be prevented. In women with breast cancer and in men with prostate cancer, who all had bone metastases, bisphosphonates (oral and i.v.) and denosumab (s.c.) reduced the risk of and delay the time of skeletal events. Bisphosphonates may also reduce bone pain and may improve quality of life. The optimal timing and duration of treatment remains undefined (Wong et al. 2012). In a large randomized study in men with bone metastases from castration-resistant prostate cancer, denosumab was better than zoledronic acid for prevention of skeletal-related events. Osteonecrosis of the jaw occurred infrequently (22 [2%] vs 12 [1%]; p = 0·09) (Fizazi et al. 2011).
- Prevention of bone metastases with osteoclastic stabilizers is currently under clinical investigation. The routine use of bisphosphonates as adjuvant treatment for patients with early breast cancer is not recommended (Wong et al. 2012). However, a number of large clinical trials investigating bisphosphonates in this setting have completed accrual and are awaiting results. A recent trial of patients with prostate cancer at risk for bone metastases showed a 4.9 month delay in the appearance of bone disease without any difference in survival, however 5% of patients on denosumab developed osteonecrosis of the jaw (Smith et al. 2012). Thus attempt at preventing the development of bone metastases is not standard of care and should be performed only within a clinical trial.

Soft tissue metastases

Many cancers can metastasize to soft tissue, but the incidence of such an event is rare - between 1 and 2% of all carcinomas. Soft tissue metastases may present in 4 different settings tabulated by decreasing order of frequency (Damron et al. 2000) (see **Table 15.3**).

1. *Presenting symptom (40%):* Soft tissue mass is the presenting sign of an occult malignancy.
2. *Solitary late (35%):* Soft tissue mass is the first sign of recurrence in the absence of disseminated disease.
3. *Disseminated disease (20%):* metastatic disease is present in various organs including soft tissue.
4. *Concurrent (5%):* Soft tissue mass and primary are present at first diagnosis.

Most patients present with a painful soft tissue mass. Often, the diagnosis can be challenging, because of the loss of differentiation of these metastases (Plaza et al. 2008). The site of implantation may

Table 15.3 Incidence of soft tissue metastases per type of primary

Primary tumor	Patients with diagnosis N	Patients with soft tissue metastases N (%)
Melanoma	41	4 (9.8)
Lymphoma	88	2 (2.3)
Lung	60	2 (3.3)
Gastrointestinal	13	1 (7.7)

Table 15.2 Treatments for hypercalcemia

Treatment	Mechanism of action	Dose	Comments	Preferred use
Saline hydration	To treat volume depletion due to hypercalcemia-induced urinary salt wasting and, in some cases, vomiting	Isotonic saline at an initial rate of 200 to 300 mL/h adjusted to maintain the urine output at 100 to 150 mL/h	Especially for symptomatic patients or patients with poor renal function	Yes
Bisphosphonates	Analogs of inorganic pyrophosphate that adsorb to the surface of bone hydroxyapatite and inhibit calcium release by interfering with osteoclast activity	Zoledronic acid 4 mg intravenously over 15 minutes every 4 weeks Pamidronate 90 mg over 120 minutes intravenously every 2 to 4 weeks	Works within 1 to 4 days Dose needs to be adjusted for decreased renal function Risk of rebound hypocalcemia is usually minimal in the hypercalcemia setting Very rare risk of jaw osteonecrosis	Yes
Denosumab	Human IgG2 monoclonal antibody that inhibits binding of the receptor activator of nuclear factor kappa-B ligand (RANKL, part of the tumor necrosis factor family) to RANK receptors located on the surface of osteoclasts and their precursors	120 mg subcutaneously every 4 weeks	No need to adjust dose for renal dysfunction	Yes
Calcitonin	Increases renal calcium excretion and decreases bone resorption via interference with osteoclast maturation	Salmon calcitonin, 4 IU/kg intramuscularly or subcutaneously every 12 hours; may increase to 6 to 8 IU/kg every six hours Nasal application does not work	Some oncologists recommend this drug as a first treatment, other do not use it Best if calcium > 14 mg/L Tachyphylaxis within 48 hours Risk of allergic reaction non negligible	May be
Glucocorticoids	Interfering with calcium absorption and metabolism	Standard high doses	More appropriate for multiple myeloma with hypercalcemia	Rarely
Gallium nitrate	Inhibition of osteoclastic bone resorption via inhibition of an ATPase dependent proton pump on the osteoclast ruffled membrane. Gallium also inhibits PTH secretion from parathyroid cells in vitro	200 mg/m^2 per day for five days intravenously	Potential for nephrotoxicity Might be a better choice for pure PTH-r induced hypercalcemia	Rarely
Miscellaneous	Plicamycin (no longer available), mithramycin, cinacalcet (for parathyroid tumors), phosphates			No

be subcutaneous or muscular. In a series of 500 patients evaluated by PET-CT for staging, 9 individuals had a total of 41 soft tissue lesions; 19 (46%) were subcutaneous and 22 (54%) were muscular lesions (Nguyen et al. 2007).

Other primaries that metastasize to soft tissue include renal cell carcinoma, breast cancer, leiomyosarcoma, and Ewing sarcoma family of tumors.

It is not possible to predict this type of recurrence, and surveillance has not been proven to prolong survival. In most cases, it is the patient who finds the tumor. The mean duration from diagnosis of soft tissue metastasis to death is less than one year (range 2–31 months). The duration of survival is longer for metastatic carcinoma of the kidney (23 months) compared to the other carcinomas (Watmough et al. 2005). Patients with solitary or oligometastases have a better prognosis.

A biopsy must be done to establish the diagnosis. A full excision is recommended when feasible. Treatment depends on the presentation. If the patient has a history of cancer and the biopsy shows a recurrence, a new staging work-up should be ordered to establish whether this is a solitary recurrence or the harbinger of widely metastatic disease. For a solitary recurrence, a localized treatment might be appropriate. In case of metastatic disease, treatment should be systemic and follow the guidelines for the primary tumor.

If the patient does not have a history of cancer, pathology should guide a tailored investigation to discover the primary disease. FDG-PET is no more sensitive than conventional studies to detect occult primaries. The mean maximal standardized uptake value of the metastatic tumors is significantly higher than that of the primary tumors, which explains the equal sensitivity of FDG-PET (Yanagawa et al. 2010). In greater than half the cases, a primary may not be found and patients have a diagnosis of unknown primary cancer (Shaffer 2003). Again, treatment depends on the histology and the extent of disease. Localized treatments include surgical resection, radiation therapy, and radiofrequency ablation.

Medical oncology

Systemic treatment is tailored to the primary cancer. Referral to a clinical trial is always appropriate.

RADIATION ONCOLOGY

The role of radiation oncology for metastatic tumors to the bone or soft tissue is largely palliative. The goal of radiation treatment is simply to decrease pain or disfunction from local mass effect on bones, nerves, or vessels. There is also a role in preventing pathologic fracture in cases where involvement of a weight bearing bone is discovered.

A new emerging role for radiation oncology is evolving with regard to oligometastatic disease (Hellman et al. 1995). Newer radiation techniques including radiosurgery to extracranial sites (stereotactic body radiotherapy – SBRT) have expanded the role of radiation therapy to include non-palliative cases. In this role, radiation therapy is used in conjunction with systemic therapy. The goal of the local radiation therapy is to reduce the overall disease burden in an effort to cure or prolong survival. Multiple phase I and phase II studies have been performed with some including spinal regions. Two examples that suggest a potential benefit are Salama from University of Chicago and Milano from Rochester University (Salama et al. 2012; Milano et al. 2012).

With regard to bone metastases, multiple studies have been performed evaluating palliation. Most randomized studies compare different dose fractionation schedules. The radiation therapy oncology group (RTOG) performed a randomized study from 1974 to 1980 that examined different radiation schedules for palliation of bone metastases. Initially, no differences were identified in pain relief (Tong et al. 1982), but reanalysis indicated that longer schedules with higher overall dose were more effective (Blitzer 1985). This issue was resolved with another randomized RTOG (9714) study comparing 8 Gy in a single fraction vs. 30 Gy in ten fractions. This demonstrated no difference in pain control, but a higher rate of re-treatment with 18% requiring re-treatment in the 8 Gy arm vs. 9% in the 30 Gy arm (Hartsell et al. 2005). In general, radiation therapy for bone metastasis is tailored to the patient with regard to prognosis, histology, performance status, and other clinical factors.

Soft tissue metastases are rare events and no specific recommendations or studies are available to guide care. For the most part, these appear as case reports or small series. In general, treatment is tailored to clinical factors with palliative intent.

Table 15.4 First line therapy for metastatic cancers (NCCN guidelines)

Primary tumor	Treatment	Comments
Lymphoma	R-CHOP	Some rare lymphomas might require specialized treatments
Melanoma	Neoadjuvant therapy followed by resection whenever possible Possible treatments: • Vemurafenib for BRAF mutation & imatinib for KIT expression • Immunotherapy (ipilimumab or IL2) • Chemotherapy (dacarbazine or platinum based regimens)	Assess BRAF and Kit
Renal cell cancer	Angiogenesis inhibition with sunitinib, pazopanib, sorafenib or bevacizumab; Temsirolimus; IL2	Resection is the first choice for a solitary lesion
Lung	Platinum-base chemotherapy Erlotinib for EGFR mutation Crizotinib for ALK *rearrangement*	Perform molecular studies for EGFR1 mutations and EML4-*ALK rearrangements*
Gastrointestinal	Chemotherapy appropriate to organ of origin	
Breast	Chemotherapy or hormonotherapy	Assess hormone receptors and ERBB2 receptor
Ewing	Systemic therapy is indicated (Chapter N)	Disease most likely systemic

CASES

Case 15.1 Metastatic renal cell carcinoma to bone and soft tissue: Unclassified renal cell carcinoma with papillary architecture

Clinical history and presentation

The patient is a 45 year old Navajo man who presents with a six month history of a left chest wall mass which was noted spontaneously. Three months prior to presentation, the patient noted a left neck mass. Both masses have progressively enlarged and recently become painful.

His past medical history is unremarkable. His family history is significant for ovarian cancer in the patient's mother.

Examination of the left chest wall reveals a greater than 10 cm firm mass that is nontender to palpation. It is immobile. The left anterior base of the neck reveals a 3-4 cm firm mass similar in consistency of the chest wall mass.

Surgical findings and comments

Open biopsy of the chest wall mass is performed.

Radiology findings

In this case, **Case figures 15.1a** and **15.1b** show two nonspecific appearing masses. One is destroying a rib and the other probably represents malignant adenopathy of the supraclavicular region. These represent an aggressive process and if the radiologist knows of the primary tumor then the diagnosis of metastatic disease is clear.

Pathology findings

Gross features

Biopsies of the neck and chest mass comprise hemorrhagic pink to red tissue aggregating to 2.9 and 5.6 cm respectively. Portions of the chest wall mass are submitted fresh to Cytogenetics and for tumor banking.

Microscopic features

Low magnification: Both biopsies reveal an epithelial tumor forming nests and papillae. Large areas of necrosis are present in both biopsies (**Case figure 15.1c**).

High magnification: The mixed papillary and nested architecture is easily appreciated at high magnification (**Case figure 15.1d**). Thin layers of tumor cells cover vascularized stromal cores. Neoplastic cells feature clear or eosinophilic cytoplasm and contain round nuclei with single prominent nucleoli. Mitotic activity is high (>20 mitoses/10 hpf), but marked nuclear atypia is absent (**Case figure 15.1e**).

Special studies: Immunohistochemistry is performed to winnow the broad array of papillary tumors. Tumor nuclei are reactive for TFE3 with weak intensity. Focal expression of CD10, RCC, and AMACR is

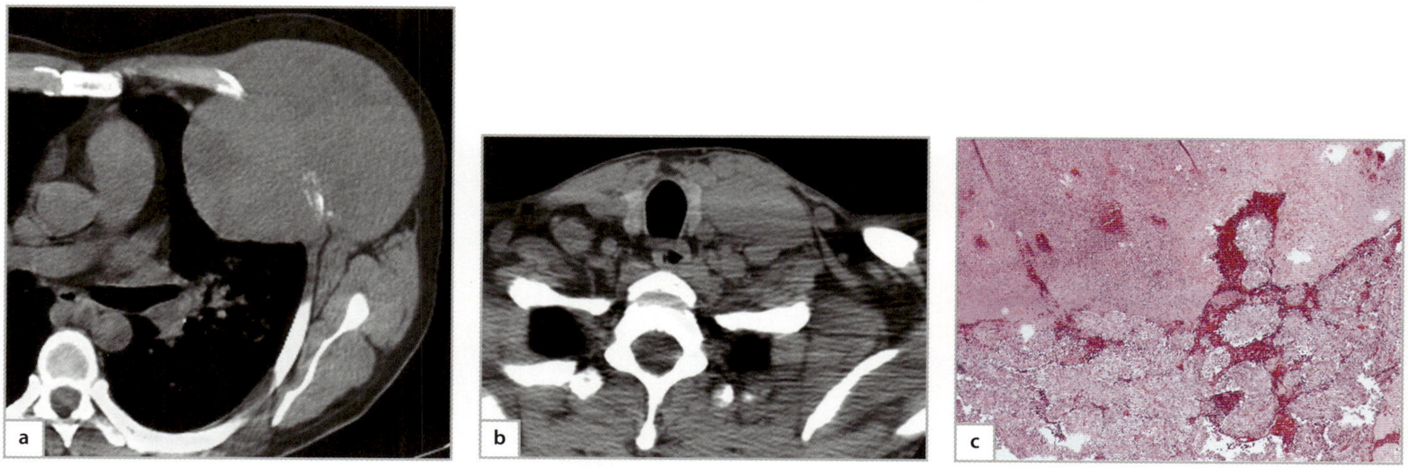

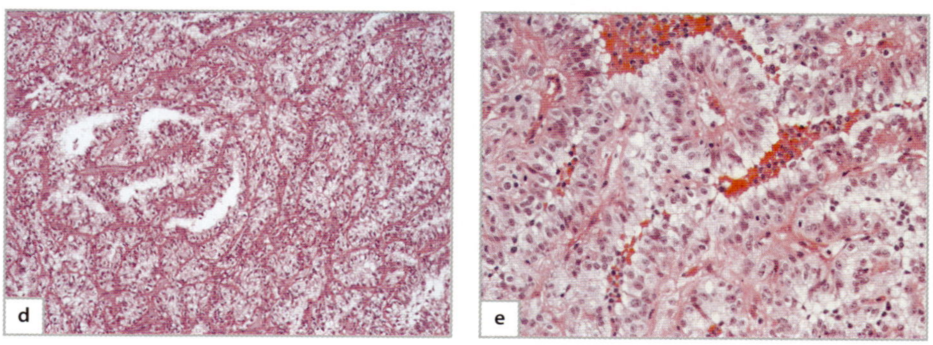

Case figure 15.1 Renal cell carcinoma metastasis. **15.1a**: Axial CT image of the chest without IV contrast in a 45 year old man shows a large, 12.3 × 12.7 × 11 cm mass destroying the left 4th rib. The mass shows no calcification and has no obvious necrosis. **15.1b**: Is an axial CT image through the neck from the same exam. This shows an oblong homogeneous soft tissue density mass measuring 2.6 × 4.8 × 3.2 cm in the left supraclavicular region consistent with a malignant, enlarged lymph node. **15.1c**: Low magnification. The tumor is uniform with a nested and papillary architecture and large areas of necrosis. **15.1d**: Medium magnification. In this area, the tumor forms nests or compressed papillae. Fibrovascular septae are prominent. **15.1e**: High magnification. The papillae are covered by a few layers of uniform, eosinophilic to clear cells. Tumor nuclei are vesicular with single nucleoli. The differential diagnosis comprises other carcinomas with a papillary to nested architecture.

also present. There is no reactivity for keratin 7, keratin 20, melanoma cocktail (HMB-45 and Melanocyte antigen) or TTF-1 (all controls are appropriately reactive).

Cytogenetics reveals a complex hypodiploid karyotype with extensive structural and numerical abnormalities in all 20 cells analyzed: 38,X,-Y,t(1;2)(q21;q21),add(1)(q12), add(4)(q13),-5,-9,-10,-11,del(12)(q22),-13,der(14)t(1;14)(q21;p11.2),add(14)(q21),-15,-16, 18,der(19)t(9;19)(q13;p13.1),add(22)p11.2),+mar[20].

Pathologic differential or, why isn't it one of the following?

Of course, imaging studies and clinical history can be invaluable in determining the source of a metastatic carcinoma with papillary architecture. Extensive pathology workups should be conducted only when clinical and radiologic findings are atypical or unhelpful.

Papillary renal cell carcinoma: Papillary renal cell carcinoma is a specific type of renal cell carcinoma with two histologic variants and a characteristic IHC and genetic profile (see **Case table 15.1a**). This patient's tumor does not conform to the typical features of papillary renal cell carcinoma from histology to genetics.

Translocation specific renal cell carcinoma: Although the morphologic features of this patient's tumor are consistent with a translocation specific renal cell carcinoma, the latter should demonstrate strong diffuse nuclear TFE3 expression, and most importantly, one of the translocations specific to this tumor type should be identifiable on karyotyping or other genetic testing (see **Case table 15.1a** Pathologic Features of Most Common Metastasizing Kidney Carcinomas). Interestingly, this patient's karyotype contains a translocation site (1q21) that may involve one of the gene partners reported in Xp11 renal cell carcinoma, *PRCC* (Klatte et al. 2012). However, no PCR or sequencing was performed to assess for *PRCC* gene involvement in this patient's carcinoma, and there was no evidence of Xp11 gene abnormalities in the karyotype.

Case table 15.1a Pathologic features of most common metastasizing kidney carcinomas

Kidney tumor	Demographics	Histology	Histopathology	IHC	Molecular genetics
Clear cell carcinoma (Conventional RCC)	90% of all renal cell carcinomas and responsible for 90% of metastases. Middle aged and older adults	Solid, alveolar, acinar or mixed pattern of clear cells with low grade up to high grade nuclei. Eosinophilic variant occurs	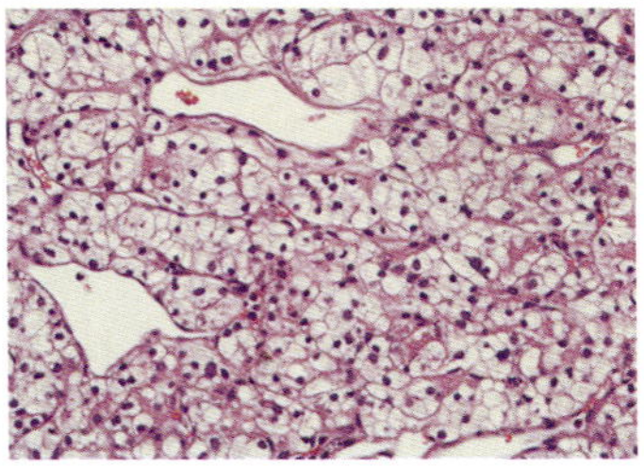	Positive: CK8, 18, 19, RCC, CD10, EMA. Negative: CK7, CK20, Usually negative: c-kit, AMACR	Frequent loss of regions 3p21, 3p12-14, 3p25 (Von Hippel-Lindau gene)
Papillary RCC	10-15% of all RCC Middle aged and older adults	Two patterns: Type 1: small round dark cells forming a single layer over papillary cores. Type 2: Large pseudostratified eosinophilic cells cover cores Cores of both types may have sclerosis, psammoma bodies, and foamy macrophages	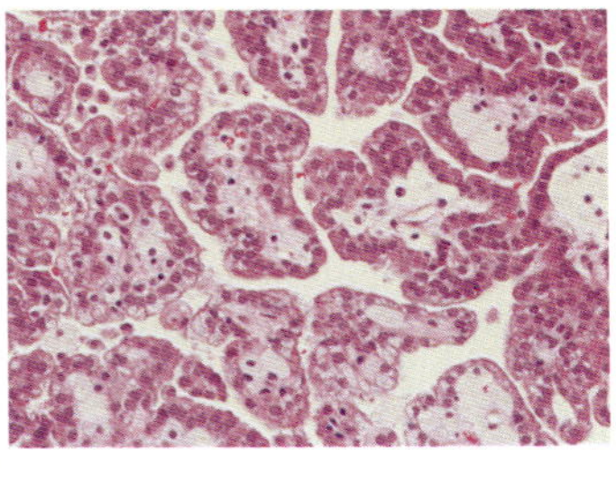	Positive: RCC, CK7, (Type 1 mostly), AMACR, e-cadherin. Uncommonly positive: CK20	Trisomies or tetrasomies of 3q, 7, 12, 16, 17, 20 and loss of Y in male patients
Chromophobe RCC	5% of all RCC Middle aged and older adults	Solid +/- focal tubules. Two cell types: large cells with distinct 'plant-like' borders smaller eosinophilic cells often with perinuclear halo	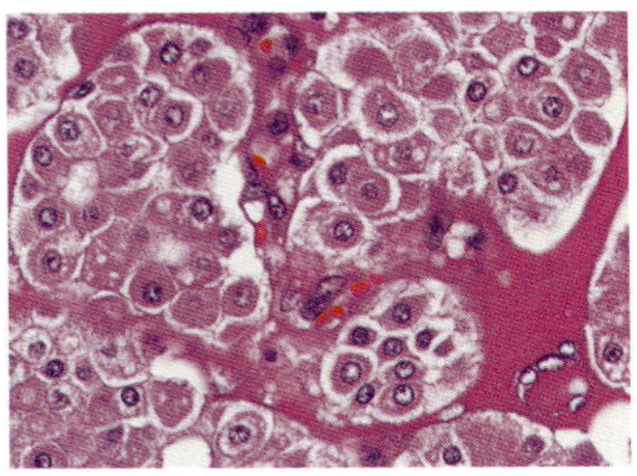	Positive: CK7 and EMA diffusely positive. Negative: CD10, S-100. Variable: RCC	Extensive chromosome loss most commonly involving 1, 2, 6, 10, 13, 17, 21
Renal cell carcinoma, unclassified	~6% of all RCC	Histology does not meet criteria of other tumors: may have multiple patterns	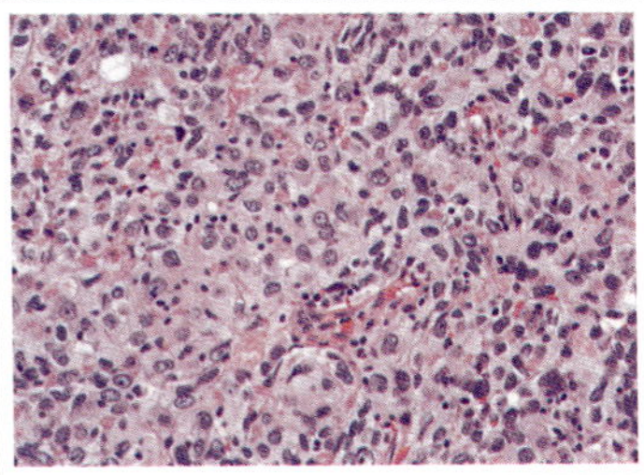	Mixed pattern of IHC reactivity	No specific genetic findings

Case table 15.1a: Continued from page 349

Kidney Tumor	Demographics	Histology	Histopathology	IHC	Molecular genetics
Translocation specific or Xp11 RCC	Rare. Children and young adults. Rare older adults	Papillary and/or alveolar or nested patterns of clear cells or eosinophilic cells with abundant cytoplasm. Psammoma bodies common	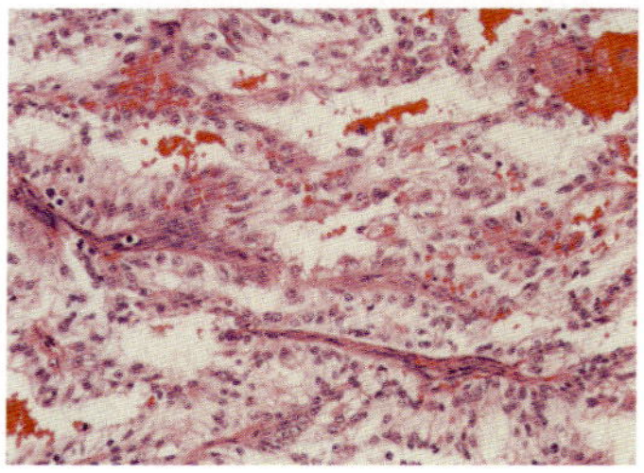	Positive: Strong diffuse nuclear TFE3 reactivity, AMACR, RCC, CD10, PAX2, PAX8. Some cases may show reactivity for HMB45 or Melan A. Negative: S-100, MiTF, Usually negative: EMA, CK7, e-cadherin	TFE3 gene fuses with one of several possible partners: t(X;17(p11;q25)(ASPL) t(X;1)(p11;q21)(PRCC) inv(X)(p11;q12) (NonO) t(X;17)(p11.2;q23)(CLTC). FISH break-apart probe sets are available and may be required to confirm the diagnosis.
Sarcomatoid RCC	An aggressive histologic pattern that can be found in other variants of RCC. Usually not pure but associated with other variants such as Clear cell RCC	High grade solid, fascicular, or storiforming pleomorphic and spindle cell tumor	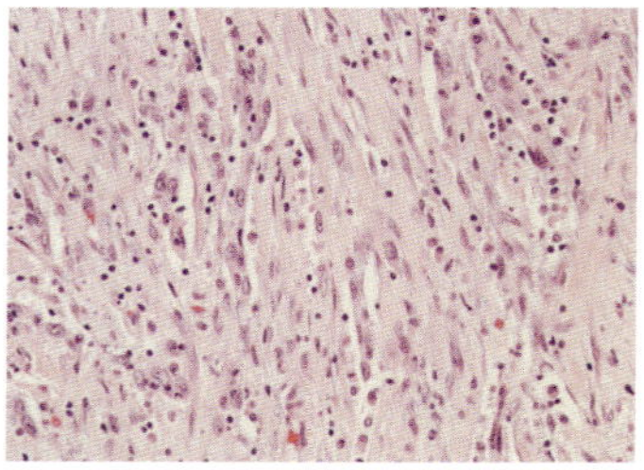	Often shows reactivity for keratins as well as vimentin	May exhibit the genetic profile of the more differentiated, non-metaplastic component

Other papillary carcinomas: Many organs may produce a carcinoma composed of papillae. Among the most common are papillary thyroid carcinoma, papillary urothelial carcinoma, papillary carcinoma of the kidney, papillary lung carcinoma, and papillary serous carcinoma of the ovary or endometrium. Of these, papillary thyroid, papillary kidney, and papillary lung carcinoma are most likely to metastasize to bone or soft tissue. Urothelial carcinoma can metastasize to mesenchymal sites, but usually the implants are high grade, non-papillary tumors.

Immunohistochemical staining helps sort through the candidates when faced with a papillary carcinoma metastatic in soft tissue or bone. Both lung and thyroid carcinoma express nuclear TTF-1, but thyroid carcinoma is also usually reactive for thyroglobulin, while most lung adenocarcinomas also express Napsin A absent in most thyroid carcinomas. Papillary serous carcinoma of the ovary seldom metastasizes to the soft tissue and skeleton but expresses estrogen receptor, WT-1, and CA-125 in most cases.

Of course, as previously noted, imaging studies and clinical history can point to the origin of the metastatic papillary-appearing carcinoma without the need for extensive, expensive pathology testing. Notoriously, however, tumors such as renal cell carcinoma may first present as a metastasis many years after the primary tumor was resected or may first present at an odd metastatic site (such as soft tissue of the thumb), and in these instances, additional pathology tests will usually be required to identify the tumor's source.

Case table 15.1b Summary pathology findings of Case 15.1

Diagnosis	Metastatic renal cell carcinoma with papillary features
Size	Two metastatic implants to rib and soft tissue of neck (probably adenopathy) Rib lesion measures: 12.5 × 11.9 × 10.4 cm
Location	Bone and soft tissue
Margin status	Not applicable- no resection attempted
Histologic grade (FNCLCC grading system)	Not applicable- this is a carcinoma not a sarcoma
Pathologic stage (AJCC TNM classification)	Stage IV

FNCLCC: Fédération Nationale des Centres de Lutte Contre le Cancer (French Federation of Cancer Centers). AJCC: American Joint Committee on Cancer

Oncology approach

Medical oncology

The patient is diagnosed with a metastatic renal cell cancer. He starts treatment with temsirolimus and remains asymptomatic for now. M-Tor pathway inhibitors and antiangiogenic agents are the treatment of choice for renal cell cancers. Treatment is based on prognosis. A poor prognosis includes 3 or more of the following anomalies: high lactate dehydrogenase, low hemoglobin, hypercalcemia, poor performance status, 3 or more sites of metastases, and less than one year between diagnosis and recurrence. Enrollment on a clinical trial is the preferred treatment recommendation. Temsirolimus belongs to category 2A evidence (Hudes et al. 2007); all other anti-angiogenics and erlotinib are category 3 evidence (Coppin et al. 2011).

Radiation oncology

Patients with soft-tissue and bone metastasis are generally treated symptomatically. Palliative radiation therapy is given in patients with pain, neurological, and/or vascular compromise. In this case, the patient had minimal pain and consequently was treated with systemic agents alone to good effect.

In patients with a small number of metastases (oligometastasis, see Hellman et al. 1995), consideration for local therapy to all sites of metastasis can be considered. A growing body of literature advocates for this approach, but so far no benefit to overall survival has been proven. Multiple phase I and phase II studies have shown that radiation therapy with newer techniques (extracranial radiosurgery or stereotactic body radiotherapy - SBRT) are safe and effective (Milano et al. 2012; Salama et al. 2012). This patient could be considered for such an approach.

Patient outcome

The patient is currently asymptomatic but with residual disease including a primary kidney tumor and lymph node and chest wall metastases.

Case 15.2 Metastatic melanoma to soft tissue

Clinical history and presentation

This patient is a 51 year old woman of fair complexion who presents with a three week history of a deeply situated left thigh mass. The mass was noted spontaneously and is asymptomatic. It has not changed significantly in size since first noted.

The patient's medical history is significant for complete excision of a small, superficial spreading, non-ulcerated melanoma from the left lower leg 21 years previously. The Breslow thickness was 0.67 mm.

Examination of the left thigh reveals an ill-defined firm mass over the medial aspect of the left thigh intimate within the deep fascia. It is non-tender on palpation, and there are no overlying skin changes. No other masses are found.

Surgical findings and comments

An open biopsy of the tumor is performed. Findings at surgery reveal a soft, fleshy mass with melanotic pigmentation.

Radiology findings

In this case, **Case fig. 15.2a** through **15.2d** shows a nonspecific mass in the proximal left thigh. The location in the neurovascular bundle could represent any number of tumors, potentially neurogenic in etiology. The location could also be seen with adenopathy related to a process distal in the extremity. The MR appearance is not specific for infection or neoplastic disease. If the primary tumor and its location were known to the radiologist, then they could suggest this is regional tumor or adenopathy recurrence. The PET shows markedly increased uptake of FDG which does not distinguish between phlegmon or neoplasia, however, no other sites of disease were found

Occasionally, melanoma and its metastases will have T1 high signal due to hemorrhage products or melanin production.

Pathology findings

Gross features

The incisional biopsy consists of firm gray tissue fragments dotted with black flecks aggregating to 1.2 cm. A small sample is submitted fresh to Cytogenetics, and additional tissue is flash frozen for tumor banking. Four cassettes are made of the remaining tissue for routine histology. **Case fig. 15.2e** is not from this patient but shows a large pigmented metastatic deposit of melanoma; the gross appearance provides a clue to the diagnosis.

Microscopic features

Low magnification: The tumor consists of nodules that in areas are cuffed by lymphocytes suggesting the tumor arose in lymph nodes and subsequently expanded extra-nodally (**Case fig. 15.2f**).

High magnification: Medium magnification reveals epithelioid cells (round cells with a moderate N/C ratio) forming back to back, solid nests (**Case fig. 15.2g**). This is a common appearance of melanoma. At high magnification, tumor cells are moderately pleomorphic in terms of nuclear size and shape, and mitotic activity is high (**Case fig. 15.2h**). Melanin pigment is spotty on microscopic review, but this irregular concentration of pigment matches the flecking noticed grossly.

Special studies: By immunohistochemistry, tumor cells diffusely express HMB-45 and Melanocyte A antigen (using a dual antibody with a red chromogen; **Case fig. 15.2i**). The malignant melanocytes are also strongly reactive for S-100 protein. These results are consistent with metastatic melanoma.

Karyotyping reveals nonspecific complex aneuploidy that is typical of melanoma. PCR is performed on DNA extracted from formalin-fixed, paraffin-embedded tissue, and subsequent pyrosequencing of codons 599-601 of the *BRAF* gene shows a mutation, V600E (*GTG>GAG* mutation). This mutation is common in non-acral cutaneous melanomas (present in up to 60% of patients) and indicates the patient may respond to Vemurafenib, a potent inhibitor of BRAF kinase (Bhatia et al. 2012).

Pathologic differential or, why isn't it one of the following?

Clear cell sarcoma (CCS): Clear cell sarcoma was once known as 'melanoma of soft parts' because it shows melanocytic differentiation. However, it is a completely independent entity that most commonly occurs in young adults and children without a skin

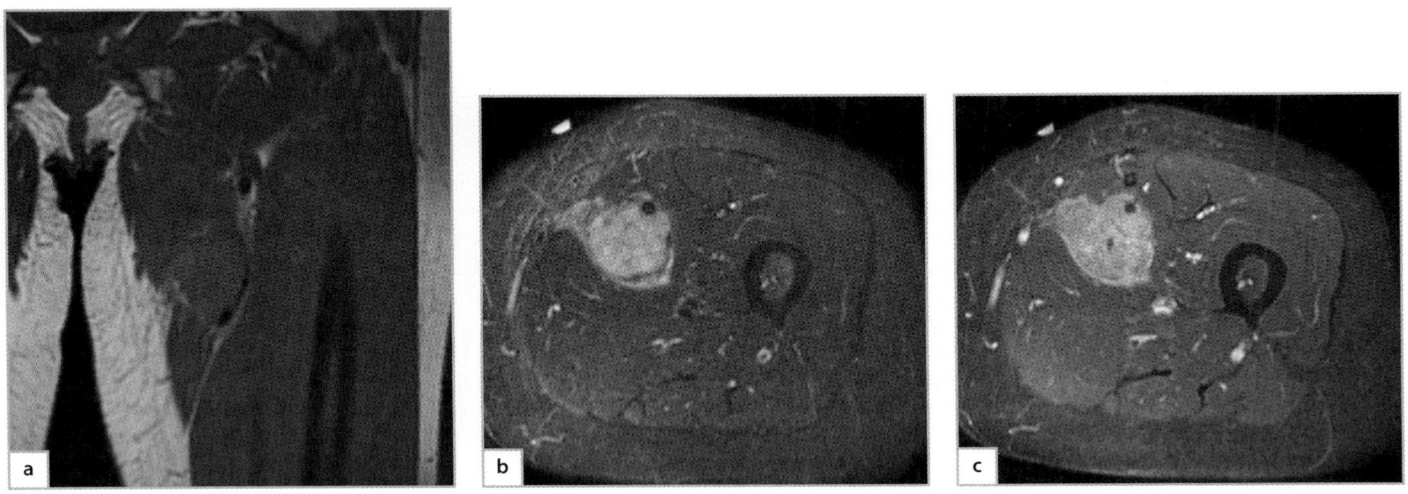

Case figure 15.2 Melanoma metastasis. MR images including; **15.2a**: Coronal T1, **15.2b**: Axial STIR, **15.2c**: Axial T1 fat saturated post-contrast. There is a 4.2 × 3.1 × 3.8 cm mass in the muscles of the adductor compartment of the thigh in this 51 year old woman. The mass shows T1 iso to slight hyper signal intensity and STIR high signal with intense diffuse enhancement. The mass surrounds the superficial femoral neurovascular bundle.

Case figure 15.2: Continued from page 351

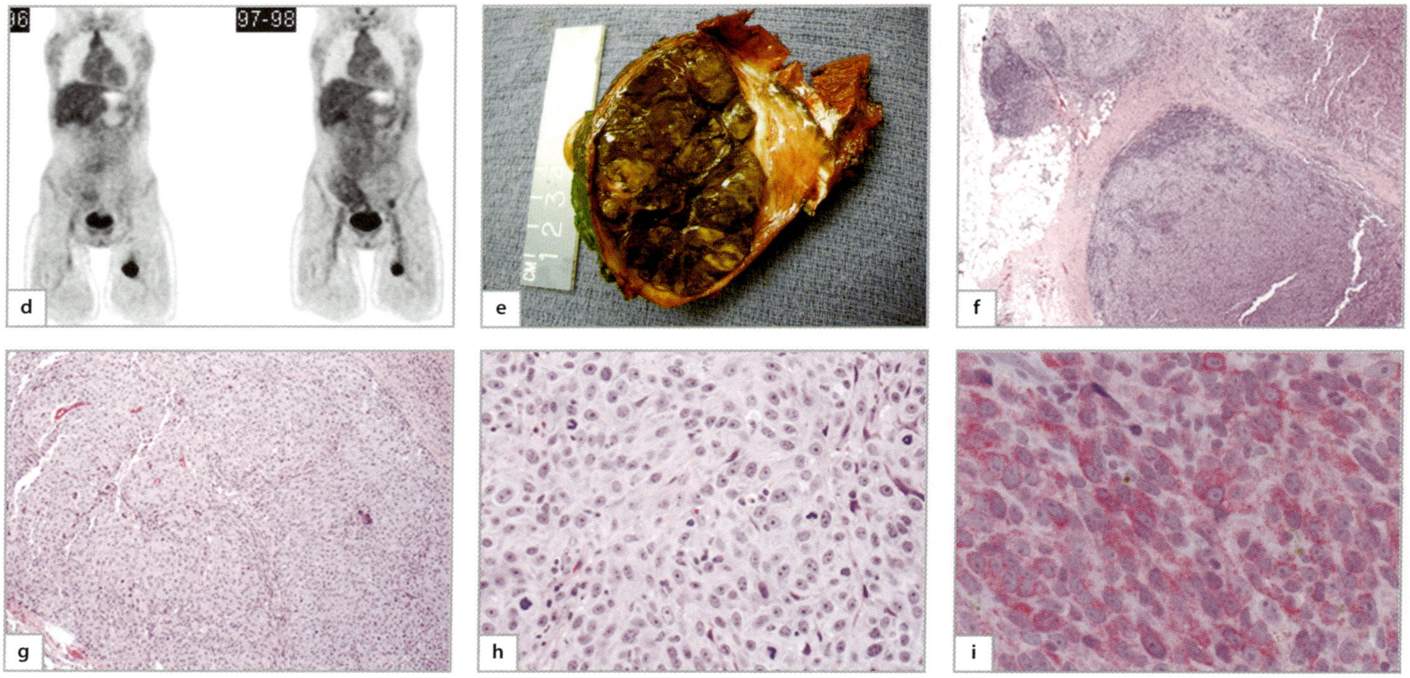

15.2d: PET image shows intense FDG uptake by the tumor. **15.2e**: Gross cross section of another patient's tumor. The deep greenish-brown color of this lobulated metastatic melanoma is highly suggestive of the diagnosis. Hemosiderin pigment can look similar, however. **15.2f**: Low magnification. At scanning view, the tumor forms nodules two of which are associated with a rim of lymphocytes. Given the location: intimate association with the femoral nerve and vessels, and the long latency period, the tumor probably metastasized to lymph nodes and subsequently invaded surrounding soft tissue. **15.2g**: Medium magnification. In this field the tumor forms adjoining nests of swirling cells. In contrast to clear cell sarcoma, an entity in the differential, tumor vascularity is inconspicuous. **15.2h**: High magnification. Malignant melanocytes often are epithelioid (rounded with central nuclei) or polygonal, as in this field. Cytoplasm is moderate in volume, and tumor nuclei are mildly pleomorphic. Many contain macronucleoli ('cherry red nucleoli'), a feature often seen in melanoma. Mitotic activity is brisk and five are detectable in this single, 400x field. Less prominent is individual cell necrosis characterized by shrunken, hypereosinophilic cells with pyknotic (dark smudgy) nuclei. **15.2i**: Dual immunohistochemical stain for HMB45 and Melanocyte A103 antigens (red chromogen), high magnification. Tumor cells show a range of reactivity from absent to strong for these melanocytic markers. The scant brown pigment in the background could represent melanin or hemosiderin. Some metastatic melanomas do not express any melanocytic markers. In these cases, clinical history, morphology, and lack of reactivity for antigens indicative of carcinoma, sarcoma or lymphoma enable the correct diagnosis.

component. The tumor is usually less pleomorphic than melanoma, the tumor cells are clear to spindled and usually lack melanin. Although tumor cells are reactive for S-100 protein, HMB-45 and Melanocyte antigen as with melanoma, genetically the two entities diverge conspicuously. Most cases of CCS contain one of two translocations involving the EWS gene: t(12;22)(q13;q12) = *EWS-ATF1* or t(2;22)(q13;q12) = *EWS-CREB1* fusion. By contrast, melanomas do not have these translocations, and often disclose a complex aneuploid karyotype without consistent recurrent abnormalities. *BRAF* mutations are absent to rare in CCS and occur commonly in cutaneous melanoma. This patients' karyotype, *BRAF* mutation status, pleomorphic pigmented tumor cells, older age and history of melanoma support the diagnosis of metastatic melanoma rather than clear cell sarcoma. Melanoma is one of the malignancies capable of late metastasis, and this patient's latency period of 21 years is unusual but not exceptional. Any patient with a history of melanoma and a new malignant tumor mass should be carefully assessed for recurrent tumor. Moreover, with new therapies for high stage melanoma, it behooves the clinical team to ensure that the correct diagnosis is rendered.

PEComa of soft tissue: Perivascular epithelioid cell tumor of soft tissue is extremely rare. It more closely resembles clear cell sarcoma than the typical, more cytologically pleomorphic melanoma. Tumor cells are clear to eosinophilic, round to spindled, and arranged in nests with prominent, intervening fibrovascular septae. Immunohistochemically, PEComas express melanocytic markers such as HMB-45 and Melanocyte A antigen with absent to sparse reactivity for S-100 protein. Importantly, tumor cells, especially spindle cell component, express muscle markers such as smooth muscle actin, calponin, and h-caldesmon (desmin is usually negative). PEComa lacks the translocations of CCS.

Case table 15.2a lists variant histologic features of metastatic melanoma.

Oncology approach

Medical oncology

Because the recurrence happens after many years, the patient's prognosis is likely to be more favorable than would otherwise be expected. She is referred to a clinical trial with a new immunotherapy agent, a programmed death-1 (PD1) antibody.

Case table 15.2a Some of the many variant histologic features of metastatic melanoma

Variant feature	Frequency	Comment	Microscopic photo
Epithelioid cells with prominent macronucleoli and scattered multinucleated giant cells	Common	With these features, in most cases, a diagnosis can be rendered without special stains	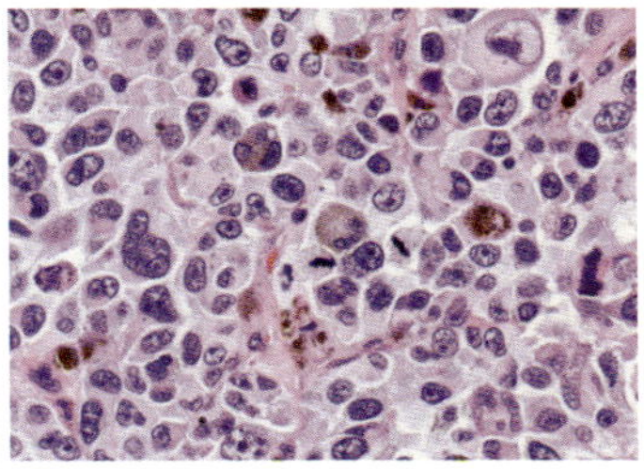
Spindle cells appearing low grade	Uncommon to rare	Spindle cells may be mixed with epithelioid cells	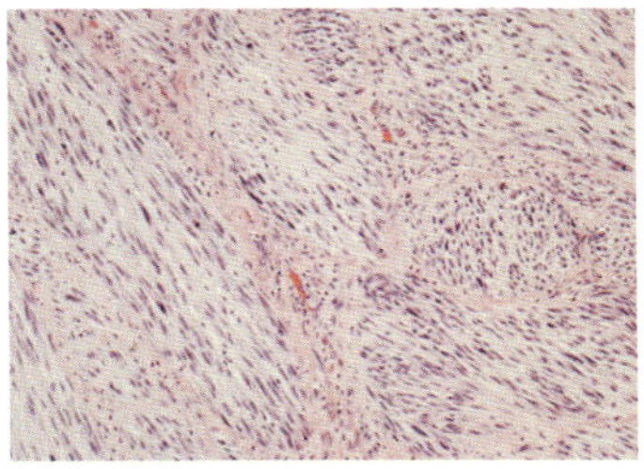
Spindle cells appearing high grade	Uncommon in pure form	May mimic sarcomas such as MPNST and synovial sarcoma among others	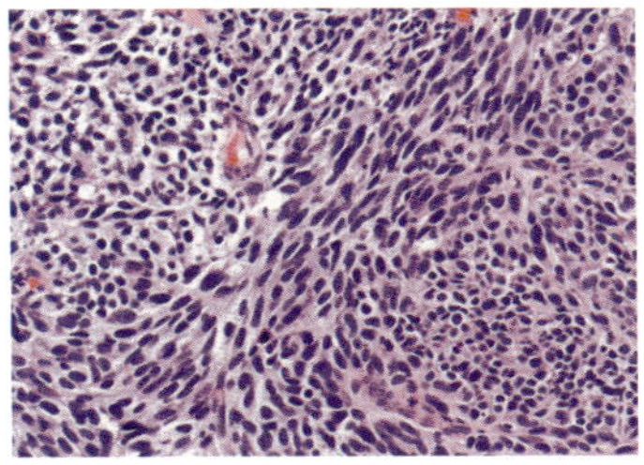
Nests of non-pigmented cells that resemble adenocarcinoma	Relatively common	Up to 2/3rds of metastatic melanoma are amelanotic	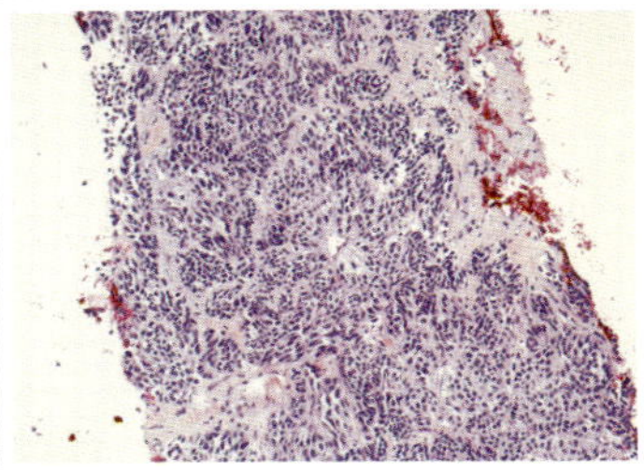
Clear cell change	Uncommon	Mimics other clear cell tumors	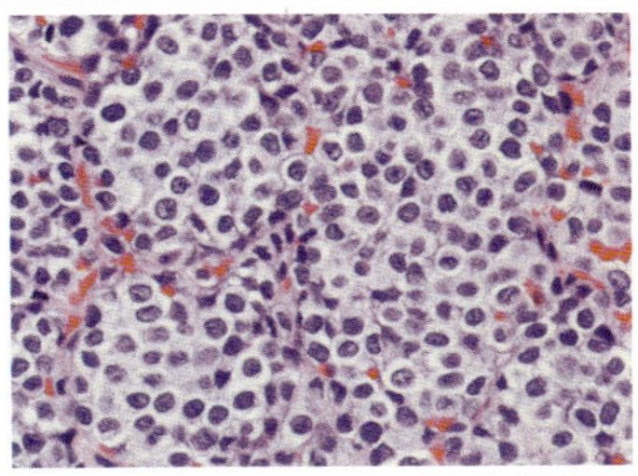
Small round blue cell variant	Uncommon	Requires immunohistochemistry to exclude lymphoma, small cell carcinoma and others	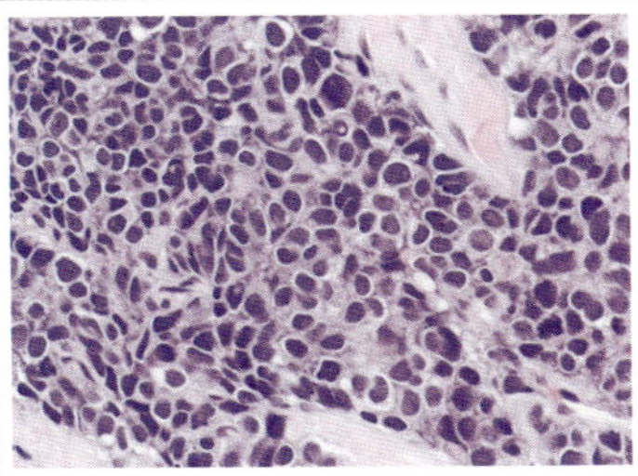

Case table 15.2a: Continued from page 353

Variant feature	Frequency	Comment	Microscopic photo
Rhabdoid alveolar pattern	Rare	Resembles other tumors with alveolar growth pattern. Rhabdoid cells are nonspecific and can be seen in sarcomas, carcinomas and melanoma	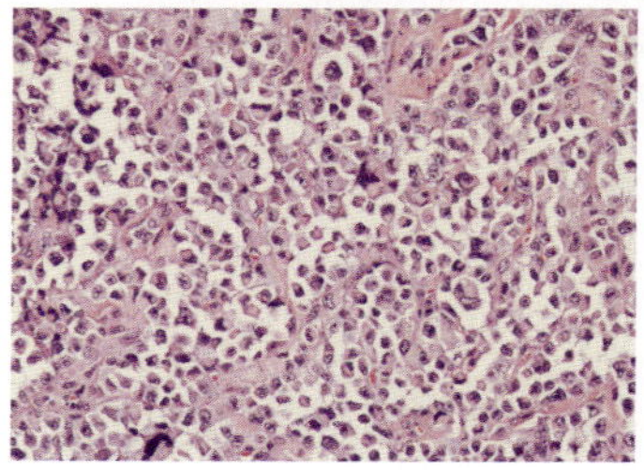
Lack of melanocytic antigen expression	Uncommon	Some metastatic melanomas may express vimentin only or vimentin and MITF. Clinical history, morphology, and lack of expression of antigens denoting other tumors is required for the diagnosis. Genetic testing may also prove useful	
Aberrant antigen expression	Rare	Rare melanomas may express desmin, keratins, or lymphoid markers. These can be challenging cases to diagnose	

Case table 15.2b Summary pathology findings of Case 15.2

Diagnosis	Metastatic melanoma
Size	4.5 cm
Location	Deep soft tissue of thigh
Margin status	Not applicable- no resection attempted
Histologic grade (FNCLCC grading system)	Not applicable- this is a melanoma not a sarcoma
Pathologic stage (AJCC TNM classification)	Stage IV1a

FNCLCC: Fédération Nationale des Centres de Lutte Contre le Cancer (French Federation of Cancer Centers). AJCC: American Joint Committee on Cancer

Until 2011, no medical treatment for melanoma conferred a survival advantage except for 5% of patients treated with interleukin 2 who achieved a complete remission (Korn et al. 2008). In 2011, two very different therapeutic approaches showed a survival advantage. The first approach is a modulation of the immune system with a CTLA4 inhibitor, the monoclonal antibody ipilimumab (Verschraegen 2012). Another immunologic approach to maintain T cell activation involves PD1 antibody, which prevents PD-1 protein from attaching to its ligand on the activated T cell thus halting down-regulation of the immune system (Simeone, et al. 2012).

The third approach targets the *BRAF* V600E mutation, present in 50% of patients, which encodes a hyperactivated tyrosine kinase protein that vemurafenib inhibits (Chapman et al. 2011). This small molecule tyrosine kinase inhibitor induces a 50% overall response rate which lasts for about 9 to 12 months. Many other kinases inhibitors are in clinical trials.

Chemotherapy remains an option with single agent for palliation or neoadjuvant chemotherapy combination to decrease the size of a potentially resectable metastatic tumor. Chemotherapy drugs include dacarbazine, temozolomide, platinum, taxanes, and vinblastine.

The newest Phase I and II trials involve combining immunotherapy with targeted drug therapy. Combinations include ipilimumab with vemurafenib and anti-PD1 antibody with vemurafenib. Initial results are highly encouraging.

This patient, who is enrolled in an anti-PD1 antibody trial, consents to needle core biopsies of her thigh mass prior to start of therapy and after 6 infusions. Predictive of her excellent response, the patient's melanoma cells produce large amounts of PD-1 protein (noted on immunohistochemistry) that the therapeutic PD1 antibody blocks from attaching to inhibitory ligands on T-cells. Following six infusions, the second biopsy of the leg mass reveals a large influx of activated T lymphocytes in the diminished tumor. By infusion #16, PET-CT scan reveals no residual tumor in the patient's thigh, and the previously PET-avid, enlarged iliac lymph node is normal in size with no increased metabolic activity.

Radiation oncology

This patient presented with a nonpainful metastasis involving the proximal left thigh with evidence of ipsilateral pelvic nodal involvement. No other sites of metastatic disease were identified. This is consistent with regional/distal spread of her initial melanoma of the left lower leg. Due to the long time interval between the initial melanoma and this regional recurrence, she likely will have a favorable outcome. Also, recurrence in the nodal region will likely be clinically of greater significance as she is less likely to die of distant metastatic disease. Consequently, I would recommend resection of gross disease followed by adjuvant radiation therapy to the bed of the metastasis and/or the nodal region. This would depend upon the pathology result of the resection.

The role of radiation therapy in the adjuvant setting for melanoma with lymph node involvement is somewhat controversial. Elective nodal radiation and adjuvant nodal radiation of patients with melanoma of the head and neck might decrease the risk of local recurrence (Bonnen et al. 2004, Ballo et al. 2003). This, however, did not translate into any obvious survival benefit. Later Agrawal and Ballo reported in a retrospective study a benefit to local recurrence and disease specific survival with adjuvant nodal radiation after therapeutic dissection (Agrawal et al. 2009). Lastly, an international randomized study demonstrated a statistical improvement in local relapse with adjuvant radiation therapy. No benefit to disease specific survival or overall survival was identified (Burmeister et al. 2012). This patient's case is not specifically a de novo melanoma with lymph node involvement. However, I would argue to treat it as such given her late regional recurrence.

In this case, the patient elected to enroll in a clinical trial and so far has had an excellent outcome.

Patient outcome

The patient has a radiologically confirmed complete response at 6 months and continues on therapy while returning full time to work. The patient's complete response in the setting of Stage IV disease provides further evidence of the efficacy of immune therapy in the treatment of selected patients with high stage melanoma.

Case 15.3 Lymphoma presenting as a solitary mass in soft tissue type: diffuse large B-cell lymphoma, not otherwise specified

Clinical history and presentation

The patient is a 67 year old man who presents with a three month history of an enlarging right buttock mass and progressive sciatic nerve palsy. He is otherwise healthy.

Past history is significant for diabetes mellitus.

Surgical findings and comments

Physical examination reveals a large, deep seated, firm tumor in the right buttock. If is fixed to underlying deep tissue. It is non-tender. Neurologic evaluation reveals diffuse weakness in the sciatic nerve distribution of the right lower extremity. Sensation is diminished over the dorsum of the right foot.

The patient is brought to surgery. A frozen section diagnosis is rendered of 'high grade malignant neoplasm' and the mass is subsequently removed.

Radiology findings

In this case, **Case figs 15.3a** through **15.3f** shows a heterogeneous complex mass of the gluteal musculature with significant adjacent inflammatory reaction. The inflammatory appearance can be seen with malignancy or an infectious process such as a phlegmon or a developing abscess. Lymphomas and metastatic carcinomas can have marked inflammatory reaction.

Interestingly, the tumor shows little enhancement without fluid signal on MRI, most likely due to high nuclear to cytoplasmic ratio seen amongst the group of small round blue cell tumors.

Pathology findings

Gross features

The resection specimen measures 17 × 15 × 8 cm. After differentially inking the outer surface, cross sections reveal a yellow to tan, fleshy to myxoid 10 × 8 × 8 cm mass located in skeletal muscle (**Case fig. 15.3g**). Sample is collected fresh for cytogenetics. Because the tumor is not immediately recognized as hematopoietic, no sample is reserved for flow cytometry, placed in AZF fixative, or used to create touch preps as is the usual protocol for 'rule out lymphoma.' Fortunately, the diagnosis could be rendered without these additional maneuvers.

Microscopic features

Low magnification: The tumor is solid, highly cellular, and infiltrates and replaces skeletal muscle (**Case fig. 15.3h**).

High magnification: At medium magnification, the tumor cells appear bluish purple because of a high N/C ratio and tight packing. The scattered ovoid eosinophilic masses are degenerating skeletal muscle fibers (**Case figure 15.3i**). Tumor cells also surround and infiltrate large nerves.

High magnification reveals a small round blue cell neoplasm with cell or nuclear molding, and high mitotic rate and atypical mitoses. Individual cell necrosis is also present (**Case fig. 15.3j**). By hematopoietic standards, the tumor cells are not small but large and atypical with immunoblastic/plasmablastic features comprising round to irregular nuclei, macronucleoli, and eosinophilic cytoplasm.

Special studies: Neoplastic cells express CD45, CD20 (**Case fig. 15.3k**), Bcl-6, and MUM-1 with a small subset positive for Bcl-2. The Ki-67 proliferation rate is very high (>90%) (**Case fig. 15.3l**). Negative results are noted for ALK-1, CD10, CD138, CD3, EBER, cytokeratins, EMA, S-100, Melan A103, and smooth muscle actin (controls are appropriately reactive). Kappa and lambda in situ hybridization results do not reveal an abnormal plasma cell population. Because the tumor cells express Bcl-6 and MUM-1, this patient's diffuse large B-cell lymphoma is of an activated or post-germinal center phenotype.

Additional biopsies and staging workup: Peripheral blood exam, bilateral bone marrow biopsies and PET-CT scans are negative for other sites of lymphoma involvement.

Pathologic differential or, why isn't it one of the following?

This case illustrates the uncommon situation of a lymphoma presenting as a solitary soft tissue mass that is clinically suggestive of sarcoma. The surgeon thoughtfully requested a frozen section before proceeding with surgery, but a diagnosis of lymphoma could not be immediately rendered. This is because the frozen sections exhibited a small round blue cell morphology which encompasses a broad list of possible diagnoses. With such a differential, only immunohistochemistry (sometimes augmented by genetic analysis) can enable accurate diagnosis. Alas, immunohistochemistry is not a technique amenable to intraoperative interpretation, as it requires several hours to complete.

However, a patient with a possible hematopoietic malignancy ideally should undergo biopsy and Pathology processing appropriate for

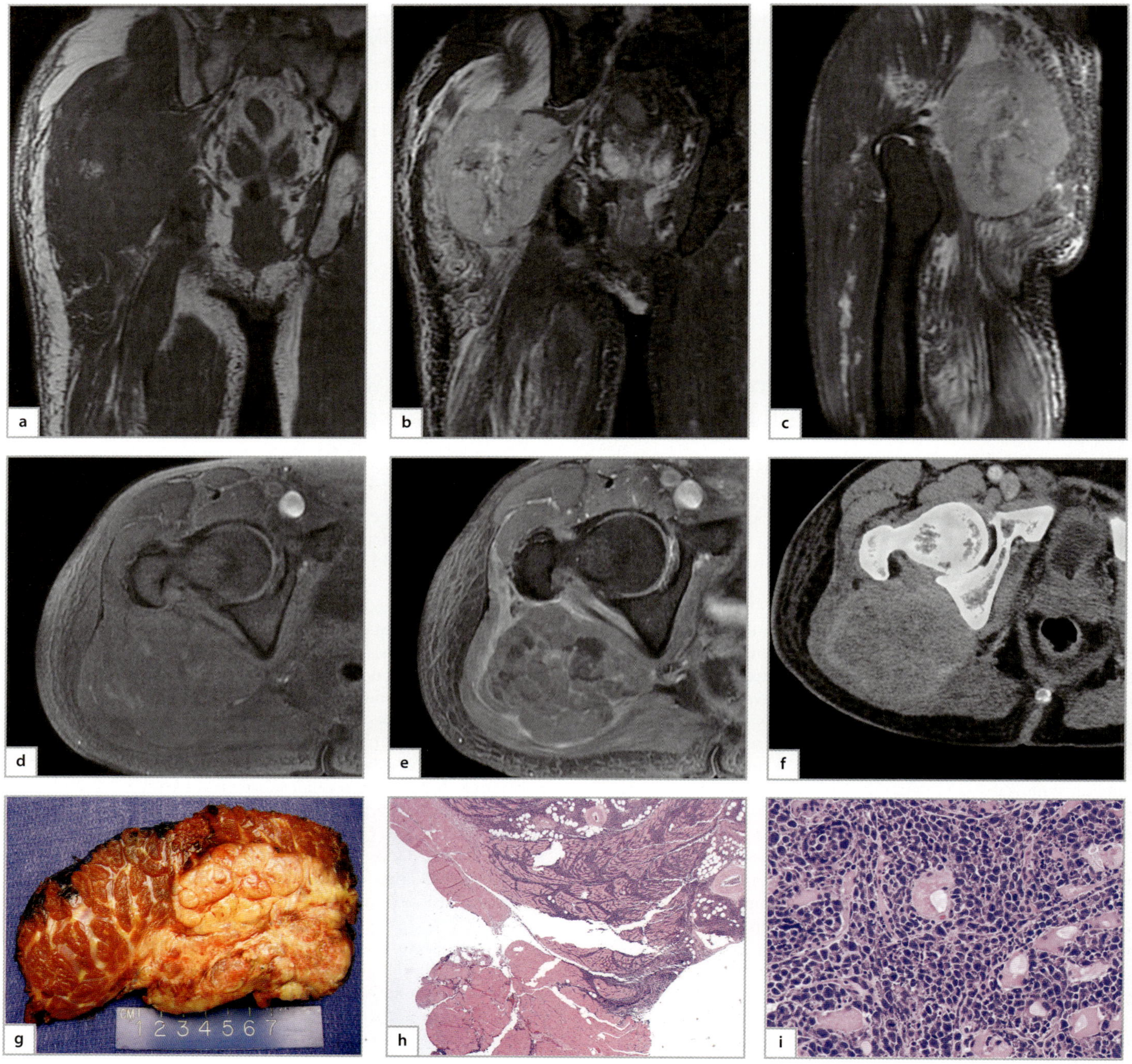

Case figure 15.3 Lymphoma of soft tissue. MR images including: **15.3a**: coronal T1, **15.3b**: Coronal STIR, **15.3c**: Sagittal T2 fat saturated, **15.3d**: Axial T1 fat saturated, **15.3e**: Axial T1 fat saturated post-contrast. The MR images of this 67 year old man show a 9.9 × 8.6 × 11.2 cm heterogeneous mass in the gluteal muscles. The mass shows extensive adjacent skin and muscle edema implying tumor infiltration or inflammatory response. The tumor is predominantly T1 iso-signal intensity with STIR heterogeneous high signal and modest heterogeneous enhancement. **15.3f**: Axial CT image post IV contrast shows modest enhancement and no calcifications. Note the adjacent soft tissue and skin edema even visible by CT imaging. **15.3g**: Gross photo of cross section. This lymphoma resembles sarcoma grossly as it is large, fleshy and multilobulated with areas of hemorrhage and chalky flecks consistent with necrosis. **15.3h**. Low magnification. Although grossly the tumor appears well circumscribed, microscopically it diffusely invades adjacent skeletal muscle. **15.3i**: Medium magnification. Atrophic, degenerated skeletal muscle fibers are surrounded by the malignant infiltrate.

Case figure 15.3: Continued from page 356

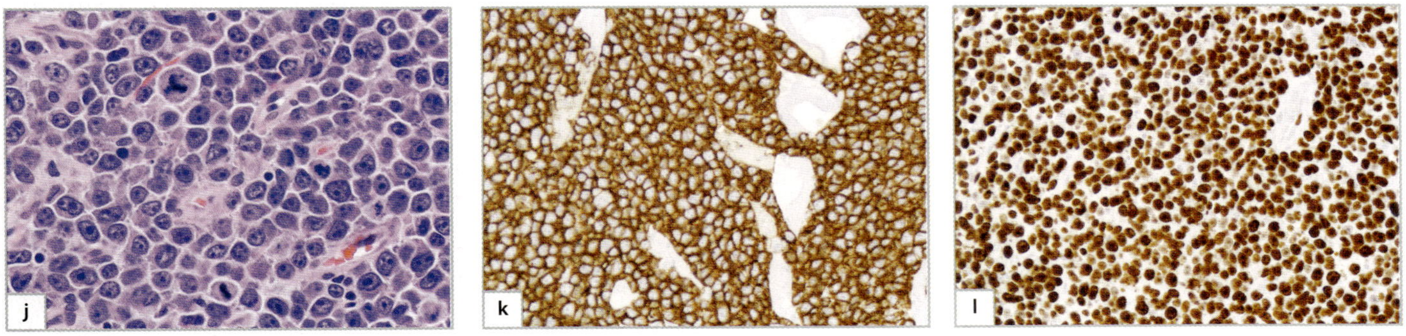

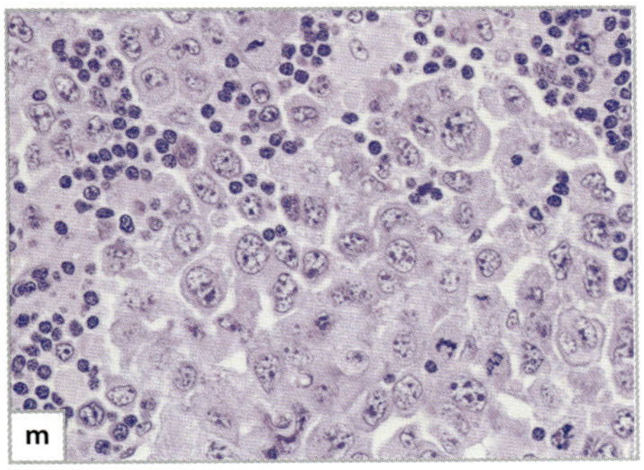

15.3j: High magnification. Tumor cells reveal a 'small round blue cell' morphology which raises several diagnostic possibilities (see text). The open chromatin pattern and subtle cell dyscohesion are consistent with but not specific for lymphoma. The high mitotic rate including atypical mitoses, relatively large size for neoplastic lymphocytes and prominent nucleoli support the diagnosis of a high grade lymphoma. **15.3k**: High magnification, CD20 immunohistochemical stain. The neoplastic lymphocytes are diffusely strongly reactive for CD20 in a membranous pattern. This is consistent with a B-cell lymphoma. **15.3l**: High magnification, Ki67 proliferation rate immunohistochemical stain. Some high grade lymphomas exhibit an astonishingly high proliferation rate: here virtually all the malignant nuclei express Ki-67, a protein expressed only in cycling cells (brown chromogen). A blood vessel with negative endothelial nuclei serves as an internal negative control. **15.3m**: Another patient's diffuse large B-cell lymphoma, anaplastic variant, high magnification. Some diffuse large B-cell lymphomas feature very large cells with multinucleation and marked nuclear pleomorphism, as in this instance. Normal lymphocytes indicate the relatively giant size of the neoplastic lymphocytes. Such cases do not fit into the category of 'small round blue cell tumor,' and extensive immunohistochemical staining may be required to achieve the correct diagnosis.

evaluation for lymphoma. This includes submitting viable fresh tissue for flow cytometry analysis. In this case, a diagnosis was ultimately made in the absence of flow studies. However, with other lymphoma subtypes, lack of flow surface marker studies could compromise the ability to render a specific diagnosis and consequently hinder or delay appropriate treatment.

Expert hematopathologist consultation is preferable when dealing with a lymphoma, leukemic infiltrate, or other hematopoietic lesion. Hematopathology is a complex field requiring advanced training, and the diagnostic and predictive testing entailed in the workup should proceed under the direction of an experienced subspecialist.

Other small round blue cell tumors: Given the patient's age and location of the mass, the most likely small round blue cell tumors in the differential consist of poorly differentiated synovial sarcoma, pure round cell liposarcoma, metastatic melanoma, metastatic poorly differentiated squamous cell carcinoma and metastatic small cell undifferentiated carcinoma. **Case table 15.3a** lists these and other small round blue cell tumors applicable to this patient's presentation and provides the key diagnostic features. In many instances, negative IHC results are as critical as positive results in ruling out an entity. Of course, in many cases, clinical history or imaging studies can be diagnostically helpful.

Other lymphomas: It is not the purpose of this text to provide a detailed review of hematopathology: excellent thick textbooks devoted to that subject assume that duty. It is enough to note that lymphomas may occur in the soft tissue and bone and may present as one or more discrete masses mimicking a sarcoma or other tumor. However, this patient's lymphoma is not classified as primary cutaneous diffuse large B-cell lymphoma, leg type, because it does not involve the skin.

Even if implausible, It is important not to exclude lymphoma as a possibility when biopsying a patient with a solitary soft tissue mass so appropriate triaging is conducted in Pathology to secure an accurate, specific and timely diagnosis. Flow cytometric and most genetic analyses require a fresh, viable sample. In the Pathology suite, a frozen section or touch imprints can be performed at the time of receipt of the biopsy to help determine the optimal testing regimen. Even on immediate evaluation for specimen triaging, a few lymphomas may mimic other tumors such as melanoma, carcinoma, or a sarcoma with epithelioid looking cells (**Case fig. 15.3m**). Clinical and radiologic features must also be considered, especially in morphologically ambiguous cases.

Oncology approach

Medical oncology

The treatment of a diffuse large B-cell lymphoma is the R-CHOP regimen, the CD20 monoclonal antibody, rituximab (Fu et al. 2008) in combination with cyclophosphamide, doxorubicin, prednisone, and vincristine (Fisher et al. 1993, Habermann et al. 2006). The patient received 6 cycles and went into a complete remission. He remains in remission without further treatment. The length of treatment depends on the bulk of the tumor (smaller or greater than 10 cm) and patient characteristics (Solal-Celigny 2006). In this case the patient has no other abnormalities and carries a favorable prognosis. Consideration of radiotherapy was discussed given the fact that this was an isolated lesion involving the sciatic nerve.

Radiation oncology

Diffuse large B-cell lymphoma that is early (Stage I or II) is generally treated with upfront R-CHOP chemotherapy followed by involved field radiation therapy (IF-XRT). The radiotherapy portion remains a controversial element. Multiple randomized studies have been performed, but two of the most commonly quoted are a study from the southwestern oncology group (SWOG 8736) and the eastern cooperative oncology group (ECOG 1484). The SWOG study compared three cycles of CHOP chemotherapy with IF-XRT to eight cycles of CHOP. Initially, this showed an overall survival benefit (Miller et al. 1998), but later analysis showed no overall survival benefit (ASH Abstract,

Case table 15.3a Differential diagnosis of small round blue cell tumors in adults presenting as a soft tissue mass with key diagnostic features

Tumor	Demographics	IHC	Genetics
Lymphoma	Uncommonly presents as a discrete mass Usually older adults	Lymphoid markers positive including: CD45, CD 19 and CD20 (for B-cells) CD3 and CD4 (for T cells); many others used for specific subtyping	Specific translocations occur in subtypes of lymphomas: refer to a hematopathology or general surgical pathology text
Synovial Sarcoma, poorly differentiated variant	Young to middle aged adults most commonly	Positive: EMA, keratins, TLE-1. Sometimes CD99, S-100 protein	t(X;18) in nearly all cases
Round cell liposarcoma	Young to middle aged adults most commonly	May be negative or only focally positive for S-100 protein. Negative for other markers	t(12;16)(q13;p11) or t(12;22)(q13;q12) in nearly all cases
Extraskeletal mesenchymal chondrosarcoma	Young adults to 40 years most commonly.	May be focally positive for S-100 protein and SOX9. Negative for lymphoid markers, TLE-1, keratins	No specific recurrent abnormalities. Usually features a complex karyotype
Ewing sarcoma family of tumors	Rare in older adults; most commonly children and adolescents	CD99 almost always positive with membranous reactivity; FLI-1 also positive in most. Negative for lymphoid markers. Some cases S-100 protein or keratin positive. Negative for TLE-1	Any of several translocations with EWSR1 gene or other TET family member t(11;22)(q24;q12) t(21;22)(q22;q12) t(7;22)(p22;q12) t(17;22)(q12;q12) and others
Merkel cell carcinoma	Older adults. Usually purely dermal. Seldom reaches a size > 5 cm; most are usually 1-2 cm	Positive for chromogranin, synaptophysin, broad spectrum keratins, neurofilament, Merkel cell polyomavirus antigen. Often positive for keratin 20 in a dot-like paranuclear pattern	No specific recurrent abnormalities
Metastatic melanoma, small round blue cell histologic variant	Middle aged to older adults most commonly	Usually reactive for at least one of the following: S-100 protein, HMB-45, Melanocyte A103, MITF	Complex aneuploid karyotype in many cases May have BRAF or ckit mutations
Metastatic small cell undifferentiated carcinoma (poorly differentiated neuroendocrine carcinoma)	Middle aged or older adults	Usually reactive for a marker consistent with neuroendocrine differentiation such as chromogranin, synaptophysin, CD56. Positive for keratins. Negative for lymphoid markers	No specific recurrent abnormalities
Metastatic poorly differentiated squamous cell carcinoma	Middle aged or older adults	Positive for p63 and/or keratins 5/6. Negative or only focally positive for neuroendocrine markers	No specific recurrent abnormalities

Case table 15.3b Summary pathology findings of Case 15.3

Diagnosis	Diffuse large B-cell lymphoma
Size	Single 10 cm lesion
Location	Deep soft tissue of buttock
Margin status	Not applicable as this is a lymphoma
Histologic grade (FNCLCC grading system)	Not applicable- this is a lymphoma not a sarcoma
Pathologic stage (AJCC TNM classification)	Not staged by AJCC system as this is a lymphoma.

FNCLCC: Fédération Nationale des Centres de Lutte Contre le Cancer (French Federation of Cancer Centers). AJCC: American Joint Committee on Cancer

Spier et al. 2004). The ECOG study compared eight cycles of CHOP with or without IF-XRT. This study showed no overall survival benefit (Horning et al. 2004). Both studies showed a benefit to disease free survival. As a result of these studies some favor radiation therapy, and some do not. Both studies incorporated patients with extranodal disease. Of note, a randomized study of patients greater than 60 years of age showed no benefit to overall or event-free survival with the addition of IF-XRT after four cycles of CHOP (Bonnet et al. 2007).

Patient outcome

The patient is currently in complete remission. The patient will be carefully followed because of risk of disease progression with spread to additional sites including lymph nodes, bone marrow and central nervous system.

Case 15.4 Metastatic Ewing sarcoma to epidural region

Clinical history and presentation

The patient is an otherwise healthy 22 year old man who presents with a three month history of a left scapular mass. The mass was noted spontaneously. It has grown progressively in size and now is excruciatingly painful.

Exam of the left shoulder reveals a large soft tissue mass over the posterior aspect of the left shoulder which is firmly fixed to the underlying scapula. He is significantly tender on palpation.

Surgical findings and comments

An open biopsy of the scapular mass is performed.

Staging work-up reveals small pulmonary metastases and increased lactate dehydrogenase in the serum.

The patient is not taken to surgery for resection of the scapular based tumor because of his Stage IV status.

Course of disease

Approximately 8 months after presentation, CT scan reveals interval development of extensive mediastinal metastasis and multifocal osseous metastases prompting re-initiation of chemotherapy. Soon thereafter, the patient presents to the Emergency Room with a chief complaint of sudden sharp chest pain, shortness of breath and numbness in his body. He is otherwise neurologically intact. He has diminished appetite. Physical exam reveals temporal wasting, and the patient is in acute distress. He is found to be neutropenic, thrombocytopenic, and also has low magnesium and phosphate levels. He is treated with Neupogen, appropriate mineral replacement therapy, oxygen, and his pain medications are adjusted.

Two days later, while in the hospital, he develops inability to move his legs and numbness below the waist prompting MRI of the thoracic and lumbar spine. Imaging reveals a T4 epidural mass severely compressing the spinal cord.

The patient and his family request treatment for his epidural mass symptoms. The neurosurgeon consults with the patient's oncologist and discusses the risks of the procedure with the patient and his family. These include death on the operating table from excessive blood loss, inability to extubate him because of diminished respiratory function, development of epidural hematoma due to his thrombocytopenia, complications of his neutropenia including fulminant sepsis, wound infection, and non-wound healing, and possibility of persistent paralysis. The patient and his family elect surgical resection.

Surgical findings and comments

Because of excessive bleeding (although the patient's platelet count was supplemented to over 100,000/ml^3), the patient remains in surgery longer than expected. A gray, soft mass is completely removed, and the patient is successfully closed and taken to the neurosurgical intensive care unit.

Radiology findings

In this case, **Case figs 15.4a** through **15.4g** shows the tragic rapid progression of disease in a patient who presents with metastatic disease to the lung and a scapular primary Ewing sarcoma. At his ten month follow up exam, there is extensive increase in the metastatic disease of the lungs, best shown on the CT image, **Case fig. 15.4g**. There is also extensive new metastatic disease of the marrow seen on the spine MR images, **Case fig. 15.4d**.There is an unusual metastasis within the spinal canal of the mid thoracic spine causing compression of the spinal cord.

Pathology findings

Gross features

The patient's epidural mass consists of multiple fragments of pale gray tissue aggregating to 1.5 cm maximally. It is submitted in entirely for routine processing (given the patient's known disease history).

Microscopic features

Low magnification: The tumor is cellular with a blue-purple appearance due to hypercellularity and low nuclear to cytoplasmic ratio of malignant cells. There are large areas of necrosis.

High magnification: High magnification reveals a relatively uniform population of cells arranged in nests and cords. Malignant cells have indistinct cell borders, clear cytoplasm, and round, normochromatic nuclei with scattered mitoses (**Case fig. 15.4h**). Comparison with the patient's original tumor biopsy reveals identical morphology.

Special studies: A PAS stain without diastase demonstrates cytoplasmic glycogen as the cause of the clear cell appearance (**Case fig. 15.4i**). Although not specific, many Ewing sarcoma tumors contain abundant intracellular glycogen. Characteristic of Ewing sarcoma family of tumors, the malignant cells express CD99 in a strong membranous pattern (**Case fig. 15.4j**).

Pathologic differential or, why isn't it one of the following?

Other small round blue cell tumors: It is possible that the patient could develop iatrogenic lymphoma in this short time frame. However, the morphology of the tumor and its immunohistochemical profile match the features of his original tumor which was also shown to be positive for an EWS translocation by FISH. It is a classic Ewing sarcoma by clinical presentation, initial imaging findings, histology, IHC, and genetics.

Oncology approach

Medical oncology

The patient is treated with the dose dense schedule of AEWS0031 (a Children Oncology Group clinical trial), off protocol because it is closed to accrual. The dose dense arm was found to improve survival (see description of the Ewing case in the Ewing Chapter). The chemotherapy consists of an alternance of vincristine, cyclophosphamide, and doxorubicin with 2 weeks later ifosfamide and etoposide. Filgrastim is administered to induce a quick marrow recovery between cycles of chemotherapy. Stem cells are collected after the third course of chemotherapy for a consolidation with autologous stem cell transplantation. Chemotherapy including the transplant is completed in 5 months, and the bed of the tumor is treated with radiation for 7 weeks (see Radiation Oncology below). Unfortunately, the tumor recurs one month after completion of the radiation with fulminant node, lung and bone metastases. One month later, despite salvage chemotherapy with cisplatin and irinotecan, the patient develops an epidural lesion compressing the thoracic cord.

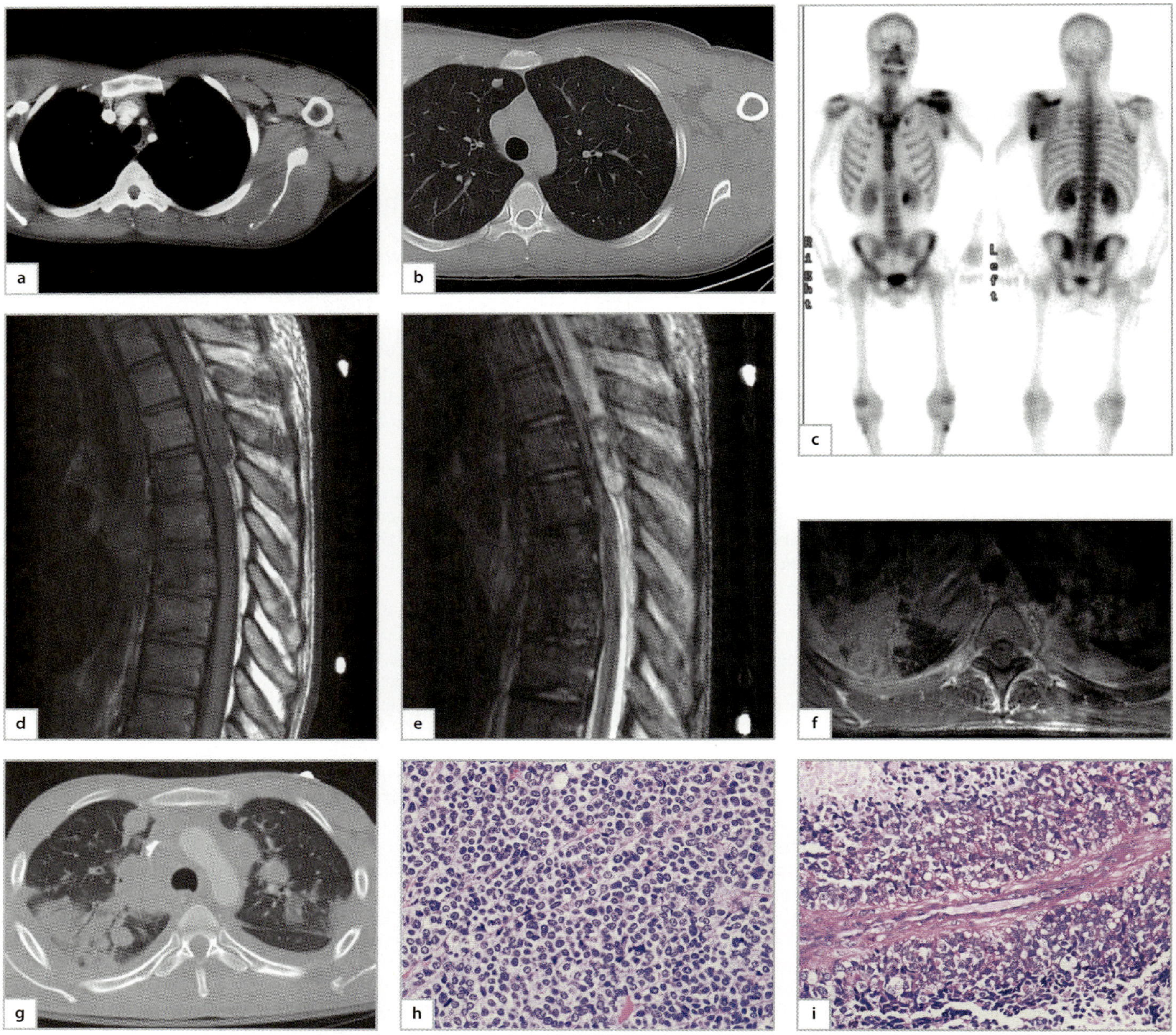

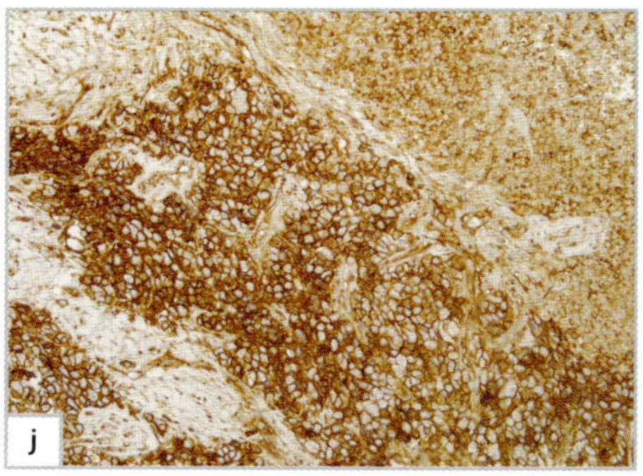

Case figure 15.4 Ewing sarcoma with metastasis. **15.4a**: Axial soft tissue window and **15.4b**: Axial bone window CT images after IV contrast. There is a destructive lesion of the left scapular body measuring 7.5 × 8.6 × 7.6 cm. The mass is slightly less dense than the surrounding muscles. Note the 9 mm nodule in the right upper lobe of the lung consistent with metastasis. The initial bone scan, **15.4c**: Shows the increased uptake of the left shoulder affecting the scapula and proximal humerus. Subsequent MR images obtained 10 months later of the spine include; **15.4d**: Sagittal T1, **15.4e**: Sagittal T2, and **15.4f**: Axial T1 fat saturated post-contrast. These show a 3.3 × 2.1 × 1 cm mass within the spinal canal at the T4 – T5 level causing significant impingement of the cord. There are also extensive metastatic infiltration of the marrow throughout the thoracic spine. There are numerous metastases of the lungs and pleura. **15.4g**: Is an axial post contrast CT scan also showing the extensive pleural and parenchymal metastasis. Note there is partial healing of the scapula from the original primary tumor. **15.4h**: Medium magnification. The tumor comprises fairly uniform small cells with clear cytoplasm disposed in vague columns and nests. Tumor nuclei are round to oval, normochromatic and lack prominent nucleoli. Mitotic activity averages 10 mitoses per 10 high magnification microscopic fields (a moderate rate). **15.4i**: PAS without diastase special stain, high magnification. Viable tumor cells clinging on either side of a blood vessel contain magenta granules consistent with glycogen. Although not specific, many Ewing sarcoma family tumors feature clear cytoplasm due to abundant glycogen. Notice the necrosis as tumor cells become egress from the feeding vessel. **15.4j**: CD99 immunohistochemical stain, medium magnification, brown chromogen. Characteristically, Ewing sarcoma tumor cells express CD99 in a strong membranous pattern. Note that the necrotic tumor cells at the upper right of the field exhibit nonspecific granular cytoplasmic staining. Since only membranous reactivity is more specific for Ewing sarcoma, this photomicrograph illustrates the importance of biopsying viable tumor in order to enable the correct diagnosis.

Case table 15.4 Summary pathology findings of Case 15.4

Diagnosis	Ewing sarcoma
Size	3.3 × 2.1 × 1 cm epidural mass
Location	Multiple metastases to lung, mediastinum skeleton and spinal cord
Margin status	Palliative resection of epidural mass is performed
Histologic grade (FNCLCC grading system)	High grade (Grade 3)
Pathologic stage (AJCC TNM classification)	Stage IV

FNCLCC: Fédération Nationale des Centres de Lutte Contre le Cancer (French Federation of Cancer Centers). AJCC: American Joint Committee on Cancer

The prognosis of patients with Ewing sarcoma is based on pretreatment factors and response to neoadjuvant chemotherapy. Favorable pretreatment factors include distal site, smaller size, younger age, female gender, normal serum lactate dehydrogenase, absence of metastases, and noncomplex cytogenetics (Cotterill et al. 2000, Rodriguez-Galindo et al. 2007). Minimal or no residual viable tumor after neoadjuvant chemotherapy confers a significantly better event-free survival compared with patients with larger amounts of viable tumor (Paulussen et al. 2001). The characteristics not considered to be adverse prognostic factors include pathologic fracture, neural differentiation and the EWS-FL1 translocation (Le Deley et al. 2010). Except for non-complex cytogenetics and excellent response to neoadjuvant chemotherapy, this patient has all the poor prognostic factors.

Radiation oncology

In this case, I would recommend surgery followed by radiation therapy for palliation. The patient's prognosis is poor and long term survival in children with bone and lung metastasis is low. Radiation therapy for spinal cord compression or cauda equine syndrome is well established. A randomized study does demonstrate the superiority of surgery followed by radiation therapy over radiation therapy alone with 84% able to ambulate in the surgery plus radiation group and 57% in the radiation only group (Patchell et al. 2005).

Patient outcome

Despite aggressive systemic therapy, the patient develops widespread bony and soft tissue metastases over the ensuing eight months, including a thoracic epidural metastasis requiring surgical decompression to attempt to alleviate paralysis. Although the epidural tumor is successfully removed by laminectomy, the patient soon develops pulmonary infiltrates consistent with pneumonia or progression of Ewing sarcoma, and he is re-intubated one day after his surgery. At a family meeting, the clinical care team informs the patient and his family of his likely inability to survive without intubation, and comfort care is described in detail. The patient and his family decide on extubation, he is started on analgesics and sedatives, and he expires several hours after extubation.

This tragic outcome is in keeping with the fate of most patients presenting with Stage IV Ewing sarcoma for which overall survival is less than 20% (Spraker et al. 2012). Unfortunately, approximately 25% of patients present with metastatic disease (van Maldegem et al. 2012).

Case 15.5 Breast carcinoma metastatic to bone

Clinical history and presentation

The patient is a 61-year-old female who presents with a recently noted right axillary mass. The mass was spontaneously noted and is asymptomatic

The patient's past medical history is significant for hypertension. There is no family history of breast or other cancer.

Physical examination reveals the left breast to be normal without masses. The right breast has a 4 × 6 cm mass in the upper outer quadrant. In the axilla, there is a 4 × 4 cm mass close to the tail of the axilla, and there is also some fullness higher up in the axilla.

Core needle biopsy of both masses is performed and is consistent with invasive ductal breast carcinoma with regional metastasis. The tumor is estrogen and progesterone receptor positive and HER-2/Neu is not overexpressed.

She is treated with neoadjuvant tamoxifen, a year later undergoes modified radical mastectomy. Three months later, she develops a right supraclavicular node that is positive on fine needle aspiration biopsy for metastatic breast carcinoma. She receives radiation therapy of the right supraclavicular area, right chest wall, and appropriate boost for seven weeks (see Radiation Oncology below).

Twenty-one months later she remains on tamoxifen and is clinically free of disease. Four months after this visit she presents with a pathologic fracture of the right humerus during normal use of the arm.

Surgical findings and comments

Open reduction and internal fixation of the fracture is performed along with bone cement augmentation of the humeral defect.

Fifteen months later the patient has stable pulmonary metastases and additional bone metastases. She has regained functional use of the right arm and shoulder with minimal pain.

Radiology findings

In this case, **Case figs 15.5a** through **15.5c** shows the evolution of bone metastatic disease over a 3 year interval. Initially, the right humeral lesion is discernible as a subtle focus of activity on the first bone scan. The patient subsequently develops a pathologic fracture through the humeral lesion with several new bone metastases. The humeral lesion shows a classic permeative destruction pattern indicative of a highly aggressive lesion.

Pathology findings

Gross features

The specimen consists of abundant curettings of bone and soft tissue aggregating to 8 × 5 × 2 cm. Six cassettes are submitted for routine histology. This includes three cassettes of bone fragments processed after decalcification. Although there is no gross photo of this patient's metastatic tumor, another patient's carcinoma metastatic to the femur

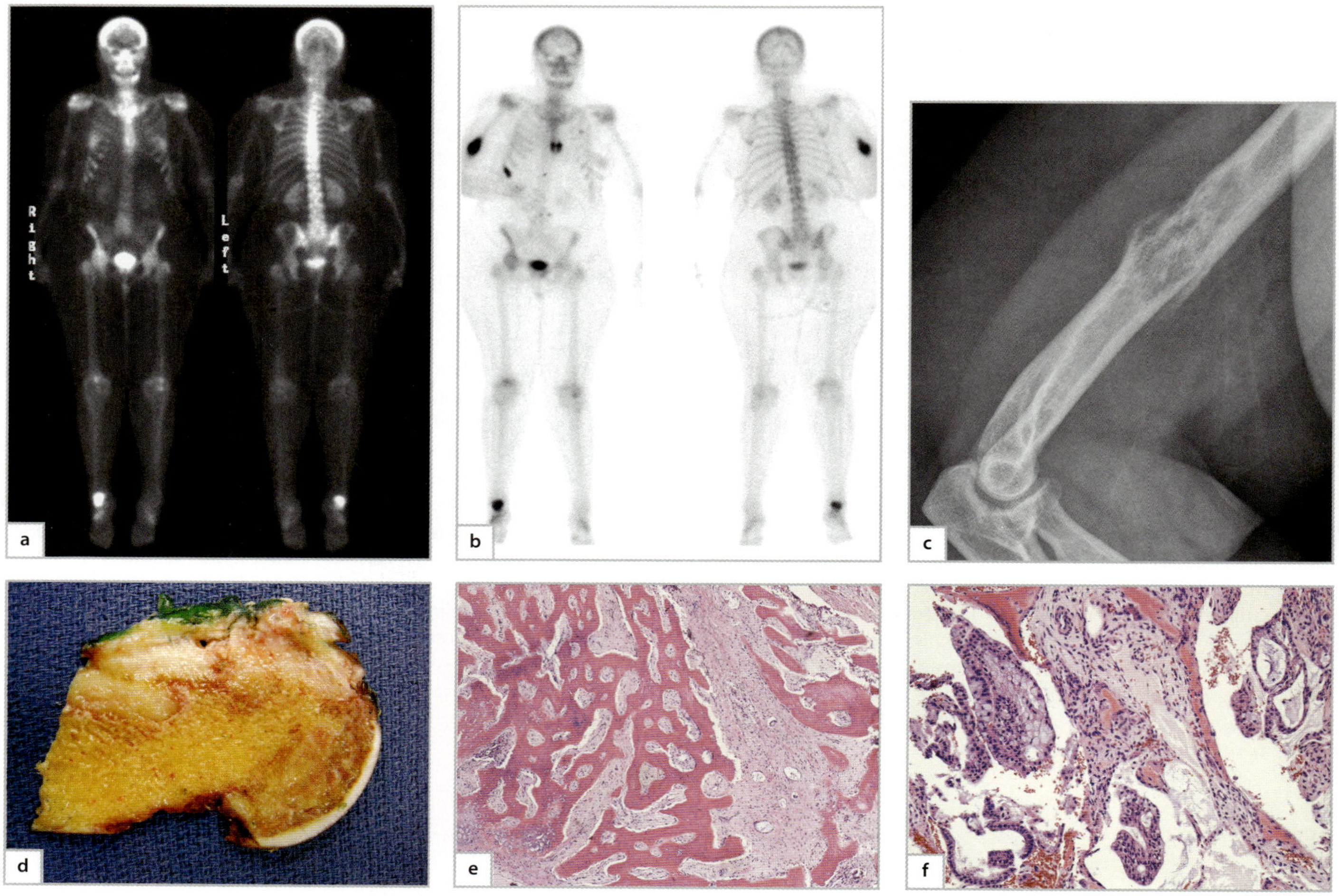

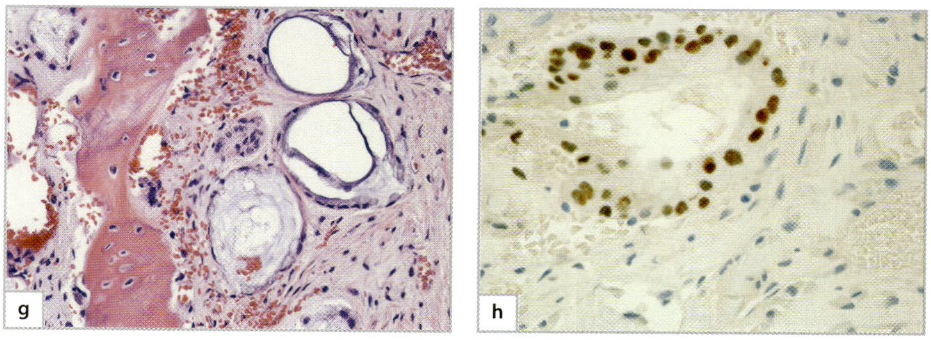

Case figure 15.5 Breast carcinoma metastasis. **15.5a**: Is the initial bone scan showing very subtle increased uptake of the mid right humeral diaphysis in this 65 year old woman. There is marked increase uptake of the right ankle, thought to be from osteoarthritis. The follow up bone scan, **15.5b**: Obtained nearly 3 years later shows marked increased uptake of the right humeral lesion. The right ankle uptake is unchanged. There are new lesions of the right 9th rib and the sternum. Radiographs taken at the time of the follow up bone scan, and **15.5c**: Lateral views show a pathologic fracture through the right humeral lesions. This metastasis measures about 6.2 × 2.6 × 3.6 cm and has permeative destruction of bone. **15.5d**: Another patient with metastatic breast carcinoma to bone, gross cross section. In this section of femur, osteolytic tumor forms soft tan nodules that destroy medullary bone and cortex (top) while less obvious osteoblastic tumor intercalates among preserved trabeculae (irregular tan glistening tumor beneath cortical bone bottom right). Close scrutiny reveals another small subcortical focus of tumor (bottom left). **15.5e**: Low magnification. The long anastomosing strands of bone in this photomicrograph are reactive and indicate an osteoblastic response to metastatic carcinoma noticeable as small cystic glands. **15.5f**: Medium magnification. The patient's tumor is well-differentiated and forms recognizable glands and papillary structures. The normal marrow is replaced by a sparse amount of metastatic tumor that is inciting a prominent fibroblastic reaction. **15.5g**: High magnification. This field captures the three main elements of the process: metastatic, mucin producing glands, fibrous to fibroblastic stroma, and reactive new bone. **15.5h**: Estrogen receptor immunohistochemical stain, high magnification, brown chromogen. Tumor cells express estrogen receptor (nuclear reactivity) consistent with metastatic breast carcinoma.

is provided as a representative macroscopic appearance of metastatic carcinoma to bone (**Case fig. 15.5d**).

Microscopic features

Low magnification: The tumor evokes an osteoblastic reaction with abundant reactive new bone (**Case fig. 15.5e**). Breast carcinoma is one of the few carcinomas that regularly forms osteoblastic metastatic deposits.

High magnification: At medium magnification, the tumor consists of glands and gland aggregates that produce abundant mucin (**Case fig. 15.5f**). Tumor cells are uniform and well-differentiated, and the surrounding marrow demonstrates a fibrotic reaction to the metastatic glands (**Case fig. 15.5g**).

Special studies: Because of the slightly unusual mucinous nature of the adenocarcinoma considering the probable origin from the patient's breast carcinoma, immunohistochemical staining is performed. Estrogen receptor is expressed in 75% of tumor cells at 2-3+ intensity (**Case fig. 15.5h**), and there is no expression of PR receptor. These results are consistent with metastatic well-differentiated mucinous carcinoma of the breast.

Pathologic differential or, why isn't it one of the following?

Other carcinomas: Without a history of a specific carcinoma, this patient's metastasis could derive from any number of primary tumors. However, breast and lung carcinoma would be the most likely candidates given the patient's age, gender, and the histologic features. Less likely candidates would include colorectal, stomach, and pancreatic primaries. Clinical history, imaging studies, and immunohistochemistry can resolve the origin of most carcinomas metastatic to the skeleton. In this case, the osteoblastic nature of the tumor on imaging also strongly suggests breast carcinoma origin. In a male, osteoblastic bone metastases would highly favor prostatic adenocarcinoma as the source.

Case table 15.5 Summary pathology findings of Case 15.5

Diagnosis	Metastatic breast adenocarcinoma
Size	4.3 × 2.8 × 2.9 cm
Location	Humerus, other bone sites and lymph node
Margin status	Negative
Histologic grade (FNCLCC grading system)	Not applicable- this is a carcinoma not a sarcoma
Pathologic stage (AJCC TNM classification)	Stage IV

FNCLCC: Fédération Nationale des Centres de Lutte Contre le Cancer (French Federation of Cancer Centers). AJCC: American Joint Committee on Cancer

Oncology approach

Medical oncology

Postmenopausal patients with hormone receptor positive tumors are best treated with hormonal manipulation (Gibson et al. 2009, Howell et al. 2005, Thurlimann et al. 2005). Drugs include non-steroidal aromatase inhibitors such as anastrozole or letrozole, steroidal aromatase inactivators such as exemestane, estrogen receptor antagonists such as fulvestrant, serum estrogen receptor modulators such as tamoxifen or toremifene, progestogens such as megestrol acetate, estrogens such as ethynyl estradiol, or androgens such as fluoxymesterone. Everolimus an M-Tor pathway inhibitor, combined with an aromatase inhibitor also improves progression-free survival in patients with hormone-receptor–positive advanced breast cancer previously treated with nonsteroidal aromatase inhibitors (Baselga et al. 2012).

However, symptomatic localized lesions should be treated with local treatments, such as surgery, radiotherapy or both as in this case. The pathologic fracture is fixed surgically and shows the disappearance of the progesterone receptor expression, while maintaining estrogen receptor expression (Bogina et al. 2011). A bone scan shows metastatic disease in the distal right tibia, right ninth rib and the sternum. The patient is switched to another hormonal therapy (Largillier et al. 2008), letrozole at 2.5 mg/day and is referred for consideration of radiation therapy. Once the radiotherapy is completed, she starts on a bisphosphonate to prevent further development of bony metastases (Gralow et al. 2009)

Radiation oncology

In this case, radiation therapy is administered following open reduction and internal fixation. This probably represents the standard approach to pathologic fracture. Recurrence following this approach can occur, but is rare. The efficacy of radiation therapy following stabilization has never been formally studied, but some reports associate recurrence with cases that did not receive radiation (Wedin et al. 1999).

Patient outcome

The patient remains on hormonal treatment without further progression of disease.

REFERENCES

Abrams HL. Skeletal metastases in carcinoma. Radiology 1950;55(4):534–8.

Agrawal S, Kane JM 3rd, Guadagnolo BA, et al. The benefits of adjuvant radiation therapy after therapeutic lymphadenectomy for clinically advanced, high-risk, lymph node-metastatic melanoma. Cancer 2009;115(24):5836–44

Applebaum MA, Worch J, Matthay KK, et al. Clinical features and outcomes inpatients with extraskeletal Ewing sarcoma. Cancer 2011;117:3027–32.

Ballo MT, Bonnen MD, Garden AS, et al. Adjuvant irradiation for cervical lymph node metastases from melanoma. Cancer 2003;97(7):1789–96.

Baselga J, Campone M, Piccart M, et al. Everolimus in postmenopausal hormone-receptor-positive advanced breast cancer. N Engl J Med 2012; 366–520-9.

Bernatchez C, Radvanyi LG, Hwu P. Advances in the treatment of metastatic melanoma: adoptive T-cell therapy. Semin Oncol 2012;39(2):215–26.

Bhatia S, Thompson JA. Systemic therapy for metastatic melanoma in 2012: dawn of a new era. J Natl Compr Canc Netw 2012;10(3):403–12.

Biermann JS, Holt GE, Lewis VO, et al. Metastatic bone disease: diagnosis, evaluation, and treatment. J Bone Joint Surg 2009;91:1518–1530.

Blitzer PH. Reanalysis of the RTOG study of the palliation of symptomatic osseous metastasis. Cancer 1985;55:1468–1472.

Bogina G, Bortesi L, Marconi M, et al. Comparison of hormonal receptor and HER-2 status between breast primary tumours and relapsing tumours: clinical implications of progesterone receptor loss. Virhows Arch 2011;459:1–10.

Bonnen MD, Ballo MT, Myers JN, et al. Elective radiotherapy provides regional control for patients with cutaneous melanoma of the head and neck. Cancer 2004;100(2):383–9.

Bonnet C, Fillet G, Mounier N, et al and Groupe d'Etude des Lymphomes de l'Adulte. CHOP alone compared with CHOP plus radiotherapy for localized aggressive lymphoma in elderly patients: a study by the Groupe d'Etude des Lymphomes de l'Adulte. J Clin Oncol 2007;25(7):787–92.

British Association of Surgical Oncology Guidelines. The management of metastatic bone disease in the United Kingdom. The Breast Speciality Group of the British Association of Surgical Oncology. Eur J Surg Oncol 1999;25(1):3–23.

Buijs JT, van der Pluijm G. Osteotropic cancers: from primary tumor to bone. Cancer Lett 2009;2373(2):177–93.

Burmeister BH, Henderson MA, Ainslie J, et al. Adjuvant radiotherapy versus observation alone for patients at risk of lymph-node field relapse after therapeutic lymphadenectomy for melanoma: a randomised trial. Lancet Oncol 2012;13(6):589–97.

Campbell BA, Voss N, Woods R, et al. Long-term outcomes for patients with limited stage follicular lymphoma: involved regional radiotherapy versus involved node radiotherapy. Cancer 2010;116:3797–806.

Caudle AS, Ross MI. Metastatectomy for stage IV melanoma: for whom and how much? Surg Oncol Clin N Am 2011;20(1):133–144.

Chapman PB, Hauschild A, Robert C, et al. Improved survival with vemurafenib in melanoma with BRAFV600E mutation. N Engl J Med 2011;364:2507–16.

Coghlin C, Murrary GI. Current and emerging concepts in tumour metastasis. J Pathol 2010;222(1):1–15.

Coleman RE. Bone cancer in 2011: Prevention and treatment of bone metastases. Nat Rev Clin Oncol 2011;9(2):76–8.

Coppin C, Kollmannsberger C, Le I, et al. Targeted therapy for advanced renal cell carcinoma (RCC): a Cochrane systemic review of published randomized trials. BHU Int 2011;108:1556–63.

Cotterill SJ, Ahrens S, Paulussen M, et al. Prognostic factors in Ewing's tumor of bone: analysis of 975 patients from the European Intergroup Cooperative Ewing's Sarcoma Study Group. J Clin Oncol 2000;18:3108–14.

Damron TA, Heiner J. Distant soft tissue metastases: a series of 30 new patients and 91 cases from the literature. Ann Surg Oncol 2000;7(7):526–34.

Damron TA, Heiner J. Management of metastatic disease to soft tissue. Orthop Clin North Am 2000;31:661–73,ix.

Divoli A, Mendonca EA, Evans JA, et al. Conflicting biomedical assumptions for mathematical modeling: The case of cancer metastasis. PLOS Comput Biol 2011;7(10):e1002132.

Dorfman, Howard D., Bogdan Dzerniak. Bone Tumors. Mosby Inc.: St. Louis, USA, 1998.

Dundr P, Povysil C, Tvrdik D. Actin expression in neural crest cell-derived tumors including schwannomas, malignant peripheral nerve sheath tumors, neurofibromas and melanocytic tumors. Pathol Int 2009;59(2):86–90.

Fidler IJ. The pathogenesis of cancer metastasis: the 'seed and soil' hypothesis revisited. Nat Rev Cancer 2003;3(6):453–8.

Fisher RI, Gaynor ER, Dahlberg S, et al. Comparison of a standard regiment (CHOP) with three intensive chemotherapy regiments for advanced non-Hodgkin's lymphoma. N Eng J Med 1993;328:1002–6.

Fizazi K, Carducci M, Smith, M, et al. Denosumab versus zoledronic acid for treatment of bone metastasesin men with castration-resistant prostate cancer: a randomized, double-blind study. Lancet 2011;377(9768):813–22.

Fu K, Weisenburger DD, Choi WW, et al. Addition of rituximab to standard chemotherapy improves the survival of both the germinal center B-cell-like and non-germinal center B-cell-like subtypes of diffuse large B-cell lymphoma. J Clin Oncol 2008;26:4587–94.

Fuxe J, Karlsson MC. TGF-β-induced epithelial-mesenchymal transition: A link between cancer and inflammation. Semin Cancer Biol 2012;22(5-6):455–61.

Gibson L, Lawrence D, Dawson, et al. Aromatase inhibitors for treatment of advanced breast cancer in postmenopausal women. Cochrane Database Syst Rev 2009;CD003370.

Gralow JR, Biemann JS, Farooki A, et al. NCCN Task Force Report: Bone Health in Cancer Care. J Natl Compr Canc Netw 2009;7 Suppl 3:S1-32; quiz S33–5.

Greenspan, Adam; Jundt, Gernot; Remagen, Wolgang. Differential Diagnosis in Orthopaedic Oncology, 2nd Edition. Lippincott Williams and Wilkins: Philadelphia, USA, 2007.

Habermann TM, Weller EA, Morrison VA, et al. Rituximab-CHOP versus CHOP alone or with maintenance rituximab in older patients with diffuse large B-cell lymphoma. J Clin Oncol 2006;24:3121–7.

Hartsell WF, Scott CB, Bruner DW, et al. Randomized trial of short- versus long-course radiotherapy for palliation of painful bone metastases. J Natl Cancer Inst 2005;97(11):798–804.

Hellman S, Weichselbaum RR. Oligometastasis, J Clin Oncol 1995;13(1):8–10.

Horning SJ, Weller E, Kim K, et al. Chemotherapy with or without radiotherapy in limited-stage diffuse aggressive non-Hodgkin's lymphoma: Eastern Cooperative Oncology Group study 1484. J Clin Oncol 2004;22(15):3032–8

Howell A, Cuzick J, Baum M, et al. Results of the ATAC (Arimidex, Tamoxifen, Alone or in Combination) trial after completion of 5 years' adjuvant treatment for breast cancer. Lancet 2005;365:60–2.

Hudes G, Carducci M, Tomczak P, et al. Temsirolimus, interferon alfa, or both for advanced renal-cell carcinoma. N Engl J Med 2007;356:2271–81.

Hung CC, Pan CC, Lin CC, et al. XP11.2 translocation renal cell carcinoma: clinical experience of Taipei Veterans General Hospital. J Chin Med Associ 2011:74(11):500–4.

Kane III JM, Finley JW, Driscoll D, et al. The treatment and outcome of patients with soft tissue sarcomas and synchronous metastases. Sarcoma 2002;6(2):69–73.

Kelly M, Lee M, Clarkson P, et al. Metastatic disease of the long bones: a review of the health care burden in a major trauma centre. Can J Surg 2012;55(2):95–8.

Klatte T, Streubel B, Wrba F, et al. Renal cell carcinoma associated with transcription factor E3 expression and Xp11.2 translocation: incidence, characteristics, and prognosis. Am J Clin pathol 2012;137(5):761–8.

Korn EL, Liu PY, Lee SJ, et al. Meta-analysis of phase II cooperative group trials in metastatic stage IV melanoma to determine progression-free and overall survival benchmarks for future phase II trials. J Clin Oncol 2008;26:527–34.

Langley RR, Fidler IJ. The seed and soil hypothesis revisited – The role of tumor-stroma interactions in metastasis to different organs. Int J Cancer 2011;128(11):2527–35.

Largillier R, Ferrero JM, Doyen J, et al. Prognostic factors in 1,038 women with metastatic breast cancer. Ann Oncol 2008;19:2012–9

Le Deley MC, Delattre O, Schaefer KL, et al. Impact of EWS-ETS fusion type on disease progression in Ewing's sarcoma/peripheral primitive neuroectodermal tumor: prospective results from the cooperative Euro-E.W.I.N.G. 99 trial. J clin Oncol 2010;28:1982–8.

Mathot L, Stenninger J. Behavior of seeds and soil in the mechanisms of metastasis: A deeper understanding. Cancer Sol 2012;103(4):626–31.

Mellman I, Coukos G, Dranoff G. Cancer immunotherapy comes of age. Nature 2011;480(7378):480–9.

Milano MT, Katz AW, Zhang H, Okunieff P. Oligometastases treated with stereotactic body radiotherapy: long-term follow-up of prospective study. Int J Radiat Oncol Biol Phys 2012;83(3):878–86.

Miller TP, Dahlberg S, Cassady JR, et al. Chemotherapy alone compared with chemotherapy plus radiotherapy for localized intermediate- and high-grade non-Hodgkin's lymphoma. N Engl J Med 1998;339(1):21–6.

Mohlendick B, Niederacher D, Stoecklein NH. From primary to secondary cancer formation – models for disseminating cancer cells. Drug Discovery Today: Disease Models 2011;8:2–3.
Monteiro J, Fodde R. Cancer stemness and metastasis: therapeutic consequences and perspectives. Eur J Cancer 2010;46(7):1198–203.
Morra L, Moch H. Periostin expression and epithelial-mesenchymal transition in cancer: a review and an update. Virchows Arch 2011;459(5):465–75.
Nakashima, Yasuaki. Bone and Soft Tissue Pathology: A Volume in the Series Foundations in Diagnostic Pathology. Chapter 24 'Metastases involving bone'. Andrew L. Folpe, Carrie Y. Inwards. Saunders Elsevier: Philadelphia, USA, 2010.
Neeman E, Ben-Eliyahua S. Surgery and stress promote cancer metastasis: New outlooks on perioperative mediating mechanisms and immune involvement. Brain Behav Immun 2013;30 Suppl:S32–40.
Nguyen NC, Chaar BT, Osman M. Prevalence and patterns of soft tissue metastasis: detection with true whole-body F-18 FDGPET/CT. BMC Med Imaging 2007:7:8.
Ollila DW, Gleisner AL, Hsueh EC. Rationale for complete metastasectomy in patients with stage IV metastatic melanoma. J Surg Oncol 2011;104(4): 420–424.
Park SI, Soki FN, McCauley LK. Roles of bone marrow cells in skeletal metastases: No longer bystanders. Cancer Microenviron 2011;4(3):237–46.
Patchell RA, Tibbs PA, Regine WF, et al. Direct decompressive surgical resection in the treatment of spinal cord compression caused by metastatic cancer: a randomised trial. Lancet 2005;366(9486):643–8.
Paulussen M, Ahrens S, Dunst J, et al. Localized Ewing tumor of bone: final results off the cooperative Ewing's Sarcoma Study CESS 86. J Clin Oncol 2001;19:1818–29.
Plaza JA, Perez-Montiel D, Mayerson J, et al. Metastases to soft tissue: A review of 118 cases over a 30-year period. Cancer 2008;112(1):193–203.
Purushotham A, Pinder S, Cariati M, et al. Neoadjuvant chemotherapy: not the best option in estrogen receptor-positive, HER2-negative, invasive classical lobular carcinoma of the breast? J Clin Oncol 2010;28:3552–4.
Rekhtman Natasha; Bishop, Justin A. Quick Reference Handbook for Surgical Pathologists. Springer-Verlag: Berlin Heidelberg, 2011.
Ribatti D, Mangialardi G, Vacca A. Stephen Paget and the 'seed and soil' theory of metastatic dissemination. Clin Exp Med 2006;6(4):145–9.
Rodriguez-Galindo C, Liu T, Krasin MJ, et al. Analysis of prognostic factors in ewing sarcoma family of tumors: review of St. Jude Children's Research Hospital studies. Cancer 2007;110:375–84.
Ruan K, Bao S, Ouyang G. The multifaceted role of periostin in tumorigenesis. Cell Mol Like Sol 2009;66(14):2219–30.
Salama JK, Hasselle MD, Chmura SJ, et al. Stereotactic body radiotherapy for multisite extracranial oligometastases. Cancer 2012;118(11):2962–70.
Shaffer K. Imaging cancer of unknown primary site. In: Kufe DW, Pollock RE, Weichselbaum RR, et al., eds Holland-Frei Cancer Medicine. 6th edition. Hamilton (ON) : BC Decker; 2003. Chapter 36a
Simeone E, Ascierto PA. Immunomodulating antibodies in the treatment of metastatic melanoma: The experience with anti-CTLA-4, anti-CD137, and anti-PD1. J Immunotoxicol 2012;9(3):241–7.
Singletary SE, Patel-Parekh L, Bland KI. Treatment trends in early-stage invasive lobular carcinoma: A report from the National Cancer Data Base. Ann Surg 2005;242:281–9.
Sleeman JP, Christofori G, Fodde R, et al. Concepts of metastasis in flux: The stromal progression model. Semin Cancer Biol 2012;22(3):174–86.
Smith MR, Saad F, Coleman R, et al. Denosumab and bone-metastasis-free survival in men with castration-resistant prostate cancer: results of a phase 3, randomized, placebo-controlled trial. Lancet 2012;379(9810):39–46
Solal-Celigny P. Follicular Lymphoma Internal Prognostic Index. Curr Treat Options Oncol 2006;7:270–5.
Spier CM, LeBlanc M, Chase EM, et al. Histologic subtypes do not confer unique outcomes in early-stage lymphoma: long-term follow-up of SWOG 8736. Blood (ASH Annual Meeting Abstracts) 2004 104: Abstract 3263.
Spraker HL, Price SL, Chaturvedi A, et al. The clone wars – revenge of the metastatic rogue state: the sarcoma paradigm. Front Oncol 2012;2:2.
Theriault RL, Theriault RL. Biology of bone metastases. Cancer Control 2012;19(2):92–101.
Thurlimann B, Keshavish A, Coates AS, et al. A comparison of letrozole and tamoxifen in postmenopausal women with early breast cancer. N Engl J Med 2005;353:2747–57.
Tong D, Gillick L, Hendrickson FR. The palliation of symptomatic osseous metastases, final results of the study by the Radiation Therapy Oncology Group. Cancer 1982;50:893–899.
van Maldegem AM, Bhosale A, Gelderblom HJ, et al. Comprehensive analysis of published phase I/II clinical trails between 1990–2010 in osteosarcoma and Ewing sarcoma confirms limited outcomes and need for translational investment. Clin Sarcoma Res 2012;2(1):5.
van Maldegem AM, Hogendoorn PC, Hassan AB. The clinical use of biomarkers as prognostic factors in Ewing sarcoma. Clin Sarcoma Res 2012;2(1):7.
Verschraegen C. The monoclonal antibody to cytotoxic T lymphocytic antigen 4, ipilimumab, in the treatment of melanoma. Cancer Manag Res 2012;4:1–8.
Watmough P, Canty S, Higgins G, et al. Soft tissues metastases from malignant tumours. J Bone Joint Surg 2005;87B Supp 1:2-3.
Wedin R, Bauer HC, Wersäll P. Failures after operation for skeletal metastatic lesions of long bones. Clin Orthop Relat Res 1999;(358):128–39.
Weng CJ, Yen GC. Chemopreventive effects of dietary phytochemicals against cancer invasion and metastasis: phenolic acids, monophenol, polyphenol, and their derivatives. Cancer Treat Rev 2012;38(1):76–87.
Weng CJ, Yen GC. Flavonoids, a ubiquitous dietary phenolic subclass, exert extensive in vitro anti-invasive and in vivo anti-metastatic activities. Cancer Metastases Rev 2012;31(1–2):323–51.
Wong MG, Stockler MR, Pavlakis N. Bisphosphonates and other bone agents for breast cancer. Cochrane Database Syst Rev 2012;2:CD003474
Yanagawa T, Shinozaki T, Lizuka Y, et al. Role of 2-deoxy-2-[F-18] fluoro-D-glucose positron emission tomography in the management of bone and soft tissue metastases. J Bone Joint Surg Br 2010;92:419–23.
Zhao E, Xu H, Wang L, et al. Bone marrow and the control of immunity. Cell Mol Immunol 2012;9(1):11–9.
(Unknown Authors] Tamoxifen for early breast cancer: an overview of the randomized trials. Early Breast Cancer Trialists' Collaborative Group. Lancet 1998;351:1451–67.

Chapter 16 Cartilaginous tumors of bones and joints

OVERVIEW

Cartilaginous tumors of bone encompass a range of tumors that either produce cartilaginous matrix (most of the lesions) or produce little hyaline cartilage-like matrix but show differentiation towards a chondrocytic cell type (two tumors, chondromyxoid fibroma and chondroblastoma). Behavior of these tumors runs from benign to very aggressive malignant tumors with a 13% five year disease specific survival (dedifferentiated chondrosarcoma). It is difficult to estimate their true incidence, because the most common tumors, enchondroma and osteochondroma, are often asymptomatic, and thus the patient never comes to a physician for evaluation.

Although most of the malignant cartilaginous tumors occur in adulthood, one particular aggressive subtype, mesenchymal chondrosarcoma, typically occurs in children and young adults. Interestingly, treatment for the malignant cartilaginous tumors (various types of chondrosarcomas) has not changed substantially in thirty years. However, with increasing knowledge of the molecular pathogenesis of these tumors, tailored chemotherapy for particular tumor types in individual patients may become feasible within the next ten years. A few such trials are ongoing (as of 2010).

Currently, the diagnosis of cartilaginous tumors of bone depends on careful review of radiologic examinations in combination with pathologic diagnosis of biopsy or resection specimens. It is well known that interobserver variability is an issue in pathologic diagnosis especially in the following particular scenarios: 1) distinguishing enchondroma from grade 1 chondrosarcoma and 2) distinguishing grade 1 from grade 2 conventional chondrosarcoma. It is still deemed clinically important to accurately differentiate grade 1 from grade 2 chondrosarcoma as surgical treatment differs. Previously, differentiating between an enchondroma and a low grade chondrosarcoma also was of clinical importance. However, at this time, the surgical approach is similar (see discussion below), and thus the distinction is not critical in terms of treatment decision-making. Unfortunately, even expert radiologic review does not resolve some of the cases with ambiguous pathology.

Despite some limitations, it will become evident that careful radiologic evaluation of cartilaginous tumors is critical, because specific imaging features can strongly support a malignant or benign (or at least low grade) diagnosis. As there are many patients with intramedullary cartilaginous lesions that most likely represent enchondromas, not all patients are biopsied. Therefore, accurate interpretation of the radiologic findings is essential with careful follow-up of those patients for whom the radiologic features are indeterminate and to periodically check patients with initially benign appearing lesions for any suspicious changes that subsequently may occur.

Table 16.1 WHO classification of cartilaginous tumors of bone and joint (2013)

Tumor	Behavior	Additional Comments
Osteochondroma	Benign	Can occur as multiple tumors (now termed multiple osteochondromas)
Chondroma a. Enchondroma b. Periosteal chondroma c. Multiple Chondromatosis	Benign	Enchondromas may occur as multiple tumors, Ollier disease and Maffucci syndrome are types of multiple chondromatosis. Malignant transformation may occur especially in multiple chondromatosis
Osteochondromyxoma	Benign*	Very rare. Associated with Carney complex. *A few may be locally aggressive (e.g. Intermediate)
Subungual exostosis	Benign	Most common in great toe Translocation specific tumor
Bizarre parosteal osteochondromatous proliferation of the hands and feet (BPOP)	Benign*	Hands and feet most commonly Specific genetic abnormalities confirm neoplastic nature *Termed benign in WHO classification but may locally recur (up to 50% of cases)
Synovial chondromatosis	Benign*	*Termed benign in WHO classification but may recur if incompletely excised Affects joints and soft tissues
Chondroblastoma	Intermediate (rarely metastasizing)	Rare
Chondromyxoid fibroma	Intermediate (locally aggressive)	Rare
Chondrosarcoma (CS) a. Central primary CS b. Central secondary CS c. Peripheral CS d. Dedifferentiated CS e. Mesenchymal CS f. Clear cell CS	Malignant*	*Chondrosarcoma, grade 1/ atyical cartilaginous tumor is intermediate (locally aggressive) in behavior. b. Arises in enchondroma, fibrous dysplasia c. Arises in an osteochondroma but rarely occurs as a primary tumor ('periosteal' and 'juxtacortical' CS) f. Rarely metastasizes and rarely transforms to a higher grade

Benign: does not recur and does not metastasize, Intermediate: can recur but does not metastasize, Malignant: can recur and can metastasize. CS: chondrosarcoma

CLASSIFICATION

The World Health Organization (WHO) classification of cartilaginous tumors of bone is provided below in **Table 16.1** (Fletcher et al. 2013). Analogous to the other chapters of this book, cartilaginous tumors are divided according to behavior: benign tumors do not recur or recur non-aggressively, and do not metastasize, intermediate tumors can recur locally aggressively and/or rarely metastasize (<5%), and malignant tumors can both recur and commonly metastasize, sometimes metastasizing only after transformation to a higher grade of tumor.

Table 16.2 lists the cartilaginous tumors of bone and joints with incidence data and histology features including representative photomicrographs of the lesions. **Table 16.3** describes non-cartilaginous tumors that may produce hyaline cartilage-like matrix.

DEMOGRAPHICS

Malignant cartilaginous tumors of bone are rare compared with tumors such as breast carcinoma, lung cancer, and prostate cancer. **Figure 16.1** illustrates the age adjusted incidence rates per 100,000 for chondrosarcoma by sex and year of diagnosis from 1993-2007 (SEER data from 13 United States registries). Although it is generally stated that chondrosarcomas are slightly more common in males, the graph reveals an approximately equal incidence in males and females for this time period spanning ~20% of the United States population.

Figure 16.2 exhibits the chondrosarcoma subtypes recorded with the 13 SEER tumor registries from 1994-2008. Clearly, the vast majority of cases are chondrosarcoma conventional type with myxoid chondrosarcoma being the second most common type. In fact, central primary chondrosarcoma accounts for approximately 90% of chondrosarcomas

Table 16.2 Cartilaginous tumors of bones/joints grouped by behavior

Tumor	Incidence	Age and sex distribution	Most common body site (in order of occurrence)	Histopathology description	
				Medium magnification	High magnification
Benign: does not recur or recurs non-aggressively and does not metastasize					
Osteochondroma	Very common	M > F; peak age is second decade	Femur (distal), humerus (proximal), tibia (proximal); not in skull	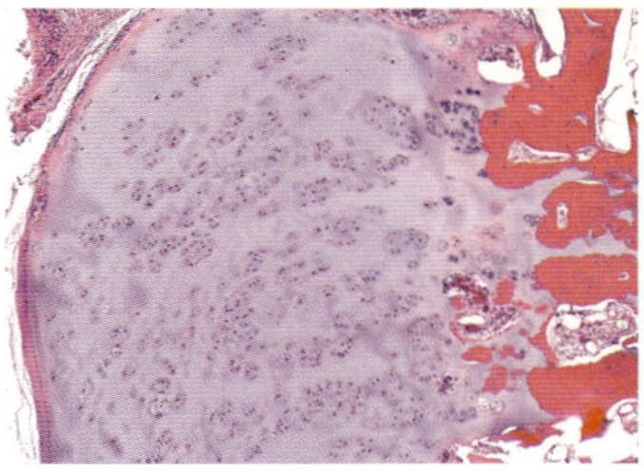	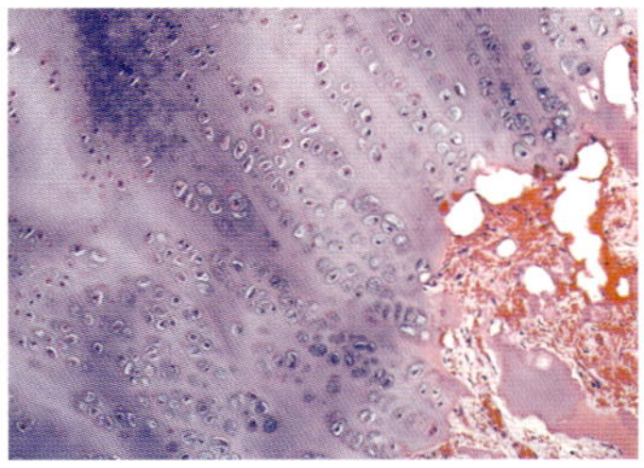
Recapitulates normal growth plate with cartilage cap and endochondral ossification at base; lesion can be flat or grow away from the normal growth plate on a bony stalk; always there is continuity with medullary cavity.					
Enchondroma	Very common	M = F; broad age distribution from teens through 7th decade	Phalanges of hand, metacarpals of hand, humerus (proximal); not in skull	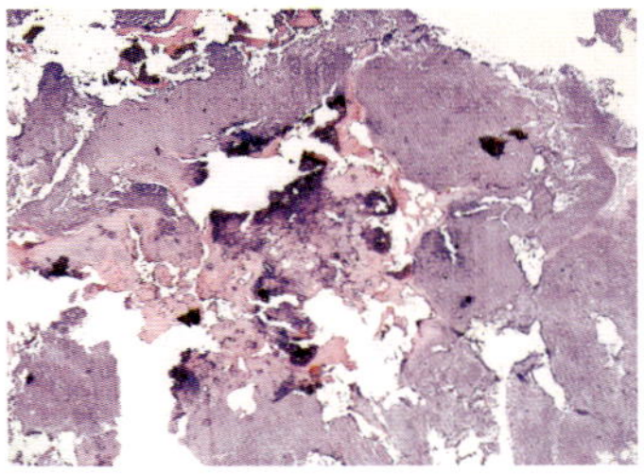	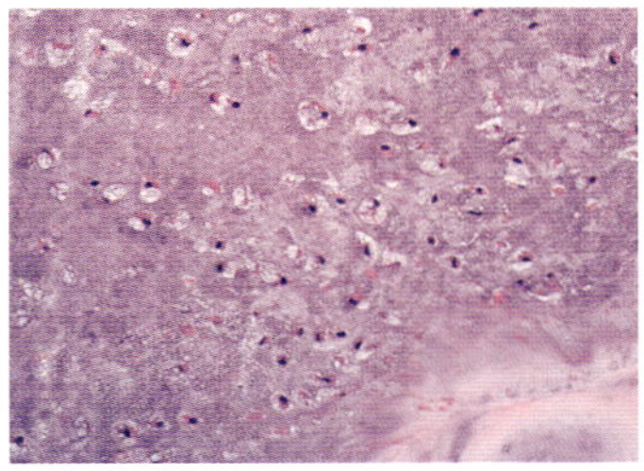
Lobules of hypocellular hyaline cartilage often with a collar of reactive bone; no invasive features.					
Osteochondromyxoma	Very rare	Occurs over broad age range in 1% of patients with Carney complex	Cranial facial bones and tibia	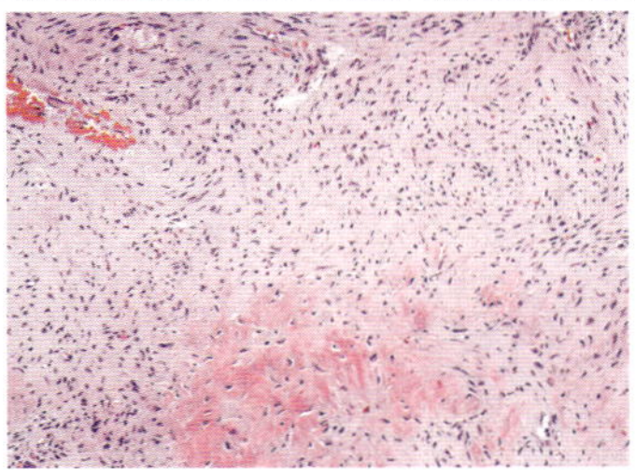	
Three main components: hypocellular myxoid spindle cell areas, hyaline cartilage nodules resembling growth plate, and osteoid and bone. May be related to chest wall hamartoma.					
Subungual exostosis	Rare	M > F Young adults most commonly	Distal phalanx of great toe at or near nail bed >> other toes and fingers (thumb and index finger)	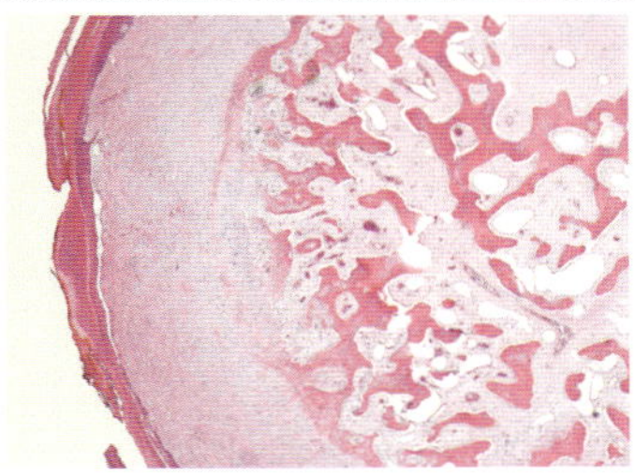	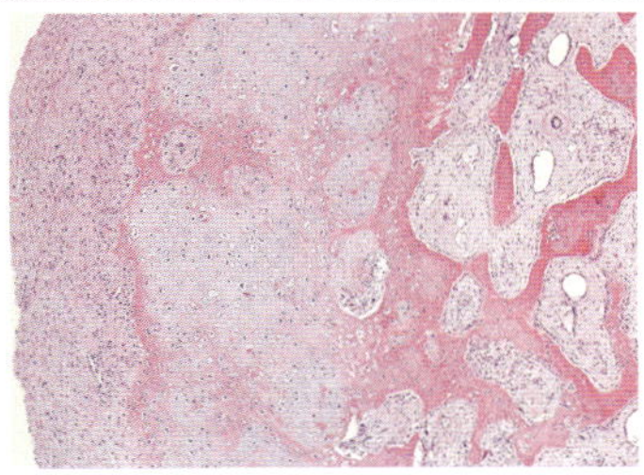
Looks like an osteochondroma with cartilaginous cap and underlying trabecular bone. Peripheral spindle cell component also present.					

Case table 16.2: Continued from page 367

<table>
<tr><th rowspan="2">Tumor</th><th rowspan="2">Incidence</th><th rowspan="2">Age and sex distribution</th><th rowspan="2">Most common body site (in order of occurrence)</th><th colspan="2">Histopathology description</th></tr>
<tr><th>Medium magnification</th><th>High magnification</th></tr>
<tr><td>Bizarre parosteal osteochondromatous proliferation of the hands and feet (BPOP)</td><td>Rare</td><td>M = F
Adolescents to young adults (20s-40s)</td><td>Proximal small bones of hands and feet; rarely long bones and cranial facial bones</td><td>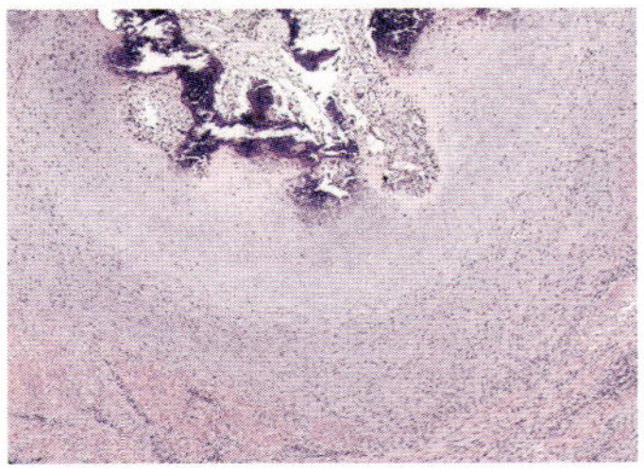</td><td>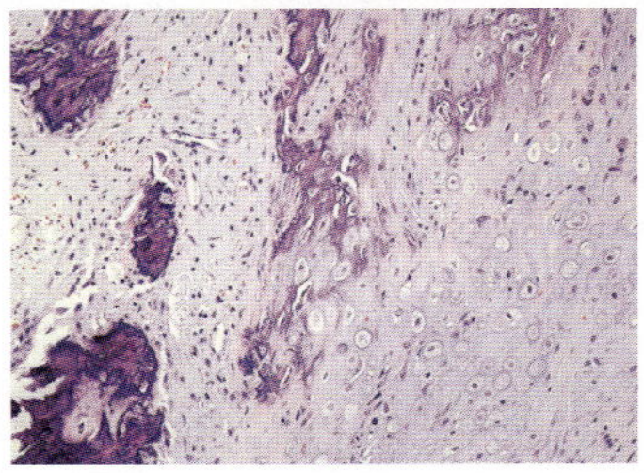</td></tr>
<tr><td colspan="6">Often disorganized mix of cartilage nodules or cap with bone and spindle cell areas. Some areas may resemble subungual exostosis/osteochondroma. Cartilage is usually hypercellular with atypia. Bone is 'blue bone' with bluish mineralization.</td></tr>
<tr><td>Synovial chondromatosis</td><td>Uncommon</td><td>M > F; most commonly in 20s -40s</td><td>Knee, hip, shoulder, elbow and ankle joints</td><td>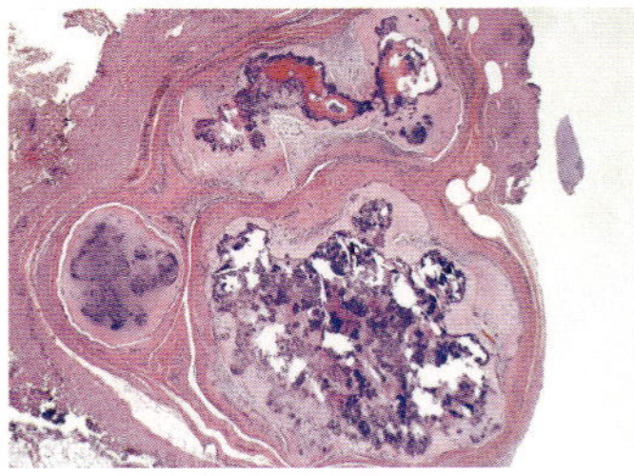</td><td>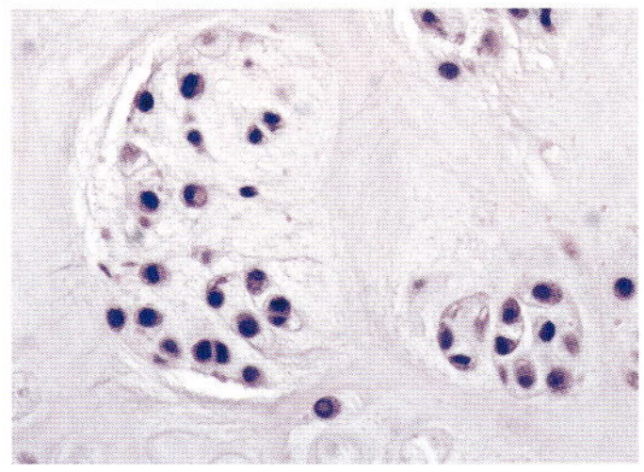</td></tr>
<tr><td colspan="6">Multiple nodules of variably cellular hyaline cartilage, floating in joint and attached to synovium; may have osteoid; more cellular than long-bone chondroma, chondrocytes often cluster.</td></tr>
<tr><td colspan="6">Intermediate: can recur locally aggressively and/or rarely metastasizes (<5%)</td></tr>
<tr><td>Chondromyxoid fibroma</td><td>Rare</td><td>M > F; broad age range but most common in decades 1-3</td><td>Knee (proximal tibia, distal femur), ankle</td><td>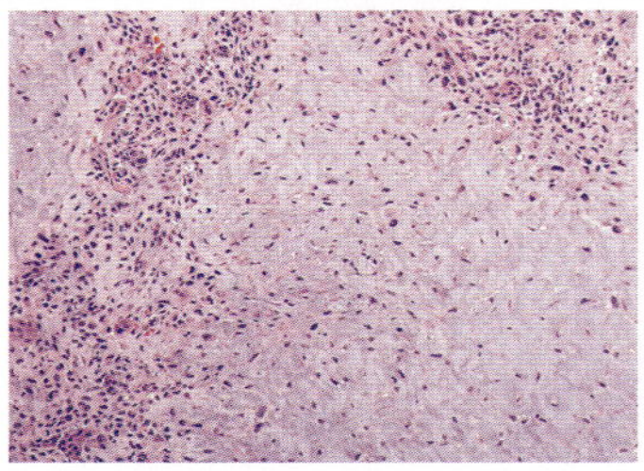</td><td>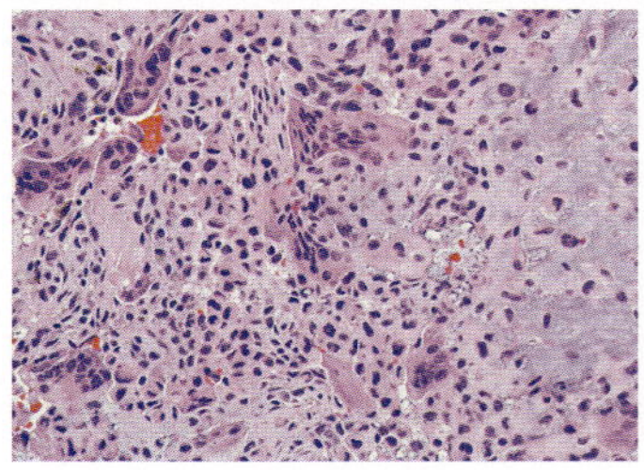</td></tr>
<tr><td colspan="6">Vaguely lobulated myxoid nodules with stellate to spindle cells; rims of lobules are cellular often with MNGCs and chondroblastoma-like cells.</td></tr>
<tr><td>Chondroblastoma</td><td>Rare</td><td>M > F; most are skeletally immature; however cases occur in middle age</td><td>Epiphysis of proximal humerus, distal femur, proximal tibia-10% occur in hands/ feet</td><td>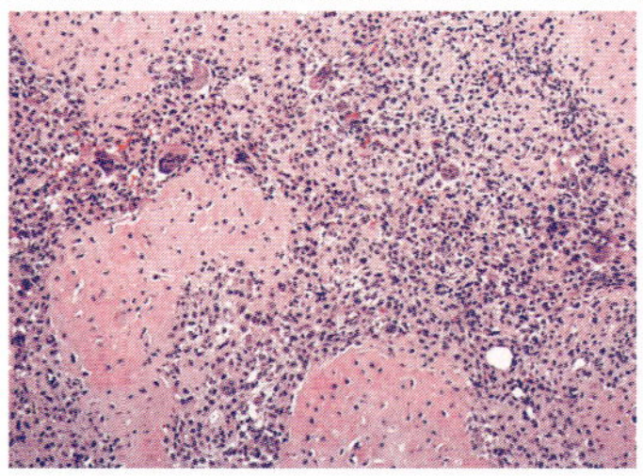</td><td>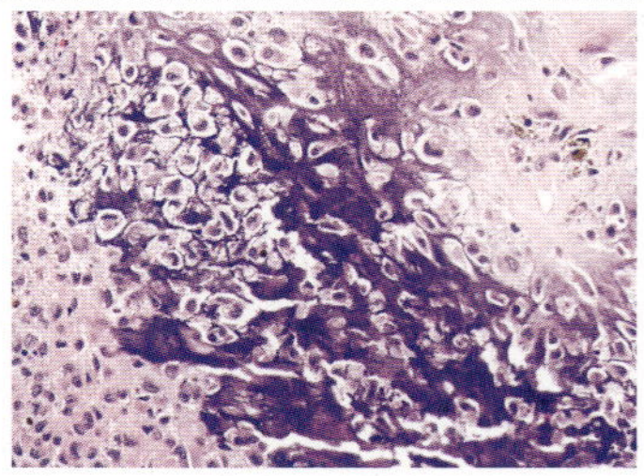</td></tr>
<tr><td colspan="6">Cellular tumor consisting of round 'chondroblast' like cells with clefted nuclei; multinucleated tumor cells and osteoclastic like giant cells present; rarely hyaline-type cartilage but often pink chondroid and 33% have 'chicken wire' calcifications.</td></tr>
<tr><td>Chondrosarcoma grade 1, central type/atypical cartilaginous tumor</td><td>Common</td><td>M > F; most in 50s and 60s; rare in childhood and adolescence</td><td>Pelvis, femur, humerus and ribs</td><td>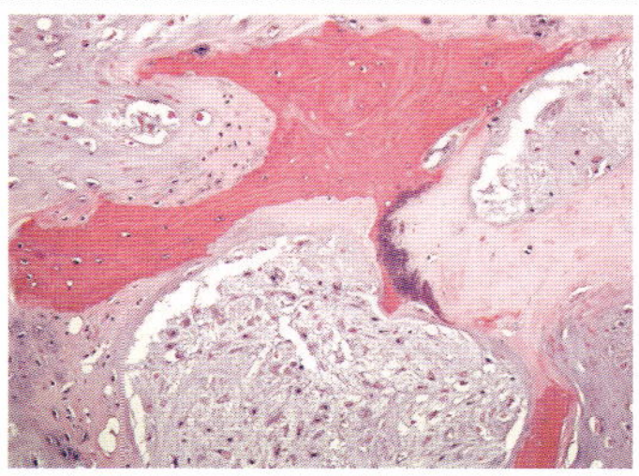</td><td>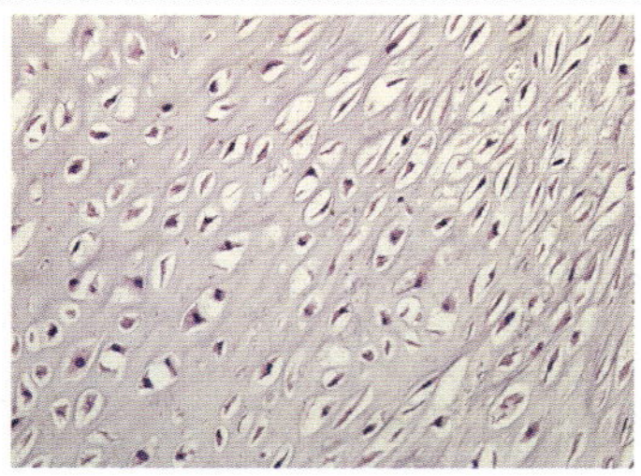</td></tr>
<tr><td colspan="6">Can look identical to enchondroma; however, may have slightly increased cellularity and mild cytologic atypia (pale nuclei with single nucleoli); cells set in hyaline cartilage like matrix.</td></tr>
</table>

Case Table 16.2: Continued from page 368

Tumor	Incidence	Age and sex distribution	Most common body site (in order of occurrence)	Histopathology description: Medium magnification	Histopathology description: High magnification
Malignant: can recur and commonly metastasizes					
Peripheral Chondrosarcoma arising in Osteochondroma	Rare	M > F; younger than patients with central CS; 30s-40s	Pelvis, humerus, scapula	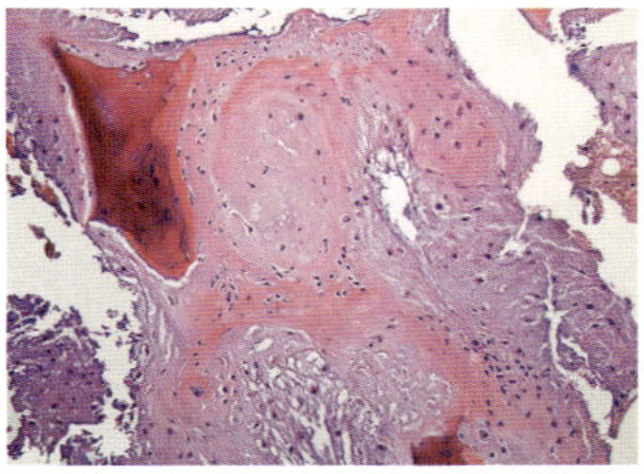	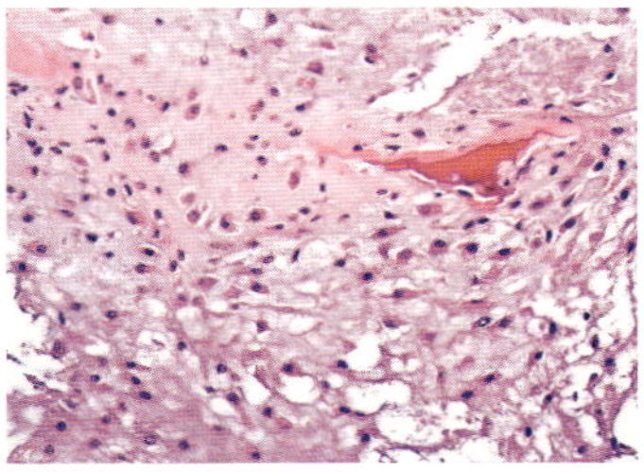
Looks like conventional type chondrosarcoma. Usually grade 1 or 2.					
Chondrosarcoma, grades 2 and 3, central type	Uncommon	M > F; most in 50s and 60s; rare in childhood and adolescence	Pelvis, femur, humerus and ribs	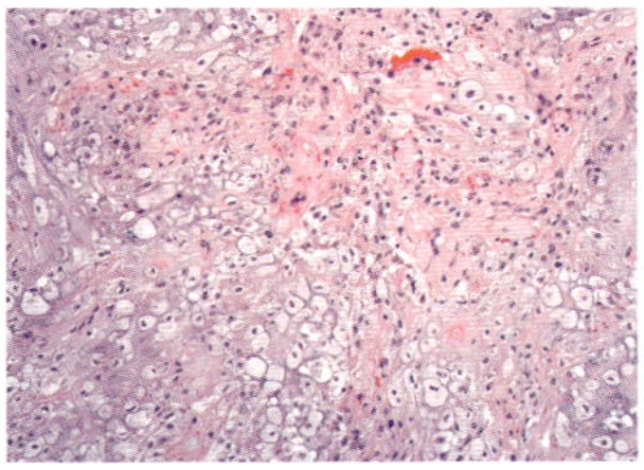	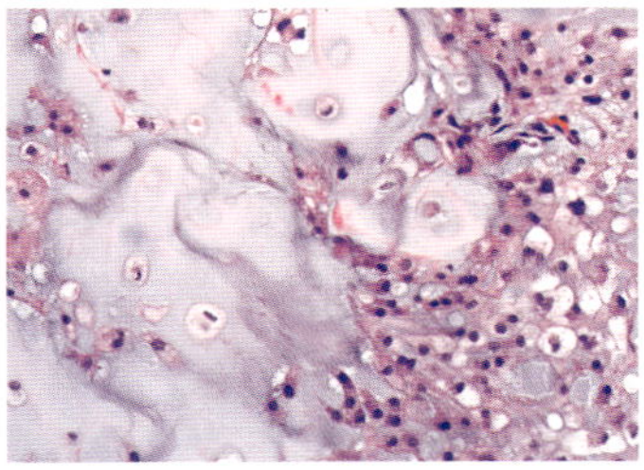
Increasing cellularity and atypia compared to grade 1 CS; rare mitotic figures, +/-necrosis; may have spindle cells and vessels in stroma between neoplastic lobules.					
Dedifferentiated chondrosarcoma	Rare	M > F; most in 50s and 60s; rare in childhood and adolescence	Femur, pelvis	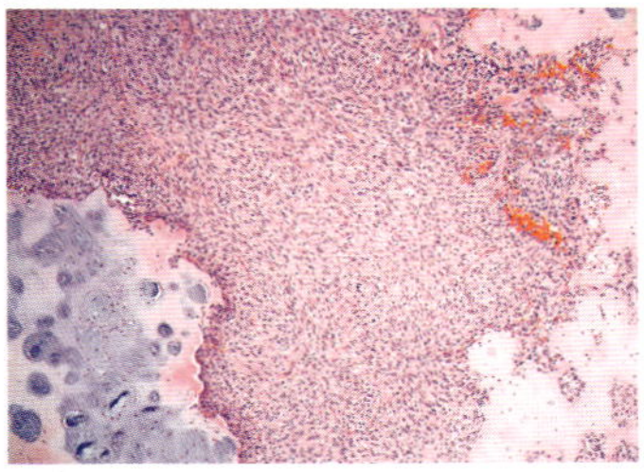	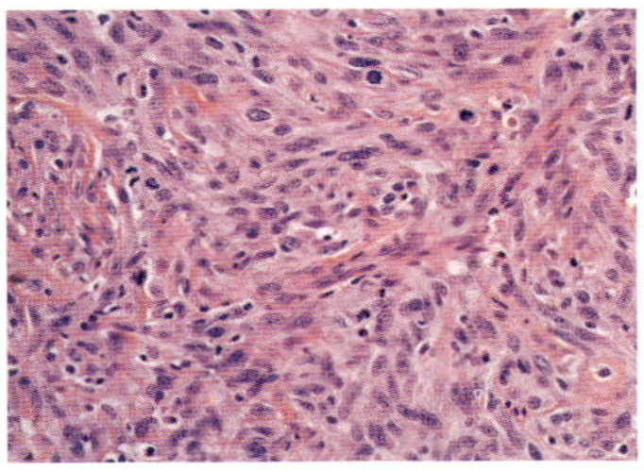
Dual appearance of CS (grade 1 or 2 usually) with abrupt transition to high grade sarcoma that is usually spindle or pleomorphic NOS, but can include osteosarcoma and others.					
Mesenchymal chondrosarcoma	Rare	M = F; most in 20s and 30s	Mandible, maxilla, femur, fibula, ribs; 30% arise in soft tissue	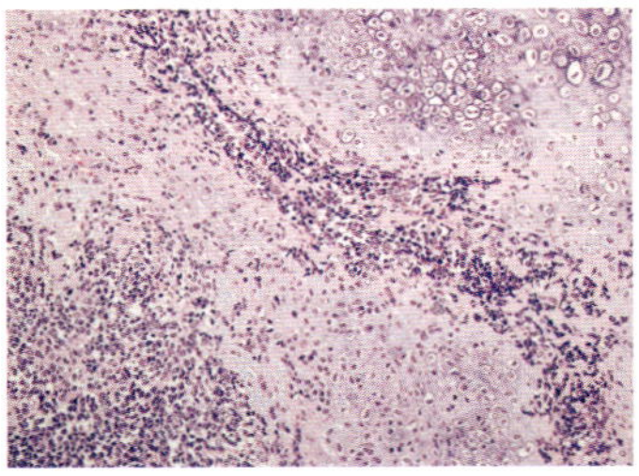	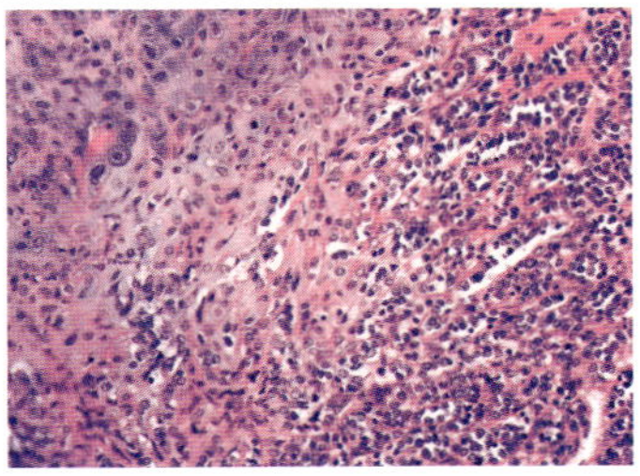
Dual appearance of small round blue cells (blastic type cells) and chondrosarcoma (usually grade 1 or 2).					
Clear cell chondrosarcoma	Very rare	M > F; most patients in 30s and 40s but also children and elderly	Proximal femur, proximal humerus, distal femur, proximal tibia	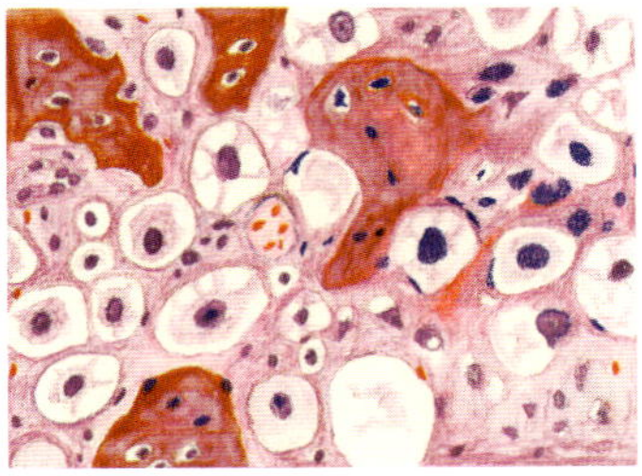	
Clear cells forming ill-defined lobules. Often with mineralization and scattered osteoid. Cartilage matrix scant. Multinucleated osteoclast like giant cells present. Mitoses and atypia only in rare cases.					

Incidence note: 'Common to very common' indicates that a medium sized practice will treat at least several to dozens of patients with the lesion annually, 'Uncommon to Rare' indicates the same practice size will treat one to two patients with the lesion every five years, 'Rare to very rare' indicates the same sized practice will see zero to one patient with the lesion every 20 years.

Table 16.3 Non-cartilaginous lesions that contain cartilage

Tumor	Incidence	Age and sex distribution	Most common body sites (in order of occurrence)	Cell types	Histopathology and special studies (if indicated)
Non-neoplastic: a benign mimicker of a neoplasm					
Fracture callus	Common	M > F except in old age; all ages	All sites varying in frequency with age	Fibroblasts, chondroblasts, endothelial cells, inflammatory cells	Hypercellular combination of immature bone and cartilage in fibroblastic tissue background. Cellular but no atypia. History can be very helpful
Chondromesenchymal hamartoma (chest wall hamartoma, vascular cartilaginous hamartoma of chest wall)	Very rare	M ≥ F; infancy rarely reported up to young adults (mid-20s)	Chest wall arising from a rib; rarely spine, sternum	Spindle cells, chondrocytes, endothelial cells, and osteoblasts/osteocytes	Hyaline cartilage nodules embedded in a highly vascular spindle cell stroma with reactive bone. Secondary ABC often present
Benign: does not recur or recurs non-aggressively and does not metastasize					
Fibrous dysplasia	Very common	M = F; Most patients are older children to young adults	Craniofacial bones, femur, tibia and ribs	Spindle cells predominantly with some chondrocytes, rare identifiable osteoblasts, and osteoclastic giant cells	Fibrous tissue in which immature bone nodules form in short curving 'alphabet' shapes mostly without rimming osteoblasts. Cartilage is present in 10% of cases. No atypia, but mitoses present
Malignant: can recur and commonly metastasizes					
Chordoma	Rare	M > F; most patients are in their 40s–60s	Sacrum/coccyx (50%), base of skull (30%) and remainder in vertebrae	Notochordal cells with bubbly clear cytoplasm (physaliphorous cells) and eosinophilic cells	Lobulated with extra-cellular and intracellular mucin, may have atypia, some have chondroid component (especially when located in the skull) Positive for S-100 protein, brachyury, and keratins
Chondroblastic osteosarcoma	Common	M > F; most patients are children or adolescents; second peak in late middle age	Long bones, pelvis	Chondrocytes and spindle to round osteoblasts, both usually with marked atypia. Osteoclastic giant cells also common	Lacelike or filigree osteoid combined with malignant hypercellular cartilage and a cellular atypical spindle cell stroma. Necrosis and atypical mitoses can be seen
Dedifferentiated liposarcoma	Uncommon	M > F; most patients are 50 and older	Extremities, (also retroperitoneum and mediastinum). Since this is a soft tissue tumor, it usually is not confused with a primary cartilaginous tumor of bone. However, it can metastasize to the bones	Can have different cell types depending on the type of dedifferentiated component but most commonly includes spindle cells, pleomorphic round and polygonal cells and lipoblasts. Inflammation can be present	Rarely can form malignant cartilage. Sometimes lower grade liposarcoma is present (lipoblasts identifiable). At least some areas look like a non-specific high grade spindle or pleomorphic sarcoma. CDK4, MDM2 usually positive. Karyotype shows giant ring and marker chromosomes
Metaplastic carcinoma (sarcomatoid carcinoma)	Uncommon	M > F except with breast primary tumors; most patients are 50 and older	Primary sites include breast, lungs, bladder, and kidney. All can metastasize to the bones and cause confusion with dedifferentiated chondrosarcoma, for example	Malignant epithelial cells and metaplastic spindle and pleomorphic cells	May uncommonly form cartilage and bone. Some areas are usually positive for epithelial markers like keratins. History can be helpful

Incidence note: 'Common to very common' indicates that a medium sized practice will treat at least several to dozens of patients with the lesion annually, 'Uncommon to rare' indicates the same practice size will treat one to two patients with the lesion every five years, 'Rare to very rare' indicates the same sized practice will see zero to one patient with the lesion every 20 years.

This is not an exhaustive list but includes those lesions that may more commonly be encountered and likely to be confused with a cartilaginous tumor of bones/joints. M: male, F: female, ABC: aneurysmal bone cyst.

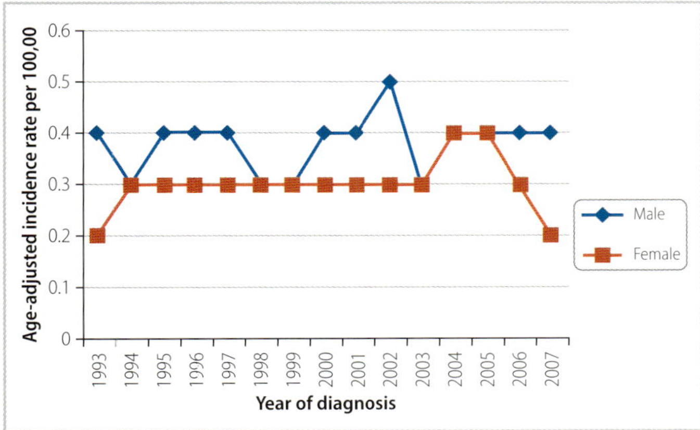

Figure 16.1 Age-adjusted incidence rates per 100,000 for chondrosarcoma by sex and year of diagnosis, 1993-2007. The number of cases reported in 13 SEER sites in the 15 year period is relatively small (n= 1862). The age adjusted incidence rate for males is only slightly higher than for females: 0.4 to 0.3 per 100,000.

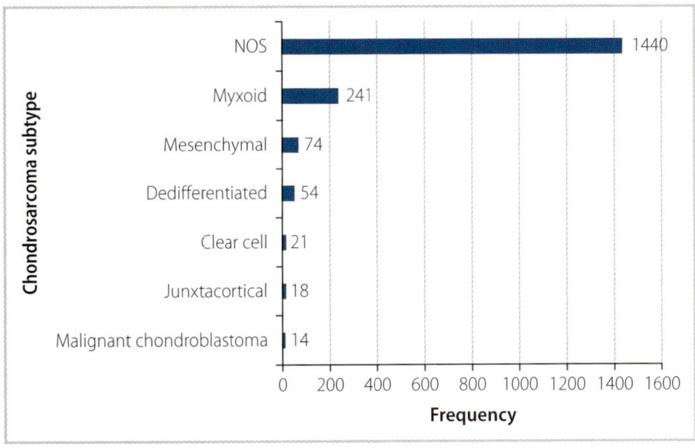

Figure 16.2 Frequency of chondrosarcoma subtypes diagnosed between 1993 and 2007 (SEER data from 13 US tumor registries). NOS (not otherwise specified) is equivalent to conventional chondrosarcoma.

according to the WHO (Fletcher et al. 2013). The SEER category of 'myxoid chondrosarcoma' is limited only to extra-osseous examples in this chapter as extra skeletal myxoid chondrosarcoma is no longer considered a type of chondrosarcoma and will be discussed later in this book in the chapter, Tumors of Uncertain Differentiation. Rarely, a central chondrosarcoma exhibits extensive myxoid change. These rare intra-medullary myxoid chondrosarcomas are reported to NOT share the genetic features of extra skeletal myxoid chondrosarcoma. The SEER Registries do not track benign cartilaginous tumors. **Table 16.4** segregates the chondrosarcomas by grade (SEER data 1993-2007): most conventional chondrosarcomas are grade 1 or 2 and close to 70% of all chondrosarcomas types are grade 1 or 2, according to these data.

Since SEER data only deal with malignant cartilaginous tumors, for perspective, the frequency of resected benign cartilaginous tumors at the University of New Mexico (2000-2010 numbers) is reported in the case presentations portion of this chapter. These numbers, although not necessarily archetypal, comprise patients having resections performed at a medium sized orthopedic oncologic surgical practice at an academic medical center.

Figure 16.3a depicts patient age by subtype of chondrosarcoma of those patients diagnosed between 1994-2008 (SEER, US data). Malignant cartilaginous tumors affect a broad age range with some tumors more common in older patients and others in younger. For example, younger individuals with malignant cartilaginous tumors develop malignant chondroblastoma and mesenchymal chondrosarcoma. By contrast, most individuals with clear cell chondrosarcoma, juxtacortical chondrosarcoma, conventional chondrosarcoma, myxoid chondrosarcoma and dedifferentiated chondrosarcoma affect increasingly older patients (see **Fig. 16.3a**) although, the age range for any one tumor type is wide.

Most of the malignant cartilaginous tumors of bone arise in the long bones, especially in the lower limbs (**Fig. 16. 3b**)

PATHOGENESIS

The relative rarity of cartilaginous tumors, especially the malignant tumors, has impaired the study of the pathogenesis of these tumors. Despite this handicap, researchers are beginning to describe repetitive genetic and molecular profiles of these tumors that relate to pathogenesis or behavior.

Table 16.4 Histologic tumor grade by chondrosarcoma type, number of cases (percent)

Chondrosarcoma subtype	Well differentiated	Moderately differentiated	Poorly differentiated	Undifferentiated; anaplastic	Unknown
	Grade I	**Grade II**	**Grade III**	**Grade IV**	
NOS	557 (39)	559 (39)	114 (8)	82 (6)	128 (9)
Juxtacortical	6 (33)	7 (39)	2 (11)	2 (11)	1 (6)
Malignant chondroblastoma	2 (14)	0 (0)	0 (0)	1 (7)	11 (79)
Myxoid	27 (11)	86 (36)	24 (10)	22 (9)	82 (34)
Mesenchymal	2 (3)	4 (5)	13 (18)	14 (19)	41 (55)
Clear cell	1 (5)	6 (29)	0 (0)	0 (0)	14 (67)
Dedifferentiated	3 (6)	4 (7)	15 (28)	26 (48)	6 (11)
All subtypes	**598 (32)**	**666 (36)**	**168 (9)**	**147 (8)**	**283 (15)**

Most chondrosarcomas, when the subtypes were combined, were moderately differentiated (grade II) (36%). After stratifying by subtype, the majority of NOS, juxtacortical and myxoid were moderately differentiated (grade II); however most malignant chondroblastoma, mesenchymal and clear cell tumors were of unknown histologic grade. The majority of dedifferentiated cases were undifferentiated (grade IV).

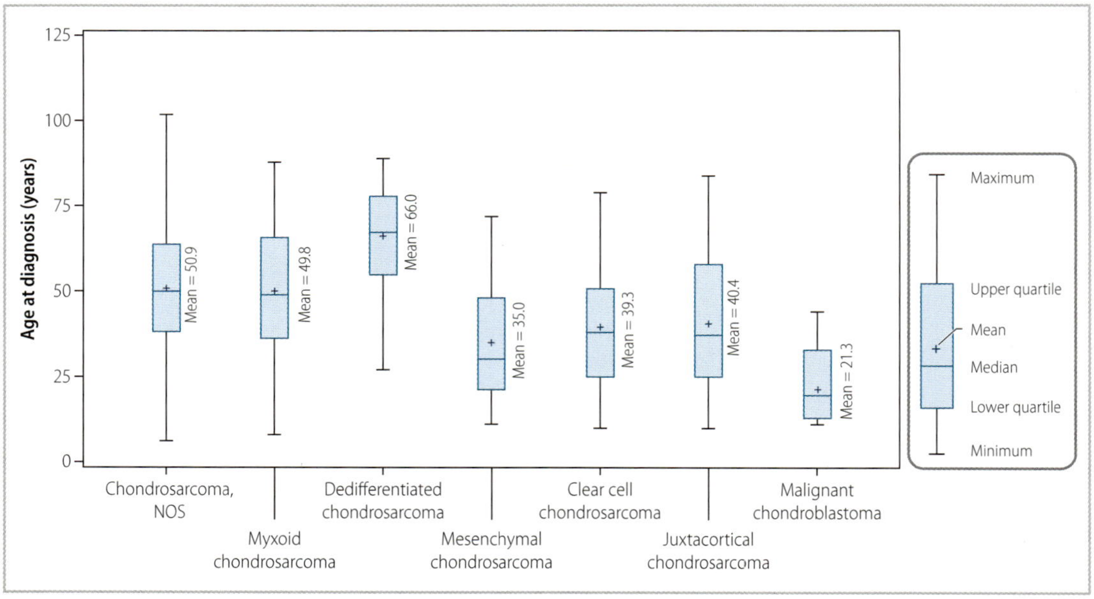

Figure 16.3a Age distribution by chondrosarcoma subtype diagnosed between 1993 and 2007. (SEER data from 13 sites in the US.) The average age of diagnosis for chondrosarcoma patients was 52.1 years; however, the ages vary widely by subtype. Although not statistically significant, it is important to note these differences in mean age at diagnosis. When chondrosarcoma was stratified by subtype, malignant chondroblastoma cases were the youngest at diagnosis (mean = 21.3 years), and cases diagnosed with dedifferentiated chondrosarcoma were the oldest (mean = 66 years).

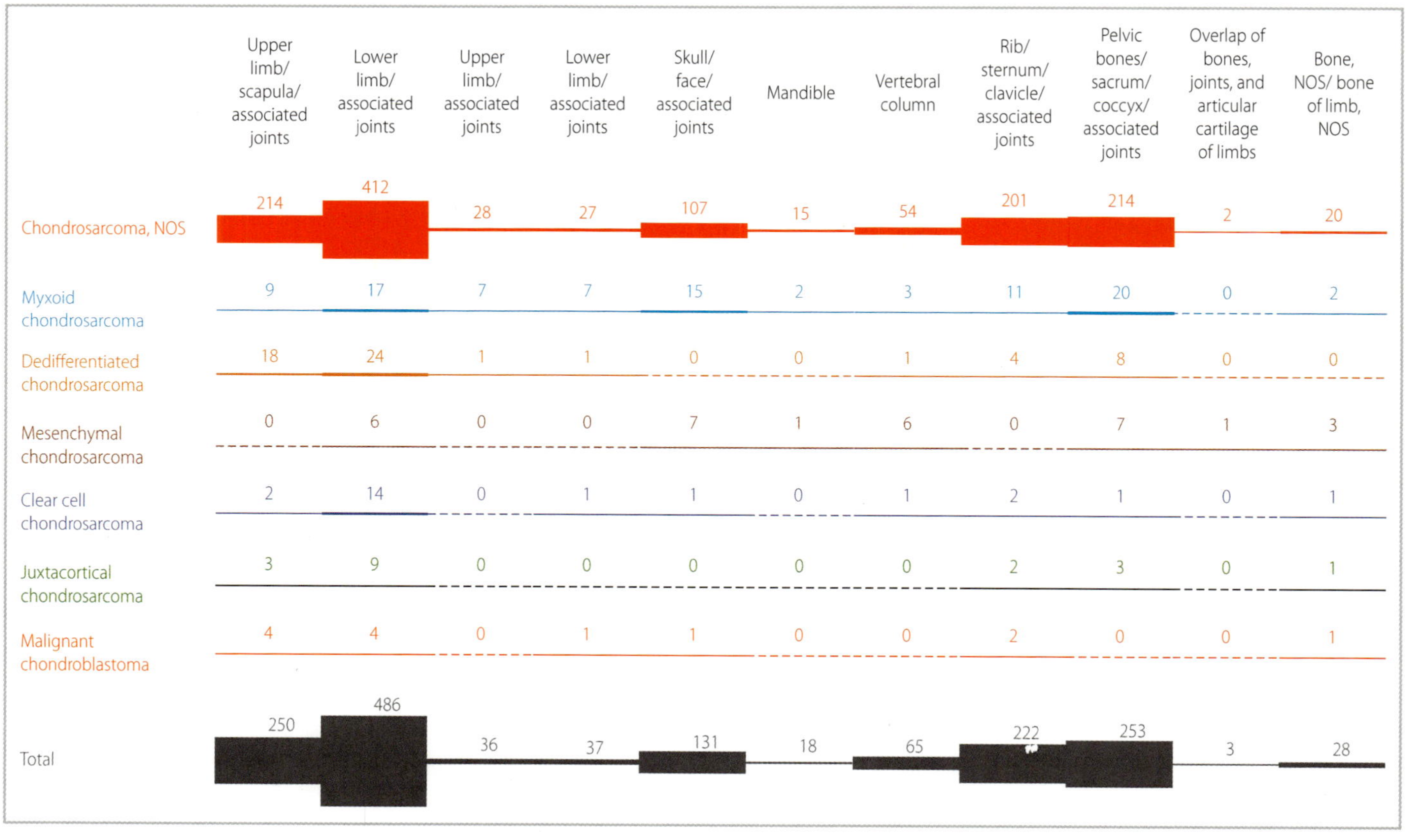

Figure 16.3b Cartilage tumors of the bone by site for cases in 13 SEER registries diagnosed between 1994 and 2008. Most of these tumors are diagnosed in the long bones, especially in the lower limbs and associated joints. Patients diagnosed with clear cell chondrosarcoma had the best prognosis compared to the other subtypes (5-year relative survival=100%). Furthermore, 94.4% of juxtacortical patients survive their cancer at least 5 years from diagnosis after adjusting for normal life expectancy. Tumors that were classified as dedifferentiated chondrosarcoma had the worst prognosis (29.3%) of all the subtypes (Case table 16.2).

The approach to studying the genetic features of cartilaginous tumors has paralleled advances in techniques in molecular biology. In particular, especially investigators from Europe have begun to characterize genetic features of cartilaginous tumors using cDNA expression analysis, fluorescence in situ hybridization, comparative genomic hybridization, PCR for loss of heterozygosity at gene loci, and immunohistochemical expression of molecules, among other techniques (Boeuf et al. 2008, Hallor et al. 2009, Romeo et al. 2007, Aigner 2002).

The impact of new techniques can be shown by the example of a standard rigorous karyotype study of 100 cartilaginous tumors. In that study, abnormal karyotypes were found in only 41/92 cartilaginous tumors (Tallini G et al. 2002). More recently, using methods that can explore genetic alterations not detectable by standard karyotyping, even karyotypically normal tumors exhibit genetic abnormalities. For example, HMGA2 locus alterations on chromosome 12q13-15 have been reported in enchondromas many of which display a normal karyotype (Bell et al. 2006). Note that the HMGA2 gene is also involved in some adipocytic tumors as well as other tumor types.

Table 16.5 lists the genetic findings of cartilaginous tumors discovered to date. Many aspects of the molecular signature of these tumors are still unknown.

Enchondromas and osteochondromas occur sporadically singly or as multiple tumors as a syndrome. The two most common enchondromatosis syndromes are Ollier disease and Maffucci syndrome. In contrast to the other major cartilaginous tumors syndrome, multiple osteochondromas, which is inherited in an autosomal dominant manner, the enchondromatosis variants are non-hereditary, meaning that seldom are multiple family members affected.

The latest theory regarding the pathogenesis of enchondromas involves abnormalities of the Indian Hedgehog signaling pathway (Chow 2007). This pathway is important in normal long bone development as it inhibits the terminal differentiation of growth plate chondrocytes. Interestingly, enchondromas are located in close proximity to former growth plates. Such a tumor could thus arise from abnormal constitutive Hedgehog signaling preventing end-stage differentiation of chondrocytes. Hence the development of an enchondroma from these continuing proliferating growth plate chondrocytes (Bovée et al. 2010).

Table 16.5 Genetics of cartilaginous tumors of bones and joints

Tumor	Chromosomal abnormality	Genes involved	Percentage of tumors with abnormality
Osteochondroma	Usually near diploid; 8q24 and 11p11-p12 mutations	*EXT1* (8q24) and *EXT2* (11p11-p12)	Majority
Enchondroma and other chondromas	Usually diploid or near diploid; may have abnormalities of 4q, 5, 7, 11, 14q, 16q22-q24, 20 and rearrangements of 6 and 12q12-15	*HMGA2* (12q15); unknown others	Unknown
Osteochondromyxoma	Diploid (four cases reported)	*PRKAR1A* (17q23-24) and *CNC2* (unknown location). Some cases also have 2p16 mutations (gene unknown)	100% of Carney complex patients have mutations. This tumor may be the intra-osseous version of the myxomas seen in Carney complex
Subungual exostosis	t(X;6)(q24-26;q15-25) +/- other abnormalities (seven cases reported)	*CO12A1* (6q13-14) *COL4A5* (Xq22)	~100%
Bizarre parosteal osteochondromatous proliferation of the hands and feet (BPOP)	t(1;17)(q32-42;q21-23) in most cases Paracentric inversions of 7q, 6q or ring chromosomes with 12 sequences also reported	Unknown	~100% for the translocation or inversions of 7q or 6q
Synovial chondromatosis	Abnormalities of 6, most commonly as loss of part or all of this chromosome, +5 in some	Unknown	Unknown
Chondromyxoid fibroma	6q12-13, 6q25 abnormalities	Unknown	Unknown
Chondroblastoma	Usually diploid or near diploid; may have abnormalities of 2q35, 3q21-q23, 5, 8, 9p, 13q, 17p13, 18q21, 19q	Possibly p53, INK4A/p16 and INK4A/p14, and RB1	Unknown
Peripheral chondrosarcoma arising in osteochondroma	Near haploid or duplications of haploid, 8q24 and 11p11-p12 mutations	*EXT1* (8q24) and *EXT2* (11p11-p12) and others	Unknown
Chondrosarcoma grade 1, central type	Usually diploid karyotype; no specific highly recurrent abnormalities	Unknown	Majority are diploid
Chondrosarcoma, grades 2 and 3, central type	Usually complex aneuploid karyotype; most have alterations of pRb pathway	Unknown	100% of grade 3 have aneuploid karyotype >50% of grade 2
Dedifferentiated chondrosarcoma	Usually complex aneuploid karyotype	Unknown	Majority
Mesenchymal chondrosarcoma	der(13;21)(q10;q10)	Unknown	Unknown
Clear cell chondrosarcoma	Usually diploid or near diploid; may have loss/changes in chromosome 9 and gain of chromosome 20	Unknown	Majority are diploid or near-diploid

Many cells in this table contain the word 'unknown' or the qualifiers 'usually' or 'may have'. Information accrues constantly, so refer to the most recent publications for updates on the genetic profiles of these tumors.

A related gene, the parathyroid hormone-Like hormone (PTHL), may be mutated in approximately 8% of enchondromas. The PTHL gene product normally down regulates the Hedgehog signaling pathway, and mutation of this gene causes abnormal constitutive Hedgehog signaling.

The morbidity conferred by deformities that occur with multiple lesions in Ollier disease (manifested as enchondromas only) and in Maffucci syndrome, (enchondromas plus benign vascular lesions, most likely spindle cell hemangiomas) is overshadowed by the potential for malignant progression in these patients: up to 35% of patients with Ollier disease and possibly up to 50% of patients with Maffucci syndrome will develop chondrosarcoma (Bovée et al. 2010).

Osteochondromas comprise a well-organized outgrowth of bone and overlying cartilage. They develop in long bones, characteristically growing opposite to the normal growth plate and ceasing growth when the normal growth plate closes. As with enchondroma, osteochondroma is considered to result from abnormal proliferating growth plate chondrocytes. Osteochondromas most commonly occur as sporadic solitary lesions, but an autosomal dominant condition known as multiple osteochondromas (previously termed hereditary multiple exostoses) does occur. Like enchondromas, osteochondromas may undergo malignant transformation to a chondrosarcoma. The risk is difficult to calculate but may be as high as 4-8% for solitary lesions and 10-36% for multiple osteochondromas patients (Altay et al. 2007, Ahmed et al. 2003). Fortunately, most secondary chondrosarcomas arising from either osteochondroma or enchondroma are histologically low grade with excellent long term survival rates in the range of 85-90%.

In prior times, the pathogenesis of osteochondromas was conjectured to be due to an abnormal physical displacement of growth plate cartilage and not due to genetic alterations as in a true neoplasm. However, more recent studies have found mutations in the genes producing proteins, exostosin-1 (EXT1) at 8q24 (65% of cases) or exostosin-2 (EXT2) at 11p11-13 (35% of cases)(Rozeman et al. 2002). As with enchondromas, the pathogenesis of osteochondromas is thought to relate to abnormal Hedgehog signaling. The proteins encoded by EXT1 and EXT2 help to form heparin sulfate proteoglycan that normally binds to Hedgehog protein ligands in the hyaline matrix of hyaline cartilage. Mutations of these two gene sites can cause a diminished amount of normal extracellular heparin sulfate proteoglycan resulting in the abnormal diffusion of Hedgehog ligands in the extracellular matrix. This is conjectured to misdirect growth plate chondrocytes to proliferate in a direction opposite to the normal (Bovée et al. 2010). Despite its elegance as an explanation, defects in Hedgehog signaling do not tell the complete story for enchondromas or osteochondromas, and work is ongoing to fill out the details of pathogenesis. For example, chondromas as a whole exhibit abnormalities of chromosomes 6, 12q12-q15, 5, 7, 17, 4q, 14q, 11, 16q22-24 and 20 more commonly than at other sites (Buddingh et al. 2003). To what degree these variable abnormalities determine chondroma development or how they may interact with Hedgehog signaling is unknown.

Chondroblastoma and chondromyxoid fibroma are the two less common benign cartilaginous tumors of bone. Chondromyxoid fibroma (CMF) appears to have abnormalities of the long arm of chromosome 6 (chromosome 6q13 and also 6q25) as a characteristic of this lesion (Bell et al. 2006). Abnormalities reported include translocations and inversions at these sites on 6q. Based on protein expression studies, CMF may contain a mix of cells with features of 1) chondrocytes, 2) myofibroblasts, and 3) a peculiar blended cell, a 'myochondroblast' (Nielsen et al. 1999).

Chondroblastoma has not been studied in great detail. However, abnormalities of chromosomes 5, 8, and recurrent breakpoints at chromosomes 2q35, 3q21-23, and 18q21 have been reported (Bell et al. 2006). In fact, whether chondroblastoma is a legitimate cartilaginous tumor has been questioned. Some researchers have suggested that chondroblastoma is more akin to an osteoblastic or osteogenic tumor than a cartilaginous tumor because of the lack of some cartilaginous specific protein expression in chondroblastoma and expression of bone specific collagen (namely lack of collagen II and instead expression of collagen I in chondroblastoma) (Soder et al. 2006). Chondroblastomas are perhaps related to hypertrophic chondrocytes/transformative osteoblastic cells (transformation of chondroblasts to osteoblasts occurs normally in the chick growing cartilage plate and may somehow also occur in chondroblastomas) (Romeo et al. 2007).

However, recent evidence supports classifying chondroblastoma as a cartilaginous tumor albeit an unusual one. A gene expression profiling study using a custom cDNA array containing ~8700 clones enriched for cartilage related genes was used to investigate the relationship between chondroblastoma, chondromyxoid fibroma, and conventional chondrosarcoma (Romeo et al. 2007). Chondromyxoid fibroma and chondroblastoma expressed genes involved in cartilage formation confirming that chondroblastoma does exhibit a cartilaginous nature at the gene expression level. In addition, recurring differences were also noted. Chondroblastoma, in contrast to chondromyxoid fibroma, down regulated expression of two molecules that are involved in the condensation of the cartilaginous matrix and its differentiation (versican and perlican). The authors of this paper speculate that the lack of expression of these two proteins results in a lack of obvious cartilaginous matrix noted in nearly all chondroblastomas (Romeo et al. 2007). This group also found that the more myxoid matrix typical of chondromyxoid fibroma may be explained by higher levels of collagen IV than usually occurs in hyaline cartilage.

An additional difference noted between chondroblastoma and chondromyxoid fibroma at the protein expression level comprises differential keratin expression. Chondromyxoid fibromas do not express keratins, while the great majority of chondroblastomas produce a range of cytokeratins, predominantly cytokeratins 8, 18, and less commonly cytokeratin 19 (Bousdras et al. 2007). Further support that chondroblastoma is rightly placed in the family of cartilaginous neoplasms is its sharing of loss of heterozygosity patterns with low grade chondrosarcoma. An evaluation of seventeen genetic markers known to be involved in mesenchymal tumors showed a similarity in loss of heterozygosity patterns at 5q, 9p, 11p, 13q, and 19q in chondroblastoma and low grade chondrosarcoma (Papachristou et al. 2006). Of note also, this study showed that the extent of genetic abnormalities (measured as the mean fractional allele loss [FAL]) was similar between chondroblastoma and chondrosarcoma. Unfortunately, the degree of allelic abnormalities did not predict behavior (Papachristou et al. 2006). Finally, chondroblastoma shares with gastrointestinal stromal tumor expression of DOG-1, although the two tumors are disparate otherwise (Akpalo et al. 2012).

The other benign cartilaginous tumors, osteochondromyxoma, subungual exostosis and bizarre parosteal osteochondromatous proliferation of the hands and feet are associated with specific genetic abnormalities (see **Table 16.5**).

Regarding malignant cartilaginous neoplasms, chondrosarcomas tend to show increasingly complex karyotypes as they progress from grade 1 (well differentiated) to grade 3 (poorly differentiated or high grade) tumors. Most low grade chondrosarcomas are near diploid, while most high grade chondrosarcomas are aneuploid with complex karyotypes. A few genes are recurrently amplified or otherwise altered in chondrosarcomas and these include the CDK4, p16 (CDKN2A) and p53 genes (Chow 2007, Gelderblom et al. 2008). An unusual feature of chondrosarcoma compared to most human malignancies is that at least some high grade central chondrosarcomas develop from duplication of an initial chromosome complement that is near haploid or slightly less than diploid, a process termed polyploidization (Hallor et al. 2009). In a comparative genomic hybridization study of 67 patients with chondrosarcoma, no independent prognostic genomic features were identified that could better anticipate outcome than increasing patient age and increasing tumor grade (Hallor et al. 2009).

Cartilaginous tumors may resemble fat tumors in that both sets of tumors recapitulate features of maturing normal adipocytes and chondrocytes, respectively. Liposarcoma cells bear a resemblance to normal adipocytes arrested in various stages of their twenty-one day maturation cycle based on overlap in molecular profiles of arrested normal fat cells with types of liposarcoma (see Chapter 5). Similarly, it appears as if both benign and malignant cartilaginous tumors can closely resemble particular stages of chondrocyte differentiation analyzed by gene expression profiles of mesenchymal stem cells arrested at specific points of chondrocyte differentiation. Mesenchymal stem cells arrested at days 0, 7, 28, and 42 of chondrogenesis and of 18 chondrosarcomas of different grades showed that the malignant tumors could be classified as prechondrogenic or chondrogenic based on an expression profile of 74 genes related to degree of differentiation of chondrocytes (Boeuf et al. 2008). Interestingly, the clustering of these 74 genes allowed discrimination between grade 1 and grade 3 chondrosarcoma but separated the grade 2 chondrosarcomas into two groups. The two groups of grade 2 chondrosarcomas included a pre-chondrogenic cluster and a chondrogenic cluster. Of note, only the grade 2 chondrosarcomas expressing a prechondrogenic profile developed metastases (6 of 10 patients with a mean follow-up of forty months), compared to none of the grade 2 chondrosarcomas in the chondrogenic cluster (0 of 8 developing metastases with a mean follow-up of 55 months). These tantalizing results suggest that gene expression profiling may provide prognostic information independent of histologic grade (however, many more cases need to be examined in a prospective manner to confirm these preliminary results)(Boeuf et al. 2008).

Mesenchymal chondrosarcoma (MCS) is characterized by a dual population consisting of primitive small round blue cells similar in appearance to Ewing sarcoma/PNET and a second component of grade 1 or 2 conventional chondrosarcoma (rarely grade 3 chondrosarcoma). There are few reports of the genetics of this tumor. One case demonstrated marked aneuploidy, and two cases showed the same chromosomal abnormality of der(13;21)(q10;q10)(Bruns et al. 2004, Gelderblom et al. 2008). Like conventional chondrosarcoma, the cartilage forming tumor cells mimic growth plate chondrocytes (Fanburg-Smith et al. 2009).

Dedifferentiated chondrosarcoma, like mesenchymal chondrosarcoma, is also biphasic and comprises areas of low grade conventional chondrosarcoma mixed with non-cartilaginous sarcoma. There is a paucity of data regarding the genetics of these tumors, but both components share identical genetic changes with additional changes in the high grade sarcomatous areas. It has not been deciphered whether the anaplastic portion of the tumor and the chondrosarcoma portion derive from a common progenitor cell or whether the anaplastic lineage arises from a more differentiated chondrocytic tumor cell (Aigner 2002). The sarcomatous component is most often histologically consistent with osteosarcoma, including chondroblastic osteosarcoma, but fibroblastic and myoid sarcomas are also reported (Dornauer et al. 2010).

Clear cell chondrosarcoma is the rarest cartilaginous tumor. Based on limited numbers of cases analyzed, it may have extra copies of chromosome 20 and loss or rearrangements of chromosome 9p (Nishio et al. 2005).

PATHOLOGY

Histologic grading of cartilaginous tumors

Benign cartilaginous tumors are not graded. The most common grading system used for malignant cartilaginous tumors is three tiered (other systems have been proposed). Conventional chondrosarcomas are graded according to cellularity, degree of cytologic atypia and mitotic activity with myxoid change notable in higher grade tumors. Necrosis is also present and tends to be a feature of higher grade chondrosarcomas but is not part of the grading system. In general, reviewing series of conventional chondrosarcomas, most tumors (approximately 60%) are grade 1 (well differentiated), 35% are grade 2 (intermediate differentiation) and a minority, 5%, are grade 3 (poorly differentiated) (Damjanov et al. 2007). Recurrent tumors can occur as a higher grade.

A caveat regarding the pathologic diagnosis of malignant cartilaginous tumors: aspects of pathologic grading of chondrosarcomas have known problems of inter-observer and even intra-observer variability (Jones et al. 2007). However, there are to date no additional laboratory tests or radiologic evaluations that can better predict outcome than the current system of combined expert radiologic and pathologic assessment by traditional microscopic evaluation, X-ray, MRI and CT evaluations. The search for factors or biomarkers that can better predict prognosis and individual response to therapy is ongoing.

Figures 16.4a through **16.4c** illustrate representative fields at similar magnification of grade 1, grade 2 and grade 3 conventional chondrosarcoma, respectively. Note the increasing cytologic atypia and cellularity of the cells as grade progresses. As these are conventional chondrosarcomas, hyaline matrix is an integral element of the tumor. Table 16.4 contains the numbers of chondrosarcoma subtype distributed according to histologic grade from the SEER registry data for 13 registries from 1993–2007. Slightly differing from the most common grade 1 - grade 3 scale system of grading chondrosarcomas, the SEER registry imparts a grade 4 (IV) to 'undifferentiated' type of chondrosarcoma. There are some limitations to the SEER data in that ~300 cases had no grading information, the initial tumor size was not collected, and the type of surgical resection also not recorded, but the data are population based and subject to careful quality control measures.

Mesenchymal chondrosarcoma and dedifferentiated chondrosarcoma are high grade tumors. Clear cell chondrosarcoma is a low grade tumor.

It is important to note that histologic grade, though imperfect, predicts risk for recurrence, metastasis and survival. Many potential biomarkers have been assessed to attempt to improve prognostication, but none so far independently improve upon the microscopic grade of tumor.

Behavior of cartilaginous tumors

Table 16.6 indicates the five year relative survival rate by chondrosarcoma type according to the SEER data collected 1993-2007. Data reported from the American College of Surgeons tumor registry of chondrosarcomas (n=9606) reveal survival rates similar to SEER reports (Damron et al. 2007). There is a large range in behavior among the malignant chondrosarcomas. The NOS chondrosarcoma subtype behavior is a combined behavior for grades I-IV. Clear cell chondrosarcoma, juxtacortical chondrosarcoma and malignant chondroblastoma

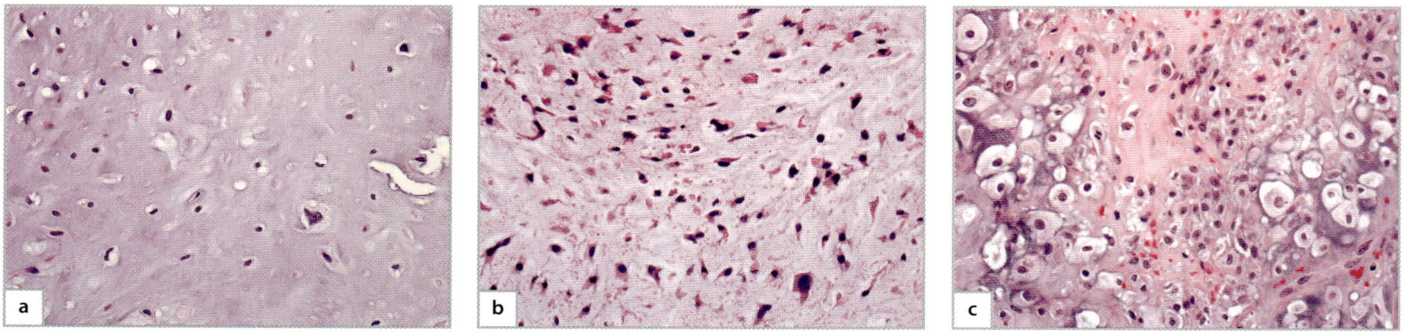

Figure 16.4 **a.** Grade 1 chondrosarcoma at high magnification. Note the hyaline cartilage matrix and relatively low cellularity. However, the chondrocytes are atypical. **b.** Grade 2 chondrosarcoma at high magnification. Tumor cells are more crowded than in the grade 1 chondrosarcoma. Atypia is noticeable. **c.** Grade 3 Chondrosarcoma at high magnification. Cellularity is high with less developed hyaline cartilage; the central cells don't sit in a hyaline matrix but merge slowly with cells that do produce matrix. A mitotic figure is also present. Tumor nuclei range from hypo- to hyperchromatic with variably prominent nucleoli.

Table 16.6 Five-year relative survival rate* by cartilage tumors of the bone type in 13 SEER registries for the years 1994 to 2008, percent survival (SE= standard error).

Tumor type	Percent survival (SE)
Chondrosarcoma, NOS	84.0% (1.40%)
Myxoid chondrosarcoma	74.2% (5.8%)
Dedifferentiated chondrosarcoma	29.3% (9.3%)
Mesenchymal chondrosarcoma	65.3% (9.6%)
Clear cell chondrosarcoma	100.0% (0.0%)
Juxtacortical chondrosarcoma	94.4% (5.7%)
Malignant chondroblastoma	86.0% (13.3%)

*Five-year survival was the chosen instead of 10 year survival due to small numbers in a few of the subtypes.

Patients diagnosed with clear cell chondrosarcoma had the best prognosis.

Cases that were classified as dedifferentiated chondrosarcoma had the worst prognosis (13.7%) of all the subtypes. These cases, as noted in Table 16.1, were more likely to be grade IV tumors.

all exhibit an excellent relative five year survival rate matching numerous reports of these tumors in the literature. By contrast, the most aggressive type of chondrosarcoma, dedifferentiated, exhibits a dismal five year relative survival rate of 15%.

Factors affecting survival include type of tumor, histologic grade, tumor size, tumor location, patient age and adequacy of resection margin. Molecular markers predicting tumor aggressiveness such as p53 mutations have not been shown to be independent of tumor grade on multivariate analysis (Rozeman et al. 2002). As work continues, there is hope that independent, accurate predictive and prognostic biomarkers will be discovered, (one possible independent prognostic 'pre-chondrogenic' gene signature was described above in the Pathogenesis section).

Special stains or tests used to diagnosis cartilaginous tumors of bone

Immunohistochemistry

1. **S-100 protein** is expressed in chondrocytes but is not specific, as many tumors are reactive for S-100 protein. Some chondroblastomas are negative for S-100 protein or only focally positive. The small round cell component of mesenchymal chondrosarcoma and the non-cartilaginous dedifferentiated regions of dedifferentiated chondrosarcoma are also negative.
2. **Keratins** are often expressed in chondroblastomas (up to 90%), including keratins 8, 18 and 19 (Bousdras et al. 2007). This can be helpful in the differential diagnosis of chondroblastoma versus chondromyxoid fibroma, as the latter is keratin negative by immunohistochemical staining.
3. **DOG1** appears to be a relatively sensitive and specific marker for chondroblastoma, as it is expressed in few other tumors other than gastrointestinal stromal tumor (GIST).
4. **Smooth muscle actin** is expressed in chondromyxoid fibroma, often diffusely and may also be expressed in chondroblastoma.
5. **FLI-1** can be useful in the differential diagnosis of mesenchymal chondrosarcoma and Ewing sarcoma/PNET in a small needle core biopsy where the two can look identical. FLI-1 is commonly detectable in Ewing sarcoma/PNET tumors and does not stain the histologically similar small round cells of mesenchymal chondrosarcoma allowing for distinction even in small samples. Another entity in the differential diagnosis on small biopsy of mesenchymal chondrosarcoma is small cell osteosarcoma. Like other cartilaginous tumors, mesenchymal chondrosarcoma expresses SOX9 while small cell osteosarcoma is negative (Fanburg-Smith et al. 2010). The small round blue cells of osteosarcoma are reactive for antibody to osteocalcin; the small round cells of mesenchymal chondrosarcoma are reportedly negative for osteocalcin expression (Fanburg-Smith et al. 2010).
6. **Galectin-1** is a lectin that is expressed in many cells and several tumor types. It may be helpful in discriminating between chondrosarcoma and chondroblastic osteosarcoma, as it appears to be negative in chondrosarcoma and positive in approximately 50% of chondroblastic osteosarcomas (by immunohistochemistry and Western blot studies)(Gomez-Brouchet et al. 2010). It may also be reactive in chondroblastoma which may not be surprising given the unusual partly osteogenic nature of this tumor (Gomez-Brouchet et al. 2010).
7. **Collagen types** can assist diagnostically and provide insight into relationship of a particular cartilaginous tumor to the normal developing chondrocyte. For example, the most prevalent collagen in cartilage, type II collagen, can help distinguish between clear cell chondrosarcoma and chondroblastoma. As both tumors are epiphyseal and overlap in age range, collagen antibody staining can be helpful diagnostically especially with small biopsies.

RADIOLOGY

Cartilage tumors offer the radiologist a unique opportunity to potentially diagnose tissue type by identifying the presence of cartilage matrix. Cartilage matrix is variably calcified, and when visible is classically described as having 'arcs and rings' of calcification. Each arc or ring typically ranges from 1 - 4 mm is size and can be identified best with plain film or CT imaging (**Fig. 16.5**). Cartilage matrix has a less specific appearance on MRI but tends to emulate the appearance of water, thus showing T1 low signal with relatively high signal on T2 and STIR sequences. There can be subtle heterogeneity to the T2 or STIR high signal which gives it a 'dirty' appearance best seen by carefully adjusting the window and level setting.

In general, the benign cartilage lesions are slow growing allowing the adjacent normal bone time to form a sclerotic margin. A sclerotic margin typically indicates a non-aggressive lesion with a so called narrow zone of transition. Benign cartilage lesions can show slow enlargement over months to years. Calcifications can also slowly develop over time. Benign cartilage lesions may have mild endosteal scalloping, although the radiologist must be careful in interpreting the significance of scalloping. Smooth endosteal scalloping resulting in fairly uniform cortical thinning is common and usually not associated with malignancy. However, cortical breakthrough or marked focalized thinning is worrisome for a nidus of aggressive or malignant tissue. Also, rapidly increasing cortical thinning may be a harbinger of histological change or a fundamentally more aggressive lesion. Non-aggressive growth on the other hand simply expands the cortex outward with minimal thinning.

Many believe that cartilage lesions warrant surveillance to monitor for the rare instance of malignant transformation. There is scant guidance in the literature for appropriate surveillance interval and method (Lohrer et al. 2010). Depending on age and clinical setting; such as size and lesion location, imaging surveillance may be performed at 6 months intervals extending to 1 or even 2 year intervals over time. At some juncture, the patient must be educated that malignant transformation is rare, and often is slow growing. The patient can be a valuable participant in the surveillance of their lesion by monitoring for new onset of unexplained pain.

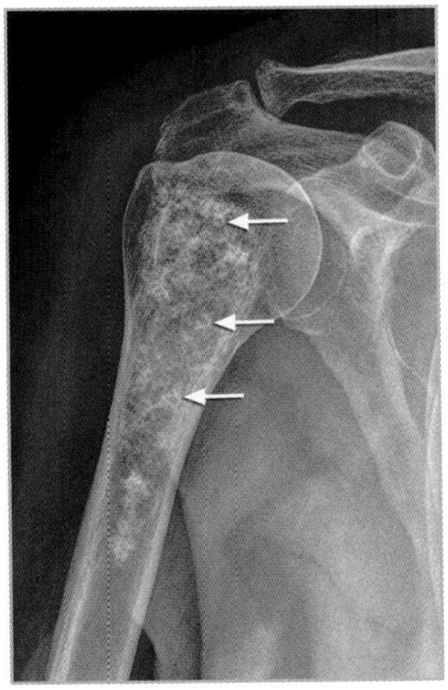

Figure 16.5 Chondrosarcoma of the humerus, AP radiograph. There is a partially calcified lesion of the proximal metaphysis. Arrows point to numerous calcified 'arcs and rings'.

The radiologists must carefully compare the lesion for ominous signs such as areas that decrease in calcification, new areas of focal erosion, cortical breakthrough or focal areas that appears to grow at a different pace. The radiologist is looking for any indication that histology or behavior has changed. Unfortunately, sometimes the transformation is dramatic and frankly malignant chondrosarcoma can be diagnosed by identifying malignant periosteal reaction, frank bone destruction or soft tissue mass.

CLINICAL PEARL

The musculoskeletal radiologist is often asked to distinguish between a bone infarct and a chondroid lesion such as an enchondroma. The bone infarct typically has more calcifications peripherally, will have a characteristic serpentine margin and on MRI may show the double line sign on T2 images. On the other hand, the enchondroma will typically have more calcification centrally, with a lobulated border and hopefully will show the characteristics of cartilage matrix. See Figures 16.6a through 16.6c for radiographs of a bone infarct.

Enchondroma

The typical enchondroma is located in the marrow space near the physeal scar. They are common in long bones. There were incidentally encountered in 2.9% of knee MR exams (Walden et al. 2008). The lesion is generally oval in shape with lobulated margins and variable calcification that may show the classic cartilage arcs and rings pattern. MRI will show variable heterogeneity depending on the degree of calcification. The non-calcified portions are typically T1 low signal with T2 and STIR high signal. There is no adjacent edema. Contrast enhancement is none or minimal. Interestingly, the enchondromas occurring in the phalanges typically do not calcify.

Multiple enchondromatosis is a rare entity where the skeleton is riddled with numerous enchondromas. The numerous lesions can lead to skeletal deformities.

Chondrosarcoma

Chondrosarcomas show a broad spectrum of appearances on imaging depending on the grade of underlying tumor and duration of disease. Imaging interpretation can be difficult and fraught with subjectivity. Often a given cartilage lesion may have inconclusive features necessitating close follow up or biopsy.

In the setting of a high grade chondrosarcoma the underlying matrix may be destroyed leaving no tissue specific radiographic findings. The mass may be quite large and usually shows non-specific MRI appearance with T1 low signal, T2 or STIR high signal and heterogeneous enhancement. Plain radiographs may show gross bone destruction with large soft tissue mass evident. With these findings, the radiologist can only diagnose a non-specific aggressive tumor. Interestingly, chondrosarcomas are usually relatively slow growing even when high grade and may cause surprisingly few symptoms. This is a common presentation for chondrosarcomas of the pelvic which can virtually replace the innominate bone and fill the pelvis by time of presentation. Despite their relatively large size and protracted time course, lung metastases do not usually appear until late in disease course. The radiologist's task with high grade chondrosarcomas is to define the extent of local disease and survey for local recurrence or distant metastasis.

The radiologist's role is more complex in the setting of the less aggressive chondroid lesions. Often there is identifiable chondroid matrix visible allowing at least the generic diagnosis of a cartilage tumor. The radiologist must determine if the lesion is an enchondroma

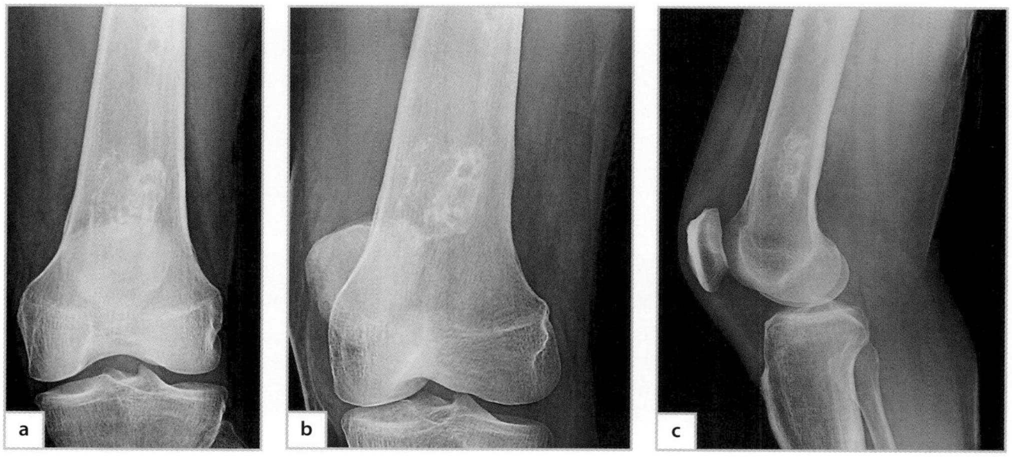

Figure 16.6 Bone infarct. **a.** Frontal, **b.** oblique and **c.** lateral views of the distal femur show the characteristic irregular serpentine sclerotic margins of a bone infarct. Note the absence of central calcifications.

where routine surveillance may be sufficient follow up. Alternatively, if the lesion has any aggressive features it warrants closer surveillance or referral to orthopedic oncology for possible tissue diagnosis. There can be significant overlap in appearance of enchondromas and low grade chondrosarcomas.

On radiographs, the radiologist should look for aggressive features such as focal erosions, erosions with abrupt margins, periosteal reaction or cortical breakthrough. Signs of histologic heterogeneity are also worrisome, such as a focus of non-calcified matrix in a cartilage lesion which is otherwise well calcified. A chondroid lesion without aggressive features can be considered an enchondroma, however, routine follow up is usually performed to establish lesion stability. Follow up imaging can be performed at 6 or 12 month intervals depending on the clinical setting. Ominous changes such as an area of matrix that loses calcification or significant increase in overall size might warrant tissue diagnosis. In general, larger cartilage lesions are more worrisome, nevertheless at this institution we do not have a specific size threshold concerning for malignancy. However, a large lesion that fills the marrow space and appears to extend or extrude into the adjacent marrow space is worrisome for more aggressive histology. These larger tumors appear to have their growth contained by cortex but have sufficiently aggressive behavior to expand through adjacent cancellous bone.

The decision to biopsy a cartilage lesion can be difficult due to the broad spectrum of appearances for cartilage tumors. Experience is invaluable as is consultation with an orthopedic oncologist as to the appropriate follow up course. Further imaging workup might include CT scan to help confirm the presence of cartilage matrix and assess for erosive or destructive features. MR imaging may help to assess for adjacent edema, total extent of tumor, expansion into adjacent marrow and presence of soft tissue tumor component. Nuclear medicine bone scan is not favored at our institution because of the lack of specificity. If a bone scan is performed, high uptake may indicate pathologic fracture or the high metabolism of malignancy. However, many cartilage lesions simply show nonspecific intermediate uptake. A cold appearance on bone scan is strongly reassuring that the cartilage lesion is benign. At our institution FDG-PET is not utilized for cartilage lesion evaluation.

Recent work by Yoo et al., 2009, studied the MR imaging differences between low grade and high grade chondrosarcomas. 93% of low grade chondrosarcomas had entrapped fat visible within the tumor, whereas only 1% of high grade chondrosarcomas showed this. Soft tissue mass was seen in 4% of low grade chondrosarcomas but was present in 79% of high grade chondrosarcomas.

Osteochondroma

Osteochondromas are interesting lesions for their classic appearance, often readily diagnosed by plain film. They are morphologically either pedunculated or sessile lesions. The pedunculated lesions commonly originate in the metaphysis of a long bone and point away from the joint. Both lesions commonly have a layer of cartilage overlying the top or tip of the lesion, described as a cartilage cap. Osteochondromas are thought to originate as a segment of the physis which became separated from the parent bone. Osteochondromas typically should not grow after skeletal maturity. The radiographic hallmark of an osteochondroma consists of smooth cortical continuity of the parent bone and the osteochondroma, and direct extension of the medullary canal of the parent bone into that of the stalk of the osteochondroma. There must be both cortical and marrow continuity.

There are benign and malignant complications associated with osteochondromas. The benign complications relate to their potential mass effect. The osteochondroma may impinge on nerves, interfere with muscle or tendon motion or may limit range of motion of a joint. Mass effect of an osteochondroma between the paired bones such as the radius and ulna can limit rotational and may also lead to pressure erosion or deformity of the adjacent normal bone. Constant soft tissue irritation can lead to development of adventitious bursa overlying the osteochondroma. On occasion, trauma may cause fracture of the pedunculated osteochondroma. These complications and symptoms alone may warrant surgical removal.

Malignant transformation of the cartilaginous cap is rare (Garrison et al. 1982, Staals et al. 2007). The development of pain is ominous; however, given the frequency of benign complications, MRI evaluation can be helpful to ascertain the cause of symptoms. Traditionally, it was thought the cartilage cap should not exceed 1 cm in thickness. However, recently, Bernard et al. 2010, studied 101 osteochondromas and developed a standard method for measuring the cap. First, the tidemark between marrow and cartilage must be visualized on CT or MRI. Then a measurement of the cartilage thickness is made perpendicular to the tidemark, excluding any crevasses of cartilage. They found benign caps measured 0.1 to 2.2 cm on MRI, and all chondrosarcomatous caps were greater than 2 cm in thickness. They suggest a 2 cm cutoff for maximum benign cartilage caps thickness.

Osteochondromyxoma

Osteochondromyxoma (OCM) is a very rare benign tumor seen in association with Carney complex. There is little published on the appearance of these tumors, and unfortunately we do not have a case to present.

Bizarre parosteal osteochondromatous proliferation

Bizarre parosteal osteochondromatous proliferation (BPOP) is a rare benign lesion characterized by a focal area of growing bone with periosteal reaction predominantly affecting the hands and feet that appears to arise from the cortex. It was initially described by Nora and is sometime known as Nora disease or lesion. The lesion can sometimes grow rapidly and may be painful and tender. The radiographic appearance may show mature bone protuberance and periosteal reaction. The lesion lacks the marrow continuity, cortical continuity and cartilage cap seen in osteochondromas. BPOP do not have normal marrow signal internally. The lesion can be peduculated but have an overall irregular shape that does not follow anatomic planes leading to its 'bizarre' appearance. BPOP is most common in the hands of patients in their 20s and 30s, primarily occurring in the proximal and middle phalanges. BPOP is described as T1 low signal with T2 high signal on the surface and irregular T2 signal internally (Gruber et. al. 2008). The differential for BPOP might include myositis ossificans, granulomatous infection, osteochondroma and surface osteosarcoma. Fortunately, surface osteosarcomas are rare in the hands and feet. Resection may be performed for these symptomatic lesions and definitive diagnosis, however, recurrence is common. We do not have a case to present.

Subungual exostosis

Subungual exostosis (SE) is a benign bone protuberance often of the tuft of the great toe characterized by mature bone and a hyaline cartilage cap. On radiographs, SE shows connection to the underlying bone. However, clear cortical and medullary continuity may not be evident which distinguishes these from osteochondromas. The differential for SE also includes BPOP which is typically more irregular appearing and involves the middle or proximal phalanges, not the subungual tuft. We do not have a case to present.

Synovial osteochondromatosis

Synovial osteochondromatosis is an uncommon process of synovial metaplasia resulting in innumerable cartilaginous bodies filling a joint. This typically involves the large joints and is monoarticular. Bursae and tendon sheaths can be involved.

The imaging appearance is variable depending on the degree of calcification and presence of effusion. CT is helpful to visualize calcified bodies and to evaluate bone erosions. MRI can show extensive cartilage bodies distending the joint. The bodies tend to be strikingly uniform in size. Synovial osteochondromatosis should not be confused with joint bodies caused by joint degeneration and osteoarthritis. The usual stigmata of degeneration such as joint space narrowing, spurs, subchondral changes are absent with synovial osteochondromatosis.

Chondroblastoma

Chondroblastoma is a relatively rare benign cartilaginous lesion typically seen in young individuals, in the epiphysis of a long bone with a sclerotic margin. CT and MRI may be helpful to better visualize cartilage matrix and assess the margin. Chondroblastomas can have a distinctive thick, solid periosteal reaction in 47% of all chondroblastomas and seen in 57% of chondroblastomas involving long bones. MRI may show adjacent edema and bone scan can show increased uptake, findings suggesting inflammatory reaction incited by the lesion (Bower et al. 1990).

Chondromyxoid fibroma

Chondromyxoid fibroma is a rare benign cartilage lesion of long bones. The lesion is usually expansile with scalloped intact margins and a paucity of calcification in the matrix. Schajowicz et al. (1971) reviewed 32 cases of chondromyxoid fibroma and showed 68% occurred in the lower extremity with 28% in the tibia. They were usually eccentric within the metaphysis and in close proximity to the physis but usually do not cross the physis. There may be the appearance of calcified septa due to the endosteal ridges and scalloping. There are usually sclerotic margins where the lesion abuts the marrow.

TREATMENT

Osteochondroma

Indications for surgical resection of an osteochondroma include pain, deformity, dysfunction, neural or vascular compromise, and occasionally cosmesis. New onset pain and growth of the osteochondroma in an adult should raise the concern for malignant degeneration (a rare late possibility in this tumor), but may also be secondary to development of a pseudo-bursa and inflammation.

Simple excision at the base of the lesion is sufficient. This is accomplished relatively easily in the pedunculated osteochondroma where insertion of a broad osteotome in the 'axilla' of the lesion excises the mass through the junction of the normal and deformed cortex. Sessile lesions may take a little more finesse. Removal of the attached normal cortex is unnecessary and raises the concern for susceptibility to fracture or the requirement for bracing or internal fixation.

Because these are not truly neoplastic lesions, recurrence *per se* does not occur. Any residual cartilaginous portion of osteochondroma left behind (a not uncommon scenario with attempted removal of a large and very sessile lesion) in the skeletally immature patient will have the capacity to grow and cause a clinical 'recurrence.'

Osteochondromyxoma

Osteochondromyxoma is a rare tumor, seen almost exclusively as part of the Carney complex (a familial lentiginous and multiorgan tumorous syndrome). These tumors are benign but locally aggressive. Complete surgical excision generally results in cure, but incomplete resection may result in recurrence.

Subungual exostosis

Subungual exostosis arises from the distal portion of the terminal phalanx of the toes, particularly the great toe, rarely from the thumb and fingers. Complete excision is generally curative.

Bizarre parosteal osteochondromatous proliferation

Bizarre parosteal osteochondromatous proliferation (BPO Por Nora's lesion) represents a rare neoplasm. Intralesional or marginal excision can result in a high rate of local recurrence (up to 50%). Wide resection results in a very low recurrence rate but often requires disabling surgery or even amputation. Because this represents a benign condition, complete local excision is recommended as the initial treatment. Recurrences may require more aggressive attempts at resection.

Chondroma (cortical chondroma, periosteal chondroma, juxtacortical chondroma)

Chondromas may generally be treated with marginal excision with a low incidence of recurrence. Extensive and multiply recurrent tumors may require more aggressive resection.

Enchondroma

Enchondromas are rarely symptomatic. If pain is present, every effort should be made to rule out other causes, including chondrosarcoma. In the rare tumor that is symptomatic, simple curettage will generally suffice and result in a low incidence of local recurrence. The defect can be filled with allograft or bone graft substitute to facilitate healing.

Lesions of the hand will frequently present with pathologic fracture. With rare exception, surgery is warranted in all solitary enchondromas of the hand to prevent fracture. If the patient presents with a pathologic fracture, the fracture is rarely displaced. The fracture should be treated conservatively and the enchondroma addressed after fracture healing.

Malignant transformation is very rare in the solitary lesion but can occur more commonly in the multiple enchondromatoses (Ollier disease, Maffucci syndrome). However if this possibility is suspected, then formal biopsy should be performed prior to any other intervention.

Low grade chondrosarcoma

Low-grade chondrosarcoma presents an area of controversy to the orthopaedic oncologist. The challenge for the multi-disciplinary team is to separate the enchondroma from chondrosarcoma based on the totality of the clinical and pathologic picture. Pain, growth, and cortical penetration appear to be the best distinguishing characteristics with an enchondroma typically demonstrating no growth, no cortical penetration, and rarely pain, while low grade chondrosarcoma may be more likely to present with one or all of these characteristics. There is recognized interobserver disparity between experienced radiologists and pathologists as seen in the Skeletal Lesions Interobserver Correlation among Expert Diagnosticians (SLICED) study group highlighting the importance of the clinical exam and consensus of a multidisciplinary team (SLICED Study Group, 2007).

Historically, the treatment for all chondrosarcomas has been wide versus radical en bloc resection. There is little doubt that this approach offers the overall lowest rate of local recurrence. There may, however, be some room here for prudence. Low-grade chondrosarcomas are slowly growing tumors and present a lower risk of metastasis, which in many cases appears relatively independent of the effectiveness of local control. An argument can be made, and recent data would tend to support, a role for extended curettage with local adjuvant therapy, either with phenol, argon beam or polymethylmethacrylate (Aarons et al. 2009). This strategy would spare the patient from a large and potentially morbid procedure often requiring complex reconstruction and generally associated with substantial functional impairment.

GRAY AREA

Because of the relatively low local aggressivity of these tumors, wide or radical resection may not be necessary to achieve adequate local control. Curettage with margin extension via adjuvant means may result in an equivalent local control rate.

Intermediate and high grade chondrosarcoma

High grade chondrosarcomas are aggressive and have a sizable risk of recurrence and metastasis. Surgical treatment offers the only hope of cure, as adjuvant treatment has demonstrated little success with these tumors. Wide surgical resection is the treatment of choice.

GRAY AREA

Some data suggests that intermediate grade chondrosarcoma tends to behave more similarly to low grade chondrosarcoma and may more appropriately be treated as such (Reith et al. 2003).

Dedifferentiated chondrosarcoma

Dedifferentiated chondrosarcoma represents a variant of chondrosarcoma (any grade) in which there is a simultaneous component of another high grade sarcoma. Surgically, this tumor is treated the same as a high grade chondrosarcoma. Adjuvant chemotherapy may have a role in treatment, particularly if the dedifferentiated component is a chemotherapy sensitive tumor.

Mesenchymal chondrosarcoma

Mesenchymal chondrosarcoma is a distinct subtype of chondrosarcoma with aggressive clinical behavior. Surgically, this tumor is treated the same as a high grade chondrosarcoma. Adjuvant chemotherapy may have a role in treatment.

Chondroblastoma

Although these tumors typically demonstrate a fairly limited growth and destruction potential, most are painful and will require treatment. Curettage with bone grafting is the treatment of choice and will generally result in a low incidence of recurrence. Axial location and/or addition of an aneurysmal bone cyst component may increase the risk of local recurrence (Ramappa et al. 2000). More aggressive treatment may be warranted in multiply recurrent or metastatic tumors.

Chondromyxoid fibroma

Most chondromyxoid fibromas can be excised or treated with local curettage and bone grafting. Wide surgical margins have been advocated for the aggressive stage 3 lesions (Campanacci et al. 1999). Age appears related to recurrence and the extent of curettage. Bone grafting appears to decrease recurrence. Recurrence is common, but with rates reported between 4-80% there is little prognostic value available for individual cases (Campanacci et al. 1999, Jaffe 1958).

Synovial chondromatosis

Synovial chondromatosis is best treated with loose body removal and synovectomy. Recurrence can occur in up to 30% of patients.

MEDICAL ONCOLOGY

There is no medical oncology indication for the following cartilaginous tumors: osteochondroma, chondroma (cortical chondroma, periosteal chondroma, juxtacortical chondroma), enchondroma, chondroblastoma, chondromyxoid fibroma, synovial chondromatosis, and low grade chondrosarcoma, osteochondromyxoma, subungual exostosis, and bizarre parosteal osteochondromatous proliferation of the hands and feet (BPOP).

Intermediate and high grade chondrosarcoma

The intermediate and high grade chondrosarcoma are generally considered to be resistant to chemotherapy due to poor vascularity, expression of multidrug resistance genes, and relative slow growth. High-grade chondrosarcomas have a high metastatic potential with a 10 year survival of 29% (Bjornsson 1998). In practice, these patients are treated with a doxorubicin based-regimen (see introduction on chemotherapy treatments). Standard chemotherapy does not affect the outcome of patients with this disease. Both standard chemotherapy and radiation therapy are ineffective to control tumor growth and should not be indicated outside of a clinical trial (Grimer 2007).

Platelet -derived growth factor receptor (PDGFR-) α and PDGFR-β have both been found to be overexpressed in chondrosarcoma. However, a recently reported phase II study of imatinib (PDGFR/KIT inhibitor) failed to show meaningful activity in the 26 patients studied (Grignani 2010). Targeting histone deacetylase as well as inhibition of the hedgehog pathway and aromatase signaling have also shown promising activity in cell line models. A study of aromatase inhibition in 10 patients with chondrosarcoma showed stable disease in the 7 evaluable patients, who were progressing prior to initiation of therapy (Gelderblom 2010). Current phase II studies are investigating the use of dasatinib (dual SRC/ABL inhibitor), as well as GDC-0449 (hedgehog antagonist).

Dedifferentiated chondrosarcoma

Dedifferentiated chondrosarcoma represents a variant of chondrosarcoma where usually low grade cartilage tumor (but could be any grade) is mixed with a high grade spindle cell sarcoma. Ten percent of all chondrosarcoma are dedifferentiated, and they are usually diagnosed in the sixth or seventh decade of life. Adjuvant chemotherapy may have a role in treatment, particularly if the dedifferentiated component is a chemotherapy sensitive sarcoma type (Dickey et al. 2004, Staals et al. 2007, Nooij et al. 2005). Most patients will develop lung metastases (90%), at which time this cancer is not responsive to chemotherapy (Mitchell et al. 2000, Staals et al. 2006). Most patients with metastases will die within the year. Medical treatment is best delivered through a clinical trial. Drugs that have been studied in vitro and in vivo include histone deacetylase, angiogenesis inhibitors, and aromatase inhibitors (Cleton-Jansen et al. 2005, Sakimura et al. 2007, Klenke et al. 2007). Incidental responses of chondrosarcomas to targeted agents have been reported with vascular endothelial growth factor antisense (Levine et al. 2006) and recombinant human Apo2L/tumor necrosis factor receptor apoptosis-inducing ligand (TRAIL) (Herbst et al. 2006).

Mesenchymal chondrosarcoma

Mesenchymal chondrosarcoma affects young adults (20-40 years old) and is mainly seen in flat bones, such as mandible, spine, pelvis, or ribs. Surgically, this tumor is treated like a high grade chondrosarcoma. Adjuvant chemotherapy may have a role in treatment, as this is the most chemotherapy sensitive chondrosarcoma (Huvos et al. 1983). In patients with localized tumors, radiation therapy should be considered after surgical resection and adjuvant chemotherapy, or concurrently with chemotherapy (Hardwood et al. 1981, Sevel 2006). More than half the patients will develop metastases. The chemotherapy of choice is similar to the one used for Ewing sarcoma. Survival at 10 years is about 30%.

RADIATION ONCOLOGY

Cartilaginous tumors represent a very heterogeneous group of tumors with a relatively indolent natural history and low risk of metastasis. This places increased importance on local control as morbidity is associated with recurrence and the toxicity of multiple local therapies. Radiation therapy for cartilaginous malignancies has generally been felt to be of limited benefit, as these tumors are felt to be radiation resistant. However, cases of higher grade malignant lesions or lesions where complete resection is not possible do benefit from radiation therapy. This is particularly true in cases of recurrence or in an area where surgical resection is prohibited. Most notably, chondrosarcomas of the base of skull or intracranial locations require radiation therapy with best results obtained using particle radiation (proton/carbon ion).

For benign tumors and low grade malignancies adjuvant radiation therapy is generally not utilized. An exception is in cases of low grade chondrosarcoma of the base of skull. The largest series reported excellent local control with surgical resection and postoperative proton therapy 98% and 99% at 5 and 10 years respectively (Rosenberg et al. 1999). Multiple reviews echo the role of proton therapy in the adjuvant treatment of base of skull chondrosarcoma. Many of these reviews are coupled with reports of chordoma, a tumor arising from notochord remnants that has similar clinical presentation but significantly worse prognosis with disease specific survival of 40-60% long term (Almefty et al. 2007). No randomized studies have been performed due to the rarity of this tumor, but enough retrospective data has been performed to suggest radiation is beneficial. Similarly, radiation therapy to other sites where complete resection is not possible is associated with benefit from radiation therapy, although this remains controversial (Koch et al. 2000, Goda et al. 2011).

For the higher grade tumors (high grade chondrosarcoma, dedifferentiated chondrosarcoma, and mesenchymal chondrosarcoma), radiation therapy should be considered in patients with localized disease, particularly in cases where a wide resection is not feasible. Local recurrence rates with high grade tumors can be high, and radiation is an attractive option to help with local control. This remains a controversial point, as no randomized data is available and retrospective data remains mixed. However, a recent article demonstrated excellent long term local control rates with 'high risk' chondrosarcoma provided gross disease was resected, but only contained eight high grade patients (Goda et al. 2011).

CASES

Case 16.1 Osteochondroma

Clinical history and presentation

The patient is an 8 year old girl who presents with her parents who are concerned about the presence of an arm mass which was first noted six months prior to presentation and has been persistent. She occasionally experiences mild pain with contact but otherwise has no symptoms.

Physical examination reveals a palpable bony mass over the posterior aspect of the proximal humerus. She has full range of motion of the shoulder.

A minimally symptomatic osteochondroma such as this patient's may be observed. Decision for removal is generally elective, based on symptoms, interference with adjacent joint motion, or cosmesis.

This patient and her parents elect for surgical excision.

Surgical findings and comments

Findings at surgery reveal a sessile osteochondroma arising from the posterior aspect of the proximal humerus and projecting into the triceps musculature. It is resected at the level of the cortex with an oscillating saw.

SURGERY GRAY AREA

Since all osteochondromas will grow proportionately to skeletal growth, a mildly symptomatic osteochondroma (particularly a sessile one) may warrant removal at an early, less symptomatic stage, if future problems are predicted as the resection may be easier.

Radiology findings

Case fig. 16.1a shows a surface lesion of the proximal humeral metaphysis. The lesion shows cortical continuity inferiorly and appears to blend with the marrow space. The MR images, **Case figs 16.1b** and **16.1c**, show the cartilage cap. **Case fig. 16.1d** shows there is no appreciable enhancement. The MR images confirm there is marrow and cortical continuity which are characteristic of osteochondromas. MRI can be helpful to evaluate osteochondromas for complications. This is a sessile osteochondroma.

For comparison of this patient's lesion with the condition of multiple osteochondromas, additional radiographs are presented. See **fig. 16.1e** for an example of a patient with multiple pedunculated osteochondromas.

Pathology findings

Gross features

The specimen is received as multiple fragments of bone with focally bulging attached gray, glistening cartilage. Representative sections are taken for microscopic review.

Microscopic features

Low magnification: Scanning the fragments at low magnification reveals a cartilaginous and bony lesion with striking zonal growth reminiscent of endochondral ossification. The lesion forms a bulging excrescence on cortical bone with a cartilaginous 'cap' and underlying columns of bone that blend into surrounding intramedullary bone trabeculae (**Case fig. 16.1f**).

High magnification: The cells forming the lesion comprise an orderly progression of perichondrial cells, chondrocytes embedded in hyaline matrix, and chondrocytes covered by new bone (**Case fig. 16.1g**). The hyaline cartilage, especially in young individuals such as this patient, recapitulates the zones of the growth plate of long bones: the outer portion of the cartilage is modestly cellular with mature chondrocytes residing in lacunae. Deeper in the cap, the chondrocytes form columns with cellular hypertrophy (**Case fig. 16.1h**). Underneath this layer, the matrix surrounding the chondrocytes begins to mineralize. Finally, endochondral ossification consisting of woven bone deposition on residual columns of calcified cartilage merges with the patient's normal medullary bone (**Case fig. 16.1i**).

Special studies: These are not performed, as the radiologic, gross and microscopic features are characteristic.

Pathologic differential or, why isn't it one of the following?

Parosteal osteosarcoma: Parosteal osteosarcoma is usually larger than osteochondroma and it lacks the orderly progression of endochondral ossification seen in osteochondroma. Usually, the cortex beneath the parosteal osteosarcoma is intact whereas the base of an osteochondroma merges into the medullary cavity of the patient's bone without an intervening cortex. Parosteal osteosarcoma also contains an atypical spindle cell stroma surrounding tumor bone.

Periosteal chondroma: This may enter the differential diagnosis of a very flat osteochondroma. However, the periosteal chondroma sits on top of an intact cortex, while the osteochondroma base merges into the medullary cavity without an intervening cortex.

Florid reactive periostitis: This lesion is generally disorganized histologically and forms over an intact cortex.

Malignant transformation of osteochondroma: One should suspect that secondary chondrosarcoma has developed in an osteochondroma when the cartilaginous cap exceeds 2.0 cm in adults. In addition, one usually finds nodules of tumor in the adjacent soft tissue. Uncommonly, an osteochondroma will be associated with its own bursa. In a few such cases, chondroid metaplasia of the synovium can result in rice bodies that can simulate soft tissue nodules of secondary chondrosarcoma. Microscopically, most chondrosarcomas arising from an osteochondroma are grade 1 or 2 and show mild to moderate increased cellularity and cytologic atypia. Attention to the cytologic atypia of the associated cartilaginous cap can help distinguish the rare osteochondroma with rice bodies in its bursa from low grade secondary chondrosarcoma with malignant soft tissue nodular extension. Rarely, high grade spindle cell sarcoma or osteosarcoma may develop (generally in the setting of multiple osteochondromas syndrome). These will commonly exhibit bone destruction and invasion of soft tissue. They will not cause the cartilaginous cap to increase in thickness, but the radiologic features otherwise will be consistent with malignancy. The average age of development of secondary chondrosarcoma is approximately 30 years which is about 15 years younger than for conventional chondrosarcoma (Dorfman and Czerniak 1998).

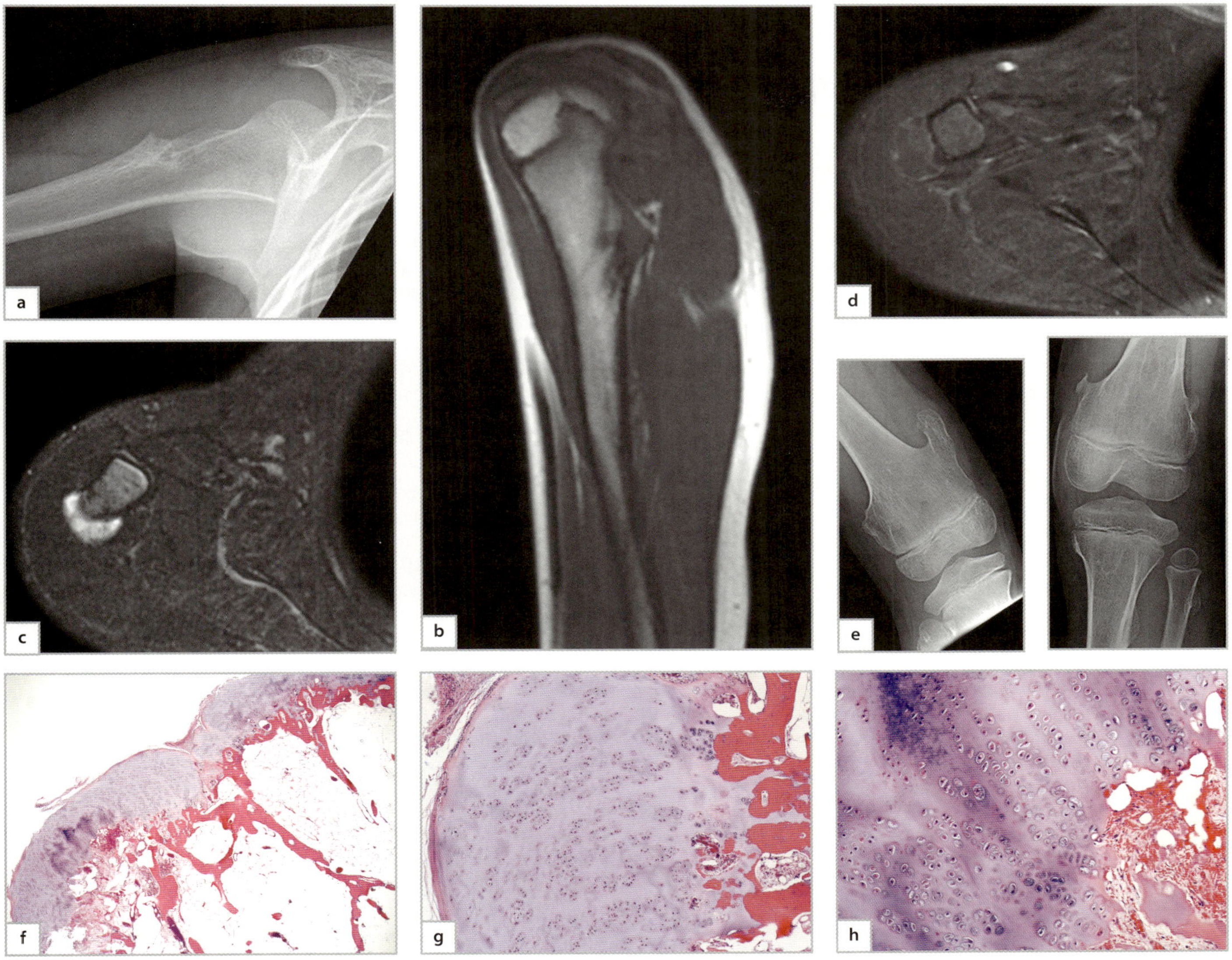

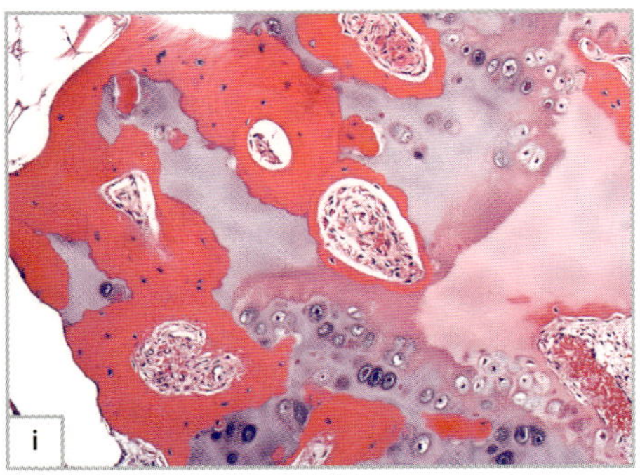

Case figure 16.1 Osteochondroma 16.1a: Lateral radiograph of the humerus. **16.1b**: Sagittal T1 weighted MR image. **16.1c**: Axial STIR MR image. **16.1d**: Axial T1 fat saturated post contrast MR image. The x-ray shows a sessile surface lesion. The MR images show marrow and cortical continuity between the parent bone and the lesion. There is negligible enhancement. **16.1e**: Osteochondromatosis: AP radiographs of both knees. There are multiple sessile and pedunculated osteochondromas around the knees. Note the pedunculated lesions point away from the joint. There is clear cortical and marrow continuity demonstrated. **16.1f**: The lesion forms a cap of cartilage bulging outward from the normal bone surface. This example does not have a prominent bony stalk. **16.1g**: Perichondrial tissue covers the top of the cap and bone forms at the base. **16.1h**: Osteochondromas can mimic the histology of the normal growth plate closely as in this area of the patient's lesion with the smaller more superficial chondrocytes at top left and the larger chondrocytes columns at bottom right recapitulating the zones of chondrocyte proliferation and hypertrophy of the epiphyseal plate. **16.1i**: The base of the osteochondroma reprises the zones of calcified cartilage and bone formation of the normal long bone growth plate. Marrow fat is noted in the left side and pink osteoid deposits on residual hyaline cartilage. Notice the small vessels flowing through channels in the bone.

Oncology approach

This is a benign lesion with no role for adjuvant therapy. However, osteochondroma are seen as sequelae of radiation therapy or radiation exposure at a young age, typically accompanied by growth retardation. Rates can be as high as 30% nine years following total body irradiation (Faraci et al. 2005).

Patient outcome

The patient is doing well four years post-surgery.

Case table 16.1 Summary pathology findings of Case 16.1

Diagnosis	Osteochondroma
Size	2.9 × 1.9 × 1.2 cm
Location	Proximal humerus
Margin status	Not assessable in this specimen and also of no clinical significance
Histologic grade	Not graded: benign
Pathologic stage (TNM classification)	Not staged: benign

Case 16.2 Enchondroma

Clinical history and presentation

The patient is a 42 year old woman who presents with a four month history of pain and swelling along the ulnar aspect of her hand. Onset was spontaneous and symptoms have been persistent.

Physical examination reveals fusiform bony enlargement of the fifth metacarpal. There is mild tenderness on bony palpation. Range of motion is uninhibited.

Pathologic fractures through enchondromas of the hand occur commonly. Surgery is indicated to decrease pain and prevent pathologic fracture.

Surgical findings and comments

Curettage of the tumor is performed along with allograft packing of the defect. At surgery, the cortex is noted to be substantially thinned and expanded, easily broached with a curette.

Radiology findings

Case fig. 16.2a shows a mildly expansile lucent lesion of the 5th metacarpal. There is no appreciable calcified matrix. There is modest, gentle appearing scalloping and thinning of the cortex. No aggressive feature is seen such as focal erosion or periosteal reaction. CT scan could be performed to assess the lesion for chondroid matrix; however, this is the typical appearance of an enchondroma in the hand which does not usually calcify.

For comparison, additional radiology findings of other enchondromas are provided. **Case figs 16.2b** (posterior-anterior radiograph) and **16.2c** (lateral radiograph) represent an enchondroma with pathologic fracture. The lesion is lucent and calcified with a suggestion of the arc and ring pattern of cartilage matrix. There is mild, gentle scalloping without focality or periosteal reaction. **Case fig. 16.2d** (posterior-anterior radiograph) shows an expansile mixed density lesion of the 3rd metacarpal. No cortical breakthrough is seen. A fifth metacarpal lesion is shown in **Case fig. 16.2e** (posterior-anterior radiograph) disclosing a mildly expansile lucent lesion without definite cartilage matrix seen. There is mild cortical scalloping.

An example of multiple enchondromatosis is depicted in **Case figs 16.2f** (Coronal T1 MR image) and **16.2g** (Coronal STIR MR image). Numerous T1 low signal, STIR high signal lesions are seen. The patient had malignant dedifferentiation of a left femoral enchondroma with recurrence and then above knee amputation. A second patient with enchondromatosis demonstrates the X-ray findings of the disease (**Case figs 16.2h**: anterior-posterior radiograph of the knee, and **16.2i**: anterior-posterior radiograph of the pelvis). There are multiple lucent lesions of the femur and tibia without cartilage matrix visible. Note mild degree of expansion and cortical thinning with some of the lesions.

Pathology findings

Gross features

The specimen is received fragmented and bloody and grossly appears fibrocartilaginous. The pieces aggregate to 2.0 cm.

Microscopic features

Low magnification: At low magnification, the tumor is roughly multinodular and consists of blue-gray hyaline cartilage lobules many of which exhibit an outer casing of bright pink osteoid (**Case fig. 16.2j**). Calcifications are present in some of the otherwise uniform nodules of cartilage (**Case fig. 16.2k**).

High magnification: At highest magnification, the lesional cells reside in lacunae and are more crowded than in enchondromas of the larger long bones (**Case fig. 16.2l**). Although the cells exhibit slight nuclear atypia (nuclear clearing with discernable nucleoli; **Case fig. 16.2m**) these features are common in enchondromas of the hands and feet and not worrisome at these locations. **Case fig. 16.2n** provides a comparison high power view of the chondrocytes present in long

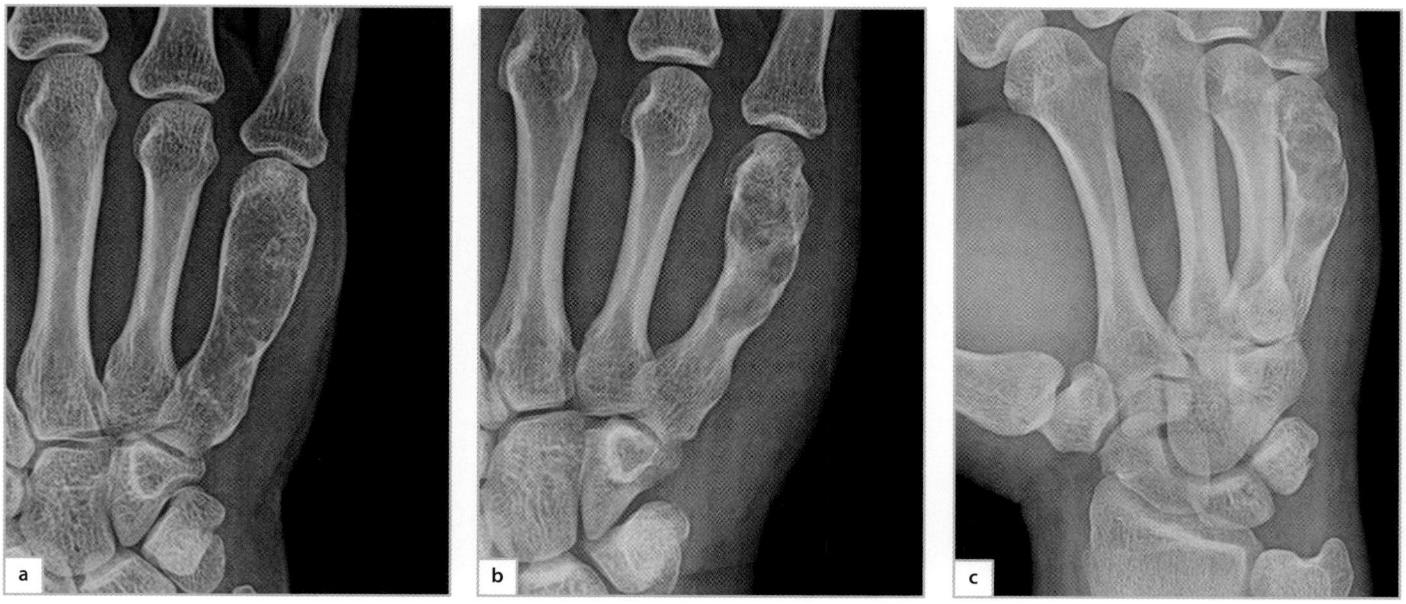

Case figure 16.2 Enchondroma. 16.2a: PA radiograph of the hand. There is a lucent, mildly expansile lesion of the 5th metacarpal lesion. No calcified matrix is seen, typical of enchondromas of the hand. There is modest scalloping without focal aggressive erosion or periosteal reaction. First additional patient with, **16.2b**: PA and **16.2c**: oblique radiographs of the hand showing a non-calcified enchondroma of the 5th metacarpal with pathologic fracture.

Case figure 16.2: Continued from page 384

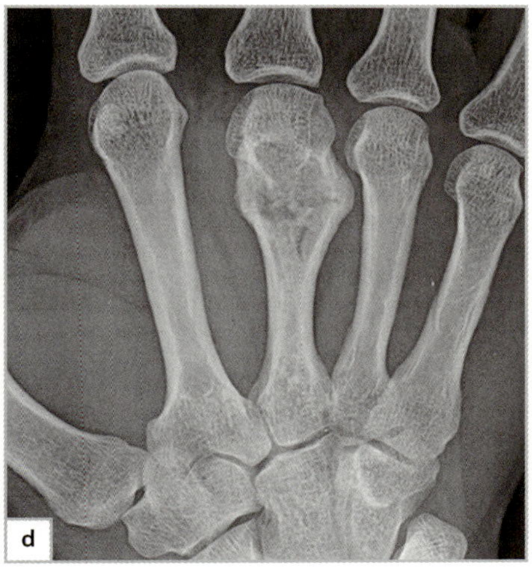

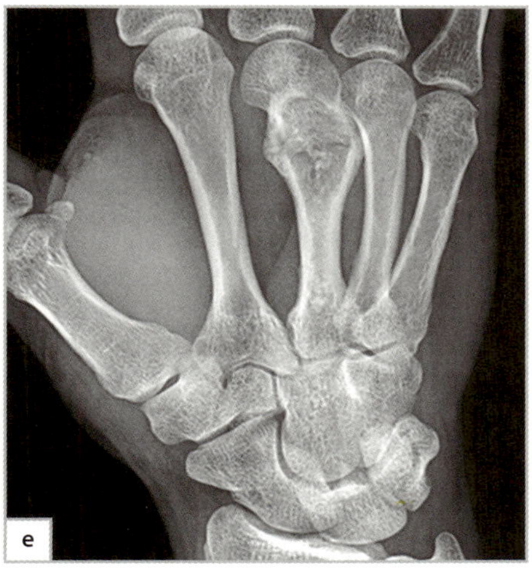

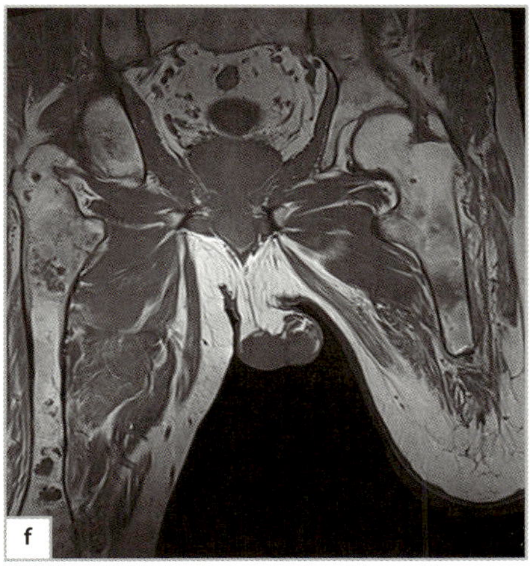

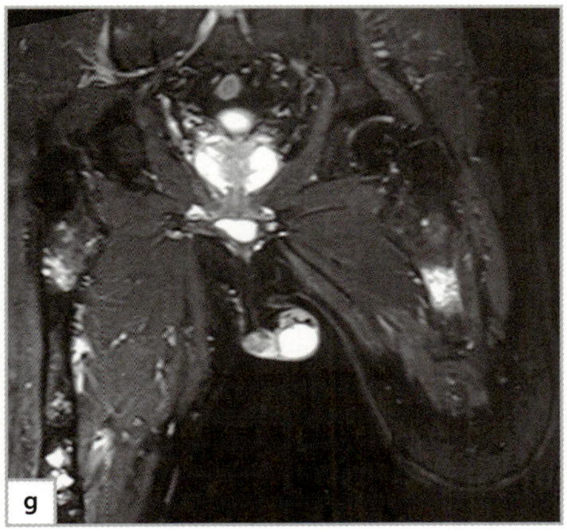

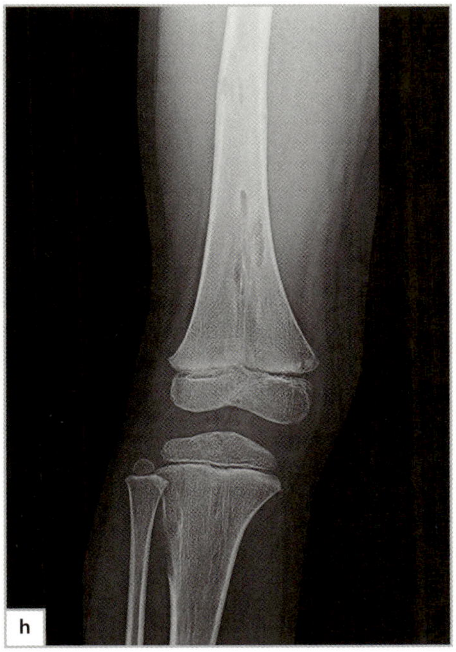

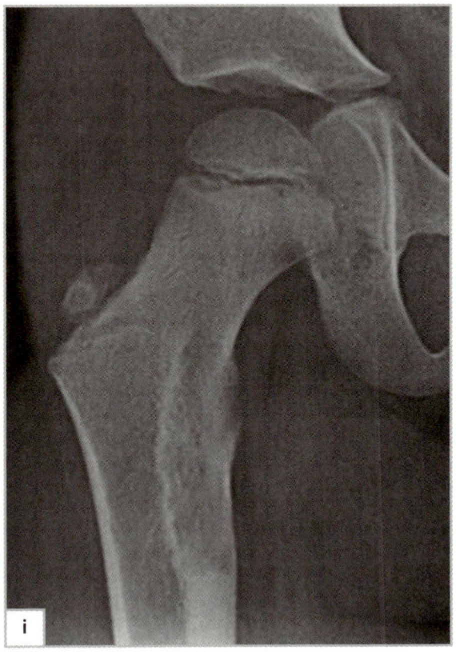

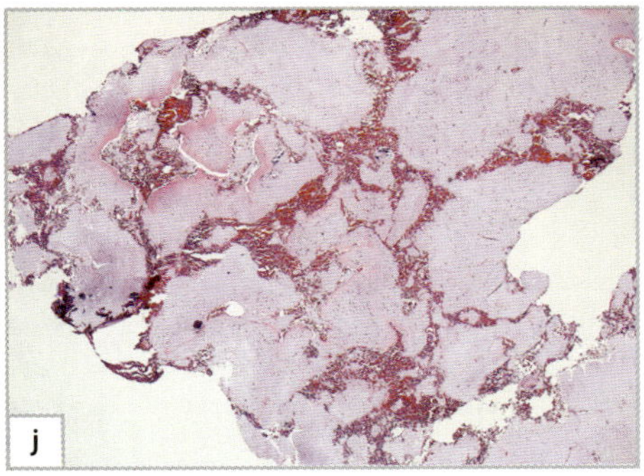

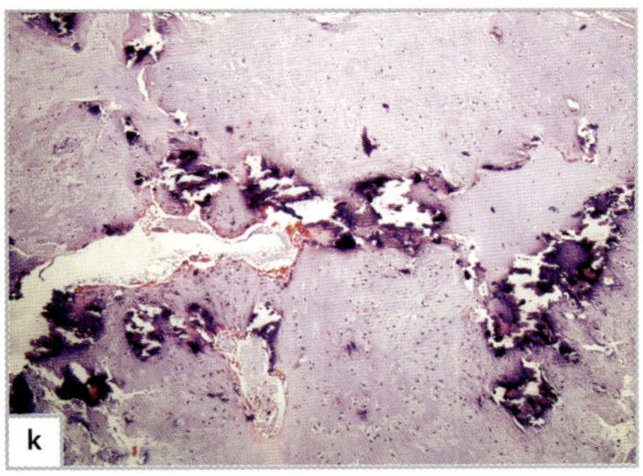

Second additional patient with a enchondroma - **16.2d:** PA radiograph and 1**6.2e:** Oblique radiograph show an enchondroma of the 3rd metacarpal with healing pathologic fracture. There may be minimal calcified matrix visible. Third additional patient with multiple enchondromatosis. **16.2f:** Coronal T1 MR image and **16.2g:** Coronal STIR MR image. There are numerous enchondromas. There was a remote previous distal femoral enchondroma that had malignant transformation requiring mid femoral amputation. Fourth patient additional patient has multiple enchondromatosis. **16.2h:** AP radiograph of the knee and **16.2i:** AP view of the pelvis. There are multiple lucent enchondromas of the femur and tibia, none show calcified matrix. **16.2j:** This curetted specimen still retains the lobular architecture of the tumor. Notice the rimming bands of pink osteoid. **16.2k:** Higher magnification reveals foci of calcification of the hyaline cartilage, a feature often appreciated on radiologic studies.

Case figure 16.2: Continued from page 385

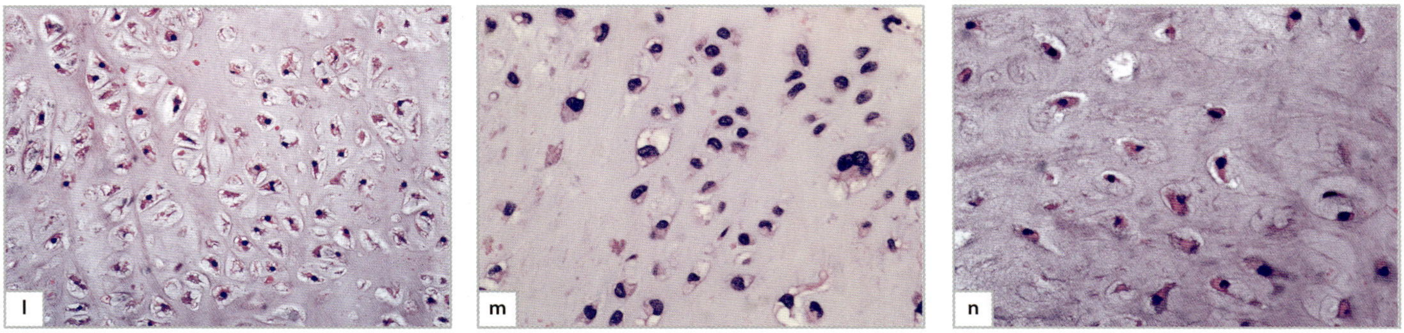

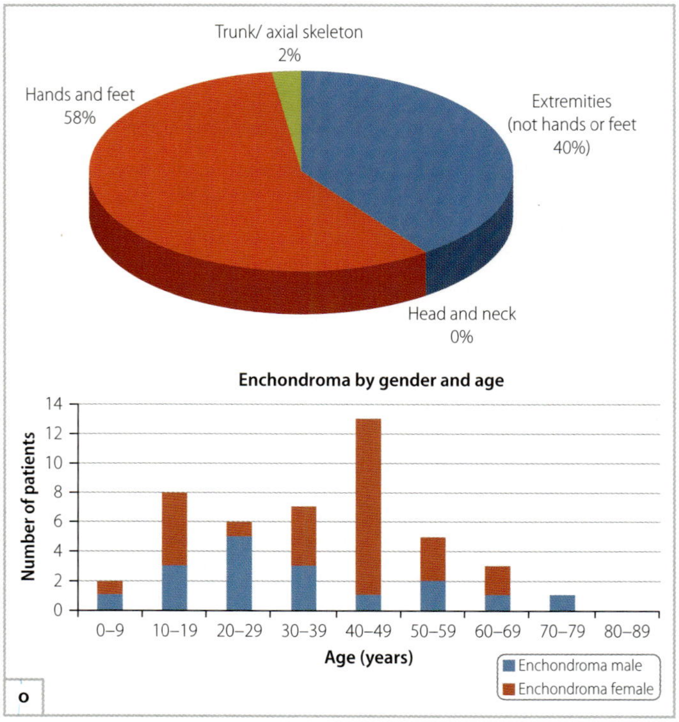

16.2l High magnification of a nodule discloses the relative mild hypercellularity of enchondromas of the hands/feet as compared to enchondromas located elsewhere. **16-2m**: The chondrocytes have relatively large pale nuclei with prominent nucleoli. In a cartilaginous neoplasm, such nuclear features are considered atypical. However, enchondromas of the hands and feet often show this degree of nuclear atypia. **16.2n**: This is a high magnification view of chondrocytes from an enchondroma in a long bone. Compared to the chondrocytes of the case, there is lower cellularity and the cells are not atypical meaning in this context that the nuclei are shrunken and hyperchromatic without discernible nucleoli. **16.2o**: Enchondromas resected at University of New Mexico Health Sciences Center 2000-2010 (n = 45)

bone enchondromas. Cellularity is lower than in finger/toe enchondromas and the chondrocytes are not atypical in that they exhibit small, condensed nuclei.

Special studies: Special stains or studies are not performed.

Pathologic differential or, why isn't it one of the following?

Low Grade Chondrosarcoma: Even before microscopic examination, it is almost a given that the lesion is *not* a chondrosarcoma. This is because chondrosarcomas of the hands and feet are rare. Unequivocal malignant features must be present radiologically to permit a diagnosis of malignancy in an intramedullary, hyaline cartilage tumor of the hands/feet. The histologic features of malignancy would require evidence of an invasive growth pattern: 1) permeation of tumor around pre-existing trabecular bone, 2) growth of tumor through Haversian canals, 3) soft tissue invasion. Without one or more of these features, rendering a diagnosis of low grade chondrosarcoma in the hand or foot would be foolhardy.

Case fig. 16.2o illustrates the patients with enchondromas resected at the University of New Mexico Health Sciences Center from 2000 through 2010. Many more patients were evaluated without surgical intervention (by a factor of ~ 10x). In the University of New Mexico series, there is a broad age range, and hands and feet are the most common sites. No cases occurred in the head/neck region.

Oncology approach

This is a benign lesion with no role for adjuvant therapy.

Patient outcome

The patient is asymptomatic and doing well five years post-surgery.

Case table 16.2 Summary pathology findings of Case 16.2

Diagnosis	Enchondroma
Size	3.4 × 1.3 × 1.4 cm
Location	5th metacarpal
Margin status	Not assessable in this curettage specimen and not of clinical significance
Histologic grade	Not graded: benign
Pathologic stage (TNM classification)	Not staged: benign

Case 16.3 Synovial chondromatosis

Clinical history and presentation

The patient is a 34 year old man who presents with a two year history of left knee pain, intermittent swelling, and periodic catching. He denies any history of trauma. The symptoms have been slowly progressive and have increasingly interfered with functional activity.

Physical examination reveals a small effusion in the knee. Palpation reveals several boggy multinodular mobile masses throughout the joint. Range of motion is limited to an arc of 10-100 degrees.

Surgical findings and comments

In this case surgery is indicated to relieve symptoms and decrease the chance of developing progressive secondary osteoarthritis.

Open arthrotomy of the knee is performed with removal of osteocartilaginous loose bodies and synovectomy. At surgery, multiple loose bodies are visualized along with nodular involvement of the synovium and moderate degenerative arthritis throughout the joint. There is a large joint effusion with large subchondral erosions and joint line spurs. Note the relative preservation of joint space.

Radiology findings

The radiographs in **Case figs 16.3a** and **16.3b** show a knee effusion, marginal erosions and preservation of joint space. No calcified joint bodies are found. The differential for this constellation of findings includes PVNS and synovial chondromatosis. The MR images, **Case fig. 16.3b** through **16.3e** show the joint is packed with innumerable oval bodies of fairly uniform size. There is minimal enhancement and no appreciable calcification or ossification which may develop later. Note that with PVNS, there would be irregular areas of low signal tissue from hemosiderin deposition (see Chapter 7, Case Presentation 7-2).

For comparison, images of a patient with synovial chondromatosis of the tendon sheath are provided. **Case fig. 16.3f** comprises AP and lateral radiographs of the foot. There are irregular clusters of soft tissue calcification with possible arc and ring matrix pattern visible. Representative MR images (**Case figs 16.3f** through **16.3i**) reveal a heterogeneous mass of the plantar forefoot, intimate with the flexor hallucis tendon. There is minimal edema and moderate heterogeneous enhancement.

Pathology findings

Gross features

The specimen comprises a 4.0 cm aggregate of nodular fibrocartilaginous tissue fragments (**Case fig. 16.3j**). The largest fragment is ovoid and partially calcified measuring 1.9 cm maximally. A portion of the specimen is sent for cytogenetic evaluation.

Microscopic features

Low magnification: At low magnification, the lesion comprises numerous discreet cartilaginous nodules embedded in soft tissue. The nodules vary in size and color ranging from blue (hyaline cartilage) to purple (calcified hyaline cartilage) to bright pink (ossification) (**Case fig. 16.3k**).

High magnification: Similar to enchondromas of the hands and feet, synovial chondromatosis (SC) commonly displays chondrocyte atypia. The degree of atypia can mimic a grade 2 chondrosarcoma in terms of cellularity, clearing or pallor of the nuclei and presence of nucleoli. Binucleate chondrocytes are common (**Case fig. 16.3l**). Some nodules slow chondrocyte clustering which is commonly seen in synovial chondromatosis and mimics the distribution of chondrocytes in normal articular hyaline cartilage (**Case fig. 16.3m**). A few other nodules exhibit a less mature appearance with diffuse distribution of the chondrocytes (**Case fig. 16.3n**).

Special studies Cytogenetics testing is performed and reveals three cells (a clone) with the karyotype: 46,XX,t(5;11)(q23;p11.2). The genetic findings of synovial chondromatosis are seldom reported, but some cases show additional chromosome 5 or chromosome 6 abnormalities (Tallini et al. 2002, Buddingh et al. 2003). The translocation of a portion of chromosome 5 in this patient's karyotype may have an equivalent effect to the extra copy of 5 reported in some cases.

Pathologic differential or, why isn't it one of the following?

Osteocartilaginous loose body: These can be multiple but float freely in the joint space. While some of the nodules in synovial chondromatosis can also float in the joint space, at least some are embedded in the synovium and may even grow in the extra-articular tendons. Other than the definitional location in synovium or tendons in synovial chondromatosis, microscopically, the two conditions can appear similar.

Chondrosarcoma arising in synovial chondromatosis: Malignant transformation of synovial chondromatosis is extremely rare. It may only be diagnosed after multiple recurrences. Of course, synovial chondromatosis itself is associated with multiple recurrences. Some SC associated chondrosarcomas may demonstrate necrosis and marked cytologic atypia with chondrocyte spindling and myxoid stroma, features usually absent in synovial chondromatosis. In the few cases of chondrosarcoma arising in synovial chondromatosis reported, the tumors formed a consolidated, calcified mass that commonly eroded adjacent bone. Chondrosarcoma arising in synovial chondromatosis is typically grade 1 or 2 (Dorfman and Czerniak, 1998).

Chart 16.3 presents the cartilaginous tumors resected at the University of New Mexico Health Sciences Center from 2000-2010. Two hundred seventy one tumors were removed. These numbers are intended to represent a medium sized, academic orthopaedic oncology practice. Although enchondromas and osteochondromas are much more common than indicated in the pie chart, judicial selection of patients for surgery leads to a relatively low intervention rate. Synovial chondromatosis is an uncommon lesion; only seven patients were surgically treated during this time period.

Oncology approach

This is a benign lesion with no role for adjuvant therapy. Rarely, this condition is associated with synovial chondrosarcoma a very rare malignancy for which radiation may be beneficial.

Patient outcome

Although at substantial risk for developing a recurrence, at 18 months after synovectomy, the patient has not had evidence of recurrent disease.

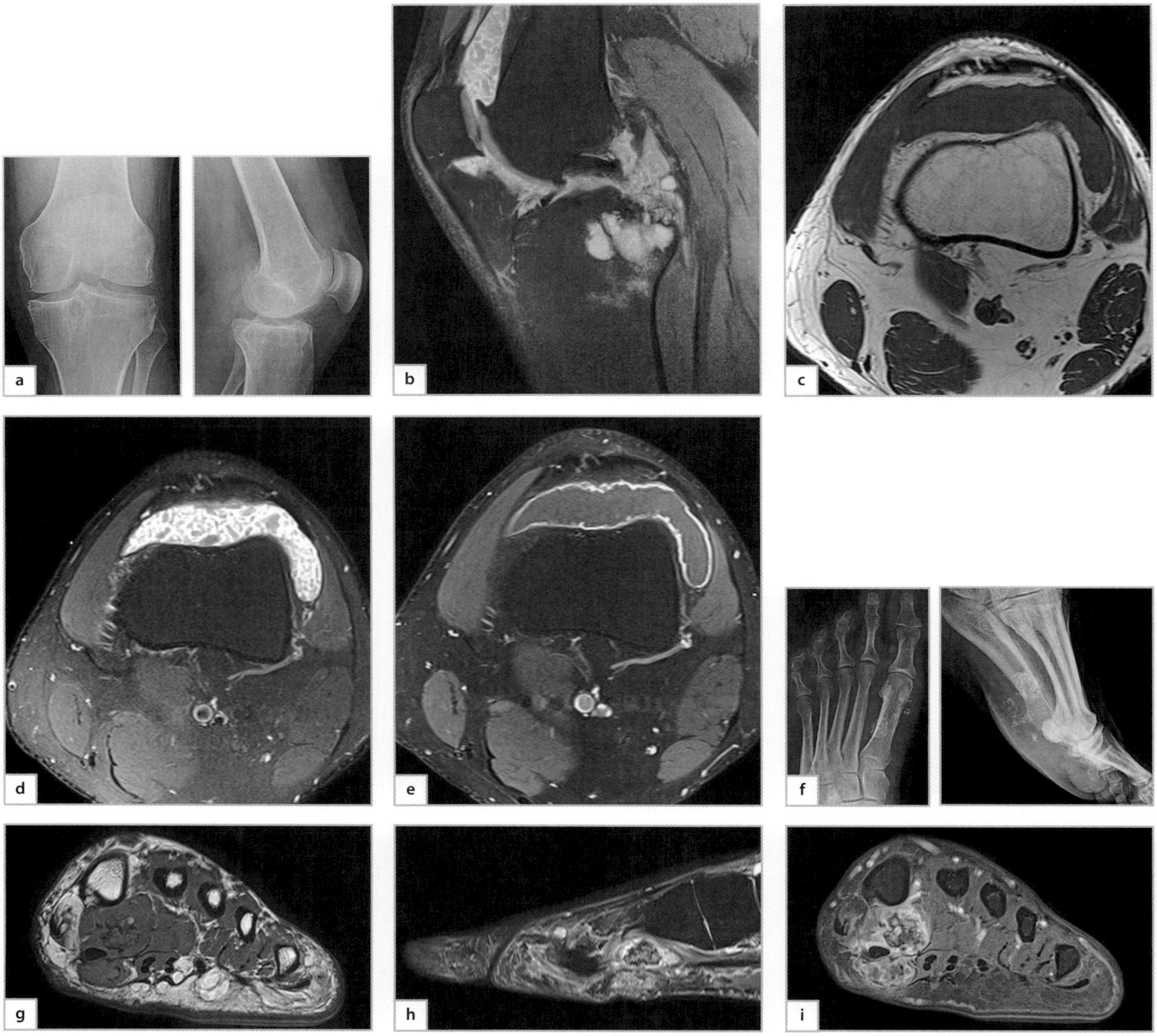

Case figure 16.3 Synovial chondromatosis 16.3a: AP and lateral radiographs of the knee. There is a large joint effusion with large subchondral erosions and joint line spurs. Note the relative preservation of joint space. **16.3b**: Sagittal proton density MR image of the knee. **16.3c**: Axial T1 MR image of the knee. **16.3d**: Axial T2 weighted MR image of the knee. **16.3e**: Axial T1 fat saturated post contrast MR image of the knee. The joint is packed with innumerable small joint bodies which show TI isointensity and low signal on PD and T2 sequences. The lesions do not enhance. **16.3f**: AP and lateral radiographs of the foot. There are irregular clusters of soft tissue calcifications with possible arc and ring matrix pattern visible. **16.3g**: Coronal T1 MR image of the foot. **16.3h**: Sagittal STIR MR image of the foot. **16.3i**: Coronal T1 fat saturated post contrast MR image of the foot. There is a heterogeneous mass of the plantar forefoot, intimate with the flexor hallucis tendon. There is minimal edema, and moderate heterogeneous enhancement.

Case figure 16.3: Continued from page 388

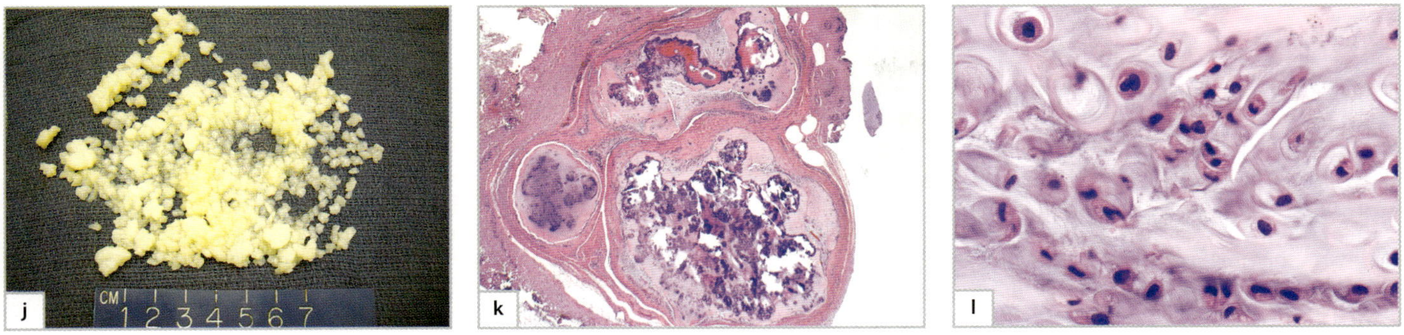

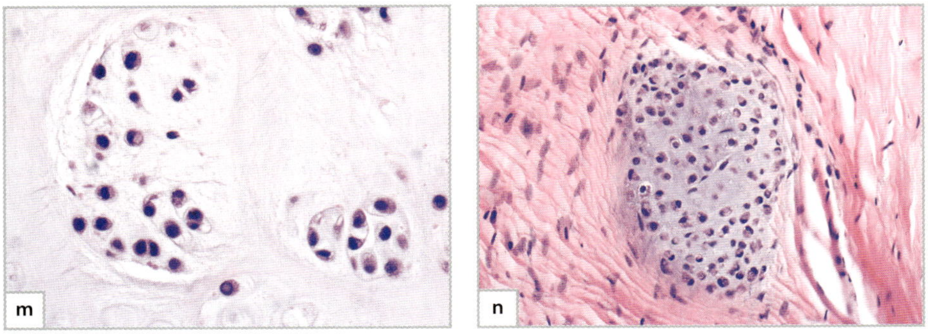

16.3j Gross appearance of resection revealing multiple glistening cartilaginous nodules. Some have coalesced. **16.3k**: Low magnification shows the range of appearances of the metaplastic nodules embedded in soft tissue. All three nodules contain hyaline cartilage, but pale pink chondroid matrix and endochondral ossification are also present. (The tears in the tissue are due to artifacts in cutting the section in the histology laboratory.) **16.3l**: High magnification reveals chondrocyte atypia akin to that seen in enchondromas located in the hands and feet. The cells have vesicular or pale nuclei with prominent nucleoli. A binucleate chondrocyte is also present. **16.3m**: In this field at high magnification, the chondrocytes cluster loosely, a common finding in synovial chondromatosis. **16.3n**: This small, developing nodule is more cellular than its larger companions and may represent a stage in the growth of these nodules from more primitive chondroblasts to mature chondrocytes with endochondral ossification.

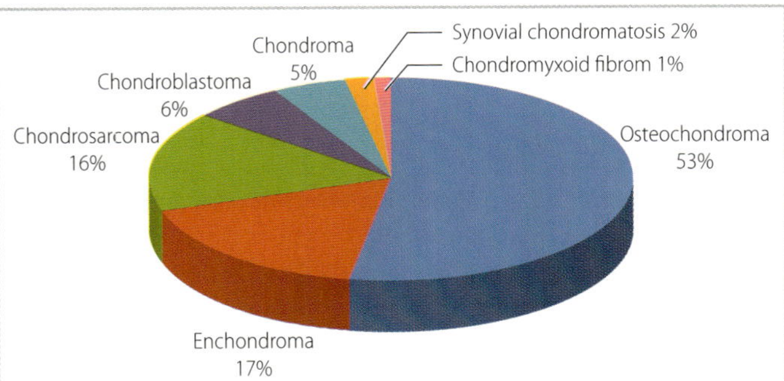

Tumor	Number of patients
Osteochondroma	144
Enchondroma	45
Chondrosarcoma	44
Chondroblastoma	16
Chondroma	13
Synovial chondromatosis	7
Chondromyxoid fibroma	2

Chart 16.3 Cartilaginous tumors resected at UNM Health Sciences Center 2000–2010 (n = 271)

Case table 16.3 Summary pathology findings of Case 16.3

Diagnosis	Synovial chondromatosis
Size	4.0 cm in aggregate
Location	Knee joint
Margin status	Negative margins; complete synovectomy performed
Histologic grade	Not graded: benign
Pathologic stage (TNM classification)	Not staged: benign

Case 16.4 Low grade chondrosarcoma

Clinical history and presentation

The patient is a 42 year old woman who presents with a two to three year history of right knee pain which began insidiously and has been persistent.

Physical examination is remarkable only for diffuse tenderness about the proximal tibia.

Pain and likely penetration of the posterior tibial cortex raise the likelihood that this lesion represents a low grade chondrosarcoma rather than an enchondroma.

Surgical findings and comments

Open biopsy is performed with abundant tissue sampling. Pathologic findings are consistent with low grade chondrosarcoma. Extended curettage is performed utilizing a power burr and polymethylmethacrylate (bone cement).

SURGERY GRAY AREA

Because of the relatively low local aggressivity of these tumors, wide or radical resection may not be necessary to achieve adequate local control. Curettage with margin extension via adjuvant means may result in an equivalent local control rate.

Radiology findings

This patient presents with a grade 1 chondrosarcoma and recurs as a grade 2 chondrosarcoma. **Case figs 16.4a** and **16.4b** are CT scan images showing a partially calcified and lytic lesion of the proximal tibia. There is erosive appearing thinning of the posterior cortex with near breakthrough. The MR images, **Case figs 16.4c** through **16.4d** confirm there is no soft tissue mass. The lesion is T1 low, STIR high signal intensity with a 'dirty' appearance typically seen with cartilage matrix. Incidentally found is a separate enchondroma of the tibial diaphysis that was stable on follow-up exams. Note the striking similarity in appearance with the metaphseal grade 1 CS.

Follow up exams show recurrent chondrosarcoma of the proximal tibial lesion. **Case fig. 16.4e** consists of AP radiographs obtained 11 months apart showing increasing lucency lateral to the area of cement packing. This is worrisome for recurrent tumor destroying adjacent bone. **Case fig. 16.4f** shows Axial T1 MR images also obtained about 11 months apart. MR images confirm there is increasing T1 low signal tissue expanding laterally consistent with growing recurrent tumor. **Case fig. 16.4g**, the Axial T1 fat saturated post contrast MR image, shows the expanding tissue area has intense heterogeneous enhancement, more than expected for post-surgical change.

Pathology findings

Gross features

The initial biopsy comprises a 4.5 cm aggregate of trabeculated, spiculated bone and gray cartilage fragments.

Five months later, repeat biopsies are obtained of a right proximal tibia tumor and right tibial shaft tumor. The gross appearance is similar to the initial specimen.

One year and nine months later, recurrent tumor at the site of the proximal tibial tumor is curetted. The recurrent tumor comprises bone and cartilage fragments mixed with blood. Some of the cartilage fragments are soft and gelatinous (**Case fig. 16.4h**).

Microscopic features

Low magnification: The first two biopsies reveal neoplastic lobulated hyaline cartilage. Like enchondroma, at least some of the lobules are encased in collars of endochondral new bone produced by the tumor (**Case fig. 16.4i**). The recurrent tumor differs even at low power, because areas are myxoid with spindling of tumor cells, and there is noticeably greater cellularity in the hyaline matrix-rich areas (**Case fig. 16.4j**).

High magnification: High magnification of the first two biopsies reveals definite invasive growth of tumor, even in the tumor of the tibial shaft which otherwise histologically could easily be mistaken for an

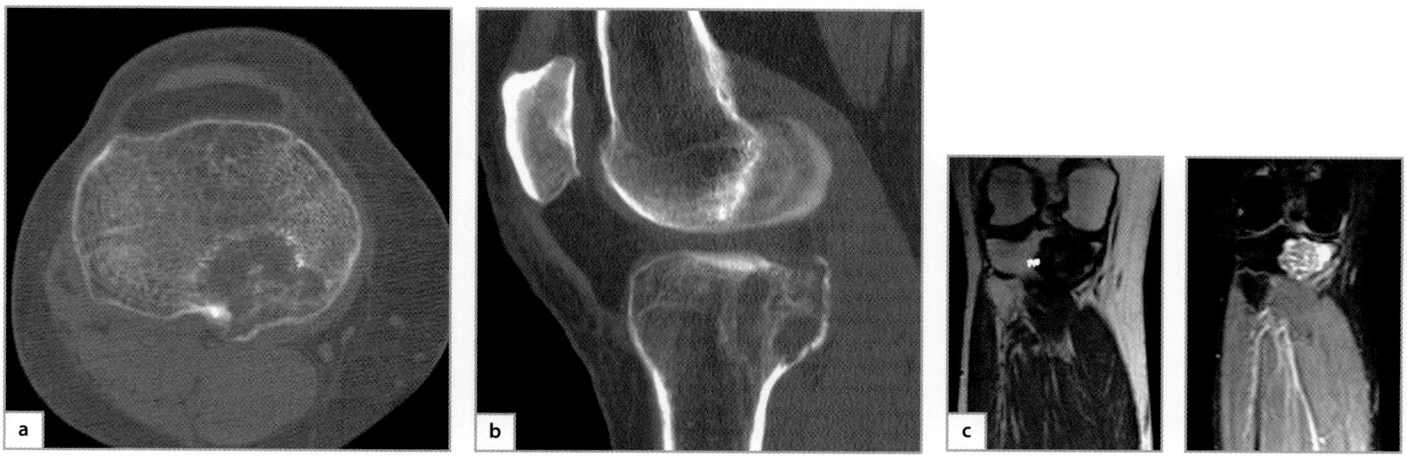

Case figure 16.4 Low grade chondrosarcoma. 16.4a: Axial CT image. **16.4b**: Sagittal reconstructed CT image. CT scan shows a partial calcified eccentric lesion of the proximal tibia. There is marked focal erosion and an area of cortical breakthrough although no soft tissue mass is yet present. There are arc and ring calcifications indicating a cartilage lesion. **16.4c**: Coronal T1 and STIR MR images at the same slice position showing the proximal metaphyseal lesion.

Case figure 16.4: Continued from page 390

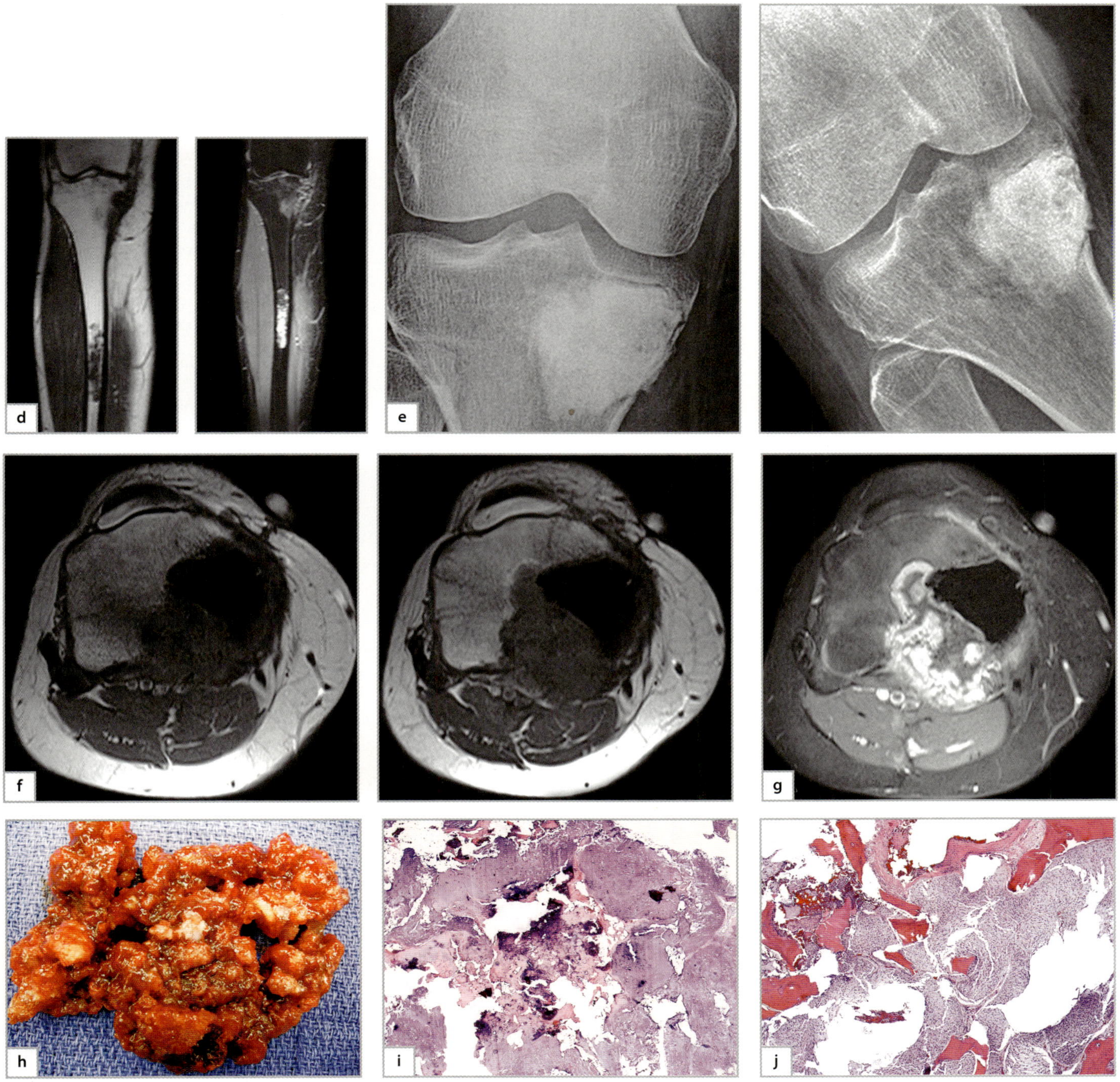

16.4d: Coronal T1 and STIR MR images showing the incidentally found diaphyseal cartilage lesion, likely an enchondroma. Note the similarity in appearance with the metaphyseal lesion. No tissue diagnosis is available for the diaphyseal lesions, however, it proved stable on follow-up exams. **16.4e:** AP radiographs obtained 11 months apart showing increasing lucency lateral to the area of cement packing. This is worrisome for recurrent tumor destroying adjacent bone. **16.4f**: Axial T1 MR images also obtained about 11 months apart. MR images confirm there is increasing T1 low signal tissue expanding laterally consistent with growing recurrent tumor. **16.4g**: Axial T1 fat saturated post contrast MR image. This shows the expanding tissue area has intense heterogeneous enhancement, much more than expected for post-surgical change, and again indicating recurrent tumor. **16.4h**: Gross specimen comprises ragged fragments of bone, cartilage, and gelatinous tumor nodules mixed with blood clot. **16.4i**: At low magnification, the tumor is composed of lobulated hyaline cartilage partially surrounded by collars of pink osteoid resembling an enchondroma. These are curettings so the tumor is fragmented. Dark areas comprise mineralized bone. **16.4j**: Tumor percolates around and partially destroys the patient's trabecular bone spicules in an invasive manner. The tumor cells are spindled and float in a myxoid matrix consistent with grade 2 features.

Case figure 16.4: Continued from page 391

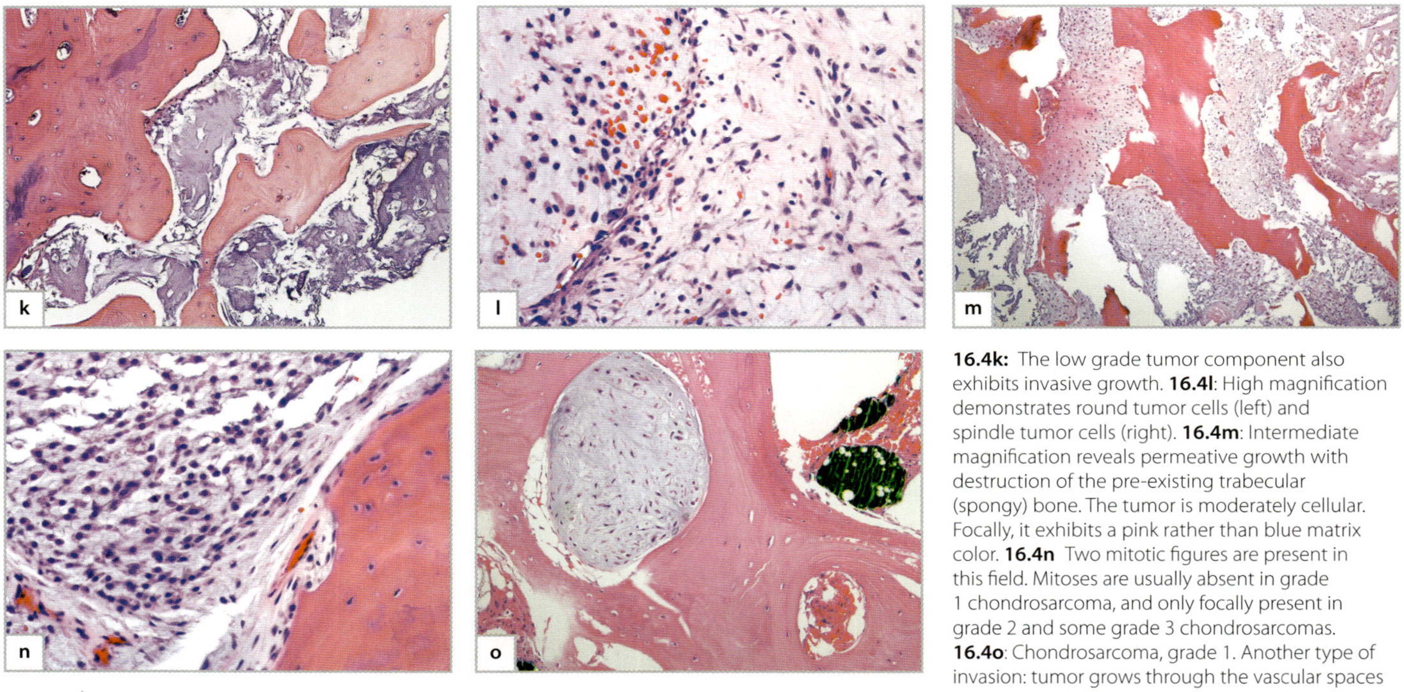

16.4k: The low grade tumor component also exhibits invasive growth. **16.4l**: High magnification demonstrates round tumor cells (left) and spindle tumor cells (right). **16.4m**: Intermediate magnification reveals permeative growth with destruction of the pre-existing trabecular (spongy) bone. The tumor is moderately cellular. Focally, it exhibits a pink rather than blue matrix color. **16.4n** Two mitotic figures are present in this field. Mitoses are usually absent in grade 1 chondrosarcoma, and only focally present in grade 2 and some grade 3 chondrosarcomas. **16.4o**: Chondrosarcoma, grade 1. Another type of invasion: tumor grows through the vascular spaces in trabecular bone analogously to invasion through Haversian canals of cortical bone.

enchondroma (**Case fig. 16.4k**). The recurrent tumor retains in areas a lobulated, low-power enchondroma like architecture, but in other regions a myxoid matrix in which are suspended round to spindled chondrocytes dominates (**Case fig. 16.4l**). Permeative destructive growth is conspicuous (**Case fig. 16.4m**). Unlike grade 1 chondrosarcoma, in this grade 2 recurrence, mitotic figures, though uncommon, can be found scattered throughout the tumor (**Case fig. 16.4n**).

Special studies: No special studies are performed.

Pathologic differential or, why isn't it one of the following?

Enchondroma: A low grade chondrosarcoma can histologically look like an enchondroma. However, a sure way to differentiate the two is to find evidence of a permeative growth pattern. The clearest marker of invasive growth is envelopment or entrapment of the patient's trabecular bone spicules by tumor as seen in **Case fig. 16.4n**. Additionally, tumor growing as plugs in Haversian canals (in cortical bone) or in vascular tunnels of trabecular bone (**Case fig. 16.4o**) also declares malignancy. Sometimes the disaggregation effected by curettage makes examination for permeative growth impossible. **Case table 16.4a** lists the features bone experts have touted as helpful in separating the two entities. This table aside, there are still patients whose tumors cannot be reliably categorized as benign or low grade malignant. Pathologists acknowledge this troublesome set by terms such as: CHUMP (cartilaginous tumor of uncertain malignant potential), low grade cartilaginous neoplasm, atypical enchondroma, hypercellular enchondroma, and chondrosarcoma

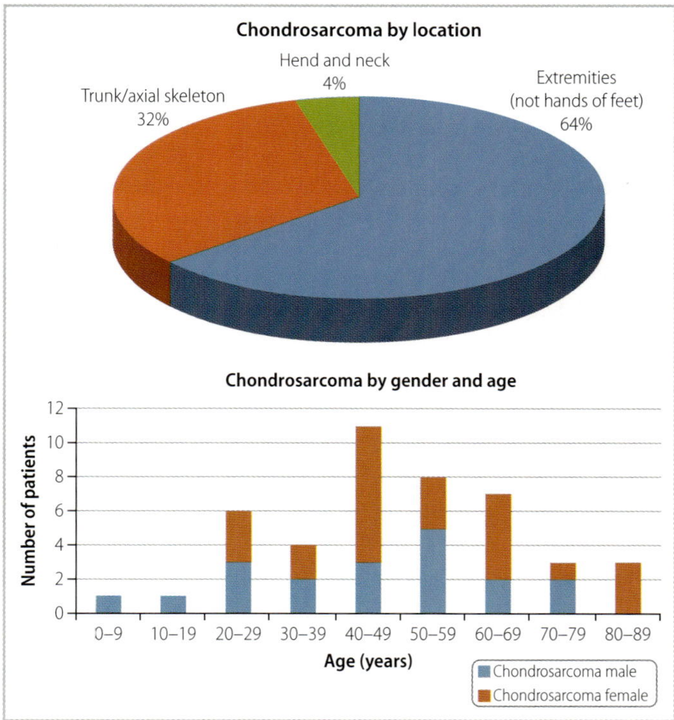

Chart 16.4 Chondrosarcomas resected at UNM health sciences center 2000–2010 (n = 44).

grade ½ among others. The WHO achnowledges this difficulty by combining chondrosarcoma, grade 1 with 'atypical cartilaginous tumors'. Treatment options are similar for diagnostically unequivocal enchondroma to CHUMP to unequivocal low grade chondrosarcoma, except for lesions in the pelvis. . Work continues to improve accuracy and reproducibility in the diagnosis of low grade cartilaginous tumors. The tumors are closely related, and in some patients with grade 1 chondrosarcoma, fragments of a classic enchondromas may also be found consistent with malignant transformation of the latter.

*Enchondromas of enchondromatosis may be more cellular with focal spindling of tumor cells and nuclear atypia.

Grade 2 chondrosarcoma: This patient actually recurs with a grade 2 chondrosarcoma. The table above describes the differences that can be seen in grade 2 versus grade 1 chondrosarcoma. This particular patient's recurrent tumor adheres closely to the Table as it contained areas of myxoid change, spindled chondrocytes, prominent vessel rich septae, nuclear atypia, hypercellularity, and mitotic figures. It is important to note, however, that some areas resembled low grade chondrosarcoma and even enchondroma. Thus, small biopsies of low to intermediate chondrosarcomas may underestimate grade since they can contain areas virtually indistinguishable from benign enchondroma or grade 1 chondrosarcoma.

Chart 16.4 presents information on 44 patients with chondrosarcomas resected at UNM Health Sciences Center from 2000-2010. Not surprisingly, given that most chondrosarcomas are conventional intramedullary in type, most patients were 40-70 years old. However, a few patients were quite young consistent with their diagnosis of mesenchymal chondrosarcoma. In accordance with the literature, most of the patients with conventional intramedullary chondrosarcoma presented with a grade 1 or 2 tumor.

Oncology approach

The patient's initial diagnosis of grade 1 chondrosarcoma does not warrant chemotherapy. Although her tumor recurs locally as grade 2 chondrosarcoma, aggressive curettage without chemotherapy is appropriate for this particular patient, as there is no evidence of metastatic disease, and the patient will be carefully followed.

Radiation oncology

Typically, low grade chondrosarcoma is managed with resection, often without a wide local excision. However, radiation therapy can be utilized in cases where multiple recurrences or where an extensive surgical resection is likely to be associated with significant morbidity. This is especially true for cases of chondrosarcoma of the base of skull. These are often grouped with the treatment for chordomas, a slow growing malignancy of notochord remnants typically involving the clivus or sacrum. Adjuvant or definitive radiation therapy is typically indicated in these cases. Multiple reports have shown that particle therapy (proton, carbon ion) may be a superior treatment option (Rosenberg et al. 1999). Consequently, radiation therapy should be considered in cases where surgery is not possible.

Patient outcome

The patient is doing well three years after aggressive curettage of her recurrent chondrosarcoma. She is regularly followed with physical exams, leg and chest radiographs.

Case table 16.4b Summary pathology findings of Case 16.4

Diagnosis	Chondrosarcoma, grade 1, recurring as chondrosarcoma grade 2
Size	3.1 × 3.7 × 2.7 cm
Location	2 lesions; shaft and metaphysis of tibia
Margin status	The lesions are aggressively curettaged. Unable to formally assess margins by microscopic review
Histologic grade	Initial tumors are consistent with grade 1 and recurrent tumor is grade 2
Pathologic stage (TNM classification)	T1/N0/M0 = Stage IA

Case table 16.4a Histologic features of enchondroma and chondrosarcoma grades 1 and 2

Histologic feature	Enchondroma	Chondrosarcoma grade 1	Chondroscarcoma grade 2
Permeative growth indicated by entrapment of trabecular bone, plugs in Haversian canals, and growth into the cavities of trabecular bone spicules	Almost always absent	Present	Present
Myxoid matrix	Absent to very focal	Can be present and multifocal	Often present
Spindling of chondrocytes	Absent to very focal	Can be present and multifocal	Often present and multifocal
Vascular septa between lobules of tumor	Absent	Present but may be focal	Present and multifocal
Peripheral reactive bone cuffing neoplastic lobules	Widespread	Often present; may be more focal	Can be absent or only focal
Cellularity	Usually low cellularity in long bone locations	Can be focally hypercellular	Hypercellularity is more widespread
Nuclear atypia (clearing or hypochromasia with nucleoli)	Usually absent or very focal in long bone locations	Usually present at least focally.	Present and usually more atypical than Grade 1 with irregular shapes and sizes
Mitotic figures	Absent in long bone locations	Usually absent or very rare	Often present but scattered

Case 16.5 Chondroblastoma

Clinical history and presentation

A 24 year old woman presents with a two year history of left anterior knee pain that began insidiously and has been persistent. The pain is increased with activity, particularly stair climbing and squatting.

Physical examination reveals no masses, swelling, or joint effusion. There is tenderness on palpation of the patella.

Surgical findings and comments

Surgery is indicated to treat symptoms and decrease bone destruction with progression of the tumor.

Curettage of the chondroblastoma is performed along with allograft packing of the defect.

Radiology findings

The radiographs in **Case figs 16.5a** and **16.5b** show a partially calcified lesion of the patella. There is a suggestion of chondroid matrix. The lesion has clearly defined sclerotic borders. There is no periosteal reaction or soft tissue component seen. The lesion location is unusual, but the patella is considered an epiphyseal equivalent. The findings of a lesion with sclerotic margins in an epiphysis should raise the consideration of chondroblastoma, especially in the presence of cartilage matrix.

Pathology findings

Gross features

The tumor is received as curetted pink to tan, glistening firm but yielding soft tissue fragments aggregating to 2 × 0.8 × 0.6 cm. A small portion is submitted for cytogenetic analysis.

Microscopic features

Low magnification: Lower magnification discloses a tumor with cellular, matrix-poor regions interspersed by hypocellular, pink, matrix-rich areas (**Case fig. 16.5c**). At medium magnification (**Case fig. 16.5d**), the pink chondroid matrix is populated by round cells identical to those in the stroma poor area.

High magnification: High magnification reveals that the rounded tumor cells have a moderate nuclear to cytoplasmic ratio and most feature discrete cell borders. Tumor giant cells as well as multinucleated osteoclastic or chondroclastic reactive cells are also present (**Case fig. 16.5e**).

Although this patient's tumor does not contain the famous chicken wire pattern of calcifications that can be seen in about one third of tumors, a comparison photo of these calcifications from another patient is provided (**Case fig. 16.5f**). Although these chicken wire calcifications are a characteristic feature of chondroblastoma, two thirds of cases do not contain them.

Special studies: The karyotype of the tumor is normal female: 46,XX. Most chondroblastomas are diploid by karyotyping (Greenspan et al. 2007).

Scattered tumor cells are positive for S-100 protein and keratins 8 and 18 (by immunohistochemistry). These results are consistent with chondroblastoma.

Pathologic differential or, why isn't it one of the following?

Giant cell tumor of bone (GCT): GCT occurs in skeletally mature bones. Therefore, patients are generally older than patients with chondroblastoma(20x-50x versus 10-25), although the age ranges overalip. Giant cell tumor of bone can appear similar to chondroblastoma histologically. However, the mononuclear cells of GCT do not contain the nuclear grooves and indentations noticeable in at least some of the chondroblastoma cells. Also, the pink chondroid matrix islands and chicken wire calcifications are absent in GCT. Giant cell tumor often displays a remarkably even distribution of giant cells, and these cells can also contain many nuclei (greater than 40). These two characteristics of GCT are not replicated by chondroblastoma. The mononuclear cells of GCT are often p63 reactive and negative for S-100 protein and keratins, the opposite pattern of reactivity in chondroblastoma. Tumor cells in chondroblastoma express DOG1 which is not expressed in the tumor cells of giant cell tumor of bone.

Chondromyxoid fibroma (CMF): CMF is seldom located in the epiphysis. It usually demonstrates a lobulated architecture with central hypocellular myxochondroid matrix and peripheral hypercellularity sometimes with scattered multinucleated giant cells in the ring of hypercellularity. It lacks a chicken wire calcification pattern, and usually the constituent cells are not rounded with nuclear indentations. CMF is positive for S-100 protein but negative for keratins.

Chondroblastoma-like osteosarcoma (CB-OS): This is truly a rare beast. Moreover, both entities can contain atypical cells and mitotic figures in these cells. CB-OS must divulge unequivocal tumor bone formation. By radiology exam, it should appear aggressive. Atypical mitotic figures and extensive necrosis may be seen. There are too few cases of chondroblastoma-like osteosarcoma to comment on the immunohistochemical features.

Solid type of aneurysmal bone cyst (solid ABC): About 20% of chondroblastomas will contain a focus of aneurysmal bone cyst as a secondary change. Therefore, it is important to extensively sample an epiphyseal tumor in a young person with ABC features, as the residual chondroblastoma may be only present in one or two sections. Areas of pink chondroid matrix, chicken wire calcifications, cells with clefted nuclei, and S-100 protein and keratin reactivity should distinguish ABC from chondroblastoma, even when both reside in the same lesion.

The age, gender and tumor skeletal location of patients with chondroblastomas resected at UNM HSC are presented in Chart 16.5. Consistent with larger series, most patients are younger, but middle-aged individuals are also affected, and most cases occur in the extremities.

Oncology approach

This is a benign lesion with usually no need for adjuvant therapy. However, rare presentations in the temporal bone may benefit from adjuvant radiation therapy.

Patient outcome

The patient is doing well 4.5 years post-surgery.

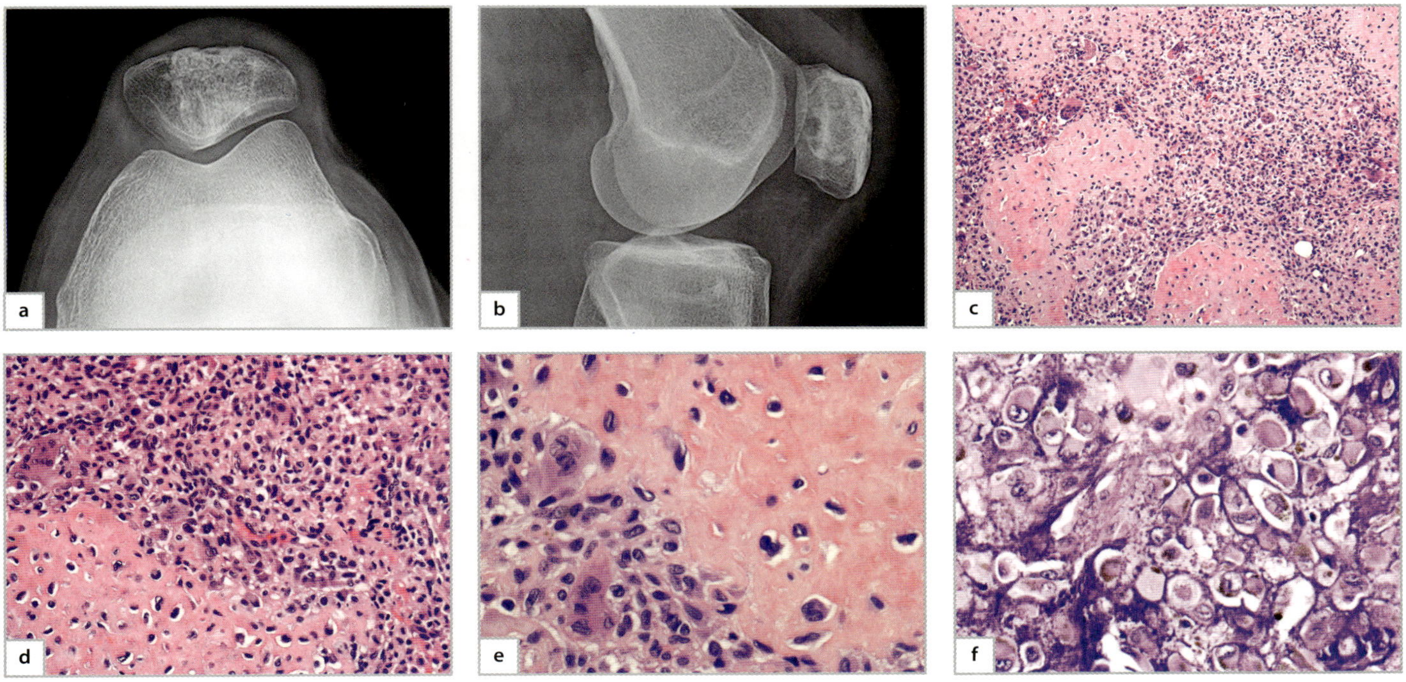

Case figure 16.5 Chondroblastoma. **16.5a**: Sunrise radiograph. There is a mixed density lesion with sclerotic borders in the patella. Chondroid matrix is difficult to visualize. Note the absence of effusion or periosteal reaction. **16.5b**: There is a mixed density lesion with sclerotic borders in the patella. Chondroid matrix is difficult to visualize. Note the absence of effusion or periosteal reaction. **16.5c**: Intermediate magnification reveals hypocellular islands of pink chondroid floating in a cellular background. **16.5d**: Slightly higher magnification (20x objective) reveals the typical high cellularity of a chondroblastoma. **16.5e**: High magnification (40x) demonstrates the round shapes of the tumor cells both in the pink chondroid and adjacent cellular area. Two giant cells are also present. The smaller, rounded tumor cells feature pale ovoid nuclei. A few exhibit nuclear grooves or clefts. **16.5f**: 'Chicken wire' like calcifications encase tumor cells. In this tumor, some cells have cytoplasmic granular brown hemosiderin pigment (40x objective).

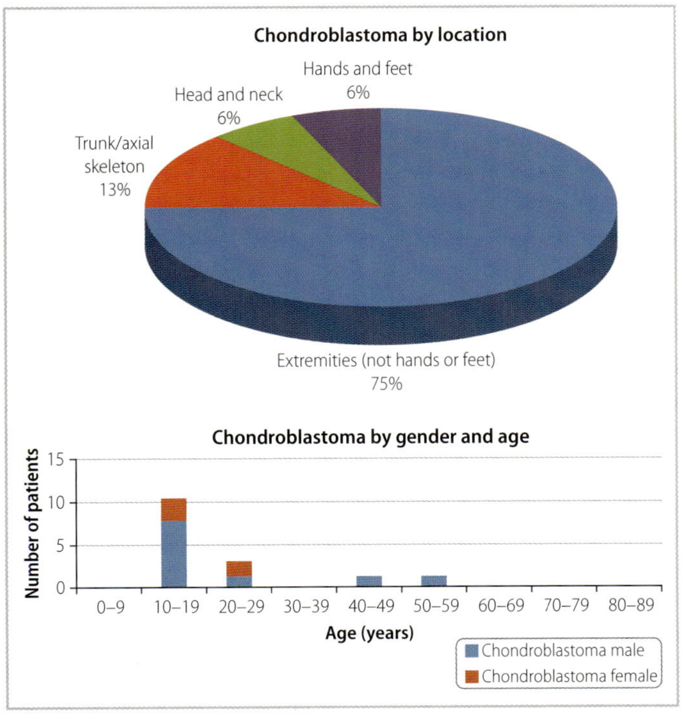

Chart 16.5 Chondroblastomas resected at University of New Mexico Health Sciences Center 2000-2010 (n = 16).

Case table 16.5a Variant histologic features of chondroblastoma

Histologic feature	Comment
Marked coarse solid calcifications	Can be associated with cell necrosis
Spindle cells	Can be prominent and merge with round cells
Marked cystic change	May be associated with only scant typical tumor
Secondary aneurysmal bone cyst formation	Blood-filled cystic spaces with no lining; may obscure residual chondroblastoma
Tumor cells containing brown granular hemosiderin pigment	May be more common in tumors with ABC change and at a particular site, the temporal-mandibular joint
Cytologic atypia	Does not correlate with worse behavior; not associated with atypical mitotic figures

Case table 16.5b Summary pathology findings of Case 16.5

Diagnosis	Chondroblastoma
Size	2.5 × 2.1 × 2.6 cm
Location	Patella
Margin status	Tumor is curetted; formal margin assessment is not possible
Histologic grade	Not graded: benign
Pathologic stage (TNM classification)	Not staged: benign

Case 16.6 Chondromyxoid fibroma

Clinical history and presentation

The patient is a 15 year old girl who presents with a right leg mass noted nine months prior and which has been prominent since. Pain occurs in the area of the mass with activity. She has no pain at rest or at night.

Physical examination reveals a fullness over the anterolateral aspect of the proximal tibia. She has tenderness to palpation over this area. Knee range of motion is normal.

Surgical findings and comments

Chondromyxoid fibromas are locally aggressive tumors and therefore treatment is indicated.

Curettage of the tumor is performed along with allograft packing of the defect.

Radiology findings

Case figs 16.6a and **16.6b** are radiographs showing an eccentric expansile lesion of the proximal tibia. There is mature appearing distal periosteal reaction. No matrix is identifiable. The MR appearance in **Case figs 16.6c** through **16.f** shows T1 low signal with high signal on STIR and T2 images. Note the 'dirty' appearance of cartilage on fluid sensitive sequences. Despite the expansion, there is no cortical break through or soft tissue mass. There is no adjacent marrow or soft tissue edema. Overall the findings indicate a non-aggressive lesion. Even though the appearance is not specific for chondromyxoid fibroma, the suggestion of cartilage matrix should guide the radiologist to include this rare benign cartilage lesion in the differential diagnosis.

Pathology findings

Gross features

Curetted fragments of bony tissue and glistening red-brown tissue are received measuring in aggregate 4.0 × 3.5 × 1.5 cm. A portion is submitted for cytogenetics and multiple cassettes for routine processing and staining.

Microscopic features

Low magnification: Low magnification reveals the classic appearance of chondromyxoid fibroma: myxoid or basophilic vaguely chondroid areas separated by zones of hypercellular tissue (**Case fig. 16.6g**). At slightly higher magnification, the basophilic chondroid matrix is juxtaposed to cellular bands that contain scattered multinucleated giant cells (**Case fig. 16.6h**).

High magnification: High magnification of the junction between myxoid matrix and cellular band reveals a pink matrix in which are suspended spindled to stellate cells; this matrix differs from the other nodules with more basophilic slightly more chondroid appearance. Cells in the cellular region include mononuclear chondroblastic-like cells and multinucleated osteoclastic or chondroclastic giant cells (**Case fig. 16.6i**). Highest magnification comparing the basophilic areas with the myxoid areas demonstrates that cells range from round (basophilic matrix) to stellate or spindled (pink myxoid matrix). There are no mitoses, and in this patient, atypia is only mild. Two unusal features of this patient's tumor include a rare focus of hyaline type cartilage (**Case fig. 16.6l**) and bone formation (**Case fig. 16.6m**). Hyaline cartilage is found in approximately 20% of CMFs and is usually only focal (Wu et al. 1998).

Special studies: The karyotype is near tetraploid with additional material of unknown origin on the long arms of two chromosome 14s and loss of chromosome 20: 89~94, XXXX, add(14)(q32), add(14)(q32)-20. The reported consistent abnormalities of CMF comprise alterations of chromosome 6 encompassing the *COL12A1* locus but not all tumors are affected (Tallini et al. 2002). It is possible that the 'unknown material' on chromosome 14 may represent portions of chromosome 6q.

Pathologic differential or, why isn't it one of the following?

Chondroblastoma (CB): The cellular areas of CMF can be indistinguishable from chondroblastoma. However, chondroblastoma does not have centrally myxoid nodules, and calcification is more prominent with the chicken wire variety specific in this setting for CB. Both tumors can exhibit pink chondroid matrix, however. Mitotic figures are absent to very rare in CMF and more commonly noted in CB. Immunohistochemically, CMF is positive for smooth muscle actin, while CB is often positive for keratins 8 and 18 and if positive for SMA, usually only focally. As both are positive for S-100 protein and SOX9 by immunohistochemistry consistent with their cartilaginous nature, these antibodies are not discriminatory. However, DOG1 expression may be seen only in CB and not CMF, based on one report (Akpalo et al. 2012). **Case fig. 16.6n** illustrates the most common locations of chondroblastoma and chondromyxoid fibroma in the adult skeleton. There is extensive overlap in particular bones including the knee and the foot. While chondroblastoma is almost always an epiphyseal tumor and chondromyxoid fibroma is metaphyseal in the long bones, larger tumors of either type may expand and obscure this site of origin.

Chondrosarcoma with extensive myxoid change: Most chondrosarcomas with extensive myxoid change are grade 2 and would also contain at least some areas of hyaline cartilage matrix material. Necrosis and mitotic figures would make CMF very unlikely. Additionally, most patients with CMF are younger than 30 years, and most patients with chondrosarcoma are older than 50 years. Cytogenetics could prove helpful in small specimens if the characteristic 6q abnormalities are present in CMF. Most grade 2 chondrosarcomas, by contrast, feature markedly aneuploid karyotypes with numerous numerical and structural abnormalities.

Chondromyxoid fibroma-like osteosarcoma: This is an extraordinarily rare tumor. Although it can simulate CMF on low magnification, higher magnification reveals atypical cells and mitotic activity as well as osteoid formation. Two cases reported in 1996 also presented with radiologic features of malignancy: bone erosion and infiltration of soft tissue (Chow et al. 1996). This patient's tumor does not have mitotic activity, significant cytologic atypia or aggressive radiologic features.

Oncology approach

This is a benign lesion with no role for adjuvant chemotherapy. Once again, the role for radiation therapy in these lesions is limited. Typically, these are managed by surgery alone. Rare presentations in the head and neck region, particularly the base of skull, may benefit from adjuvant radiation therapy.

Patient outcome

Although a 15% recurrence rate is reported, this patient has no evidence of tumor at 2 years post curettage with careful follow-up. (Most recurrences occur within the first two years.)

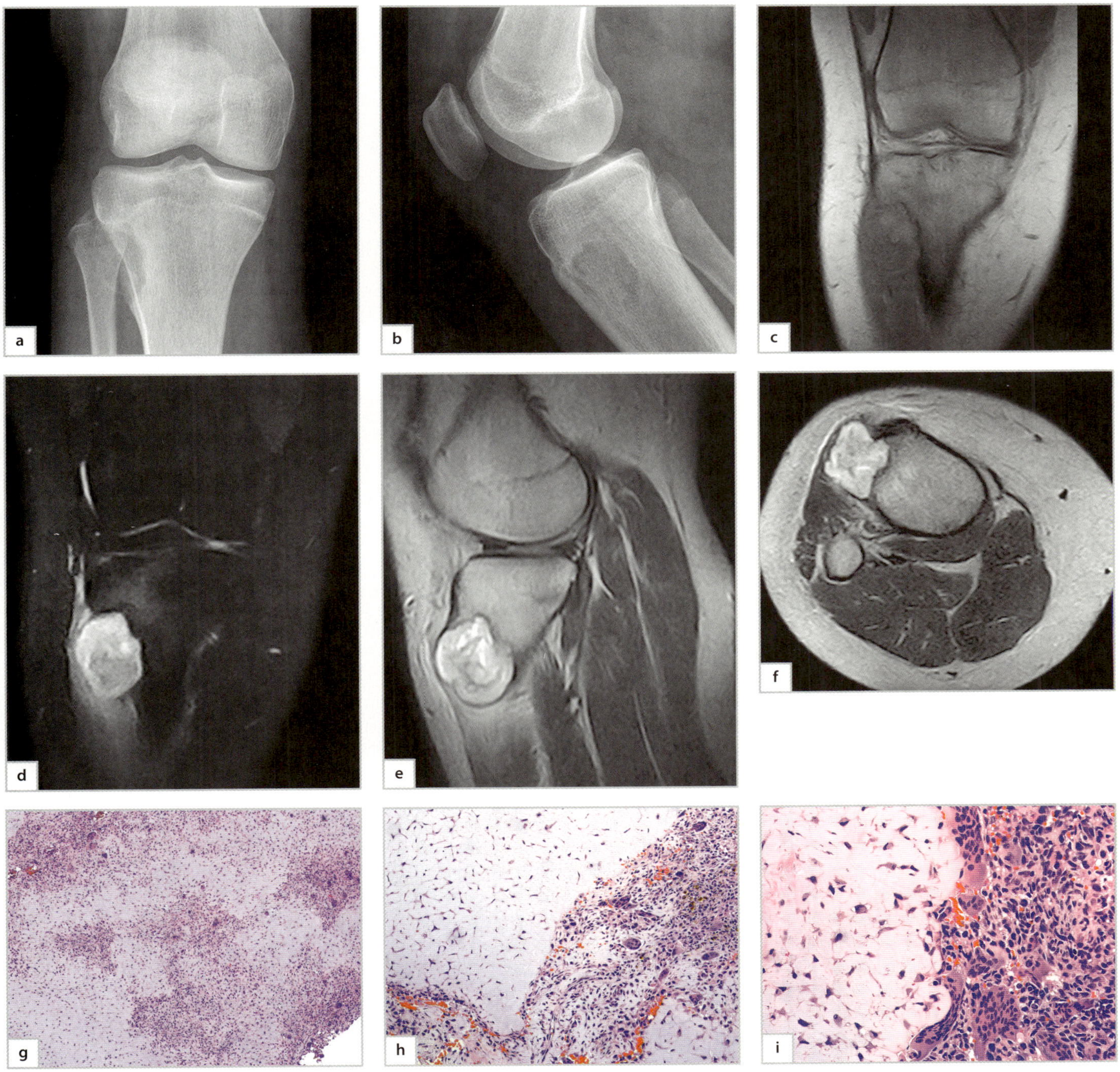

Case figure 16.6 Chondromyxoid fibroma. **16.6a**: AP and **16.6b**: Lateral radiograph of the knee show a predominantly lucent, expansile, eccentric lesion of the proximal tibia. There is mature periosteal buttressing distal to the lesion. Cartilage matrix is not visible. **16.6c**: Coronal T1 MR image. **16.6d**: Coronal STIR MR image. **16.6e**: Sagittal T2 MR image. **16.6f**: Axial T2 MR image. MR images show the lesion is T1 isointense and is high signal on the T2 and STIR images. Note the heterogeneous, 'dirty' appearance of the cartilage. There is no soft tissue mass or adjacent edema of the marrow or soft tissues seen in this chondromyxoid fibroma.. **16.6g**: The tumor comprises forms ill-defined, hypocellular lobules with intervening cellular areas. **16.6h**: Medium magnification. Myxochondroid regions are separated by bands of cellular tissue that contain multinucleated giant cells and rounded cells reminiscent of chondroblastoma. **16.6i**: The interface between the matrix rich lobules and cellular regions is usually sharp, as in this photomicrograph. Stellate to spindle cells reside in the pale gray chondroid matrix while multinucleated osteoclast (or chondroclast) type giant cells hug the perimeter.

Case figure 16.6: Continued from page 397

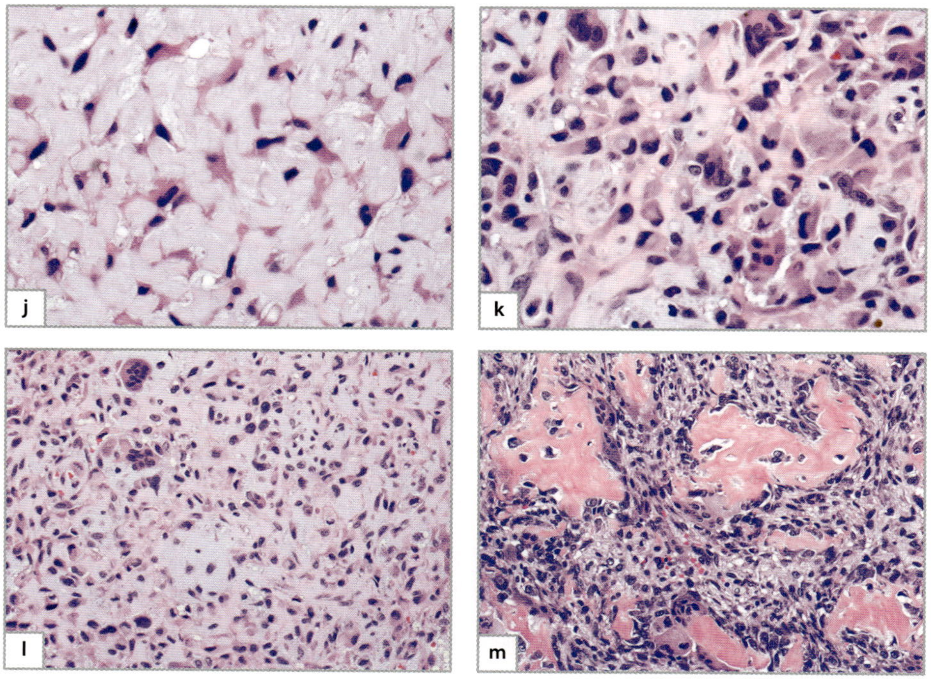

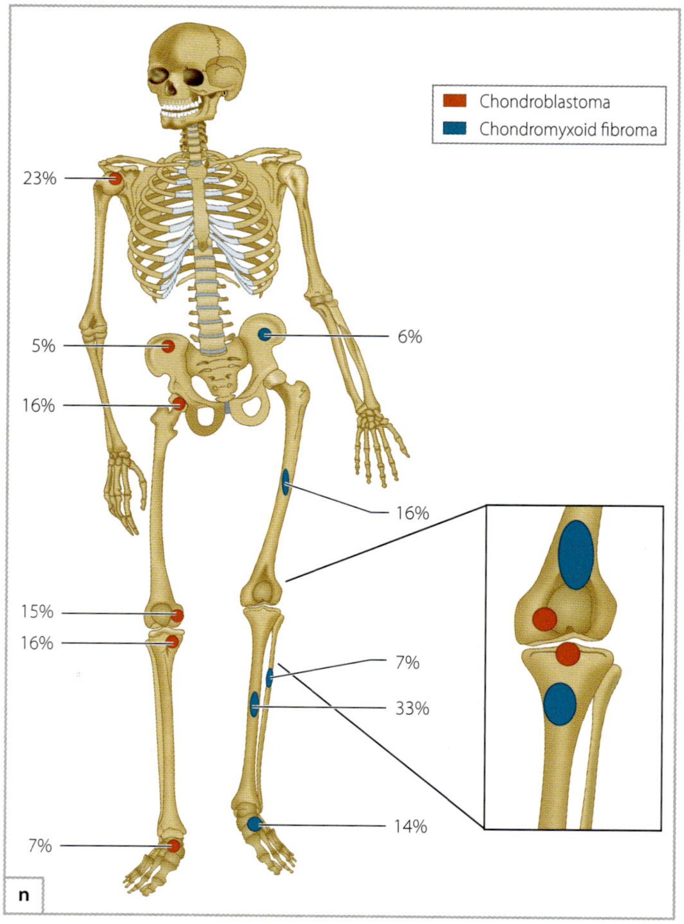

16.6j: The stellate and spindle cells suspended in myxoid or chondroid matrix (the latter in this photomicrograph) are mildly variable in nuclear shape. Some cases exhibit more prominent atypia that is of no clinical significance. **16.6k**: The interlobular cellular regions imitate the appearance of chondroblastoma with round chondroblast-like cells and interspersed multinucleated osteoclast-like giant cells. **16.6l**: High magnification. Two small lobules in this patient's tumor appear more like hyaline cartilage than the others. Hyaline cartilage lobules containing cells set in lacunar spaces are unusual in CMF (no more than 15% of cases). **16.6m**: Medium magnification. An area of new bone formation is present. This may be occurring secondary to microfracture through the bone at the site of the tumor. Such new bone formation is unusual in CMF. **16.6n**: Skeletal location of chondromyxoid fibroma and chondroblastoma. The most common sites affected are depicted in this drawing of the adult skeleton. (Numbers are derived from several textbooks of skeletal tumors; see bibliography).

Case table 16.6 Summary pathology findings of Case 16.6

Diagnosis	Chondromyxoid fibroma
Size	3.5 × 2.4 × 2.8 cm
Location	Proximal tibia
Margin status	Tumor is curetted; formal margin assessment is not possible
Histologic grade	Not graded: benign
Pathologic stage (TNM classification)	Not staged: benign

Case 16.7 Chondrosarcoma (high grade)

Clinical history and presentation

The patient is a 53 year old man who presents with a two year history of right hip pain which began insidiously and has been slowly progressive. He denies a history of antecedent trauma. Pain is increased with activity but also occurs at rest and awakens him at night.

Physical examination reveals no mass. He has mild tenderness on palpation of the right greater trochanter. He has full range of motion of the right hip but has pain localized to the groin and lateral hip on extremes of rotation.

Surgical findings and comments

Open biopsy is performed and the findings are consistent with low grade chondrosarcoma. Following confirmation of the final pathology, extended curettage is performed with a burr along with polymethylmethacrylate (bone cement) for margin enhancement and defect reconstruction, along with internal fixation. Final pathology from the resection reveals areas of high grade tumor. Following the change in pathologic grade, the patient is later returned to surgery for wide resection of the involved proximal femur and limb salvage surgery consisting of proximal femoral replacement.

SURGERY GRAY AREA

Chondrosarcoma, even high grade, is a slowly growing tumor and patients can often present with a long and fairly benign history of symptoms.

SURGERY GRAY AREA

In chondrosarcoma, even an open biopsy with substantial tissue harvest can result in a sampling error, missing areas of higher grade tumor. Sequential interventions must be planned with this possibility in mind.

Radiology findings

Case fig. 16.7a radiograph shows a predominantly lucent lesion with a small irregular sclerotic area. No clear cartilage matrix is seen. The lesion has a focal area of erosion medially. The lesion is somewhat worrisome because of its large size and the presence of apparent heterogeneous histology shown by the calcified and uncalcified areas. The MR images, **Case figs 16.7b** through **16.7d**, confirm the large size but show no cortical breakthrough or soft tissue mass. The T1 low signal and STIR high signal is non-specific. There is fairly intense enhancement along the endosteal margin of the lesion. The bone scan, **Case fig. 16.7e** shows intense uptake of the proximal portion with only mild uptake of the distal portion. Again, this indicates heterogeneous tissue with the proximal portion having high metabolic activity worrisome for an aggressive lesion. Unfortunately, without visible cartilage matrix, the radiologist can only diagnose a lesion with some worrisome aggressive features, and perhaps direct the biopsy to the proximal area where the highest metabolic activity is seen.

Pathology findings

Gross features

The initial biopsies comprise curetted fragments of pink-tan to red-brown soft tissue measuring in aggregate 6.5 × 6.5 × 0.8 cm. A portion of the sample is sent to cytogenetics. A diagnosis of chondrosarcoma, grade 1 to 2 is rendered.

The second curettage specimen performed about two months after the first contains more tissue, aggregating to 11.0 cm. At this point, a diagnosis of chondrosarcoma, grade 3, is made.

Ten months later, the tumor is widely resected including a portion of the femur. The chondrosarcoma measures 24 × 6 × 5 cm, is intramedullary and extends through the cortex into surrounding skeletal muscle and fibroadipose tissue. It is soft and fleshy with a gray glistening to hemorrhagic appearance. Separately submitted biopsies of synovium are negative for tumor. Resection margins are negative but two are close at approximately 0.5 cm. The tumor persists as a mixture of histologic grades 2 and 3.

The third curettage biopsy performed two years two months after the initial biopsy consists of an 8 × 7 × 3 cm aggregate of gelatinous to necrotic tissue fragments. A portion is submitted for cytogenetic evaluation. The tumor is histologic grade 3 with 40% necrosis.

Two more curettages are performed at the right hip for palliative purposes at approximately two years 5 months and two years nine months after the initial biopsy. These comprise locally recurrent tumor aggregating to 8 cm and 6 cm, respectively. Both specimens are 50% necrotic.

Microscopic features

Low magnification of first curettage: Diagnosis of the initial biopsy is grade 1 to 2 chondrosarcoma. The tumor forms abundant hyaline cartilage matrix and infiltrates and destroys trabecular bone (**Case fig. 16.7f**). Cellularity varies from low to moderate, the latter consistent with foci of grade 2 tumor (**Case fig. 16.7g**). In this biopsy, no grade 3 areas are found.

High magnification of first curettage: Atypia comprises slightly enlarged hypochromatic nuclei with prominent nucleoli (**Case fig. 16.7g**). Necrosis and mitotic activity are absent.

Remaining specimens from this patient

Low magnification: The patient's additional specimens comprise predominantly grade 3 chondrosarcoma with intermingled lower grade tumor. At low power, the tumor is cellular with only focal areas of chondroid matrix (**Case fig. 16.7h**).

High magnification: Consistent with a grade 3 chondrosarcoma, the appearance of the tumor varies from regions producing hyaline cartilage gray matrix and pink chondroid matrix (**Case fig. 16.7i**) to areas with less matrix production (**Case fig. 16.7j**) to areas of myxoid matrix and dispersed stellate cells appearing like a cellular chondromyxoid fibroma (**Case fig. 16.7k**). Mitotic figures are identified, with rare high power fields containing two division figures. Necrosis is also present.

Special studies: Tumor is collected for cytogenetic analysis from the second curettage. The karyotype is typical of grade 3 chondrosarcoma: aneuploid with multiple structural and numerical abnormalities including the abnormalities of the short arm of chromosome 9. Structural abnormalities of 9p are recurrent in chondrosarcomas.

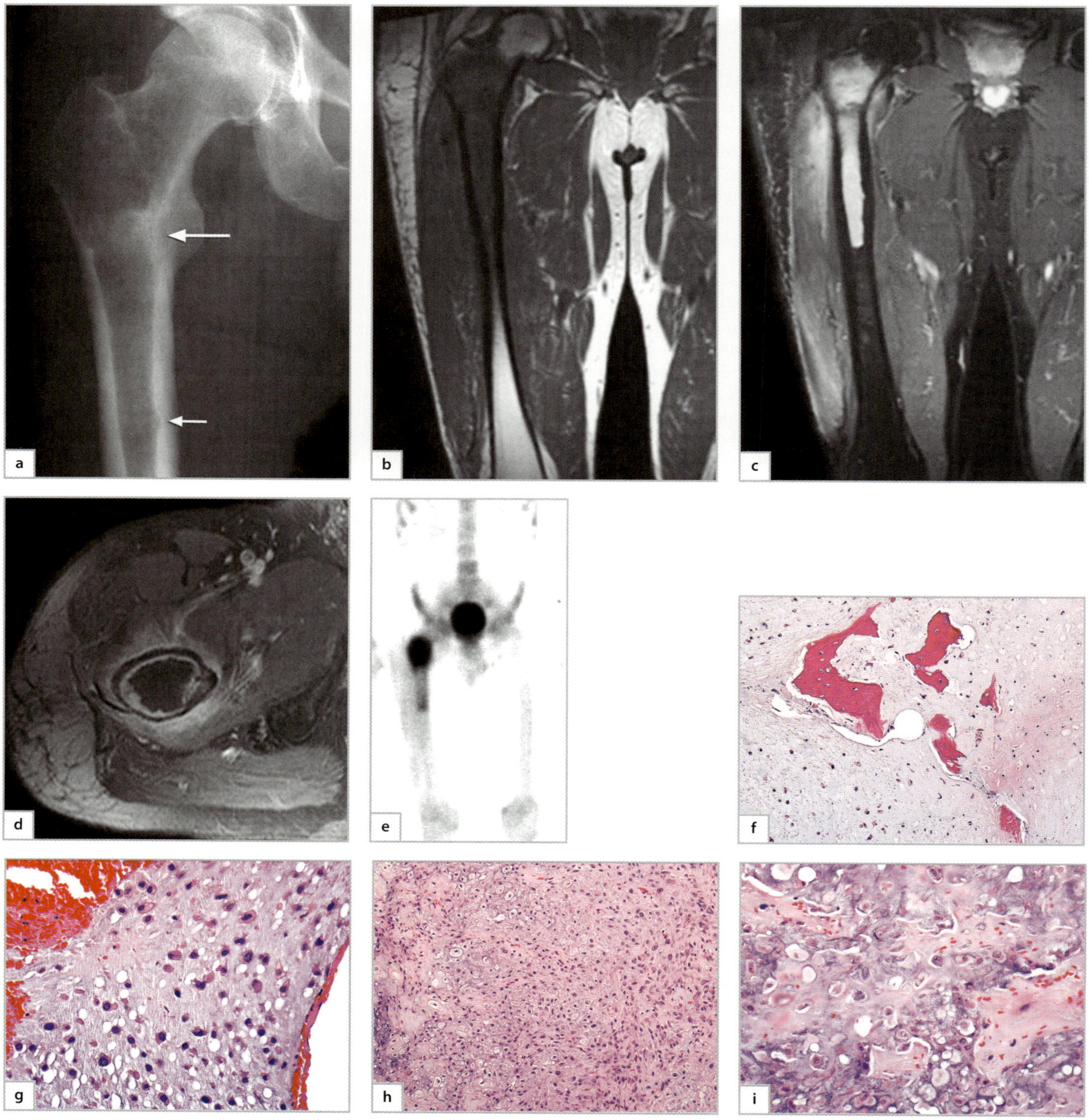

Case figure 16.7 Chondrosarcoma, high grade. **16.7a**: AP radiograph of the hip. There is abnormal irregular calcification, long arrow, without definite arc or ring pattern. There is focal endosteal scalloping, short arrow. **16.7b**: Coronal T1 weighted MR of the hip. **16.7c**: Coronal STIR MR of the hip. **16.7d**: Axial T1 fat saturated post contrast MR of the hip. MR images shows the lesion is quite extensive and has the typical T1 low signal, STIR high signal appearance of cartilage. The margins of the lesion enhance intensely. **16.7e**: AP view of the bone scan. The proximal portion of the lesion has intense uptake, as no pathologic fracture is seen, this implies histological heterogeneity of the lesion as well as an area of high metabolic activity. **16.7f**: Low magnification. Within a single tumor, the grade of a chondrosarcoma can vary tremendously. This patient's tumor has areas of grade 1 chondrosarcoma, as seen in this field. Although cellularity and atypia is mild enough to qualify for an enchondroma, malignant behavior is clear: the tumor infiltrates and destroys the patient's trabecular bone. **16.7g** Chondrosarcoma, grade 2, medium magnification. In this field, the tumor assumes the look of a grade 2 chondrosarcoma with moderately increased cellularity and nuclear atypia. **16.7h**: Low magnification. Grade 3 tumor includes areas with little chondroid matrix production. Notice in this field only a few cells residing in lacunae; most of the cells lack this feature of well-developed hyaline cartilage matrix. **16.7i**: High magnification. The matrix in a chondrosarcoma can appear grayish blue (most closely resembling hyaline cartilage) or pink. Both forms are termed 'chondroid' and are present in this photo.

Case figure 16.7: Continued from page 400

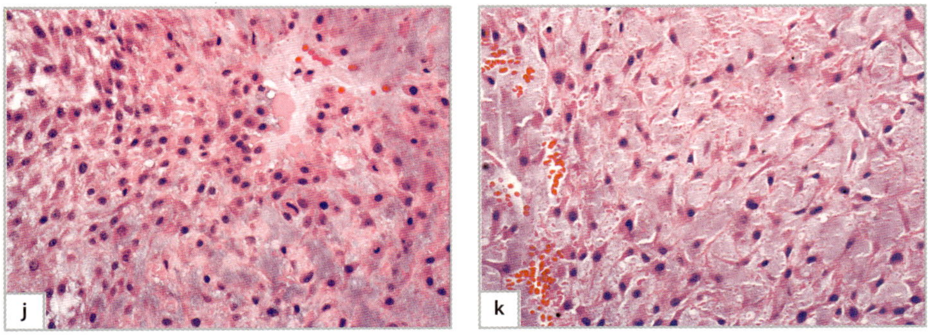

16.7j: Chondrosarcoma, grade 3, high magnification. Sparse chondroid matrix is seen. The tumor cells are eosinophilic with indistinct cell borders and round nuclei that range from hypo- to hyperchromatic. **16.7k**: High magnification. Higher grade chondrosarcomas are often plethoric in microscopic appearance. In this field, the patient's tumor mimics the myxoid matrix with floating stellate tumor cells of chondromyxoid fibroma.

Pathologic differential or, why isn't it one of the following?

Chondrosarcoma grade 2: Although the initial biopsy curettage was generous in volume, areas of grade 3 chondrosarcoma were not sampled. Chondrosarcomas may show heterogeneity in grade within one tumor, as was the case with this patient's tumor. The grade 3 areas are too cellular with loss of matrix production, areas of necrosis and mitotic activity to be considered grade 2. **Case table 16.7a** describes the histologic features that determine the grade of conventional chondrosarcoma. These features are not quantifiable and thus do not result in more than 'good' concordance among expert musculoskeletal pathologists. Nevertheless, they are predictive of behavior in most cases.

Chondroblastic osteosarcoma: A diagnosis of chondroblastic osteosarcoma should be made when osteoid, often cytologically atypical osteoid, is present in addition to areas of malignant cartilage. It is the pattern and type of new bone that is diagnostic. Even grade 2 chondrosarcoma can elicit a reactive new bone response that cuffs the edges of the chondroid tumor nodules. However, this reactive bone has an orderly appositional growth and is not formed by large, hyperchromatic, irregularly shaped osteoblasts. Some of this appositional bone may also feature rimming small osteoblasts consistent with reactive bone. Occasionally, reactive bone may form in chondrosarcoma that does not cup the edges of cartilaginous tumor nodules. This bone too should appear cytologically and architecturally benign. By contrast, the osteoid of chondroblastic osteosarcoma is irregular in deposition scattering haphazardly among malignant cartilage areas or forming an infiltrating lacelike network. There are no rimming osteoblasts in the osteosarcomatous new bone, and the osteoblasts in the bone matrix are usually at least slightly atypical. Immunohistochemistry may be of value in the differential, as the lectin, galectin-1, seems to be expressed in chondroblastic osteosarcoma (even in the chondroid areas) and not in chondrosarcoma (Gomez-Brouchet et al. 2010).

Oncology approach

Medical oncology

This patient is diagnosed after incisional biopsy with a right proximal femur chondrosarcoma, grade 1 to 2. The patient is treated on an NCI sponsored protocol (NCT00096213: Intralesional Resection in Treating Patients with Chondrosarcoma of the Bone), and undergoes curettage approximately two months after initial biopsy.

While the patient's original biopsy demonstrated a grade 1 to 2 tumor, the more complete sampling in the curettage specimen demonstrates areas of grade 1 and 2 but also areas of grade 3 chondrosarcoma. Indeed, a review of the radiologic studies was more consistent with a chondroid neoplasm such as high-grade chondrosarcoma.

Ten months after curettage, the patient has a local recurrence and undergoes a resection of the right proximal femur. A 25 cm tumor is resected with clear margins.

Case table 16.7b Summary pathology findings of Case 16.7

Diagnosis	Chondrosarcoma, grade 3
Size	24 × 6 × 5 cm
Location	Proximal femur
Margin status	Margins are negative but two are close at ~0.5 cm each.
Histologic grade	Grade 3 using a 3-tiered system = high grade
Pathologic stage (TNM classification)	T2/N0/M0 at the time of resection = Stage IIB; he later develops metastases to the lungs and mediastinum

Case table 16.7a Histologic grading of conventional chondrosarcoma

Feature	Grade 1 CS	Grade 2 CS	Grade 3 CS
Matrix	Abundant, well-developed	Often abundant; commonly myxoid areas present	Chondroid often sparse, myxoid areas may be common
Cellularity	Relatively low but usually higher than most long gone enchondromas	Moderately cellular; cell density may increase at the periphery of tumor lobules	Highly cellular
Necrosis	Almost always absent	Focal to abundant	Commonly abundant
Nuclei	Most small and dark; a few larger and pale with nucleoli	Usually twice the size of normal chondrocyte nuclei, may be irregularly shaped and hyperchromatic or large and pale (vesicular) with nucleoli	Markedly pleomorphic with hyperchromasia or hypochromasia and nucleoli. May have multinucleated pleomorphic cells
Mitoses	Absent to rare	Scattered mitoses are common; usually less than 2/10 high power microscopic fields (hpf)	Mitoses usually >2/10hpf May be atypical

CS: chondrosarcoma, hpf: high power microscopic field. (From Cancer Grading Manual, 2007 edited by Ivan Damjanov and Fang Fan).

Approximately eight months later, he develops metastatic disease to the mediastinal lymph nodes and the lungs and receives treatment on study with perifosine without success (NCT00401388: A Trial of Perifosine in Patients with Chemo-Insensitive Sarcomas), then on another study NCT00441467: Safety and Efficacy Study of Glufosfamide in Previously Treated Advanced Soft Tissue Sarcoma, again without success.

Six months after identification of his metastatic lung disease, the primary tumor recurs again, and for palliative purpose, another curettage of the lesion is done. The patient also tries a macrobiotic diet, which seems to coincide with a reduced rate of cancer growth.

Two months after the curettage, the patient is treated with doxorubicin 60 mg/m^2 q 3 weeks and receives 2 doses, with control of the metastases but not of the primary lesion, which grows further. Another palliative resection is done four months after curettage preceded by preoperative radiation to reduce the pain. The patient has no improvement and the primary lesion regrows again. The last palliative curettage is performed three months after the preceding procedure. A new karyotype shows non-clonal evolution with many more chromosome anomalies.

The patient opts for hospice care and dies approximately three years after his initial presentation.

This case typically illustrates the lack of response of high grade chondrosarcoma to chemotherapy. According to the NCCN guidelines, this patient participated in two clinical trials of potential novel agents for sarcoma. Both drugs were shown to be either inactive (perifosine) (Knowling et al. 2006) or toxic (glufosfamide) in this patient population (D'Amato et al. 2008).

In a series of 46 patients with grade 1 and 2 chondrosarcomas, (25 men and 21 women) with a mean age of 43 years (range, 17-79 years) and a minimum follow-up of 32 months (range, 32-312 months), 23 of the tumors were intracompartmental (Enneking A); of these, 19 were grade 1 and 4 were grade 2. The other 23 tumors were extracompartmental (Enneking B); of these, 4 were grade 1 and 19 were grade 2. Twenty-five patients underwent an intralesional resection, 18 had a wide resection, and three had amputations. The disease-free survival rate was 90%. None of the patients with grade 1 tumor died. Two patients with grade 2 tumor died among 10 patients with a recurrence. For lesions with radiographic characteristics of intracompartmental grade 1 chondrosarcoma, intralesional resection followed by electrocauterization and cement may be the best treatment. The NCI study should soon confirm these results. When the imaging suggests an aggressive (Grade 2 or 3) chondrosarcoma, wide resection is indicated (de Camargo et al. 2010).

Radiation oncology

While a complete resection is the most important factor to prevent local recurrence, adjuvant radiation therapy is of benefit in preventing local recurrence in high grade chondrosarcoma. This can be seen in the study by Goda, et al., which showed local control rates of 94-100% in with adjuvant radiation in extra-cranial cases with an R0 or R1 resection (Goda et al.). There is also clear benefit in cases of head and neck cases due to difficulty in getting complete resection. In this case, the patient developed metastatic disease before adjuvant radiation. Subsequently, only palliative radiotherapy was administered, which was of limited benefit due to disease volume. With his metastatic disease, the patient had multiple local recurrences which caused symptoms and required multiple surgeries. This case is a good example of the importance of local control. Recurrent or high grade chondrosarcoma should be considered for adjuvant radiation therapy.

Patient outcome

The patient succumbs to disease three years after presentation after enduring repeated local recurrences and lung and mediastinal metastases.

Case 16.8 Dedifferentiated chondrosarcoma

Clinical history and presentation

The patient is a 55 year old man admitted to the hospital with a four day history of right hip pain and inability to ambulate. He denies a history of trauma.

Physical examination reveals painful range of motion of the right hip.

Surgical findings and comments

Open biopsy is performed with prophylactic internal fixation to prevent propagation of the pathologic fracture noted on radiologic imaging.

Following confirmation of the final pathology, wide resection is performed with limb salvage surgery consisting of proximal femoral replacement.

Radiology findings

The lateral radiograph, **Case fig. 16.8a** shows a lucent lesion with pathologic fracture of the proximal femur. There is sunburst periosteal reaction extending anteriorly from the femur indicating soft tissue spread in a highly aggressive bone tumor. There is probable calcified matrix visible in the proximal portion of the lesion with arc and ring appearance.

This could be confirmed with a CT scan; however, this was not performed. The MR images, **Case figs 16.8b** through **16.8f**, show a large soft tissue component, bone destruction and heterogeneous enhancement. The areas without enhancement may be necrotic tissue or may represent non-enhancing cartilage matrix. These findings are of a highly aggressive lesion originating in bone, the presence of cartilage matrix indicates the diagnosis of a higher grade chondrosarcoma.

Pathology findings

Gross features

The initial biopsies comprise fragments of firm gray to hemorrhagic material aggregating to 7.5 × 5.7 × 1.3 cm. The tumor is diagnosed as consistent with dedifferentiated chondrosarcoma.

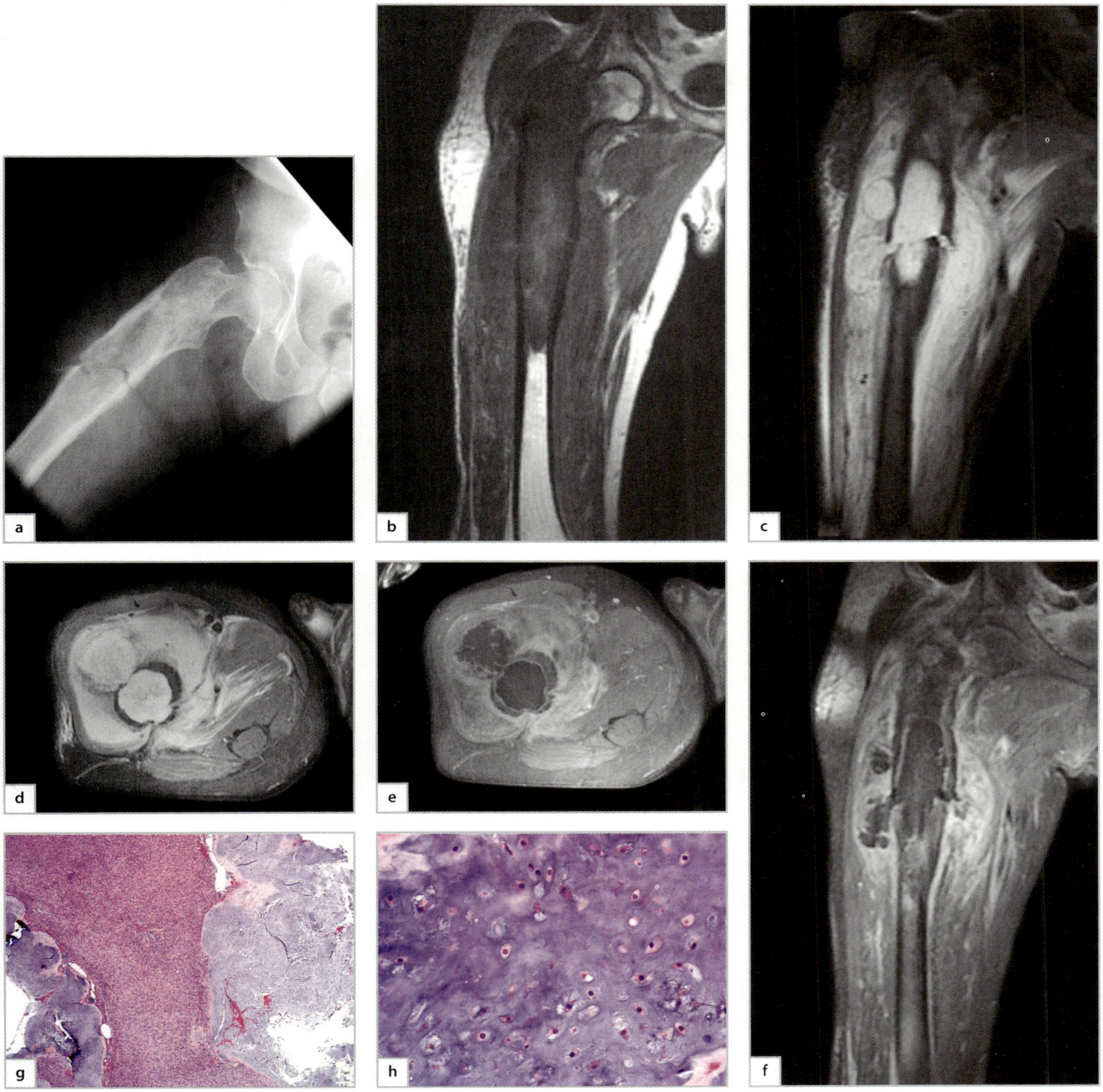

Case figure 16.8 Dedifferentiated chondrosarcoma 16.8a: Lateral radiograph of the right hip. **16.8b**: Coronal T1 MR image. **16.8c**: Coronal STIR MR image. **16.8d**: Axial STIR MR image. **16.8e**: Axial T1 fat saturated post-contrast. **16.8f**: Coronal T1 fat saturated post-contrast. The radiograph shows a pathologic fracture through the proximal femoral lesion. There is 'sunburst' periosteal reaction indicating tumor has invaded through the cortex, out in to the soft tissues. There is questionable arc and ring calcified matrix visible. MR images show a destructive lesion expanding through the cortex into the soft tissues. There are areas of enhancing tumor. The large areas of non-enhance tissue indicate necrosis or cartilage matrix.

Case figure 16.8: Continued from page 403

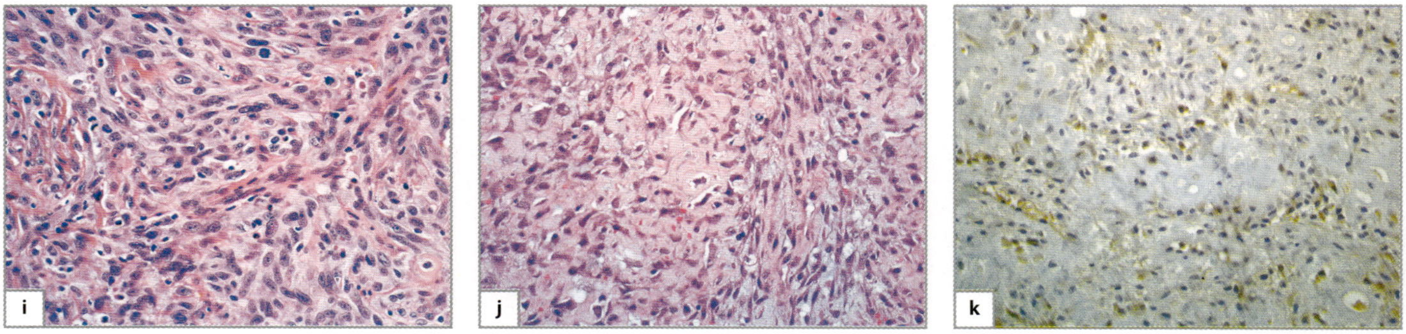

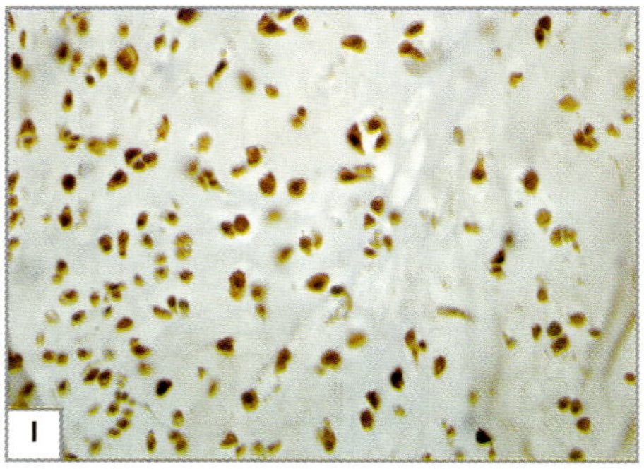

16.8g: Low magnification. The tumor exhibits the characteristic sharp zonation of lower grade hyaline cartilage matrix-producing chondrosarcoma, and high grade sarcoma. **16.8h**: Dedifferentiated chondrosarcoma, medium magnification. The cartilaginous portion of the tumor appears low grade with abundant chondroid matrix and low cellularity (identical to grade 1 conventional chondrosarcoma). **16.8i**: High magnification. The dedifferentiated part of this patient's tumor comprises a non-specific high grade spindle cell sarcoma (other sarcomas such as osteosarcoma, rhabdomyosarcoma, and angiosarcoma, may also constitute the 'dedifferentiated' component). Notice the mitotic figures. **16.8j**: Dedifferentiated chondrosarcoma, high magnification. In this field, the tumor cells produce a dense pink collagenous stroma. Mineralization, well-defined edges, and cells set in lacunae would be convincing for osteoid; those features are absent. **16.8k**: High magnification. The dedifferentiated component shows no expression of S-100 protein by immunohistochemistry. **16.8l**: Dedifferentiated chondrosarcoma, high magnification. The cartilaginous component, as expected, is strongly reactive for S-100 protein by immunohistochemistry.

Wide resection of the tumor occurs approximately 1 month later. The tumor is large at 28 × 15 × 14 cm and is centered in the right proximal femur with extension into the soft tissues of the thigh. Surgical margins are negative and all >1.0 cm from tumor. Lymphovascular invasion is absent, and two lymph nodes are likewise negative for tumor.

Because of recurrent local tumor, the patient undergoes hemipelvectomy six months after the wide resection. The recurrent tumor measures 6.4 × 4.7 × 3.4 cm and is located in the soft tissue lateral to the hip joint metal endoprosthesis. The tumor mass is gray-white and lobulated and is hemorrhagic, necrotic and mucoid on cross-sectioning. Surrounding the femoral endoprosthesis is a cavity filled with blood clot and necrotic appearing tissue measuring 30 × 8 × 8 cm. Surgical margins are clear by 3 cm. Five pelvic lymph nodes are negative for tumor.

Microscopic features

Low magnification: The tumor abruptly transitions from relatively low grade hyaline cartilage areas to high grade spindle cell sarcoma (**Case fig. 16.8g**).

High magnification: The malignant cartilage is histologically compatible with grade 1 chondrosarcoma (**Case fig. 16.8h**). However, the dedifferentiated component is high grade and predominantly comprises a non-specific spindle cell proliferation with nuclear atypia and mitotic activity (**Case fig. 16.8i**). Mineralized, unequivocal osteoid is not identified; however, some cells form a dense collagenous stroma (**Case fig. 16.8j**).

Special studies: S-100 protein expression is examined by immunohistochemistry. The areas of spindle cell sarcoma are negative for S-100 protein (**Case fig. 16.8k**), and, as expected, the cartilaginous lobules are strongly positive (**Case fig. 16.8l**).

Pathologic differential or, why isn't it one of the following?

Chondroblastic osteosarcoma: This tumor has intermixed high grade cartilage and malignant bone. Although the dedifferentiated portion of dedifferentiated chondrosarcoma can comprise chondroblastic osteosarcoma, low grade to intermediate grade cartilage nodules will be present, and there is usually a sharp interface between the lower grade cartilaginous component and the dedifferentiated chondroblastic osteosarcoma component. A galectin-1 antibody stain may be useful in that it stains chondroblastic areas of chondroblastic osteosarcoma and not the cartilaginous regions of dedifferentiated chondrosarcoma.

High grade spindle cell sarcoma, not otherwise specified: The presence of at least focal low grade malignant cartilage excludes the diagnosis of high grade spindle cell sarcoma.

Case table 16.8 Summary pathology findings of Case 16.8

Diagnosis	Dedifferentiated chondrosarcoma
Size	28 × 15 × 14 cm
Location	Proximal femur
Margin status	Margins are negative by >1.0 cm
Histologic grade	Grade 3 (high grade) using a 3 tiered system, Grade 4 using a 4 tiered system
Pathologic stage (TNM classification)	T2/N0/M0 at time of wide resection = Stage IIB; the patient later develops lung metastases and malignant pleural effusions

Oncology approach

Medical oncology

Eight months later, after resection of this proximal femur dedifferentiated chondrosarcoma, the patient presents with shortness of breath and is diagnosed with bilateral pleural effusions. Bilateral drainage catheters are placed to improve the respiratory function. The pleural effusion contains malignant cells of sarcoma origin. The patient is too ill for chemotherapy treatment and is treated with palliative care only.

Radiation oncology

Similar to high grade chondrosarcoma, dedifferentiated chondrosarcoma may also benefit from adjuvant radiation. As with other chondroid tumors, surgery is the mainstay of therapy. However, adjuvant radiation may enhance local control. This case is a good example. The patient underwent wide local resection, but did not undergo adjuvant radiation therapy due to adherence issues. Unfortunately, he had a local recurrence necessitating hemipelvectomy and leg amputation. The patient subsequently developed lung metastases with a malignant effusion.

Patient outcome

The patient dies within one month after developing symptomatic malignant pleural effusions and approximately nine months after his initial presentation of hip pain and inability to ambulate. Sadly, most patients with dedifferentiated chondrosarcoma die within two years of initial presentation.

Case 16.9 Mesenchymal chondrosarcoma

Clinical history and presentation

The patient is a 31 year old man who presents with a six month history of right hip pain. He denies any history of trauma. The pain has been slowly progressive and has increasingly interfered with functional activity.

Physical examination reveals a fullness of the right lateral pelvic area but no discrete definable mass. He is tender on palpation diffusely throughout the area of fullness. He has full range of motion of the hip but pain throughout the range.

Surgical findings and comments

Open biopsy is performed.

Due to the massive size of this tumor with involvement of the sacrum, it is concluded that limb salvage cannot be performed with satisfactory function of the salvaged limb and adequate margins. Therefore, an amputative hemipelvectomy with hemisacrectomy with wide surgical margins is performed. Definitive surgery demonstrates a grade 3/3 chondrosarcoma with 0/3 lymph nodes. The primary tumor size is 14.5 × 10 × 10 cm. All margins are negative; the closest margin is 0.2 cm to the tumor.

Radiology findings

Case figs 16.9a through **16.9e** shows a very large mass originating in the iliac bone, destroying it and spreading into the adjacent soft tissues. There are irregular calcified portions; some show cartilage matrix appearance with arc and rings visible. The MR images, **Case figs 16.9b** through **16.9e**, show the mass is T1 low signal with STIR high signal and heterogeneous intense enhancement. The appearance clearly indicates a high grade aggressive sarcoma, given the cartilage matrix, a chondrosarcoma is the likely diagnosis.

Pathology findings

Gross features

The initial biopsy specimen comprises gray, slightly yielding soft tissue mixed with blood clot aggregating to 4.8 × 3.5 × 0.6 cm. A portion is reserved and sent to Cytogenetics. A diagnosis of mesenchymal chondrosarcoma is rendered.

Approximately one week after the initial biopsy, the patient undergoes right hemipelvectomy as noted in the Surgical Findings and Comments. A 14.5 × 10 × 10 cm firm, white tumor involves the majority of the ilium and part of the sacrum and it erodes through the iliac crest. The femoral head is not involved. The margins are negative, but one margin is close at ~ 0.2 cm. Tumor is grossly noted to invade the internal iliac vein. Three lymph nodes are negative for tumor.

Microscopic features

Low magnification: The patient's tumor contains large swathes of small round blue cells in which nodules of neoplastic cartilage are strewn (**Case fig. 16.9f**). The low magnification of the small round blue cell component exhibits dilated, angulated 'staghorn' vessels, a feature often seen in mesenchymal chondrosarcoma (but not specific or pathognomonic for it) (**Case fig. 16.9g**).

High magnification: Some of the cartilaginous nodules feature the degree of cellularity and atypia consistent with grade 2 chondrosarcoma (**Case fig. 16.9h**). The small round blue cells are aptly named (**Case fig. 16.9i**). Lymphovascular invasion is identified (**Case fig. 16.9j**).

Special studies: The tumor cells embedded in hyaline cartilage matrix are strongly positive for S-100 protein expression by immunohistochemistry, while the small round blue cells are negative (**Case fig. 16.9k**). Cytogenetics is unsuccessful, as the tumor cells fail to grow in culture.

Pathologic differential or, why isn't it one of the following?

Small cell osteosarcoma: Small cell osteosarcoma must exhibit osteoid production. This type of osteosarcoma can also produce cartilage, so the presence of cartilage does not differentiate the two sarcomas. Cells of both tumors may be spindled. Often, the round cell areas of mesenchymal chondrosarcoma exhibit a hemangiopericytomatous vessel pattern (eg, angulated, dilated medium-sized blood vessels that look vaguely like deer antlers) that is not seen in small cell osteosarcoma..

Ewing sarcoma/PNET: Ewing sarcoma/PNET does not contain cartilage as mesenchymal chondrosarcoma does. In small biopsies, FISH for evidence of translocation of the EWS gene can be performed. There have been no reports of EWS gene translocations in mesenchymal chondrosarcoma.

Dedifferentiated chondrosarcoma: Both dedifferentiated and mesenchymal chondrosarcoma are biphasic in which one portion

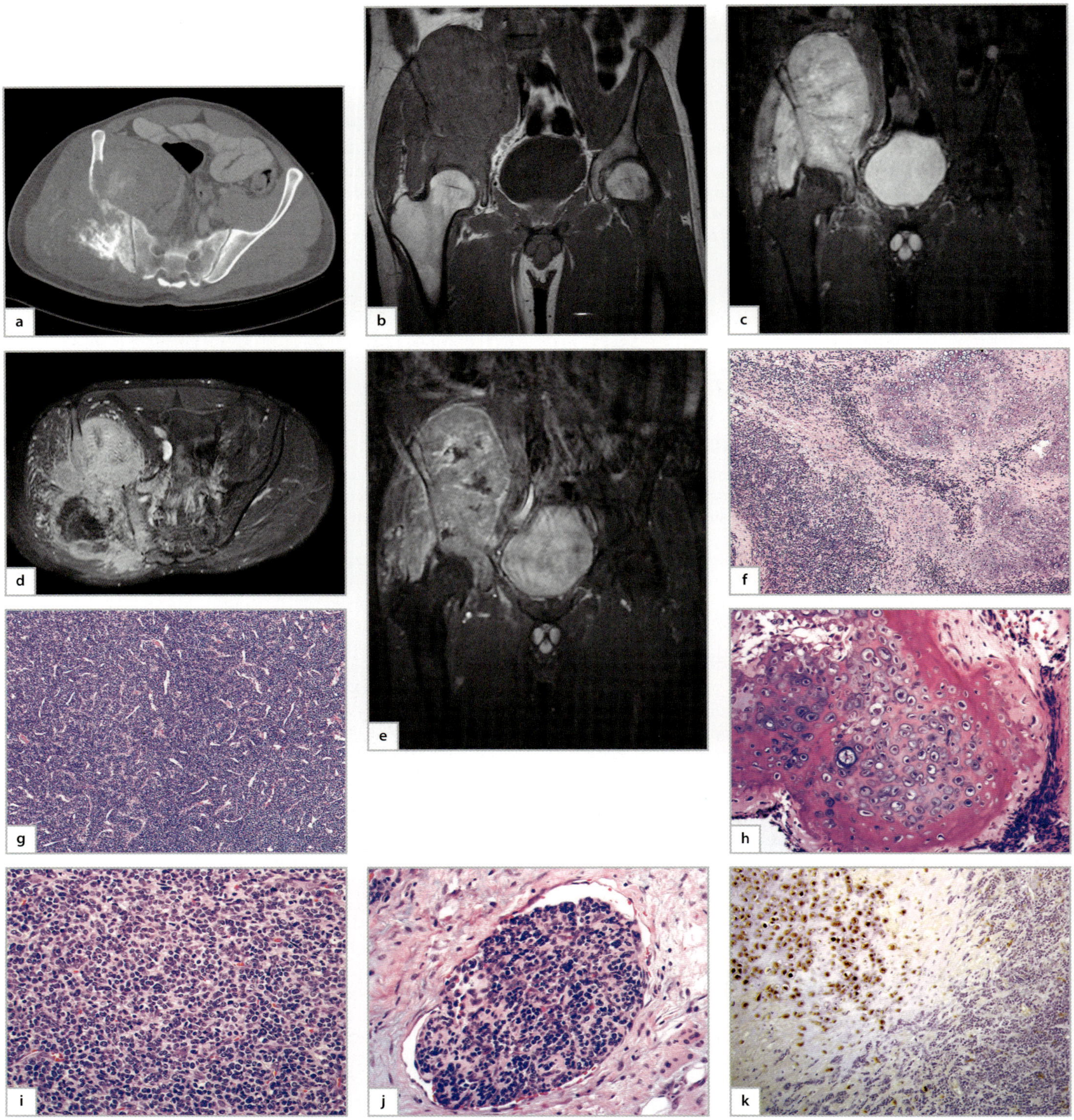

Case figure 16.9 Mesenchymal chondrsarcoma. **16.9a**: Axial CT image of the pelvis. **16.9b**: Coronal T1 MR image. **16.9c**: Coronal STIR MR image. **16.9d**: Axial T1 fat saturated post-contrast. **16.9e**: Coronal T1 fat saturated post-contrast MR image. The CT scan image shows a destructive lesion of bone expanding into the soft tissues of the pelvis and gluteal musculature. There is irregular calcification with chondroid matrix appearance. The MR images show a large mass originating and destroying the iliac bone. There is heterogeneous enhancement with small non-enhancing areas indicating matrix or necrotic areas. **16.9f**: Low magnification. The tumor is biphasic comprising: 1) hyaline cartilage nodules and 2) sheets of small round blue cells. **16.9g**: Low magnification. Commonly, the small round blue cells will exhibit a hemangiopericytomatous vascularity; e.g., the short, dilated, thin-walled vessels are angulated like 'staghorns'. This pattern is not specific to mesenchymal chondrosarcoma, but it is usually absent in Ewing sarcoma/PNET, an entity in the histologic differential on small biopsies when the cartilage component is not sampled. **16.9h**: Medium magnification. In this field, the neoplastic cartilage exhibits the cellularity and atypia of grade 2 conventional chondrosarcoma. Notice the compressed band of small round blue cells on the right. **16.9i**: High magnification. The small round blue cells appear blastic with little cytoplasm and uniform round nuclei. The blue appearance at low power is due to the high density of the cell nuclei with little intervening cytoplasm. This photo could derive from any small round blue cell tumor. **16.9j**: Medium magnification. Vascular invasion is present with a nest of tumor cells filling a thin-walled vein. **16.9k**: High magnification. By immunohistochemistry, as expected, S-100 protein labels tumor cells in the chondroid area (brown stain is positive), the round cell component is strikingly negative.

consists of relatively low grade hyaline-cartilage producing chondrosarcoma (resembles grade 1 or grade 2 conventional chondrosarcoma). Generally, the high grade component of dedifferentiated chondrosarcoma consists of non-specific spindle cell or pleomorphic sarcoma, osteosarcoma, or rarely, rhabdomyosarcoma or angiosarcoma. These patterns would appear distinctly different histologically from the small round blue cells of mesenchymal chondrosarcoma.

Case table 16.9 Summary pathology findings of Case 16.9

Diagnosis	Mesenchymal chondrosarcoma
Size	14.5 × 10 × 10 cm
Location	Ilium and portion of sacrum
Margin status	Negative; closest margin is 0.2 cm
Histologic grade	Grade 3 (high grade)
Pathologic stage (TNM classification)	T2/N0/M0 = IIB at the time of resection; he later develops peritoneal and cervical spine metastases

Oncology approach

Medical oncology

Six months after resection, peritoneal metastases are found on pelvic MRI scan, but the patient is then lost to follow-up for 4 months. He returns to the clinic with increased pain and is found with the same peritoneal metastases and a new spinal canal involvement of L5-S1, and C3. He is treated on a clinical study with a combination of gemcitabine, docetaxel, and bevacizumab. He does not respond to this chemotherapy, and the treatment is changed to standard doxorubicin and ifosfamide. He has a near complete response after 6 cycles with ossification of several lesions by CT scan.

Ten months later he develops another recurrence in the peritoneum, the bones, and the primary site, and is treated with 5 courses of irinotecan and temozolomide with stable disease. He then receives palliative radiotherapy on the primary lesion and the cervical spine for pain control and is then referred to hospice.

Radiation oncology

Surgery is the primary treatment with the role of chemotherapy and radiation therapy poorly defined. In cases of close or positive margins and re-excision is not feasible, radiation should be considered. In this case, the patient presents with locally advanced disease and undergoes amputative surgery and chemotherapy. The patient develops metastatic disease and receives palliative radiation therapy to the neck.

Patient outcome

Eighteen months after initial diagnosis, the patient dies in hospice.

REFERENCES

Aarons C, Potter BK, Adams SA, et al. Extended intralesional treatment versus resection of low-grade chondrosarcomas. Clin Orthop Relat Res 2009;467:2105–2111.

Ahmed AR, Tan TS, Unni KK, et al. Secondary chondrosarcoma in osteochondroma: report of 107 patients. Clin Orthop Relat Res 2003;(411):193–206.

Aigner T. Towards a new understanding and classification of chondrogenic neoplasias of the skeleton–biochemistry and cell biology of chondrosarcoma and its variants. Virchows Arch 2002;441(3):219–30.

Akpalo H, Lange C, Zustin J. Discovered on gastrointestinal tumour (DOG1): a useful immunohistochemical marker for diagnosis of chondroblastoma. Histopathol 2012;60:1099–1106.

Almefty K, Pravdenkova S, Colli BO, et al. Chordoma and chondrosarcoma: similar, but quite different, skull base tumors. Cancer 2007;110(11): 2457–67.

Altay M, Bayrakci K, Yildiz Y, et al. Secondary chondrosarcoma in cartilage bone tumors: report of 32 patients. J Orthop Sci 2007;12(5):415–23.

Armah HB, McGough RL, Goodman MA, et al. Chondromyxoid fibroma of rib with a novel chromosomal translocation: a report of four additional cases at unusual sites. Diagn Pathol 2007;2:44.

Bacchini P, Inwards C, Biscaglia R, et al. Chondroblastoma-like osteosarcoma. Orthopedics 1999;22(3):337–9.

Bell WC, Klein MJ, Pitt MJ, et al. Molecular pathology of chondroid neoplasms: part 1, benign lesions. Skeletal Radiol 2006;35(11):805–13.

Bernard SA, Murphey MD, Flemming DJ, et al. Improved Differentiation of benign osteochondromas from secondary chondrosarcomas with standardized measurement of cartilage cap in CT and MR imaging. Radiology 2010;255(3):857–865.

Bjornsson J, Mcleod RA, Unni KK, et al. Primary chondrosarcoma of long bones and limb girdles. Cancer 1998;83(10):2105–19.

Boeuf S, Kunz P, Hennig T, et al. A chondrogenic gene expression signature in mesenchymal stem cells is a classifier of conventional central chondrosarcoma. J Pathol 2008;216(2):158–66.

Bousdras K, O'Donnell P, Vujovic S, et al. Chondroblastomas but not chondromyxoid fibromas express cytokeratins: an unusual presentation of a chondroblastoma in the metaphyseal cortex of the tibia. Histopathol 2007;51(3):414–6.

Bovée JV, Hogendoorn PC, Wunder JS, et al. Cartilage tumours and bone development: molecular pathology and possible therapeutic targets. Nat Rev Cancer 2010;10(7):481–8.

Brower AC, Moser RP, Kransdorf MJ. The frequency and diagnostic significance of periostitis in chondroblastoma. Am J Roentgenol 1990;154:209–314.

Bruns J, Fiedler W, Werner M, et al. Dedifferentiated chondrosarcoma--a fatal disease. J Cancer Res Clin Oncol 2005;131(6):333–9.

Buddingh EP, Naumann S, Nelson M, et al. Cytogenetic findings in benign cartilaginous neoplasms. Cancer Genet Cytogenet 2003;141(2):164–8.

Campanacci M, Bertoni F, Bacchini P, et al. Bone and Soft Tissue Tumors: Clinical Features, Imaging, Pathology and Treatment, 2nd ed. New York: Springer 1999:265–278.

Chen C, Zhou H, Wei F, et al. Increased levels of hypoxia-inducible factor-1α are associated with Bcl-xL expression, tumor apoptosis, and clinical outcome in chondrosarcoma. J Orthop Res 2011;29(1):143–51.

Chow WA. Update on chondrosarcomas. Curr Opin Oncol 2007;19(4):371–6.

Cleton-Jansen AM, van Beerendonk HM, Baelde H,J et al. Estrogen signaling is active in cartilaginous tumors: Implications for antiestrogen therapy as treatment option of metastasized or irresectable chondrosarcoma. Clin Cancer Res 2005;11:8028–8035.

Collins MS, Koyama T, Swee RG, et al. Clear cell chondrosarcoma: radiographic, computed tomographic, and magnetic resonance findings in 34 patients with pathologic correlation. Skeletal Radiol 2003;32(12):687–94.

Corradi D, Bacchini P, Campanini N, et al. Aggressive clear cell chondrosarcomas: do distinctive characteristics exist?: a report of 4 cases. Arch Pathol Lab Med 2006;130(11):1673–9.

D'Amato GZ, Verschraegen CF, Cranmer LD, et al. Preliminary efficacy and safety results of glufosfamide (GLU) in relapsed soft tissue sarcoma: Results of a phase II trial. J Clin Oncol 2008;26 suppl;abstr 10591.

Damjanov I, Fang F, eds. Cancer Grading Manual. New York: Springer, 2007.

Damron TA, Ward WG, Stewart A. Osteosarcoma, chondrosarcoma, and Ewing's sarcoma: National Cancer Data Base Report. Clin Orthop Relat Res 2007;459:40–7.

Dantonello TM, Int-Veen C, Leuschner I, et al. Mesenchymal chondrosarcoma of soft tissues and bone in children, adolescents, and young adults: experiences of the CWS and COSS study groups. Cancer 2008;112(11):2424–31.

de Camargo OP, Baptista AM, Atanásio MJ, et al. Chondrosarcoma of bone: lessons from 46 operated cases in a single institution. Clin Orthop Relat Res 2010;468(11):2969–75.

Dickey ID, Rose PS, Fuchs B, et al. Dedifferentiated chondrosarcoma: The role of chemotherapy with updated outcomes. J Bone Joint Surg Am 2004;86–A:2412–2418.

Donati D, Yin JQ, Colangeli M, et al. Clear cell chondrosarcoma of bone: long time follow-up of 18 cases. Arch Orthop Trauma Surg 2008;128(2):137–42.

Dornauer K, Söder S, Inwards CY, et al. Matrix biochemistry and cell biology of dedifferentiated chondrosarcomas. Pathol Int 2010;60(5):365–72.

Fanburg-Smith JC, Auerbach A, Marwaha JS, et al. Reappraisal of mesenchymal chondrosarcoma: novel morphologic observations of the hyaline cartilage and endochondral ossification and β-catenin, Sox9, and osteocalcin immunostaining of 22 cases. Hum Pathol 2010;41(5):653–62.

Garrison RC, Unni KK, McLeod RA, et al. Chondrosarcoma arising in osteochondroma. Cancer 1982;49(9):1890–7.

Gelderblom H, Hohenberger P, Bovee JV. Aromatase inhibition in patients with recurrent and/or metastatic chondrosarcoma (CS). Journal of Clinical Oncology, 2008 ASCO Annual Meeting Proceedings (Post-Meeting Edition). Vol 26, No 15S (May 20 Supplement), 2008:10542

Giuffrida AY, Burgueno JE, Koniaris LG, et al. Chondrosarcoma in the United States (1973 to 2003): an analysis of 2890 cases from the SEER database. J Bone Joint Surg Am 2009;91(5):1063–72.

Goda JS, Ferguson PC, O'Sullivan B, et al. High-risk extracranial chondrosarcoma: Long-term results of surgery and radiation therapy. Cancer 2011 Jan 18.

Gomez-Brouchet A, Mourcin F, Gourraud PA, et al. Galectin-1 is a powerful marker to distinguish chondroblastic osteosarcoma and conventional chondrosarcoma. Hum Pathol 2010;41(9):1220–30.

Greenspan A, Jundt G, Remagen W. Differential Diagnosis in Orthopaedic Oncology, 2nd ed. Philadelphia: Lippincott Williams and Wilkins, 2007

Grignani P, Palmerini E, Stacchiotti S, et al. A phase II trial of imatinib (IM) in relapsed, nonresectable chondrosarcoma (CS) expressing platelet-derived growth factor receptor-α or -β (PDGFR-α/PDGFR-β): An Italian Sarcoma Group study. Cancer 2011;117(4):826–31.

Grimer RJ, Gosheger G, Taminiau A, et al. Dedifferentiated chondrosarcoma: prognostic factors and outcome from a European group. Eur J Cancer 2007;43(14):2060–5.

Gruber G, Giessauf C, Leithner A, et al. Bizarre parosteal osteochondromatous proliferation (Nora lesion): a report of 3 cases and a review of the literature. Can J Surg 2008;51(6):486–489.

Hallor KH, Staaf J, Bovée JV, et al. Genomic profiling of chondrosarcoma: chromosomal patterns in central and peripheral tumors. Clin Cancer Res 2009;15(8):2685–94.

Harwood AR, Krajbich JI, Fornasier VL. Mesenchymal chondrosarcoma: A report of 17 cases. Clin Orthop Relat Res 1981;(158):144–148.

Herbst RS, Mendolson DS, Ebbinghaus S, et al. A phase I safety and pharmacokinetic (PK) study of recombinant Apo2L/TRAIL, an apoptosis inducing protein in patients with advanced cancer. J Clin Oncol 2006;24(suppl 18):Abstract 3013.

Hicks J. USCAP Specialty Conference, case 2: chondroblastic osteosarcoma with features resembling chondromyxoid fibroma. Pediatr Dev Pathol 2005;8(1):67–73.

Huvos AG, Rosen G, Dabska M, et al. Mesenchymal chondrosarcoma. A clinicopathologic analysis of 35 patients with emphasis on treatment. Cancer 1983;51:1230–1237.

Itälä A, Leerapun T, Inwards C, et al. An institutional review of clear cell chondrosarcoma. Clin Orthop Relat Res 2005;440:209–12.

Jones KB, Buckwalter JA, McCarthy EF, et al. Skeletal Lesions Interobserver Correlation among Expert Diagnosticians (SLICED) Study Group. Reliability of histopathologic and radiologic grading of cartilaginous neoplasms in long bones. J Bone Joint Surg Am 2007;89(10):2113–2123.

Kilpatrick SE, Inwards CY, Fletcher CD, et al. Myxoid chondrosarcoma (chordoid sarcoma) of bone: a report of two cases and review of the literature. Cancer 1997;79(10):1903–10.

Klenke FM, Abdollahi A, Bertl E, et al. Tyrosine kinase inhibitor SU6668 represses chondrosarcoma growth via antiangiogenesis in vivo. BMC Cancer 2007;7:49.

Knowling M, Blackstein M, Tozer R, et al. A phase II study of perifosine (D–21226) in patients with previously untreated metastatic or locally advanced soft tissue sarcoma: A National Cancer Institute of Canada Clinical Trials Group trial. Invest New Drugs 2006;24(5):435–9.

Koch BB, Karnell LH, Hoffman HT, et al. National cancer database report on chondrosarcoma of the head and neck. Head Neck 2000;22(4):408–25.

Lersundi A, Mankin HJ, Mourikis A, et al. Chondromyxoid fibroma: a rarely encountered and puzzling tumor. Clin Orthop Relat Res 2005;439:171–5.

Levine AM, Tulpule A, Quinn DI, et al. Phase I study of antisense oligonucleotide against vascular endothelial growth factor: Decrease in plasma vascular endothelial growth factor with potential clinical efficacy. J Clin Oncol 2006;24:1712–1719.

Lohrer L, Vordemvenne T, Neuber M, et al. Enochondroma of the hand - treatment and long-term outcome. Z Orthop Unfall 2010;148(6):709–715.

Mitchell AD, Ayoub K, Mangham DC, et al. Experience in the treatment of dedifferentiated chondrosarcoma. J Bone Joint Surg Br 2000;82:55–61.

Mohler DG, Chiu R, McCall DA, et al. Curettage and cryosurgery for low-grade cartilage tumors is associated with low recurrence and high function. Clin Orthop Relat Res 2010;468(10):2765–73.

Nielsen GP, Keel SB, Dickersin GR, et al. Chondromyxoid fibroma: a tumor showing myofibroblastic, myochondroblastic, and chondrocytic differentiation. Mod Pathol 1999;12(5):514–7.

Nishio J, Reith JD, Ogose A, et al. Cytogenetic findings in clear cell chondrosarcoma. Cancer Genet Cytogenet 2005;162(1):74–7.

Nooij MA, Whelan J, Bramwell VH, et al. Doxorubicin and cisplatin chemotherapy in high-grade spindle cell sarcomas of the bone, other than osteosarcoma or malignant fibrous histiocytoma: A European Osteosarcoma Intergroup Study. Eur J Cancer 2005;41:225–230.

Ostrowski ML, Johnson ME, Truong LD, et al. Malignant chondroblastoma presenting as a recurrent pelvic tumor with DNA aneuploidy and p53 mutation as supportive evidence of malignancy. Skeletal Radiol 1999;28(11):644–50.

Papachristou DJ, Goodman MA, Cieply K, et al. Comparison of allelic losses in chondroblastoma and primary chondrosarcoma of bone and correlation with fluorescence in situ hybridization analysis. Hum Pathol 2006;37(7):890–8.

Ramappa AJ, Lee FY, Tang P, et al. Chondroblastoma of bone. J Bone Joint Surg Am 2000;82A(8):1140–1145.

Reith JD, Horodyski MB, Scarborough MT. Grade 2 chondrosarcoma: stage I or stage II tumor? Clin Orthop Relat Res 2003;(415):45–51.

Riedel RF, Larrier N, Dodd L, et al. The clinical management of chondrosarcoma. Curr Treat Options Oncol 2009;10(1–2):94–106.

Romeo S, Oosting J, Rozeman LB, et al. The role of noncartilage-specific molecules in differentiation of cartilaginous tumors: lessons from chondroblastoma and chondromyxoid fibroma. Cancer 2007;110(2):385–94.

Rosenberg AE, Nielsen GP, Keel SB, et al. Chondrosarcoma of the base of the skull: a clinicopathologic study of 200 cases with emphasis on its distinction from chordoma. Am J Surg Pathol 1999;23(11):1370–8.

Rozeman LB, Hogendoorn PC, Bovée JV. Diagnosis and prognosis of chondrosarcoma of bone. EJ Molec Diagno 2002;2(5):461–72.

Sakimura R, Tanaka K, Yamamoto S, et al. The effects of histone deacetylase inhibitors on the induction of differentiation in chondrosarcoma cells. Clin Cancer Res 2007;13:275–282.

Schajowicz F, Gallardo H. Chondromyxoid fibroma of bone, a clinico-pathological study of thirty-two cases. J Bone Joint Surg Br 1971;53(2):198–216.

Schwartz HS, Zimmerman NB, Simon MA, et al. The malignant potential of enchondromatosis. J Bone Joint Surg Am 1987;69(2):269–74.

Sevel D. Mesenchymal chondrosarcoma of orbit. Br J Ophthalmol 1974;58:882–887.

Sharma H, Jane MJ, Reid R. Chondromyxoid fibroma of the foot and ankle: 40 years' Scottish bone tumour registry experience. Int Orthop 2006;30(3):205–9.

Söder S, Oliveira AM, Inwards CY, et al. Type II collagen, but not aggrecan expression, distinguishes clear cell chondrosarcoma and chondroblastoma. Pathology 2006;38(1):35–8.

Staals EL, Bacchini P, Bertoni F. Dedifferentiated central chondrosarcoma. Cancer 2006;106:2682–2691.

Staals EL, Bacchini P, Mercuri M, et al. Dedifferentiated Chondrosarcomas arising in preexisting osteochondromas. J Bone Joint Surg Am 2007;89(5):987–93.

Streitbürger A, Ahrens H, Balke M, et al. Grade I chondrosarcoma of bone: the Münster experience. J Cancer Res Clin Oncol 2009;135(4):543–50.

Tallini G, Dorfman H, Brys P, et al. Correlation between clinicopathological features and karyotype in 100 cartilaginous and chordoid tumours. A report from the Chromosomes and Morphology (CHAMP) Collaborative Study Group. J Pathol 2002;196(2):194–203.

Walden MJ, Murphey MD, Vidal JA. Incidental enchondromas of the knee. AJR 2008;190(6):1611–5.

Wu CT, Inwards CY, O'Laughlin S, et al. Chondromyxoid fibroma of bone: a clinicopathologic review of 278 cases. Hum Pathol 1998;29(5):438–46.

Yoo HJ, Hong SH, Choi JY, et al. Differentiating high-grade from low-grade chondrosarcoma with MR imaging. Eur Radiol 2009;19:3008–3014.

FURTHER READING

Bullough, PG. Orthopaedic Pathology, 5th ed. Maryland Heights: Mosby, 2010
Dorfman HD, Czerniak B. Bone Tumors. St Louis: Mosby, 1998
Folpe AL, Inwards CY (Eds). Bone and Soft Tissue Pathology. A volume in the series: Foundations in Diagnostic Pathology. Goldblum JR (series ed). Philadelphia: Elsevier Saunders, 2010.
Fletcher CDM, Bridge JA, Hogendoorn P, Mertens F (eds). WHO Classification of Tumours of Soft Tissue and Bone, 4th ed. Lyon: IARC Press, 2013.
Gelderblom H, Hogendoorn P, Dijkstra SD, et al. The clinical approach towards chondrosarcoma. The Oncologist 2008;13(3):320–329.
Jaffe HL. Chondromyxoid Fibroma. Tumors and Tumorous Conditions of the Bones and Joints. Philadelphia: Lea & Febiger, 1958;203–213.
Marco RA, Gitelis S, Brebach GT, Healey JH. Cartilage tumors: evaluation and treatment. J Am Acad Orthop Surg 2000;8(5):292–304.
Weiner SD. Enchondroma and Chondrosarcoma of bone: clinical, radiologic, and histologic differentiation. Instr Course Lect 2004;53:645–9.

Chapter 17 Osteogenic tumors of bone

OVERVIEW

These are tumors that produce osteoid (unmineralized bone matrix) and/or fully mineralized bone. They range from benign tumors that can spontaneously regress (osteoid osteoma) to highly aggressive malignant sarcomas (secondary osteosarcoma).

Corresponding to the behavior of the tumors, treatment ranges from minimal such as administration of non-steroidal anti-inflammatory agents (osteoid osteoma) to radical surgery with systemic therapy (many cases of conventional osteosarcoma). Improvements in survival for osteosarcoma stalled in the 1990s when it reached a high of 70% long-term, overall survival. With advances in molecular medicine, insights in osteosarcoma genesis are suggesting new gene targeted and immunotherapy approaches that may save the 30% of osteosarcoma patients who currently die of their disease.

CLASSIFICATION

Table 17.1 lists the World Health Organization (WHO) Classification of osteogenic tumors of bone (2013).

DEMOGRAPHICS

Osteoma

Osteomas are usually asymptomatic. They may be present in a substantial portion of the adult population based on being commonly found on imaging for other reasons. Those occurring in the calverial, facial, and gnathic bones occur with no gender predilection. Those occurring in the spine, pelvis, and long bones more commonly are found in men. The latter are termed enostoses or bone islands.

Osteoid osteoma

Osteoid osteoma is relatively common and accounts for 11% of all benign bone tumors (third most common benign bone tumor and 3% of all bone tumors) (Lee et al. 2006). A broad age range is affected from infancy to old age, but most patients are adolescents and young adults. Osteoid osteoma is more common in males by a ratio of 3:1 (Lee et al. 2006).

Osteoblastoma

Osteoblastoma is noticeably less common than osteoid osteoma and comprises less than 1% of all benign bone tumors. It likewise occurs over a wide age range, but most patients are in their second to fourth decades (mean age is 20 years) (Baker et al. 2010). Males are twice as commonly affected as females (Folpe et al. 2010).

Osteosarcoma

Osteosarcoma is the most common malignant bone tumor (if one excludes myeloma). Even so, the incidence pales by comparison with more common tumors such as lung, prostate and breast cancer. The incidence varies slightly worldwide and peaks in two age groups. Osteosarcoma of childhood/adolescence affects 3-4.5 individuals/million/year, drops to 1-2 individuals/million/year in the 25-59 year old age range, and increases again in patients older than 60 years with a rate of 1.5-4 individuals/million/year (Savage et al 2010). Parosteal osteosarcoma and small cell osteosarcoma occur in a slightly older age group than conventional (intramedullary high grade) osteosarcoma (less common in adolescents and more common in young adults). Additionally, parosteal osteosarcoma occurs with slightly greater frequency in females. This contrasts with the other variants of osteosarcoma which show a slight predominance in males.

Table 17.1 WHO classification of osteogenic tumors of bone (2013)

Tumor	Behavior	Additional comments
Osteoma	Benign	Called enostosis or bone island when occurring outside the skull
Osteoid osteoma	Benign	Relatively common. Often with a distinctive presentation of pain at night relieved by aspirin or NSAIDS
Osteoblastoma	Intermediate (locally aggressive)	Rare. Several histologic subtypes
Conventional osteosarcoma	Malignant	Most common type of osteosarcoma. High grade. Several histologic subtypes including chondroblastic, fibroblastic, and osteoblastic
Periosteal osteosarcoma	Malignant	Uncommon. Medium risk for malignant behavior
Parosteal osteosarcoma	Malignant	Low risk for malignant behavior: Rate of metastasis (<5%) in absence of dedifferentiation
Telangiectatic osteosarcoma	Malignant	Rare. May mimic ABC on radiology
Small cell osteosarcoma	Malignant	Extremely rare. Some cases show rearrangements of EWS gene
Low grade central osteosarcoma	Malignant	Rare. Low risk of malignant behavior
High grade surface osteosaroma	Malignant	Rare
Secondary osteosarcoma	Malignant	Most occur in older adults. Causes include prior radiation therapy, long-standing metal implant, prior chemotherapy

ABC: aneurysmal bone cyst. NSAIDS: non-steroidal anti-inflammatory drugs. Medium risk malignant: risk of metastasis is lower than for conventional osteosarcoma but higher than for low grade central osteosarcoma or parosteal osteosarcoma. Low risk malignant: very low risk of metastasis in the absence of dedifferentiation (transformation to a high grade osteosarcoma).

Using Surveillance, Epidemiology and End Results (SEER) data from 13 US tumor registries for the 15 years spanning 1994 through 2008, the average annual incidence rate is 1.9 per million for osteosarcoma NOS, 0.4 per million for chondroblastic osteosarcoma, 0.2 per million for parosteal osteosarcoma and fibroblastic, 0.1 per million for telangiectatic osteosarcoma and osteosarcoma in Paget disease of bone, and 0.0 per million for small cell, central, intraosseous well differentiated and periosteal osteosarcomas. Three of these types differ by sex. Females have a 1.6 times higher incidence rate of parosteal osteosarcomas than males. Additionally, females have a 28% lower rate of osteosarcoma NOS and a 31% lower rate of chondroblastic osteosarcoma compared to males. The number of cases reported in 13 SEER registries is shown in **Figure 17.1**.

The mean ages for osteosarcoma types are under 35 years old except for those patients diagnosed with osteosarcoma in Paget disease of bone (mean age = 71.4 years). **Figure 17.2** depicts the age distribution of osteosarcomas using SEER registry data (1994-2008; 13 registries in US).

Pathogenesis/etiology

Table 17.2 lists the genetic abnormalities found thus far in osteogenic tumors of bone. This is an evolving area of research and thus may be significantly out of date by the time of publication. Nonetheless, it offers a starting point and snapshot of the state of knowledge as of 2013. Of course, genetic changes can explain the pathophysiology and pathogenesis of a tumor; what ultimately causes the genes to alter may be unknown. Epigenetic irregularities may also theoretically contribute to tumor formation, while the perturbers of epigenetic regulation may be undeciphered.

Osteoma

Osteoma (enostosis, bone island) seems to be a hamartomatous proliferation in the great majority of cases. Multiple osteomas/enostoses may occur in two syndromes (Gardner and Buschke-Ollendorff) (Baumhoer et al. 2013).

Osteoid osteoma

Osteoid osteoma is a bona fide neoplasm based on the finding of monoclonality in a number of case reports including repetitive involvement of chromosome 22q (Folpe et al. 2010). The cause is not known.

Osteoblastoma

As with osteoid osteoma, the cause of osteoblastoma is unknown. Osteoblastoma is basically a 'super-sized' version of osteoid osteoma. In many cases, the two are histologically indistinguishable. Size is what differentiates the two entities: osteoblastomas are at least 2 cm in size, and osteoid osteomas are smaller. However, osteoblastoma is more protean in morphology than osteoid osteoma with variants that are markedly cystic, show degenerative changes, or epithelioid (among others; see Case presentations within this chapter for a list of osteoblastoma morphologic appearances).

Osteosarcoma

Like other sarcomas, many cases of osteosarcoma (OS) develop as a result of the interplay of environment and genes. Known environmental risk factors include radiation exposure (implicated in approximately 2% of osteosarcomas) and exposure to chemicals or fibers including methylcholanthrene, chromium salts, beryllium oxide, zinc beryllium silicate, aniline dyes and asbestos (Broadhead et al. 2011).

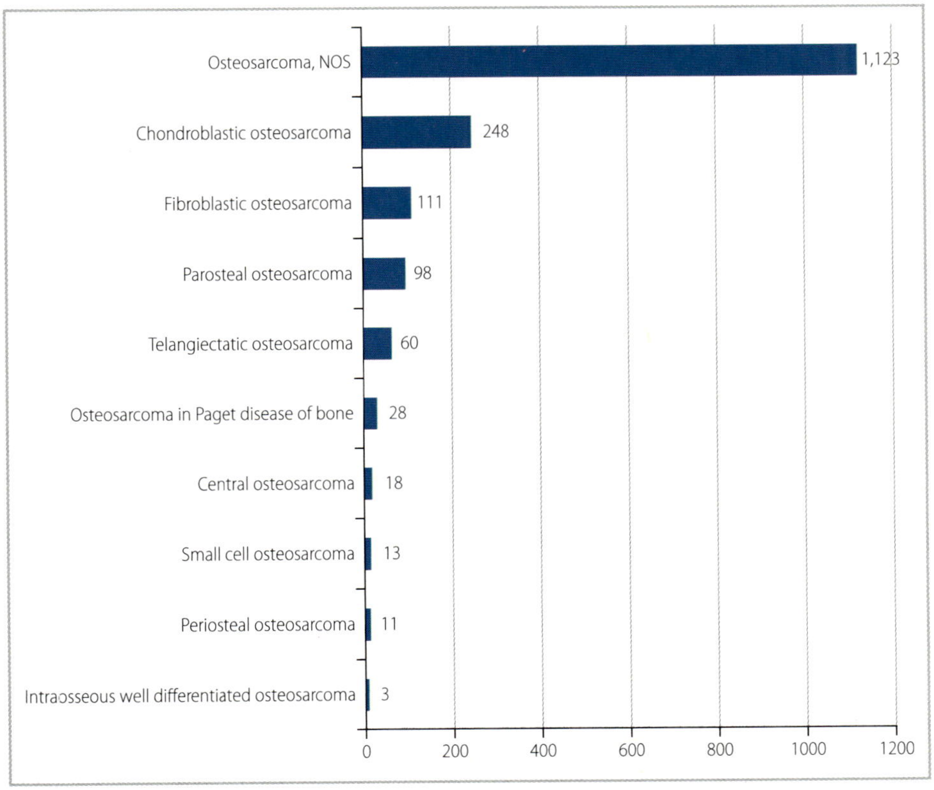

Figure 17.1 Frequency of osteogenic bone tumor types in 13 SEER registries between the years 1994 and 2008.

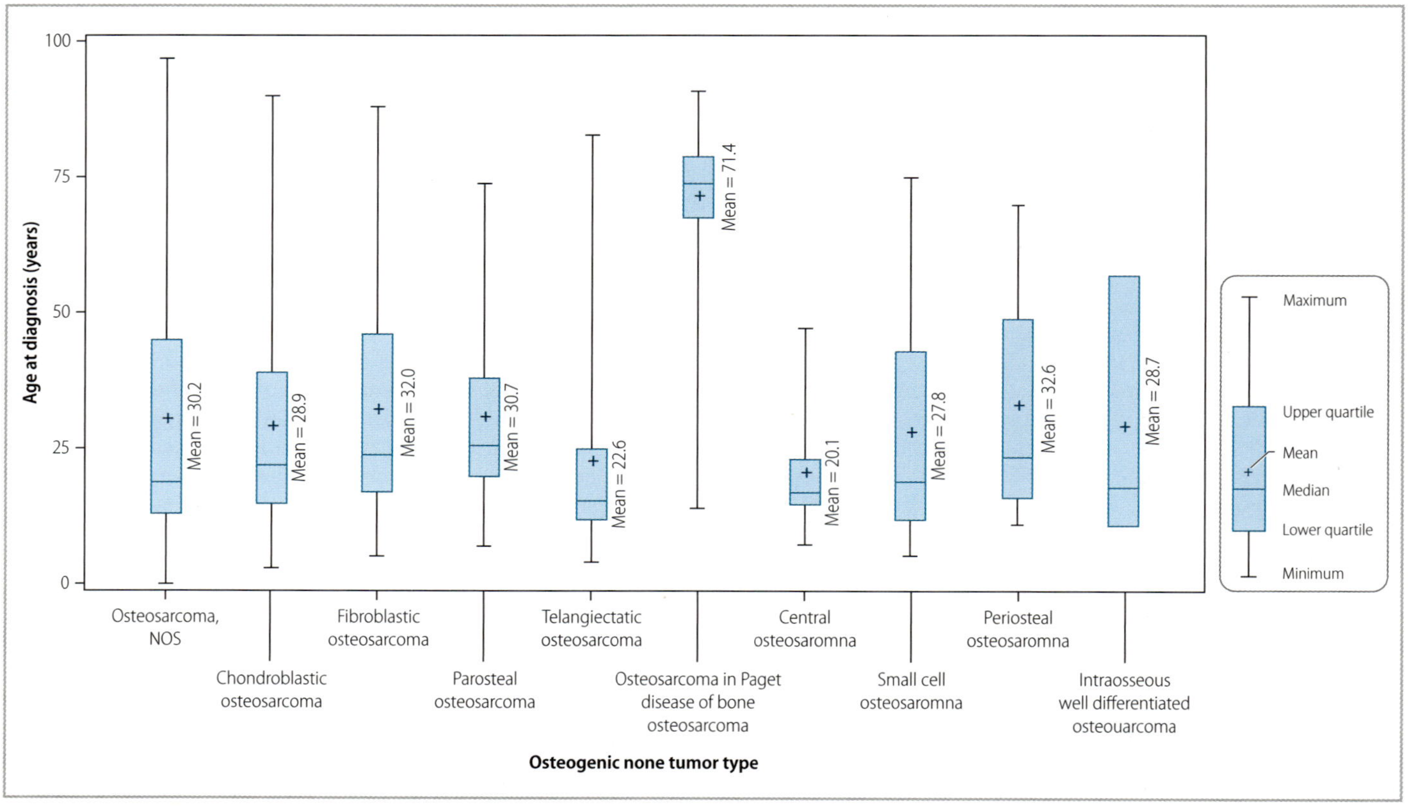

Figure 17.2 Age distribution of osteosarcoma types in 13 SEER registries during the time period 1994-2008 (N=1,713).

Table 17.2 Genetics of osteogenic tumors of bone

Tumor	Chromosomal abnormality	Genes involved	Percentage of tumors with abnormality
Osteoma	Multiple lesions may be associated with Gardner syndrome (especially in the jaws) or Buschke-Ollendorff syndrome	*APC* (5q21) (Gardner syndrome) *LEMD3* (12q14) (Buschke-Ollendorff syndrome)	<5% estimated Most cases are sporadic hamartomas
Osteoid osteoma	Consistent abnormalities of 22q and 17q. However, most cases show a normal karyotype. [few cases studied]	Unknown	Unknown
Osteoblastoma	May have a complex karyotype including translocations with no recurring, specific abnormalities. [few cases studied]	Unknown	Unknown
Conventional osteosarcoma	Complex aneuploid karyotype with extensive numerical and structural abnormalities. Some recurring sites involved (but not universal to all cases) include gain of 1 and loss of material on 6, 9, 10, 13 and 17. Rearrangements or copy number changes most commonly affect: 1p11-13, 1q11-12, 1q21-22, 3q26, 6p, 8q, 11p14-15, 12q12-13 14p11-13, 14q24-qter, 15p1-13, 17p including 17p11.2-p12, and 19q12-13	Multiple genes have been studied. Most likely, there is heterogeneity in gene abnormalities across individual tumors Genes reported to be abnormal are *p53*, *BRCA1*, *RB1*, DNA helicases, with Amp of *Myc*, O-E of *FOS*, *JUN*, *IGF-I* and *II*, *TGF-β*, *CTGF*, *PTHrP*, *PTH*, *DTHR1*, *PDGF1*, among many others	70% have complex aneuploidy ~20% have p53 mutations ~20% have LOH of *BRCA1*
Periosteal osteosarcoma	Complex aneuploid karyotype	Presumed similar to conventional osteosarcoma	Presumed similar to conventional osteosarcoma
Parosteal osteosarcoma	Ring chromosomes composed of multiple copies of 12q13-15	Amplified *CDK4* and *MDM2*	Majority have ring chromosomes. Majority have *CDK4* and *MDM2* amplification
Telangiectatic osteosarcoma	Same changes as in conventional osteosarcoma	Same changes as in conventional osteosarcoma	Same as for conventional OS
Small cell osteosarcoma	[few cases studied] Three way translocation in one case t(6;16;17). One case of t(11;22)(q24;q12) and one case of t(11;22)(p11;q12) have been reported, although some investigators exclude tumors with *EWSR1* translocations from the small cell osteosarcoma category	*p53* and others Possibly *EWSR1*, *CREB3L1*	Unknown
Low grade central osteosarcoma	Same ring chromosomes as for parosteal osteosarcoma. Some may also have 6p abnormalities	Amplified *CDK4* and *MDM2*	Majority have ring chromosomes. Majority have *CDK4* and *MDM2* amplification

Table 17.2: Continued from page 412

Tumor	Chromosomal abnormality	Genes involved	Percentage of tumors with abnormality
High grade surface osteosaroma	Complex aneuploid karyotype. A few have ring and marker chromosomes comprising amplified 12q13-15 indicating transformation from a low grade osteosarcoma	Same as for conventional OS. Plus a few have amplified *CDK4* and *MDM2*	Majority have complex aneuploidy. ~10% have amplified *CDK4* and *MDM2*
Secondary osteosarcoma	Most have complex aneuploid karyotype	May be similar to conventional osteosarcoma	May be similar to conventional osteosarcoma

Amp: amplification, O-E: over-expressed, LOH: loss of heterozygosity, OS: osteosarcoma.

See References for papers and texts pertaining to this table. This static list of genetic abnormalities must be viewed in the context of continuing discovery and refinement of genetic findings.

Certain inherited syndromes or disorders also place patients at risk for osteosarcoma; these include Li-Fraumeni syndrome, hereditary retinoblastoma, and Diamond-Blackfan anemia, among others (see **Table 17.3** for a more detailed list). However, proportionally, these account for very few cases of osteosarcoma.

The majority of tumors develop during periods of rapidly proliferating bone occurring naturally in childhood and adolescence. Paget's disease also stimulates bone growth, and it is estimated that 50% of osteosarcoma cases arise in the background of this unnatural bone growth stimulator (Savage et al. 2010).

Consistent with the idea that risk for OS increases in a setting rich in growth factors and mitotically active osteoblast progenitor cells (the milieu of normal bone growth and Paget's disease), osteosarcoma occurs with greater frequency in males and taller individuals (on average, longer growth spurts involving more bone volume).

Osteosarcoma may also arise at the site of a metal implant, chronic osteomyelitis or a benign tumor such as fibrous dysplasia or osteoblastoma. Similar logic pertains as for growth spurts: increased cell turnover causes an increased risk of sarcomatous transformation.

Population based studies of single nucleotide polymorphisms indicate that patients with certain specific, naturally occurring variants of specific genes may be at increased risk for development of osteosarcoma. These genes include TNF-α, VDR (vitamin D receptor), IGF2R, TGF-β, FAS, and a gene (or genes) at chromosome locus 8q24 (Savage et al. 2010).

PATHOLOGY

Table 17.4 provides brief descriptions of the demographics, body site, and histology of these tumors. The photomicrographs are

Table 17.3 Genetic or inherited disorders associated with an increased risk for osteosarcoma

Condition	Prevalence of disorder	Genes involved	Chromosome site	Inheritance pattern	Other associated tumors
Li- Fraumeni Syndrome	Rare (1/20,000)	p53 = tumor protein *p53*	17p13.1	Autosomal dominant	Breast CA, adrenocortical CA, bronchioloalveolar CA, STS including RMS, NST, HEME
Hereditary retinoblastoma	Rare	*RB1* = retinoblastoma 1	13q14.2	Autosomal dominant	Retinoblastoma, STS
Diamond blackfan anemia	Rare	Ribosomal protein genes such as RPS19, RPL5 and others	Multiple	Autosomal dominant	HEME
Familial Paget's disease	Rare	Multiple	18q21, 5q31, 5q35, others	Autosomal dominant	Chondrosarcoma
Neurofibromatosis type 1	Relatively common (1/4000)	*NF1* = neurofibromin	17q11	Autosomal dominant in 50%; 50% sporadic new mutation	Neurofibromas, MPNST; GIST, NST, HEME, CA. Risk for OS is controversial and most likely low
Rothmund Thompson syndrome	Very rare	*REQL4* = RecQ protein-like 4, DNA helicase	8q24.3	Autosomal recessive	CA, HEME, NST, GermCT
Werner syndrome	Very rare	*WRN* = Werner syndrome, RecQ helicase-like	8p12	Autosomal recessive	STS
Bloom syndrome	Very rare	*BLM* = Bloom syndrome, RecQ helicase-like	15q26.1	Autosomal recessive	None other than OS
Mazebraud syndrome	Very rare	*GNAS1* = guanine nucleotide-binding protein α stimulating activity polypeptide 1	20q13	Sporadic	Polyostotic fibrous dysplasia, Intramuscular myxomas
McCune-Albright syndrome	Rare	*GNAS1*= guanine nucleotide-binding protein α stimulating activity polypeptide 1	20q13	Sporadic	Polyostotic fibrous dysplasia

CA: carcinoma, OS: osteosarcoma, RMS: rhabdomyosarcoma, NST: nervous system tumors, HEME: hematopoietic tumors including lymphoma, and/or leukemia and/or myelodysplastic syndrome, GermCT: germ cell tumors, STS: soft tissue sarcoma

Table 17.4 Osteogenic tumors of bone grouped by behavior

Tumor	Incidence	Age and sex distribution	Body site (in order of occurrence)	Histopathology description including IHC Medium magnification	High magnification
Benign: does not recur or recurs non-aggressively and does not metastasize					
Osteoma (enostosis, bone island)	Unknown but probably common	Adults most commonly. M=F in skull. M>F elsewhere	Skull (all bones) Spine, pelvis, long bones	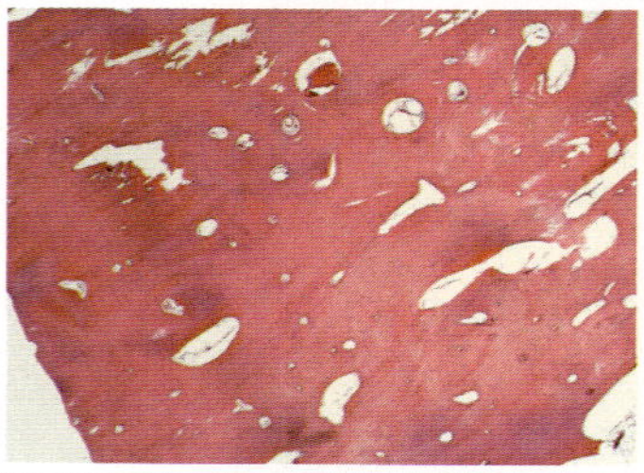	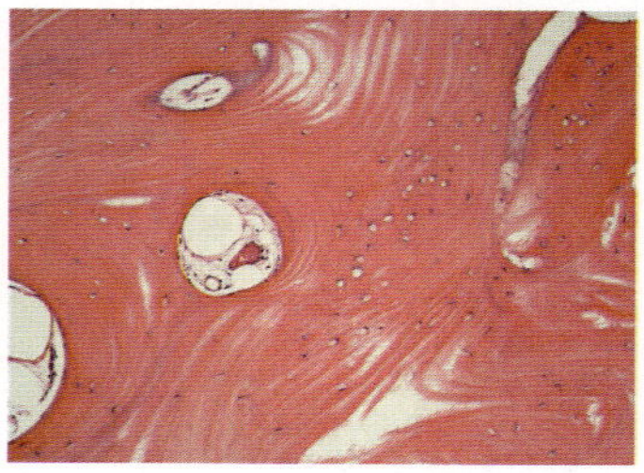
Osteoma: sharply defined lesion of lamellar bone with sometimes cellular stroma and prominent osteoblasts and osteoclasts. Bone is compact and/or spongiotic. Enostosis (bone island): discrete nodule of compact bone located in the medulla of spine, pelvis, or long bones					
Osteoid osteoma	Common	Most patients are 5-25 years. M > F by 3-4:1	Metadiaphysis of femur and tibia, spine, hands and feet and rarely elsewhere. Rarely intra-articular or subperiosteal	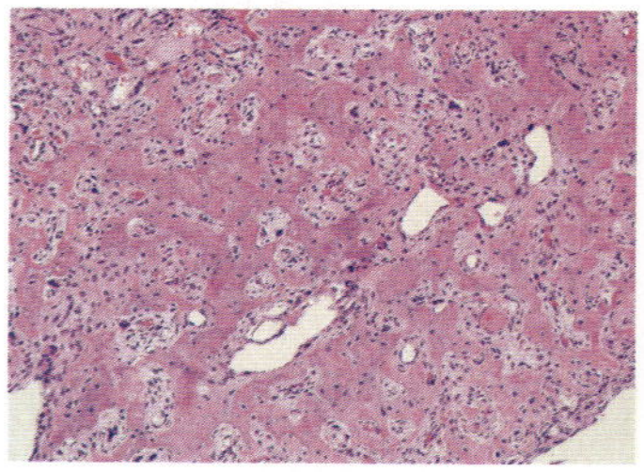	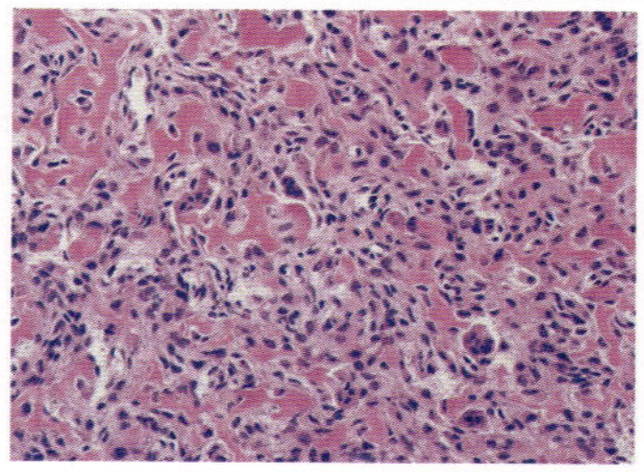
Zonal pattern with central nidus of dense woven tumor bone covered by prominent osteoblasts with a vascular stroma and reactive bone perimeter. Osteoclasts common. No cytologic atypia, no invasion of surrounding normal bone. Cartilage extremely rare. Must be less than 2.0 cm in diameter. S-100 IHC stain commonly shows intratumoral nerve fibers.					
Intermediate: can recur locally aggressively and/or rarely metastasizes (<5%)					
Osteoblastoma	Rare	Broad age range but most patients 10-30 years. M > F by 2:1	Spine (dorsal elements most commonly) and sacrum, mandible, femur, tibia, ribs, calverium, but any bone can be involved	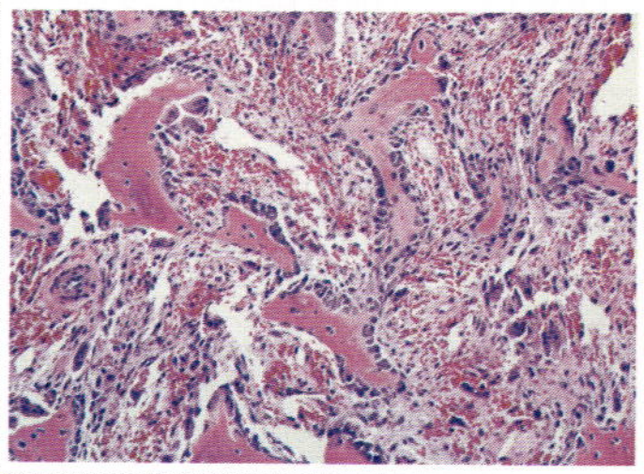	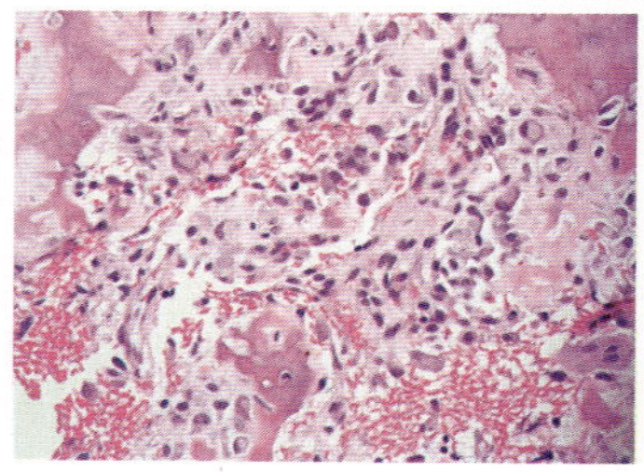
Can look exactly like osteoid osteoma except > 2 cm in diameter. Variants include 'aggressive OB' with large epithelioid osteoblasts, cystic OB (with secondary ABC change), pseudomalignant OB (with degenerative cytologic atypia). Cartilage rare. No intratumoral nerve fibers.					
Parosteal osteosarcoma	Rare	Most patients are young to middle aged adults (mean of 33 years). F > M	Distal posterior femur, proximal tibia, humerus >> other bones	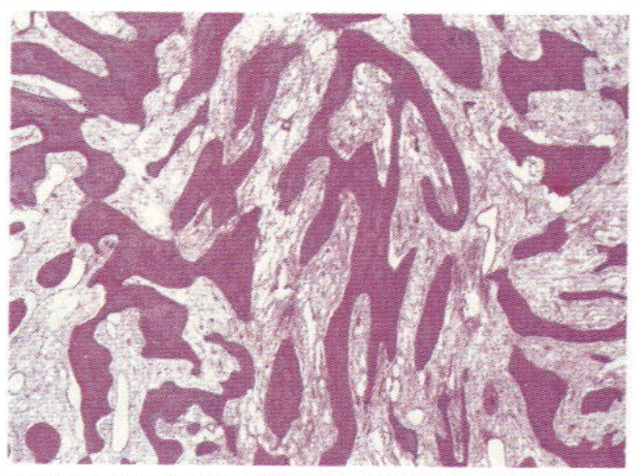	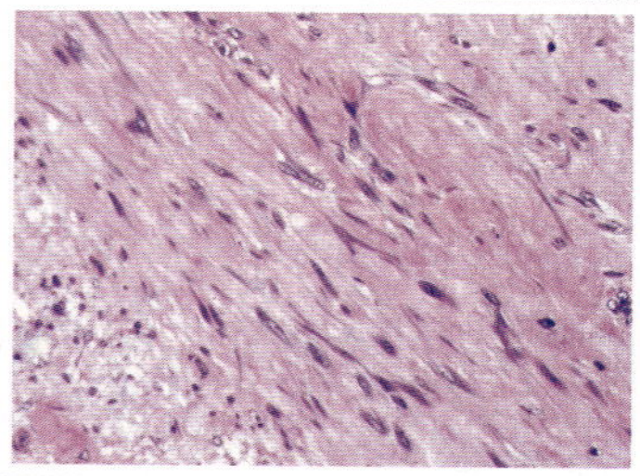
Histologically low grade with long parallel arrays of woven (and rarely lamellar) tumor bone. Osteoblastic rimming of the tumor bone may be present. Stroma is usually moderately cellular with elongate spindle cells and few mitoses. Malignant cartilage is present in 50% and may be intermixed or present as an outer cap mimicking osteochondroma. Most cases positive for CDK4 and MDM2 by IHC.					

Table 17.4: Continued from page 414

Tumor	Incidence	Age and sex distribution	Body site (in order of occurrence)	Histopathology description including IHC	
				Medium magnification	High magnification
Low grade central osteosarcoma	Rare	Most patients are adolescents and young adults. M = F	Distal femur, proximal tibia, other long bones > flat bones. Tumor arises in medullary cavity	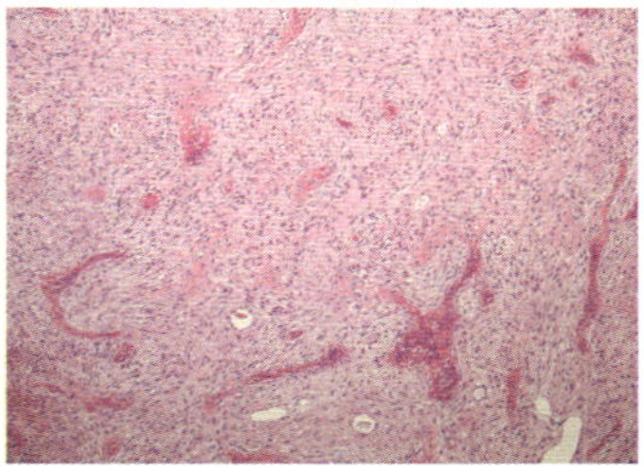	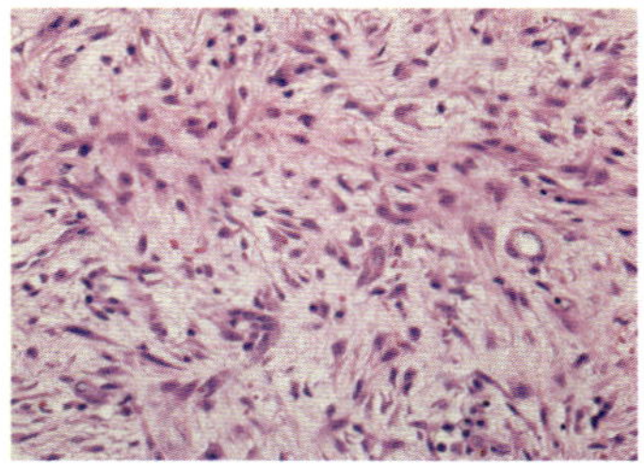
Mildly to moderately cellular spindle cell matrix with tumor osteoid and bone that may grow in long parallel arrays of woven or lamellar bone (like parosteal OS) or as the 'Chinese character' tumbled, irregular bone shapes in fibrous dysplasia. Tumor cartilage may be focally present. Many cases positive for MDM2 and CDK4 by IHC.					
Malignant: can recur and commonly metastasizes					
Conventional osteosarcoma	Common	Most patients are adolescents and young adults. M > F	Distal femur, proximal tibia, proximal humerus, then other long bones; gnathic bones and axial skeleton progressively more common in older patients. Metaphysis (90%), diaphysis (9%), epiphysis (1%)	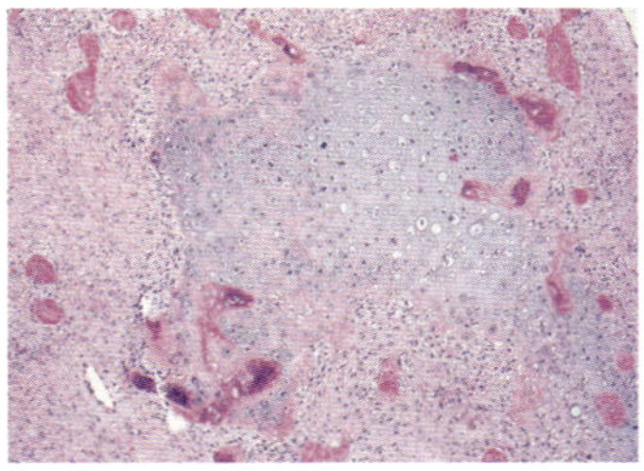	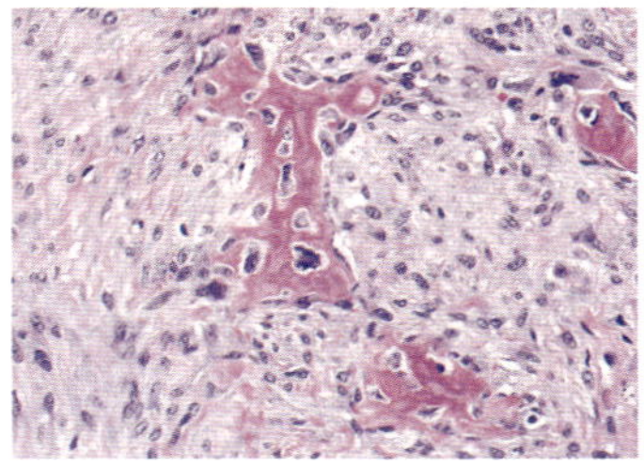
High grade tumor with three main histologic variants: osteoblastic, chondroblastic, and fibroblastic. All tumors must form neoplastic osteoid or bone (mineralized osteoid). Cytologic atypia is marked. Necrosis is often present. Mitoses usually easy to find with atypical forms. Tumor invades normal bone. Neoplastic bone does not have rimming osteoblasts. Osteoid and osteoblasts often express osteocalcin by IHC Osteoblasts also express SATB2. IHC is otherwise polyphenotypic.					
Periosteal osteosarcoma	Rare	Most patients are adolescents and young adults. M > F	Tibia, femur, humerus >> other long bones, pelvis, mandible, clavicle. Most are diaphyseal with a few metaphyseal/ diaphyseal	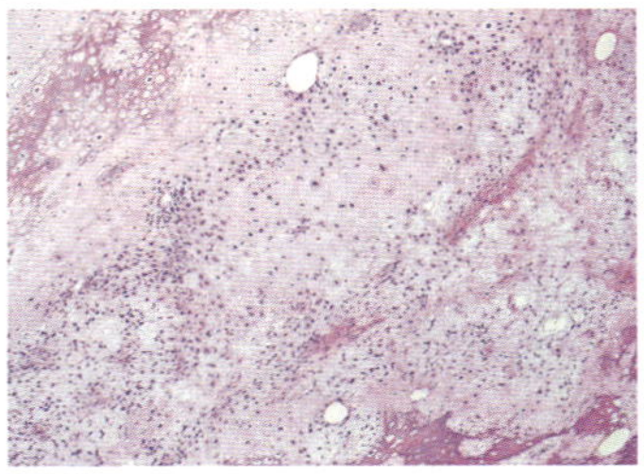	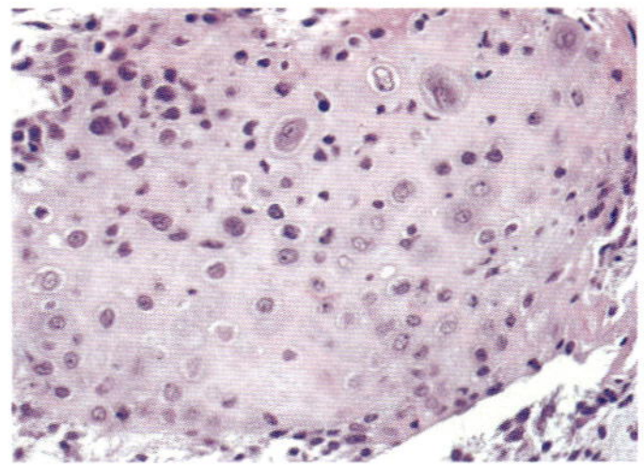
Predominantly chondroblastic with foci of intermediate grade osteosarcoma. Lobules of malignant cartilage merge with foci of osteoid. Periphery may contain more lacelike osteoid set in myxoid spindle cell stroma. Malignant osteoblasts express nuclear SATB2 by IHC.					
Telangiectatic osteosarcoma	Rare	Most patients are children to young adults (mean age 16 years). M > F	Distal femur, proximal tibia, proximal humerus, proximal femur; rare in other bones Almost always metaphyseal	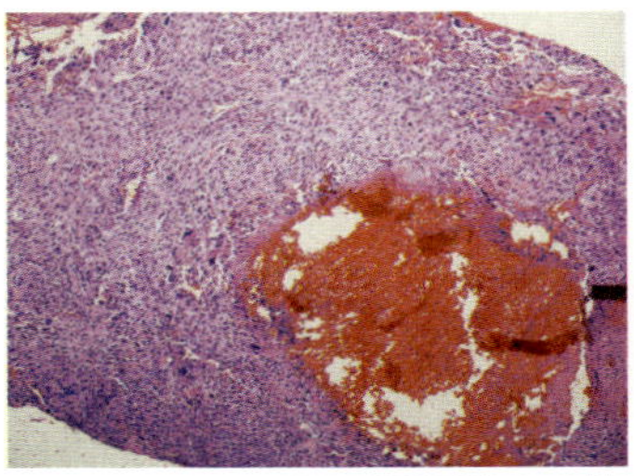	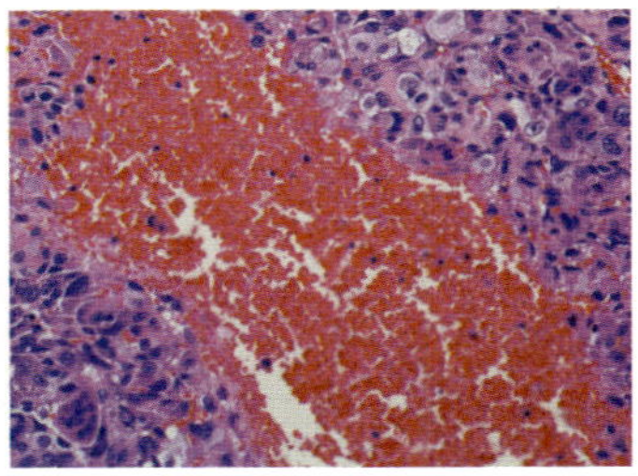
High grade malignant osteoblasts and many osteoclasts line blood- filled cavities. Cavities may be septated. A few solid areas may be present between smaller hemorrhagic cysts. Tumor osteoid is often focal and lacelike. Histologic features of pathologic fracture commonly seen. Malignant osteoblasts express nuclear SATB2 by IHC.					

Table 17.4: Continued from page 415

Tumor	Incidence	Age and sex distribution	Body site (in order of occurrence)	Histopathology description including IHC Medium magnification	High magnification
Small cell osteosarcoma	Very rare	Most patients are teens to adults up to age 40 years (slightly older average age than for conventional OS). M > F	Metaphysis of long bones > pelvic bones, spine and ribs	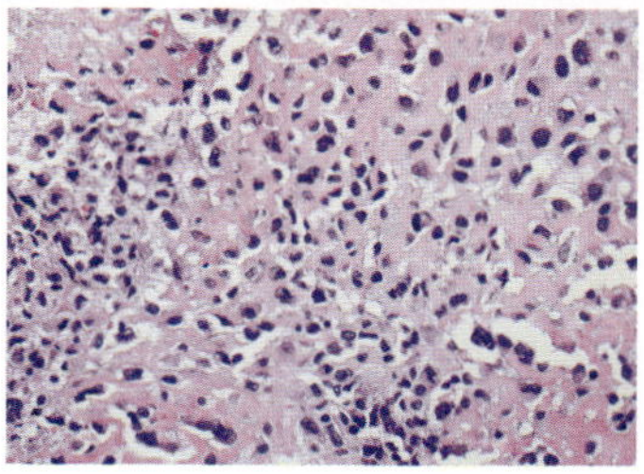	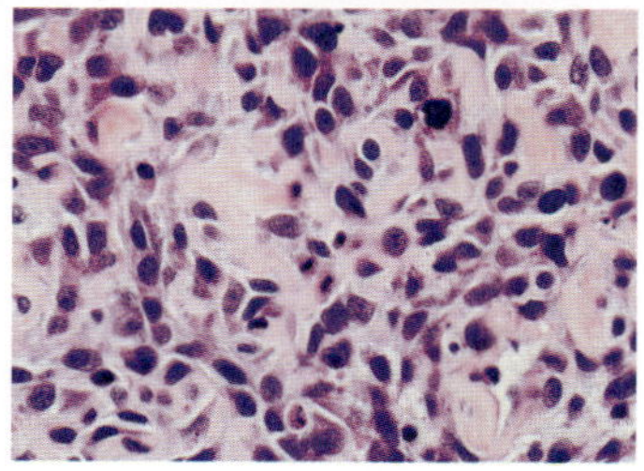
Small cells that may be round or spindled mixed with prominent lacelike osteoid. Osteoblasts may be smaller and round (Ewing sarcoma-like) larger and round (large cell lymphoma-like) or short and spindled (spindle cell variant). CD99 may be positive but only rarely in a membranous pattern. Mitoses and necrosis common. Polyphenotypic but also osteonectin and osteocalcin (50%) positive. Currently unknown whether tumor cells express nuclear SATB2 by IHC.					
High grade surface osteosaroma	Rare	Most patients are adolescents to young adults. M > F	Femur, humerus, tibia, other long tubular bones >> axial skeleton, craniofacial bones	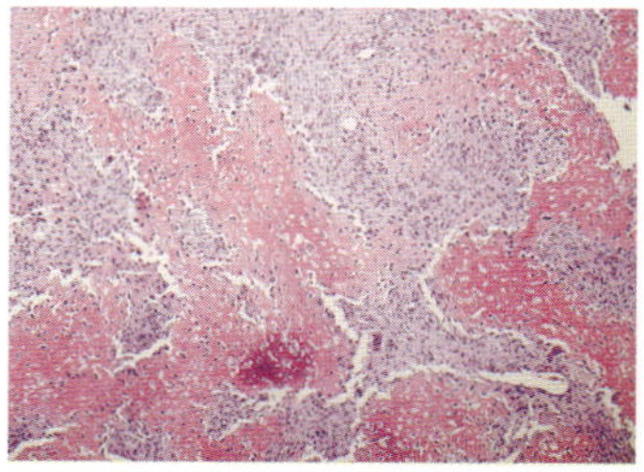	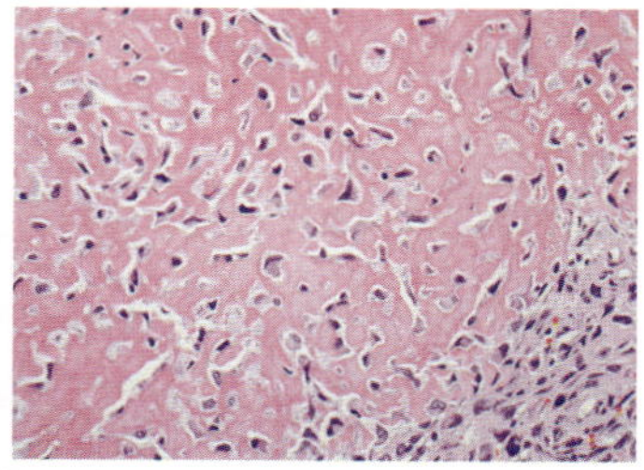
Same histology as conventional osteosarcoma. Usually has more high grade fibroblastic areas than periosteal OS. A few cases may be positive for CDK4 and MDM2 consistent with dedifferentiation from a lower grade tumor. Lower grade tumor may also be present on routine histology.					
Secondary osteosarcoma	Rare	Middle aged to older adults, but may occur in young adults after childhood radiation therapy. M > F	Femur, humerus, tibia, other long tubular bones > pelvis, skull and scapula	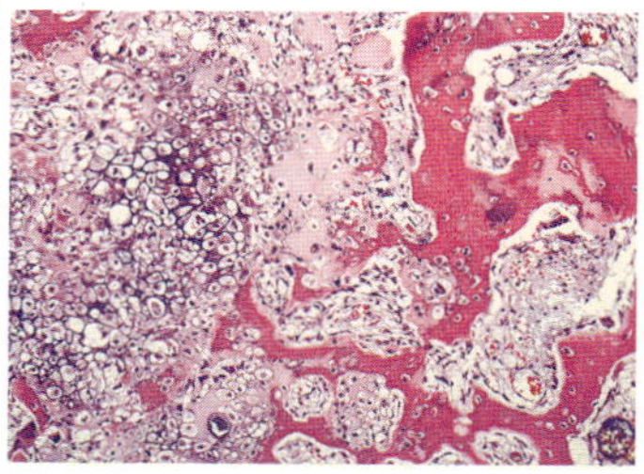	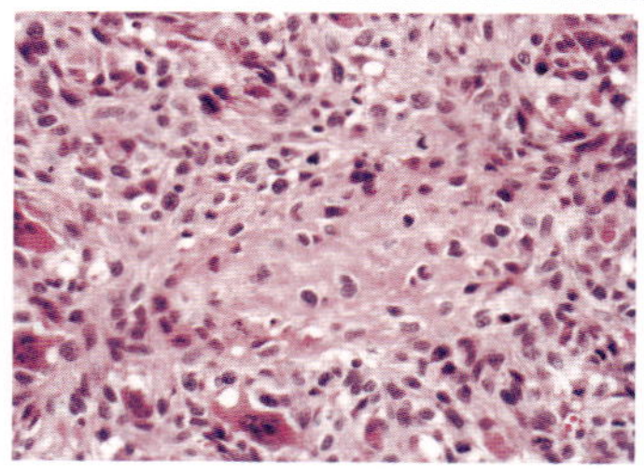
Same histology and polyphenotypic IHC reactivity as in conventional OS. (Polyphenotypic IHC expression includes cases with EMA, keratins, muscle markers, and/or S-100 expression). Osteocalcin is more specific than osteonectin for identifying osteoblasts and osteoid (stains 80% of cases). SATB2 is another specific IHC marker of osteoblastic differentiation.					
M: male, F: female, OS: osteosarcoma, IHC: immunohistochemistry, ABC: aneurysmal bone cyst.					
Incidence Note: 'Common to very common' indicates that a medium sized practice will treat at least several to dozens of patients with the lesion annually, 'Uncommon to rare' indicates the same practice size will treat one to two patients with the lesion every five years, 'Rare to very rare' indicates the same sized practice will see zero to one patient with the lesion every 20 years.					

representative and do not necessarily capture all the appearances of the lesions. More expansive views of some tumors are provided in the Case presentations portion of the chapter. According to SEER registry data, most osteosarcomas are diagnosed in the long bones, especially in the lower limbs (**Fig. 17.1**).

Histologic grading

Osteoma

Osteoma is benign and therefore is not graded. However, it may exhibit stromal hypercellularity and prominent osteoblastic rimming that could be mistaken for osteoid osteoma or osteoblastoma.

Osteoid osteoma

Osteoid osteoma is a benign tumor and therefore is not graded. Hypercellularity may be present, but cytologic atypia is absent.

Osteoblastoma

Osteoblastoma is also a benign tumor and not graded. However, some histologic variants can feature prominent atypia that is degenerative (smudgy, enlarged, hyperchromatic nuclei) or contain large, epithelioid osteoblasts that aggregate in sheets. These appearances may be alarming. Reassuringly, the tumor is sharply circumscribed from surrounding bone and does not invade Haversian canals, atypical mitoses are absent, and the mitotic rate is usually lower than would be seen in a high grade osteosarcoma (the type of osteosarcoma in the differential). Furthermore, the osteoid produced by the tumor is rimmed by osteoblasts, a finding only exceptionally seen in osteosarcoma.

Osteosarcoma

Low grade osteosarcomas include low grade central osteosarcoma and parosteal osteosarcoma. These tumors may demonstrate

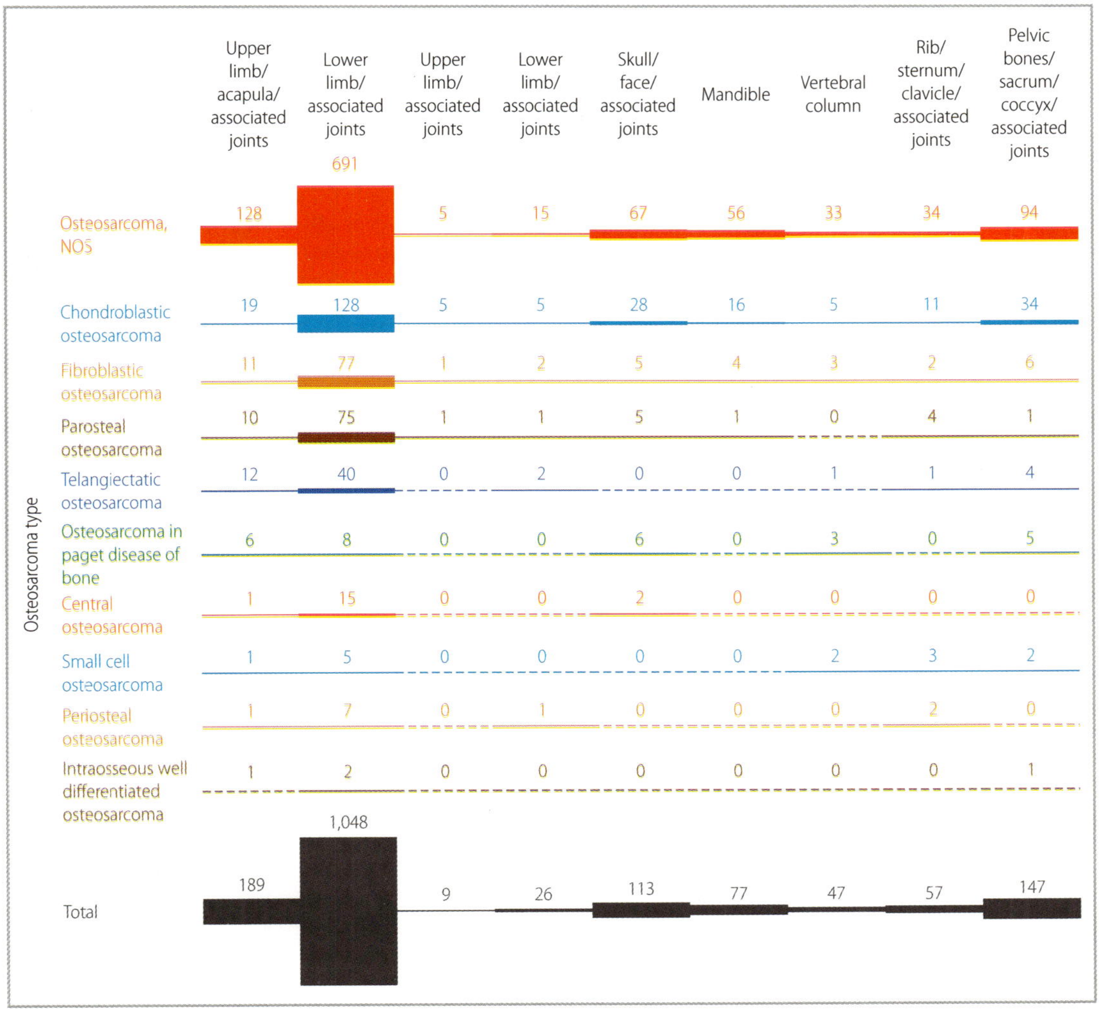

Figure 17.3 Osteosarcoma types by site for cases in 13 SEER registries diagnosed between 1994 and 2008.

minimal cytologic atypia but will irregularly invade normal bone in a malignant fashion. Clues to the diagnosis of parosteal osteosarcoma include long parallel arrays of tumor bone and up to moderate cellularity of the spindle cell stroma. Mitotic activity may be low without atypical mitoses. These tumors would be considered Grade 1. Grade 2 tumors exhibit moderate nuclear atypia including moderate range in nuclear size and shape and will generally feature readily identifiable mitotic figures. Grade 3 tumors are very cellular, contain areas of markedly pleomorphic cells or cells with a blastic, undifferentiated, monotonous appearance (as in small cell osteosarcoma), and mitotic rates are often high with scattered atypical mitoses. Fields of necrosis are usually seen in grade 3 tumors and often can be spotted in grade 2 tumors, also. Conventional osteosarcoma may be osteoblastic, fibroblastic, or chondroblastic, and the grades of the tumor may vary within a single lesion. In many tumors, the neoplastic cells residing within osteoid or bone may show less atypia than the tumor cells in the surrounding fibrous or cartilaginous areas with a smaller overall size. This phenomenon is termed 'normalization'. The grade of the tumor should be assessed from the most atypical areas of the lesion.

Behavior

Osteoma

Osteoma is benign but may cause nasal obstruction when occurring in the sinuses. Extracranial osteomas are seldom symptomatic and do not predispose to fracture or arthritis.

Osteoid osteoma

Osteoid osteoma is a benign tumor with no risk of metastasis or dedifferentiation. Many tumors may be managed by use of oral NSAIDs or by radio-ablation. The local recurrence rate is approximately 5%.

Osteoblastoma

Osteoblastoma is a benign tumor that is treated by surgical excision. Patients may experience progressive pain but not usually the distinct pattern of nocturnal pain alleviated by aspirin or NSAIDs that is associated with osteoid osteoma. When occurring in the spine, osteoblastoma may cause scoliosis. It does not metastasize except in exceptionally rare instances of dedifferentiation to osteosarcoma. The local recurrence rate is approximately 20%.

Osteosarcoma

Behavior is most dependent on tumor stage and histologic grade. Parosteal osteosarcoma and low grade central osteosarcoma have a very good five year survival of >90% and a local recurrence rate of 7% with only rare patients developing metastases (Dujardin et al. 2011). Dedifferentiation to high grade osteosarcoma occurs in 15% to 30%, and in such tumors, metastasis is much more likely resulting in a prognosis that may be only slightly better than conventional high grade osteosarcoma (Schwab et al. 2008). Periosteal osteosarcoma also overall has a better outcome than conventional osteosarcoma with survival rates up to 89% (at 5 years) and 83% (at 10 years) (Grumer et al. 2005).

Beyond high stage and high histologic grade, additional adverse prognostic factors include multi-centricity (with synchronous tumors behaving worse than metachronous tumors: median survival of 14 months versus 43 months in one recent series), age over 40 years, male sex, association with Paget's disease, association with prior radiation, proximal extremity or axial location, soft tissue extension, inadequate surgical margins, local recurrence, and less than 90% tumor necrosis after neoadjuvant chemotherapy (Corradi et al. 2011, Savage et al. 2010).

In spite of accurate staging and grading, surprisingly, a significant number of patients in the conventional high grade osteosarcoma category do not require chemotherapy to achieve long term survival. Identifying this 18% of patients is currently not possible but will most likely be eventually based on molecular genetic discriminators of behavior that form a 'low risk gene signature' (Niswander et al. 2010). Analysis of altered cell pathways in osteosarcoma is ongoing and holds the promise not only of improved prognostication and prediction but also targeted gene therapy. Future laboratory assessment of osteosarcoma will undoubtedly expand beyond microscopic review to include gene expression profiling, possibly tumor proteome analysis, and evaluation of gene-level changes in response to therapy. With a brisk pace of advancement in osteosarcoma molecular genetic research, it is an exciting time to be a pathologist, an impatient time to be an oncologist, and a warily hopeful time to be a patient.

Additional laboratory testing

Immunohistochemistry

Osteoma, osteoid osteoma and osteoblastoma are usually diagnosed without the aid of immunohistochemistry because of characteristic radiologic and pathologic findings. An unusual feature of osteoid osteoma is the presence of nerve twigs in the tumor and in the immediately surrounding reactive perimeter. These can be identified by virtue of expression of neurofilament or S-100 protein. As nerve fibers are not seen in most other bone tumors, this finding may be of diagnostic assistance.

High grade osteosarcoma exhibits reactivity for a range of immunohistochemical markers that may include in some cases keratin, smooth muscle actin, S-100 protein (especially in chondroid and cartilaginous areas) and epithelial membrane antigen. This can cause diagnostic confusion with other tumors such as metastatic carcinoma, myogenic sarcoma chondroblastoma or chondrosarcoma. Thus, it is imperative that tumor-produced osteoid and/or bone be found to enable the correct diagnosis. Osteoid can be confused with collagen deposition, as both are orange-red intercellular deposits (on standard hematoxylin and eosin-staining). Differences in architecture can aid in distinguishing the two materials (see Case Presentations portion of this chapter for examples). Osteocalcin expression in osteoblasts and in osteoid can also strongly support the diagnosis of osteosarcoma versus a sarcoma with collagen deposits resembling osteoid (Fanburg-Smith et al. 1997). Nuclear SATB2 expression is a new marker reported to be specific and sensitive for osteoblast differentiation (Conner et al. 2013).

Reactivity with antibodies to CDK4 and MDM2 is expected in low grade osteosarcomas that may easily be mistaken for a benign lesion such as fibrous dysplasia. This is diagnostically extremely helpful, especially in the setting of small biopsies, as benign bone lesions in the histologic differential of low grade OS are negative for these markers (Yoshida et al. 2010, Dujardin et al. 2011). High grade osteosarcomas arising from low grade OS also appear to express CDK4 and MDM2 in contrast to de novo high grade OS which is almost always negative for these markers (Yoshida et al. 2012).

Routine cytogenetics

Cytogenetics is not usually obtained in osteoma or osteoid osteoma. Only a few cases of osteoid osteoma have been karyotyped, and several have shown alterations of chromosome 22q, although most cases reported have a normal karyotype.

As with osteoid osteoma, there are relatively limited data regarding the karyotypes of osteoblastoma. However, complex karyotypes involving translocations and other changes have been reported but with no consistent findings (Baker et al. 2010). While not helpful in the differential diagnosis of osteoblastoma from osteosarcoma which also often displays a complex karyotype, other entities in the differential of some osteoblastomas such as primary aneurysmal bone cyst and giant cell tumor of bone can be excluded because of characteristic karyotypes commonly seen in these lesions (*USP6* fusion genes in 70% of ABC and telomeric associations in many cases of GCT).

Molecular genetics

Investigators throughout the world are focusing on altered cell pathways to develop targeted gene therapy that is effective and tailored to the individual patient. Areas being studied in osteosarcoma (and that have been studied for up to 35 years) include specific oncogenes, tumor suppressor genes, transcription factors, cell cycle controllers, receptor tyrosine kinases and growth factors, and genes implicated in: anoikis (the death of cells on detachment from basement membranes or matrix), apoptosis, angiogenesis, cell adhesion and migration, tumor stromal invasion, chemotherapy resistance, and osteoclastogenesis (Broadhead et al. 2011, Hameed et al. 2011).

Many proteins or gene abnormalities have been reported to be predictive of behavior, but none have proven clinically useful to date. This may change with more controlled prospective trials scrupulously linking outcome with specific laboratory results.

RADIOLOGY

Introduction

There are three characteristic matrices visible by radiography; cartilage with its arc and ring appearance, fibrous tissue with ground glass appearance and osteoid which has a cloud like calcification pattern. The presence of osteoid indicates new bone formation and may be a benign finding of healing bone after fracture or heterotopic ossification from soft tissue hematoma. However, osteoid and new bone formation can also be seen with osteogenic tumors. The visualization of new bone formation varies with its mineralization. Osteoid mineralization depends on maturity, tumor aggressiveness, necrosis and patient general health.

Osteoid osteoma

Osteoid osteoma has a characteristic clinical presentation and imaging appearance. The patient often complains of deep seated bone pain that is worse at night but is rapidly relieved with salicylate medication. The patient usually is 10 to 35 years old. They commonly occur in long bones; particularly the femoral neck and tibia. Osteoid osteomas can also occur in the spine and are associated with scoliosis with concavity on the side of the lesion. Radiographs typically show a lucent lesion, called the nidus, in the cortex with exuberant adjacent periosteal reaction and cortical thickening. The nidus is usually less than 1.5 cm, larger lesions are likely osteoblastomas. Sometimes, there is a punctate central calcification within the lucent nidus. There may be adjacent soft tissue edema. Bone scan shows marked increase uptake indicative of the lesions intense inflammation. Intra-articular lesions have no periosteal reaction and show less cortical buttressing because there is no periosteum within the joint. MRI will show a T1 low signal, T2 or STIR high signal nidus. The nidus can enhance intensely and there is marked marrow and soft tissue edema adjacent to the lesion.

The imaging modality of choice is CT because the bone and periosteal reaction are well shown, and the nidus is optimally identified. Radiofrequency ablation (RF) is becoming the treatment of choice for osteoid osteoma and non-complicated osteoblastoma, (Liberman et al. 2010). This is typically performed with CT imaging guidance with the patient under conscious sedation. In a study of 38 patients with osteoid osteoma (34 patients) and osteoblastoma (4 patients) treated with RF ablation, 97% had complete remission of pain after a single treatment. One patient needed a second treatment before achieving complete remission of symptoms (Liberman et al. 2010).

Using thin slice CT scans, there is a new sign associated with osteoid osteoma described in recent literature. 79.6% of osteoid osteomas in long bones had a blood vessel entering or in close proximity to the nidus. (Yaniv et al. 2011). Additionally, thin vascular grooves extend from the periosteum down to the tumor nidus in 73.8% of patients, with 96.6% specificity for osteoid osteoma. These vascular groves are less than 1 mm in diameter and best demonstrated with thin slice CT technique (2-3 mm slice) (Lui et al. 2011).

Osteoblastoma

Osteoblastoma is a histologically similar tumor to osteoid osteoma and may be difficult to differentiate them at pathology. Traditionally osteoblastoma and osteoid osteoma are distinguished radiographically by size, with the osteoblastoma being greater than 1.5cm. 31% of osteoblastomas occur in the spine, 19% occur in the jaw, 24% occur in the femur or tibia. In the long bones, 76% occurred in the diaphysis and 24% in the metaphysis. None occurred in the epiphysis. 83% showed well defined margins. 64% had lucent nidus and only half of tumors had abundant sclerotic reaction surrounding the lesion. 75% showed cortical expansion. When osteoblastomas occur in the spine, 64% are exclusively in the posterior elements, 24% involved the vertebral body and the posterior elements and only 14% were entirely in the vertebral body. Osteoblastomas occur in adolescents and young adults with a mean age of 20 years (range, 6 months to 75 years). 84% of patients have pain, and only 7% have relief with aspirin (McLeod et al. 1976). Osteoblastomas show aggressive features such as cortical expansion and destruction in 39% of cases with malignant features seen in 12%, (Lucas et al. 1994). But usually, they are sharply marginated with a peripheral rind of sclerotic bone.

The differential for osteoblastoma includes osteoid osteoma, osteosarcoma, aneurysmal bone cyst, and giant cell tumor. A cortical lesion with lucent nidus and marked periosteal reaction and cortical buttressing smaller than 1.5 cm should be an osteoid osteoma. The osteoid osteoma is usually more symptomatic. Osteosarcoma is not well marginated and does not have a sclerotic rim but often has a soft tissue mass. Occasionally, an aggressive osteoblastomas may have osteoid formation and no sclerotic margin mimicking the appearance of an osteosarcoma. There can be significant overlap in the appearance of osteoblastomas and aneurysmal bone cysts because both can show marked expansion and exuberant periosteal reaction. Fortunately, both are benign entities treated with enbloc resection. Giant cell tumor (GCT) should be distinguishable from osteoblastoma on location because GCT occurs in the epiphysis of long bones, not the metaphysis. Likewise, osteoblastoma occurs in the vertebral body of the spine, not the posterior elements. Also, giant cell tumors do not have sclerotic margins whereas the typical osteoblastoma will.

Osteosarcoma

Introduction

Osteosarcoma (OS) is the dreaded malignancy of bone. OS is the most common malignancy of bone and generally occurs in the long bones around the knee of young and adolescent patients. Previously, the prognosis was poor; however substantial improvements have been won largely due to the advent of combination chemotherapy. There are several variants (**Table 17.1**) all characterized by the presence of malignant bone formation, seen on imaging as osteoid production. Their appearance is quite variable ranging from a mostly cystic, markedly expansile and hemorrhagic tumor as seen with telangiectatic subtype to the mostly sclerotic, ivory appearance seen in some parosteal osteosarcoma.

Conventional osteosarcoma

The typical appearance of the conventional subtype of osteosarcoma is that of a destructive lytic lesion with aggressive periosteal reaction and osteoid formation. This typically occurs in a long bone metaphysis around the knee, most commonly in the distal femur. However, any bone can be affected. The periosteal reaction is often disrupted by the tumor expanding into the soft tissues. The marrow is often involved and extends significantly beyond the area of involvement shown by radiography. The radiographic appearance is usually diagnostic of osteosarcoma, however, MR imaging is helpful to show the overall tumor extent, hence, the entire bone of origin should always be imaged. Chest CT scan is necessary for staging the lung, the usual site of distant metastases.

Telangiectatic osteosarcoma

Telangiectatic osteosarcoma (TOS) accounts for approximately 6.8% of all OS cases. 17% present with metastatic disease, with lung the most common site of spread at presentation (Weiss et al. 2007). In a series of 40 TOS patients (Murphey et al. 2003), 68% of patients were male, and the mean age at presentation was 24 years. The lower extremity is involved in 77% of cases with the femur being most commonly affected (50% of all patients). The metaphysis is involved in 83% of cases, and 83% of these, also showing extension to the epiphysis. Radiographs show geographic bone destruction in 94%, with motheaten or permeative destruction in the remaining 6%. Radiographs were only able to demonstrate matrix mineralization in about half of patients and it was subtle in all cases. CT exams showed cortical destruction in 92%, with soft tissue mass in 76%. Predictably, CT was better able to show osteoid mineralization in 85% of cases. MR imaging showed marrow involvement in 100% of cases and hemorrhage was seen in 96% with fluid-fluid levels in 74%. MR showed cortical destruction and soft tissue mass in 89%. Post-contrast MR images showed 100% had thick peripheral and septal enhancement with nodular enhancing areas.

The prognosis of TOS has improved substantially and approaches conventional OS prognosis. TOS classically shows an aggressive, destructive lesion of the metaphysis with marked expansion of bone and a soft tissue mass. Cross sectional imaging will show that most of the lesion (>90%) is comprised of multiple hemorrhagic and cystic spaces (Murphey et al. 2003). These cystic areas often show fluid-fluid levels related to the hemorrhage products. There may only be minimal mineralized osteoid because so much of the tumor is necrotic or hemorrhagic (Yarmish et al. 2010). CT is best to detect any mineralized osteoid.

The classic differential for TOS is an aneurysmal bone cyst (ABC) which typically also shows marked expansion with multiple hemorrhagic and cystic areas. The ABC may have marked cortical thinning due to the expansion of the lesion but should not show cortical breakthrough or any soft tissue mass. Hence, cross sectional imaging with MRI and/or CT are crucial to distinguish between these lesions. MR is best suited to evaluate for soft tissue extension or mass, whereas CT is best to assess the cortex for erosion and whether there is full thickness cortical break through. Given the gravity of diagnosis, the radiologist should not hesitate to perform both CT and MR if necessary. Of course, both lesions can present with pathologic fracture which will significantly complicate interpretation of the cross sectional imaging as the fracture causes hematoma and healing response in the adjacent soft tissues which can mimic or obscure a true soft tissue mass. Careful history and close interval imaging follow up may be required to distinguish ABC from TOS.

Parosteal osteosarcoma

There are three surface osteosarcoma variants including periosteal, high grade, and parosteal osteosarcoma.

Parosteal OS is the most common of the surface osteosarcomas and is unique among osteosarcomas for having a better prognosis and presenting with an indolent course. These have a propensity for occurring on the posterior distal femur (Samardziski et al. 2009) and present later in life, during the third and fourth decades. Parosteal OS appears as a variably calcified irregular mass which is closely associated with or originates from the metaphysis. The most common pattern of calcification is localized and homogeneous occurring in approximately 43% of cases. The pattern of calcification does not appear to correlate with degree of malignancy (Lindell et al. 1987). This gives the appearance of an ivory mass next to bone. There may be a partial cleft separating the mass from the parent bone; however there is a stalk or region of continuity with the cortex. There is scant if any periosteal reaction. The differential includes benign entities such as osteochondromas, myositis ossificans, or an osteoma. Osteochondroma has a characteristic appearance with cortical and marrow continuity with the parent bone. This is usually clear on radiography, but cross sectional imaging is sometimes required to definitively show these features and to assess complications of osteochondromas. CT scan can be very helpful in differentiating myositis ossificans from parosteal OS. In myositis ossificans (MO), the densest and most mature bone is on the periphery and the lesion is separate from the adjacent bone. With parosteal OS, the densest calcification is central and there is attachment to the adjacent bone cortex.

Periosteal osteosarcoma

In a series of 40 patients (Murphey et al. 2004), the periosteal OS uniformly appeared as a broad-based soft tissue mass with cortical attachment. There is cortical thickening in 83%, with cortical erosion in 93%. Perpendicular periosteal reaction (so called hair on end appearing periosteal reaction, see **Case fig. 17.3a** in Case 17.3) is seen in 95% of cases. These commonly involve the diaphysis of a long bone, particularly the tibia and femur. There are low density areas of the tumor on CT in 25% of cases related to the high water content associated with the cartilage portions. Similarly, MR will show T1 low signal and T2 high signal of the water in cartilage. Marrow invasion can be difficult to ascertain and was only seen in one patient (2.5%) with periosteal OS, however, reactive marrow changes were seen in 23% (Murphey et al. 2004). True medullary invasion was characterized on MR imaging as having marrow tumor in continuity with the soft tissue tumor mass.

High grade surface osteosarcoma

High grade surface OS (HGSOS) is rare, accounting for only 0.4% of all osteosarcoma (Yarmish et al. 2010). HGSOS invades the marrow in 43% of cases (Murphey et al. 2004). HGSOS predominates in men (76%) and has a mean age at presentation of 21 years. In another series (Staals et al. 2008), all lesions were located in the lower extremity with the femoral diaphysis being the most common location, and 68% of cases involved the diaphysis. The majority of these tumors showed dense to moderate mineralization. HGSOS tends to surround the bone of origin and showed an average extent of circumferential involvement of 53%. Cross sectional imaging showed marrow involvement in 48%. Interestingly, 24% of cases, the HGSOS mimicked parosteal OS with metaphyseal location and dense well defined bone production. Also, in 12% of cases, HGSOS mimicked periosteal OS with diaphyseal location and a more lucent lesion. The 5 year survival rate is about 82% (Staals et al. 2008). Traditionally, HGSOS was considered to have a worse prognosis, more recent data suggest a similar prognosis to conventional OS.

The differential diagnosis for bone surface malignancy includes the three surface osteosarcomas; periosteal, parosteal, and high grade surface osteosarcomas, as well as juxtacortical chondrosarcoma and Ewing sarcoma. Juxtacortical chondrosarcoma occurs in the metaphysis of older patients and tends not to show perpendicular periosteal reaction. Ewing sarcoma is common in the diaphysis but rarely spares the medullary space. Also, calcification of the soft tissue mass and perpendicular periosteal reaction is unusual for Ewing sarcoma at presentation. Parosteal osteosarcoma affects an older population and the lesion has a strong propensity for the posterior distal femur. Parosteal OS may have a cleft of separation from the parent bone but is attached to the cortex. In parosteal OS, there is usually no perpendicular periosteal reaction. High grade surface OS is more similar in appearance to periosteal OS. High grade surface OS is more likely to invade the marrow, surround more of the parent bone and will not show high water content appearance of cartilage on CT and MRI (Murphey et al.2004).

Dedifferentiated parosteal OS is a rare subtype. These may result from transformation of a previous conventional parosteal OS that has had multiple recurrences. Areas of lucency may occur in the superficial or deep portions of the tumor and may indicate dedifferentiation (Lindell et al. 1987).

Secondary osteosarcoma

Secondary osteosarcoma has the same radiologic appearance as conventional OS but occurs in the setting of pre-existing disease or risk factor. Predisposing conditions include prior radiation exposure, Paget disease, chronic osteomyelitis, familial retinoblastoma (deficient oncogene suppressor on chromosome 13), bone infarct, fibrous dysplasia and osteogenesis imperfecta. In a large series of osteosarcomas (Huvos et al. 1983), 5.5% were secondary to long standing Paget disease. The most common sites of involvement in descending order were pelvis, humerus and femur. Unrelenting pain and swelling were symptoms at presentation in 85%. Two thirds of cases presented with a lytic lesion while the remaining patients showed mixed density lesions. The incidence of Pagetic osteosarcoma appears to be decreasing with an increased age of presentation (Mangham et al. 2009). Unfortunately, the prognosis remains poor.

Malignant transformation associated with chronic osteomyelitis is rare. The most common histology is squamous cell cancer, which has been reported to occur in 0.23 – 0.5% of cases, however, sarcomas can occur rarely (Behrooz et al. 1979). There is a broad range of sarcomas that can occur in chronic osteomyelitis with case reports describing fibrosarcoma, angiosarcoma, rhabdomyosarcoma, and osteosarcomas.

The diagnosis of post-radiation sarcomas (PRS) must meet 4 criterion: (1) the histology of the original tumor and the PRS must be different; (2) The PRS must occur within the radiation field; (3) the latent period is at least 4 years from completion of radiation and discovery of the new tumor; (4) the patient does not have a genetic syndrome such as Li-Fraumeni (germline mutations of the p53 tumor suppressor gene), or Rothmund – Thomson (mutations of the *RECQL4* helicase gene on 8q24). PRS represent 3% of all sarcomas and has an average latent period of 13.6 years (Bjerkehagen et al. 2009). In this series, osteosarcoma occurred in 24% of cases and was the second most common post-radiation sarcoma, after 'malignant fibrous histiocytoma'. The incidence of PRS is about 0.1% (Inoue et al. 2000).

Long standing fibrous dysplasia can have sarcomatous transformation in 0.5% to 4.4 % of cases. The range of malignancies includes osteosarcoma (53%), fibrosarcomas (33%) and chondrosarcomas (13%). Of the fibrous dysplasia patients who developed sarcomas, 73% had polyostotic disease. The malignant transformation tended to occur in the cystic expansive portion of fibrous dysplasia (Xu et al. 1996, Taconis et al. 1988).

Small cell osteosarcoma

Small cell osteosarcoma (SCOS) is a rare subtype of osteosarcoma comprising about 1% of cases. The femur is the most commonly occurring site. In a series of 72 patients, 40% had radiographic appearance similar to Ewing's sarcoma or lymphoma (Nakajima et al. 1997). Distinguishing SCOS from these 2 diseases can be difficult for the radiologist because all three entities will present as a lytic lesion with soft tissue mass and a paucity of calcification.

Low grade central OS

LGCOS is a rare subtype of OS that can mimic the appearance of fibrous dysplasia. In a series of 99 cases, LGCOS had variable appearance on radiographs with mixed lytic and sclerotic components, and varying amounts of thick and coarse trabeculations (Andresen et al. 2004). LGCOS usually affects the metaphysis of a long bone, particularly involving the lower extremity in two thirds of cases with femur being the most common site. Soft tissue tumor extension was present in 33% of cases (Yu et al. 2010), but another larger series showed 100% had soft tissue extension and mass at presentation (Andresen et al. 2004). Thus cross sectional imaging may prove valuable in distinguishing LGCOS from fibrous dysplasia as the former will have cortical breakthrough and a soft tissue mass. The mean patient age is 31 years and periosteal reaction is seen in 33% of cases (Yu et al. 2010). The overall prognosis of LGCOS is better than the one of conventional OS.

SURGERY

Osteoid osteoma

These tumors have been successfully treated with non-steroidal anti-inflammatory medications (NSAIDs). It appears that the tumors may 'burn out' after three to four years of conservative management. NSAIDs do not appear to influence regression of the tumor *per se* but, in many cases, will render them asymptomatic during this period.

For patients who do not obtain satisfactory relief with NSAIDs, or in those who are prevented from chronic use of the medications due to adverse reactions, surgical treatment is an option. Many patients will opt for surgical treatment rather than a prolonged course of NSAIDs.

These tumors have a low rate of local recurrence following simple curettage. The surgical challenge in these tumors is less related to the simple curettage, but rather (1) the difficulty often involved in identifying the nidus; and (2) surgical morbidity which may be required in gaining access to the nidus in particularly difficult anatomic locations such as the femoral neck or spine.

Historically, several different modalities have proven helpful in localizing the tumor intra-operatively including fluoroscopy and radioisotope scanning.

More recently, CT guided radiofrequency ablation has demonstrated a very high success rate with low risk of local recurrence and low morbidity.

Osteoblastoma

Marginal resection of these tumors results in a low rate of local recurrence. Recurrence rate is higher in the spine secondary to the difficulty of obtaining satisfactory tumor removal in this location. Since the posterior elements of the spine represent the most common location of this tumor, en bloc resection is often preferred to minimize the risk of recurrence and adequately decompress the spinal canal.

Osteosarcoma

Osteosarcoma (conventional high grade medullary type)

Wide surgical resection of the bone and involved surrounding soft tissue, along with neoadjuvant chemotherapy is the treatment of choice for this high grade bone sarcoma.

Surface osteosarcoma (parosteal and periosteal osteosarcoma)

Wide surgical resection is indicated. With low grade tumors, risk of local recurrence and metastasis is extremely low with satisfactory margins. With high grade tumors, treatment and prognosis are the same as with conventional types. A distinction was previously made with these tumors regarding intramedullary involvement. Any surface osteosarcoma with intramedullary extension was felt to behave clinically in a manner similar to conventional osteosarcoma. This belief is no longer favored, and therefore treatment and prognosis is currently believed to be directly related to tumor grade alone.

MEDICAL ONCOLOGY

Osteoid osteoma

Osteoid osteoma is benign and not treated with chemotherapy.

Osteoblastoma

Osteoblastoma is a benign disease and treated surgically without the need for chemotherapy. There are only case reports of malignant dedifferentiation of osteoblastoma, and the diagnostic criteria for osteosarcoma would then apply as well as the treatment options.

Osteosarcoma

The three most common anatomical sites where osteosarcoma grows are the extremities, the pelvis, and the face. Flat bones (pelvis, ribs, skull) might also degenerate into osteosarcomas, especially in patients with Paget's disease or in patients treated for retinoblastoma in infancy. Rarely, the disease can have an extraosseous anatomic origin, which is mainly seen in adults. The prognosis is much worse in older adults (Mirabelloet al. 2009).

Osteosarcoma treatment approach is multidisciplinary and for most cases involves a combination of surgery and chemotherapy. Chemotherapy is usually given first neoadjuvantly, to assess the response of the cancer against the treatment, then adjuvantly for weeks after surgery. The most important prognostic factor is response to neoadjuvant chemotherapy, which is measured in percentage of necrosis seen microscopically on the resected specimen (Rosen et al. 1982). Patients have a favorable prognostic when the necrosis is greater than 90%. All other patients have a poor prognosis and require an adjustment in chemotherapy drugs and dosing in the postoperative setting. However, patients who receive no chemotherapy do worse than patients who are treated with chemotherapy, independently of the necrosis assessment.

Osteosarcoma of the extremities

It is a disease of adolescents, and usually starts in the growing metaphyseal plates. Chemotherapy is given for high grade disease. For lower grade, surgery alone might be sufficient. Randomized studies could not establish the better regimen.

Neoadjuvant chemotherapy should employ the most active drugs upfront. The current standard is a combination of cisplatin and doxorubicin every 3 weeks or high dose methotrexate (with or without doxorubicin and cisplatin) prior to surgical resection. There is a debate about the use of methotrexate, especially in adults where this combination could have significant renal toxicity. However, in order to achieve effective anticancer activity, the serum level of methotrexate must reach 1,000 micromolar (10^{-3}M) at the completion of the high-dose methotrexate infusion for 4 to 6 hours. Leucovorin rescue therefore starts later and hydration should be given to eliminate the methotrexate after sufficient exposure (Rosen et al. 1995). With these regimens, limb salvage procedures are possible in about 50% of cases (Bielack et al. 1999). At surgery, all primary metastases should be removed, whenever surgically feasible. A good histological response (>90% tumor necrosis) should be noted in about 40-60% of patients. If greater than 90% necrosis is observed in the primary tumor, the same regimen is usually continued in the postoperative settings. Less toxic chemotherapy might be appropriate (Rosen et al. 1985).

If less necrosis is observed, ifosfamide and high dose methotrexate (12 g/m^2 per course with leucovorin rescue) might be added. Various other combinations including dose dense (Lewis et al. 2007), continuous administration (Bielack et al. 1999), dose modulations, route of chemotherapy administration (Ferrari et al. 1999), and other agents such as ifosfamide (6 to 18 g/m^2 per course), bleomycin, cyclophosphamide, and actinomycin-D have been tested without conclusive results (Souhami et al. 1997). The scheduled duration of chemotherapy ranges from 9 to 38 weeks.

Survivals at 5 and 10 years of patients who do not have metastatic disease at diagnosis are about 65% and 55% respectively (Allison et al. 2011). Two-third of relapses occurs within 2 years, and almost all relapses are seen within the first 5 years. It is important that intensive multi-agent chemotherapy and delayed surgery be used to maximize good outcome. Tumor size, anatomical site, and response to chemotherapy correlated with outcome. In patients who are metastatic at diagnosis, the outcome is much poorer, with about 10-15% survivors at 4 years (Bacci et al. 2003).

Osteosarcoma of other bones

The principles are the same as in the osteosarcoma of the extremities. Radiation therapy might be considered for difficult anatomical area, such as head and neck or pelvis.

New therapies for osteosarcoma

Muramyl tripeptide phosphatidyl-ethanolamine (MTP) is a synthetic lipophilic analog of muramyl dipeptide, which is a component of the cell wall of Bacille Calmette-Guerin. MTP is encapsulated in liposomes, which help to activate monocytes and macrophages, which then become tumoricidal. Rodent xenograft models and spontaneous canine osteosarcomas are sensitive to MTP (MacEwen et al. 1989). MTP in combination with chemotherapy enhances event-free survival (EFS) and overall survival in newly diagnosed patients with osteosarcoma (Meyers et al. 2008). The addition of MTP to chemotherapy improved 6-year overall survival from 70% to 78% (P = .03) with a hazard ratio for overall survival of 0.71 (95% CI, 0.52 to 0.96).

The receptor activator of nuclear factor κB ligand (RANKL/TNFSF11) is expressed in metastatic bone cancer cells and has been suggested to play a key role in cell migration and metastatic behavior. Increased RANKL expression is related to a poor response to preoperative chemotherapy (P = 0.03) and associated with inferior survival (Lee et al. 2011). Denosumab, a RANKL inhibitor has not yet been tested in osteosarcoma.

Her2 is overexpressed in a small percentage of osteosarcoma. The Children's Oncology Group has completed a randomized study of the addition of traztuzumab to chemotherapy. Results have not been reported to date.

Osteosarcoma variants

Besides the high grade conventional type osteosarcomas (about 90% of cases), other variants have been described. These are the telangiectatic (5%), the small cell (1%), the low grade central, the secondary (after radiation or Paget disease), the parosteal, the periosteal, and the high grade surface variants.

The telangiectatic, the small cell, the secondary, and the high grade surface variants are treated like the conventional high grade osteosarcoma. Osteosarcomas secondary to radiation are a therapeutic challenge, but should receive a similar chemotherapy treatment. They are quite resistant to chemotherapy.

The low grade central, the parosteal, and the periosteal variants are usually not treated with chemotherapy, although the optimal medical treatment for the periosteal variant, an intermediate grade lesion, has not been defined. **Table 17.5** lists the current neoadjuvant chemotherapy regimens and **Table 17.6** lists the current adjuvant chemotherapy regimens for those patients whose tumors exhibit less than 90% necrosis.

RADIATION ONCOLOGY

Osteoid osteoma and osteoblastoma

Osteoid osteomas and osteoblastomas are generally less aggressive variants of osteogenic tumors. Some consider both to be variants of the same disease with osteoid osteoma being a smaller version of osteoblastoma. While radiation therapy is never used for osteoid osteoma, its use for osteoblastoma is controversial. Case reports have described the successful use of radiation therapy for osteoblastoma in which surgery is not possible.

Osteosarcoma

There are different pathologic types of osteosarcomas, but these differences do not influence the indications for radiation therapy.

Table 17.5 Chemotherapy regimens for neoadjuvant chemotherapy of osteosarcoma

Regimens	Drugs	Doses	Schedules
Rosen, T-10	Methotrexate/leucovorin rescue[1]	12 g/m^2	Days 1, 8, 15, 22 Days 63 and 70 Days 98 and 105
	Bleomycin	15 mg/m^2/day	Days 42 and 43
	Cyclophosphamide	600 mg/m^2/day	Days 42 and 43
	Actinomycin-D	600 micrograms/m^2/day	Days 42 and 43
	Doxorubicin	30 mg/m^2/day	Days 78, 79, 80
Bacci, every 4 weeks × 2	Methotrexate/leucovorin rescue	8 g/m^2	Day 1
	Cisplatin	120 mg/m^2	Day 7 Intra-arterial[2] infusion for 72 hours
	Doxorubicin	60 mg/m^2	Day 9
	Doxorubicin	25 mg/m^2/day	Days 1-3
Souhami, every 3 weeks × 3	Cisplatin	100 mg/m^2	Day 1, continuous infusion

1 It is the serum concentration of methotrexate that is essential to obtain a good necrosis of the primary tumor

2 Not used anymore

Table 17.6 Chemotherapy regimens for adjuvant chemotherapy of osteosarcoma with <90% necrosis

Regimens	Drugs	Doses	Schedules
Rosen, T-10 for 3 cycles of 56 weeks	Doxorubicin	30 mg/m^2/day	Days 1 & 2, 22 & 23
	Cisplatin	120 mg/m^2/day	Days 1, 22
	Bleomycin	15 mg/m^2/day	Days 42 and 43
	Cyclophosphamide	600 mg/m^2/day	Days 42 and 43
	Actinomycin-D	600 micrograms/m^2/day	Days 42 and 43
Bacci, for 3 cycles of 68 days each	Doxorubicin	45 mg/m^2/day	Days 1 and 2
	Ifosfamide/Mesna	2 g/m^2/day × 5 days	Days 21 to 25
	Methotrexate/leucovorin rescue	8 g/m^2	Day 42
	Cisplatin	40 mg/m^2/day × 3 days	Days 48 to 50
	Etoposide	120 mg/m^2/day × 3 days	Days 48 to 50
Souhami, every 3 weeks × 3	Doxorubicin	25 mg/m^2/day	Days 1-3
	Cisplatin	100 mg/m^2	Day 1, continuous infusion

Note: Doses are susceptible to change in newer studies.

Even though surgery is the mainstay of treatment for osteosarcoma, radiation therapy has been used for cases in which complete surgical resection is not possible. This includes instance, in which surgery is not possible due to location of tumor, medical co-morbidities of the patient or patient refusal of surgery. A review of 31 patients who refused surgery for osteosarcoma was reported (Machak et al. 2003). These patients underwent external beam radiation therapy to a median dose of 60 Gy (range 40-68 Gy). The mean local progression free survival at 5 years was 56%. Eighty six percent of these surviving patients without local disease progression had excellent limb function (Machak et al. 2003). The optimal radiation dose is not well defined. Nonetheless, the highest radiation dose possible up to 70 Gy without compromising surrounding critical structures should be used.

CASES

Case 17.1 Osteoid osteoma

Clinical history and presentation

The patient is a 16 year old boy who presents with a one year history of groin pain. Symptoms began spontaneously and have progressively increased since onset. He relates pain which awakens him at night. He experiences complete and total relief of the pain with ibuprofen, but symptom relief is of short duration.

Physical examination is remarkable only for groin pain with extreme internal rotation.

Surgical findings and comments

The patient is offered treatment options including conservative NSAID management, operative curettage, or percutaneous ablation. He opts for CT guided ultrasound ablation which is performed successfully.

SURGERY GRAY AREA

Osteoid osteomas are benign tumors with limited growth potential. Most appear to spontaneously involute after a period of years. Treatment with chronic NSAIDs until symptoms resolve is an appropriate alternative to invasive removal, but many patients would prefer a definitive procedure to prolonged treatment with these medications. Surgical curettage results in a high degree of cure, but there can be substantial morbidity associated with localizing and removing the tumor, particularly in a precarious location such as the femoral neck. Percutaneous ultrasound ablation has provided a minimally invasive alternative to surgery with excellent results.

Radiology findings

The patient (**Case figs 17.1a** through **17.1h**) has a diaphyseal cortical lesion with marked cortical buttressing and extensive periosteal reaction. The lucent nidus is difficult to visualize due to the extent of sclerotic reaction. The differential includes stress fracture, but no fracture line lucency seen; and bone abscess, but no serpentine tract is evident. CT is unavailable, but would be the next best exam to confirm nidus morphology and to plan for radiofrequency ablation.

Three additional cases of osteoid osteoma are presented. The first additional case (**Case figs 17.1i** through **17.1l**) shows a subtle lucent lesion of the proximal tibial metaphysis. This case shows some of the variability of osteoid osteoma as there is only modest sclerotic reaction with no periosteal reaction. The CT fortunately shows the cortical nidus well. The second additional case (**Case fig. 17.1m**) shows a classic intra-articular lesion where no periosteal reaction is expected as there is no periosteum. Also note that the intra-articular osteoid osteomas tend to have less sclerotic reaction. The third additional case of osteoid osteoma, **Case figs 17.1n** through **17.1o**, shows a faint thin lucent tract extending from the nidus to the surface of the cortex consistent with a tiny vessel. This is a recently described sign of osteoid osteomas seen on thin section CT scans.

Pathology findings

Gross features

The curettage specimen comprises hemorrhagic soft tissue with intermixed minute bone fragments aggregating to 1.5 cm. The entire specimen is decalcified and submitted for routine processing and staining.

Microscopic features

Low magnification: Low magnification reveals a cellular, bone forming tumor intermixed with normal trabecular bone spicules (**Case fig. 17.1p**). Because this is a curettage specimen, it is not possible to assess whether the lesion has an abrupt border or permeative border with surrounding non-neoplastic reactive bone and normal bone.

High magnification: Medium magnification of the nidus reveals abundant osteoid with scant interspersed stroma (**Case fig. 17.1q**). On polarization, the osteoid shows the typical irregular hashwork of collagen fibers consistent with immature, unmineralized bone matrix

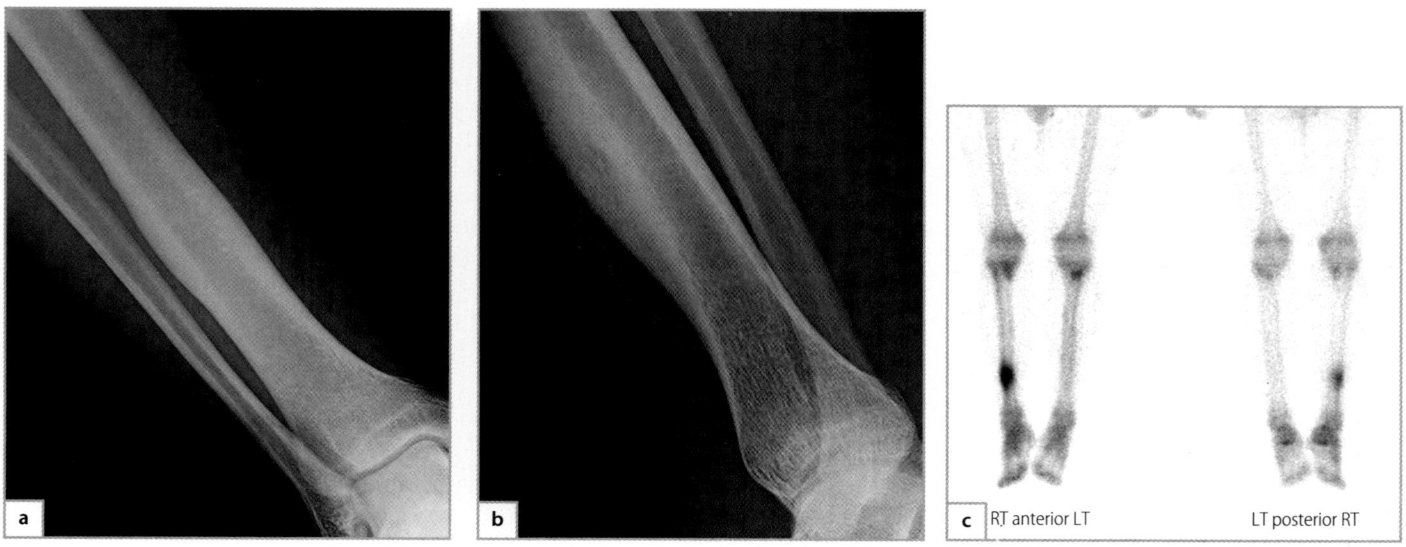

Case figure 17.1 Osteoid osteoma 17.1a: Anteroposterior and **17.1b**: Lateral radiographs of the distal tibia and fibula. **17.1c**: Tc99 MDP bone scan.

Case figure 17.1: Continued from page 424

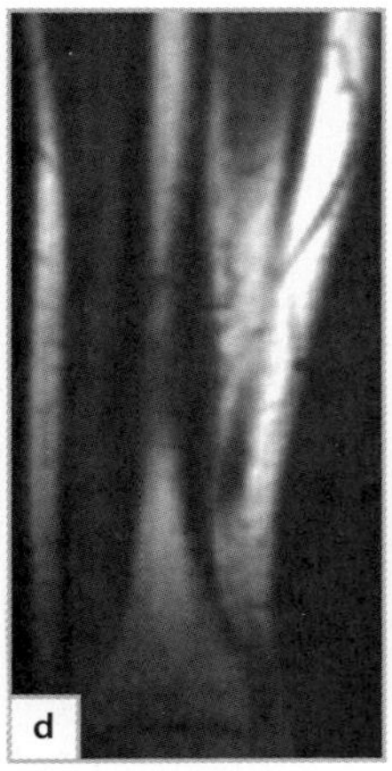

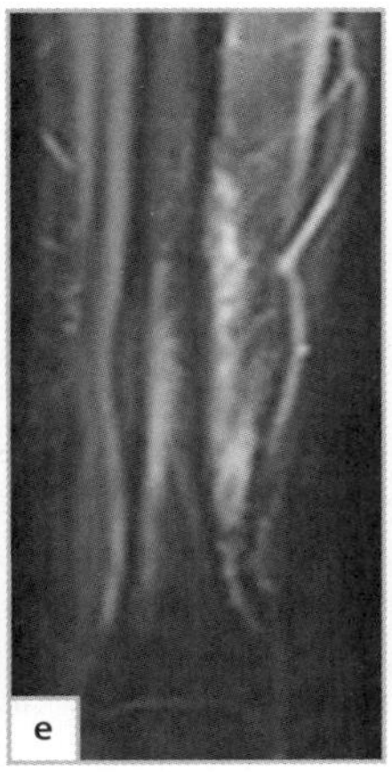

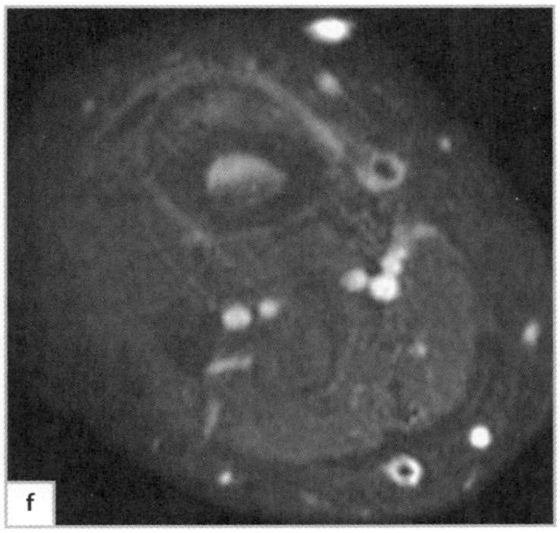

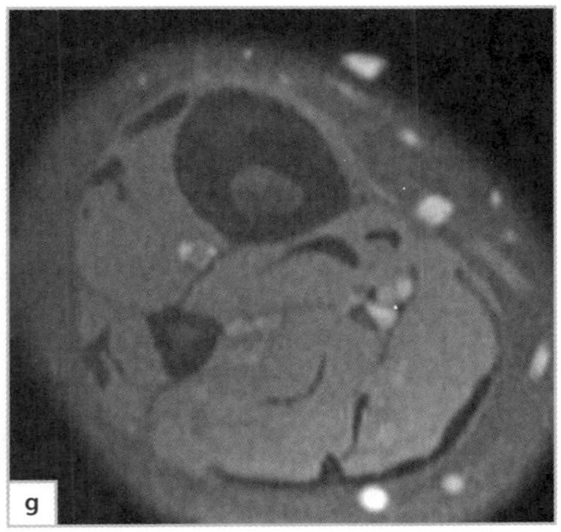

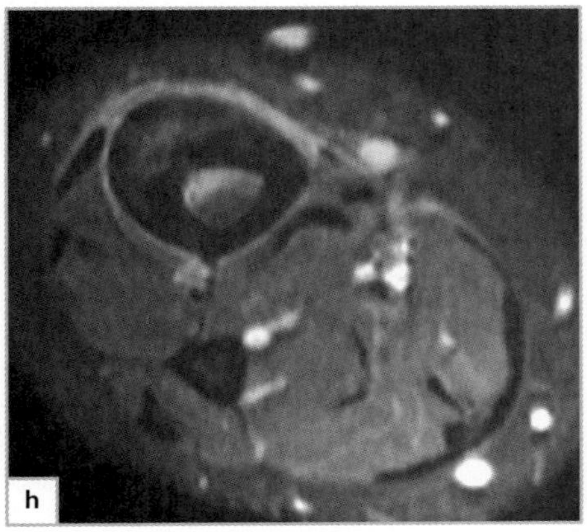

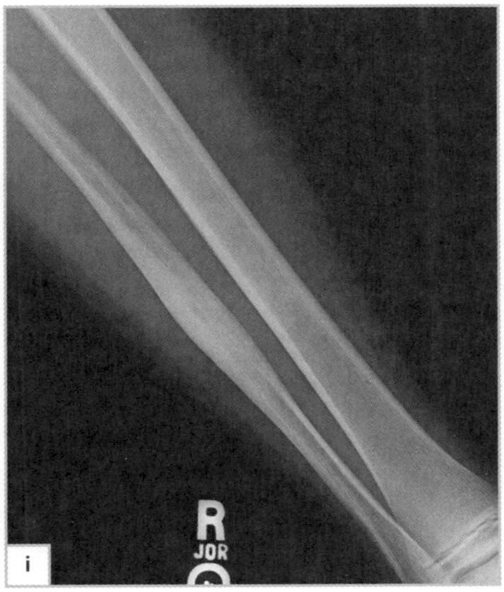

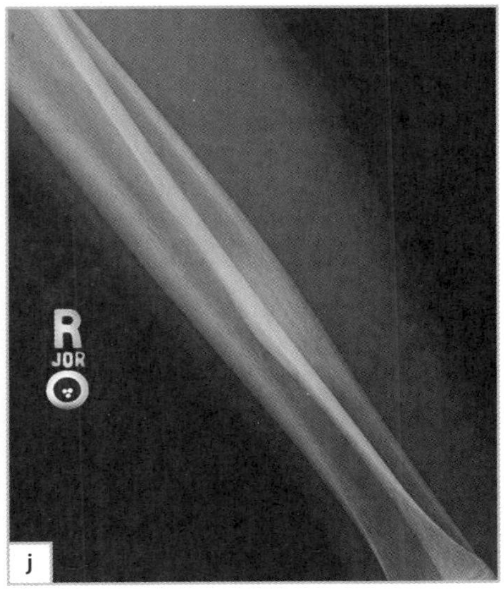

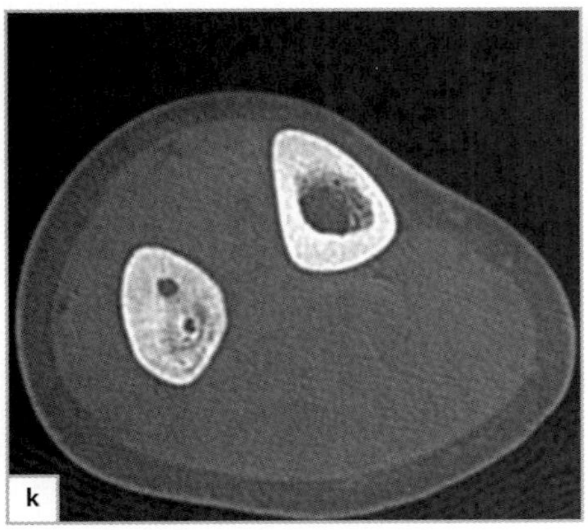

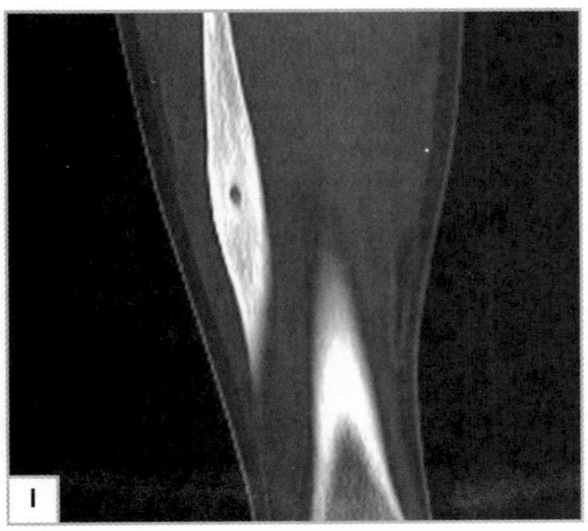

17.1d Coronal T1, **17.1e**: Coronal STIR, **17.1f**: Axial STIR, **17.1g**: Axial T1 fat saturated, **17.1h**: Axial T1 fat saturated post-contrast. The plain radiographs in this 16 year old boy show a sclerotic expansile lesion of the distal tibial cortex. There is smooth, mature appearing periosteal reaction with a small central lucent area, the nidus. The lesion has marked increase uptake on bone scan. The MR images show the cortical thickening and only a suggestion of the central nidus. The lesion has significant soft tissue and marrow edema suggesting inflammation. There is only modest enhancement despite the apparent inflammation. *Osteoid osteoma three additional cases.* The first additional case has **17.1i**: Anteroposterior and **17.1j**: Lateral radiograph of the tibia and fibula of an 11 year old girl. **17.1k**: Axial and **17.1l**: Coronal CT reformation images. These show a sclerotic expansile lesion of the fibula. The radiographs show subtle central lucent nidus much better shown with CT scan. There is no soft tissue component. The second osteoid osteoma additional case.

Case figure 17.1: Continued from page 425

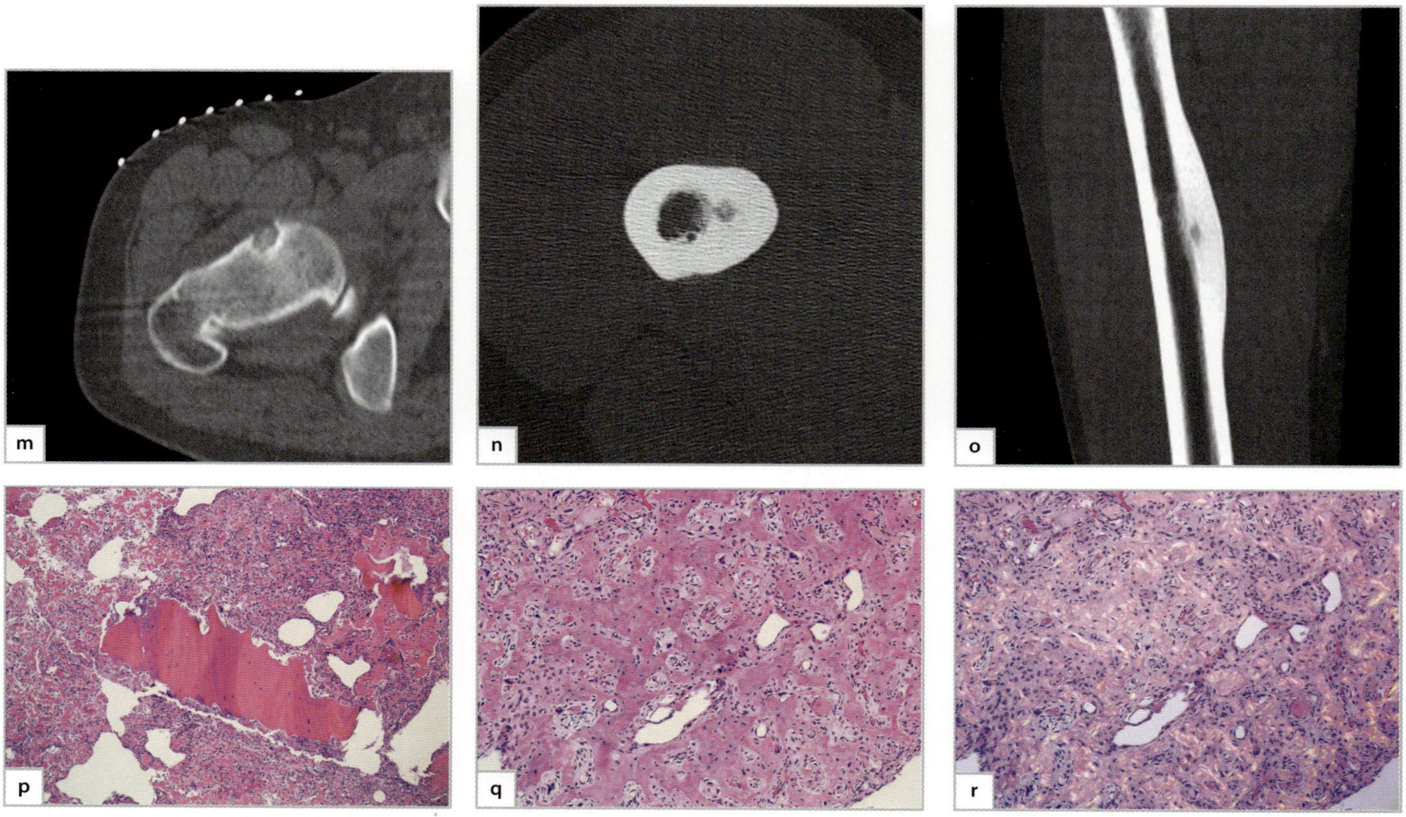

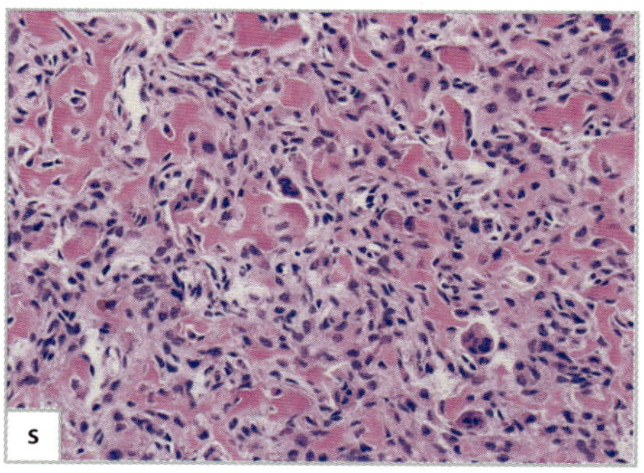

17.1m Axial CT images of this 16 year old boy show an irregular lucent cortical lesion of the femoral neck. There is partial central calcification of the nidus. There is an overlying marking grid for targeting of radiofrequency ablation. There is no periosteal reaction due to the intra-articular location. Note also the absence of cortical buttressing. The third bonus case of osteoid osteoma; **17.1n**: Axial and **17.1o**: Coronal reformation CT images show a cortical lesion with smooth periosteal reaction and cortical buttressing in this 17 year old young woman. There is a central lucent nidus with a subtle tiny feeding vessel extending from the nidus to the cortical surface. This is a recently described sign of osteoid osteoma. **17.1p**: Low magnification of presented patient's lesion. This is a cellular tumor with fine seams of osteoid intermixed with reactive bone and normal patient trabecular bone (consistent with a curettage specimen). **17.1q**: Medium magnification. Tumor osteoid forms interconnected ribbons. Vascular stroma fills the spaces between the osteoid ribbon. **17.1r**: Medium magnification, same field as Figure 17.1p. Under polarization, the collagen fibers forming the bulk of the tumor osteoid are choppy, misaligned, and of varying thickness consistent with woven (immature) bone. **17.1s**: Osteoid osteoma, high magnification. Neoplastic osteoblasts extrude osteoid in an irregular pattern. Osteoblastic rimming is present, and osteoclasts resorb newly laid down osteoid. While the lesion is cellular, there is no cytologic atypia.

(**Case fig. 17.1r**). High magnification of another area shows runnelly osteoid with mixed osteoblasts and osteoclasts and no cytologic atypia (**Case fig. 17.1s**). Surface osteoblasts rimming the osteoid are not conspicuous but are present focally consistent with a bone producing tumor that is not an osteosarcoma.

Special studies: Because the clinical history, radiologic features and histologic appearance are classic, no special studies are performed. However, S-100 or NSE IHC staining can identify nerve fibers in the stroma of osteoid osteoma and can be a useful adjunct diagnostic feature in small biopsies or in cases of non-classic radiologic findings.

Pathologic differential or, why isn't it one of the following?

Osteoblastoma: Many osteoblastomas are histologically indistinguishable from osteoid osteoma. Tumors greater than 2.0 cm in diameter are diagnosed as osteoblastoma.

Stress fracture: Radiologic features and clinical history help with this differential. The mix of inflammation, reactive fibrosis, acute hemorrhage and immature cartilage associated with a fracture are absent.

Chronic osteomyelitis: Osteomyelitis can induce reactive new bone in the infected area. However, areas of inflammation (characteristically plasma cells), fibrosis, and resorbing, dead, host bone are also present.

Osteosarcoma: The thick, corded, web-like pattern of osteoid deposition present in this patient's tumor can be seen in osteosarcoma. However, an osteosarcoma that had the degree of cellularity present in this patient's specimen would also exhibit nuclear pleomorphism, mitotic activity (and often atypical mitotic figures) and usually also necrosis. Moreover, only rarely does osteosarcoma demonstrate rimming osteoblasts on tumor osteoid.

Case table 17.1 Summary pathology findings of Case 17.1

Diagnosis	Osteoid osteoma
Size	1.0 cm
Location	Femur, neck
Margin status	This is a curettage specimen and therefore, the margin is not assessable
Histologic grade	Not graded: tumor is benign
Pathologic stage	Not staged: tumor is benign

Oncology approach

Medical oncology

This is a benign lesion that does not require chemotherapy.

Radiation oncology

The patient undergoes CT guided ultrasound ablation and appears to be cured. There is no role for radiation therapy.

Patient outcome

Five years following the procedure, the patient is asymptomatic, has a normal hip, and no clinical or radiographic evidence of recurrence.

Case 17.2 Osteoblastoma

Clinical history and presentation

A nine year old boy presents with a 4-5 month history of low back pain which was spontaneous in onset and has been slowly progressive. He denies an antecedent history of trauma. Pain is described as a constant dull ache, poorly related to activity. He has been unable to participate in sports over the past three months due to the pain. Pain awakens him at night. Pain is localized to the low back but radiates down the anterior aspect of the right thigh to the knee. He denies paresthesias, numbness, or weakness.

Surgical findings and comments

Unlike osteoid osteoma, osteoblastoma typically demonstrates slow but progressive growth. As these tumors frequently occur in the posterior elements of the spine, associated scoliosis and nerve root or spinal canal impingement occurs commonly. Marginal resection of the tumor results in a low risk of recurrence; however when the tumor is located in the spine, removal often needs to include spinal cord or nerve root decompression which may result in potential instability of the spine. For these reasons, operative resection of the tumor is performed along with decompression of the spinal canal and short segment posterior spinal fusion in this patient.

Radiology findings

The case presented (**Case figs 17.2a** through **17.2e**) shows a typical, although quite large, spinal osteoblastoma with associated scoliosis and the complications of extension into the neuroforamina and early encroachment of the spinal canal. Differential includes giant cell tumor which is usually in the vertebral body. The presence of an intact sclerotic rim also militates against giant cell tumor and other aggressive lesions such as osteosarcoma.

Two additional cases of osteoblastoma are presented involving the femur (**Case figs 17.2f** through **17.2j**) and the humerus (**Case figs 17.2k** through **17.2o**). The femoral lesion is in the epiphysis and the differential of giant cell tumor should be considered, however GCT would not have a sclerotic margin. There are aggressive features such as reactive changes of the periosteum, marrow edema and soft tissues edema with a joint effusion. Yet, the lesion has a sclerotic margin indicating indolent behavior. This juxtaposition of aggressive and non-aggressive findings can be seen with osteoid osteoma or osteoblastoma; given the size, osteoblastoma is favored in this case. The additional case of osteoblastoma in the humerus has all the classic features of an osteoid osteoma, except it is too large. This osteoblastoma is cortically based with a central lucent nidus and extensive adjacent cortical and periosteal reaction.

Pathology findings

Gross features

The specimen consists of hemorrhagic fibrous and bony tissue aggregating to 5.5 cm. The lesion is generously sampled in five cassettes.

Microscopic features

Low magnification: Low magnification of the solid areas of tumor reveal interconnecting, curving bands of osteoid arising from a hemorrhagic and edematous, fibrovascular background (**Case fig. 17.2p**). Other regions feature blood-filled cavities consistent with secondary aneurysmal bone cyst formation (**Case fig. 17.2q**).

High magnification: Higher magnification of a solid area shows classic features including irregular bony trabeculae surfaced by prominent plump osteoblasts and scattered osteoclasts (**Case fig. 17.2r**). Characteristically, the stroma is hypervascular (**Case fig. 17.2s**). An unusual finding is the presence of neoplastic hyaline cartilage which can be seen rarely in osteoblastoma and osteoid osteoma (**Case fig. 17.2t**).

Special studies: Because the radiologic and clinical features match the histology and meet the diagnostic criteria for osteoblastoma, no special studies are performed. For quality control purposes, the slides are sent to a national expert in bone tumor surgical pathology. That consultant agrees with the diagnosis of osteoblastoma with secondary aneurysmal bone cyst change and an unusual cartilaginous component.

Pathologic differential or, why isn't it one of the following?

Osteoid osteoma: As noted for Case 17.1, osteoid osteoma and osteoblastoma may have identical histologic features. Osteoid osteoma may occur in the spine although less frequently than osteoblastoma (see **Case fig. 17.2u** demonstrating the most common locations of osteoid osteoma and osteoblastoma in the skeleton).

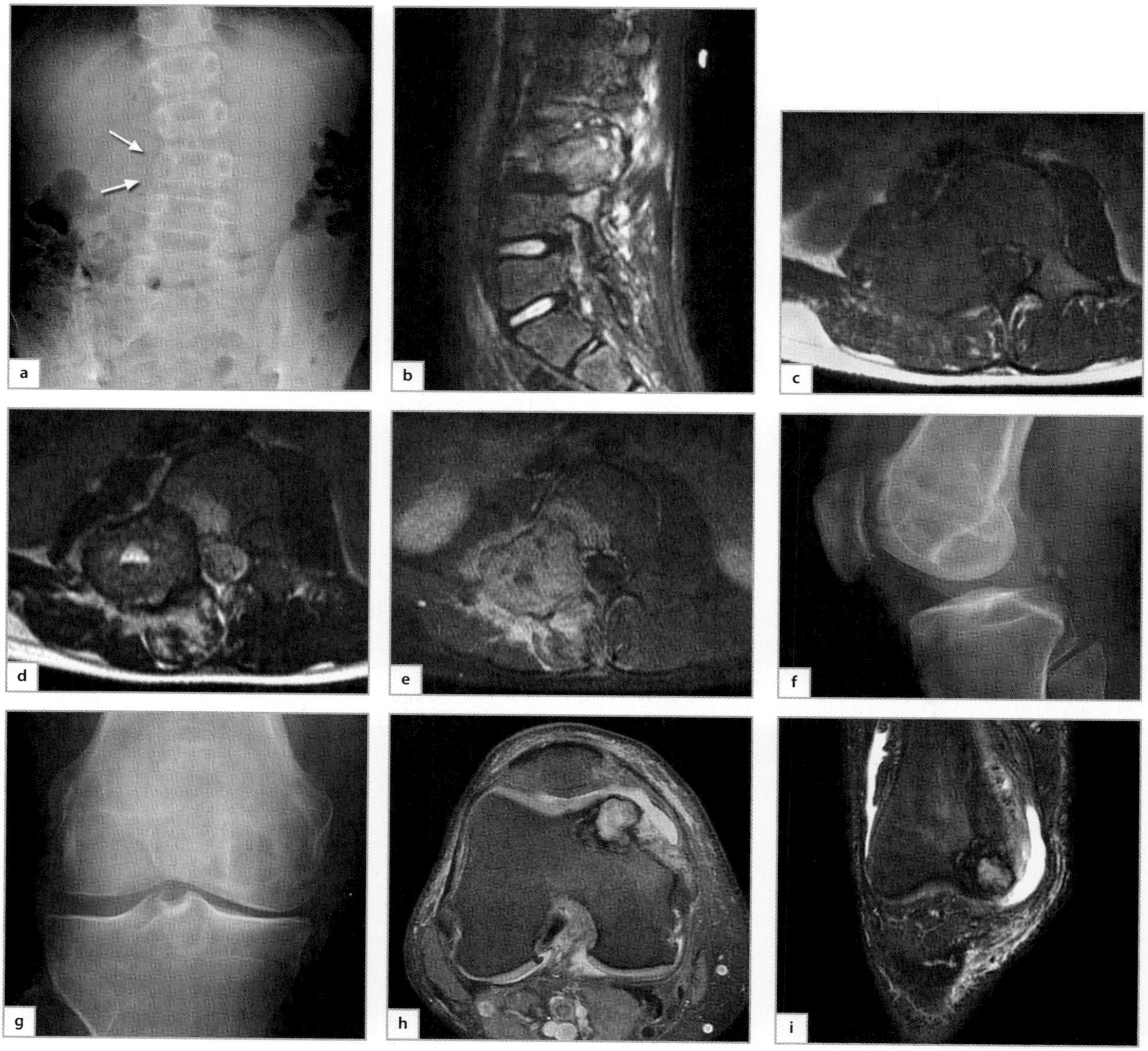

Case figure 17.2 Osteoblastoma 17.2a: Anteroposterior radiograph of the lumbar spine shows a scoliosis convex to the left. There is partial absence of the right L3 pedicle, arrows. **17.2b**: Sagittal STIR MR image. **17.2c**: Axial T1 MR image. **17.2d**: Axial T2 MR image. **17.2e**: Axial T1 fat saturated post-contrast MR image. MR imaging shows a complex expansile lesion of the right L3 pedicle partial extending into the vertebral body in this 10 year old boy. There is an irregular but intact sclerotic margin with T1 low signal and heterogeneous T2 signal. There is intense fairly uniform enhancement. Note the early encroachment on the right aspect of the spinal canal and the frank obliteration of the right L3-4 neuroforamina. *Two additional cases involving the femur and humerus.* **17.2f**: Lateral and **17.2g**: Frontal radiographs of the knee show a lucent lesion with thin irregular sclerotic margins involving the femoral epiphysis in this 61 year old man. There is no visible osteoid or periosteal reaction. There is a small knee joint effusion. **17.2h**: Axial PD fat saturated MR image. **17.2i**: Coronal STIR MR image.

Case figure 17.2: Continued from page 428

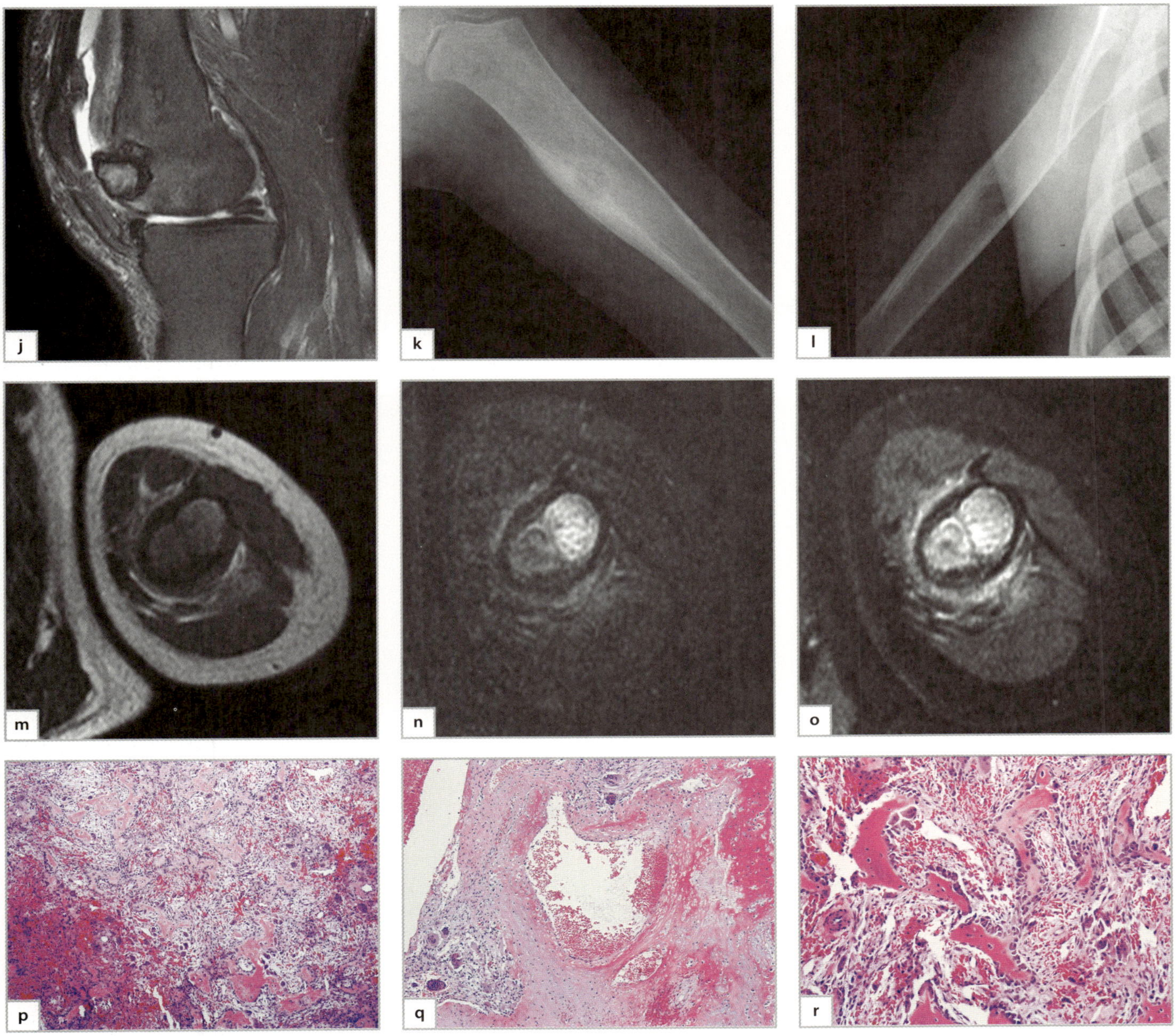

17.2j: Sagittal T2 fat saturated MR images show a cortical mass measuring 2.6 × 2 × 2.6 cm of the distal femur. There is expansion and a low signal margin correlating with the sclerotic margin seen on radiographs. The lesion causes moderate adjacent marrow edema. Second additional osteoblastoma case: **17.2k**: Anteroposterior and **17.2l**: Lateral radiographs of the humerus. **17.2m**: Axial T1 MR image. **17.2n**: Axial STIR MR image. **17.2o**: axial T1 fat saturated post-contrast. Radiographs show a lucent lesion measuring 1.6 × 1.0 × 1.2 cm in the cortex of the mid humeral diaphysis of this 3 year old boy. There is extensive adjacent periosteal reaction and cortical buttressing. There is intense lesion nidus enhancement with moderate adjacent edema and enhancement of the soft tissues. **17.2p**: Low magnification of presented patient's tumor. The tumor resembles osteoid osteoma with irregular, anastomosing bands of osteoid and a hemorrhagic, edematous stroma. **17.2q**: Medium magnification. Secondary hemorrhagic cystic degeneration consistent with aneurysmal bone cyst is present. Secondary ABC is a fairly common occurrence in osteoblastoma. Note the fibrosis, osteoclasts, and irregular osteoid formation typical of ABC. **17.2r**: High magnification. Osteoblasts and a few osteoclasts crowd together on the surfaces of the neoplastic osteoid. This osteoblastic rimming (sometimes with osteoclasts intermingled) is a typical finding in osteoblastoma and osteoid osteoma that is seldom seen in osteosarcoma.

Case figure 17.2: Continued from page 429

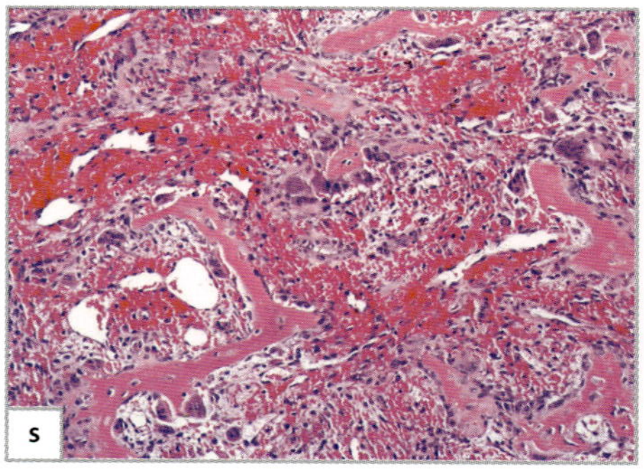

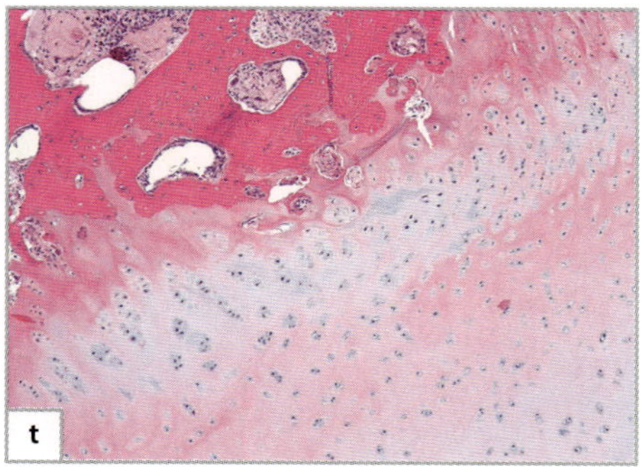

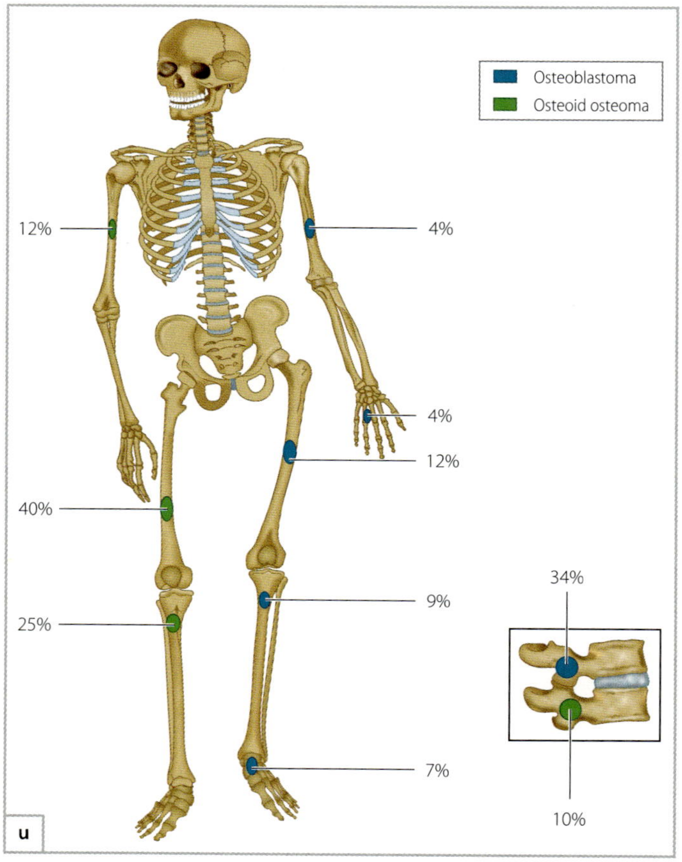

17.2s: Medium magnification. Dilated, thin walled vessels figure prominently in the stroma. Both osteoblastoma and osteoid osteoma exhibit a hypervascular stroma. **17.2t**: Medium magnification. This patient's tumor also contains neoplastic cartilage which is rarely seen in osteoblastoma and osteoid osteoma. Its presence should prompt careful consideration of other entities in the differential such as osteosarcoma or chondrosarcoma with pathologic fracture. **17.2u**: Common skeletal sites involved by osteoid osteoma and osteoblastoma.

Osteosarcoma: Osteosarcoma only rarely contains tumor osteoid or bone with prominent rimming osteoblasts, a feature characteristic of osteoblastoma (and osteoid osteoma). Nuclear atypia, atypical mitotic figures, and necrosis are commonly seen in osteosarcoma and are absent in osteoblastoma, although the latter may have a moderate mitotic rate of several mitoses/10 high power magnification fields (averaged across multiple sets of 10 hpf). Osteosarcoma is permeative meaning it will invade around adjacent trabecular bone and grow into Haversian canals. Osteoblastoma does not show this destructive invasive behavior. Both osteoblastoma and osteosarcoma may break through the cortex of the bone, and osteoblastoma can do this especially when it occurs in the small bones of the hands and feet. However, osteosarcoma seldom occurs in the hands and feet, and osteoblastoma usually induces an outer shell of reactive new bone once it breaches cortical bone. This would not be seen in osteosarcoma.

Aneurysmal bone cyst (ABC): Secondary ABC may develop in an osteoblastoma as has occurred with this patient's tumor. Primary ABC fairly frequently involves the spine and also has a preference for the posterior elements. However, ABC does not contain the broad areas of interconnecting curving bone trabeculae set in a fibrovascular stroma.

'Aggressive' osteoblastoma: Most aggressive osteoblastomas are on the larger side (4 cm or greater). The primary distinction from conventional osteoblastoma lies in the neoplastic cells. Histologically, this variant is formed by large epithelioid (round cells with sharp cell borders) osteoblasts that are two to three times the size of normal osteoblasts. These cells have round nuclei with prominent nucleoli. The cytoplasm also often displays a perinuclear clear zone (hof) consistent with a pronounced Golgi apparatus. The mitotic rate can be high, but there are no atypical mitotic figures. This tumor must be distinguished from 'osteoblastoma-like' like osteosarcoma. The latter exhibits some cytologic atypia and grows invasively into surrounding bone.

Case table 17.2b summarizes the histologic variants of osteoblastoma.

Oncology approach

Medical oncology

This is a benign if sometimes locally aggressive neoplasm that is not treated by chemotherapy.

Radiation oncology

The patient undergoes operative resection which is usually curative. There is no role for radiation therapy.

Case table 17.2a Summary pathology findings of Case 17.2

Diagnosis	Osteoblastoma
Size	5.5 cm
Location	Lumbar spine, posterior elements and right pedicle of L2
Margin status	The tumor is curetted and therefore margins are not assessable
Histologic grade	Not graded: tumor is benign
Pathologic stage	Not staged: tumor is benign

Case table 17.2b Variant histologic features of osteoblastoma

Feature	Frequency	Comment
Secondary aneurysmal bone cyst change	Common	In addition to classic areas of osteoblastoma, blood-filled cavities are present and the septae and rims feature fibroblasts, osteoclasts, and linear deposits of osteoid
'Aggressive' variant	Rare	Large, epithelioid osteoblasts with central to eccentric pale nuclei and prominent nucleoli must be the dominant tumor cell. These cells may form groups or sheets between coarse osteoid seams
'Pseudomalignant' variant	Rare	Degenerative nuclear atypia is present similar to that seen in 'ancient' schwannoma (some tumor cell nuclei are hyperchromatic, enlarged, and smudgy.)
Multifocal or multinodular osteoblastoma	Rare	One tumor has multiple growth centers with interposed reactive bone or spindle cell stroma
Cementoblastoma	Uncommon	Osteoblastoma of the jaws; usually very ossified with neoplastic bone radiating away from a tooth root
Neoplastic cartilage	Rare	Hyaline cartilage is focally present

Patient outcome

Three years postoperatively, the patient is leading a normal life with no evidence of tumor recurrence.

Case 17.3 Conventional osteosarcoma

Clinical history and presentation

The patient is a 14 year old boy who presents with a one month history of leg pain which began insidiously and has been slowly progressive. Pain increases with activity but also occurs at rest and awakens him at night.

On physical examination he is noted to ambulate with an antalgic gait. He has mild fusiform swelling of the proximal leg with mild tenderness on palpation over the proximal tibia. Knee range of motion occurs from -5 degrees extension to 100 degrees of flexion. Extremes of motion are associated with pain in the proximal leg.

Surgical findings and comments

Work-up reveals a tumor of the proximal tibia as well as lung lesions suspicious for metastatic disease.

Open biopsy of the tibia tumor is performed revealing high grade conventional osteosarcoma.

Three months following initiation of neoadjuvant chemotherapy, wide resection of the proximal tibia is performed. Reconstruction is done with a metallic proximal tibial replacement and rotating hinge total knee arthroplasty. Postoperatively, chemotherapy is administered.

A biopsy of one of the patient's pulmonary nodules is also performed.

Radiology findings

Three cases of conventional osteosarcoma are presented. The first case (**Case figs 17.3a** through **17.3g**) and first bonus case (**Case figs 17.3h** through **17.3l**) both show the typical destructive lesion with osteoid formation involving the metaphysis of a long bone in a teenaged patient. Both cases have a soft tissue mass and show the classic 'hair-on-end' appearance of highly aggressive malignant periosteal reaction. The presence of osteoid in such an aggressive lesion makes the diagnosis of osteosarcoma.

The second bonus case (**Case figs 17.3m** through **17.3n**) is also a conventional osteosarcoma; however it presents without many of the characteristic features. The lesion is best seen on the anteroposterior view (**Case fig. 17.3m**) and only shows mottled lucency of permeative destruction. There is no calcifying osteoid, soft tissue mass, cortical destruction or periosteal reaction. Despite the aggressive destructive behavior of osteosarcomas, they can be occult or very subtle lesions on radiographs. In this case, the radiologist can only diagnose an aggressive lesion causing the permeative destruction. Tissue diagnosis is needed, as the differential includes infection and sarcoma.

Pathology findings

Gross features

The biopsy comprises curetted fragments of bone and hemorrhagic soft tissue 3.0 cm in aggregate.

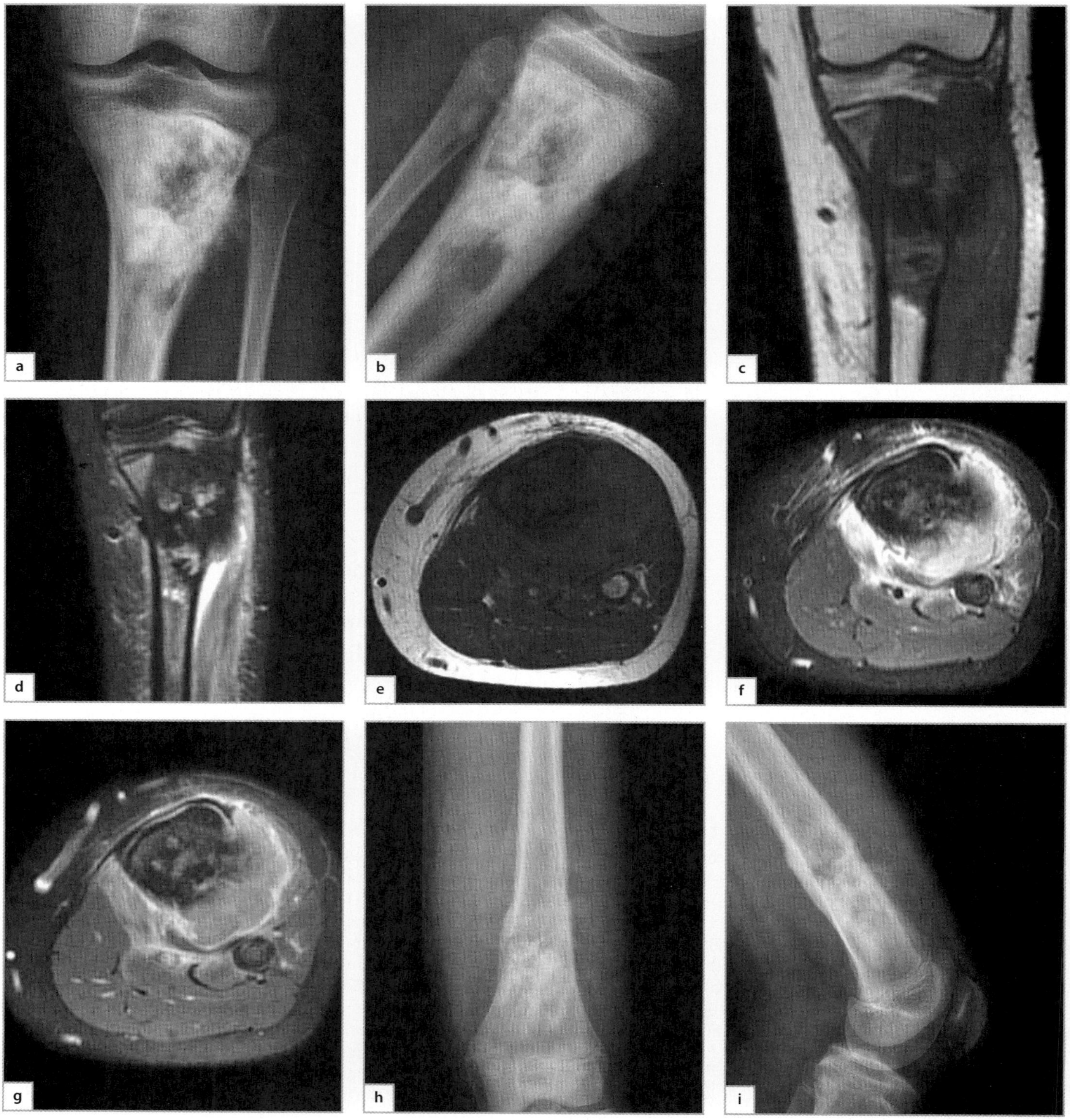

Case figure 17.3 Conventional osteosarcoma 17.3a: Anteroposterior and **17.3b**: Lateral radiographs of the knee in the 14 year old male patient. **17.3c**: Coronal T1 MR image, **17.3d**: Coronal STIR MR image, **17.3e**: Axial T1 MR image, **17.3f**: Axial STIR MR image, **17.3g**: Axial T1 fat-saturated post-contrast MR image. The radiographs show an aggressive, destructive lesion of the proximal tibial metaphysis. There is osteoid production and hair-on-end periosteal reaction (17.3a) along the lateral aspect of the proximal tibia. This is aggressive periosteal reaction. The MR images show the lesion extends into the proximal tibial epiphysis and distally into the tibial diaphysis. There is cortical destruction with contiguous adjacent soft tissue mass. The soft tissue portion shows only modest, heterogeneous enhancement likely from underlying calcification of the osteoid. Note also the adjacent soft tissue edema and reaction to the presence of the tumor. **17.3h** through **17.3l**: First additional case. **17.3h**: Anteroposterior and **17.3i**: Lateral radiographs of the knee in a 13 year old male patient. There is an aggressive destructive lesion of the distal femoral metaphysis. Again, we see osteoid formation and the highly aggressive periosteal reaction with hair-on-end appearance.

Case figure 17.3: Continued from page 432

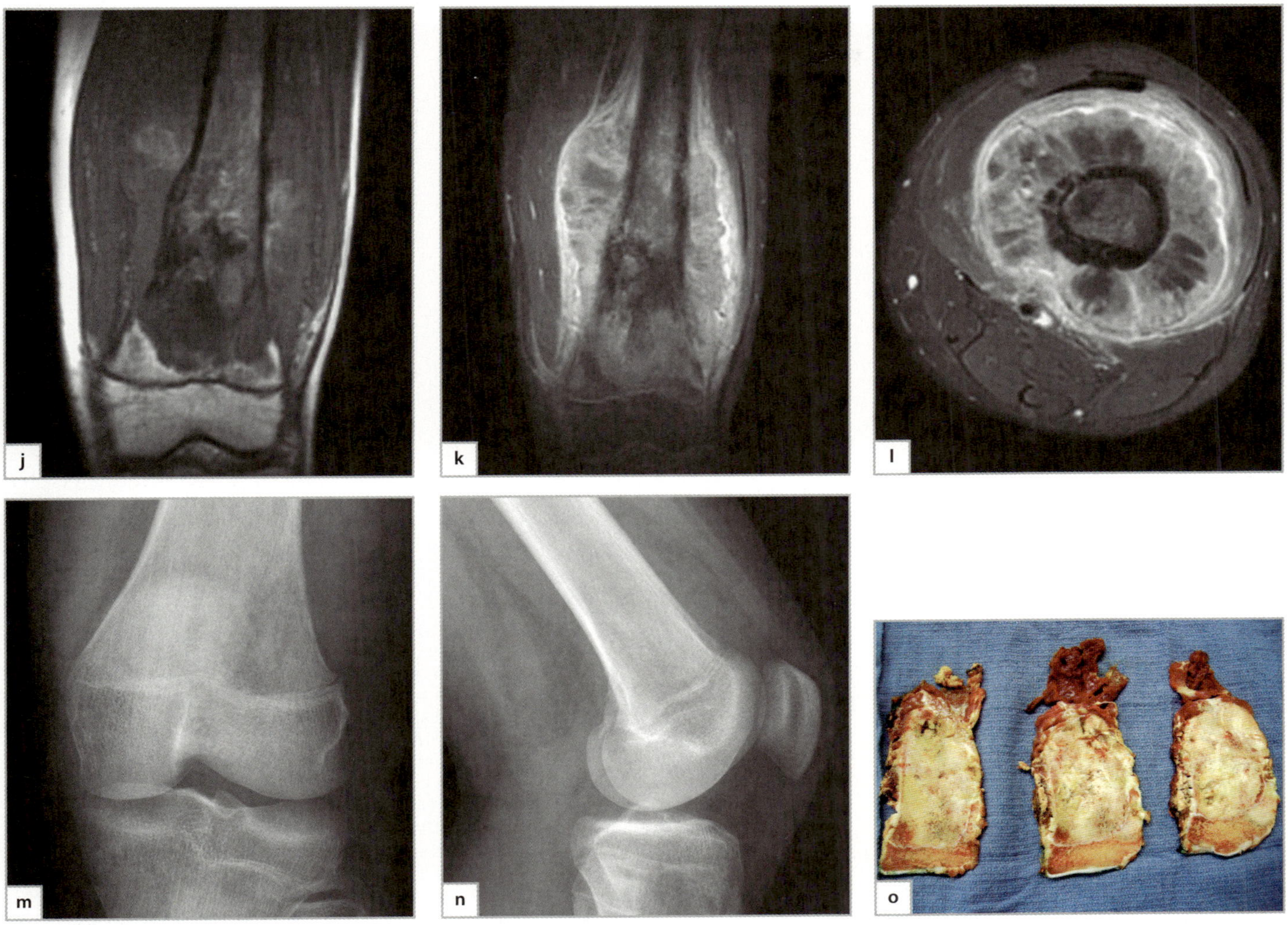

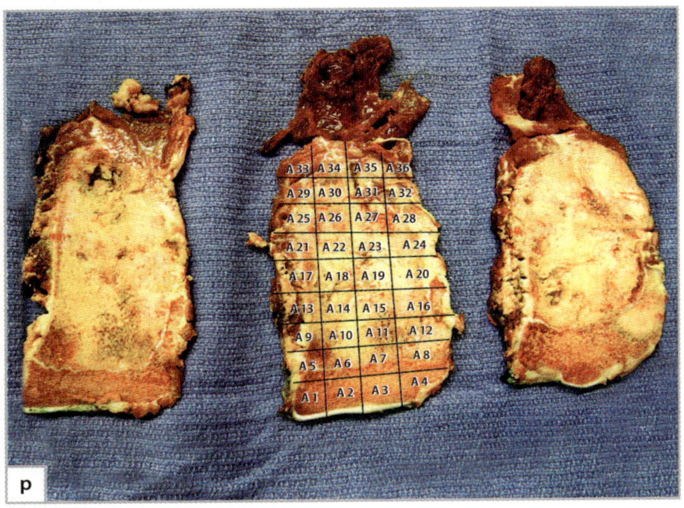

17.3j: Coronal T1 MR image, **17.3k**: Coronal STIR MR image and **17.3l**: Axial T1 fat-saturated post-contrast MR image show the cortical destruction with soft tissue tumor. Note again, the heterogeneity of enhancement with non-enhancing areas likely due to necrosis or calcified osteoid. Also, there is adjacent soft tissue edema and reaction. **17.3m** and **17.3n**: Second additional case. Case figure 17.3m, anteroposterior and Case figure 17.3n, lateral radiographs of the knee in a 16 year old male patient. The lateral view shows only subtle area of decreased density in the distal femoral metaphysis. The AP view shows an area of mottled lucency indicating permeative destruction. Note the absence of soft tissue mass or clear cortical destruction. No calcifying osteoid or periosteal reaction is yet evident. **17.3o**: Gross dissection of the presented patient's resected tumor. Three longitudinal sections of the proximal tibia reveal an aggressive tumor that focally involves the epiphysis and extends into the diaphysis. The tumor is tan to yellow with focal hemorrhagic areas. It breaks through cortical bone and extends into soft tissue. **17.3p**: Map of sections taken to assess for necrosis. A grid map of the tumor is made to indicate the location of the sections taken for microscopic assessment of necrosis. This is the standard procedure for osteosarcomas treated with neoadjuvant chemotherapy.

Case figure 17.3: Continued from page 433

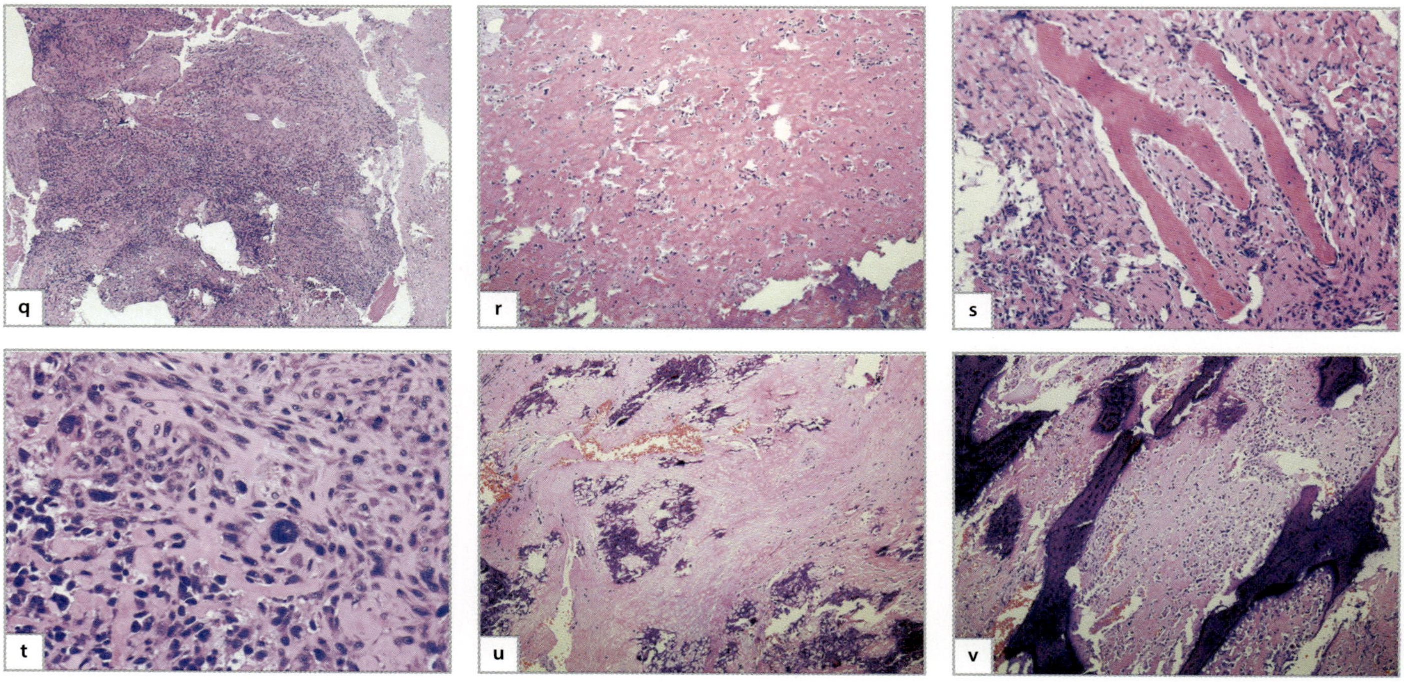

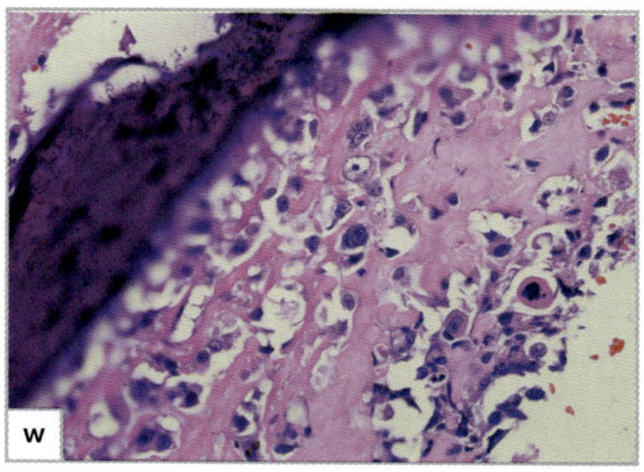

17.3q: Low magnification. The biopsy consists of chunks of viable tumor of varying cellularity. **17.3r**: Medium magnification. In this field, tumor osteoid grows as a hypocellular sheet with scant intervening stromal tissue. An osteosarcoma composed entirely of these sheets would be called the sclerotic osteoblastic variant of conventional osteosarcoma. **17.3s**: Medium magnification. The tumor engulfs and erodes residual normal trabecular bone spicules. **17.3t**: Biopsy at high magnification. Pleomorphic tumor cells show marked variation in nuclear shape and size and are hyperchromatic. Some tumor cells are multinucleated. Note the mitotic figure. The matrix is most convincing for osteoid in the lower left corner with tumor cells adhering to cylinders of pink substrate (tumor osteoblasts making osteoid). **17.3u**: Resection post neo-adjuvant therapy. This patient responded well to neo-adjuvant chemotherapy with 97% necrosis. In this field, the partially mineralized tumor osteoid is virtually acellular due to dropout necrosis of malignant cells. **17.3v**: Resection post neo-adjuvant therapy, medium magnification. Numerous sections reveal rare foci of histologically viable tumor as seen here. The tumor grows between host bone spicules. **17.3w**: Resection post neo-adjuvant therapy, high magnification. Viable tumor cells float in lacunae of neoplastic osteoid. Only one cell appears non-viable with a shrunken, condensed (pyknotic) blob-like nucleus and glassy, hyper-eosinophilic cytoplasm.

The resection consists of a 15 × 9.6 × 6.5 cm portion of proximal tibia, proximal fibula, scant soft tissue and an ellipse of skin. The specimen is oriented, differentially inked, and carefully cut in serial 0.5 cm slices with a band saw yielding 12 slices. The cut sections reveal a metaphyseal, medullary centered 10.1 × 5.5 × 4.2 cm tan to yellow tumor with areas of hemorrhage and softening consistent with necrosis. The tumor extends across the epiphysis and breaches the cortex, but no discrete, definitive soft tissue tumor deposits are identified. It is located 0.5 cm to 2.6 cm from all margins. Sections representing all margins are submitted.

With patient consent, tumor is harvested for a Children's Oncology Group research protocol and for local biospecimen banking. Three slices encompassing the greatest tumor area are gridded out carefully in order to allow for assessment of percent necrosis. A map is drawn to indicate the location of tumor according to cassette submitted for processing (**Case figs 17.3o** and **17.3p**). All cassettes containing bone are decalcified.

Microscopic features

Biopsy

Low magnification: The biopsy yields abundant tumor tissue that is composed of cellular areas mixed with osteoid bands (**Case fig. 17.3q**) and hypocellular areas composed of sclerotic tumor osteoid (**Case fig. 17.3r**). Although the specimen is fragmented due to curetting, it shows obvious erosion of normal bone trabeculae and marrow permeation by tumor (**Case fig. 17.3s**).

High magnification: Pleomorphic spindle to round tumor cells are embedded in swirling, pasty osteoid (**Case fig. 17.3t**). Mitoses are evident.

Resection

Low magnification: A careful review of all gridded sections yields a figure of 97% necrosis (**Case fig. 17.3u**). (Necrosis equal to or greater than 90% indicates an excellent response to neoadjuvant chemotherapy.)

High magnification: Only rare areas contain histologically viable tumor (**Case figs 17.3v** and **17.3w**).

Lung biopsy: A wedge resection from the right lung contains a small focus of non-caseating granulomatous inflammation. There is no evidence of viable or necrotic tumor. However, radiologic impression and response to chemotherapy indicates the patient did present with lung metastases.

Case figure 17.3: Continued from page 434

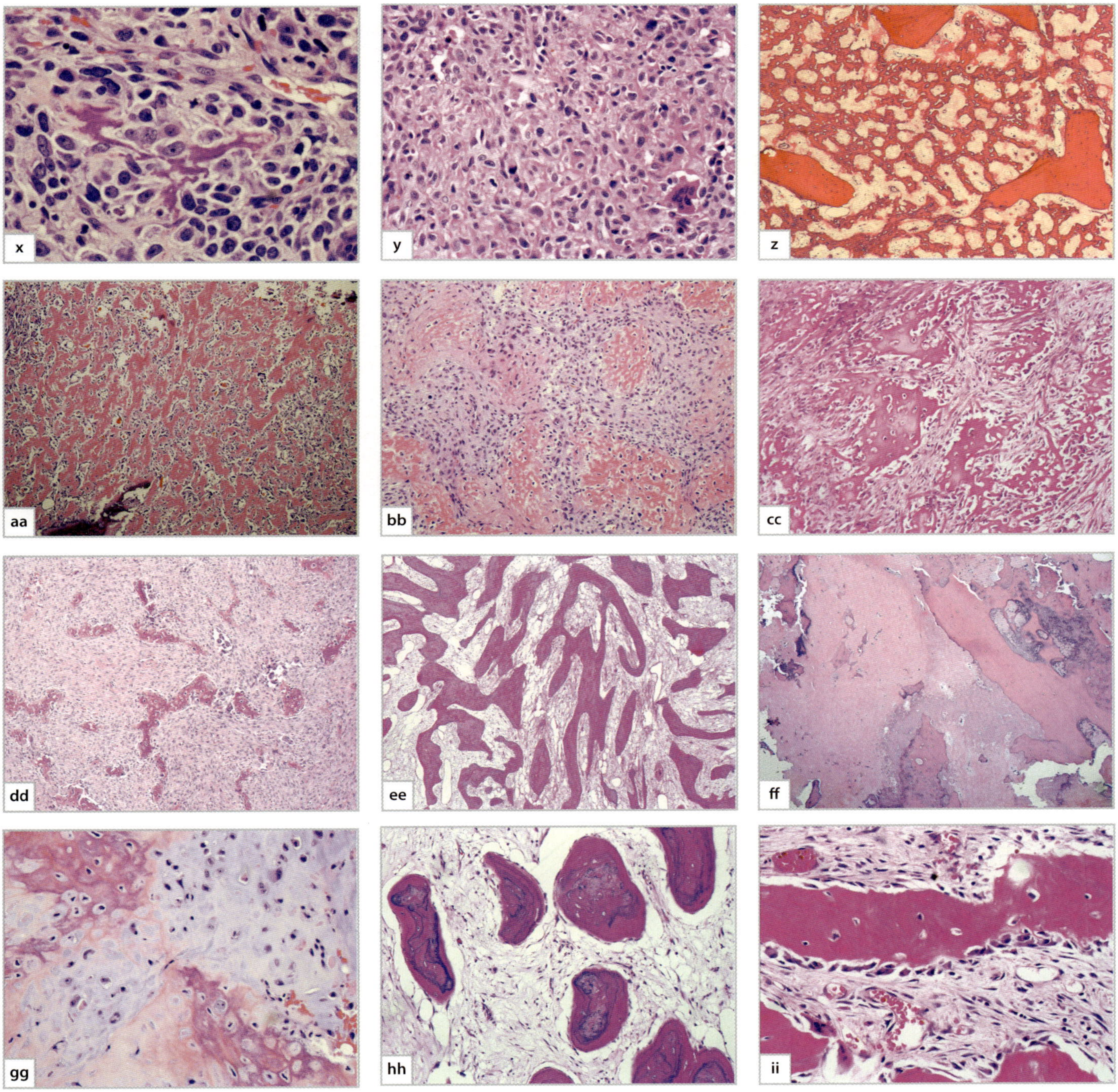

Variant appearances of tumor osteoid (Figures 17.3x through 17.3ii): **17.3x:** Filamentous mineralizing osteoid, high magnification. **17.3y**: More extensive filamentous osteoid, medium mag. **17.3z**: Lacelike osteoid/bone with residual normal trabeculae, Low magnification. **17.3aa**: Coarse fusing bands of osteoid, low magnification **17.3bb**: Blobby, spongy osteoid, medium mag. **17.3cc**: Bristly osteoid with tentacular extensions, medium mag. **17.3dd**: Scattershot irregular osteoid resembling fibrous dysplasia, low magnification. **17.3ee**: Elongate streaming osteoid common in parosteal osteosarcoma, low magnification. **17.3ff**: Dense nearly acellular osteoid with residual normal eroded trabeculae, medium mag. **17.3gg**: Endochondral type tumor osteoid, higher mag. **17.3hh**: Pagetoid tumor bone with numerous irregular cement lines. **17.3ii**: Tumor osteoid with rimming osteoblasts (from a lung met of low grade OS).

Special studies: Cytogenetics is attempted on the initial biopsy but is unsuccessful (sarcomas can be difficult to grow in culture). Fungal (Gomori methenamine silver) and AFB (acid fast bacillus) stains on the wedge resection of lung with granulomatous inflammation are negative for microorganisms.

Pathologic differential or, why isn't it one of the following?

There is no practical differential for this tumor, as it shows osteoid production and high grade nuclear features perfect for conventional osteosarcoma. Moreover, the patient's age, location in the metadiaphyseal region of the tibia, and radiologic findings are concordant with a diagnosis of high grade, intramedullary (conventional) osteosarcoma.

One cannot make a diagnosis of osteosarcoma without confirming bone or osteoid formation by tumor cells. It can be challenging to distinguish osteoid from dense collagen, especially in a small biopsy. Fortunately, in most cases, osteoid is focally mineralized to bone which is very helpful diagnostically, or its architecture is characteristic: filamentous to lacelike, inter-anastomosing coarser cords, irregular trabeculae without osteoblastic rimming, trabeculae with multiple, irregular, haphazard cement lines mimicking Paget's disease, or broad sheets with tumor cells floating in lacunae. **Case figs 17.3xx** through **17.3ii** provides examples of these patterns. In small biopsy specimens where the osteoid is scant and it is difficult to discern typical architecture, antibody staining for osteocalcin may be of diagnostic use, as it will label the osteoid of 80% of osteosarcomas and the osteoblasts of ~90% of osteosarcomas (Fanburg-Smith et al. 1999). SATB2 is another nuclear marker of osteoblastic differentiation that may be diagnostically helpful (Conner et al. 2013). To allow distinction from malignant osteoid or tumor bone, reactive bone should be surfaced with osteoblasts. It will not exhibit the particular neoplastic architecture of tumor osteoid or intimate association with pleomorphic tumor cells (recall that the most atypical cells are often located in the stroma and commonly show 'normalization' or less atypia as they become embedded in tumor osteoid).

This patient's tumor is an obvious conventional osteosarcoma with abundant malignant osteoid and bone. It is an example of the osteoblastic variant of conventional OS. **Case table 17.3a:** lists variants of intramedullary osteosarcoma. Most are histologic variants of conventional osteosarcoma and behave similarly. Three medullary-based tumors are not considered conventional OS variants: telangiectatic osteosarcoma, small cell osteosarcoma, and low grade central osteosarcoma. Small cell osteosarcoma is so rare it requires a national expert to confirm the diagnosis. Its exact defining features have not been firmly established.

Case table 17.3a Histologic variants of intramedullary osteosarcoma

Variant	Frequency	Description	Comment
Osteoblastic	Common (~50%)	Abundant tumor osteoid Architecture of osteoid can be filigree, lacelike, and/or puddled	Conventional OS histologic variant (Grade 2-3)
Chondroblastic	Common (~50%)	Tumor matrix is predominantly chondroid or cartilage	Conventional OS histologic variant (Grade 2-3)
Fibroblastic	Uncommon (~25%)	Tumor is mostly composed of spindle cells with scant osteoid +/- tumor cartilage	Conventional OS histologic variant (Grade 2-3)
High grade undifferentiated pleomorphic sarcoma-like (malignant fibrous histiocytoma-like)	Rare	Tumor mimics high grade pleomorphic sarcoma with only scant amounts of osteoid +/- tumor cartilage	Conventional OS histologic variant (Grade 2-3)
Osteoblastoma-like	Rare	Tumor has trabecular or thick irregular lacelike osteoid mimicking osteoblastoma	Conventional OS histologic variant (Grade 2-3)
Sclerosing osteoblastic	Rare	Extremely dense, hypocellular osteoid in sheets	Conventional OS histologic variant (Grade 2-3)
Giant cell rich	Uncommon	Tumor has abundant osteoclast-like giant cells	Conventional OS histologic variant (Grade 2-3)
Chondromyxoid fibroma-like	Rare	Tumor mimics chondromyxoid fibroma	Conventional OS histologic variant
Chondroblastoma-like	Rare	Tumor mimics chondroblastoma	Conventional OS histologic variant
Clear cell	Rare	Tumor osteoblasts exhibit clear cytoplasm (usually due to glycogen)	Conventional OS histologic variant
Epithelioid	Rare	Tumor osteoblasts are round with distinct cell borders mimicking epithelial cells	Conventional OS histologic variant (Grade 2-3)
Mixed	Common	Approximately equal amounts of other conventional OS types such as mixed chondroblastic and osteoblastic	Conventional OS histologic variant (Grade 2-3)
Small cell	Very rare	Tumor is composed of small round or spindled cells (smaller than the usual malignant OS cells) with extensive lacelike osteoid	These are very rare and not well defined. Relationship to Ewing sarcoma not firmly established. Needs expert consultation for diagnosis. (Grade 2-3)
Telangiectatic	Rare	Tumor comprises blood filled cavities lined by pleomorphic tumor cells. Osteoid is present but scant.	Same prognosis as conventional high grade OS. (Grade 2-3)
Low grade central	Rare	Can mimic the long parallel arrays of woven or lamellar tumor bone of parosteal OS or can mimic the appearance of fibrous dysplasia	Rare. Significant percentage (15-30%) may dedifferentiate to high grade conventional OS (Grade 1)

Case table 17.3b Summary pathology findings of Case 17.3

Diagnosis	Osteosarcoma, conventional type
Size	10.1 × 5.5 × 4.2 cm
Location	Tibia, left proximal metaphysis
Margin status	Negative; all margins approximately 1.0 cm from tumor
Histologic grade (AJCC bone sarcoma grading)	High grade (grade 3-4)
Pathologic stage (AJCC TNM classification)	IVA (any grade, any size, N0, lung mets only)
AJCC = American Joint Committee of Cancer	

Oncology approach

Medical oncology

Because the patient is a teenager with a conventional osteosarcoma, he is enrolled on a Children's Oncology Group protocol (COG AOST0331). He receives a standard three-drug induction regimen consisting of 2 cycles of cisplatin and doxorubicin along with four cycles of methotrexate (MAP). After surgical resection, the histological response of the primary sarcoma is measured as a 97% necrosis, which places him in the good responder group. The suspicious lung lesions, although not diagnosed as osteosarcoma after a pulmonary biopsy, have also regressed. He is then randomized to continue the MAP standard of care instead of the experimental therapy which is pegylated interferon alfa-2b as maintenance therapy after MAP (MAPifn). The doses are A=doxorubicin 37.5 mg/m^2/day. Days 1-2; P= cisplatin 60 mg/m^2/day Day 1, 2; M= methotrexate 12 g/m^2/day with folinic acid rescue, on day 4.

He tolerates the treatment well and remains in remission after 3 years. The study schema is shown below.

Neoadjuvant chemotherapy

Week	1	2	3	4	5	6	7	8	9	10
Drug	AP			M	M	AP			M	M

Surgery on week 11

Adjuvant chemotherapy

Week	12	13	14	15	16	17	18	19	20	21
Drug	AP			M	M	AP			M	M
Week	21	22	23	24	25	26	27	28	29	
Drug	M	A		M	M	A		M	M	

Radiation oncology

The primary tumor is treated with wide resection and reconstruction. With the addition of adjuvant chemotherapy, the patient is fortunately disease free years later. No radiation therapy is recommended.

Patient outcome

The patient remains in remission three years after initiation of treatment.

Case 17.4 Telangiectatic osteosarcoma

Clinical history and presentation

The patient is a ten year old girl who sustained a fracture of the femur after a collision which occurred while playing kickball. On further questioning, she does recall mild activity related pain in the thigh which had been present several weeks prior to the injury. The fracture was treated with open reduction and internal fixation with a plate and screws. Over the next three months, she developed a progressively enlarging soft tissue mass in the thigh, increasing pain, and a progressively destructive bone lesion on radiographs.

Physical examination reveals pronounced fusiform swelling of the thigh with tenderness on palpation.

Surgical findings and comments

Open biopsy is performed with finding of telangiectatic osteosarcoma.

Following a pre-operative course of neoadjuvant chemotherapy, the patient undergoes wide resection of the femoral tumor, including the associated hardware from the prior surgery, and allograft reconstruction.

One year later she develops a local recurrence in the thigh which is widely resected. Six months later she undergoes pulmonary metastatectomy after CT scan reveals pulmonary metastases.

Radiology findings

Our case (**Case figs 17.4a** through **17.4m**) is of a 10 year old girl who presented with a mid diaphyseal pathologic fracture. Unfortunately, the subtle lucency (**Case fig. 17.4a**) distal to the fracture indicating an underlying destructive lesion was not recognized. The immediate postoperative films show successful open reduction and internal fixation of the fracture, (**Case figs 17.4c** and **17.4d**). On routine follow up exam, the films (**Case figs 17.4e** and **17.4f**) show a large soft tissue mass of the distal femoral metadiaphysis. The patient was then referred to an orthopedic sarcoma specialist.

The next set of radiographs, (**Case figs 17.4g** and **17.4h**) was obtained after several rounds of chemotherapy. There is progression of bone destruction with new foreshortening of the hardware indicating the bone is disintegrating and the repair is collapsing. There is some maturing bone along the proximal and distal aspect of the soft tissue mass, perhaps from healing response. The MR exam (**Case figs 17.4i** through **17.4m**) was performed at the time of this last set of radiographs and shows a heterogeneous aggressive soft tissue mass. There is only modest enhancement visible probably related to the extensive necrosis and hemorrhage. This difficult case underscores the importance of maintaining constant vigilance for subtle underlying lesions when encountering fractures in otherwise healthy individuals.

Pathology findings

Gross features

The biopsy comprises multiple red to brown fragments of soft tissue with interspersed flecks of bone aggregating to 3.5 cm. A frozen section is performed, and the diagnosis rendered is 'high grade malignancy

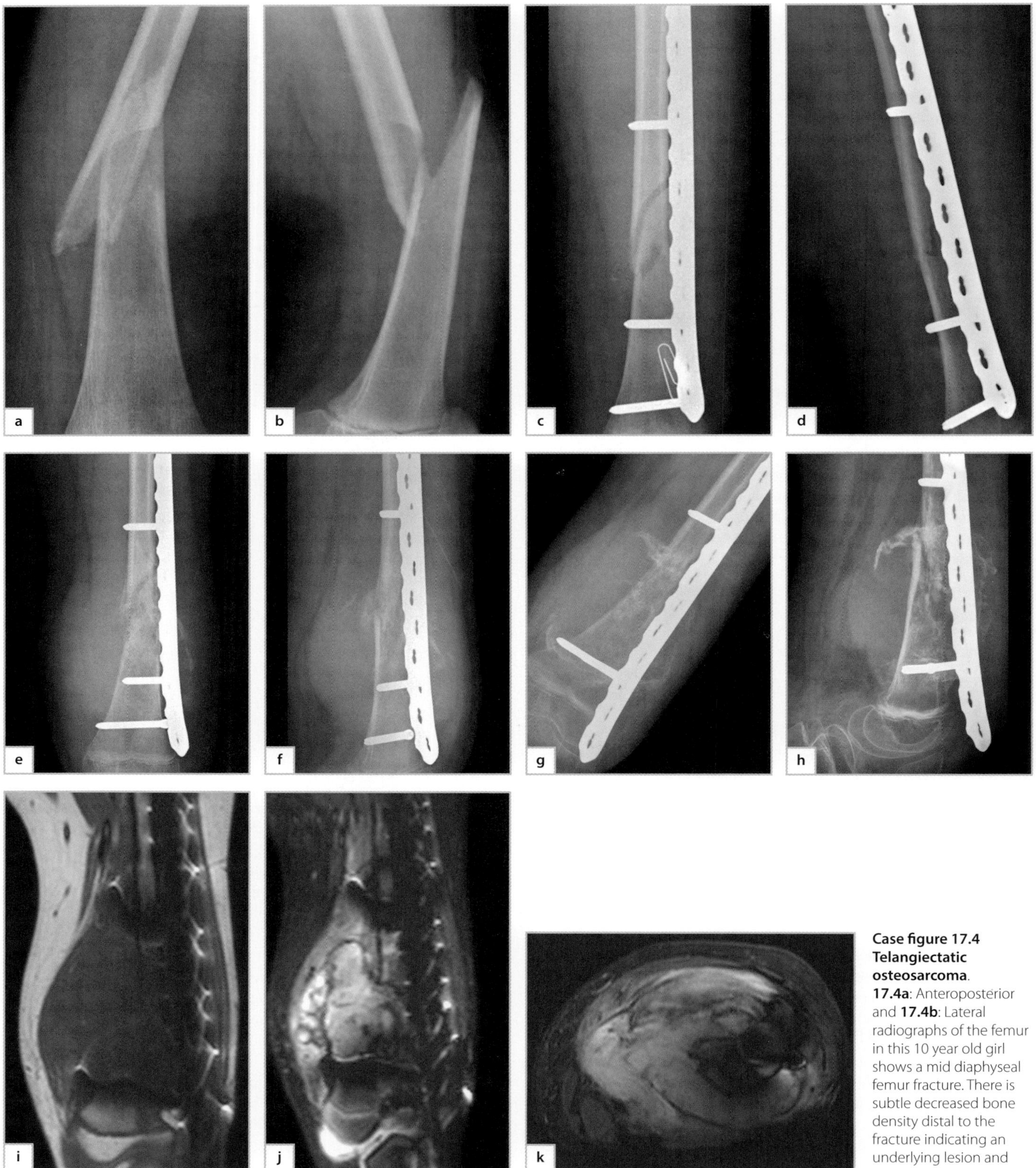

Case figure 17.4 Telangiectatic osteosarcoma. **17.4a**: Anteroposterior and **17.4b**: Lateral radiographs of the femur in this 10 year old girl shows a mid diaphyseal femur fracture. There is subtle decreased bone density distal to the fracture indicating an underlying lesion and a pathologic fracture. Unfortunately, this was not diagnosed at time of fracture. The initial follow up films. **17.4c**: Anteroposterior and **17.4d**: Lateral radiographs show internal fixation hardware with excellent alignment and early healing response. On subsequent follow-up, several weeks after initial ORIF. **17.4e**: anteroposterior and **17.4f**: Lateral radiographs show an obvious soft tissue mass with permeative destruction of the femur and discontinuous periosteal reaction. Clearly, there is a highly aggressive underlying lesion, no tumor osteoid is seen. The next set of radiographs, **17.4g**: Anteroposterior and **17.4h**: Lateral films, show a new pathologic fracture with hardware migration. There is some maturing bone seen along the superior margin of the soft tissue mass probably related to chemotherapy response. The MR images taken at the time of this last set of radiographs include **17.4i**: Coronal T1, **17.4j**: Coronal STIR, **17.4k**: axial STIR.

Case figure 17.4: Continued from page 438

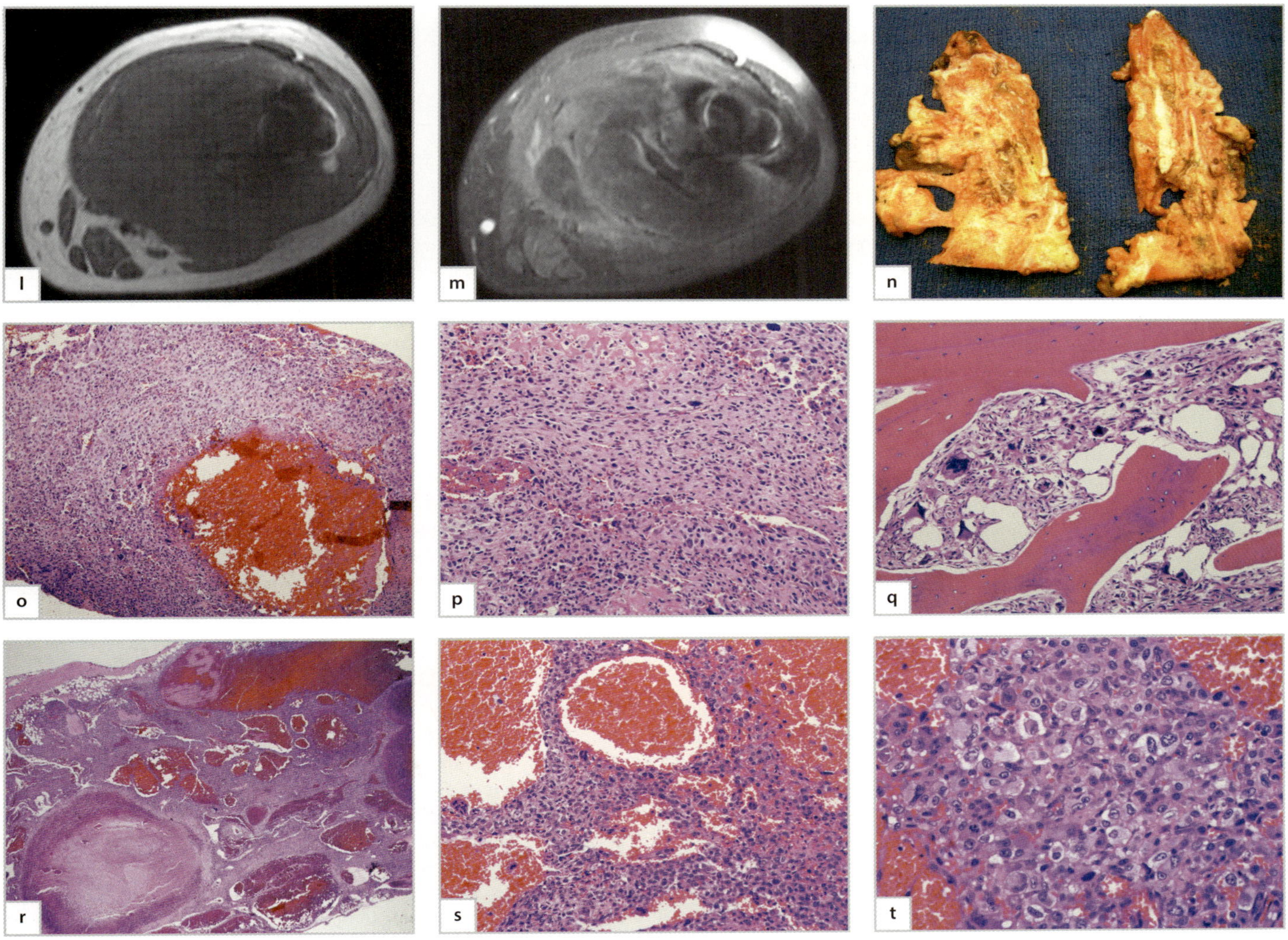

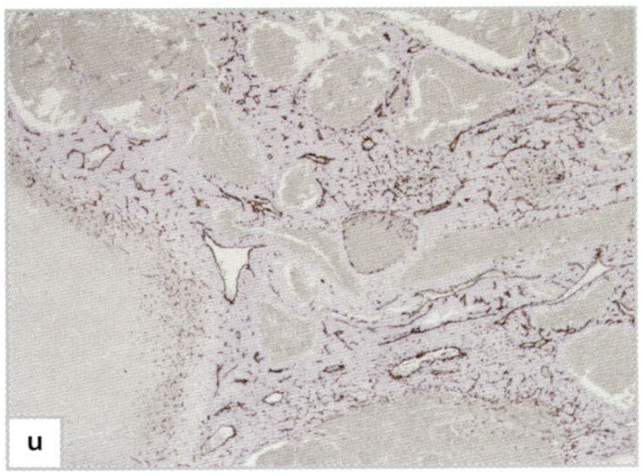

17.4l Axial T1, **17.4m**: Axial T1 fat saturated post-contrast images. The image quality is limited by the metallic hardware components. Nevertheless, the large soft tissue mass is demonstrated measuring 12 × 8.1 × 10.4 cm. The mass is T1 low signal and STIR high signal and shows only minimal heterogeneous enhancement. The lack of abundant enhancement is probably related to extensive areas of hemorrhage, fluid and necrosis. **17.4n**: Gross photo of cut resection specimen, metal rod removed. Cut section reveals a yellow to green, cystic to solid tumor occupying the medullary cavity and extending into adjacent soft tissue. **17.4o**: Initial biopsy, medium magnification. The tumor fragments consist primarily of solid sheets of pleomorphic cells with a few scattered blood-filled cysts. **17.4p**: Initial biopsy, medium magnification. The tumor contains a few areas of lace-like, unequivocal tumor osteoid (top and bottom of field). **17.4q**: Resection post neo-adjuvant therapy, medium magnification. Only a few areas (~2%) remain of viable tumor. **17.4r**: Low magnification. Classic appearance of telangiectatic osteosarcoma with multiple blood-filled cavities. **17.4s**: Medium magnification. The blood cysts have only a few floating tumor cells. Osteoid is scant in the entire tumor, and there is none in this field. **17.4t**: High magnification. The malignant cells look a bit like histiocytes with a round shape, frothy cytoplasm, and eccentrically located, pale ovoid to reniform nuclei. They are too pleomorphic for histiocytes, however. Notice the atypical mitotic figure and intermixed osteoclasts. **17.4u**: CD34 immunohistochemical stain, medium magnification. CD34 expression is limited to true vessels (highlighted by brown chromogen), while the inner surfaces of the cystic spaces are negative. This confirms the non-vascular nature of the large hemorrhagic cavities.

consistent with sarcoma'. Some of the specimen is submitted for cytogenetic analysis.

The resection consists of the left distal femur and associated soft tissues including skeletal muscle with metal rod in place. The margins are differentially inked and the specimen is sectioned fresh in 0.5 cm thick, sagittal slices. The tumor is large (8.5 cm maximally), centered in the medullary cavity of the metaphysis and invades the soft tissues extensively. On cut section, the tumor varies from firm and white to soft and cystic with yellow necrotic areas (**Case fig. 17.4n**). One complete longitudinal section is gridded out and submitted in entirety, and representative margins are also submitted (total number of cassettes processed: 27).

The soft tissue metastasis is located in yellow lobulated adipose tissue, measures 4.2 cm in maximum dimension, and is spongy, red-brown, septated and hemorrhagic. Samples are collected fresh for karyotyping and tissue banking.

Microscopic features

Biopsy

Low magnification: The tumor is mostly solid with a few cavities filled by blood (**Case fig. 17.4o**). It is possible that crushing induced by curettage collapses some of the hemorrhagic cysts rendering them less conspicuous than in the later metastasis specimen which is excised intact with a rim of surrounding fat.

High magnification: At higher magnification, the biopsy discloses unequivocal osteoid formation consistent with osteosarcoma (**Case fig. 17.4p**). Marked pleomorphism is present.

Resection

Low magnification: Careful gridding of the specimen reveals 98% necrotic tumor.

High magnification: Very scant viable tumor remains (**Case fig. 17.4q**).

Soft tissue metastasis

Low magnification: The soft tissue metastasis is removed intact and cross sections reveal the classic, numerous blood filled cavities of telangiectatic osteosarcoma (**Case fig. 17.4r**).

High magnification: At higher magnification, only a few tumor cells float in the hemorrhagic cysts; most are concentrated in the walls and septae (**Case fig. 17.4s**). The round tumor cells have ovoid to reniform, variably folded, hypochromatic nuclei and frothy cytoplasm; consequently, some appear histiocytoid (resembling histiocytes). Many nuclei are eccentrically located. Scattered osteoclast-like giant cells and mitotic figures are present (**Case fig. 17.4t**).

Special studies: A CD34 immunohistochemical stain marks numerous vessels in the tumor. Notably, there is no CD34 reactive, inner lining to the large cavities (**Case fig. 17.4u**). This confirms the impression that the large blood-filled structures are not vessels but cysts.

Karyotyping was attempted twice but yields a normal 46,XX result from the initial biopsy and two non-clonal aberrations from the metastasis sample (46,XX,-20+r and 46,XXt(3;4)(q29;q21). Most cases of telangiectatic osteosarcoma demonstrate a complex aneuploid karyotype similar to conventional osteosarcoma (Fletcher et al. 2002).

Pathologic differential or, why isn't it one of the following?

Conventional osteosarcoma (OS): Conventional osteosarcoma does not contain the large number of hemorrhagic cysts surrounded by viable tumor characteristic of telangiectatic OS. Hemorrhagic areas can occur in conventional OS, but they usually form in areas of necrosis or fibrosis. Osteoclasts may be abundant in telangiectatic OS and may aggregate around the blood-filled cavities. However, the giant cell rich variant of conventional OS lacks the hemorrhagic cysts of telangiectatic OS.

Case table 17.4 Summary pathology findings of Case 17.4

Diagnosis	Telangiectatic osteosarcoma
Size	8.5 × 6.9 × 6.5 cm
Location	Femur, left distal, metaphysis
Margin status	Negative; closest margin is 0.5 cm,
Histologic grade (AJCC bone sarcoma grading)	High grade (grade 3-4)
Pathologic stage (AJCC TNM Classification)	IIB (histologic high grade, T2 = tumor > 8 cm, N0, M0)

AJCC = American Joint Committee of Cancer

Aneurysmal bone cyst (ABC): Both ABC and telangiectatic OS feature small and large cysts filled with blood. However, similarities end at low magnification, because high magnification reveals the markedly pleomorphic tumor cells of telangiectatic OS which are absent in ABC. Atypical mitotic figures may also be identified in telangiectatic OS and are not seen in aneurysmal bone cyst.

Oncology approach

Medical oncology

Because the patient is a child with a variant osteosarcoma, she is enrolled on a Children's Oncology Group protocol (COG AOST0331). She initially receives a standard three-drug induction regimen consisting of 2 cycles of cisplatin and doxorubicin along with four cycles of methotrexate (MAP). Again, after surgical resection, the histological response of the primary sarcoma is measured as a 98% necrosis, which places her in the good responder group. She is then randomized to the experimental therapy with pegylated interferon alfa-2b as maintenance therapy after MAP (MAPifn). The doses are A= doxorubicin 37.5 mg/m²/day, days 1-2. P=cisplatin 60 mg/m²/day, days 1 and 2. M=methotrexate 12 g/m²/day with folinic acid rescue. PegIFN=pegylated interferon alfa-2b 0.5-1.0 micrograms/kg/week.

She tolerates the treatment well and remains in remission after 3 years. The study schema is shown below.

Neoadjuvant chemotherapy

Week	1	2	3	4	5	6	7	8	9	10
Drug	AP			M	M	AP			M	M

Surgery on week 11

Adjuvant chemotherapy

Week	12	13	14	15	16	17	18	19	20	21
Drug	AP			M	M	AP			M	M
Week	22	23	24	25	26	27	28	29	30	102
Drug	A		M	M	A		M	M	PegIFN	

In the telangiectatic variant, local recurrence has been found to be more common than metastases. Telangiectatic osteosarcomas have vascular spread and also metastasize to the bones and lungs. Unfortunately, this patient recurs locally and in the lungs. The local recurrence is excised and she then starts on another COG study (AOST0221) of a salvage regimen with inhaled Sargramostim (GM-CSF). Her lung metastases are resected after two courses of GM-CSF and she then continues to receive inhaled therapy for one year.

This case illustrates the fact that patients who recur with lung metastases have a chance of cure with appropriate management. One should thus avoid a nihilistic approach. In fact, it is the local recurrence, usually associated with poor margins, that bears the worse outcome.

Radiation oncology

The patient undergoes an initial wide resection after neoadjuvant chemotherapy and a second wide resection for local recurrence. She later develops metastatic disease to the lung which is resected. She has no evidence of disease years later. Radiation therapy is not indicated.

Patient outcome

Three years following the pulmonary metastectomy, the patient remains in remission.

Case 17.5 Periosteal osteosarcoma

Clinical history and presentation

The patient is a 15 year old boy who presents with a two year history of a bony tibial mass which was noted spontaneously and has progressively enlarged. He denies a history of trauma. Over the past several months the mass has become mildly tender.

Physical examination reveals a prominent bony mass over the anterior aspect of the tibia. It is intimately associated with the underlying bone. There is mild tenderness on palpation.

Surgical findings and comments

Open biopsy is performed revealing periosteal osteosarcoma of intermediate grade.

Three months following initiation of neoadjuvant chemotherapy, wide resection of the tibial tumor is performed. Reconstruction of the leg is accomplished with an intercalary allograft.

Radiology findings

This case of periosteal OS (**Case figs 17.5a** through **17.5g**) shows the classic features of a broad based lesion of a diaphysis with irregularity, thickening and erosion of the cortex. Our case has fairly extensive calcifying osteoid which may obscure underlying periosteal reaction. The 'hair-on-end' periosteal reaction is suggested on the axial CT image (**Case fig. 17.5c**). Although marrow invasion is unusual and can be confused with benign marrow reaction, this case shows enhancing tumor and calcifying osteoid contiguous with the soft tissue mass through the breach in the cortex. There is tumor continuity into the marrow space indicates true marrow invasion.

Two additional cases of surface osteosarcoma are presented. The additional case of periosteal osteosarcoma (**Case figs 17.5h** through **17.5l**) is somewhat unusual for its metadiaphyseal location. There is otherwise a typical appearance with irregular cortical thickening and hair-on-end periosteal reaction. The MR shows clearly the origin is from the cortex and also shows there is no marrow involvement.

The additional case of *parosteal osteosarcoma* (**Case figs 17.5m** through **17.5p**) shows the typical location of the posterior distal femoral metaphysis. The lesion originates from the cortex. The axial images show a subtle possible cleft of separation from the cortex along the posterior metaphysis. CT scan might better have shown a cleft of separation but was not performed. These two bonus cases of surface osteosarcomas are similar in being calcified surface lesion with reactive changes worrisome for malignancy. The periosteal OS is typically diaphyseal and has periosteal reaction. The parosteal OS is characteristically located at the posterior distal femur and, although the calcification is variable, it is typically more dense or even ivory like and there is usually little if any periosteal reaction. Parosteal OS may have a partial thin cleft of separation with a connecting stalk to the bone of origin.

Pathology findings

Gross features

The biopsy consists of a 2 cm aggregate of red soft tissue with interspersed firm gray particulates.

The resection consists of proximal to mid tibia with associated soft tissues. The specimen is sectioned fresh in serial 0.5 cm slices along the long axis of the tumor. Cross sections reveal a single, 9 × 3 × 2 cm tumor that forms a mushroom-like, surface mass over the diaphysis. The base of the tumor merges into thickened, reactive cortical bone. The medullary cavity focally is involved by tumor. The osteosarcoma exhibits a firm central, gray-white semi-translucent to pink granular appearance. Its convex outer border consists of a peripheral rim of soft tan tumor tissue covered by a thin slip of non-neoplastic fibrous tissue.

Microscopic features

Biopsy

Low magnification: The tumor comprises lobulated neoplastic cartilage set in a myxoid, spindle cell stroma (**Case fig. 17.5q**). Some of the cartilage is calcified.

High magnification: This myxoid spindle cell matrix contains a scattered nodule of neoplastic osteoid (**Case fig. 17.5r**). The finding of malignant osteoid establishes the diagnosis of osteosarcoma rather than chondrosarcoma.

Resection

The patient has an adequate response to neoadjuvant therapy, as 90% of the sarcoma is determined to be necrotic upon careful histologic review. The following photos derive from residual, histologically viable tumor.

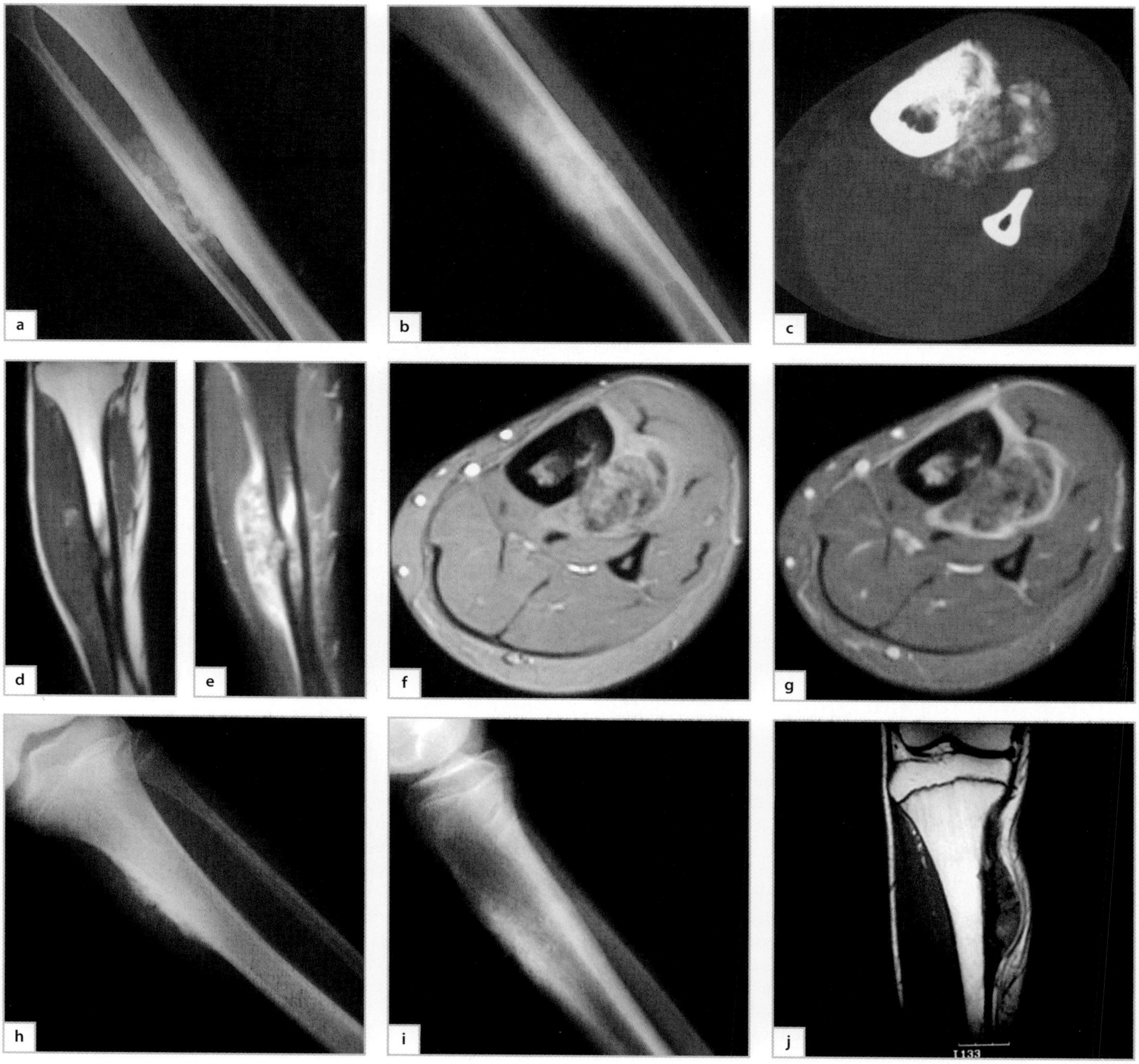

Case figure 17.5 Periosteal osteosarcoma. **17.5a** Anteroposterior and **17.5b**: Lateral radiographs of this patient show an osteoid producing tumor between the tibia and fibula. There is periosteal reaction, cortical thickening and surface irregularity of the tibia indicating this is the bone of origin. **17.5c**: Axial CT scan shows there is cortical destruction and involvement of the marrow space. The tumor is comprised of extensive osteoid with variable mineralization. MR images including: **17.5d**: Coronal T1, **17.5e**: Coronal STIR, **17.5f**: Axial T1 fat saturation and **17.5g**: Axial T1 fat saturation post-contrast. The MR images show a 9 × 2.3 × 3 cm T1 isointense, STIR high signal heterogeneous mass with rim enhancement. There is cortical destruction and areas of low signal corresponding with areas of calcification. The coronal STIR sequence (Case fig. 17.5e) shows high signal extending proximal and distal to the area of cortical destruction. This could simply represent reactive change; however, post-contrast images (Case fig. 17.5g) show enhancing tumor extending into the marrow with areas of calcified tumor osteoid replacing the marrow. *Additional case of periosteal osteosarcoma*. **17.5h**: Anteroposterior and **17.5i**: Lateral radiographs of the leg show a osteoid producing lesion of the proximal tibial metadiaphysis with cortical irregularity and thickening. The MR images: **17.5j**: Coronal T2.

Case figure 17.5: Continued from page 442

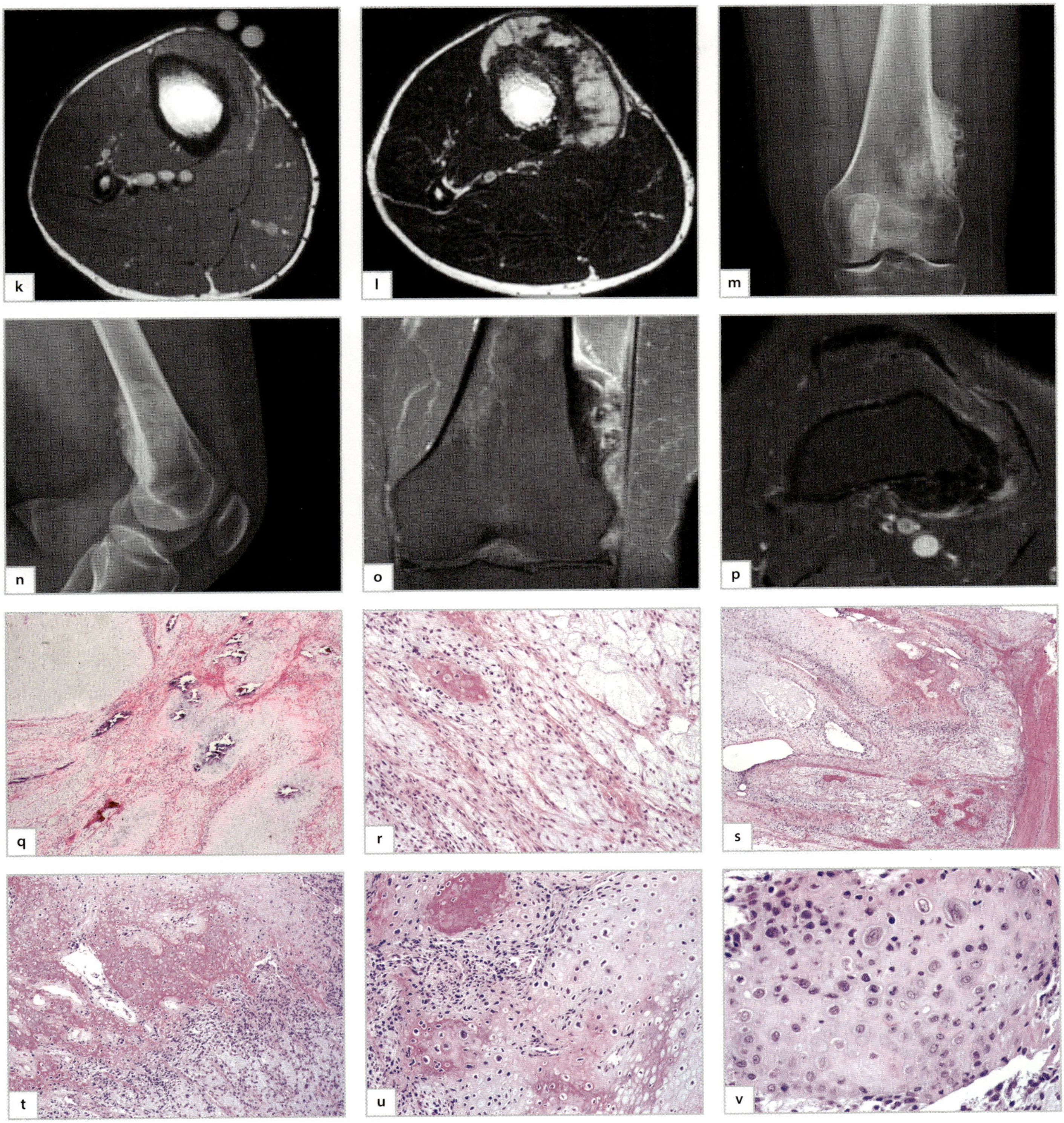

17.5k: Axial T1, **17.5l**: Axial T2 show a surface mass with T1 isointense and T2 heterogeneous signal. The cortex is irregular and thickened. There is no cortical breakthrough and the marrow signal appears normal without evidence of invasion. There are low signal areas probably from calcified matrix. The final additional case is a parosteal osteosarcoma to contrast with the above periosteal osteosarcoma case. **17.5m**: Anteroposterior and **17.5n**: Lateral radiographs show an irregular densely calcified mass intimate to the posterolateral aspect the distal femoral metaphysis in this 32 year old woman. MR images include: **17.5o**: Coronal and **17.5p**: Axial T1 fat saturated post-contrast images show mass originating from the femoral cortex. No cortical breakthrough or marrow invasion seen. The mass is predominantly low signal probably related to the dense calcification. Minimal enhancement is seen within the mass with intense adjacent soft tissue enhancement proximal to the lesion perhaps from mechanical irritation as no infiltrative features are seen. The axial images show a suggestion of a thin posterior cleft separating the mass from the cortex.

Case figure 17.5: Continued from page 443

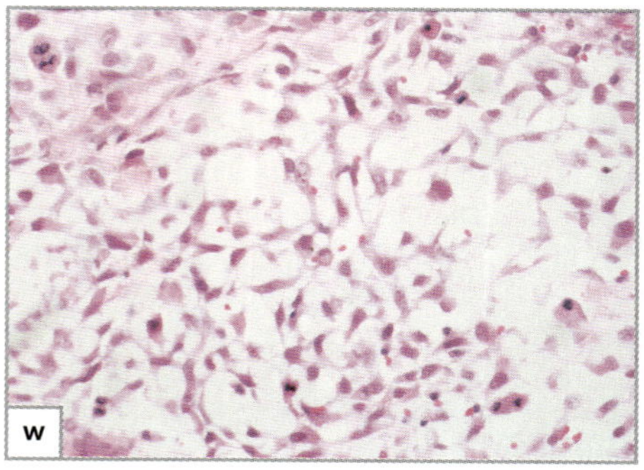
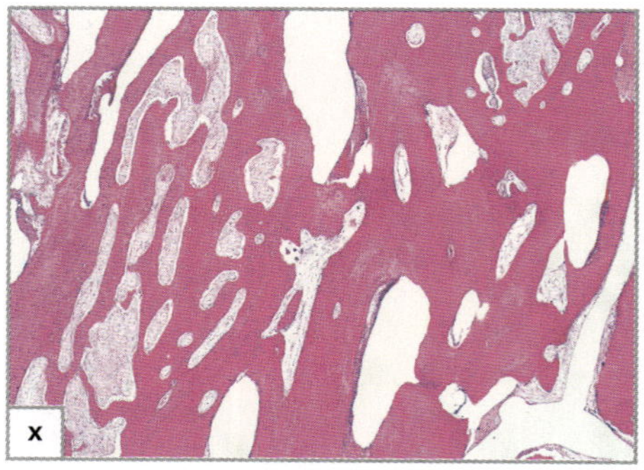
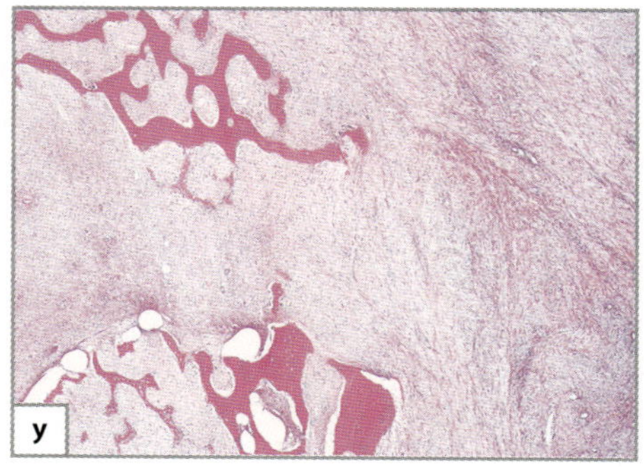
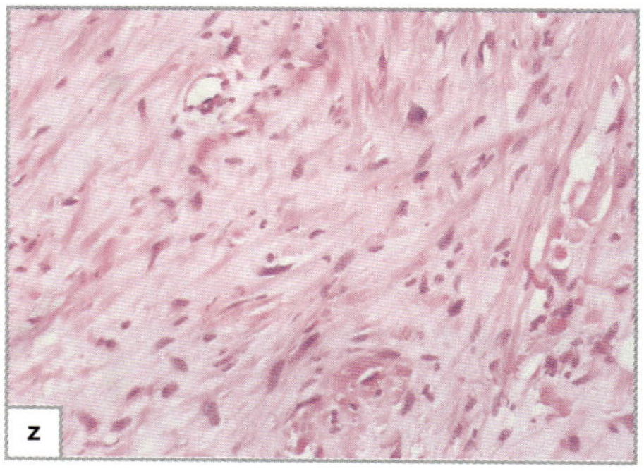

17.5q Biopsy at low magnification. The incisional biopsy contains lobulated cartilage embedded in a myxoid, spindle cell stroma. Mineralized, areas are present (cracked, open areas with drop-out of most the calcified material). These could represent calcified cartilage or neoplastic bone. **17.5r**: Biopsy at higher magnification. Unequivocal tumor osteoid (upper left corner) forms abruptly from a myxoid, spindle cell background. **17.5s**: Resection at low magnification. This field is classic for periosteal osteosarcoma. A column of cartilage forms pink osteoid at its base reminiscent of endochondral ossification. In addition, small nodules of tumor osteoid arise abruptly from the myxoid spindle cell matrix reminiscent of intramembranous ossification. **17.5t**: Resection at medium magnification. Osteochondroid matrix at the base of a broad column of cartilage. It is not possible to find a sharp margin between fully formed osteoid and cartilage undergoing ossification. **17.5u**: Periosteal osteosarcoma, resection at higher magnification. Here the cartilage changes from gray to bright pinkish red (upper nodule) consistent with conversion to osteoid. **17.5v**: Resection at high magnification. The neoplastic cartilage is hypercellular with striking variation in tumor nuclear size and shape. This is equivalent to grade 3 chondrosarcoma. **17.5w:** Resection at high magnification. The myxoid spindle cell matrix is composed of spindled to polygonal cells that display a high mitotic rate. A myxoid spindle cell matrix is frequently seen in periosteal osteosarcoma. *Comparison case of parosteal osteosarcoma.* **17.5x**: Low magnification. In contrast to periosteal osteosarcoma, the bone and osteoid of parosteal OS is abundant, often aligned in long parallel rows, and may mature to lamellar bone. Neoplastic cartilage can be present in parosteal OS but is usually scant and of low histologic grade. **17.5y**: Medium magnification. In contrast to periosteal osteosarcoma, the matrix is relatively hypocellular and fibrotic. **17.5z**: High magnification. The fibrotic matrix of parosteal osteosarcoma is only mildly atypical and of relatively low cellularity.

Low magnification: Typically, periosteal osteosarcoma contains a myxoid spindle cell matrix with abrupt formation of tumor osteoid, and lobules or columns of hyaline cartilage that mineralize and gradually convert to osteoid mimicking endochondral bone formation. All these features are present in **Case fig. 17.5s**.

High magnification: The osteoid can form at the periphery of cartilage columns in close association with spindle cell matrix (**Case fig. 17.5t**), or it can develop in a blotchy fashion from malignant cartilage (**Case fig. 17.5u**). The neoplastic cartilage demonstrates the cellularity and pleomorphism of a grade 3 (high grade) chondrosarcoma (**Case fig. 17.5v**). At high magnification, the spindle cell matrix is very mitotically active with atypical division figures also easily identified (**Case fig. 17.5w**).

Special studies: Because the clinical presentation, radiologic imaging and histologic features are classic for periosteal osteosarcoma, no special studies are performed.

Pathologic differential or, why isn't it one of the following?

Parosteal osteosarcoma: Both periosteal OS and parosteal OS are surface tumors that most commonly involve many of the same bones. However, parosteal osteosarcoma is lower grade, primarily osteoblastic and fibroblastic (**Case figs 17.5x** through **17.5z**), and will have radiologic imaging distinctive from periosteal osteosarcoma (see Radiology discussion). In addition, many cases of parosteal osteosarcoma are reactive for CDK4 and MDM2 by immunohistochemistry. Neoplastic cartilage is often present in parosteal osteosarcoma, but it is of lower grade than in periosteal osteosarcoma and forms a minor component of the tumor.

Conventional osteosarcoma, chondroblastic variant: Conventional chondroblastic osteosarcoma will be centered in the medullary cavity of the bone. Otherwise, it could look histologically identical to periosteal osteosarcoma. **Case fig. 17.5aa** depicts the common skeletal locations of conventional and surface osteosarcomas.

Juxtacortical chondrosarcoma: This tumor tends to occur in older individuals. It usually does not elicit a pronounced periosteal reaction as is characteristic of periosteal osteosarcoma. The grade of the malignant cartilage is low with mild cytologic atypia and cellularity. Most importantly, it does not form neoplastic osteoid or bone.

Oncology approach

Medical oncology

In this case, the patient was not treated on a COG protocol, but received the same neoadjuvant chemotherapy as the other two patients. However, the degree of necrosis observed was only 90%, which still had put him in a favorable category 14 years ago, although the percentage of necrosis defining good outcome has become more stringent with time. After surgical resection, the same chemotherapy regimen was continued and the tumor did not recur.

There is a debate whether neoadjuvant and/or adjuvant chemotherapy is improving outcome or not, because periosteal osteosarcoma tends to be a localized disease. In a retrospective study, chemotherapy administration was in fact associated with a worse prognosis, but because the study was retrospective it is probable that the patients

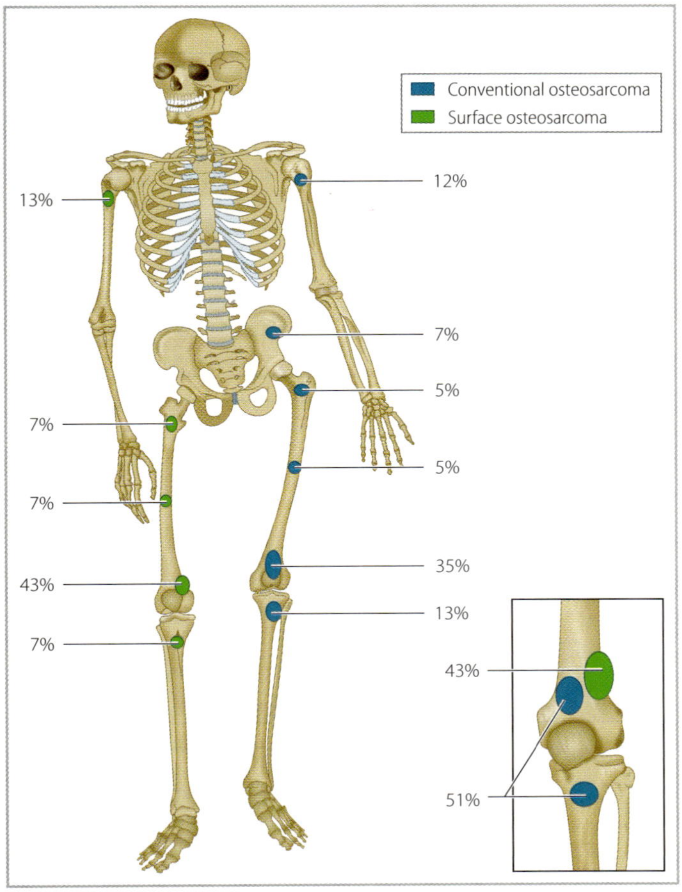

Case figure 17.5aa Common skeletal locations of conventional osteosarcoma and surface osteosarcoma.

Case table 17.5 Summary pathology findings of Case 17.5

Diagnosis	Periosteal osteosarcoma
Size	9 × 3 × 2 cm
Location	Tibia, proximal
Margin status	Negative; all margins > 1.0 cm from tumor
Histologic grade (AJCC bone sarcoma grading)	High grade (grade 3-4)
Pathologic stage (AJCC TNM classification)	IIB (histologic high grade, T2 = tumor > 8 cm, N0, M0)

AJCC = American Joint Committee of Cancer

presenting with more advanced disease were the ones receiving chemotherapy, thus biasing the outcome computation. Randomized studies are needed to establish the efficacy of chemotherapy in this osteosarcoma subtype. Local recurrence is in fact the only clinical feature statistically associated with a worse outcome.

Radiation oncology

After neoadjuvant chemotherapy followed by wide resection and reconstruction, the patient is disease free years later. Therefore, no radiation therapy is indicated.

Patient outcome

Fourteen years following diagnosis, the patient remains in remission with a normally functioning leg.

REFERENCES

Allison DC, Carney SC, Ahlmann ER, et al. A meta-analysis of osteosarcoma outcomes in the modern medical era. Sarcome 2012: epub article ID:704872

Andresen KJ, Sundaram M, Unni KK, et al. Imaging features of low-grade central osteosarcoma of the long bones and pelvis. Skeletal Radiol 2004;33(7):373–9.

Bacci G, Briccoli A, Rocca M, et al. Neoadjuvant chemotherapy for osteosarcoma of the extremities with metastases at presentation: recent experience at the Rizzoli Institute in 57 patients treated with cisplatin, doxorubicin, and a high dose of methotrexate and ifosfamide. Ann Oncol 2003;14(7):1126–34.

Bacci G, Picci P, Ferrari S. Primary chemotherapy and delayed surgery for non-metastatic telangiectatic osteosarcoma of the extremities. Results in 28 patients. Eur J Cancer 1994;30A(5):620–6.

Bacci G, Longhi A, Versari M, et al. Prognostic factors for osteosarcoma of the extremity treated with neoadjuvant chemotherapy: 15-year experience in 789 patients treated at a single institution. Cancer 2006;106(5):1154–61.

Behrooz AA, Wirth CR, Colman N. Fibrosarcoma arising from chronic osteomyelitis. J Bone Joint Surg 1976;58(1):123–5.

Bielack S, Kempf-Bielack B, Schwenzer D, et al. Neoadjuvant therapy for localized osteosarcoma of extremities. Results from the Cooperative osteosarcoma study group COSS of 925 patients. Klin Padiatr 1999;211(4):260–70.

Bjerkehagen B, Smeland S, Walberg L, et al. Radiation-induced sarcoma: 25-year experience from the Norwegian Radium Hospital. Acta Oncol 2008;47(8):1475–82.

Brandal P, Bjerkehagen B, Bruland OS, et al. Synchronous and metachronous skeletal osteosarcomas: the Norwegian Radium Hospital experience. Acta Oncologica 2009;48:1165–1172.

Broadhead ML, Clark JCM, Myers DE, et al. The molecular pathogenesis of osteosarcoma: a review. Sarcoma 2011; article 959248, 12 pages.

Cesari M, Alberghini M, Vanel D, et al. Periosteal osteosarcoma: a single institution experience. Cancer 2011;117:1731–1735.

Corradi D, Wenger DE, Bertoni F, et al. Multicentric osteosarcoma: a clinicopathologic and radiographic study of 56 cases. Am J Clin Pathol 2011;136:799–807.

Debelenko LV, McGregor LM, Shivakumar BR, et al. A novel EWSR1-CREB3L1 fusion transcript in a case of small cell osteosarcoma. Genes Chromosomes Cancer 2011;50:1054–1062.

Dujardin F, Nguyen Binh MB, Bouvier C, et al. MDM2 and CKD4 immunohistochemisty is a valuable tool in the differential diagnosis of low-grade osteosarcomas and other primary fibro-osseous lesions of the bone. Mod Pathol 2011;24:624–637.

Fanburg-Smith JC, Brathauer GL, Miettinen M. Osteocalcin and osteonectin immunoreactivity in extraskeletal osteosarcoma: a study of 28 cases. Hum Pathol 1999;30:32–38.

Ferrari S, Mercuri M, Picci P, et al. Nonmetastatic osteosarcoma of the extremity: results of a neoadjuvant chemotherapy protocol (IOR/OS-3) with high-dose methotrexate, intraarterial or intravenous cisplatin, doxorubicin, and salvage chemotherapy based on histologic tumor response. Tumori 1999;85(6):458–64.

Ferrari A, Dileo P, Casanova M, et al. Rhabdomyosarcoma in adults: a retrospective analysis of 171 patients treated at a single institution. Cancer 2003;98(3):571–580.

Grimer RJ, Bielack S, Flege S, et al. Periosteal osteosarcoma--a European review of outcome. Eur J Cancer 2005;41(18):2806–11.

Hayes-Jordan A, Andrassy R. Rhabdomyosarcoma in children. Current Opinion Pediatrics 2009;21(3):373–378.
Huvos AG, Butler A, Bretsky SS. Osteogenic sarcoma associated with Paget's disease of bone. A clinicopathologic study of 65 patients. Cancer 1983;52(8):1489–95.
Inoue YZ, Frassica FJ, Sim FH, et al. Clinicopathologic features and treatment of post-irradiation sarcoma of bone and soft tissue. J Surg Oncol 2000;75(1):42–50.
Klein MJ, Siegal GP. Osteosarcoma anatomic and histologic variants. Am J Clin Pathol 2006;555–581.
Krailo M, Ertel I, Makley J, et al. A randomized study comparing high-dose methotrexate with moderate-dose methotrexate as components of adjuvant chemotherapy in childhood nonmetastatic osteosarcoma: a report from the Childrens Cancer Study Group. Med Pediatr Oncol 1987;15(2):69–77.
Lee JA, Jung JS, Kim DH, et al. RANKL expression is related to treatment outcome of patients with localized, high-grade osteosarcoma. Pediatr Blood Cancer 2011;56(5):738–43
Lee EL, Shafi M, Hui JHP. Osteoid osteoma: a current review. Journal Pediatric Orthopaedics 2006;26:695–700.
Lewis IJ, Nooij MA, Whelan J, et al. Improvement in histologic response but not survival in osteosarcoma patients treated with intensified chemotherapy: a randomized phase III trial of the European Osteosarcoma Intergroup. Natl Cancer Inst 2007;99(2):112–28.
Lindell MM, Shirkhoda A, Raymond AK, et al. Parosteal osteosarcoma: Radiologic-pathologic correlation with emphasis on CT. AJR 1987;148:323–328.
Liu PT, Kujak JL, Roberts CC, et al. The Vascular Groove Sign: a new CT finding associated with osteoid osteomas. Am J Roentgenol 2011:196; 168–173.
Lucas DR, Unni KK, McLeod RA, et al. Osteoblastoma: clinicopahtologic study of 306 cases. Hum Pathol 1994;25(2):117–134.
Lucas DR. Osteoblastoma. Arch Pathol Lab Med 2010;134(10):1460-1466.
Machado I, Alberghini M, Giner F, et al. Histopathological characterization of small cell osteosarcoma with immunohistochemistry and molecular genetic support: a study of 10 cases. Histopathol 2010;57:162–166.
MacEwen EG, Kurzman ID, Rosenthal RC, et al. Therapy for osteosarcoma in dogs with intravenous injection of liposome-encapsulated muramyl tripeptide. J Natl Cancer Inst 1989;81:935–938.
Mangham DC, Davie MW, Grimer RJ. Sarcoma arising in Paget's disease of bone: declining incidence and increasing age at presentation. Bone 2009;44(3):431–6.
McLeod AJ, Zornoza J, Shirkhoda A. Leiomyosarcoma: computed tomographic findings. Radiol 1984;152(1):133–136.
McLeod RA, Dahlin DC, Beabout JW. The spectrum of osteoblastoma. Am J Roentgenol 1976;126(2):321–325.
Meyers PA, Schwartz CL, Krailo MD, et al. Osteosarcoma: the addition of muramyl tripeptide to chemotherapy improves overall survival--a report from the Children's Oncology Group. J Clin Oncol 2008;26(4):633–8.
Mirabello L, Troisi RJ, Savage SA. Osteosarcoma incidence and survival rates from 1973 to 2004: Data from the Surveillance, Epidemiology, and End Results Program. Cancer 2009;115(7):1531–1543.
Murphey MD, Jelinek JS, Temple TH, et al. Imaging of periosteal osteosarcoma: radiologic-pathologic comparison. Radiol 2004;233:129–138.
Murphey MD, wan Jaovisidha S, Temple HT, et al. Telangiectatic osteosarcoma: radiologic-pathologic comparison. Radiol 2003;229(2):545–53.
Nakajima H, Sim FH, Bond JR, et al. Small cell osteosarcoma of bone. Review of 72 cases. Cancer 1997;79(11):2095–106.
Papathanassiou ZG, Megas P, Petsas T et al. Osteoid osteoma: diagnosis and treatment. Orthopedics 2008;31:1118–1127.
PosthumaDeBoer J, Witlox MA, Kaspers GJL, van Royen BJ. Molecular alterations as target for therapy in metastatic osteosarcoma: a review of literature. Clin Exp Metastasis 2011;28:493–503.
Rosen G, Caparros B, Huvos AG, et al. Preoperative chemotherapy for osteogenic sarcoma: selection of postoperative adjuvant chemotherapy based on the response of the primary tumor to preoperative chemotherapy. Cancer 1982;49(6):1221–30.
Rosen G, Nirenberg A. Neoadjuvant chemotherapy for osteogenic sarcoma: a five year follow-up (T-10) and preliminary report of new studies (T-12). Prog Clin Biol Res 1985;201:39–51.
Rosen G, Forscher CA. Modern Therapy for Osteogenic Sarcoma: Reinventing the Wheel at the Mayo Clinic - The Damron/Pritchard Article Reviewed. Oncol 1995:9(4).
Samardziski M, Zafiroski G, Tolevska C, et al. Parosteal osteosarcoma. Bratisl Lek Listy 2009;110(4):240–244.
Savage SA, Mirabello L. Using epidemiology and genomics to understand osteosarcoma etiology. Sarcoma 2011;2011:548151.
Simmons M, Tucker AK. The radiology of bone changes in rhabdomyosarcoma. Clin Radiol1978;29(1):47–52.
Souhami RL, Craft AW, Van der Eijken JW, et al. Randomised trial of two regimens of chemotherapy in operable osteosarcoma: a study of the European Osteosarcoma Intergroup. Lancet 1997 27;350(9082):911–7.
Staals EL, Bacchini P, Bertoni F. High-grade surface osteosarcoma: a review of 25 cases from the Rizzoli Institute. Cancer 2008;112(7):1592–99.
Taconis WK. Osteosarcoma in fibrous dysplasia. Skeletal Radiol 1988;17(3):163–70.
Weiss, A, Khoury JD, Hoffer FA, et al. Telangiectatic osteosarcoma: The St Jude Children's Research Hospital experience. Cancer 2007;109(8):1627–37.
Xu D, Luan H, Zhan A, et al. Spontaneous malignant transformation of fibrous dysplasia. Chin Med J 1996;109(12):941–5.
Yaniv G, Shabshin N, Sharon M, et al. Osteoid osteoma – the CT vessel sign. Skeletal Radiol 2011;40(10):1311–1314.
Yarmish G, Klein MJ, Landa J, et al. Imaging characteristics of primary osteosarcoma: nonconventional subtypes. Radiographics 2010;30(6):1653–72.
Yoshida A, Ushiku T, Motoi T et al. Immunohistochemical analysis of MDM2 and CDK4 distinguishes low-grade osteosarcoma from benign mimics. Mod Pathol 2010;23:1279–1288.
Yoshida A, Ushiku T, Motoi T et al. MDM2 and CDK4 immunohistochemical coexpression in high grade osteosarcoma: correlation with a dedifferentiated subtype. Am J Surg Pathol 2012;36:423–431.
Yu H, Li H, Wang CF, Zhu XZ. Low-grade central osteosarcoma: a clinicopathologic analysis of nine cases. Zhonghua Bing Li Xue Za Zhi 2010;39(11):726–6.

FURTHER READING

Folpe AL, Inwards CY (eds). Bone and Soft Tissue Pathology. A volume in the series: Foundations in Diagnostic Pathology. Goldblum JR (series ed). Philadelphia: Elsevier Saunders, 2010.
Dorfman HD, Czerniak B. Bone Tumors. St Louis: Mosby, 1998.
Fletcher CDM, Bridge JA, Hogendoorn P, Mertens F (eds). World Health Organization Classification of Tumours of Soft Tissue and Bone, 4th Ed. Lyon: IARC Press, 2013.

Chapter 18 Fibrogenic tumors of bone

OVERVIEW

Two tumors form this World Health Organization (WHO) category: desmoplastic fibroma and fibrosarcoma of bone. Both tumors were originally described well before routine use of immunohistochemistry and sophisticated genetic analysis. Consequently, in the ensuing decades, many of these tumors, especially those conforming to the histologic definition of fibrosarcoma, were revealed upon additional newer testing to comprise other distinct entities such as osteoid-poor fibroblastic osteosarcoma or intra-osseous versions of leiomyosarcoma, synovial sarcoma, malignant peripheral nerve sheath tumors, myofibrosarcoma, and others. This shrinking incidence of primary fibrosarcoma of bone parallels the similar contraction affecting fibrosarcoma of soft tissue (Bahrami et al. 2010). Nonetheless, rare, adult intra-osseous tumors composed of spindled cells arranged in streaming fascicles and herringbone patterns that fail to express specific markers and lack specific genetic findings typical of other tumors are yet categorizable as primary fibrosarcoma of bone.

Some fascicular spindle cell sarcomas of bone may arise in the setting of prior irradiation, in longstanding Paget disease or as a dedifferentiated component of another tumor. Whether all these tumors, which resemble each other under the microscope, actually resemble each other genetically or genetically match the sporadically occurring 'fibrosarcoma of bone' is not known. Most likely, some of the fibrosarcomas of bone currently diagnosed represent a polyglot bunch that do not define a specific category but instead are only superficially alike. When faced with such a tumor, the pathologist must vigorously exclude specific tumor types to ensure the patient is appropriately treated. 'Fibrosarcoma of bone' is a diagnosis of last resort.

Desmoplastic fibroma, a benign but locally aggressive intra-osseous tumor that histologically mimics desmoid-type fibromatosis (DTF) has always been rare. Accumulating data suggest it is NOT the exact bony equivalent of DTF. Desmoplastic fibroma too, must be carefully and rigorously assessed in pathology, as it is also a diagnosis of exclusion. Perhaps the most common misdiagnoses of desmoplastic fibroma occur when a soft tissue fibromatosis erodes into bone and is misconstrued as arising in bone or when a small biopsy of fibrous dysplasia fails to disclose tumor bone spicules. Careful radiologic-pathologic correlation prevents these errors.

CLASSIFICATION

Table 18.1 lists the fibrogenic tumors of bone.

DEMOGRAPHICS

Desmoplastic fibroma

According to the WHO, desmoplastic fibroma occurs equally in males and females and presents in adolescence or early adulthood.

Fibrosarcoma of bone

The largest series of primary fibrosarcoma of bone (n=130 patients diagnosed from 1918 to 1973 at Memorial Sloan-Kettering Cancer Center) reported an equal sex distribution and an age range of 4 to 83 years with a mean of 38 years (no patients had a pre-existing benign bone condition) (Huvos et al. 1975). A subsequent review of 92 patients treated at the Mayo Clinic from 1910-1995 also found an equal gender distribution and nearly identical age involvement: mean of 38 years and range of 8-84 years (Papagelopoulos et al. 2000). However, at least some of these tumors most likely represent other entities such as leiomyosarcoma, myofibrosarcoma, low grade fibromyxoid sarcoma, synovial sarcoma, MPNST, solitary fibrous tumor and osteoid-poor fibroblastic sarcoma.

After confirming absence of specific genetic findings (such as t(X;18) of synovial sarcoma) or telltale immunohistochemical findings (such as diffuse, strong, multiple muscle marker expression as in leiomyosarcoma of bone), a 'fibrosarcoma of bone' is most likely to be diagnosed in an adult in the 4th to 6th decade of life. Fascicular spindle cell sarcomas without specific diagnostic IHC or genetic features and high cytologic grade may also be diagnosed as 'undifferentiated high grade spindle cell sarcoma, not otherwise specified'. These occur more commonly in middle aged to elderly adults. Cases associated with pre-existing conditions such as prior radiation therapy for Ewing sarcoma or chronic osteomyelitis may occur in younger individuals.

PATHOGENESIS/ETIOLOGY

Desmoplastic fibroma

Although it may histologically appear similar to a desmoid-type fibromatosis (DTF), desmoplastic fibroma is likely a distinct tumor

Table 18.1 Fibrogenic tumor of bone WHO Classification (2013)

Tumor or lesion	Behavior	Additional comments
Desmoplastic fibroma	Intermediate (locally aggressive)	Very rare: 0.12% of primary bone tumors Diagnosis of exclusion
Fibrosarcoma of bone	Malignant	Rare: < 5% of primary malignant bone tumors Diagnosis of exclusion Some cases may represent poorly differentiated spindle cell sarcomas that are not characterized by specific genetic findings and should be termed 'high grade spindle cell sarcoma not otherwise specified' ~25% of FS of bone are associated with other conditions such as prior irradiation or Paget disease

Malignant: can recur and commonly metastasizes. Benign: does not recur or recurs non-aggressively and does not metastasize. Intermediate: can recur aggressively and/or rarely metastasizes (<5%)

with no close relationship to DTF. There is no association with colonic polyps (associated with intra-abdominal desmoids and mutations of the *APC* gene). More importantly, desmoplastic fibromas only rarely express nuclear β-catenin and do not carry activating mutations of the β-catenin gene as is found in the majority of soft tissue fibromatoses (Hauben et al. 2005, Ng et al. 2005). However, some cases of desmoplastic fibroma share chromosomal abnormalities commonly seen in DTF including trisomy 8 and/or trisomy 20 (Bridge et al. 1996).

A desmoplastic fibroma-like tumor (bland, intra-osseous spindle cell tumor with collagen production and no bone formation) has been described in the jaws of patients with tuberous sclerosis (Vargas-Gonzalez et al. 2004). Whether this is truly a desmoplastic fibroma or a distinctive, benign low grade spindle cell tumor unique to tuberous sclerosis is not known.

Desmoplastic fibroma of the gnathic bones must be distinguished from odontogenic fibroma which behaves less aggressively but which can histologically mimic desmoplastic fibroma. DF typically causes cortical bone destruction, seldom involves the maxilla and usually affects younger patients (Ikeshima et al. 2005). Distinguishing the two is not trivial, as treatment is ostectomy for odontogenic fibroma and more extensive resection for desmoplastic fibroma.

FIBROSARCOMA OF BONE

Fibrosarcoma-like tumors of bone may occur as a radiation induced sarcoma, in the setting of longstanding Paget disease, as the dedifferentiated component of a chondrosarcoma or ameloblastic fibroma, at the site of prior curettage of a benign bone tumor, or in association with chronic osteomyelitis, bone infarct, fibrous dysplasia, or hereditary bone dysplasia (Staals et al. 2007, Sopta et al. 2008, Picci et al. 2011, Sharma et al. 2006, Mavrogenis et al. 2012, Fletcher et al. 2002).

True fibrosarcoma of bone may be related to osteosarcoma and is usually treated as such. However, at the molecular genetic level, the two may be significantly dissimilar. A recent genetic study of carefully immunohistologically weeded cases found gain of the PDGF-β gene (22q12.3-q13.1) as the most common aberration (3 of 5 cases; Hattinger et al. 2004). As the authors note, PDGF-β is abnormal in other tumors including dermatofibrosarcoma protuberans where it fuses with the collagen 1A1 gene (on 17q21). A single case report of a fibrosarcoma arising in the iliac bone of a 10 year old girl reported a ring chromosome 6 as the only abnormality (Hallor et al. 2007). An array comparative genomic hybridization study of 13 cases showed some fairly consistent losses (6q,8p,9p,10,13q, and 20p) and gains (1q, 4q,5p,8q,12p,15q,16q,17q,20q,22q and Xp)(Niini et al. 2010). In this last study, IHC expression of PDGF-β and/or PDGF-α was found in 12 of 17 samples.

PATHOLOGY

Table 18.2 briefly describes the two fibrogenic tumors of bone according to incidence, body site, and pathologic features.

Table 18.2 Fibrogenic tumors of bone

Tumor	Incidence	Age and sex	Body site (in order of occurrence)	Histopathology description including IHC	
				Medium magnification	High magnification
Intermediate: can recur locally aggressively and/or rarely metastasizes (<5%)					
Desmoplastic fibroma	Very rare	Adolescents to young adults most commonly, middle aged adults Male = Female	Long bones, mandible, pelvis, skull; rarely elsewhere	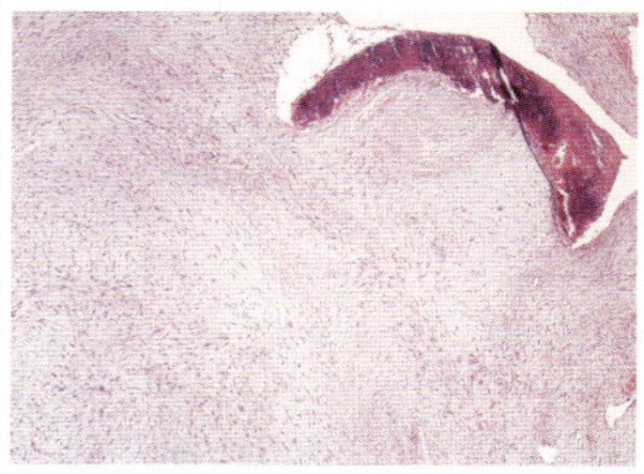	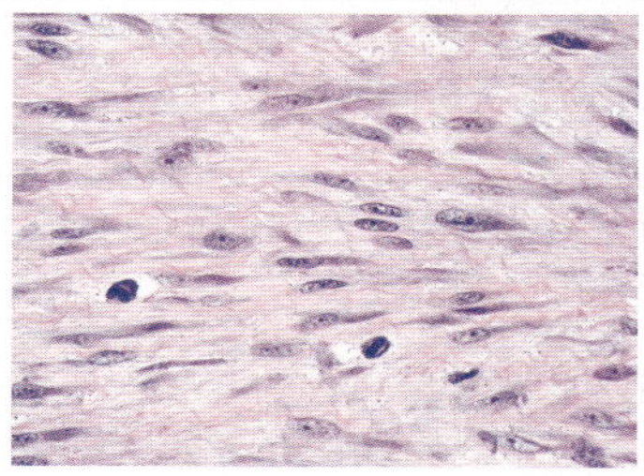
Mildly to moderately cellular spindle cell tumor arranged in loose intersecting fascicles often with abundant collagen. Myxoid background may be focally present. Rare cases have numerous hyaline cartilage nodules. There is no nuclear atypia and only rare mitotic figures. Tumor nuclei may be ovoid, plump spindled, or elongate spindled, and cell borders are usually indistinct. Nucleoli are usually inconspicuous. Tumor is infiltrative and locally destructive often breaking through cortex. Mast cells are commonly intermingled. IHC: Most cases express SMA, either focally or diffusely and of low to moderate intensity (the tumor is considered a myofibroblastic neoplasm). Rare cases also focally express desmin. Nuclear β-catenin expression is absent in nearly all cases. ER and CyclinD1 are not expressed.					
Malignant: can recur and can metastasize					
Fibrosarcoma of bone	Very rare	Middle aged to older adults most commonly but broad age range including children Male = Female	Long bones, especially femur (~60% of cases), humerus, tibia, pelvis; rarely elsewhere	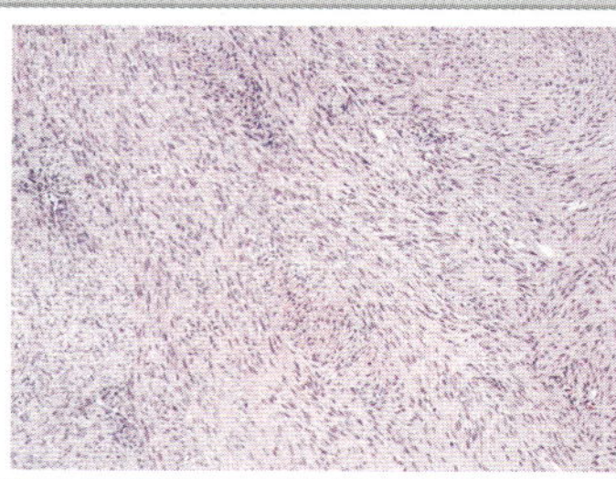	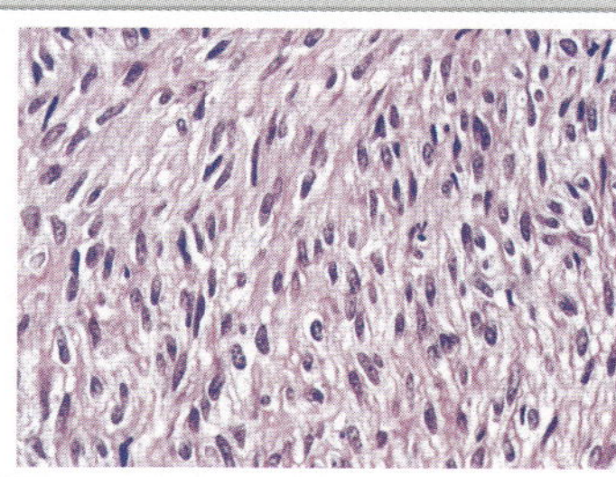
Fascicular and herringbone arrangement of spindled tumor cells with mild to moderate nuclear atypia and scant mitotic activity. Rare cases show increased nuclear pleomorphism, more mitoses, and necrosis while retaining the fascicular architecture. Some cases show focal or diffuse fibrosis. Focal myxoid stroma may be present. Tumor is infiltrative and may break through cortex. IHC: Many cases show weak or focal reactivity for SMA. 60-100% express PDGF or PDGFR. There is no reactivity in fibrotic matrix for osteopontin or osteocalcin and no nuclear expression of SATB2.					
Incidence Note: 'Common to very common' indicates that a medium sized practice will treat at least several to dozens of patients with the lesion annually, 'Uncommon to rare' indicates the same practice size will treat one to two patients with the lesion every five years, 'Rare to very rare' indicates the same sized practice will see zero to one patient with the lesion every 20 years.					

Histologic grading

Desmoplastic fibroma

Desmoplastic fibroma is not graded, as it is not a malignant tumor. However, three cases of malignant transformation of DF have recently been reported. These three cases showed a desmoplastic fibroma component in association with high nuclear grade, pleomorphic tumor cells and additionally, in two cases, malignant osteoid consistent with transformation to osteosarcoma (Min et al. 2010, Takazawa et al. 2003, Abdelwahab et al. 2002).

Rare cases may produce abundant hyaline cartilage nodules and, together with large size and extension into soft tissue, mimic a low grade chondrosarcoma. However, nuclear atypia, necrosis and mitotic activity are absent (Bahk et al. 2003, Callahan et al. 2006).

Fibrosarcoma of bone

High grade cytologic features are uncommon in fibrosarcoma of bone. Reviews of FS of bone published before 2000 included many tumors with marked nuclear pleomorphism and concordant loss of fascicular architecture, but most experts today consider such primary bone sarcomas 'undifferentiated high grade pleomorphic sarcomas.' The current concept of FS of bone comprises spindle cell, fascicular tumors of predominantly low to intermediate nuclear grade (mild to moderate nuclear pleomorphism); only rarely does fibrosarcoma of bone contain cells of marked nuclear atypia while definitionally retaining a pure fascicular spindle cell appearance.

For this tumor, mild nuclear atypia is characterized by minimal variation in nuclear size and shape, with fine chromatin and inconspicuous nucleoli. Moderate nuclear atypia is attained by greater variation in nuclear size often accompanied by hyperchromaticity and increased mitotic activity. Marked nuclear atypia in FS of bone includes great variety in nuclear size, some variation in nuclear shape and hyperchromasia with coarse chromatin. Mitoses in Grade 3 FS of bone are often numerous (>10/10 hpf).

Behavior

Desmoplastic fibroma

Desmoplastic fibroma commonly shows aggressive local growth with cortical break breakthrough and extension into surrounding soft tissues in 15-30% of cases. Exceptional cases of transformation to undifferentiated pleomorphic sarcoma or osteosarcoma have been reported (Abdelwahab et al. 2002, Takazawa et al. 2003, Min et al. 2010. However, most examples of this rare tumor, do not metastasize and do not undergo dedifferentiation.

Fibrosarcoma of bone

Both low and high grade fibrosarcoma may locally recur with incomplete excision. High grade fibrosarcoma is associated with an increased risk for distant metastasis and death (10 year survival of 80% versus 34% for high versus low grade) (Folpe et al. 2010). Metastatic sites include lungs and skeleton.

Additional laboratory testing

Immunohistochemistry: Desmoplastic fibroma often expresses smooth muscle actin, labeling 10 to >50% of cells with intensity ranging from weak to strong. Less commonly, desmin is focally reactive. These findings are similar to those seen in desmoid-type fibromatosis. Nuclear β-catenin reactivity is discrepant between the two tumors. Only rare desmoplastic fibromas exhibit aberrant nuclear expression of β-catenin which instead is observed in approximately 70-90% of desmoid-type fibromatoses (Hauben et al. 2005). One third of desmoid-type fibromatoses express estrogen receptor, but ER is not detectable in desmoplastic fibroma (Hauben et al. 2005). Cyclin D1 may also be overexpressed in desmoid-type fibromatoses (especially in cases with nuclear β catenin accumulation), but such overexpression is not detected in desmoplastic fibroma (Hauben et al. 2005). Desmoplastic fibroma should not express MDM2 or CDK4 as is observed in many cases of low grade osteosarcoma.

Fibrosarcoma of bone may show focal or weak reactivity for smooth muscle actin (Folpe et al. 2010). Unlike most osteosarcomas, it does not express osteopontin or osteonectin in tumor matrix, an absence of reactivity that may be diagnostically helpful (Hattinger et al. 2004). In one study, all cases expressed PDF-β protein, PDF-β receptor, and/or PDGF-α receptor (Hattinger et al. 2004). A more recent study confirmed IHC expression of PDGFR-α or PDGFR-β in 71% of cases (12/17) (Niini et al. 2010). This is not a unique finding in fibrosarcoma of bone, as some osteosarcomas, pleomorphic undifferentiated sarcoma, and Ewing sarcoma family of tumors also express PDGF proteins or receptors.

Routine cytogenetics and molecular genetics: Desmoplastic fibroma may show trisomies of chromosomes 8 and or 20 similar to desmoid-type fibromatosis (Bridge et al. 1996; three cases analyzed). It appears to lack mutations of the β-catenin gene, *CTNNB1*, which are detectable in ~50% of desmoid-type fibromatoses (Hauben et al. 2005). A hemizygous deletion of five genes at 11q13 accompanied by der(19)t(11;19)(q13;p13) was recently reported in a tumor arising in the femur of a 20 year old woman (Trombetta et al. 2012).

As with desmoplastic fibroma, only a few studies of the genetics of fibrosarcoma of bone have been published. Thus far, there are no consistent recurrent findings that allow distinction from osteosarcoma or pleomorphic high grade undifferentiated sarcoma of bone. Nine cases analyzed by comparative genomic hybridization (CGH) and selected rtPCR revealed DNA sequence copy number changes in 70% with losses outnumbering gains. The most common changes were gain of 22q (*PDGF-β* gene) and 8q24 (*MYC* gene) both revealed on microarray and rtPCR analysis (Hattinger et al. 2004). A case of FS with a ring chromosome 6 with loss of material distal to 6p25 and 6q14 as the sole abnormality was recently reported (Hallor et al. 2007, karyotyping, FISH and CGH performed). An additional 11 patients with FS of bone assessed by CGH revealed DNA sequence copy number changes in most with some overlap between cases in losses and gains at particular sites. Genes involved at some of the sites included *KIT, PDGFR-α, KDR, IGF1R, CHD1L and CDKN2A* (Niini et al. 2010). Compared with the other studies, this group confirmed losses at 6q and gains at 8q and 22q as more common events (among others). The differences in these studies may be due to slightly different histologic criteria for the diagnosis of FS of bone, differences in methodology and relatively low numbers of analyzed cases. Whether the cases studied had pre-existing factors such as prior irradiation was not indicated in the two series (Hattinger et al. 2004, Niini et al. 2010). It is also possible that FS of bone does not carry a specific recurrent genetic abnormality but shows a mixture of findings with some changes occurring more commonly than others (such as PDGF and PDGFR overexpression and deletion of *CDKN2A*).

RADIOLOGY

Desmoplastic fibroma

Desmoplastic fibroma (DF) is a very rare benign bone tumor occurring in young adults and is comprised of fibroblasts and collagen. The lesion can be locally aggressive and with time, cortical breakthrough can occur. Radiographically, the lesions are commonly in the medullary space of the metaphysis and cause mild bone expansion and cortical thinning (Gebhardt et al. 1985). Classically, DF can show internal trabeculation, septations or struts. This is not a specific appearance, and the differential includes giant cell tumor, fibrous dysplasia and aneurysmal bone cyst. A more aggressive DF could appear similar to a malignant lesion.

In a series of 95 cases of DF radiographs showed coarsened ridge-like trabeculae 63%, cortical breakthrough 53%, and an overall sclerotic margin in 46% (Frick et al. 2005). Approximately 60% involved long bones predominantly in and around the metaphysis, and 61% were centrally located in the long bone. The remaining lesions involved, in descending order, the pelvis, calcaneus, mandible, vertebrae and skull base. MR imaging (only of 14 patients) showed T1 iso-signal or hypointense signal to adjacent muscle in all cases. Eighty-nine percent of cases were predominantly (greater than 75% of the lesion volume) T2 low signal on conventional spin echo sequences. This is an unusual appearance for a lytic lesion which usually would have T2 high signal from fluid or edema in the lytic portion. They report prominent but somewhat heterogeneous enhancement. Unfortunately, we do not have a case of DF to present. Nevertheless, DF should be considered if an expansile metaphyseal lesion with prominent strut like trabeculae is encountered. The presence of T2 low signal within the lytic portion of the lesion suggests fibrous material and would support the diagnosis of DF.

Fibrosarcoma of bone

Secondary fibrosarcoma of bone can be seen with long standing osteomyelitis, fibrous dysplasia, bone infarct, Paget disease, and after radiation therapy among others. On the other hand, primary fibrosarcoma of bone is rare with little imaging literature available. Fibrosarcoma is an aggressive tumor and radiographically will show moth-eaten or permeative bone destruction (Papagelopoulos et al. 2002). MR appearance would likely show T1 isosignal intensity with heterogeneous T2 signal and have intense enhancement. Necrotic areas, would likely show non-enhancement with fluid signal on MR images. Areas with extensive fibrous tissue content would likely appear as T2 low signal.

SURGERY

Desmoplastic fibroma

Because these are nearly always benign tumors with no real potential for metastasis (except in exceptional dedifferentiation cases), conservative surgery is indicated where appropriate. However, similar to desmoid-type fibromatosis, recurrences are frequent and frustrating. Those tumors behaving aggressively or associated with recurrence are better treated with wide resection.

Fibrosarcoma of bone

This tumor represents a sarcoma with metastatic potential and therefore any grade tumor should be treated with wide resection.

MEDICAL ONCOLOGY

Desmoplastic fibroma

This tumor is benign, although could have a tendency to recur if not resected with wide resection. There is no standard medical treatment for recurrent disease.

Fibrosarcoma of bone

Because it is such a rare disease, there are no published chemotherapy studies of fibrosarcoma of bone. By analogy with osteosarcoma, chemotherapy is often offered to patients with Stage IIB and III disease and contains a combination of doxorubicin and cisplatin. Case reports of chemotherapy describe a generally poor prognosis but some clinical benefit in selected cases (Waddell, et al. 1999).

RADIATION ONCOLOGY

Case reports have been published in the literature showing that radiation is effective for patients with desmoplastic fibroma who refuse surgical excision. Radiation therapy is an option for cases in which complete surgical resection is not possible. Doses used for extraskeletal desmoid tumors should be considered for desmoplastic fibroma of bone.

Fibrosarcoma of bone should be treated with complete surgical resection. Similar to other bone tumors, radiation therapy may be considered for palliation or for close/positive margins when further surgery is not an option. Reports in the literature on the use of radiation therapy for fibrosarcoma of bone are rare.

REFERENCES

Abdelwahab IF, Klein MJ, Hermann G, et al. Osteosarcoma arising in a desmoplastic fibroma of the proximal tibia. Am J Roentgenol 2002;178:613–615.

Bahk W-J, Kang Y-K, Lee A-H, et al. Desmoid tumor of bone with enchondromatous nodules, mistaken for chondrosarcoma. Skeletal Radiol 2003;32:223–226.

Bahrami A, Folpe AL. Adult-type fibrosarcoma: A reevaluation of 163 putative cases diagnosed at a single institution over a 48 year period. Am J Surg Pathol 2010;34:1504–13.

Böhm P, Kröber S, Greschniok A, et al. Desmoplastic fibroma of the bone. A report of two patients, review of the literature, and therapeutic implications. Cancer 1996;78(5):1011–1023.

Bridge JA, Meloni AM, Neff JR et al. Deletion 5q in desmoid tumor and fluorescence in situ hybridization for chromosome 8 and/or 20 copy number. Cancer Genetics Cytogenetics 1996;92:150–1.

Callahan KS, Eberhardt SC, Fechner RE, et al. Desmoplastic fibroma of bone with extensive cartilaginous metaplasia. Ann Diag Pathol 2006;10:343–346.

Frick MA, Sundaram M, Unni KK, et al. Imaging findings in desmoplastic fibroma of bone: distinctive T2 characteristics. Am J Roentgenol 2005;184(6):1762–1767.

Gebhardt MC, Campbell CJ, Shiller AL, et al. Desmoplastic fibroma of bone. A report of eight cases and review of the literature. J Bone Joint Surg Am 1985;67(5):732–47.

Hallor KH, Heidenblad M, Brosjo O, et al. Tiling resolution array comparative genomic hybridization analysis of a fibrosarcoma of bone. Cancer Genet Cytogenet 2007;172:80–83.

Hattinger CM, Tarkkanen M, Benini S, et al. Genetic analysis of fibrosarcoma of bone, a rare tumour entity closely related to osteosarcoma and malignant fibrous histiocytoma of bone. Eur J Cell Biol 2004;83:483–491.

Hauben EI, Jundt G, Cleton-Jansen A-M, et al. Desmoplastic fibroma of bone: an immunohistochemical study including β-catenin expression and mutational analysis for β-catenin. Hum Pathol 2005;36:1025–1030.

Huvos AG, Higinbotham NL. Primary fibrosarcoma of bone. A clinicopathologic study of 130 patients. Cancer 1975;35:837–47.

Ikeshima A, Utsonomiya T. Case report of intra-osseous fibroma: a study on odontogenic and desmoplastic fibromas with a review of the literature. J Oral Sci 2005;47:149–157.
Mavrogenis AF, Pala E, Guerra G, et al. Post-radiation sarcomas. Clinical outcome of 52 patients. J Surg Onc 2012;105:570–6.
Min HS, Kang HG, Lee J-H, et al. Desmoplastic fibroma with malignant transformation. Ann Diag Pathol 2010;14:50–55.
Ng TL, Gown AM, Barry TS, et al. Nuclear β-catenin in mesenchymal tumors. Mod Pathol 2005;18:68–74.
Niini T, Lopez-Guerrero JA, Ninomiya S, et al. Frequent deletion of CDKN2A and recurrent coamplification of KIT, PDGFRA, and KDR in fibrosarcoma of bone – an array comparative genomic hybridization study. Genes Chromosomes Cancer 2010;49:132–143.
Papagelopoulos PJ, Galanis E, Frassica FJ, et al. Primary fibrosarcoma of bone. Outcome after primary surgical treatment. Clinl Ortho Rel Res 2000;373: 88–103.
Papagelopoulos PJ, Galanis EC, Trantafyllidis P, et al. Clinicopathologic features, diagnosis, and treatment of fibrosarcoma of bone. Am J Ortho 2002;31:253–7.
Picci P, Sieberova G, Alberghini M, et al. Late sarcoma development after curettage and bone grafting of benign bone tumors. Eur J Radiol 2011;77:19–25.
Rastogi S, Varshney MK, Trikha V, et al. Desmplastic fibroma: a report of three cases at unusual locations. Joint Bone Spine 2008;75:222–225.
Sharma H, Mehdi SA, MacDuff E, et al. Paget sarcoma of the spine: Scottish Bone Tumor Registry experience. Spine 2006;31:1344–50.
Sopta J, Dordevic A, Tulic G, Mijucic V. Dedifferentiated chondrosarcoma: our clinicopathological experience and dilemmas in 25 cases. J Can Res Clin Onco 2008;134:147–52.
Staals EL, Bacchini P, Mercuri M, Bertoni F. Dedifferentiated chondrosarcomas arising in preexisting osteochondromas. J Bone Joint Surg Am 2007;89:987–93.
Takazawa K, Tsuchiya H, Yamamoto N, et al. Osteosarcoma arising from desmoplastic fibroma treated 16 years earlier: a case report. J Ortho Sci 2003;8:864–868.
Trombetta D, Macchia G, Mandahl N, et al. Molecular genetic characterization of the 11q13 breakpoint in a desmoplastic fibroma of bone. Cancer Genetics 2012;205:410–413.
Vargas-Gonzalez R, San Martin-Brieke W, Gil-Orduna C, et al. Desmoplastic fibroma-like tumor of maxillofacial region associated with tuberous sclerosis. Pathol Onco Res 2004;10:237–239.
Waddell AE, Davis AM, Ahn H, et al. Doxorubicin-cisplatin chemotherapy for high-grade nonosteogenic sarcoma of bone. Comparison of treatment and control groups. Can J Surg 1999;42:190–9.

FURTHER READING

Folpe AL, Inwards CY (Eds). Bone and Soft Tissue Pathology. A volume in the series: Foundations in Diagnostic Pathology. Goldblum JR (series ed). Philadelphia: Elsevier Saunders, 2010.
Fletcher CDM, Krishnan Unni K, Mertens F (Eds). World Health Organization Classification of Tumours. Pathology and Genetics Tumours of Soft Tissue and Bone. Lyon: IARC Press, 2013.

Chapter 19 'Fibrohistiocytic' tumors of bone

OVERVIEW

This frail category of tumors was trimmed in the 2013 World Health Organization (WHO) classification of bone tumors analogous to reductions in the WHO classification of 'fibrohistiocytic' tumors of soft tissue. The problem lies with the name which naturally suggests that the lesions in this group are composed of fibrohistiocytes. Unfortunately, no such cell is known to exist (see Chapter 7 for more detail about the nomenclature history of 'fibrohistiocytic' tumors). Despite the name handicap, the category is retained to include one tumor: non-ossifying fibroma/benign fibrous histiocytoma of bone. Although excised from this category, undifferentiated pleomorphic sarcoma of bone is also described in this chapter as it is still referred to as 'malignant fibrous histiocytoma' by some clinicians and researchers. The 2013 WHO classification of bone tumors lists undifferentiated pleomorphic high grade sarcoma as a type of miscellaneous bone tumor.

Figure 19.1 illustrates the possible origins of pleomorphic undifferentiated high grade sarcoma , formerly known as 'malignant fibrous histiocytoma', both those primary to the bone and those primary to soft tissue.

CLASSIFICATION

Non-ossifying fibroma (NOF) is currently considered by some experts to be a reactive process rather than a monoclonal neoplasm. It is histologically identical to benign fibrous histiocytoma of bone. The latter differs from NOF in that it is extremely rare, occurs in unusual bone sites such as flat bones as well as the long bones, is non-metaphyseal, and it almost always affects older patients. Some expert pathologists question the existence of benign fibrous histiocytoma of bone and contend that it may represent an involuted giant cell tumor of bone or a reactive process.

Table 19.1 comprises the current WHO classification of 'fibrohistiocytic' tumors of bone. More common synonyms are included.

DEMOGRAPHICS

Non-ossifying fibroma

This lesion is confined to the pediatric age group with most patients in the age range of 5–20 years. It is common and often undiagnosed, as small lesions tend to be asymptomatic. Perhaps 35% of children harbor NOFs (Nielsen et al. 2013).

Benign fibrous histiocytoma

An extremely rare tumor that may occur slightly more commonly in women than men. In nearly all cases the patients are adults. All bones may be affected including the axial skeleton. Location is non-metaphyseal.

Undifferentiated high grade pleomorphic sarcoma of bone

This tumor may affect a broad age of patients, but most are older than 50 years. Approximately 15% develop in the setting of radiation therapy (range of 2–14 years later) (Huvos et al. 1986), bone infarct, metallic implant or Paget's disease (Dorfman et al. 1998).

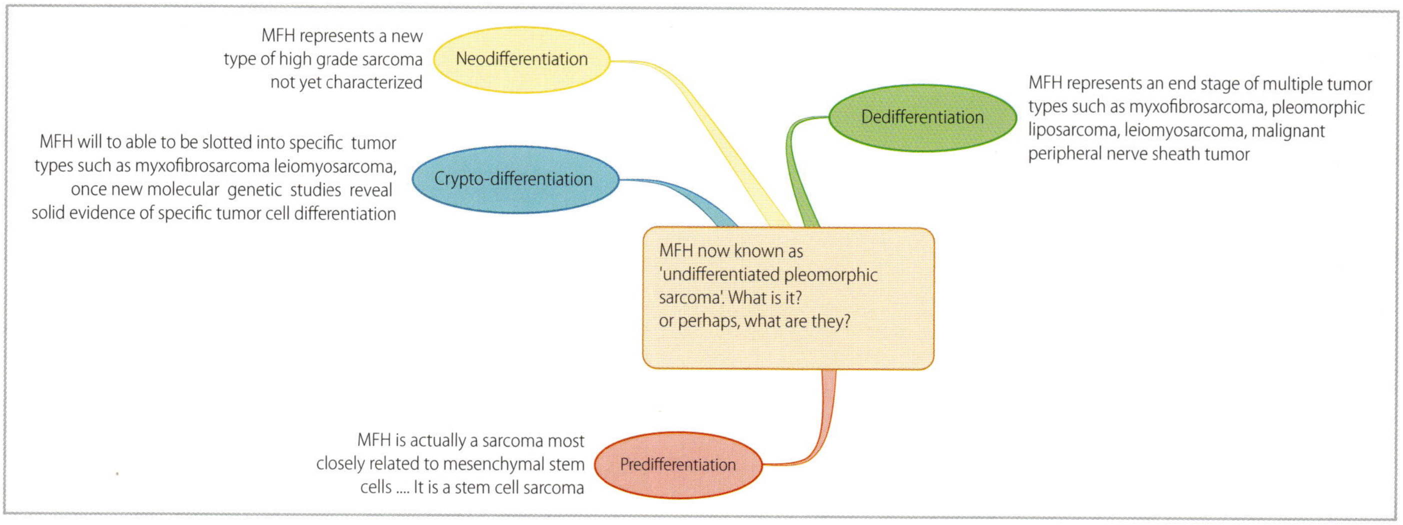

Figure 19.1 Malignant fibrous histiocytoma (MFH) differentiation theories. More than one may be found to be correct as MFH'may encompass multiple different tumors. Thus far, dedifferentiation is the most supported theory that will most likely explain most examples.

Table 19.1 WHO classification of 'fibrohistiocytic' tumors of bone and non-ossifying fibroma (2013)

Tumor or lesion	Behavior	Additional comments
Non-ossifying fibroma (NOF, fibrous cortical defect, metaphyseal fibrous defect)/ benign fibrous histiocytoma (BFH, fibroxanthomas, fibrous xanthoma, xanthofibroma, xanthogranuloma)	Benign	The lesion is called 'fibrous cortical defect' or 'metaphyseal fibrous defect' if it is small. NOF may not be a neoplasm but could represent a reparative response that sometimes occurs during excessive metaphyseal remodeling in long bone development BFH is microscopically identical to NOF but occurs usually in older adults and in non-metaphyseal locations. Also unusual bone sites such as flat bones and pelvic bones may be involved. Some tumors contain abundant foamy macrophages and have been called variations of names referring to the reactive xanthomatous histiocyte component
'Malignant fibrous histiocytoma' now termed 'Undifferentiated high-grade pleomorphic sarcoma of bone'	Malignant	This tumor is renamed to indicate that it is *not* a fibrohistiocytic differentiated tumor but an undifferentiated sarcoma. The renaming of this tumor has also occurred in the classification of soft tissue tumors. The 2013 WHO classification places it in the group, 'Miscellaneous tumors' of bone

Benign: does not recur or recurs non-aggressiveliy and does not metastasize. Intermediate: can recur aggressively and/or rarely metastasizes (<5%). Malignant: can recur and commonly metastasizes

PATHOGENESIS

Non-ossifying fibroma

This lesion is conjectured to represent a common developmental defect that appears when long bone metaphyses are remodeled. A fibrous cortical defect is seen in up to 30% of individuals with unfused growth plates (Dorfman et al. 1998). This percentage approaches the frequency of fibrocystic changes in the adult female breast (the commonality of which led to the revision of the entity's name from fibrocystic 'disease' to fibrocystic 'change').

Not uncommonly, multiple sites in one bone or in multiple bones may be affected. A rare syndrome, Jaffe-Campanacci syndrome, is defined by multifocal non-ossifying fibromas, café au lait spots and mental retardation. There may be some overlap of Jaffe-Campanacci syndrome with Type 1 neurofibromatosis (Colby et al. 2003).

Only rare non-ossifying fibromas have been examined genetically. Three reports cite clonal abnormalities which differ from each other in findings (Brassesco et al. 2010). In addition to being characteristic of neoplasms, clonal abnormalities may occasionally be seen in non-neoplastic tissue and as an artifact of long term cell culture. Further study of additional cases would be informative to determine if indeed non-ossifying fibroma actually is a lesion of characteristic genetic abnormalities.

Benign fibrous histiocytoma

As noted previously, this is an extremely rare lesion that is histologically identical to non-ossifying fibroma. It can also mimic involutional changes in giant cell tumor of bone, and many cases of benign fibrous histiocytoma may actually represent completely involuted giant cell tumors with no residual giant cell tumor left for evaluation. Obviously, in a case without residual giant cell tumor, it is difficult to prove such a relationship.

Undifferentiated high-grade pleomorphic sarcoma of bone

Approximately 20% of these tumors arise in the setting of pre-existing alteration to the bone such as with radiation therapy, bone infarct, metallic implant, or Paget's disease (see Chapter 17). These four antecedents are associated with a variably chronic stimulatory effect on mesenchymal cells that in a few patients may lead to the growth of a clone of malignant cells. There are no known specific factors predisposing to the development of the 80% of undifferentiated high-grade pleomorphic sarcoma of bone that are not associated with radiation, infarct, implant or Paget's disease. At least 90% of cases disclose a complex aneuploid karyotype with multiple gains and losses of whole chromosomes and chromosome regions; the most common sites of gains and losses are also seen in osteosarcoma and fibrosarcoma of bone (Tarkkanen et al. 2006).

PATHOLOGY

Table 19.2 lists the fibrohistiocytic tumors of bone with incidence data and histology features including representative photomicrographs of the lesions.

Histologic grading

Non-ossifying fibroma

This lesion is not graded, as it is benign and considered possibly a reactive process. However, uncommonly, it can feature scattered, slightly atypical spindle cells with nuclear enlargement and nucleoli. Additionally, necrosis can occur, most likely secondary to pathologic fracture. However, marked nuclear pleomorphism and atypical mitotic figures are absent.

Benign fibrous histiocytoma of bone

This is a low grade lesion of spindle cells arrayed in a cartwheel or basket-weave arrangement (storiform growth) with intermixed inflammatory cells. The inflammatory cells may exceed the number of spindle cells and can include xanthomatous macrophages. When the xanthoma cells predominate, the tumor has been termed: xanthofibroma, fibroxanthoma, and fibrous xanthoma, among others. Non-ossifying fibromas with similar heavy infiltrates of xanthomatous macrophages can also be given these alternative names of which all represent slightly different appearances of the same entity. Benign fibrous histiocytoma does not exhibit marked cytologic pleomorphism, and mitotic figures are of normal configuration.

Undifferentiated high-grade pleomorphic sarcoma of bone

Similar to the benign fibrous histiocytoma, this tumor comprises a storiform arrangement of spindle cells. However, the tumor cells exhibit marked nuclear pleomorphism (which includes coarse granular chromatin, irregularly distributed chromatin, and irregularly shaped hyperchromatic or vesicular nuclei with prominent, sometimes misshapen nucleoli), and some cells may lose the spindle shape and appear more polygonal. Often dispersed throughout the tumor are multinucleated tumor cells (osteoclasts can also be present but are easily distinguished from the markedly abnormal tumor giant cells). Necrosis, both geographic and affecting individual cells, and mitotic activity are prominent. Atypical mitotic figures are also common.

Lesion behavior

Non-ossifying fibroma (fibrous cortical defect, metaphyseal fibrous defect):

This is a benign lesion. It may result in pathologic fracture.

Table 19.2 Fibrohistiocytic tumors/lesions of bone (the current WHO classification combines NOF and BFH and eliminates the term 'malignant fibrous histiocytoma of bone'. This tumor is now called undifferentiated high-grade pleomorphic sarcoma of bone' and is considered a 'miscellaneous tumor of bone' by the 2013 WHO classification)

Tumor or lesion	Incidence	Age and sex distribution	Most common body site (in order of occurrence)	Histopathology description including IHC: Medium magnification	Histopathology description including IHC: High magnification
Benign: does not recur or recurs non-aggressively and does not metastasize					
Non-ossifying fibroma (fibrous cortical defect, metaphyseal fibrous defect)	Common	5–20 years Male > female Does not occur in adults	Metaphysis of: distal femur, proximal tibia, distal tibia. Less common in proximal humerus, distal radius	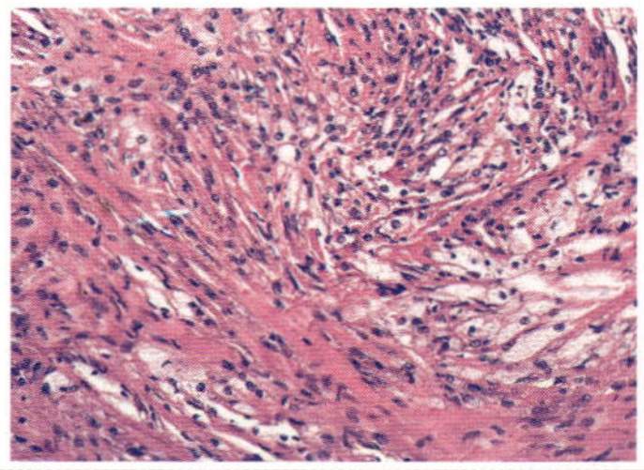	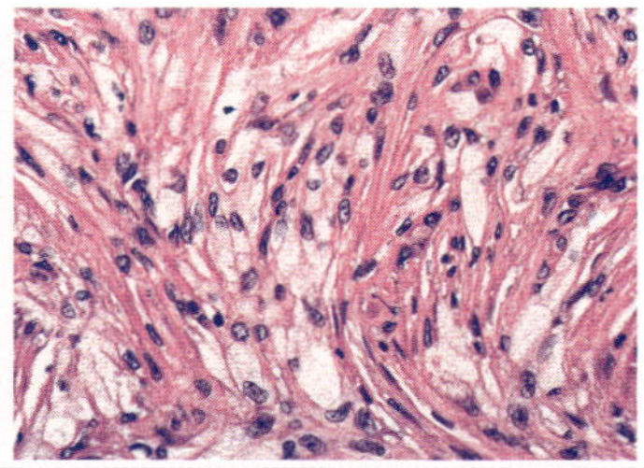
Storiforming spindle cell lesion with intermixed inflammatory cells and often reactive woven bone spicules. May have slight cytologic atypia and mitoses with hemorrhage, osteoclasts and hemosiderin. Spindle cells may be smooth muscle actin positive; usually desmin negative.					
Benign fibrous histiocytoma of bone (xanthoma, xanthofibroma, fibrous xanthoma of bone)	Rare	Adults; rarely children	Ilium, ribs, central intramedullary lesion of diaphysis of long bones	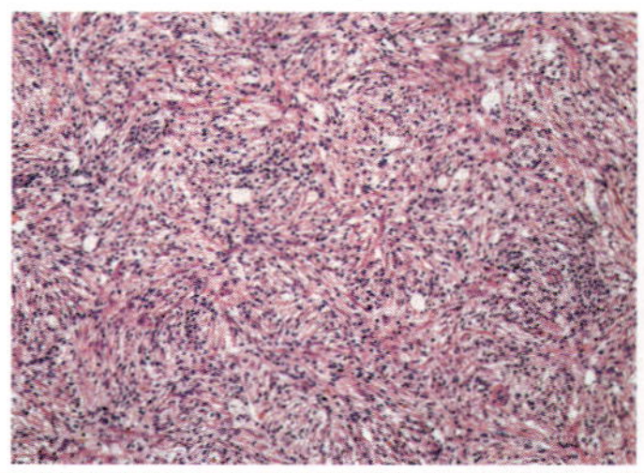	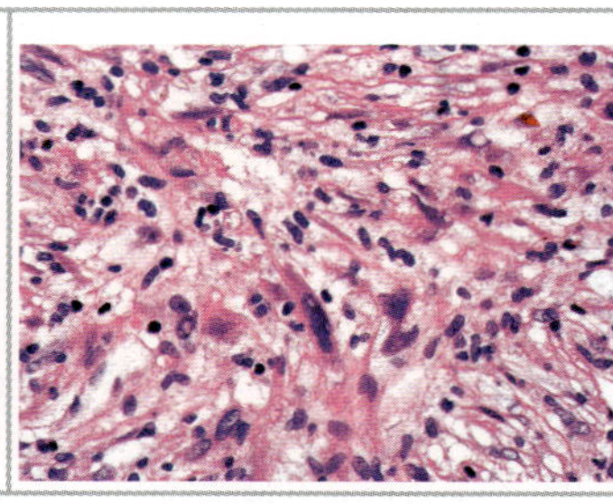
Looks identical to Non-ossifying fibroma. Some cases have marked infiltrates of foamy macrophages (xanthoma cells or xanthomatous macrophages). IHC as for non-ossifying fibroma.					
Malignant: can recur and commonly metastasizes					
'Malignant fibrous histiocytoma' of bone = Undifferentiated high grade pleomorphic sarcoma of bone	Rare	Mostly older adults. Some young adults are post-radiation therapy for pediatric bone sarcomas	Femur, ilium, tibia, humerus. Metaphysis more common than diaphysis	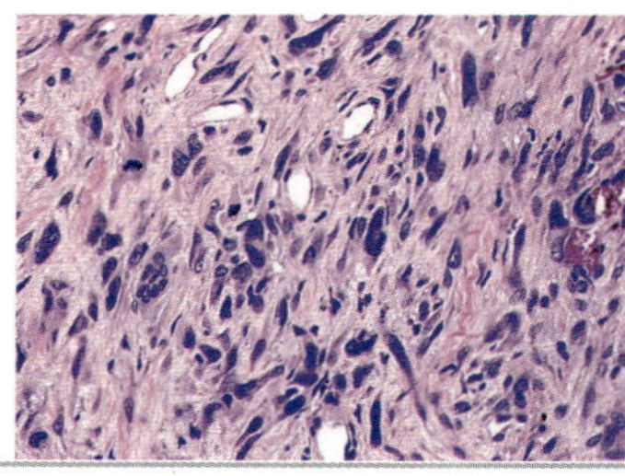	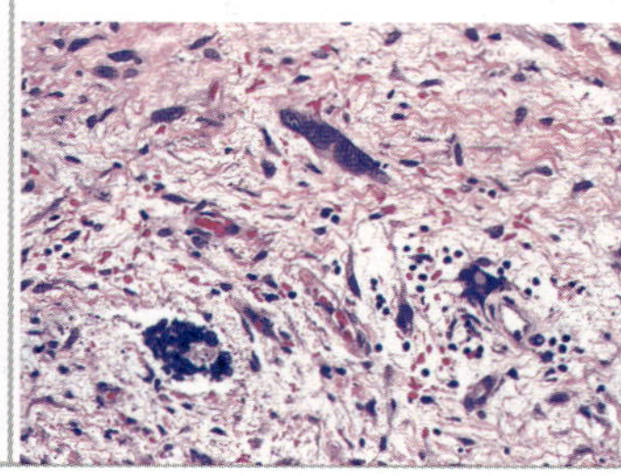
Often storiforming pattern of spindle cells and pleomorphic polygonal cells with tumor giant cells, necrosis, hemorrhage, and often many mitoses, some atypical. Looks identical to 'MFH' of soft tissue, pleomorphic type. IHC is negative for specific differentiation. No malignant bone.					
Incidence Note: 'Common to very common' indicates that a medium sized practice will treat at least several to dozens of patients with the lesion annually, 'Uncommon to rare' indicates the same practice size will treat one to two patients with the lesion every five years, 'Rare to very rare' indicates the same sized practice will see zero to one patient with the lesion every 20 years.					

Benign fibrous histiocytoma

This is a benign lesion that does not recur.

Undifferentiatd high-grade pleomorphic sarcoma of bone

This high grade sarcoma behaves similarly to adult conventional osteosarcoma. The five year survival rate is approximately 60% after resection and chemotherapy (Jeon et al. 2011).

RADIOLOGY

The radiology literature has interchangeable terms for non-ossifying fibroma, fibrous cortical defect, fibrous histiocytoma and fibroxanthoma. Typically, the lesions larger than 3 cm are called non-ossifying fibroma, while the smaller lesions are designated fibrous cortical defect. The appearances are similar with radiographs showing a lucent, eccentric, metaphyseal lesion with mild scalloping and ridges evident. There is no periosteal reaction and no appreciable matrix, although these lesions tend to heal over time with sclerotic and then isodense filling in. The radiographic appearance is usually diagnostic, and cross sectional imaging is not typically needed. The MR appearance in fact may lend confusion due to the heterogeneous signal of a non-ossifying fibroma. Occasionally, cross sectional imaging may be helpful to confirm the presence of a pathologic fracture.

Undifferentiated high-grade pleomorphic sarcoma of bone (previously termed 'malignant fibrous histiocytoma' of bone) is a very rare tumor. Imaging is nonspecific but shows an aggressive, destructive lesion. There is heterogeneous signal and heterogeneous enhancement.

SURGERY

Non-ossifying fibroma

Non-ossifying fibromas represent a self-limited neoplasm. The overwhelming majority are asymptomatic in the absence of pathologic fracture. All will resolve after skeletal maturity. Indications for surgical intervention include: (1) prior pathologic fracture, (2) predicted high risk of impending pathologic fracture, and (3) persistent pain in the absence of fracture or impending fracture. Treatment consists of curettage and bone grafting.

GRAY AREA

Predicting risk of pathologic fracture is difficult in these lesions. Small non-ossifying fibromas occasionally present with fracture while many large ones do not. Suggestion has been made for operative intervention in those lesions which occupy > 50% of the transverse diameter of the bone on both anteroposterior and lateral radiographs and those longer than 33 mm in the weight-bearing bones (femur and tibia) (Arata et al. 1981). Others have found this method unreliable (Easley and Kneisl 1997).

Pathologic fractures, when they occur, are rarely displaced. The fracture will heal with closed treatment, but the non-ossifying fibroma will rarely resolve, and therefore the risk of future fracture is not mitigated. For non-displaced fractures, allowing the fracture to heal prior to curettage facilitates an easier procedure without the need for internal fixation.

Recurrence after curettage is unusual but is directly related to the degree of skeletal maturity. Young children may exhibit a higher recurrence rate whereas those near skeletal maturity will rarely recur.

Undifferentiated high-grade pleomorphic sarcoma of bone

The treatment of this high grade sarcoma mimics that of osteosarcoma with a similar response rate. Wide surgical resection along with chemotherapy is indicated.

MEDICAL ONCOLOGY

These tumors may arise de novo or secondary to previous irradiation (Huvos et al. 1986), benign bone lesions such as giant cell tumor, fibrous dysplasia, Paget's disease, bone infarcts or cysts, or even osteomyelitis. Without chemotherapy, most patients develop metastatic disease to the lungs within 2 years, but lymph node metastases are not uncommon (Spanier et al. 1975). After pathologic diagnosis on a biopsy, treatment is analogous to the one of osteosarcoma with pre and post-surgical chemotherapy administration (See Chapter 17). Undifferentiated high-grade pleomorphic sarcoma of bone originating from the bones seems to be more sensitive to chemotherapy than the ones originating from soft tissue, which are much more common. Because of the known lymph node metastatic potential, lymphadenectomy, or perhaps a sentinel lymph node dissection, should be done at the time of surgical excision.

Neoadjuvant chemotherapy helps salvage limbs in up to 90% of patients (Bacci et al. 1998). Ninety percent or greater of tumor necrosis is observed in a quarter of the patients and linked to improved disease free survival. More than half the patients remain alive at 5 years.

In a European registry of 125 patients, there were 74 male, 51 female with a median age of 34 years (Bielack et al. 1999). The tumor originated in the long bones in all patients but 6. Chemotherapy was used in about 80% of patients. A third of the patients relapsed. The 5-year disease-free survival was above 50%. About one third of patients had a favorable response to preoperative chemotherapy with greater than 90% necrosis, among these, only one patient relapsed. Chemotherapy regimens involved a doxorubicin based combination with ifosfamide and/or cisplatin. The combination of doxorubicin and cisplatin was formally tested in an EORTC clinical study recruiting 41 patients. The regimen consisted of doxorubicin 25 $mg/m^2/d$ on days 1 through 3 and cisplatin 100 mg/m^2 by 4-hour intravenous infusion on day 1 every 3 weeks for six cycles. Patients had to be chemotherapy naïve and have measurable disease in the primary or metastatic setting. Surgery was offered to operable patients. The study confirmed a limb salvage rate of 80% in this mixed population, with a 42% rate of tumor necrosis greater than 90%, and a 5-year survival rate of 59% (Bramwell et al. 1999).

RADIATION ONCOLOGY

Clinically, many institutions treat these as they would treat an adult osteosarcoma. However, the optimal treatment of these lesions has not been defined. One of the largest studies performed was a retrospective survey of the European Musculoskeletal Oncologic Society, which reviewed 125 cases. Of these cases, fifteen selectively received radiation therapy with a local control rate of 93% (14/15). Local control without radiation therapy was 95% (104/110) (Bielack et al. 1999). It is unclear whether there is a role for radiation therapy in the management. However, there may be a role in cases where good surgical margins cannot be obtained. In these cases, adjuvant radiation therapy may result in local control rates similar to patients with wide margins. Clearly, control of distant disease is the issue with this particular cancer. Of interest, prior radiation appears to be a risk factor for development of this malignancy. Huvos, et al., found that 15% (20/130) of undifferentiated high-grade pleomorphic sarcomas of bone at their institution were radiation induced.

CASES

Case 19.1 Non-ossifying fibroma

Clinical history and presentation

The patient is a 15-year-old boy who presents with a one year history of lateral leg pain. Pain occurs with activity. He denies rest or night pain.

Physical examination reveals mild tenderness on palpation over the proximal fibular diaphysis. No soft tissue swelling or mass is identified.

Due to the painful nature of the lesion and its potential risk for pathologic fracture, surgery is offered as an option to the family. The family agrees to proceed as the boy wishes to participate in athletics.

Surgical findings and comments

Surgical exploration reveals thinned cortical bone containing a rust colored neoplasm within the bone. Curettage and allograft packing are performed.

Radiology findings

Case figs 19.1a and **19.1b** show a lucent scalloped lesion without identifiable matrix. The margins are sharply defined and sclerotic. This indicates a non-aggressive lesion. The cortical thinning is modest without periosteal reaction or breakthrough. MRI images **Case figs 19.1c** and **19.1d** show uniform T1 low signal and a margin of high signal on STIR.

Typically, the radiographic appearance is characteristic and no further diagnostic imaging is needed. Occasionally, surveillance radiographs at 6–12 month intervals can be reassuring in equivocal cases or to monitor for risk of pathologic stress fracture. These follow-up films should show slow sclerotic and then isodense healing and filling in of the lesion, until it disappears. MR usually is not needed but can confirm there is no soft tissue component or occult fracture.

Refer also to **Case figs 19.1e** through **19.1l** for other examples of patients with non-ossifying fibromas.

Pathology findings

Gross features

The specimen comprises irregular fragments of bone and hemorrhagic tan soft tissue. It is entirely submitted for microscopic review in four cassettes.

Microscopic features

Low magnification: Sections reveal a cellular lesion without necrosis but with foci of hemorrhage (**Case fig. 19.1m**).

High magnification: Medium magnification demonstrates swirls of spindle cells with a collagenous background (**Case fig.19.1n**) or with areas of new bone formation (**Case fig. 19.1o**). Bone spicule surfaces are covered by osteoblasts. The swirls of spindle cells feature interspersed osteoclast-like giant cells (**Case fig. 19.1p**) and also contain sprinkles of lymphocytes (**Case fig. 19.1q**). Pathology terms used to describe these short, broad intercalating fascicles are 'storiform' or 'basket-weave' pattern. The lesion contains multiple cell types including spindle cells, osteoclasts, osteoblasts rimming new bone, lymphocytes and xanthomatous (foamy) macrophages (**Case fig. 19.1r**). There is no cytologic atypia, and a few mitoses are found in the spindle cells, but none are atypical.

Special studies: No special studies are performed because the lesion is histologically classic and consistent with the patient's clinical history and imaging findings.

Pathologic differential or, why isn't it one of the following?

Giant cell tumor of bone (GCT): Reparative areas can be seen in giant cell tumor of bone that looks identical to non-ossifying fibroma (NOF). This should not be surprising, as many experts believe that non-ossifying fibroma is not actually a monoclonal neoplasm but a reactive process that occurs in some individuals during bone growth that can resemble other reactive processes. Both giant cell tumor of bone and non-ossifying fibroma contain osteoclastic giant cells and commonly feature reactive bone. However, giant cell tumor of bone should have diagnostic areas that comprise evenly distributed, often abnormally large osteoclasts set in a bed of mononuclear ovoid or spindle cells with nuclear features similar to the nuclei in the giant cells. These mononuclear cells usually express p63 (evaluated by immunohistochemistry). Furthermore, non-ossifying fibroma occurs in the metaphysis or diaphysis and does not involve the epiphysis: giant cell tumor of bone almost always shows at least some involvement of the epiphysis. Patients with NOF are usually under the age of 20 years; GCT of bone rarely occurs in an immature

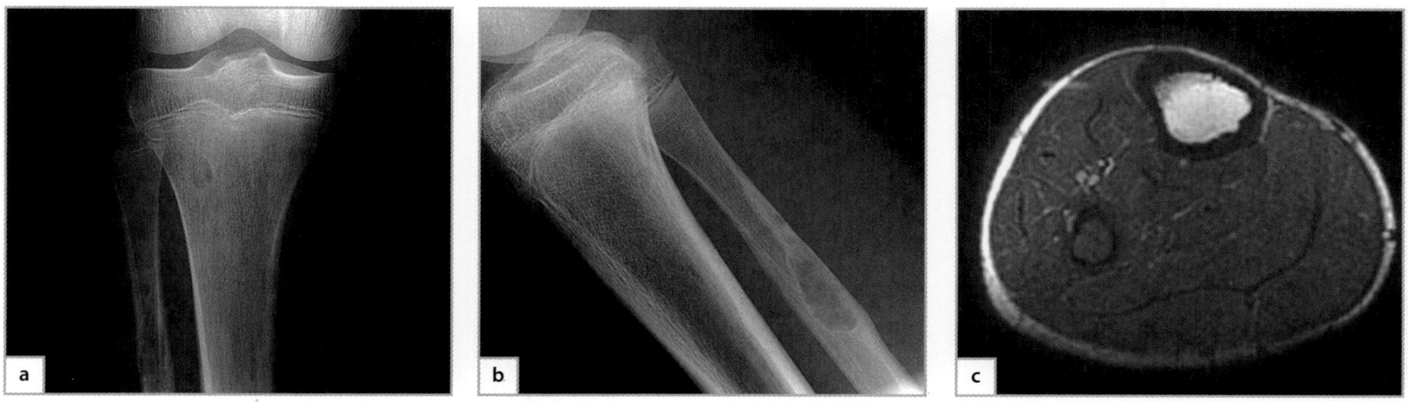

Case figure 19.1 Non-ossifying fibroma. 19.1a: Anteroposterior knee radiograph, **19.1b**: Lateral knee radiograph. **19.1c**: Axial T1 MR image.

Case figure 19.1: Continued from page 456

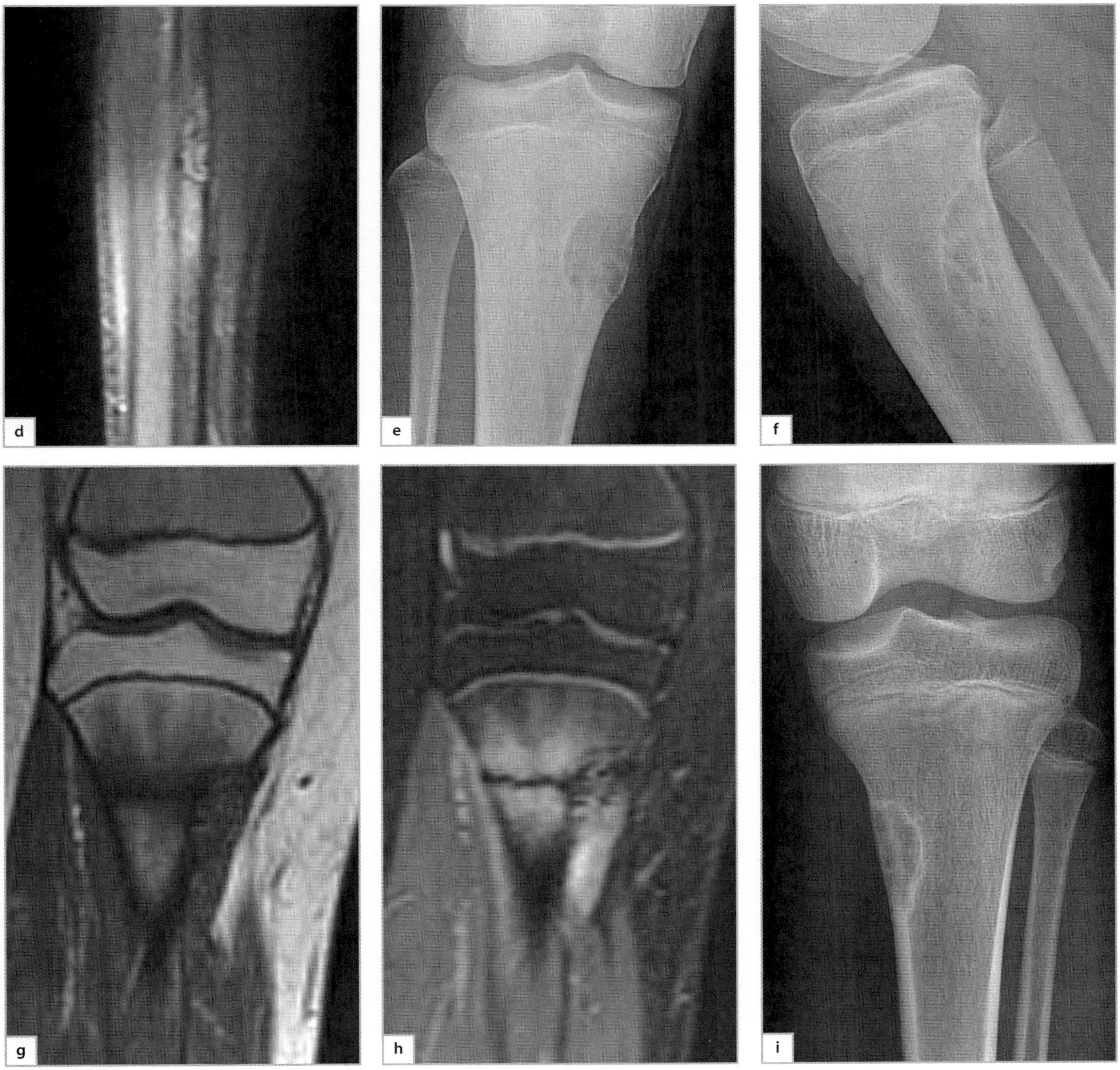

19.1d: Sagittal STIR MR image. This patient has two non-ossifying fibromas (NOF) involving the proximal tibial metaphysis and the proximal fibular diaphysis. The fibular NOF shows the characteristic eccentric, lucent lesion with mild cortical expansion and scalloped well defined margins. MRI appearance shows T1 low signal and modest STIR increased signal along the margin. See also 19.1e through 19.1l for three additional cases of non-ossifying fibroma. **19.1e**: Antero-posterior and **19.1f**: Lateral radiograph of the knee. **19.1g**: Coronal T1 MR image. **19.1h**: Coronal STIR MR image. This proximal tibial NOF has a pathologic fracture best seen with MR imaging. Note the expanded cortex has uniform mild cortical thinning. **19.1i**: antero-posterior. **19.1j**: Lateral close-up radiographs of the tibia and fibula. Note the sclerotic margin with uniform thickness and gentle scalloped contour of the proximal tibial metaphyseal lesion. **19.1k**: Antero-posterior and **19.1l**: Lateral radiographs of the knee. This femoral NOF shows healing sclerotic healing of the superior aspect of the lesion. This will eventually show radiographic isodense fill in and disappear. **19.1m**: Non-ossifying fibroma at low magnification. The lesion is hypercellular without necrosis. **19.1n**: Non-ossifying fibroma at medium magnification. This area is more collagenized imparting an eosinophilic hue. Tumor cells whirl in a basket-weave or 'storiform' pattern typically of this lesion and BFH. **19.1o**: Non-ossifying fibroma at medium magnification. Despite its name, new bone formation is not uncommon in non-ossifying fibromas, especially in cases with secondary pathologic fracture. In this field, osteoblasts rim the bone spicules, a reassuring feature usually consistent with reactive rather than malignant bone formation.

Case figure 19.1: Continued from page 457

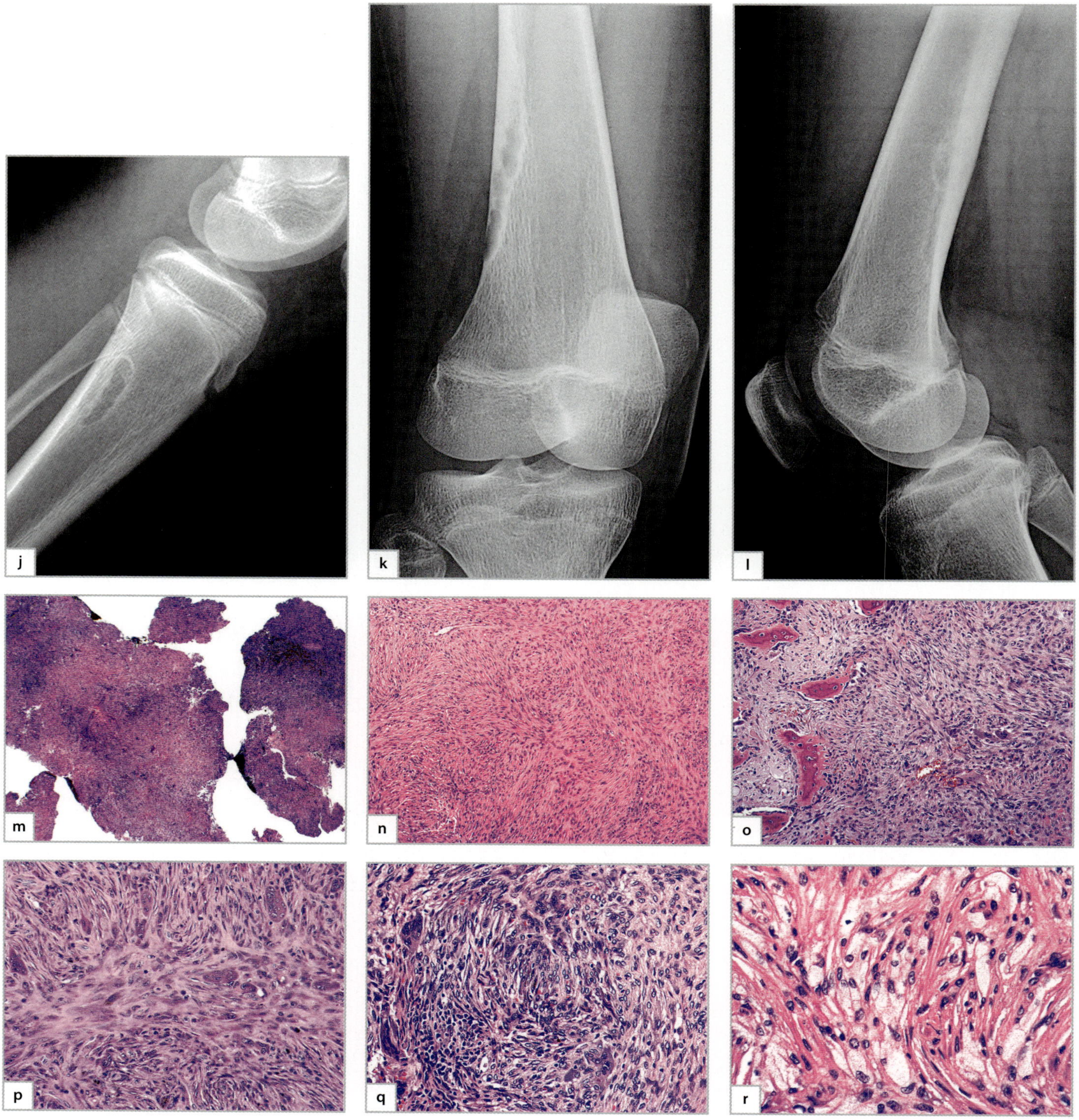

19.1p: Non-ossifying fibroma at higher magnification. The storiforming arrangement of lesional spindle cells is accentuated in this area. Synonyms for storiform include 'cartwheel' or 'basket-weave' pattern and all describe the architecture formed by intercalating thick, short streams of spindle cells. **19.1q**: Non-ossifying fibroma, medium magnification. Notice the interspersed osteoclasts and small dark lymphocytes among the plump spindle cells. **19.1r**: Non-ossifying fibroma, high magnification. The streaming spindle cells, most likely closely related to fibroblasts, feature pale, cytologically bland nuclei and inconspicuous cell borders. Mixed among the spindle cells are pale round, foamy macrophages. These reactive cells (also called xanthomatous macrophages) can accrue in large numbers in NOF.

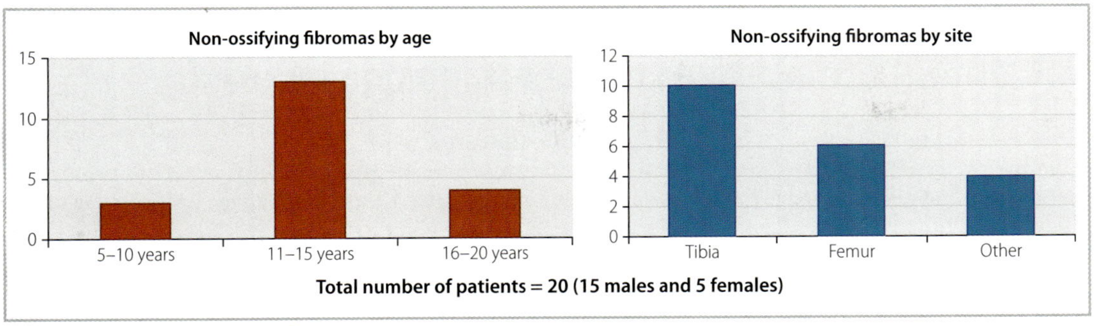

Chart 19.1: Non-ossifying fibromas resected at University of New Mexico 2000–2010. Total number of patients = 20 (15 males and 5 females).

bone before the epiphysis closes. Although usually not necessary, genetic evaluation can prove useful, as most GCT (especially those located in the long bones) show telomeric associations (end to end fusion of whole chromosomes). Sporadic, non-ossifying fibroma is not associated with any specific genetic abnormalities.

Solid type aneurysmal bone cyst (solid ABC): The solid type of ABC may be confused histologically with non-ossifying fibroma because both contain a mixture of spindle cells and inflammatory cells and often contain woven bone. Areas of hemorrhage can be present in both. A storiform growth pattern is more prominent in non-ossifying fibroma. Patient age range and site in the skeleton overlap. However, most primary ABC feature fusions of the *USP6* gene, so genetic evaluation can be diagnostically helpful. In practice, radiologic features enable distinction of the two entities.

Brown tumor of hyperparathyroidism: This lesion looks identical to giant cell reparative granuloma which in turn looks identical to solid type ABC. NOF usually features a more distinctly storiform architecture. Moreover, clinical history, serological studies and radiologic examinations should distinguish the two lesions.

Fibrous dysplasia (FD): Occasional cases of NOF may contain extensive reactive new bone and mimic superficially fibrous dysplasia. However, the new bone of non-ossifying fibroma often features many rimming osteoblasts unlike most of the woven bone in fibrous dysplasia, and osteoclasts are usually present unlike most cases of FD. Radiologic features also help to differentiate the two lesions.

Case table 19.1 Summary pathology findings of Case 19.1

Diagnosis	Non-ossifying fibroma (fibrous cortical defect)
Size	3 × 3 × 2 cm
Location	Proximal diaphysis of fibula
Margin status	Not applicable; lesion is curetted
Histologic grade	Not applicable; this is a benign lesion
Pathologic stage	Not applicable; this is a benign lesion

Chart 19.1 provides the bone location and patient age of twenty non-ossifying fibromas curetted at UNM from 2000–2010. These findings are consistent with those reported in the literature: patients are under age 20 years, and most occur in the tibia or femur.

Oncology approach

Medical oncology

This is a benign lesion with no role for adjuvant therapy.

Radiation oncology

There is no role for radiation in the treatment of non-ossifying fibroma, a benign tumor.

Patient outcome

The patient has had no recurrence six years after the procedure.

Case 19.2 Undifferentiated high grade pleomorphic sarcoma, radiation-induced (malignant fibrous histiocytoma of bone, radiation induced)

Clinical history and presentation

The patient is a 24-year-old female with a history of Ewing's sarcoma of the right ilium treated with chemotherapy and radiation at age 13. One year prior to presentation she developed chronic osteomyelitis in the irradiated bone, confirmed by biopsy and cultures, for which she had been unsuccessfully treated. She subsequently develops increasing pain, and imaging studies reveal increased bone destruction and a large associated soft tissue mass.

Physical examination reveals a chronic sinus draining purulent fluid and a large soft tissue mass surrounding the ilium.

Staging CT scan of the thorax discloses multiple bilateral pulmonary nodules.

Surgical findings and comments

Malignant fibrous histiocytoma of bone

Open biopsy of the lesion proves consistent with undifferentiated high-grade pleomorphic sarcoma of bone ('malignant fibrous histiocytoma' of bone that is radiation induced).

Radiology findings

Case figs 19.2a through **19.2e** show an aggressive, destructive and expansile mass of the right hemipelvis. There is a large soft tissue tumor component extending into the pelvis and into the gluteal muscles. The CT image, **Case fig. 19.2f** shows the permeative destruction of bone. The lesion appears to originate in bone and expands out into the soft tissues. The presence of hip effusion suggests there may be tumor invasion of the joint. There are cystic areas showing fluid-fluid levels and large areas of non-enhancing tissues which may represent necrosis or matrix. None of the imaging appearance is specific; the radiologist can only identify location and extent of the lesion and affirm its highly aggressive behavior.

Pathology findings

Gross features

The biopsy specimen comprises multiple fragments of hemorrhagic pink soft tissue aggregating to 2.8 cm in maximum dimension. A portion is submitted fresh to Cytogenetics.

Microscopic features

Low magnification: The specimen contains areas of necrotic soft tissue and bone intermixed with hemorrhage and cellular tumor (**Case fig. 19.2g**).

High magnification: Medium magnification of the viable tumor consists of streaming spindle to polygonal cells with intermixed inflammation (**Case fig. 19.2h**). Markedly pleomorphic tumor cells are appreciated at high magnification, and mitoses are numerous (**Case fig. 19.2i**).

Special studies: The karyotype is clonal and triploid with complex numerical and structural abnormalities including whole chromosome losses and gains with partial deletions and additions. A complex aneuploid karyotype is characteristic of undifferentiated high grade pleomorphic sarcomas. Because of the patient's history of Ewing sarcoma/PNET that was treated without surgery, fluorescence in situ hybridization (FISH) is performed to evaluate the tumor for presence of the EWS gene translocation. The FISH test, using a break-apart probe for the EWS gene, is negative.

Pathologic differential or, why isn't it one of the following?

Osteosarcoma, high grade: High grade osteosarcoma and undifferentiated pleomorphic sarcoma of bone can exhibit the same degree of cytologic atypia, necrosis, and mitotic activity. However, by definition, osteosarcoma must contain foci of malignant bone production, whereas undifferentiated high-grade pleomorphic sarcoma of bone must not. Both sarcomas usually also demonstrate a complex aneuploid karyotype.

Other differentiated primary sarcoma of bone: Most strict definitions of (undifferentiated high grade pleomorphic sarcoma of bone) do not allow for extensive immunohistochemical expression of markers that would suggest a specific line of differentiation. In other words, any high grade tumor of bone that is extensively positive for neural markers, muscle markers, or other specific proteins is no longer considered

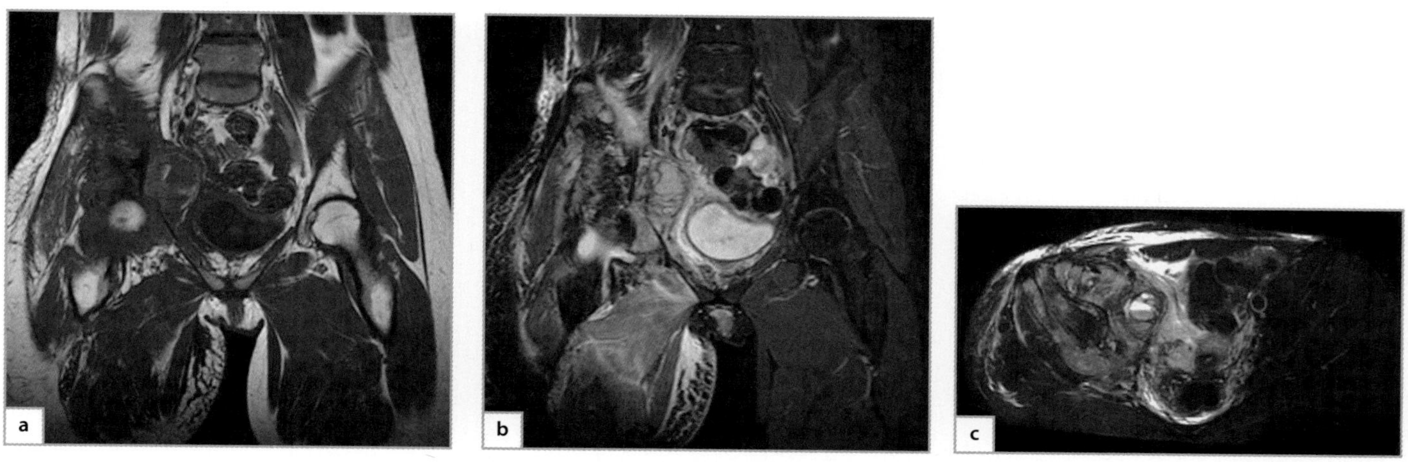

Case figure 19.2. Undifferentiated high grade pleomorphic sarcoma of bone (malignant fibrous histiocytoma of bone). 19.2a: Coronal T1 MR image. **19.2b**: Coronal STIR MR image, **19.2c**: Axial STIR MR image.

Case figure 19.1: Continued from page 460

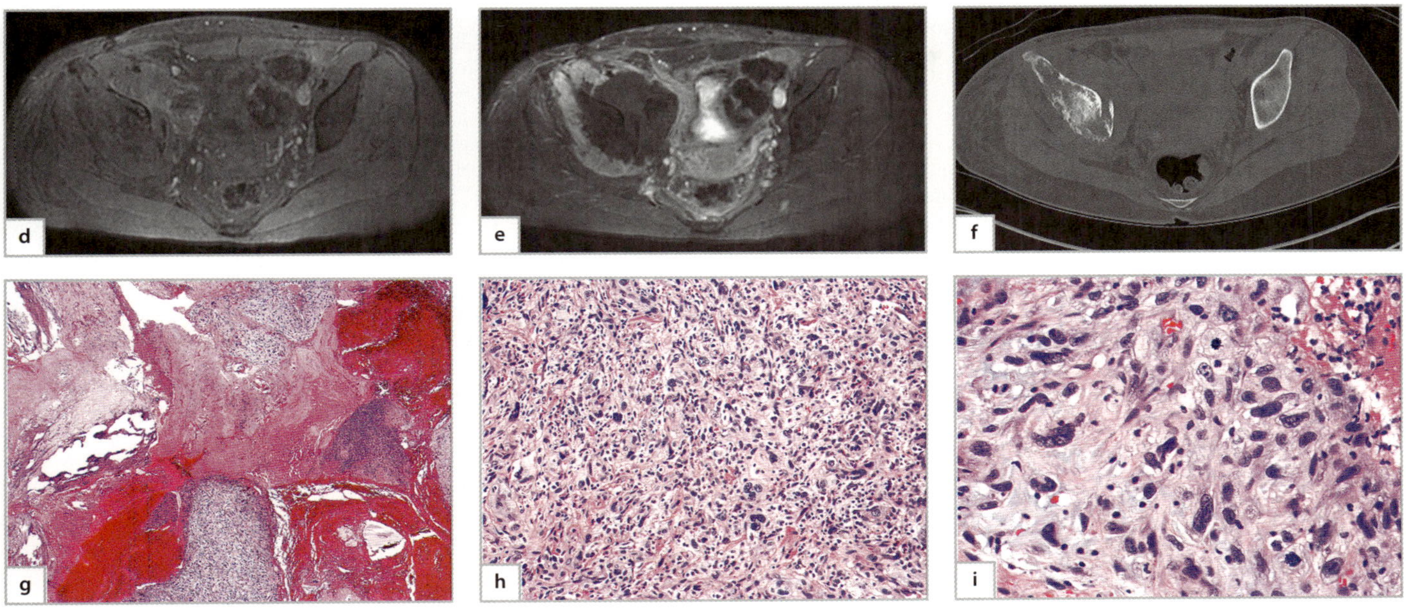

19.2d: Axial T1 fat saturated MR image, **19.2e**: Axial T1 fat saturated post-contrast, **19.2f**, Axial CT scan. The MR images show a heterogeneous destructive lesion expanding from the iliac bone into the pelvis and gluteal musculature. Much of the tumor does not show enhancement suggesting there is extensive necrosis indicative of a high grade tumor. CT scan image shows the moth eaten appearance of an infiltrating, destructive tumor. **19.2g**: Undifferentiated high grade pleomorphic sarcoma of bone ('Malignant fibrous histiocytoma' of bone) , low magnification. Typical for a radiation-induced sarcoma, the tumor exhibits large areas of necrosis and hemorrhage. **19.2h**: Undifferentiated high grade pleomorphic sarcoma of bone ('Malignant fibrous histiocytoma' of bone) , medium magnification. The tumor is highly cellular with marked variation in cell size. Inflammation is also present. **19.2i**: Undifferentiated high grade pleomorphic sarcoma of bone ('Malignant fibrous histiocytoma' of bone) , high magnification. A closer view of the pleomorphic tumor cells discloses varying cell and nuclear shapes and sizes. Two mitoses can be identified consistent with a high proliferation rate.

Case table 19.2 Summary pathology findings of Case 19.2

Diagnosis	Undifferentiated high grade pleomorphic sarcoma (malignant fibrous histiocytoma of bone)
Size	>10 cm
Location	Right ilium
Margin Status	Not applicable; lesion is not resected
Histologic grade AJCC classification of bone tumors, 2003	High grade (G4 = undifferentiated)
Pathologic stage AJCC staging	T2/N0/M1 = Stage IV (patient has lung metastases at presentation)

For comparison, from the period of 2000-2010, only three patients with malignant fibrous histiocytoma were treated at UNM. Two were younger patients with malignant fibrous histiocytoma developing at least 5 years post radiation therapy for Ewing sarcoma, and one patient was 20 years post metallic implant placement for fracture.

an undifferentiated sarcoma but would be instead labeled malignant peripheral nerve sheath tumor, high grade leiomyosarcoma or high grade myofibroblastic sarcoma, etc.

Oncology approach

Medical oncology

Doxorubicin-based chemotherapy is initiated but the patient develops rapidly progressive disease and she is referred to hospice. In this case, chemotherapy needs to be weighed against the risk of neutropenic fever and sepsis in a patient with chronic infection.

Radiation oncology

Undifferentiated high-grade pleomorphic sarcomas of bone are rare tumors typically treated similarly to osteosarcoma. It is unclear whether there is a role for radiation therapy in the management of this sarcoma. However, there may be a role in cases where good surgical margins cannot be obtained. In these cases, adjuvant radiation may help to achieve local control. Typically, the failure pattern is distant, which is likely one reason the role of radiation therapy has not been better defined. In this case, palliative radiation therapy was administered to the pelvis due to the presence of metastatic disease.

Of note, this patient developed a radiation-induced undifferentiated high-grade pleomorphic sarcoma of bone eleven years after definitive treatment of a Ewing's sarcoma of right ilium which included adjuvant radiation therapy. Treatment of Ewing's sarcoma with radiation leads to some of the highest rates of radiation induced malignancies, second only to retinoblastoma in incidence. Kuttesch, et al. (1996) showed a dose response for the development of radiation induced secondary sarcomas in patients with Ewing's sarcoma. This was found to be associated with then dose of radiation. In an analysis of 266 patients, those receiving less than 48 Gy had no radiation induced malignancies, those receiving between 48–60 Gy had less than a 5% risk of secondary malignancy, and those treated to greater than 60 Gy had greater than 10% risk of developing a secondary malignancy at 10 years. The majority of these cancers are high grade sarcomas. Also of interest, Huvos, et al. 1986 found that 15% (20) of their series of 130 malignant fibrous histiocytomas of bone were radiation induced.

Patient outcome

She expires from her disease six months after diagnosis of post-radiation undifferentiated high-grade pleomorphic sarcoma.

REFERENCES

Arata MA, Peterson HA, Dahlin DC. Pathological fractures through non-ossifying fibromas. J Bone Joint Surg Am 1981;63:980–988.
Bacci G, Picci P, Mercuri M, et al. Neoadjuvant chemotherapy for high grade malignant fibrous histiocytoma of bone. Clin Orthop 1998;346:178–89.
Bielack SS, Schroeders A, Fuchs N, et al. Malignant fibrous histiocytoma of bone: a retrospective EMSOS study of 125 cases. European Musculo-Skeletal Oncology Society. Acta Orthop Scand 1999;70:353–60.
Bramwell VH, Steward WP, Nooij M, et al. Neoadjuvant chemotherapy with doxorubicin and cisplatin in malignant fibrous histiocytoma of bone: a European Osteosarcoma Intergroup study. J Clin Oncol 1999;17:3260–9.
Brassesco MS, Valera ET, Engel EE, et al. Clonal complex chromosome aberration in non-ossifying fibroma. Pediatr Blood Cancer 2010;54:764–767.
Colby RS, Saul RA. Is Jaffe-Campanacci syndrome just a manifestation of neurofibromatosis type 1? Am J Med Genet A 2003;123A:60–63.
Dahlin D, Unni K, Matsuno T. Malignant (fibrous) histiocytoma of bone fact or fancy? Cancer 1977;39(4):1508–1516.
Dorfman DH, Czerniak B. Bone Tumors. St Louis: Mosby, 1998
Easley ME, Kneisl JS. Pathologic fractures through non-ossifying fibromas: is prophylactic treatment warranted? J Pediatr Orthop 1997;17:808–813.
Huvos AG, Woodard HQ, Heilweil M. Post-radiation malignant fibrous histiocytoma of bone. Am J Surg Pathol 1986;10:9–18.
Jeon D-G, Song WS, Kong CB, et al. MFH of bone and osteosarcoma show similar survival and chemosensitivity. Clin Orthop Relat Res 2011;469: 584–590.
Kuttesch JF Jr, Wexler LH, Marcus RB, et al. Second malignancies after Ewing's sarcoma: radiation dose-dependency of secondary sarcomas. J Clin Oncol 1996;14(10):2818–25.
Spanier SR, Enneking WF, Enriquez P. Primary malignant fibrous histiocytoma of bone. Cancer 1975;36:2084–2098.
Tarkkanen M, Larramendy ML, Bohling T, et al. Malignant fibrous histiocytoma of bone: analysis of genomic imbalances by comparative genomic hybridization and c-myc expression by immunohistochemistry. Eur J Cancer 2006;42:1172–1180.

FURTHER READING

Betsy M, Kupersmith LM, Springfield DS. Metaphyseal fibrous defects. J Am Acad Orthop Surg 2004;12:89–95.
Quinn RH, Ricci A. Malignant fibrous histiocytoma. In: Orthopaedic Knowledge Update: Musculoskeletal Tumors. Menendez L, ed. American Academy of Orthopaedic Surgeons 2002, p203–209.
Wittig JC, Villalobos CE. Malignant fibrous histiocytoma. In: Orthopaedic Knowledge Update: Musculoskeletal Tumors 2. Schwartz H, ed. American Academy of Orthopaedic Surgeons 2007, p197–198.

Chapter 20 Ewing sarcoma family of tumors of bone

OVERVIEW

Ewing sarcoma represents the quintessential 'small round blue cell tumor' which refers to the histological appearance of a variety of tumors of which Ewing sarcoma is a prime example. The small round blue cell appearance is consistent with a primitive, relatively undifferentiated or blastic cell characterized by a small to medium size, high nuclear to cytoplasmic ratio due to scant cytoplasm, round uniform nuclei, and solid growth.

The informal histologic description of 'small round blue cell tumor' summons a broad differential. In the pediatric age group, the list most commonly includes certain lymphomas, rhabdomyosarcoma, Ewing sarcoma, Wilms tumor and neuroblastoma. In adults, the Ewing sarcoma differential encompasses slightly different entities including various lymphomas, small cell undifferentiated carcinoma (also called poorly differentiated neuroendocrine carcinoma), poorly differentiated carcinoma, melanoma, and poorly differentiated synovial sarcoma, among others.

Ewing sarcoma has yet to be defined in terms of cell of origin and route of differentiation, although researchers are closing in on identifying these. This chapter discusses Ewing sarcoma of bone; however, up to 15% of these tumors arise in soft tissues. Soft tissue examples emulate the morphologic, immunohistochemical, and molecular characteristics of the intraosseous cases to a large degree.

New molecular technologies are identifying the pathways altered by tumor fusion transcripts some of which proffer new therapeutic targets, and Ewing sarcoma, with its list of fusion genes, is in need of targeted therapy. Patients with Ewing sarcoma often relapse decreasing overall five year survival to only 70% (van Maldegem et al. 2012, Kelleher et al. 2012).

CLASSIFICATION

Originally, Ewing sarcoma (EWS) was considered a discrete entity distinct from primitive neuroectodermal tumor (PNET) and Askin tumor. However, with knowledge gained from genetic studies identifying the same translocations in all three entities combined with recognition of overlapping morphology and behavior, these tumors are now considered one spectrum of a single entity. The recommended appellation for all three is now Ewing sarcoma family tumors (ESFT) emphasizing their relatedness while acknowledging the most common family member.

DEMOGRAPHICS

Ewing sarcoma of bone is the second most common pediatric malignant bone tumor comprising approximately 30% of all primary bone tumors in children (Gamberi et al. 2011). The tumor is most common in adolescents and affects males slightly more frequently then females. It is rare in patients of African or Asian descent (Hameed et al. 2011, Worch et al. 2011).

Surveillance Epidemiology and End Results (SEER) data were evaluated from 13 registries during a 15-year period (1994-2008) to assess the incidence of Ewing sarcoma (ICDO-3 code is 9260/3). In the US, the average annual incidence rate is 1.1/million and the number of cases reported in 13 SEER registries for the designated time period is 625. Females (incidence rate=0.8/million, n=220) are almost half as likely to be diagnosed with Ewing's sarcoma family tumors of the bone as males (incidence rate=1.3/million, n=405).

The age range for Ewing sarcoma of bone patients at diagnosis is wide, but patients are generally diagnosed at a younger age (adolescence). The mean age at diagnosis for Ewing sarcoma of bone is 20.2 years old according to 13 SEER registries' data. The age distribution of Ewing's sarcoma of bone (as noted in SEER data) is shown in **Figure 20.1**.

Ewing sarcoma (classic morphology) far outnumbers primitive neuroectodermal tumor (PNET), another member of the ESFT.

PATHOGENESIS

Ewing sarcoma

Ewing sarcoma is the archetypal translocation specific sarcoma. Intriguingly, the fusion transcript products of the translocations, of which there are a variety in Ewing sarcoma family of tumors (ESFT), are insufficiently oncogenic of themselves. Although the transcripts are required for specific Ewing morphology and protein expression

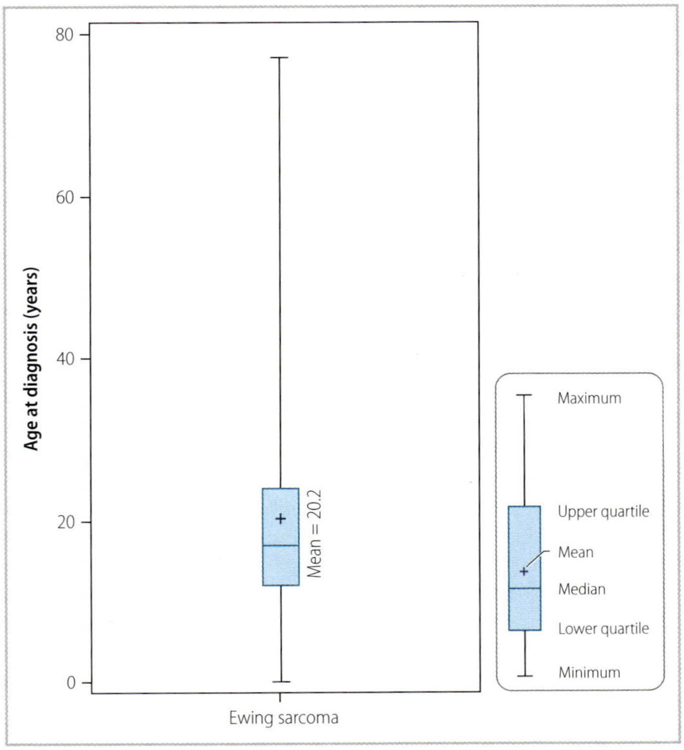

Figure 20.1 Age distribution of ewing sarcoma of bone among cases in 13 SEER registries 1994-2008 (N=625).

profile, additional molecular alterations are required for tumor to develop (Toomey et al. 2010).

The Ewing sarcoma gene (EWSR1 at 22q12) is a member of the TET family of genes which code for RNA-binding proteins of uncertain but most likely critical function (Sankar et al. 2011). This family includes FUS and TAF15 as well as EWSR1 (Szuhai et al. 2012). The great majority of patients with ESFT exhibit translocations of EWSR1 with a member of the ETS family of transcription factors, most commonly FLI1 (11q24) (Machado et al. 2011). The abnormal fusion protein interferes with cell proliferation and survival (activation of IGF1, MYC, NKX2,TOPK), enables escape from growth inhibition, senescence and apoptosis (inhibition of p21p57$_{KIP,}$TGFþR2,IGFþp3) and affects upregulation of genes required in neural tube and neural crest development, among others (Hameed et al. 2011, Kovar 2011).

Other rare fusions that lead to the Ewing sarcoma family of tumor phenotype and behavior include fusions that replace the EWSR1 gene with a fellow member of the TET (also known as FET) family, FUS (FUS/ERG, FUS/FEV) or comprise completely different gene fusions (DRD4/NUT and CIC/DUX4) (Machado et al. 2011).

Some expert sarcoma researchers and practitioners only apply the label ESFT to tumors with EWSR1-ETS family gene fusions or FUS-ETS gene family fusions (Machado et al. 2011, Szuhai et al. 2012, Sankar et al. 2011). Tumors with small round blue cell morphology and some IHC characteristics of ESFT but with the non-ETS gene fusions are often termed: 'Ewing sarcoma-like tumors'. These latter tumors may prove to behave like ESFT and respond to the same therapy, but the number of these Ewing sarcoma-like tumors is very small, and definitive determination of best moniker and treatment awaits accrual of more patients for study.

The mechanisms of action of the novel *EWSR1* fusions with non-ETS gene family members are not entirely known. However, for example, the *NFATc2* gene fusion with EWSR1 may result in alternate pathway stimulation culminating in Ewing sarcoma phenotype (Szuhai et al. 2009). Interestingly, patients reported with the *EWSR1/NFATc2* gene fusion were all older than 18 years and had complete rearrangements between chromosomes 20 and 22 resulting not only in translocation but in a fourfold amplification of the EWSR1/NFATC2 fusion site (Szuhai et al. 2009).

A novel t(4;22)(q31;q12) in extraskeletal Ewing's sarcoma fuses EWSR1 with the SMARCA5 gene (Sumegi et al. 2011). This is the first report of an EWSR1 fusion partner gene that has a completely different role than the ETS family of genes in that it encodes for a chromatin remodeling and spacing factor rather than a transcription factor. Thus, the mechanism of action of this fusion product leading to extraskeletal Ewing sarcoma is presumed to be much different than in the *EWSR1-ETS* fusions (Sumegi et al. 2011).

It is important to recognize that the EWSR1 gene on 22q12 is not exclusively translocated in ESFT. It is a fusion partner in multiple other mesenchymal tumors, including low grade malignant lesions (angiomatoid fibrous histiocytoma) as well as rare lymphomas (acute myeloid leukemia) and even tumors with epithelial differentiation including myoepithelioma and myoepithelial carcinoma. However, the ETS family of fusion partners only manifests as the Ewing sarcoma phenotype other than for a rare instance of acute myeloid leukemia (Romeo et al. 2010, Flucke et al. 2011, Szuhai et al. 2012, Thway et al. 2012).

It is uncertain why the *EWSR1* gene is a popular fusion partner in such a broad diversity but predominantly mesenchymal set of tumors. The EWSR1 protein product is vital to normal transcription and is thus ubiquitously expressed. Because of its continuous active state of transcription, it may be prone to translocations because it is constantly being transcribed or it may also possess sequence motifs that predispose it to non-allelic, homologous recombination (Toomey et al. 2010). The fusion products of the EWSR1 tumors (not just the Ewing sarcoma family of tumors) usually results in the fusion of the N-terminal transcription activating domain of *EWSR1* to the C-terminal DNA binding domain of the fusion partner which leads to the generation of a novel transcription factor (Romeo et al. 2010). In fact, eighteen different chimera transcripts are described just for the EWSR1-FLI1 fusion product alone indicating the complexity of the molecular fusion findings of the Ewing sarcoma family of tumors. Importantly, the fusion partners and the intragenic sites of fusion within a specific fusion partner do not seem to have prognostic significance.

Rarely, as is the case with the EWSR1/NFATC2 fusion, amplification and not just translocation of the fusion gene may play a supportive role in development of the tumor (Szuhai et al. 2012).

In addition to the fusion transcript present in ESFT, on karyotyping, many tumors also disclose copy number alterations including gains and losses of partial or whole chromosomes (Toomey et al. 2010). These additional changes are speculated to play a key role in ESFT oncogenesis.

Thus, the Ewing sarcoma family of tumors can be characterized by several specific, altered transcription factors created by the fusion of the *EWSR1* gene (or uncommonly the related *FUS* gene) with an ETS family member, although rare alternate, non-ETS, non-transcription factor fusion partners are described. As noted, the non-ETS partners may not be ESFT but only 'Ewing sarcoma-like tumors'. They may prove to be unusual genetic ESFT or distinctive tumors.

The cell that develops into the Ewing sarcoma family of tumors may represent a mesenchymal stem cell or progenitor cell that differentiates partially along neuroectodermal lines or it may represent a truly undifferentiated mesenchymal cell that has neuroectodermal differentiation imposed on it by the fusion transcript (Toomey et al. 2010).

Although hundreds if not thousands of genes are dysregulated by the EWS-FLI1 translocation in Ewing sarcoma, several common, vital cellular pathways are adversely affected suggesting possible sources for targeted therapy (Kovar et al. 2012). **Tables 20.1** and **20.2** describe the genetic alterations in the Ewing sarcoma family of tumors and compare them with other tumors harboring an *EWSR1* fusion.

PATHOLOGY

Table 20.3 lists the incidence, histologic features and immunohistochemical profile of the Ewing sarcoma family of tumors. Notably, approximately 10-15% of these tumors may occur in the soft tissue, most commonly in children and young adults with a similar slight male predominance (as occurs in the primary osseous tumors). The extraosseous sites for the Ewing sarcoma family of tumors include lung, mediastinum, retroperitoneum abdominal cavity, deep soft tissue and skin. The morphologic spectrum spectra and genetic findings of the extraosseous ESFT closely match those of the bone tumors with a few possible gene fusion exceptions. For example, the EWSR1/NFATc2 gene fusion and amplification has thus far only been found in soft tissue (Szuhai et al. 2009) (see **Table 20.1**).

Body site locations according to the SEER registry data from 1994 through 2008 are provided in **Figure 20.2**. Basically, the majority of these tumors are diagnosed in the bones of the lower limbs, pelvis, sacrum, and coccyx.

The diagnosis of the Ewing sarcoma family of tumors relies on integrating clinical, radiologic, routine histology, immunohistochemistry, and especially molecular findings. Almost without exception, the diagnosis of Ewing sarcoma cannot be rendered if genetic studies

Table 20.1 Genetics of Ewing sarcoma family of tumors (includes Ewing sarcoma, atypical Ewing sarcoma and peripheral neuroectodermal tumor [PNET]) and Ewing sarcoma-like tumors (small round blue cell tumors without ETS fusion partner)

Tumor	Chromosomal abnormality	Genes involved	Percentage of tumors with abnormality	Function of gene fusion	Immunophenotype	Body site
Ewing sarcoma family of tumors (ETS family of gene partners fusing with EWSR1)	t(11;22)(q24;q12)	*EWSR1-FLI-1*	85-90%	Any one of these fusions of *EWSR1* with an ETS gene results in an aberrant transcription factor that abnormally represses or upregulates hundreds of genes	CD99 +: 95% (membranous reactivity). FLI-1 +: 85-90%. Caveolin-1 +: 95%. S-100 +: 30%. Pan Keratin +: 20%. Chromogranin, Synaptophysin, NSE +: cases with PNET morphology. Neurofilaments +: 20% of PNET cases. Rare desmin +: 1%	Intraosseous in 85%. Deep soft tissue, visceral, or superficial in 15%. ETV1, E1AF, and FEV fusion transcript tumors may be primarily extraosseous
	t(21;22)(q22;q12)	*EWSR1-ERG*	5-10%			
	t(7;22)(p22;q12)	*EWSR1-ETV1*	<1%			
	t(17;22)(q12;q12)	*EWSR1-ETV4 (E1AF)*	<1%			
	t(2;22)(q33;q12)	*EWSR1-FEV*	<1%			
	t(2;22)(q31;q12)	*EWSR1-SP3*	Rare	Fusion protein most likely works by deregulating DNA transcription	CD99 + focal weak. NSE, NF: + but focal weak (n=1)	Stage IV in skin, bones, viscera
Ewing sarcoma-like tumors	t(1;22)(p36.1;q12) Paracentric inversion of 22q12	*EWSR1-PATZ1 (ZSG, ZNF278)*	Rare	May function as an aberrant transcription factor. May also require loss of wild type ZSG allele for tumorigenesis	CD99 – Desmin, keratins, synaptophysin, and NSE all + (DSRCT-like reactivity) (n=1)	Chest wall soft tissue
	t(6;22)(p21;q12)	*EWSR1-POU5F1 (OCT4)*	Rare	Aberrant transcription factor similarly modulating at least some of the same genes as in the *EWSR1-ETS* gene fusions	CD99 -; S-100 +, NSE + (n=1)	Intraosseous
	t(4;22)(q31;q12)	*EWSR1-SMARCA5*	Rare	Fusion protein deregulates normal DNA transcription by altering accessibility of DNA to transcription factors	CD99+; synaptophysin, NSE also +; desmin – (n=1)	1 soft tissue
	Ring chromosome with amplification of translocated segments	*EWSR1-NFATc2*	Rare	Aberrant transcription factor that shares some features of ETS family of gene fusion partners	CD99 +; desmin -, S-100 -, NSE - (n=4)	3 intraosseous 1 soft tissue
	t(4;19)(q35;q13)	*CIC-DUX4*	Rare	Aberrant transcription factor whose targets include *ETV5* and *ETV1* (ETS genes)	CD99 focal weak + (n=2)	2 soft tissue
	t(18;19)(q23;q13.2)	Unknown	Rare	Unknown; may have relationship to *CIC-DUX4* fusion cases	CD99 focal weak +; FLI-1 and NSE + (n=1)	1 soft tissue
	Intrachromosomal fusion of Xp11.4 and Xp11.22	*BCOR-CCNB3*	Rare	Specifics not known but modulates a different set of genes (especially morphogenesis of skeletal system) than EWSR1-ETS gene fusions. Associated copy number alterations also are distinctive	CD99 focal membranous (n=8), focal cytoplasmic (n=8), --- (n=3). CCNB3 strong diffuse nuclear (n=18/18)	19 intraosseous 5 soft tissue
Ewing sarcoma family of tumors with FUS (TLS) not EWSR1 fusion [ETS gene partners with FUS (TLS) (like EWSR1, a member of the FET [TET] gene family and closely related to EWSR1)]	t(16;21)(p11q22)	*FUS (TLS)-ERG*	Rare	Aberrant transcription factor that functions similarly to EWSR1-ETS family gene fusions	CD99 + in all (n=5) but one case was weak and patchy. One case with focal smooth muscle actin expression	3 chest wall soft tissue 1 intraosseous 1 visceral (kidney)
	t(2;16)(q35;p11)	*FUS (TLS)-FEV*	Rare		CD99 + diffuse strong (n=1)	1 intraosseous

Table 20.1: Continued from page 465

Tumor	Chromosomal abnormality	Genes involved	Percentage of tumors with abnormality	Function of gene fusion	Immunophenotype	Body site
Additional copy number alterations in Ewing sarcoma family of tumors	Gains: 1q, 1q21, 1q21-32, 1q22-qter, 2, 2q, 4p4q, 5, 5p, 7 7p21.1-p11.2, 7q, 8, 8p, 8q, 8q11.21-q22.3, 8q23-q24, 8q24.11-q24.21 12, 12p, 12q, 12q12-q15, 12q13.2-q14.1, 12q14.1-q15, 14, 14q, 14q11.2 17q21, 18, 20, 20p, 20q, 20q11.23-q13.33, 21q22.3, 22q11.21	Unknown BUT one of the above listed specific fusions is also present	Ranges from 5% to 80% per gene site, but relatively few cases tested (including primary tumors, metastatic tumors, and cell lines) using various techniques such as CGH, karyotyping, SNP microarray Affy 100k	These gains and losses are those seen in EWSR1-FLI1 gene fusion cases. The most common are: gain of 8 (50% of Ewing Sarcomas) gain of 1q (25% of ES cases) and loss of 16q (25% of ES cases). The specific effects of these CNA are unknown	CD99, FLI1, Caveolin-1 positive (same protein immunoprofile as EWSR1-FLI1 tumors)	Not specifically tracked per gene site but presumed same distribution as for EWSR1-FLI1 rearranged tumors
	Losses: 1p, 1p13-1p36.3, 3p, 7q11.2, 9p, 9p21, 10, 16q, 16q22.3 17p, 17p13-11.2, 19, 19p, 19q, Y	Unknown (except CDKN2A gene at 9p21.3) BUT one of the above listed specific fusions is also present	Ranges from 8% to 63% per gene site, but relatively few cases tested (including primary tumors, metastatic tumors, and cell lines) using various techniques such as CGH, karyotyping, SNP microarray Affy 100k)		CD99, FLI1, Caveolin-1 positive (same protein immunoprofile as EWSR1-FLI1 tumors)	Not specifically tracked per gene site but presumed same distribution as for EWSR1-FLI1 rearranged tumors

CGH: comparative genomic hybridization. SNP: nucleotide polymorphism. Affy 100k: Affymetrix gene chip 100k.

NF: neurofilaments antibody. NSE: neuron specific enolase antibody. See References for papers and texts pertaining to this table. This static list of genetic abnormalities must be viewed in the context of continuing discovery and refinement of genetic findings.

Table 20.2 Other tumors that contain EWSR1 translocations (gene fusions)

Tumor	Tumor category	Tumor behavior	Chromosomal abnormality	Genes involved	Number of tumors with abnormality
Desmoplastic small round cell tumor	Uncertain differentiation	Malignant	t(11;22)(p13;q12)	*EWSR1-WT1*	Majority
			t(21;22)(q22;q12)	*EWSR1-ERG*	Minority
Clear cell sarcoma	Melanocytic	Malignant	t(12;22)(q13;q12)	*EWSR1-ATF1*	Majority
			t(2;22)(q34;q12)	*EWSR1-CREB1*	Minority
Angiomatoid fibrous histiocytoma	Uncertain differentiation	Intermediate	t(12;22)(q13;q12)	*EWSR1-ATF1*	Minority
			t(2;22)(q34;q12)	*EWSR1-CREB1*	Majority
Extraskeletal myxoid chondrosarcoma	Uncertain differentiation	Malignant	t(9;22)(q22;q12)	*EWSR1-NR4A3*	Most common translocation in ESMCS
Small cell osteosarcoma	Osteoblastic	Malignant	t(11;22)(p11;q12)	*EWSR1-CREB3L1*	Unknown
Myxoid/round cell liposarcoma	Adipocytic	Malignant	t(12;22)(q13;q12)	*EWSR1-DDIT3*	Uncommon
Myoepithelioma of soft tissue, skin, and bone and one case of malignant myoepithelioma	Myoepithelial	Benign (one case was malignant)	t(1;22)(q23;q12)	*EWSR1-PBX1*	~50% have one of these EWSR1 translocations
			t(19;22)(q13;q12)	*EWSR1-ZNF44*	
			t(6;22)(p21;q12)	*EWSR1-POU5F1*	
			t(12;22)(q13;q12)	*EWSR1-ATF1*	

Table 20.2: Continued from page 466

Tumor	Tumor category	Tumor behavior	Chromosomal abnormality	Genes involved	Number of tumors with abnormality
Primary pulmonary myxoid sarcoma	Unknown	Malignant	t(2;22)(q34;q12)	*EWSR1-CREB1*	Majority (n= 7 of 9 cases)
Hyalinizing clear cell carcinoma of salivary glands	Epithelial	Malignant	t(12;22)(q13;q12)	*EWSR1-ATF1*	Majority (n= 18 of 22 cases)
Mucoepidermoid carcinoma of salivary glands	Epithelial	Malignant	t(6;22)(p21;q12)	*EWSR1-POU5F1*	Unknown
Hidradenoma of skin	Epithelial	Benign	t(6;22)(p21;q12)	*EWSR1-POU5F1*	Unknown
Acute lymphoblastic leukemia	Hematopoietic	Malignant	t(12;22)(p13;q12)	*EWSR1-ZNF384*	Unknown

Some of these tumors also have additional genetic abnormalities including chromosomal gains, losses, and translocations not involving EWSR1. See References for papers and texts pertaining to this table. This static list of genetic abnormalities must be viewed in the context of continuing discovery and refinement of genetic findings. It is very possible that additional tumors and translocations involving EWSR1 will continue to be reported.

Table 20.3 Pathologic features of Ewing sarcoma family of tumors of bone

Tumor	Incidence	Age and sex distribution	Body site (in order of frequency)	Histopathology description including IHC: Medium magnification	Histopathology description including IHC: High magnification
Ewing sarcoma family of tumors (ESFT): Ewing sarcoma, typical or classic type; atypical Ewing sarcoma; primitive (or peripheral) neuroectodermal tumor (PNET)	Common	Broad age range from infancy to elderly, but most common in older children and adolescents M slightly > F Rare in persons of Asian or African descent	Bone: long bones, pelvis, other bones, rare in hands/feet 10-15% of Ewing Sarcoma Family of Tumors occurs in soft tissue, skin, and viscera Body site may be associated in some cases with a specific fusion transcript	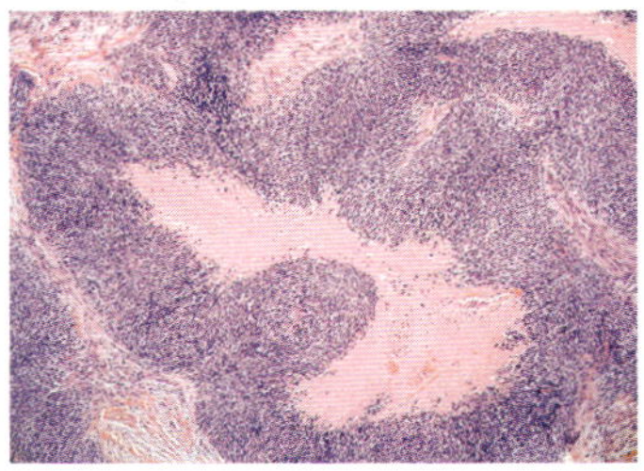	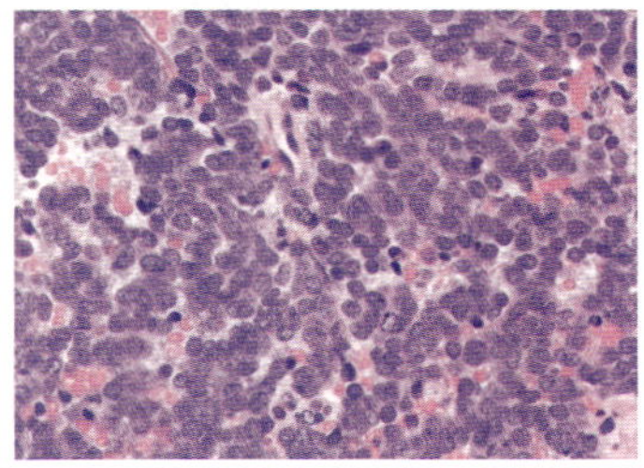
				Ewing sarcoma (classic or typical): Sheets of small round blue cells with a high N/C ratio and relatively uniform round nuclei with inconspicuous nucleoli and usually low mitotic rate. May show serpiginous perivascular preservation with necrosis between vascularized bands. Some cells may have scant clear cytoplasm (due to glycogen).	
				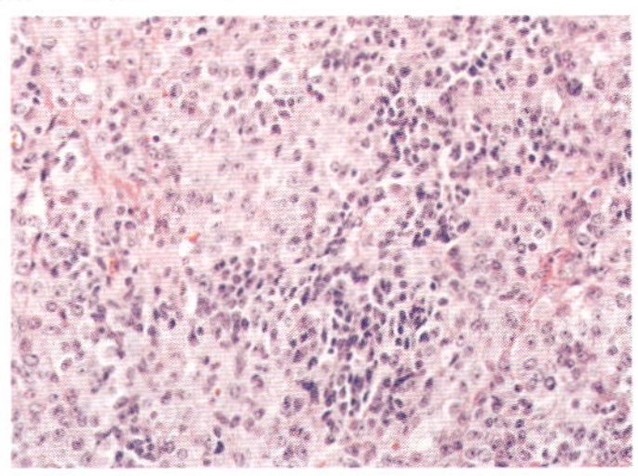	
				Atypical Ewing sarcoma: Several variants including large cell (larger cells with more cytoplasm and nuclei with nucleoli), adamantinoma-like with nests of epithelium (sometimes comprising squamous cells) embedded in otherwise typical tumor, spindle cell variant, rhabdoid cell variant, sclerosing variant with extensively hyalinized stroma, desmoplastic variant, HPC-like variant, diffusely desmin reactive variant.	
				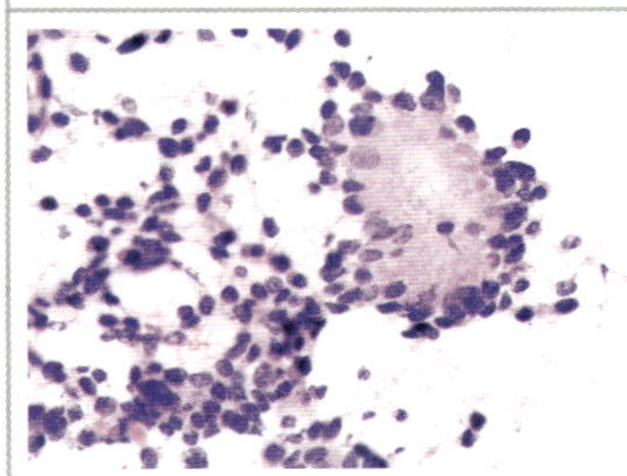	
				PNET: Sheets of small round blue cells with interspersed Homer-Wright true rosettes. Spindled tumor cells may be present. Tumor cells may be larger with more cytoplasm than typical ES. IHC: CD99 positive; NF, NSE, chromogranin, synaptophysin commonly positive.	

M: male, F: female. Incidence Note: 'Common to very common' indicates that a medium sized practice will treat at least several to dozens of patients with the lesion annually, 'Uncommon to rare' indicates the same practice size will treat one to two patients with the lesion every five years, 'Rare to very rare' indicates the same sized practice will see zero to one patient with the lesion every 20 years. Benign: does not recur and does not metastasize. Intermediate: can recur but does not metastasize. Malignant: can recur and can metastasize.

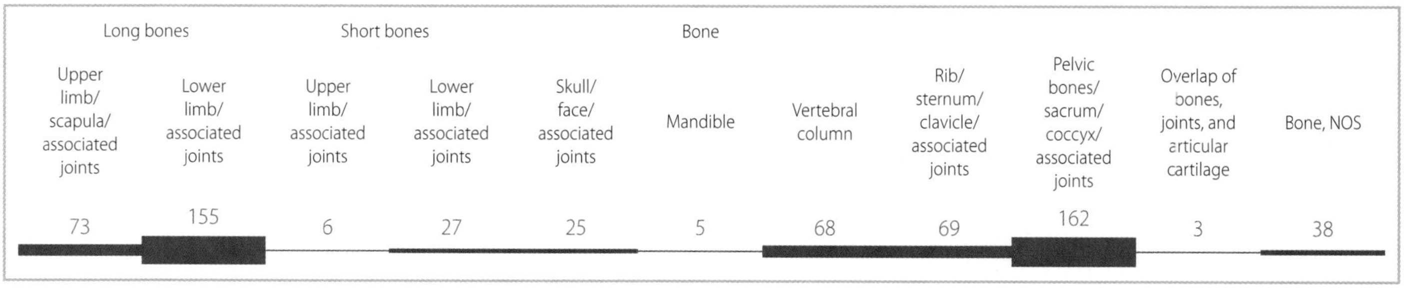

Figure 20.2 Ewing sarcoma of the bone by site for cases in 13 SEER registries diagnosed between 1994 and 2008.

fail to reveal a characteristic gene translocation (Gamberi et al. 2011; Parham 2010).

Immunohistochemistry can be immensely helpful in excluding other tumors in the differential diagnosis of Ewing sarcoma such as desmoplastic small round cell tumor, alveolar rhabdomyosarcoma, poorly differentiated synovial sarcoma, neuroblastoma, metastatic Wilms tumor, and lymphoma. The antibody most commonly used to diagnose Ewing's sarcoma is CD99 which detects the protein product of the MYC2 gene. Although membranous reactivity is found in more than 90% of Ewing's sarcomas, its expression is not limited to the ESFT, and so it is not entirely specific. Additional antibodies expressed in ESFT are FLI1 (friend leukemia integration 1 transcription factor) which is expressed in approximately 70–80% of cases, and the most recent suggested antibody to use is Caveolin-1 which is expressed in the large majority of cases (approximately 95%) including cases that are nonreactive for CD99 (Thway 2011). Unfortunately, none of these antibodies are specific for the Ewing sarcoma family of tumors, but absence of reactivity would be highly unusual and strongly suggests another diagnosis.

Molecular genetic diagnosis of Ewing sarcoma family of tumors is facilitated by the ready availability of a break apart FISH probe for the EWSR1 gene. However, evidence of EWSR1 translocation is not by itself specific for Ewing sarcoma and does not capture all cases, as noted previously in the pathogenesis discussion (Ganas et al. 2009). FISH using the break apart probe set thus serves as a strong adjunctive diagnostic add by confirming that the EWSR1 is translocated, but the specific fusion partner is not identified. Because the EWSR1 gene is translocated in quite a few tumors other than ESFT, presence of translocation must be evaluated in the context of the morphologic, immunohistochemical, radiologic, and clinical findings.

RT-PCR is a method by which specific fusion partners can be detected in Ewing sarcoma family of tumors. However, this molecular expedition can require multiple assays due to the panoply of fusion partners and is further complicated by several possible breakpoints within each candidate gene.

It might be possible to render a diagnosis of Ewing sarcoma in the absence of corroborating FISH or RT-PCR but only when all other parameters superbly fit the diagnosis (Gamberi et al, 2011, Thway 2011). In practical terms, for many national treatment protocols, molecular genetic confirmation is required for enrollment. At the University of New Mexico, within the last 12 years, 95% of Ewing sarcoma family tumors were genetically tested and demonstrated corroborating karyotypic and/or FISH evidence of EWSR1 gene translocation.

BEHAVIOR

All members of the ESFT are malignant. There is no difference in survival that can be ascribed to the PNET subtype, nor do the various translocations specifically affect survival (Sankar et al. 2011). Many variables have been investigated for prognostic value. Thus far, tumor size greater than 8 cm, presence of metastases at diagnosis, and less than 90% necrosis after neoadjuvant therapy are the only prognostic factors that have been verified in multiple studies (van Maldegem et al. 2012). However, other adverse prognostic factors that have been proposed but not independently validated in multiple studies include elevated serum lactate dehydrogenase level, axial tumor location, age greater than 15 years, gain of chromosome 8 or 1q and/or loss of chromosome 16q, overall increase of more than 3–5 copy number alterations (Toomey et al. 2010, Hallinger et al. 2002). Other potential promising biomarkers currently being investigated include 9p21 locus alterations, levels of heat shock proteins, telomerase related markers, interleukins, tumor necrosis factors, and VEGF proteins, total lymphocyte count, and Ki67 proliferation index (van Maldegem et al. 2012, Kovar et al. 2012).

One third of patients with apparently localized disease at presentation will experience distant relapse indicating that ESFT micro metastasizes (Hameed et al. 2011). Five year survival of patients with localized disease and treated with modern protocols is 70-85%, while overall survival plunges to 20% if metastatic disease is discovered at presentation. Relapsed or refractory disease is associated with a 10% survival (Kelleher et al. 2012).

Patients whose treatment includes neoadjuvant therapy must be followed long term given the increased risk for hematologic, mesenchymal and epithelial malignancies in these individuals (Schiffman et al. 2011; Longhi et al. 2012).

RADIOLOGY

Ewing sarcoma is a highly malignant tumor of bone affecting children and young adults that typically presents with a large soft tissue mass. Ewing sarcoma usually involves the diaphysis of a long bone, rib and the flat bones of the pelvis and shoulder girdle. Ewing sarcoma is extra-skeletal in about 10-15% of cases (Pradhan 2011). Ewing sarcoma patients may present with constitutional symptoms of fever, malaise and elevated sedimentation rate leading clinicians to think the aggressive bone lesion is due to osteomyelitis.

The radiographic findings of Ewing can be surprisingly subtle or may show a large destructive lesion. In a series of 22 patients with extra-skeletal Ewing sarcoma (O'Keefe 1990), no calcifications were seen.

Cross sectional imaging is important to demonstrate the large soft tissue component and the true extent of the marrow involvement. Ewing has a non-specific appearance with T1 isointensity and high signal on fluid sensitive sequences with variable enhancement.

SURGERY

Local control with these tumors is provided after neoadjuvant of chemotherapy. Wide surgical resection is the preferred local treatment modality. Radiation therapy provides local control rates approaching that of surgery, however the risk of secondary malignancy is particularly high in association with the t(11,22)(q24;q12) translocation. Radiation is certainly a reasonable alternative in unresectable tumors, situations where tumor resection would cause unreasonable morbidity, or in palliative cases. Surgery also confers the added benefit of allowing pathologic analysis and quantification of tumor necrosis following neoadjuvant chemotherapy, which has proven helpful in adjusting prognosis and determining the best postoperative chemotherapy regiment. Pulmonary metastectomy is indicated when all metastatic lesions can be removed and the primary lesion is amenable to local control.

GRAY AREA

The presence of a pathologic fracture sustained prior to or during the initial course of treatment does not necessarily preclude limb salvage surgery, particularly if the fracture is minimal displaced and there has been a good clinical response to chemotherapy.

MEDICAL ONCOLOGY

Ewing sarcoma genetics

ESFTs are aggressive diseases that typically present as rapidly growing masses and rapidly metastasize to lung, bone, and other organs. Because resection or radiation of the primary tumor seems to promote metastatic development, a multidisciplinary approach using neoadjuvant chemotherapy to kill microscopic metastatic disease has substantially improved survival. Definitive local control is then essential to eradicate the primary tumor (surgery or radiotherapy or both), followed by adjuvant chemotherapy to decrease the risk of recurrence.

Tumors with an *EWSR1* translocation might develop a variety of paraneoplastic syndromes, similar to what is observed in patients with small cell lung cancer (Guran et al. 2009, Verschraegen 2009). While these paraneoplastic manifestations must be medically addressed as part of the multidisciplinary approach, they usually resolve with optimal cancer therapy.

Chemotherapy for localized disease

All regimens described below are concurrent with definitive treatment of the primary tumor using surgery and/or radiation, usually within the first 12 weeks of starting chemotherapy. For the detailed protocols, the reader is referred to the publications of each study.

The first Intergroup Ewing Sarcoma Study (IESS) tested the addition of doxorubicin (VACA) to the actinomycin-D, cyclophosphamide, and vincristine (VAC) combination (Jaffe et al. 1976). There was a significantly better 5-year relapse-free survival (60%) with the VACA than with VAC (24%) (Nesbit et al. 1990). The second IESS (IESS-II) tested high-dose cyclophosphamide and showed an increased 5-year survival rate from 63% to 77% (Burgert et al. 1990). IESS-III studied the alternans of ifosfamide and etoposide with VACA (vincristine, doxorubicin, cyclophosphamide, and actinomycin D) with an increased 5-year survival from 61% to 72% (Grier et al. 2003). The next study tested a dose intense schedule with cytokine support. In this prospective randomized trial for 568 patients with localized ESFT, treatment was given every 2 weeks with filgrastim support in the experimental arm. The does dense administration was feasible with a median average day for retreatment of 15 days and no additional toxicities. Event-free survival at a median of 3 years was 65% for the control arm compared to 76% for the biweekly regimen demonstrating the superiority of schedule intensive treatment (Womer et al. 2008). This is currently the standard of care for treatment of localized ESFT.

One promising regimen is the dose intense VIDE (vincristine, ifosfamide, doxorubicin, and etoposide), which also allow a collection of stem cell for storage and possible use upon relapse (Strauss et al. 2003). Almost 90% of patients obtain a remission with this chemotherapy combination (**Table 20.4**).

Another regimen added a platinum analog. The combination of ifosfamide, carboplatin, and etoposide (ICE) with vincristine, doxorubicin, and cyclophosphamide (VAC), with dose intensification, was studied in 18 patients with high-risk ESFT, including some with one site of metastases. The addition of ICE improved the remission rate up to 90% with an estimated 3-year overall survival rate of 67% (Milano et al. 2006).

Actinomycin-D was dropped from ESFT regimens because it is not a crucial component when ifosfamide and etoposide are added (Miser et al. 2004).

Metastatic disease

The treatment of patients with metastatic disease remains dismal. Among metastatic patients treated in the IESS-III study, there was no significant difference in five year disease-free survival (22%)

Table 20.4 Chemotherapy regimens for localized EWS

Regimens	Drugs	5-year relapse-free survival	References
VA*CA	Vincristine Doxorubicin Cyclophosphamide Actinomycin-D	About 60%	Nesbit et al. 1990
V A*IA	Vincristine Doxorubicin Ifosfamide Actinomycin-D	Same as VACA	Paulussen et al. 2008
IE/V A*CA	Ifosfamide Etoposide Vincristine Doxorubicin Cyclophosphamide/Actinomycin-D	About70%	Grier et al. 2003
IE/V A*C (schedule intensification)	Ifosfamide Etoposide Vincristine Doxorubicin Cyclophosphamide	About 75% (3 years)	Womer et al. 2008
VIDE	Vincristine Ifosfamide/Doxorubicin Etoposide	NR	Strauss et al. 2003

A* stands for Adriamycin, which is a synonym for doxorubicin, the current generic name for the drug between the treatment groups (Grier et al. 2003). Therefore, more intensive chemotherapy approaches have been tested, using autologous stem cell transplant and lung radiation. The Euro-EWING 99 R3 study consisted of six cycles of vincristine, ifosfamide, doxorubicin, and etoposide (VIDE), one cycle of vincristine, actinomycin-D, and ifosfamide (VAI), local treatment (surgery and/or radiotherapy), and high-dose busulfan-melphalan followed by autologous stem-cell transplantation. The event-free survival at 3 years is 27% (Ladenstein et al. 2010). Other non-controlled studies of autologous stem cell transplantation showed more optimistic results with overall survival up to 50%, especially in patients who first responded to standard chemotherapy (Drabko et al. 2005, Fraser et al. 2006, Oberlin et al. 2006). Newer agents, such as topotecan, irinotecan, gemcitabine and others have been tested in clinical trials with mixed results (Padhye et al. 2010). All patients with metastatic Ewing sarcoma should be enrolled on a clinical trial.

Future therapies

The unique ESWR1 fusion genes, transcripts, and protein products provide targets for more specific therapies (reviewed in (Herrero-Martin et al. 2011)). EWS-FLI1 binding to RNA helicase A is associated with oncogenic function. YK-4-279, a small molecule inhibitor, blocks RNA helicase A binding to EWS-FLI1. The correlative effects are an induction of apoptosis and a reduction of xenograft growth in EWS models. The drug is currently under GMP manufacturing at the NCI (RAID program) (Erkizan et al. 2009). Other less specific cellular pathway drivers, such as VEGFR, IGFR1, and others are now being tested in clinical trials with minor benefits (Borinstein et al. 2011).

RADIATION ONCOLOGY

The data for radiation therapy (RT) in Ewing's sarcoma (ES) comes from multiple cooperative group studies performed in the pediatric population. Overall management follows the currently open Children's Oncology Group AESW-1031 study which consists of chemotherapy for approximately 1 year, with local therapy taking place at week 13. This consists of limb-sparing surgery without RT in patients with negative margins. However, certain locations, such as the spine, pelvis, and skull are less amenable to gross tumor resection, and therefore RT is the primary local treatment for these patients. RT is also used post-operatively in cases where there are close margins, gross residual disease, or positive lymph nodes. The dose is 45 Gy in 25 fractions to the pre-chemotherapy tumor volume, followed by a boost of 10.8 Gy in 6 fractions to areas of gross disease or post-chemotherapy tumor extent. Involved but resected nodal chains receive 50.4 Gy in 28 fractions, while gross nodal disease is treated similar to primary gross tumor.

There are no phase III studies directly comparing surgery and RT. Multiple retrospective analyses demonstrate superior local control with surgery, likely due to favorable selection bias. In general, the surgery cohorts typically have smaller tumor sizes and more favorable anatomical locations, which are associated with overall better prognosis. The CESS-86 study (Paulussen et al. 2001) reported 100% local control in patients receiving surgery, 95% for surgery and post-operative RT, and 86% for radiation alone as the local modality. The same group conducted a larger analysis of 1,058 patients from multiple trials of localized ES (Schuck et al. 2003). Local failure was 26% with definitive RT, versus 7.5% with surgery as the primary modality.

CASES

Case 20.1 Ewing sarcoma

Clinical history and presentation

The patient is a seven year old girl who presents with an eight month history of left hip pain. Her pain initially began following a fall but then resolved. Four months prior to presentation she again sustained a fall with acute onset pain in the left buttock which has been persistent. Physical examination is unremarkable.

Surgical findings and comments

Needle biopsy is consistent with Ewing sarcoma. Due to the extensive nature of the initial tumor, amputative hemipelvectomy is felt to be the procedure of choice. Although the patient and family are in agreement, they make a preoperative request to attempt limb-salvage if possible after assessment of chemotherapy response intra-operatively. At surgery, residual viable tumor is confirmed to be encasing the external iliac vessels. Therefore, the decision is made to proceed with amputation.

Radiology findings

This case, **Case fig. 20.1a** through **20.1d**, shows a large destructive mass of the left iliac wing with intense heterogeneous enhancement. The overall appearance is not specific; however, a large mass originating from a flat bone or diaphysis in a child or adolescent is likely Ewing sarcoma.

We present two additional cases of Ewing sarcoma. **Case figs 20.1e** through **20.1i** shows an aggressive destructive mass of the distal tibial metaphysis. The metaphyseal location is somewhat unusual; however, the very large soft tissue mass relative to bone lesion size is common. The second additional case, **Case fig. 20.1j** through 20-1p, has the more classic diaphyseal location with large soft tissue mass. Ewing sarcoma can present with minimal bone abnormality despite the large aggressive lesion. This case shows only modest periosteal reaction, seen best on lateral radiograph and has a mild scalloped or 'saucerized' appearance of the medial femoral cortex. A differential for these cases might include osteosarcoma with minimal calcified osteoid, or lymphoma which can also present with a very large soft tissue mass relative to the size of the bone lesion. Lymphoma and Ewing sarcoma can also present with constitutional symptoms that might lead to misdiagnosis of a bone lesion as osteomyelitis. These are all highly aggressive lesions that need definitive tissue diagnosis.

Pathology findings

Gross features

The needle core biopsy of the 'pelvic mass' consists of five, translucent filamentous fragments of soft tissue with a caliber of less than 1 mm and length up to 5 mm. Since the specimen is received fresh, a small portion is submitted to Cytogenetics, and the rest is processed for routine histology.

A separate specimen is sent from Surgery immediately prior to the hemipelvectomy. It is labeled 'pelvic scar tissue' and comprises a 3.5 cm fragment of fibrous tissue. A portion is frozen at the time of surgery with an intraoperative diagnosis of 'positive for tumor, consistent with Ewing sarcoma.'

After receipt of the frozen section diagnosis, the surgeon proceeds with hemipelvectomy. The resection is a left hemipelvectomy including the left ilium, partial pubic bone and partial ischium in addition to the entire left leg. Careful sectioning reveals a 5.9 × 1.3 × 1.9 cm area of soft, partially cystic to mucoid yellow tissue replacing normal trabecular bone of the ilium. Next to the abnormal appearing bone is possible soft tissue extension of this process. Here the periosteal-soft tissue interface is indistinct and grossly fibrotic (**Case fig. 20.1q**). The acetabulum is grossly uninvolved. A representative slice of involved ilium is gridded out in 40 cassettes to assess neoadjuvant therapy-induced percent necrosis. Additional sections of all margins and multiple lymph nodes are also sampled for histologic review.

Microscopic features

Incisional biopsy

Low magnification: The specimen consists of skeletal muscle infiltrated by a small round blue cell tumor (**Case fig. 20.1r**).

High magnification: The relatively small round tumor cells form loose clusters that infiltrate around degenerated skeletal muscle fibers (**Case fig. 20.1s**).

Special studies: Although the biopsy is scant, immunohistochemical staining is possible. Tumor cells exhibit strong membranous reactivity for CD99 which is the expected finding for Ewing sarcoma family of tumors (**Case fig. 20.1t**). Tumor cells also express FLI-1 in a nuclear pattern and caveolin-1 in a combined membranous cytoplasmic pattern, and there is no reactivity for CD45 (a general lymphoma marker) or desmin (a muscle marker that is usually positive in rhabdomyosarcoma).

The patient's karyotype is normal consistent with fibroblast overgrowth and is not considered representative of the tumor cell population.

However, fluorescence in situ hybridization using a dual color break-apart probe for the EWSR1 gene is positive and reveals a split signal in tumor cell nuclei consistent with translocation of one EWSR1 allele (**Case fig. 20.1u**). This provides genetic evidence of EWSR1 translocation. The diagnosis of Ewing sarcoma is rendered, because the histomorphology, IHC profile, FISH result, clinical and radiologic findings all are highly consistent with an ESFT profile.

Bilateral bone marrow biopsies: Bilateral iliac crest bone marrow core and aspiration biopsies are performed. The left iliac crest biopsies reveal clusters of monotonous round cells on the touch preparation (**Case fig. 20.1v**) and in the sections of the needle core biopsy (**Case fig. 20.1w**) consistent with Ewing sarcoma. The right iliac crest biopsies are negative for tumor. The patient's tumor is located primarily in the left iliac crest, so the finding of tumor cell nests on the left side bone marrow samples is not surprising and in this patient does not upstage the disease.

Tumor resection (left hemipelvectomy)

Low magnification and high magnification of pelvic scar tissue: The first specimen sent from the surgeon labeled 'pelvic scar tissue' contains a few aggregates of residual tumor (**Case fig. 20.1x**). The tumor cells are larger with clear cytoplasm (**Case fig. 20.1y**) compared to adjacent lymphocyte clusters (**Case fig. 20.1z**), although the differences are subtle.

Low magnification of main resection specimen: Greater than 90% of the tumor is necrotic consistent with an excellent response to neoadjuvant therapy (**Case fig. 20.1aa** with normal bone marrow for comparison in **Case fig. 20.1bb**).

Special studies: No special studies are performed on the resection specimen, as the biopsy established the diagnosis.

Additional cases

For completion, a few additional photos of other patients' Ewing sarcomas are presented. Because it could cause diagnostic confusion, it is important to recall that up to 20% of ESFT express keratins (**Case fig. 20.1cc**), and as many as 30% may express S-100 protein in both a nuclear and cytoplasmic pattern (Fisher et al. 2011). Rarely, ESFT may also express desmin, TFE3 or MiTF (Barisella et al. 2010). In these cases, membranous CD99 reactivity, typical histopathology, expected molecular findings, and classic clinical and radiologic presentation enable the correct diagnosis.

An unfortunate long term consequence affecting survivors of Ewing sarcoma is treatment induced sarcoma which may occur in up to ~5% of patients after 20 years and which carries a poor prognosis (Longhi et al. 2012). These tumors may present as a mild radiologic abnormality for which the differential includes reactive fibrosis or inflammation, and they may appear deceptively bland on biopsy (**Case fig. 20.1dd**). Repeat biopsies, in conjunction with continuing, growing imaging abnormalities, may be required before the diagnosis can be made (**Case figs 20.1ee** and **20.1ff**).

Second malignancy after treatment for Ewing sarcoma includes osteosarcoma, spindle cell sarcoma, not otherwise specified, high grade pleomorphic sarcoma and less commonly other specific sarcomas, but various carcinomas and hematologic malignancies are also increased (Goldsby et al. 2008). By ten to 20 years after initial treatment, patients with ESFT are more likely to develop a second malignant neoplasm than recurrent tumor (Longhi et al. 2012). Females may be at greater risk than males in developing second malignant tumors (secondary malignancies, however, include breast carcinoma). Patients surviving Ewing sarcoma exhibit a five fold increased risk for development of a solid malignancy compared to age and sex matched controls (Goldsby et al. 2008). Patients with radiation therapy are at particular risk, and the risk may rise as radiation dosage rises (Schiffman et al. 2011).

ESFT patients may also develop hematologic malignancies such as acute myeloid leukemia. Hematologic malignancies tend to present within the first three to five years following treatment, while solid tumors manifest most commonly after 8-10 years (Schiffman et al. 2011).

Pathologic differential or, why isn't it one of the following?

For this patient, a seven year old girl with a large pelvic bone centered mass and no evidence of disease elsewhere, the histologic differential is fairly narrow:

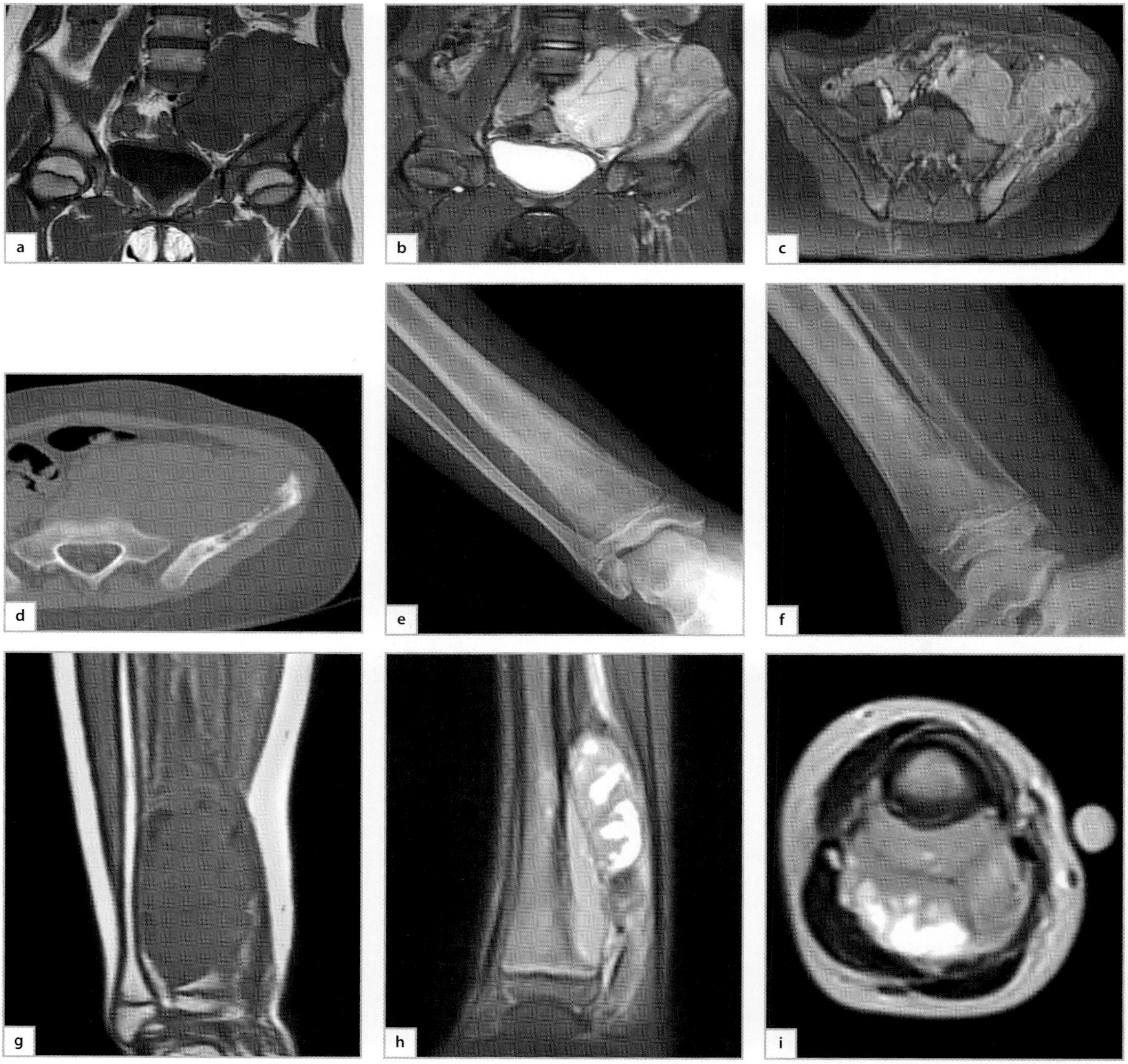

Case figure 20.1 Ewing sarcoma. MR images including. **20.1a**: Coronal T1, **20.1b**: Coronal STIR, **20.1c**: Axial T1 fat saturated post-contrast. **20.1d**: Axial CT without IV contrast. This 7 year old girl has a 7.0 × 9.3 × 9.8 cm mass originating in the left iliac bone with a very large soft tissue component displacing bowel as the tumor spreads into the pelvis. The mass is T1 isointense to muscle and high signal on STIR with intense enhancement. The CT scan shows bone destruction with mild periosteal reaction. There is no soft tissue calcification, or osteoid seen. *Radiologic findings of two additional cases of Ewing sarcoma. Figures 20.1e through 20.1i is a Ewing sarcoma of a 10 year old girl with a distal tibial metaphyseal lesion.* **20.1e**: Anteroposterior and **20.1f**: Lateral radiographs show laminated periosteal reaction and hair-on-end periosteal reaction of the distal tibial metaphysis. The lateral view shows a large soft tissue mass is associated. The MR images include; **20.1g**: Coronal T1, **20.1h**: Sagittal STIR, **20.1i**: Axial T2. There is a large soft tissue mass measuring 4.3 × 4.0 × 9.5 cm with fairly homogeneous T1 isointense and T2 high signal intensity. No contrast was given in this case. *Case figs 20.1j through 20.1p is the second additional case involving the femoral diaphysis of a 16 year old boy.*

Case figure 20.1: Continued from page 472

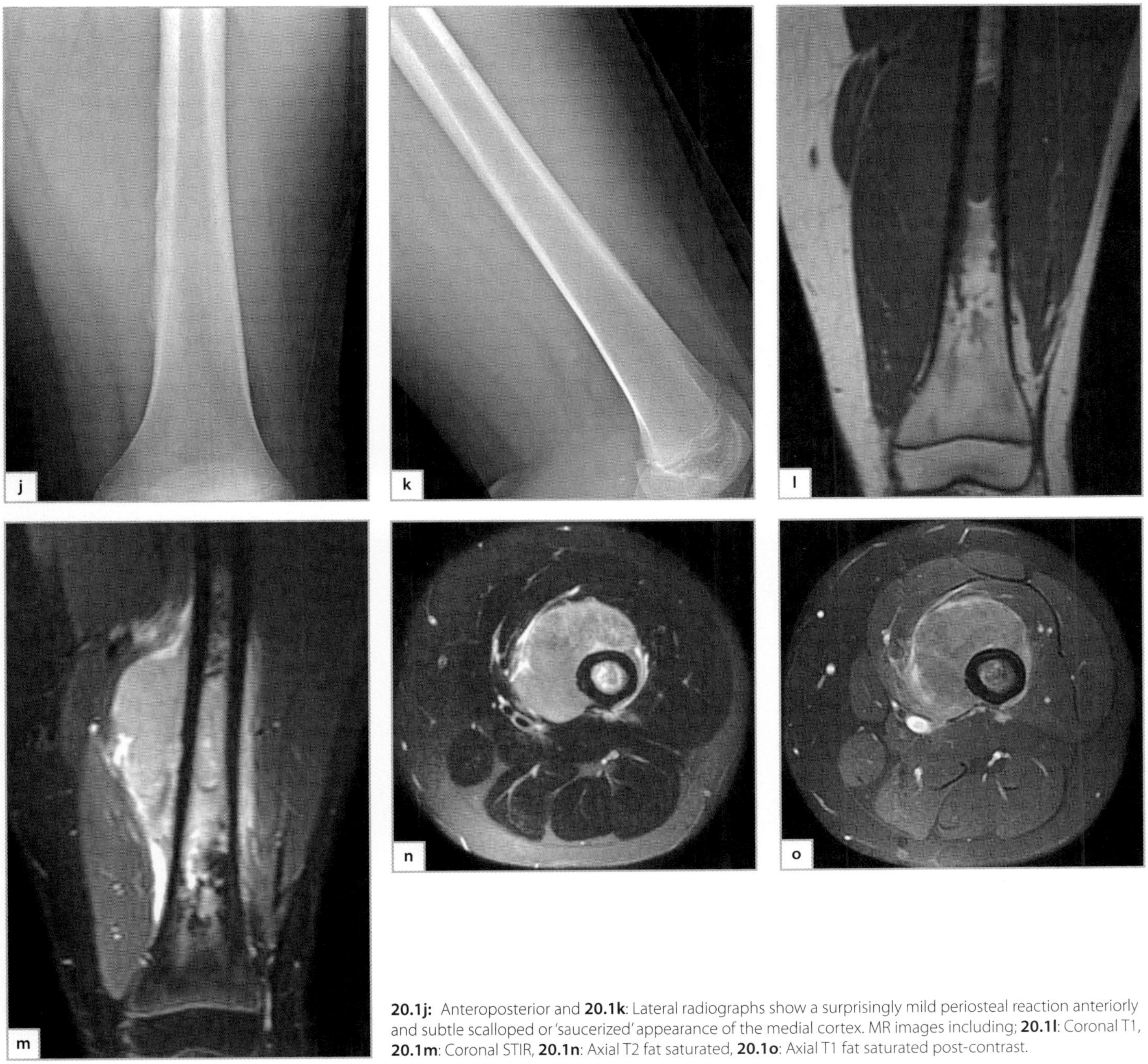

20.1j: Anteroposterior and **20.1k**: Lateral radiographs show a surprisingly mild periosteal reaction anteriorly and subtle scalloped or 'saucerized' appearance of the medial cortex. MR images including; **20.1l**: Coronal T1, **20.1m**: Coronal STIR, **20.1n**: Axial T2 fat saturated, **20.1o**: Axial T1 fat saturated post-contrast.

Lymphoma: The histologic appearance may be very similar to this patient's tumor. However, ES cells tend to be a little more cohesive, a bit larger, and cytoplasmic clearing is more frequent in Ewing sarcoma (due to glycogen) than in malignant lymphocytes. Some lymphomas are CD99 reactive. However, lymphoid markers are also reactive such as CD45, CD3, TdT etc. These markers are absent in ES. Some patients with intraosseous lymphoma also present with splenomegaly and lymphadenopathy which would be a highly unusual presentation for ESFT.

Small cell osteosarcoma: By definition, small cell osteosarcoma must contain recognizable tumor osteoid. Rare cases have been described with EWSR1 gene fusions. These latter may represent ESFT with divergent differentiation, but such EWSR1 fusion cases are currently a controversial entity.

Mesenchymal chondrosarcoma (MCS): A needle core biopsy may miss the diagnostically helpful neoplastic hyaline cartilaginous component of mesenchymal chondrosarcoma. MCS can express

Case figure 20.1: Continued from page 473

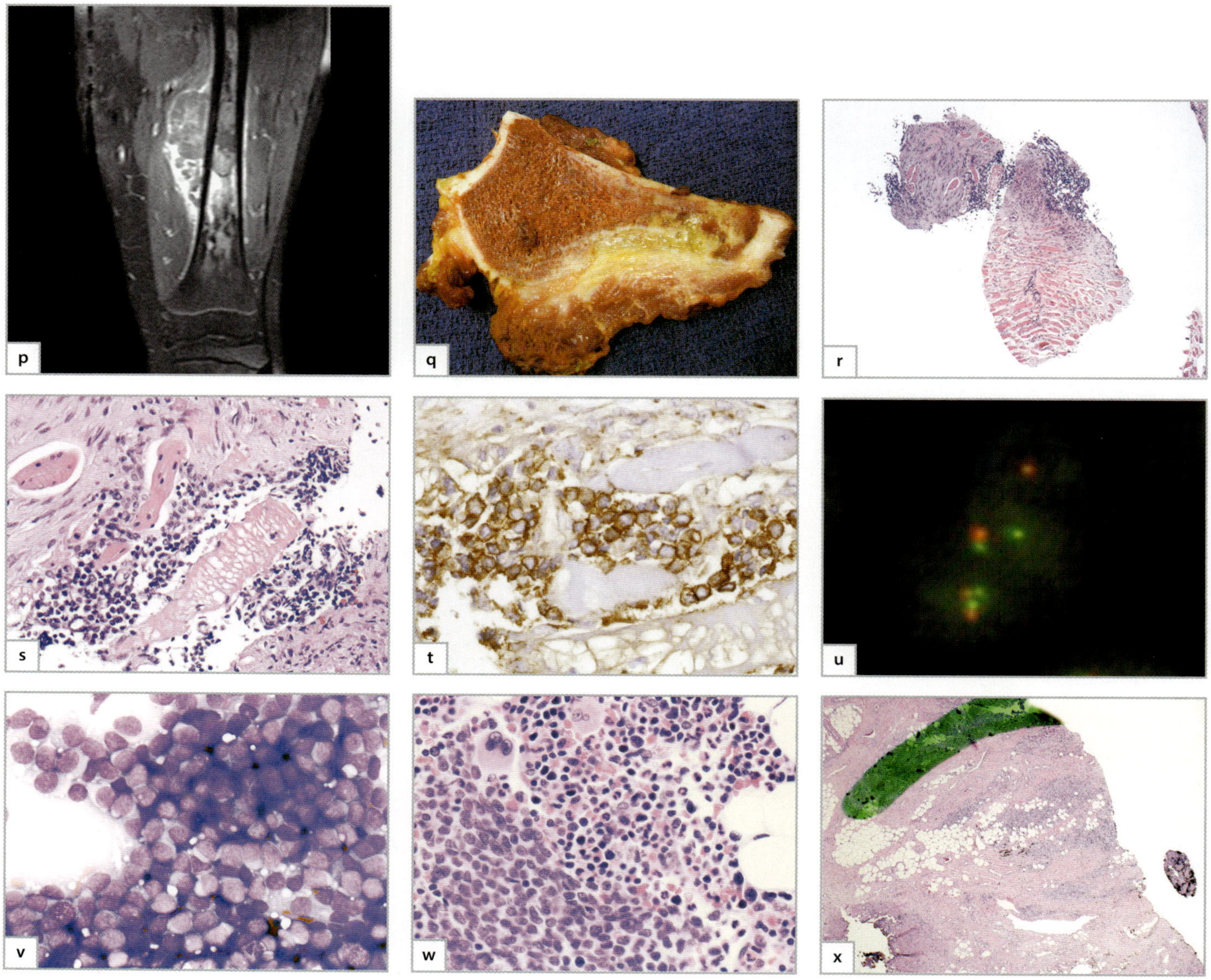

20.1p: Coronal T1 fat saturated post-contrast. The soft tissue mass measures 5.3 × 6.7 × 12.3 cm and is much larger than the area of bone disease seen on radiography. The MR images also show extensive marrow disease. This Ewing sarcoma again shows the non-specific appearance of T1 isointensity with T2 and STIR high signal. Note the modest enhancement possibly related to the high degree of cellularity as opposed to the usual necrosis or matrix production seen in other high grade sarcomas. **20.1q**: Gross photo of cross section of ilium post neo-adjuvant therapy. The site of prior tumor is indicated by mottled trabecular bone and a linear area of translucent yellow mucoid change that obscures the cortical/trabecular bone interface. A band of subjacent soft tissue is fibrotic consistent with therapy induced change in extraosseous tumor. **20.1r**: Needle core biopsy of pelvic mass, low magnification. Skeletal muscle fragments are infiltrated by nests of small, dense, blue appearing tumor cells. **20.1s**: Needle core biopsy of pelvic mass, high magnification. Loosely cohesive, small round blue tumor cells infiltrate around degenerating skeletal muscle fibers. The background is fibroblastic consistent with tumor induced stromal response andr rhabdomyonecrosis. **20.1t**: Needle core biopsy, CD99 immunohistochemical stain, high magnification. The tumor cells demonstrate strong membranous expression of CD99 (MIC2 gene product). This is a characteristic but not entirely specific for ESFT. **20.1u**: FISH (fluorescence in situ hybridization) for EWSR1 translocation, high magnification. Two nuclei are present; one with normal closely apposed EWSR1 signals. The adjacent nucleus reveals a split signal (one red and one green dot) widely spaced and one set of non-split signals. The split indicates that one allele of the EWSR1 gene has been translocated to another distant site. It confirms EWSR1 gene translocation but does not identify the specific gene partner. **20.1v**: Touch preparation of left iliac crest bone marrow aspiration, Wright-Giemsa stain, high magnification. The striking monotony of the tumor cells is apparent. The histologic category of 'small round blue cell tumor' aptly describes the patient's tumor cells. **20.1w**: Left iliac crest bone marrow biopsy, high magnification. Tumor cells form a crescent at lower left of uniform blue cells compared with the patient's normal hematopoietic bone marrow cells. Two large normal megakaryocytes contrast with the small size of the sarcoma cells. **20.1x**: 'Pelvic scar tissue' low magnification. Tissue submitted for frozen section contains residual foci of viable tumor (green ink marks the blue aggregates of malignant cells embedded in fibroadipose tissue).

Case figure 20.1: Continued from page 474

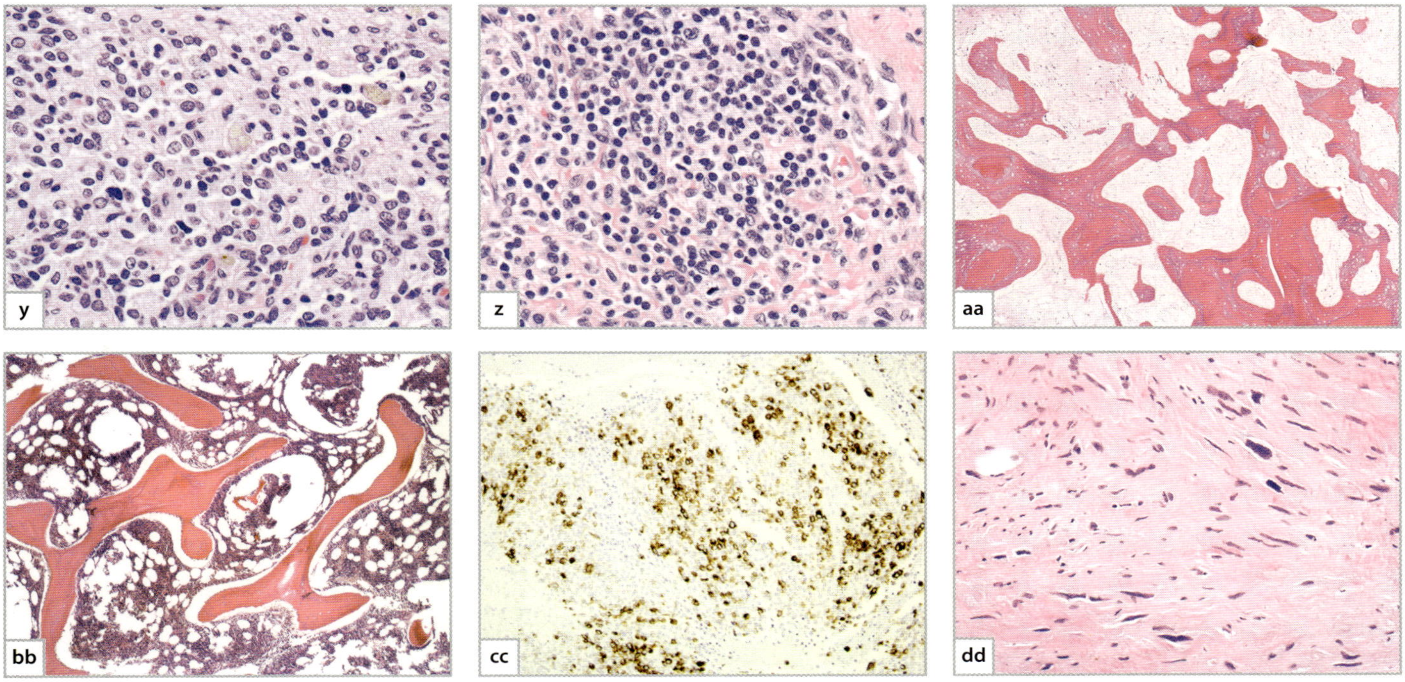

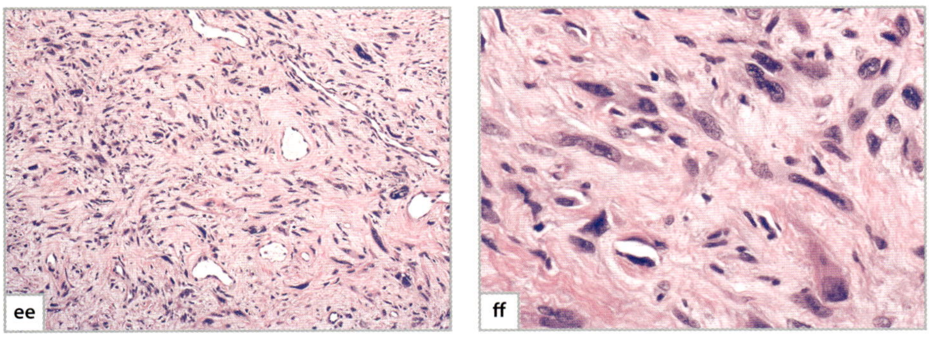

20.1y: 'Pelvic scar tissue' tumor at high magnification. Tumor cells mingle with reactive histiocytes. The histiocytes have pale brown cytoplasm, while the sarcoma cells have indistinct cytoplasm and appear to float in open spaces. **20.1z**: 'Pelvic scar tissue' reactive lymphocytes at high magnification. By comparison with the patient's tumor cells, reactive lymphocytes are smaller with more condensed chromatin (darker nuclei). Both the patient's sarcoma cells and her normal lymphocytes can be described as 'small round blue cells', so the differences are subtle. **20.1aa**: Iliac bone post neoadjuvant therapy, low magnification. The patient has an excellent response to neoadjuvant treatment with greater than 95% tumor necrosis. In this field, the area of former tumor shows slightly thickened trabecular bone and fibrosis and edema of the marrow without viable tumor cells. **20.1bb**: Iliac bone post neoadjuvant therapy, normal bone at low magnification. The patient's normal bone contrasts with the areas previously involved by tumor. Bone trabeculae are thinner than in the treated tumor site, and hematopoietic and marrow fat are normal in ratio and appearance. **20.1cc**: CAM 5.2 keratin immunohistochemical stain, medium magnification of another case. A significant minority of ESFT may express unexpected markers such as keratins (as in this tumor) or S-100 protein. This can be diagnostically confusing. **20.1dd**: Post-treatment sarcoma in third patient with Ewing sarcoma, medium magnification, first biopsy. A small percentage of Ewing sarcoma patients develop a second malignancy. In this case, the second malignancy occurred 11 years following the patient's initial surgery and neoadjuvant therapy. Radiologically, it manifested as a new density at the site of prior surgery. This biopsy shows a hypocellular spindle cell population. Scattered cells have larger nuclei. The differential diagnosis includes post-radiation fibrosis with radiation induced reactive atypia versus sarcoma. **20.1ee**: Post-treatment sarcoma in third patient with Ewing sarcoma, medium magnification, second biopsy. A second biopsy performed six months later due to advancing radiologic abnormalities, reveals a more cellular lesion with more marked variation in nuclear size. **20.1ff**: Post-treatment sarcoma in third patient with Ewing sarcoma, high magnification, second biopsy. The second biopsy contains areas of unequivocal malignant cells, and a diagnosis of post-treatment high grade spindle cell sarcoma, not otherwise specified, is rendered. Supporting the impression of sarcoma, the lesion eroded bone, demonstrated mitotic activity with rare atypical mitotic figures, and overexpressed p53 (by immunohistochemistry).

CD99, like nearly all cases of ES. However, it lacks any of the ESFT gene fusions. It often exhibits a hemangiopericytomatous architecture which is only rarely seen in ES.

Metastatic alveolar rhabdomyosarcoma (A-RMS): A-RMS has a propensity to metastasize to bone marrow. Tumor cells may resemble the ES small round blue cell except that the nuclei are usually more pleomorphic, and mitotic activity and individual cell apoptosis are more prominent. Multinucleated tumor cells are not uncommon in A-RMS and absent in ESFT. Some cells may show signs of muscle differentiation with strap, tadpole or spider shapes and deeply eosinophilic cytoplasm. Cross striations may even be detectable in scattered cells. By IHC, rhabdomyoblasts express desmin and myogenin and may sometimes express CD99. Desmin is only rarely expressed in ESFT, and myogenin is not expressed. Molecular analysis differentiates the two entities because of distinctly different fusion genes (see **Case table 20.1b**).

Case table 20.1a lists the histologic variety notable in Ewing sarcoma family of tumors. An expanded differential diagnosis of ESFT is provided in **Case table 20.1b**. This covers the most likely entities in the pathologic differential of pediatric and adult ESFT of bone and soft tissue.

Oncology approach

Medical oncology

After needle core biopsy reveals Ewing sarcoma, the patient undergoes a bone scan, a total body PET CT, an echocardiogram, an electrocardiogram, pelvic films, and a chest X-ray. Bilateral bone marrow biopsies and aspirates are performed, and a central line is placed.

The patient is enrolled in AEWS0031, a Children Oncology Group study, and randomized to the interval compression arm with the standard chemotherapy agents. During chemotherapy, she undergoes a hemipelvectomy as part of the multidisciplinary protocol. She has 2 residual foci of Ewing sarcoma in the bed of the tumor. Adjuvant chemotherapy as described by the Children Oncology Group protocol is continued, and the patient completes the prescribed treatment. She is free of disease after completion of the therapy. Preliminary results of the experimental intensive chemotherapy of this AEWS0031 study showed a favorable outcome.

Radiation oncology

As the patient undergoes radical surgery with negative margins and absence of lymph node involvement, radiation therapy is not recommended.

Patient outcome

Six months postoperatively, the patient is doing well with no evidence of local recurrence or metastatic disease.

Case table 20.1a Histologic variants and variant features of Ewing sarcoma family of tumors

Feature or variant	Frequency	Comment
Classic type	85%	Even in straightforward cases, molecular confirmation is desirable or required (the latter for patient entry into various national treatment protocols)
Atypical types:	10%	Large cell type is the most common of the variant histologic types
Large cell type with open nuclei and prominent nucleoli		
Adamantinoma-like with islands of keratin positive epithelium		Adamantinoma-like variant often occurs at the same body sites as adamantinoma
Spindle cell type with fascicles of spindle cells		Foci of classic histology may be present to aid in the diagnosis
Fibrotic or hyalinized type with abundant fibrous stroma mimicking sclerosing rhabdomyosarcoma		
Clear cell type with abundant glycogenated cytoplasm		
Epithelioid cell type		
Rhabdoid cell type		
HPC-like with numerous staghorn or antler horn vessels		
PNET (numerous Homer-Wright rosettes; pseudorosettes also often present).	5%	There is a continuum between classic ES and PNET. Some authors require Homer-Wright rosettes in 20% or greater of tumor sections plus expression of IHC neural markers (such as NSE, NF, GFAP, Leu-7, S-100 protein) to qualify the ESFT as PNET

Case table 20.1b Differential diagnosis of small round blue cell tumors in children and adults

Tumor	Typical clinical findings	Typical distinguishing microscopic findings	Typical IHC results	Typical genetic results	Comments
Ewing sarcoma family of tumors in bone or soft tissue	Long bone diaphysis or pelvic bones Soft tissue, visceral and skin sites also. Children to young adults most commonly	Uniform small round blue cells with high N/C ratio disposed in sheets (classic type)	CD99: membranous + in >90% of cases. Caveolin-1: + (95%). FLI-1: + (85%)	t(11;22): EWSR1-FLI-1 gene fusion in 85-85-90% t(21; 22): EWSR1-ERG gene fusion in 5-10% Rare other gene fusions	Direct sequencing may be necessary for cases with rare fusions Cases with unusual features require scrupulous attention to differential diagnosis
Pediatric tumors in differential					
Small cell Osteosarcoma	Metaphysis of long bones most commonly. Most patients adolescents. F slightly > M	Uniform small round blue cells but with tumor osteoid production (may be scant). Short spindle cell type also occurs	CD99: membranous + in some cases. Osteonectin, osteocalcin + in most cases (not used often)	Rare cases of EWSR1 gene fusions described. Most are negative for EWSR1 gene fusions	Malignant tumor osteoid is the best diagnostic clue
Mesenchymal chondrosarcoma	Craniofacial bones, ribs, vertebrae, pelvis. Also occurs in soft tissue including meninges. Most C in teens. M = F	Uniform small round blue cells with interspersed hyaline cartilage nodules. May have spindle cells, bone, and osteoid. Common HPC vascular pattern	CD99: may be positive in small round cell component. Cartilage is S-100 positive.	Negative for EWSR1 gene fusions or other recognized ESFT fusions. No specific genetic findings to date	Tumor cartilage and lack of EWSR1 fusion are best diagnostic clues

Case table 20.1b: Continued from page 476

Tumor	Typical clinical findings	Typical distinguishing microscopic findings	Typical IHC results	Typical genetic results	Comments
Pediatric undifferentiated sarcoma, round cell type	Soft tissues of trunk and proximal extremities. Children up to mid-adolescence most commonly	Small round blue cells in sheets	May be CD99 focally positive. Nestin, ckit, S-100 may be positive	Negative for EWSR1 gene fusions or other recognized ESFT fusions. Negative for synovial sarcoma and RMS genetic findings	Diagnosis of exclusion. This group may be whittled down as more cases are reviewed genetically
Metastatic neuroblastoma	May metastasize to bone and soft tissue and thus enter the differential with ESFT. Most patients are infants to 2 years old; rare beyond age 8 years	Small round blue cells (neuroblasts) but may also show neuropil, Schwann cell and ganglion cell differentiation	CD99 negative. CD56, NB84 and CD44 positive. Synaptophysin positive. Chromogranin commonly positive. S-100 positive in Schwann cells	Negative for EWSR1 gene fusions. Molecular studies may show MYCN amplification, 1p deletion or 17q gain	Patient often has a history of neuroblastoma
Metastatic wilms tumor	May metastasize to bone and ST and thereby enter the differential with ESFT Most patients are infants to 8 years; rare beyond age 16 years	Up to three components: primitive small round cell blastema, primitive epithelium and mesenchyme including spindle fibrous areas but also possibly muscle, cartilage and bone	CD99 negative. WT-1 positive in blastema and primitive epithelial areas. CD56 positive in blastema. Epithelial markers positive in epithelium	Negative for EWSR1 gene fusions or other recognized ESFT fusions. May have 11p13 mutation or deletion (WT1 gene). Trisomy 12 relatively common	Patient often has a history of Wilms tumor
Desmoplastic small round cell tumor	Abdominal or thoracic cavity (peritoneal surfaces). Adolescents most commonly. M >> F	Small round blue cells set in a fibrotic or fibroblastic stroma. May have obvious epithelial differentiation and spindle cells	WT-1 positive. CD99 negative. Also commonly positive for desmin, S-100 protein, keratins, and NSE	Negative for specific recognized ESFT fusions. However, most cases exhibit t(11;22) = EWSR1-WT1 gene fusion	Body site location overlaps minimally with ESFT IHC and molecular results are best clues to diagnosis, but FISH using EWSR1 break apart probe will not distinguish between the two
Rhabdomyosarcoma, alveolar or high grade embryonal types	Soft tissues of head and neck, extremities, and viscera in children to young adults	Small round blue cells in alveolar or solid patterns. There is more atypia and mitotic activity in RMS than in usual ESFT. Myoid differentiation may be apparent	CD99 may be positive. Myogenin and desmin positive. Myo-D1 and myoglobin may also be positive	Negative for EWSR1 gene fusions or other recognized ESFT fusions. 80-90% of A-RMS demonstrate t(2;13) = *PAX3-FKHR* or t(1;13) *PAX7-FKHR* gene fusions. E-RMS has no specific consistent genetic findings	Molecular results are best clues to diagnosis in cases with no myoid differentiation. Rare ESFT may have diffuse desmin expression but none show myogenin reactivity
Extra-renal rhabdoid tumor	Infants to young children <10 years most commonly. Soft tissues of head and neck most common	Sheets of round cells most of which have intracytoplasmic eosinophilic hyaline globules. High mitotic rate and apoptosis >> ESFT. A small cell variant has been described with little cytoplasm	CD99 uncommonly positive. Loss of normal nuclear INI-1 expression in almost all cases. Often positive for keratins; sometimes for desmin or actin; vimentin is often dot-like. CD34 negative	Negative for EWSR1 gene fusions or other recognized ESFT fusions. 22q deletions or translocations (*INI-1/SMARCB1* gene)	A few ESFT have many rhabdoid cells. However, diagnostic ESFT gene fusions are also present. INI-1 loss of expression is best diagnostic clue, since many tumors may have foci of rhabdoid cells
Lymphoblastic lymphoma	Most common in adolescents, mostly thymus, lymph nodes and spleen	Small round blue cells without nuclear molding. Usually more mitotically active than classic ESFT. Discohesive	CD99 usually positive. Lymphoid markers positive also (CD45, TdT, CD3, CD34 depending on subtype)	Various translocations. NOT EWSR1 gene fusions or other recognized ESFT fusions	Most cases are T-cell type
Adult tumors in differential					
Some Lymphomas	Middle aged to older adults most commonly	Discohesive uniform small round blue cells	Some cases are CD99 positive. However, lymphoid markers are also positive	Except for acute myeloid leukemia, hematopoietic malignancies are negative for EWSR1 gene fusions or other recognized ESFT fusions Many lymphomas have specific genetic findings that are diagnostically helpful	IHC results are most helpful diagnostic clues to quickly separate lymphoma from ESFT. Additional molecular studies may be needed to subtype the lymphoma or for prognosis or prediction Patients may have splenomegaly and lymphadenopathy

Case table 20.1b: Continued from page 477

Tumor	Typical clinical findings	Typical distinguishing microscopic findings	Typical IHC results	Typical genetic results	Comments
Melanoma (small round cell morphology)	Middle aged to older adults most commonly	One variant consists of small round blue cells without melanin pigment.	CD99 negative. Positive for melanoma markers (HMB45, MelanA, MiTF)	Negative for EWSR1 gene fusions or other recognized ESFT fusions. Karyotype often complex B-raf and c-kit mutations also occur	Patient may have a history of melanoma. S-100 protein reactivity is usual in melanoma but is also present in up to 30% of ESFT. Rare cases of PNET are MiTF positive
Carcinoma, small cell undifferentiated (poorly differentiated neuroendocrine CA)	Middle aged to older adults often with a heavy cigarette smoking history. Lung location most common	Small round blue cells in loose groups or sheets. Nuclear molding is blatant. May have prominent nuclear fragility. Mitoses and apoptosis more prominent than in classic ES. Tumor giant cells may be present	CD99 negative. Keratins, synaptophysin chromogranin positive. Lung cases, in particular, may be TTF-1 reactive	Exceptional cases reported to have EWSR1 gene fusions	Some ESFT are chromogranin and synaptophysin positive. A few small cell carcinomas also contain a squamous cell or adenocarcinomatous component
Carcinoma, poorly differentiated NOS	Middle aged to older adults most commonly	Small round blue cells in loose groups or sheets	CD99 negative. Positive for epithelial markers	Negative for EWSR1 gene fusions or other recognized ESFT fusions	Various types dependent on body site such as sinonasal undifferentiated carcinoma, etc
NUT midline carcinoma	Young to middle aged adults but children are also affected. Midline including upper aerodigestive tract, mediastinum, bladder and pelvic bones	Small round blue cells in sheets. Abrupt nests of squamous cells commonly present	Keratin, CEA and sometimes CD34 positive. New NUT antibody being tested: may be highly specific	Negative for EWSR1 gene fusions or other recognized ESFT fusions. Most cases have t(15;19) = *BRD4-NUT*	Associated with very poor prognosis (most patients DOD by 1 year post diagnosis). Does not respond to ESFT type therapy. Incidence may be widely underestimated. FISH is necessary for diagnosis
Synovial sarcoma, small cell, poorly differentiated	Young to middle aged adults most commonly. Deep soft tissues but also visceral and rarely intraosseous	Small round blue cells disposed in sheets similar to ESFT	CD99 rarely positive. TLE-1 positive in most cases (not entirely specific). EMA, keratins often positive	Negative for EWSR1 gene fusions or other recognized ESFT fusions. Almost all cases have t(X;18) = *SS18-SSX1* or *SS18-SSX2* or *SS18-SSX4* Rare t(X;20) = *SS18L1-SSX1*	S-100 may be positive just as in ESFT. Molecular testing is almost always performed for synovial sarcoma diagnosis
Proximal type epithelioid sarcoma	Young to middle aged adults at limb girdles most commonly	Tumor cells are usually more vesicular with more prominent nucleoli than in most ESFT. Rhabdoid cells sometimes seen	CD99 negative. Keratins, EMA, usually positive. Some are actin positive CD34 positive (50%). Some cases show loss of INI-1 expressio	Negative for EWSR1 gene fusions or other recognized ESFT fusions. 22q deletions or translocations (INI-1/SMARCB1 gene) including t(10;22). Abnormalities of 18q11	Most difficult differential is with extrarenal rhabdoid tumor rather than ESFT Molecular results are best diagnostic clue

Case table 20.1c Summary pathology findings of Case 20.1.

Diagnosis	Ewing sarcoma
Size	9.8 × 9.3 × 7 cm (original size prior to neoadjuvant therapy)
Location	Ilium, predominantly left iliac crest with extension into soft tissue
Margin status	Negative, all greater than 1.0 cm
Histologic grade (FNCLCC grading system)	High grade (Grade 3)
Pathologic stage (AJCC TNM classification)	IIB = high grade tumor > 8 cm without lymph node involvement or metastases (T2/N0/M0)

FNCLCC: Fédération Nationale des Centres de Lutte Contre le Cancer (French Federation of Cancer Centers). AJCC: American Joint Committee on Cancer

REFERENCES

Alaggio R, Bisogno G, Rosato A, et al. Undifferentiated sarcoma: does it exist? A clinicopathologic study of 7 pediatric cases and review of literature. Hum Pathol 2009;40:1600–1610.

Barisella M, Collini P, Orsenigo M, et al. Unusual myogenic and melanocytic differentiation of soft tissue pPNETs: an immunohistochemical and molecular study of 3 cases. Am J Surg Pathol 2010;34:1002–1006.

Barr FG, Womer RB. Molecular diagnosis of Ewing family tumors, too many fusions…? J Mol Diagn 2007;9(4):437–40.

Bert T, Kalsaas A-H, Buechner J, et al. Ewing sarcoma-peripheral neuroectodermal tumor of the kidney with a FUS-ERG fusion transcript. Cancer Genet Cytogenet 2009;194:53–57.

Borinstein SC, Barkauskas DA, Krailo M, et al. Investigation of the insulin-like growth factor-1 signaling pathway in localized Ewing sarcoma: a report from the Children's Oncology Group. Cancer 2011;117:4966–76.

Burgert EO Jr, Nesbit ME, Garnsey LA, et al. Multimodal therapy for the management of nonpelvic, localized Ewing's sarcoma of bone: intergroup study IESS-II. J Clin Oncol 1990;8:1514–24.

Debelenko LV, McGregor LM, Shivakumar BR, et al. A novel EWSR1-CREB3L1 fusion transcript in a case of small cell osteosarcoma. Genes Chromosomes Cancer 2011;50:1054–1062.

Deng F-M, Galvan K, de la Rosa G, et al. Molecular characterization of an EWSR1-POU5F1 fusion associated with a t(6;22) in an undifferentiated soft tissue sarcoma. Cancer Genet 2011;204:423–429.

Drabko K, Zawitkowska-Klaczynska J, Wojcik B, et al. Megachemotherapy followed by autologous stem cell transplantation in children with Ewing's sarcoma. Pediatr Transplant 2005;9:618–21.

Erkizan HV, KongY, Merchant M, et al. A small molecule blocking oncogenic protein EWS-FLI1 interaction with RNA helicase A inhibits growth of Ewing's sarcoma. Nat Med 2009;15:750–6.

Fisher C, Mentzel T, Montgomery EA, et al (Eds). Diagnostic Pathology Soft Tissue Tumors. Salt Lake City: AMIRSYS, 2011.

Flucke U, Palmedo G, Blandenhorn N, et al. EWSR1 gene rearrangement occurs in a subset of cutaneous myoepithelial tumors: A study of 18 cases. Mod Pathol 2011;24(11):1444–1450.

Folpe AL, Goldblum JR, Rubin BP, et al. Morphologic and Immunophenotypic Diversity in Ewing Family Tumors: A study of 66 genetically confirmed cases. Am J Surg Pathol 2004;29(8):1025–1033.

Fraser CJ, Weigel BJ, Perentesis JP, et al. Autologous stem cell transplantation for high-risk Ewing's sarcoma and other pediatric solid tumors. Bone Marrow Transpl 2006;37:175–81.

Gamberi G, Cocchi S, Benini S, et al. Molecular diagnosis in Ewing family tumors: The Rizzoli Experience – 222 consecutive cases in four years. J Mol Diagn 2011;13(3):313–24.

Gill S, McManus AP, Crew AJ, et al. Fusion of the EWS gene to a DNA segment from 9q22-31 in a human myxoid chondrosarcoma. Genes Chromosomes Cancer 1995;12:307–10.

Goldsby R, Burke C, Nagarajan R, et al. Second solid malignancies among children, adolescents, and young adults diagnosed with malignant bone tumors after 1976. Follow-up of a Children's Oncology Group Cohort. Cancer 2008;113(9):2597–604.

Grier HE, Krailo MD, Tarbell NJ, et al. Addition of ifosfamide and etoposide to standard chemotherapy for Ewing's sarcoma and primitive neuroectodermal tumor of bone. N Engl J Med 2003;348-694–701.

Guran T, Turan S, Ozkan B, et al. Cushing's syndrome due to a non-adrenal ectopic adrenocorticotropin-secreting Ewing's sarcoma in a child. J Pediatr Endocrinol Metab 2009;22:363–8.

Hallinger CM, Potschger U, Tarkkanen M, et al. Prognostic impact of chromosomal alterations in Ewing tumors. British J Cancer 2002;86:1763–1769.

Hameed M, Dorfman H. Primary malignant bone tumors-recent developments. Semin Diagn Pathol 2011;28(1):86–101.

Herrero-Martin D, Fourtouna A, Niedan S, et al. Factors Affecting EWS-FLI1 Activity in Ewing's sarcoma. Sarcoma 2011;2011:352580.

Jaffe N, Paed D, Traggis D, et al. Improved outlook for Ewing's sarcoma with combination chemotherapy (vincristine, actinomycin D and cytophosphamide) and radiation therapy. Cancer 1976;38:1925–30.

Kelleher FC, Thomas DM. Molecular pathogenesis and targeted therapeutics in Ewing sarcoma/primitive neuroectodermal tumours. Clin Sarcoma Res 2012;2(1):6.

Kawamura-Saito M, Yamazaki Y, Kaneko K, et al. Fusion between CIC and DUX4 up-regulates PEA3 family genes in Ewing-like sarcomas with t(4;19)(q35;q13) translocation. Hum Mol Genet 2006;15:2125–2137.

Kovar H. Dr. Jekyll and Mr. Hyde: The two faces of the FUS/EWS/TAF15 protein family. Sarcoma 2011;Epub Article ID837474.

Kovar H, Alonso J, Aman P, et al. The first European interdisciplinary Ewing sarcoma research summit. Front Oncol 2012;2:54.

Ladanyi M, Gerald W. Fusion of the EWS and WT1 genes in the desmoplastic small round cell tumor. Cancer Res 1994;54:2837–40.

Ladenstein R, Potschger U, Le Deley MC, et al. Primary disseminated multifocal Ewing sarcoma: results of the Euro-EWING 99 trial. J Clin Oncol 2010;28:3284–91.

Longhi A, Ferrari S, Tamburini A, et al. Late effects of chemotherapy and radiotherapy in Osteosarcoma and Ewing sarcoma patients. The Italian Sarcoma Group Experience (1983-2006). Cancer 2012;118(2):5050–9.

Machado I, Llombart-Bosch A. Myogenic Differentiation in Ewing Sarcoma Family of Tumors. Letters to the Editor. Am J Surg Pathol 2011;35(3);464; Author reply 464–5.

Machado I, Noguera R, Mateos EA, et al. The many faces of atypical Ewing's sarcoma. A true entity mimicking sarcomas, carcinomas and lymphomas. Virchows Arch 2011;458(3):281–290.

Mastrangelo T, Modena P, Tornielli S, et al. A novel zinc finger gene is fused to EWS in small round cell tumor. Oncogene 2000;19(33):3799–3804.

Milano GM, Cozza R, Ilari I, et al. High histologic and overall response to dose intensification of ifosfamide, carboplatin, and etoposide with cyclophosphamide, doxorubicin, and vincristine in patients with high-risk Ewing sarcoma family tumors; the Bambino Gesu Children's Hospital experience. Cancer 2006;106:1838–45.

Miser JS, Krailo MD, Tarbell NJ, et al. Treatment of metastatic Ewing's sarcoma or primitive neuroectodermal tumor of bone: evaluation of combination ifosfamide and etoposide-a Children's Cancer Group and Pediatric Oncology Group Study. J Clin Oncol 2004;22:2873–6.

Nesbit ME Jr., Gehan EA, Burgert EO Jr., et al. Multimodal therapy for the management of primary, nonmetastatic Ewing's sarcoma of bone: a long-term follow-up of the First Intergroup Study. J Clin Oncol 1990;8:1664–74.

Ng TL, O'Sullivan MJ, Pallen CJ, et al. Ewing sarcoma with novel translocation t(2;16) producing an in-frame fusion of FUS and FEV. J Mol Diag 2007;9(4):459–463.

Oberlin O, Rey A, Desfachelles AS, et al. Impact of high-dose busulfan plus melphalan as consolidation in metastatic Ewing tumors: a study by the Societe Francaise desCancers de l'Enfant. J Clin Oncol 2006;24:3997–4002.

O'Keeffe F, Lorigan JG, Wallace S. Radiological features of extraskeletal Ewing sarcoma. Br J Radiol 1990;63(750):456–60.

Padhye B, McCowage G. Chemotherapy regimens in newly diagnosed and recurrent Ewing sarcoma in children and young adults. Cancer Forum 2010;34(3).

Parham DM. Modern diagnosis of small cell malignancies in children. Surg Pathol Clin 2010;3:515–551.

Paulussen M, Ahrens S, Dunst J, et al. Localized Ewing tumor of bone: final results of the cooperative Ewing's Sarcoma Study CESS 86. J Clin Oncol 2001:19(6):1818–29.

Paulussen M, Craft AW, Lewis I, et al. Results of the EICESS-92 Study: two randomized trials of Ewing's sarcoma treatment—cyclophosphamide compared with ifosfamide in standard-risk patients and assessment of benefit of etoposide added to standard treatment in high-risk patients. J Clin Oncol 2008;26:4385–93.

Pierron G, Tirode F, Lucchesi C, et al. A new subtype of bone sarcoma defined by BCOR-CCNB3 gene fusion. Nat Genet 2012;44:461–467.

Pradhan A, Grimer RJ, Spooner D, et al. Oncological outcomes of patients with Ewing's sarcoma: is there a difference between skeletal and extra-skeletal Ewing's sarcoma? J Bone Joint Surg Br 2011;93(4):531–6.

Riccardi GF, Stein C, de la Roza G, et al. Newly described translocation t(18;19)(q23;q13.2) in abdominal wall soft-tissue tumor resembling Ewing sarcoma/primitive neuroectodermal tumor. Cancer Genetics and Cytogenetics 2010;201:1–5.

Romero S, Dei Tos AP. Soft tissue tumors associated with EWSR1 translocation. Virchows Arch 2010;456(2):219–234.

Romero S, Dei Tos AP, Hogendoorn PCW. The clinical impact of molecular techniques on diagnostic pathology of soft tissue and bone tumours. Diag Histopathol 2012;18(2):81–85.
Sankar S, Lessnick SL. Promiscuous partnerships in Ewing's sarcoma. Cancer Genet 2011;204:351–365.
Schiffman JD, Wright J. Ewing's sarcoma and second malignancies. Sarcoma 2011;2011:736841
Schuck A, Ahrens S, Paulussen M, et al. Local therapy in localizated Ewing tumors: results of 1058 patients treated in the CESS 81, CESS 86, and EICESS 92 trials. Int J Radiat Oncol Biol Phys 2003;55(1):168–77.
Shing DC, McMullan DJ, Roberts P, et al. FUS/ERG gene fusions in Ewing's tumors. Cancer Research 2003;63(15):4568–4576.
Spraker HL, Price SL, Chaturvedi A, et al. The clone wars – revenge of the metastatic rogue state: the sarcoma paradigm. Front Oncol 2012;2:2.
Strauss SJ, McTiernan A, Driver D, et al. Single center experience of a new intensive induction therapy for Ewing's family of tumors: feasibility, toxicity, and stem cell mobilization properties. J Clin Oncol 2003;21:2974–81.
Sumegi J, Nishio J, Nelson M, et al. A novel t(4;22)(q31;q12) produces an EWSR1-SMARCA5 fusion in extraskeletal Ewing sarcoma/primitive neuroectodermal tumor. Mod Pathol 2011;24(3):333–42.
Szuhai K, Cleton-Jansen AM, Hogendoorn PCW, et al. Molecular pathology and its diagnostic use in bone tumors. Cancer Genetics 2012;205(5):193–204.
Szuhai K, IJszenga M, de Jong D, et al. The NFATc2 Gene is involved in a Novel Cloned Translocation in a Ewing sarcoma variant that couples its function in immunology to oncology. Clin Cancer Res 2009 1;15(7): 2259–2268.
Tanas MR, Goldblum JR. Fluorescence in situ hybridization in the diagnosis of soft tissue neoplasms: A review. Avd Anat Pathol 2009;16(6):383–391.
Thway K. Primitive round cell neoplasms. Surg Pathol Clin 2011;4:799–818.
Thway K, Fisher C. Tumors with EWSR1-CREB1 and EWSR1-ATR1 Fusions: the Current Status. Am J Surg Pathol 2012;36(7):e1–e11.
Toomey EC, Schiffman JD, Lessnick SL. Recent advances in the molecular diagnosis of Ewing's sarcoma. Oncogene 2010;29:4504–4516.
van Maldegem AM, Bhosale A, Gelderblom HJ, et al. Comprehensive analysis of published phase I/II clinical trials between 1990-2010 in osteosarcoma and Ewing sarcoma confirms limited outcomes and need for translational investment. Clin Sarcoma Res 2012;2(1):5.
van Maldegem AM, Hogendoorn PCW, Hassan AB. The clinical use of biomarkers as prognostic factors in Ewing sarcoma. Clin Sarcoma Res 2012;2(1):7.
Verschraegen C. Unraveling the mystery of a supraclavicular mass. Oncology (Williston Part) 2009;23:721–3.
Womer R, West D, Krailo M, et al. Chemotherapy intensification by interval compression in localized Ewing sarcoma family tumours (ESFT). J Clin Oncol 2008;26S:A10504.
Worch J, Cyrus J, Goldsby R, et al. Racial differences in the incidence of mesenchymal tumors associated with EWSR1 translocation. Cancer Epidemiology Biomarkers Prevention 2011;20:449–453.
Zucman J, Delattre O, Desmaze C, et al. EWS and ATF-1 gene fusion induced by t(12;22) translocation in malignant melanoma of soft parts. Nat Genet 1993;4:341–5.

FURTHER READING

Fisher C, Montgomery EA, Thway K. Biopsy Interpretation Series: Biopsy Interpretation of Soft Tissue Tumors. Philadelphia: Walters Kluwer/Lippincott Williams and Wilkins, 2011.
Klein MJ. Ewing sarcoma. In: Folpe AL, Inwards CY, eds. Bone and Soft Tissue Pathology. A volume in the series: Foundations in Diagnostic Pathology. Goldblum JR (series ed). Philadelphia: Elsevier Saunders, 2010.
Dorfman HD, Czerniak B. Bone Tumors. St Louis: Mosby, 1998.
Maheshwari AV, Cheng EY. Ewing sarcoma family of tumors. J Am Acad Orthop Surg 2010;18:94-107
Fletcher CDM, Bridge JA, Hogendoorn P, Mertens F (eds). World Health Organization Classification of Tumours of Soft Tissue and Bone, 4th Ed. Lyon: IARC Press, 2013.

Chapter 21 Hematopoietic tumors of bone

OVERVIEW

Three malignant hematopoietic proliferations compose this World Health Organization (WHO) category: plasma cell myeloma, solitary plasmacytoma of bone, and primary non-Hodgkin lymphoma of bone. These may create tumorous masses that may be mistaken for other lesions such as metastatic carcinoma or osteomyelitis. However, at least in the case of myeloma, serum and urine studies can provide a clue to the diagnosis, the patients often have other disease-related manifestations, and radiologic findings are often highly suggestive.

Expert hematopathologist review is strongly advised in the initial workup biopsy and any follow-up biopsies of patients with plasma cell myeloma , plasmacytoma and malignant lymphoma of bone. The field of hematopathology merits its status as a subspecialty in anatomic pathology because of its complexity, evolving classification systems, and heavy dependence on sophisticated ancillary testing (which may only be available at larger medical centers). Some national research protocols require central review of the diagnostic material, but all patients with these lesions can benefit from hematopathologist involvement in their care.

CLASSIFICATION

Table 21.1 lists the hematopoietic tumors of bone.

DEMOGRAPHICS

Plasma cell myeloma (PCM)

Plasma cell myeloma is the most common primary malignant bone tumor. About 20,000 new cases are diagnosed per year in the US, and this number will rise as a larger segment of the population ages. The disease is more common in men, and a racial distribution also prevails with Africans then Caucasians then Asians affected. The median age at diagnosis is 69 years (Chesi et al. 2011). Only rarely are individuals under the age of 40 affected (3% of patients) (Slovak 2011). It is a disease of old age.

Lymphoma of bone

This designation does not refer to a specific subtype of lymphoma but instead consists of any lymphoma that predominantly produces a mass lesion in bone. Four circumstances lead to this finding: 1) the lymphoma involves only one skeletal site with or without regional lymph node involvement, 2) multiple skeletal sites are involved without nodal or visceral involvement, 3) the patient presents with a bone lesion, but work-up reveals extensive extra-osseous disease beyond regional lymph nodes, 4) the patient has a known lymphoma and presents with a new skeletal lesion (Fletcher et al. 2002). Most hematopathology experts consider Circumstances 1 and 2 as true 'primary lymphoma of bone'. With this narrowed definition, lymphoma of bone comprises approximately 5% of all extranodal lymphomas (Fletcher et al. 2002).

SEER data for plasma cell myeloma and lymphoma of bone

Surveillance, Epidemiology and End Results (SEER) data were evaluated from 13 US registries during a 15 year period (1994-2008). This section focuses on two histologic types (with the ICDO-3 code presented parenthetically): plasmacytoma/multiple myeloma (9731/3 and 9732/3) and diffuse large B-cell lymphoma (DLBCL; 9680/3). The tumors presented here are limited to the bone. However, it is probable that some of the DLBCL reported in bone in the SEER data represent cases of disseminated disease with secondary tumorous osseous involvement.

The average annual incidence rate is 1.8 per million for plasmacytoma/multiple myeloma, and 1.2 for diffuse large B-cell lymphoma. Females have about half the incidence rate of plasmacytoma/multiple myeloma compared with males (1.2 per million compared to 2.5 per million). Similarly, females are less likely to be diagnosed with diffuse large B-cell lymphoma compared to males (1.0 per million compared to 1.5 per million).

The number of cases reported in 13 SEER registries is shown in **Figure 21.1**. The mean ages at diagnosis for plasmacytoma/multiple myeloma and diffuse B-cell lymphoma of the bone are similar (63.6 years and 57.5 years, respectively). **Figure 21.2** depicts the age distribution of these tumors.

Most of the plasmacytoma/multiple myeloma tumors are diagnosed in the vertebral column, and most of the diffuse large B-cell lymphoma tumors were diagnosed in the lower long bones and associated joints (**Fig. 21.3**).

Table 21.1 Hematopoietic tumor of bone (WHO classification 2013)

Tumor or lesion	Behavior	Additional comments
Plasma cell myeloma and Solitary plasmacytoma of bone	Malignant	Commonest primary malignant bone tumor Part of a family of 'plasma cell dyscrasias' that range from simple serologic abnormalities only to highly aggressive malignant disease including a leukemic component Complex genetic findings
Primary non-Hodgkin lymphoma of bone	Malignant	These are lymphomas that cause a destructive bone appearance on imaging Most are diffuse large B cell lymphomas
Benign: does not recur or recurs non-aggressively and does not metastasize. Intermediate: can recur aggressively and/or rarely metastasizes (<5%) Malignant: can recur and can commonly metastasize.		

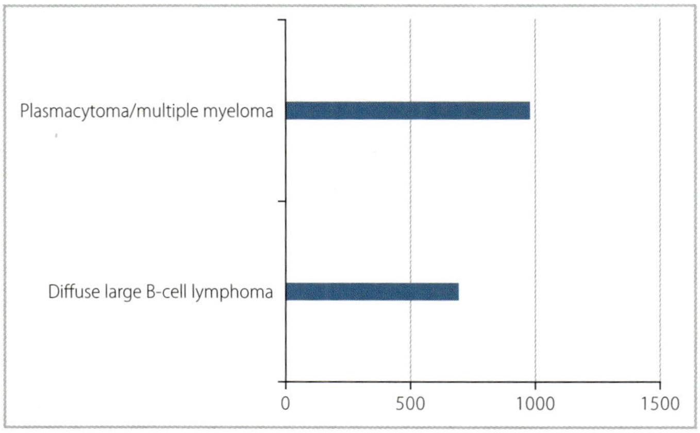

Figure 21.1 Frequency of hematopoietic bone tumor types in 13 SEER registries between the years 1994 and 2008 (only DLBCL is assessed, as it is responsible for 80-92% of primary and secondary bone lymphomas). (some of the DLBL include secondary involvement of the skeleton (exact percentage not extractable.)

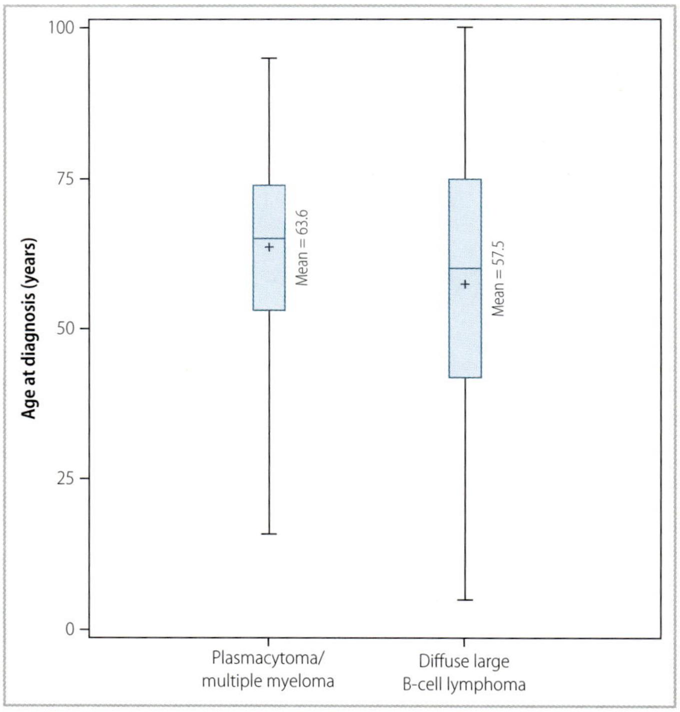

Figure 21.2 Age distribution of hematopoietic bone tumor types among cases in 13 SEER registries during the time period 1994-2008 (N=1,667).

PATHOGENESIS/ETIOLOGY

Plasma cell myeloma

Most multiple myelomas are preceded in the patient by a plasma cell monoclonal gammopathy of undetermined significance (MGUS) or by smoldering multiple myeloma (SMM). Three variants of MGUS are present in 4% of Caucasians over the age of 50 years. This is significant, because 1% of these patients develop lymphoma or PCM per year (Chesi et al. 2011). SMM carries a risk of progression of 10% per year for the first five years (Slovak 2011).

Plasma cell myeloma is a highly complex disease genetically, with a mix of abnormalities affecting important cell pathways that may occur synchronously, linearly, and often variably in subpopulations of the neoplasm. The initiating event is thought to occur with chromosomal translocations arising from abnormal immunoglobulin class switch recombinations (Morgan et al. 2012). Additional aberrant genetic events including copy number abnormalities, DNA hypomethylation, and acquired mutations lead to symptomatic disease, the ability for malignant cells to survive outside the bone marrow environment, and plasma cell leukemia. Patients may expire of other complications of disease before they progress to extra-osseous lesions and a leukemic phase.

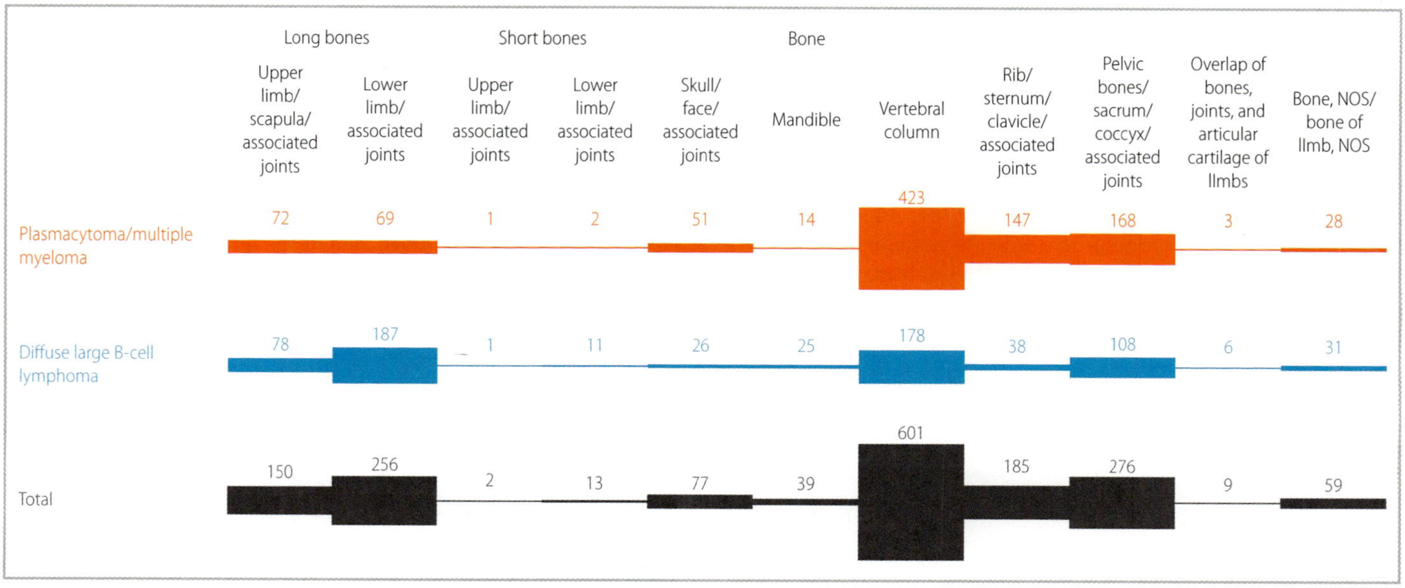

Figure 21.3 Hematopoietic bone tumors by site for cases in 13 SEER registries diagnosed between 1994 and 2008.

Lymphoma of bone

The etiology of primary lymphoma of bone is unknown and most likely is multifactorial. Chronic osteomyelitis has been proposed as one predisposing factor along with other causes of chronic inflammation (McGrory et al. 1999).

Although theoretically any lymphoma may cause a mass lesion in the skeleton, in reality 80-92% of primary non-Hodgkin lymphoma of bone consist of diffuse large B cell lymphomas (Li et al. 2010, Mikhaeel 2012). Others that uncommonly create an intra-osseous mass lesion include anaplastic large cell lymphoma, lymphoblastic lymphoma, follicular lymphoma, extra-nodal marginal zone lymphoma, mantle cell lymphoma, transformed MALT, Burkitt lymphoma, T cell lymphoma, and nodular sclerosing and mixed cellularity variants of Hodgkin lymphoma (Li et al. 2010, Alencar et al. 2010).

While most primary lymphomas of bone involve sites of persistent substantial hematopoiesis including the femur, pelvic bones, vertebra, and humerus, Hodgkin lymphoma preferentially affects flat bones and vertebra (Li et al. 2010). When the long bone is involved the lesion is usually metaphyseal or diaphyseal (Mikhaeel 2012). Generally, true primary lymphoma of bone most commonly affects the appendicular skeleton, while secondary lymphoma affects the axial skeleton.

Rarely, leukemias may cause a mass lesion in the skeleton. Leukemias most likely to do so comprise acute and chronic myelogenous leukemia (AML and CML).

PATHOLOGY

Table 21.2 briefly describes the two hematopoietic tumors of bone according to incidence, body site, and pathologic features.

Histologic grading

Plasma cell myeloma

Grading in PCM is not of major clinical significance. High grade lesions such as the plasmablastic or anaplastic PCM usually manifest cytogenetic or serologic findings of high risk disease; however plasmablastic histology does have independent prognostic significance (Lorsbach et al. 2011). Nonetheless, morphology plays a minimal role in risk stratification of PCM (Mahindra et al 2012).

Lymphoma of bone

When encountering a primary lymphoma of bone, the pathologist must subtype the lymphoma. The specific type of lymphoma reveals key prognostic and predictive information. As most primary

Table 21.2 Pathology features of hematopoietic tumors of bone

Tumor	Incidence	Age and sex distribution	Body site	Histopathology description: Medium magnification	Histopathology description: High magnification
Malignant					
Plasma cell myeloma	Common	Older adults for MM (only 3% are under age 40) with most 50-80 years old Solitary plasmacytoma occurs in slightly younger adults M > F by 2:1 Blacks > Whites > East Asians	Multiple lesions of skull, spine, pelvis, proximal femur, proximal humerus	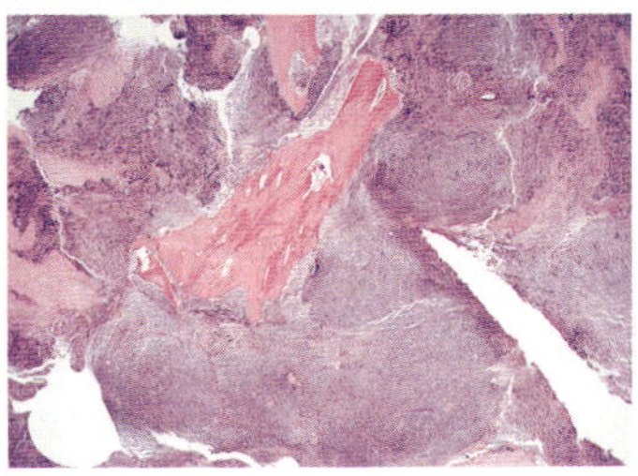	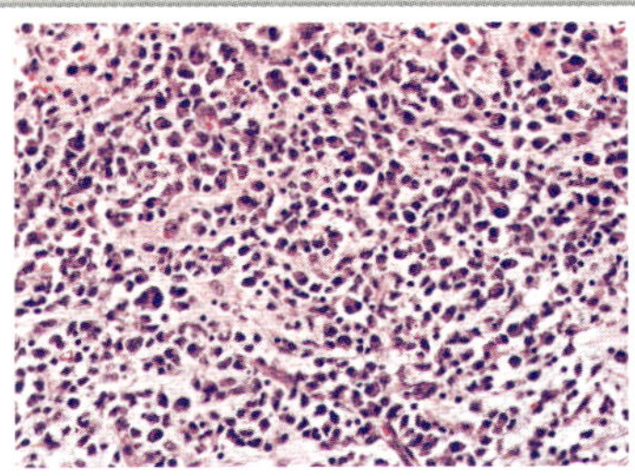
When presenting as one or more lytic (rarely blastic) bone lesions: sheets of tumor cells. Most cases show cytologic features of plasma cells: small to medium sized round cells with eccentric nuclei with a clock-face chromatin pattern and eosinophilic cytoplasm with or without perinuclear clearing (Hof) and Dutcher bodies (nuclear pseudoinclusions). Mott cells, Russell bodies and amyloid may also be present. High grade forms include: Plasmablastic variant that is less recognizable as PCM as lesional cells have vesicular nuclei and large nucleoli. Anaplastic variant is also cytologically pleomorphic and does not show plasmacytic features. There is also a small lymphocyte like variant and a variant with crystal storing-histiocytes. Leukemic phase also occurs. Rarely may be associated with other lymphomas. >90% of cases of plasma cell myeloma have M protein in serum and/or urine assisting in the diagnosis (IgG, IgA, or light chains only). Solitary plasmacytoma has no or little M-protein detected in serum or urine.					
Primary non-Hodgkin lymphoma of bone (mainly comprising diffuse large B-cell lymphoma presenting in bone)	Rare	Most common in mid 40s-mid 60s but broad age range. M slightly > F	Long bones, spine, pelvis. Rarely in acral bones and non-pelvic flat bones. When in long bones, usually located in metaphysis and/ or diaphysis	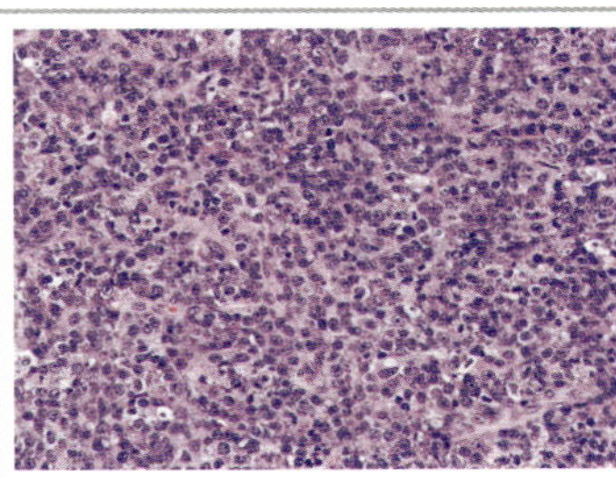	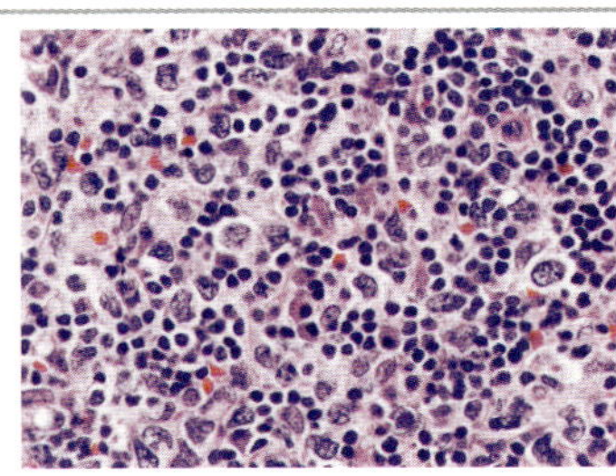
(Description is only for DLBCL) Permeative growth of relatively large malignant lymphoid cells often arranged in sheets. Some cases may have only scattered malignant cells dispersed among reactive inflammatory cells. Malignant cells most often have noncleaved nuclei with moderate pleomorphism and may have prominent nucleoli. Background stroma may be fibrotic. Cell variations include round cells with multilobated nuclei, cells with cleaved nuclei, clear cells, signet ring like cells, and spindled cells					
M: male, F: female, IHC: immunohistochemistry, DLBCL: diffuse large B cell lymphoma Incidence note: 'Common to very common' indicates that a medium sized practice will treat at least several to dozens of patients with the lesion annually, 'Uncommon to rare' indicates the same practice size will treat one to two patients with the lesion every five years, 'Rare to very rare' indicates the same sized practice will see zero to one patient with the lesion every 20 years					

lymphomas of bone are diffuse large B-cell lymphomas, this is considered an 'aggressive' histology. However, response to chemotherapy is very good to excellent with high five year overall survival rates.

Behavior

Plasma cell myeloma

Multiple myeloma is not a curable disease. Overall survival ranges from less than one year for aggressive cases to greater than 10 years. New therapies such as thalidomide, lenalidomide and bortezomib have enabled 20% of patients to survive more than 10 years (Slovak 2011).

Prognostic factors currently assessed include age, tumor burden, renal function, serum LDH, β-2 microglobulin, and albumin levels, functional status, and specific cytogenetic findings of which there are a host (Slovak 2011). However, a molecular classification system is currently under development that will more optimally risk stratify patients. It is anticipated that identification of specific pathway aberrations will enable more adept targeted therapy, understanding that the drugs used in a single patient may alter as resistant clones emerge. Clonal evolution is common in PCM.

Lymphoma of bone

The most important predictors of outcome are the subtype of lymphoma and stage of disease. However, other series suggest performance status and level of LDH also predict overall survival (Lal et al. 2008). In an earlier compilation, the five year overall survival was 61% (Heyning et al. 1999). A more recent review of 53 patients with primary lymphoma of bone report a progression free survival of 83% at four years (Alencar et al. 2010).

Additional laboratory testing

Immunohistochemistry

Immunohistochemical staining profiles of plasma cell myeloma and an abbreviated panel for the majority of primary lymphomas of bone are presented in **Table 21.3**.

Routine cytogenetics and molecular genetics

Some of the major genetic findings of multiple myeloma and primary lymphoma of bone are presented in **Table 21.4**.

Table 21.3 Immunohistochemistry profile of plasma cell myeloma and primary lymphoma of bone (DLBCL) with IHC differential diagnosis clues

Entity	Most common IHC and CISH findings	Less common IHC findings	Differential diagnosis comments
Plasma cell myeloma	CD138+(~100%) MUM1/IRF4+ (~100%), CD38+, VS38c+ (~100%) CD19-, CD45 often - EMA often positive Light chain restricted (CISH and FC)	CD56 (60-90%), CD117 (+/-), CD20+ (10-20%) CD28 (30%)	**Limited panel of IHC (CD138) is used with CISH in lesions with overt plasma cell features.** Most cases of high grade PCM are a progression of known, low grade disease. **Lymphoplasmacytic lymphoma:** most express IgM heavy chain (found in only 1% of PCM), CD138 only focally positive, surface light chain expression **Plasmablastic lymphoma:** EBV positive; most patients HIV+ DLBCL and anaplastic large cell lymphoma enter the differential with high grade PCM. **DLBCL:** CD45+, CD19+, CD20+, high Ki-67 **Anaplastic large cell lymphoma:** CD30+, CD15-, CD2,4 or5+, ALK= (60-85%); may have focal weak CD138 positivity
Diffuse large B-cell lymphoma presenting as primary bone lymphoma	CD45+ (~100%) pan-B cell markers (CD19,20,22,79a,PAX5)+, sIg often positive, Ki-67 >40-50%	CD10, CD15, Bcl-6, Bcl-2 variable	Plasmablastic myeloma: as above plus serologic and urine findings help distinguish the two Anaplastic lymphoma: as above Metastatic carcinoma: keratin positive; negative for CD20, CD45 Sarcoma: negative for CD20, CD45 Melanoma: positive for melanocytic antigens such as S-100, HMB45, MelanA. Negative for CD45, CD20

IHC: immunohistochemistry. CISH: chromogenic in situ hybridization. FC: flow cytometry. sIg: surface immunoglobulin

Table 21.4 Selected genetic findings of plasma cell myeloma and diffuse large b-cell lymphoma (the two major hematopoietic tumors of bone)

Tumor	General abnormality	Genes or chromosomes involved	Percentage of tumors with abnormality
Plasma cell myeloma (PCM)	*IGH* (immunoglobulin heavy chain locus: 14q32) translocations including t(4;14), t(6;14), t(11;14), t(14;16), t(14;20)	*FGFR3/MMSET (4p153), CCND3 (6p21), CCND1 (11q13), MAF (16q23), MAFB (20q11)*	~30%
	Hyperdiploidy	Trisomies of 3,5,7,9,11,15,19 and 21	~57%
	Secondary events including CNA, DNA hypomethylation and acquired mutations	Gains of 1q (*CKS1B, ANP32E*), 12p, 17q Deletions of 1p (*CDKN2C, FAF1, FAM6C*), 6q, 8p, 13 (*RB1, DIS3*), 14q (*TRAF3*), 16q (*CYLD,WWOX*) Abnormalities of cell cycle genes, apoptosis genes, plasma cell differentiation, RNA editing, abnormal DNA repair, proliferation Epigenetic abnormalities of multiple genes. Translocations involving MYC (8q24)	40% (1q) 30% (1p), 33% (6q), 8p (25%),13 (45%), 14q(45%), 16q(35%) Varying percentages and proportions in individual tumors and as tumors progress
Lymphoma of bone (mainly comprising diffuse large B-cell lymphoma presenting in bone: only DLBCL findings reported in this table)	t(14;18)(q32;q21) Other various abnormalities	*IGH-BCL2* *BCL6* and *MYC* and others DNA microarray reveals three types: germinal center type, activated peripheral B-cell type, and type resembling Hodgkin lymphoma	30% (follicular origin type) Type resembling Hodgkin lymphoma is primarily mediastinal in location

CNA: copy number alterations

See References for papers and texts pertaining to this table. This static list of genetic abnormalities must be viewed in the context of continuing discovery and refinement of genetic findings.

RADIOLOGY

Plasma cell myeloma

Imaging has played an important role in the assessment of disease with the number of osteolytic lesion comprising a part of the Durie and Salmon staging system for multiple myeloma (MM) tumor burden. As of 2012, the International Myeloma Working Group still considers radiographic skeletal survey as the 'gold standard' for imaging workup. However, they recognize radiographic sensitivity can be limited and there is significant inter-exam and interobserver variability. A myeloma lesion must replace at least 30% of the trabecular bone before being detectable on radiography. Furthermore, it is the presence of cortical erosion that renders a myeloma lesion most visible for diagnosis and hence will be more consistent for follow up comparison. The radiographic survey is arduous for the patient who may have significant skeletal pain and must be positioned for multiple views of the skull, axial skeleton and the proximal aspect of each extremity. At our institution, we also include anteroposterior views of the distal extremities resulting in a total of 22 radiographs. Even with a determined radiologist, consistent comparison between exams is difficult due to slight differences in projection and variation in radiographic exposure. Another factor potentially complicating radiographic interpretation is the numerous benign causes of osteopenia such as steroid use, advanced age, poor nutrition and disuse which may have similar appearance to disseminated MM.

Alternatively, MR imaging can be used for survey of the skeleton. MM lesions are usually highly conspicuous as they are T1 low signal against a background of normal high signal fatty marrow. The lesions show variable appearance on fluid sensitive sequences (T2 fat saturation and STIR) but are typically isosignal or high signal intensity on these sequences. The specificity of MR is poor as numerous marrow lesions and infiltrating processes will have similar appearance. Hence, MR should be employed for staging and follow up, not primary diagnosis in MM. There are four patterns of marrow disease on MRI; normal, micronodular, focal pattern and diffuse pattern. Gadolinium contrast is typically not needed unless there is concern for a soft tissue mass such as a vertebral lesion with possible extension into the spinal canal. Indeed, MR is the definitive imaging modality for evaluating the spine for myeloma lesions as well as assessing compression fractures and encroachment into the spinal canal. Granulocyte colony-stimulating factor (GCSF) can cause red marrow recrudescence which if exuberant may be indistinguishable from diffuse MM disease burden. MR imaging should therefore be delayed at least 4 weeks after GCSF treatment.

Using advanced whole body MR imaging equipment, Ghanem and coworkers showed total imaging time for skeletal survey with MRI ranged from 12-15 minutes versus 15-45 minutes for an 8 view radiographic survey (Ghanem et al. 2006). In their study, there were three false positive radiographic surveys that were correctly identified as having normal marrow on MRI. In 19% of cases, MRI and radiography were discordant. Approximately half of these patients had false negative radiographic surveys, and MR correctly showed disease in all of these patients. The authors conclude MR is more sensitive and specific than radiographic survey and should be used as an alternative staging procedure.

PET can have a useful imaging role for patients with MM. PET/CT is more sensitive for diagnosing extramedullary disease and can find additional lesion in 30% of patient thought to have solitary plasmacytoma based on MRI. However, PET/CT fails to find MR detected spine and pelvis lesions in 30% of newly diagnosed patients. PET/CT is also useful to assess for lesion response to therapy. A resolving lesion will show return to fatty marrow on MR imaging and will have decreasing uptake on PET/CT (Hanrahan et al. 2010).

Traditionally, TC99 bone scan is not used for workup of MM as most lesions do not show increased uptake.

Lymphoma of bone

Primary lymphoma of bone (PLB) is a rare malignancy. In up to 94% of cases the lymphoma is non-Hodgkin (Mulligan et al. 1999). PLB most commonly affects the metadiaphysis of long bones, particularly around the knee joint. On radiographs, PLB shows lytic destruction in 70% of cases, and of the remainder, most show mixed lytic and blastic lesions. The lytic portion of the lesion has a permeative or moth-eaten pattern in 74%. Approximately half of patients show periosteal reaction which usually had an aggressive interrupted pattern. On CT imaging, approximately half show cortical destruction. On MRI, the lesions show isointensity or mild hyperintensity on T1 with heterogeneous signal on T2 weighted images. Soft tissue masses are evident in all patients as seen by MRI. This overall appearance is non-specific for diagnosis but does indicate an aggressive lesion.

There are a few unusual findings found with PLB; sequestra are seen in 16% of cases and tumor extension across the joint into another bone are seen in 4% of cases. Also, PLB is purely blastic in only 2% of cases while in metastatic lymphoma of bone it is seen in 14% of cases. This probably is related to the rarity of primary Hodgkin lymphoma of bone. Mulligan describes two imaging patterns that are suggestive of PLB, although these patterns are not common (Mulligan et al. 1999). The first pattern is a discordant appearance between the normal radiographs and an accompanying markedly abnormal bone scan or MRI. This pattern is seen in 5% of cases. The second pattern is a marrow lesion with large soft tissue mass but relative preservation of the intervening cortex. These two imaging patterns may be caused by a lesion which is more infiltrative than destructive.

SURGERY

Plasma cell myeloma

Although considered a 'primary' bone tumor, for practical purposes multiple myeloma is treated in the same manner as metastatic bone disease. Because this tumor tends to be quite sensitive to systemic treatment and localized radiation therapy, a more conservative approach is often indicated. Patients with limited local and spinal disease can often be treated successfully without surgery. Pathologic fractures of the spine without instability or neurologic compromise will often do well with conservative therapy. However, patients with impending or real pathologic fractures, particularly of the weight bearing appendicular skeleton, often require surgical stabilization in a manner similar to the treatment for metastatic bone lesions. Patients with pathologic fracture of the spine with instability and/or neurologic compromise will generally require surgical intervention as well.

GRAY AREA

Controversy exists regarding the entity plasmacytoma. The preponderance of current evidence would tend to support that this disease process is a precursor to multiple myeloma and, in fact, most patients who present initially with an isolated focus of disease will progress to systemic disease over time. For those who believe plasmacytoma is a separate and potentially curable disease, wide surgical resection may be indicated.

Lymphoma of bone

Like multiple myeloma, lymphoma of bone tends to respond well to systemic treatment, localized radiation therapy, and therefore more conservative measures. Indications for operative intervention are the same as stated above for multiple myeloma and the treatment also reflects that of metastatic bone disease. Like multiple myeloma, surgery plays no role in the treatment of the disease *per se* but rather is related to treatment for palliative care or stabilization of bony lesions or pathologic fractures while undergoing definitive treatment with other modalities.

MEDICAL ONCOLOGY

Plasma cell myeloma

A solitary plasmacytoma can occur in an osseous or extraosseous site. Once the diagnosis is established after a biopsy, a full staging work-up must rule out the presence of disseminated disease. This includes bone and bone marrow biopsies. The treatment of a solitary plasmacytoma is radiation, regardless of the site of origin. Surgery is an adjunct to radiation. There is no role for medical oncology treatment when the lesion is solitary (Kilciksiz, et al. 2012). Follow-up consists of blood and urine tests to monitor the disappearance of the paraprotein (Warsame, et al. 2012). The tests include a complete blood cell count, serum creatinine, albumin, and calcium, serum quantitative immunoglobulin and protein electrophoresis, serum immunofixation electrophoresis, and serum free light chain assay. Urine analyses include a 24 hour collection for total protein quantity, a urine protein electrophoresis, and a urine immunofixation electrophoresis. An annual bone survey is usually indicated. If a recurrence is suspected, a full work-up to rule out disseminated disease is indicated.

Multiple myeloma

A complete discussion of the therapeutic approaches for multiple myeloma is beyond the scope of this book, as these patients are treated by oncologist specialists of malignant hematological diseases. A brief summary is proffered.

Multiple myeloma is a malignant disease of the bone marrow, where maligant plasma cells develop. These cells secrete monoclonal proteins (M-protein) in the serum and/or the urine (Chesi, et al. 2011, Kyle, et al. 2009). Initial presentation could be a progression from an asymptomatic monoclonal production (monoclonal gammopathy of undetermined significance (MGUS) or a smoldering myeloma) to a dramatic presentation with hypercalcemia, renal failure or bone fractures. Multiple myeloma is sensitive to chemotherapy, but responses are usually transient. New treatment approaches with biologiccal agents have changed the course of this disease to a more indolent one. Patients must be selected upfront for possible autologous stem cell transplant, depending on comorbidities and age. Candidates for transplant should be treated with a marrow sparring regimen, while non transplant candidate could be treated with more suppressive chemotherapies up front (Munshi, et al. 2011).

Table 21.5 describes the most common regimens for multiple myeloma (Rajkumar 2011, Rajkumar, et al. 2011).

Deep venous thrombosis and pulmonary embolism are major side effects of thalidomide and lenalidomide. Lenalidomide causes more myelosuppression, and thalidomide causes more sedation. Peripheral neuropathy and thrombocytopenia are major side effects of bortezomib.

Lymphoma of bone

Primary bone lymphoma (PBL) is a distinct uncommon clinicopathological entity, comprising 5% of all non-Hodgkin lymphomas (Freeman, et al. 1972) and 3% of all bone malignancies (Limb, et al. 1994). The median age at presentation is in the fifth or sixth decade of life, with a male preponderance. Early-stage disease presentation is very common.

Most patients (80%) present with intermediate grade lymphoma that originates in the long bones of the extremities (Beal, et al. 2006) or the spine (Ramadan, et al. 2007). About 80% are diffuse large-cell lymphomas. International Prognostic Index (IPI) and age, but not primary site or pathological fracture at presentation determines the prognosis.

Radiation therapy previously gave good local control, but there was a substantial risk of systemic failure (Dosoretz, et al. 1983). Improved survival rates were reported with the use of combined modality therapy versus radiation therapy alone (Fidias, et al. 1999, Miller, et al. 1998, Rathmell, et al. 1992, Zinzani, et al. 2003). Today, optimal treatment consists in the combination of chemotherapy with cyclophosphamide, doxorubicin, vincristine and prednisone plus rituximab (R-CHOP) (Alencar, et al. 2010). This treatment yields a 3-year progression-free survival of 88% compared to 52% for chemotherapy alone (Ramadan, et al. 2007).

With modern chemotherapy (**Table 21.6**), the role of radiation therapy has changed to an adjuvant to chemotherapy, especially for

Table 21.5 Treatments for multiple myeloma

Induction regimens prior to transplantation	Patients over age 65 or with significant comorbidities	Treatment for relapse
Thalidomide–dexamethasone	Melphalan and prednisone	Any combinations that has not been used in first line
Bortezomib-based regimens	Bortezomib-based regimens	
Lenalidomide–dexamethasone	Lenalidomide-based regimens	

Table 21.6 Primary bone lymphoma series with treatment outcomes according to specific chemotherapy regimen

Reference	Years	No. of patients	Findings
Zinzani, et al. 2003	1982–1998	52	Improved DFS with chemotherapy (with or without radiation therapy)
Rathmell, et al. 1992	1967–1988	27	Improved DFS with CMT versus RT alone
Fidias, et al. 1999	1970–1995	37	Improved DFS and OS with CMT compared to RT alone in historical controls
Beal, et al. 2006	1963–2003	82	Improved OS with CMT versus single modality treatment
Ramadan, et al. 2007	1983-2005	131	Improved DFS with R-CHOP versus CHOP alone
Alencar, et al. 2010	2000- 2007	52	No difference for chemotherapy versus CMT R-CHOP better

PBL: primary bone lymphoma. RT: radiation therapy. CMT: combined modality therapy. DFS: disease-free survival. R-CHOP: cyclophosphamide, doxorubicin, vincristine and prednisone plus rituximab. OS: overall survival.

patients who present with spinal cord compression or those who have residual disease at the end of chemotherapy.

RADIATION ONCOLOGY

Hematopoietic tumors include plasmacytoma and primary lymphoma of bone. Solitary plasmacytomas can be located in bone or in soft tissue. These can potentially be cured with radiation therapy. Involved field radiation therapy to a dose of between 45 and 50 Gy is recommended. Local control is usually at least 90%. Unfortunately, approximately one third of extraosseous lesions still progress to multiple myeloma and two thirds of osseous lesions progress to multiple myeloma. Multiple myeloma is disseminated plasmacytoma. Symptomatic multiple myeloma lesions can effectively be palliated by radiation therapy. Doses of between 10 and 30 Gray are used.

Primary lymphoma of bone comprises rare instances in which the lymphoma arises in the bone. Non-Hodgkin lymphoma is much more common than Hodgkin lymphoma. The most common type of non-Hodgkin lymphoma in this situation is diffuse large B cell lymphoma. Treatment is determined by the specific type of lymphoma. Early stage diffuse large B cell lymphoma of bone is treated by both chemotherapy and radiation therapy while late stage disease is treated with chemotherapy alone. When radiation therapy is indicated, at least 30 Gy of involved field radiation therapy is used. A multicenter retrospective study of early stage primary lymphoma of bone showed a 5-year survival of 76% and local control of 92% (Cai et al. 2012).

CASES

Case 21.1 Plasma cell myeloma

Clinical history and presentation

The patient is a 65 year old man who presents with a two month history of right leg pain. Symptoms began insidiously and have been progressive. Pain is increased with activity and relieved with rest.

Physical examination reveals tenderness on palpation over the proximal aspect of the right tibia. No soft tissue swelling or mass is identified.

Radiographs reveal a destructive lesion of the proximal tibia.

Surgical findings and comments

Due to the aggressive appearance of the lesion as well as the risk of pathologic fracture, surgical exploration is elected. At surgery, a destructive hemorrhagic lesion is identified consistent with malignancy. Curettage of the tumor is performed; the defect is reconstructed with PMMA and internal fixation.

Radiology findings

Our patient, **Case figs 21.1a** through **21.1d** has multiple lytic lesions of the skeleton detected several months after his initial presentation of a destructive lesion of the proximal tibial shaft. Because of the multiple lesions, the radiologic differential includes metastatic disease and multiple myeloma. The absent pedicle on radiographs is a classic finding due to tumorous destruction. The CT images also clearly demonstrate cortical destruction. The right scapular lesion and the left pubic ramus lesion both exhibit the typical lytic appearance of multiple myeloma. The scapular lesion may not be detectable by radiography due to the relative preservation of cortex.

We present three additional cases demonstrating the imaging spectrum of multiple myeloma. **Case figs 21.1e** through **21.1g**, show a lesion of the proximal fibula in a 59 year old woman which proved to be solitary and thus plasmacytoma. The MR images show enhancement indicating the tumor is solid, and there is expansion with extensive destruction of the fibular cortex indicating an aggressive lesion. Imaging is not specific, but the aggressive features indicate tissue diagnosis is warranted.

Case figs 21.1h through **21.1j** show moderate vertebral body compression fractures of T5 and T11 in a 74 year old man. The radiographic appearance is not alarming, and the fractures would likely be attributed to benign osteoporosis related insufficiency fractures. However, the MR images show uniform T1 low signal replacing the entire body of T5 and T11 without appreciable edema seen with T2 imaging. Typically, a benign compression fracture will have greater involvement of one vertebral body endplate with heterogeneous marrow edema signal and possibly adjacent soft tissue edema if the fracture is acute. Discerning benign from malignant compression fracture is difficult. In this case, the uniformity of the complete vertebral body marrow signal replacement favors underlying neoplasia.

Case figs 21.1k through **21.1n** are selected radiographs from a skeletal survey in a 57 year old woman. The skull films, **Case figs 21.1k** and **21.1l**, show numerous sharply defined lucent areas in the calvarium often described as 'punched out' appearing. This is a classic appearance for multiple myeloma. The right humerus film, **Case fig. 21.1m**, reveals numerous lytic lesions and areas of endosteal scalloping indicating extensive disease. The pelvis, **Case fig. 21.1n**, reveals several lytic lesions of the proximal femurs and the left ischial tuberosity. Without appropriate history to guide interpretation, these lesion may be missed or would be attributed to osteoporosis that is somewhat advanced for age. One could also envision how overlying bowel gas could easily lead to a false negative interpretation when searching for lucent or lytic lesion of multiple myeloma.

Pathology findings

Gross features

The curettage of the tibial lesion consists of 5 × 4 × 0.8 cm in aggregate of friable gray tissue mixed with adipose and bone fragments. Samples are collected for cytogenetics, flow cytometry, and tissue banking. The remainder is submitted in seven cassettes with five fixed in 10% neutral buffered formalin and two in AZF.

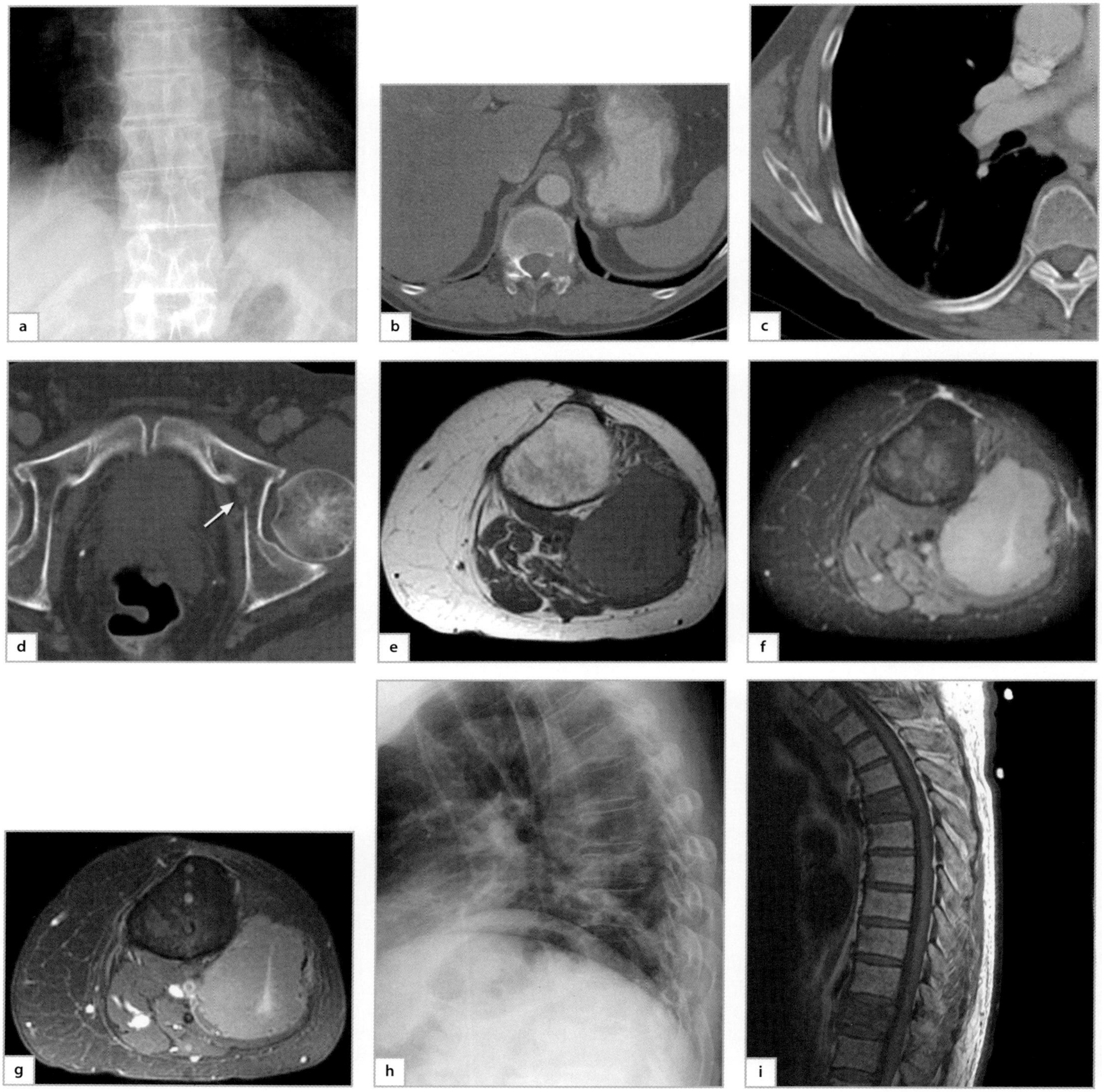

Case figure 21.1 Multiple myeloma. 21.1a: Anteroposterior radiograph of the thoracic spine in a 65 year old man shows the missing left T12 pedicle. **21.1b**: Axial CT scan image with IV contrast shows a lucent lesion destroying the left T12 pedicle corroborating the radiograph finding. **21.1c**: Shows a lytic lesion of the left scapula and **21.1d**: shows a lytic lesion destroying the medial cortex of the left superior pubic ramus. We present three additional cases of multiple myeloma. **21.1e**: Axial T1, **21.1f**: Axial STIR, and **21.1g**: Axial T1 fat saturated post-contrast of a 59 year old woman. There is a 4.9 × 5.7 × 4.6 cm mass destroying the proximal fibula. The mass is T1 iso-signal intensity and moderately high STIR signal intensity with modest enhancement. The next case is a 74 year old man who has two mild compression fractures of T5 and T12 seen on lateral chest view. **21.1h**: No lytic focus or fracture line or cortical step-off seen. The MR images: **21.1i**: Sagittal T1.

Case figure 21.1: Continued from page 488

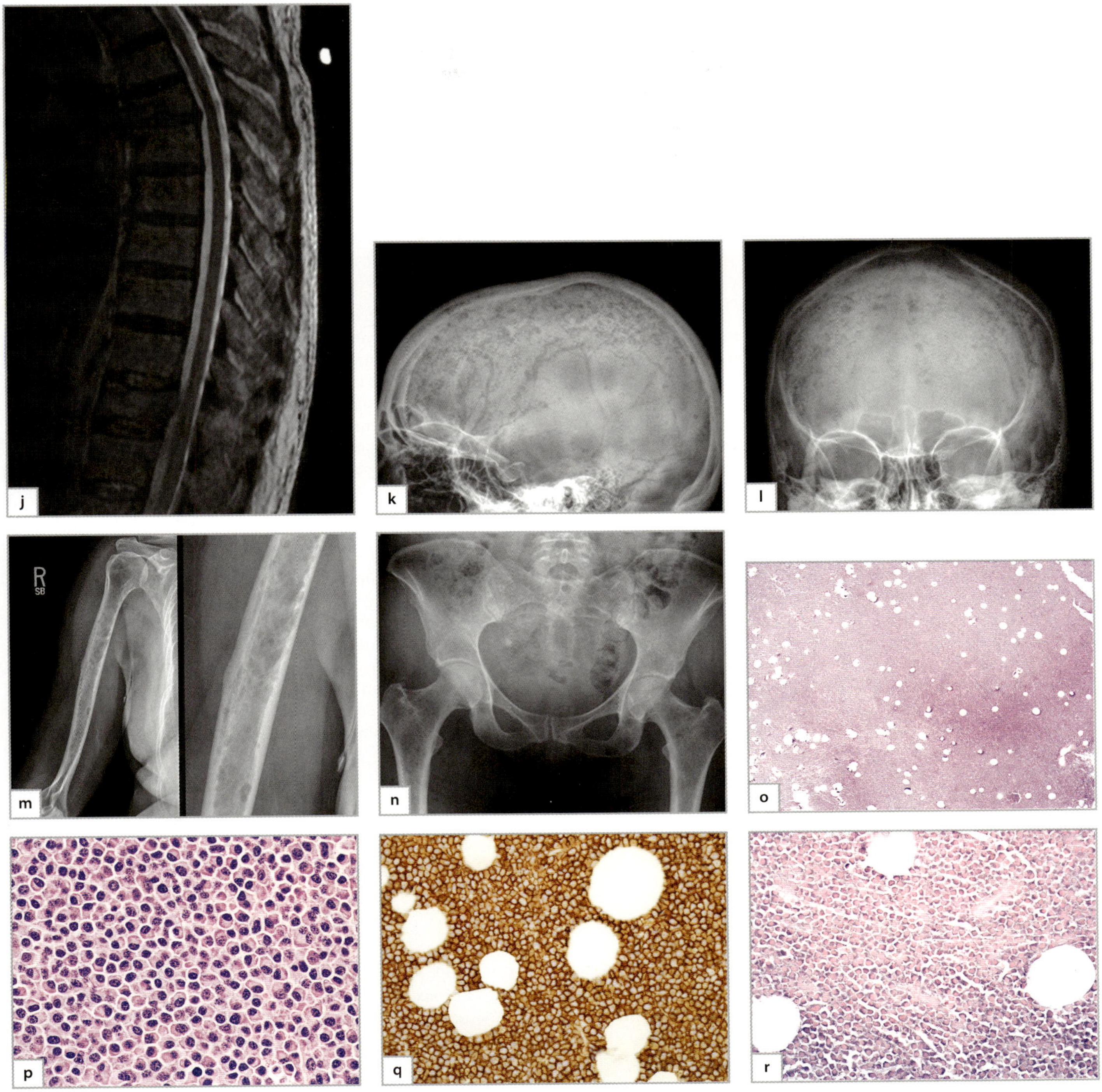

21.1j: Sagittal T2 show uniform T1 low signal of these two vertebral bodies. There is minimal T2 high signal of these vertebral bodies and no adjacent soft tissue edema. The final case involves a 57 year old woman with selected radiographs from a radiographic skeletal survey. **21.1k**: Lateral. **21.1l**: Anteroposterior skull radiographs show numerous sharply defined lytic lesions of the calvarium. **21.1m**: Is an AP view with close-up showing numerous sharply defined lytic lesions with multiple areas of endosteal scalloping involving the entire humeral diaphysis. **21.1n**: Is an anteroposterior view of the pelvis showing several small lytic lesions of the proximal femurs and a lytic lesion of the left ischial tuberosity. **21.1o**: Low magnification. The tumor destroys trabecular bone and forms sheets of cells effacing normal marrow architecture. Scattered residual marrow fat cells are widely dispersed. **21.1p**: Medium magnification. Tumor cells resemble normal plasma cells with pale eosinophilic cytoplasm, eccentrically located nuclei, and a clock-face chromatin distribution. Mitotic activity is low, and pleomorphism is minimal. **21.1q**: Medium magnification, CD138 IHC stain. As expected, CD138 is diffusely expressed with strong intensity in the neoplastic cells (brown chromogen). **21.1r**: Medium magnification, chromogenic in situ hybridization, kappa light chain. The reaction is pale, but all cells express kappa light chain consistent with a monoclonal plasma cell proliferation.

Case figure 21.1: Continued from page 489

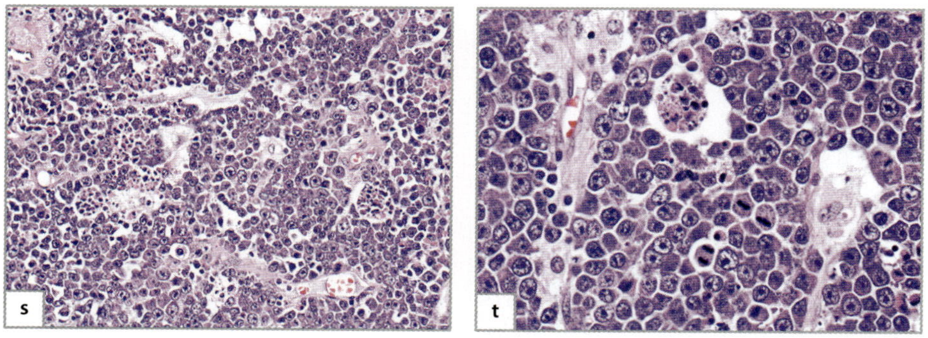

21.1s: Contrasting patient with plasmablastic myeloma, medium magnification. This patient has a high grade plasma cell myeloma with foci of necrosis and tingible body macrophage strewn among the malignant cells. **21.1t**: Contrasting patient with plasmablastic myeloma, high magnification. High grade plasma cell myelomas lack morphologic similarity to normal plasma cells. Here the malignant cells demonstrate vesicular nuclei with prominent nucleoli and a high rate of individual cell necrosis and mitotic activity. Such tumors often behave more aggressively and usually exhibit genetic poor prognostic features also.

Microscopic features

Low magnification: The lesion consists of sheets of cells that destroy trabecular bone with only scant, scattered marrow adipocytes remaining (**Case fig. 21.1o**).

High magnification: To a remarkable degree, the patient's neoplastic tumor cells appear similar to normal plasma cells. Tumor cells feature pale, glassy eosinophilic cytoplasm and eccentric nuclei resulting in a moderate N/C ratio. The nuclei exhibit a 'clock face' distribution of chunky chromatin (**Case fig. 21.1p**). Mitotic activity and necrosis are minimal.

Special studies: Virtually all PCM express CD138, and this tumor does so diffusely and with strong intensity (**Case fig. 21.1q**). The tumor is kappa light chain restricted by chromogenic in situ hybridization (**Case fig. 21.1r**) indicating monoclonality. However, the assay is suboptimal (repeated twice with appropriately reactive controls). Flow cytometry confirms kappa restriction. Flow cytometry may underestimate the level of tumor involvement due to dilution effects and increased fragility of the malignant plasma cells (Lorsbach 2010).

The patient's karyotype is not obtained due to lack of malignant cell growth in culture. FISH testing is negative for t(4;14), and there is no evidence for deletion of 11q22.3, 13q14.3, 13q34, or 17p13.1 in the cells examined. There is no evidence for the CCND1/IgA associated with t(11;14).

The patient's serum and urine reveal an M protein (IgG light chain) by immunoelectrophoresis.

Contrasting patient with plasmablastic type of plasma cell myeloma: For comparison, a patient with a high grade plasma cell myeloma is also presented. At medium magnification, the malignant cells form loosely cohesive sheets as in the patient's lesion (**Case fig. 21.1s**). High magnification reveals neoplastic plasmablasts, larger, more primitive cells with vesicular nuclei and prominent nucleoli (**Case fig. 21.1t**). Mitotic activity is high, and individual cell necrosis is prominent which as prompted the presence of scattered, tingible body macrophages. These cells do not betray a morphologic relationship to plasma cells, in contrast to the presented patient's well differentiated tumor. In cases of plasmablastic myeloma and anaplastic myeloma, additional studies (flow cytometry, extended IHC staining, FISH and CISH) are required to confirm the diagnosis of plasma cell myeloma.

Pathologic differential or, why isn't it one of the following?

Chronic osteomyelitis: Some cases of PCM do not consist of effacing sheets of atypical plasma cells but instead consist of clusters of mildly atypical plasma cells that could mimic a chronic inflammatory process. Bone destruction can occur in both diseases along with reactive new bone formation. Chronic osteomyelitis often also demonstrates marrow fibrosis and acute inflammation with spicules of necrotic bone surrounded by mixed inflammatory cells. In challenging cases, immunohistochemistry and flow cytometry will disclose the diagnostic monoclonal nature of the plasma cell infiltrate in PCM. By CISH, the kappa to lambda ratio of plasma cells in chronic osteomyelitis is normal or mildly elevated (~3:1).

In most cases, solitary plasmacytoma usually grows as sheets of malignant cells with plasmacytic histology, making the diagnosis straightforward.

Another type of lymphoma: Some plasma cell myelomas do not contain cells resembling normal mature plasma cells (so-called Marschalko morphology). Variants that may cause confusion with other lymphomas include small lymphocyte-like PCM, plasmablastic PM, and anaplastic PM. Small lymphocyte-like PCM expresses CD138, lacks surface light chain expression and usually expresses cyclin D1 in contrast to lymphoplasmacytic lymphoma (Lorsbach 2010). Most patients with plasmablastic lymphoma are HIV+, and the malignant cells are EBV+.

Metastatic carcinoma: Some plasma cell myelomas are anaplastic and can mimic metastatic carcinoma. EMA and CD138 may be expressed in both PCM and metastatic carcinoma. However, IgG light chain restriction and MUM1/IRF4 reactivity confirm the diagnosis of PCM, as both are absent in metastatic carcinoma.

Metastatic melanoma: Higher grade PCM may be difficult to distinguish from non-pigmented, metastatic melanoma which can also consist of round, dyscohesive cells with prominent macronucleoli, a high mitotic rate, and individual cell necrosis. IHC will distinguish the two, however, because melanoma expresses melanocytic markers S-100 protein, HMB45, MelanA103, and/or MIT-F while PCM lacks these antigens and shows light chain restriction and reactivity for CD138, CD38, and MUM1. However, both malignancies may express VS38c (recognizes p63) and CD56.

Oncology approach

Medical oncology

Two months after the initial surgical procedure, follow-up reveals progression of disease to multiple myeloma with detection of M protein in serum and urine samples and development of new bone lesions. The patient is randomized on the following protocol 'Phase III trial of lenalidomide and low dose dexamethasone versus bortezomib, lenalidomide and low dose dexamethasone for induction, in patients with previously untreated multiple myeloma without an intent for immediate autologous stem cell transplant.' He receives 6 cycles of

Table 21.1 Summary pathology findings of Case 21.1

Diagnosis	Solitary osseous plasmacytoma that evolves in two months to multiple myeloma
Size	5 cm
Location	Tibia, proximal shaft
Margin status	Not applicable: this is a curettage specimen of a hematopoietic malignancy
Histologic grade (Bartl et al.)	Non-high grade by the Bartl grading system. Currently, risk stratification for PCM relies primarily on stage and identification of high risk genetic abnormalities and not on morphologic grade
Pathologic stage (International staging system for myeloma)	International staging system for myeloma combines laboratory and clinical findings to generate the stage of disease. The patient is stratified into Stage I, II, or III after meeting the diagnostic criteria for multiple myeloma. Levels of serum β-2 microglobulin (with some contribution from serum albumin) determine the stage

the triple chemotherapy on the bortezomib arm (Moreau, et al. 2012). Despite this regimen, he requires an autologous stem cell transplant (Matsui, et al. 2012, Sheppard, et al. 2012) with melphalan 200 mg/m^2 as a conditioning regimen, followed by maintenance lenalidomide (Ludwig, et al. 2012) and zoledronic acid (Modi, et al. 2012). The patient obtains a complete remission after autologous stem cell transplant.

A solitary plasmacytoma does not require medical treatment. However, if the disease becomes metastatic, patients are treated like any other patient with multiple myeloma (Mahindra, et al. 2012).

Radiation oncology

Palliative radiation therapy is delivered to the right tibial lesion.

Patient outcome

Twenty-six months following autologous stem cell transplantation, the patient is noted to be in complete remission. The patient has been placed on bisphosphonates and is followed quarterly with an office appointment, complete blood count, serum protein electrophoresis and serum chemistries including creatinine. He will also undergo an annual skeletal survey.

Case 21.2 Diffuse large b cell lymphoma presenting as lymphoma of bone

Clinical history and presentation

The patient is a 51 year old woman who presents with a four month history of right shoulder pain.

Physical examination demonstrates a palpable firm mass in the proximal right humerus and anterior deltoid. The mass is non-tender. Range of motion of the shoulder is limited to approximately 50% of normal in all planes and is associated with pain.

Imaging studies reveal a destructive lesion of the proximal humerus with large associated soft tissue mass.

Surgical findings and comments

Open biopsy of the soft tissue mass is performed.

The patient is treated with systemic chemotherapy and localized radiation therapy to the humerus.

Three months following biopsy, the patient sustains a fracture of the right humerus. The fracture is treated conservatively and heals.

Radiology findings

This patient, **Case figs 21.2a** through **21.2g**, is first evaluated with radiographs that disclose a very subtle decreased density of the proximal right humerus that could be easily missed. By comparing with the normal left shoulder, one can appreciate the subtle loss of bone density. The actual extent of the tumor comes as a surprise on MR. This pattern of near normal radiographs with extensive tumor on MR or bone scan is seen in 5% of PLB. It is common for bone lymphoma to present with an extensive soft tissue tumor component.

Typically, primary bone lymphoma will cause permeative bone destruction. In this case, the destruction only becomes apparent on the ten month follow-up radiographs.

Pathology findings

Gross features

The curettage consists of fragments of tan to fatty tissue aggregating to 3 × 1.8 × 0.8 cm. A portion of firm tissue is submitted for flow cytometry, and the remainder is fixed in formalin or AZF.

Microscopic features

Low magnification: Lower magnification reveals sheets of cells that efface normal bone marrow architecture (**Case fig. 21.2h**).

High magnification: High magnification reveals relatively large, round cells with indistinct cell borders and moderate size variation of nuclei (**Case fig. 21.2i**). Most nuclei contain macronucleoli, and chromatin is coarse. The background is sclerotic. Cellular debris consistent with individual cell necrosis is present. Mitoses are frequent (>15/10hpf).

Special studies: Consistent with B-cell differentiation, the malignant lymphoid cells are diffusely strongly positive for CD20 (**Case fig. 21.2j**). The tumor cells lack CD3 (a T-cell marker) (**Case fig. 21.2k**), CD5 and CD43. Additional expressed antigens include CD10 (**Case fig. 21.2l**), Bcl-2, and Bcl-6. Approximately 90% of the malignant lymphoid cells express Ki67 consistent with a high proliferation index (**Case fig. 21.2m**). Flow cytometry identifies a highly atypical lambda-light chain restricted B-cell population expressing CD19, CD20, CD10 and Bcl-6 consistent with DLBCL of follicular origin.

Comparison patients with primary lymphoma of bone: Lymphomas are fragile cells and susceptible to crushing. In this patient, 90% of the biopsy is uninterpretable (**Case fig. 21.2n**). However, 10% of the

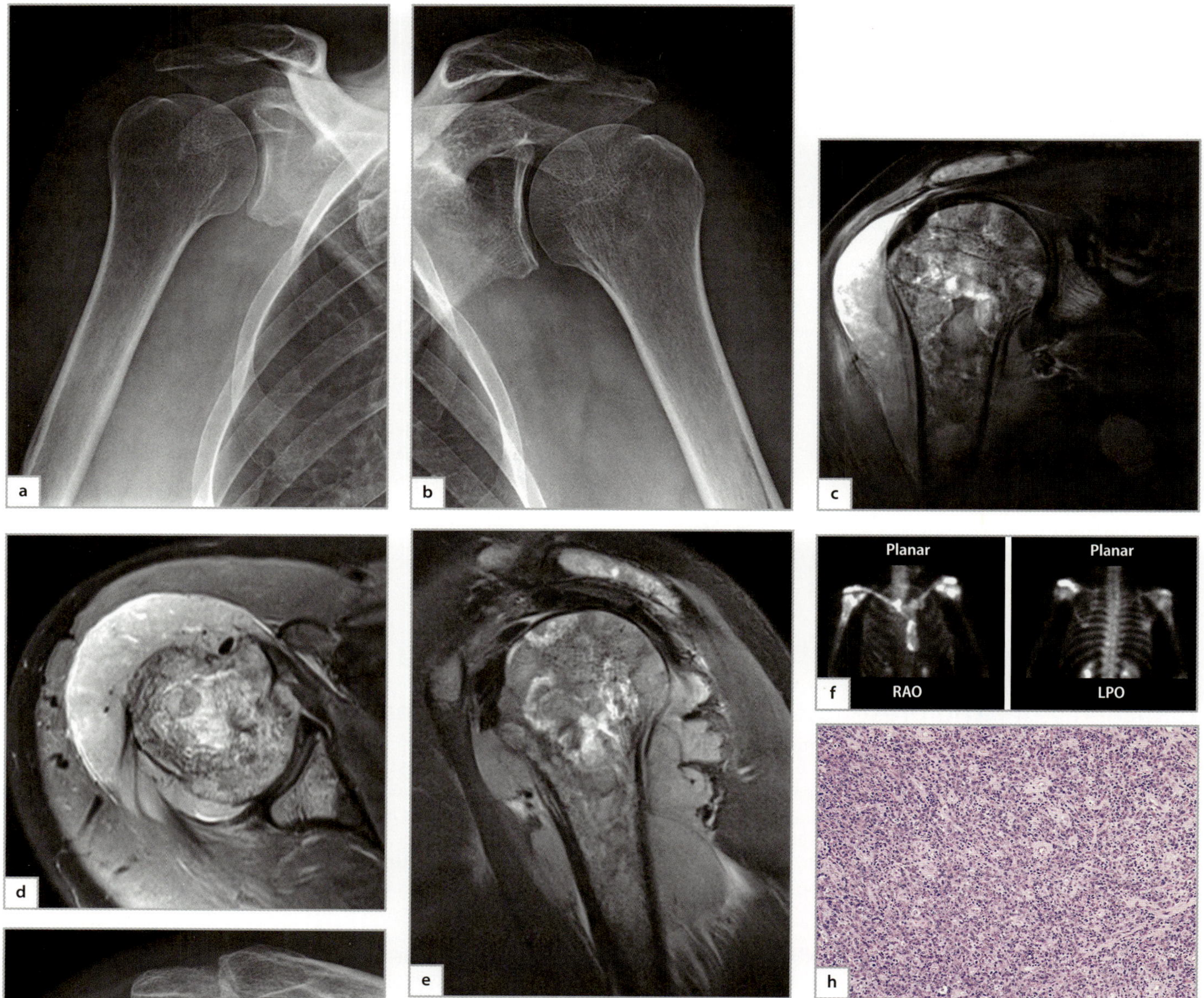

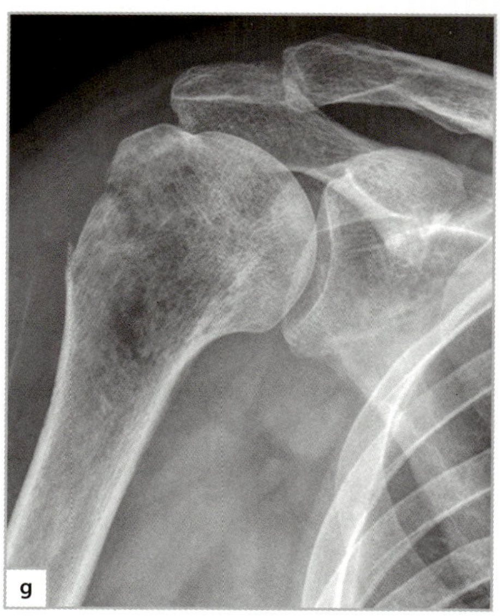

Case figure 21.2 Lymphoma of bone. **21.2a**: Internal rotation radiograph of the right shoulder shows very subtle decreased density of the proximal humerus. This is appreciable by comparing with the normal left humerus radiograph, **21.2b**: Internal rotation view of the normal left shoulder. MR images including: **21.2c**: Coronal T2 fat saturated, **21.2d**: Axial PD fat saturated and **21.2e**: Sagittal T2 fat saturated. These show an infiltrating lesion of the proximal humerus with extensive soft tissue mass. There are several enlarged axillary lymph nodes. The cortex is surprisingly intact given the extent of the soft tissue mass. This explains the near normal appearance of the humerus on radiographs. The nuclear medicine bone scan, **21.2f**: Shows significant increased uptake. The follow up radiograph, **21.2g**: obtained 10 months later shows permeative destruction of the humerus with pathologic fracture. **21.2h**: AZF fixation, lower magnification. The malignant process effaces normal bone marrow and replaces it with sheets of neoplastic cells. Small, hyalinized blood vessels are embedded in the tumor.

Case figure 21.2: Continued from page 492

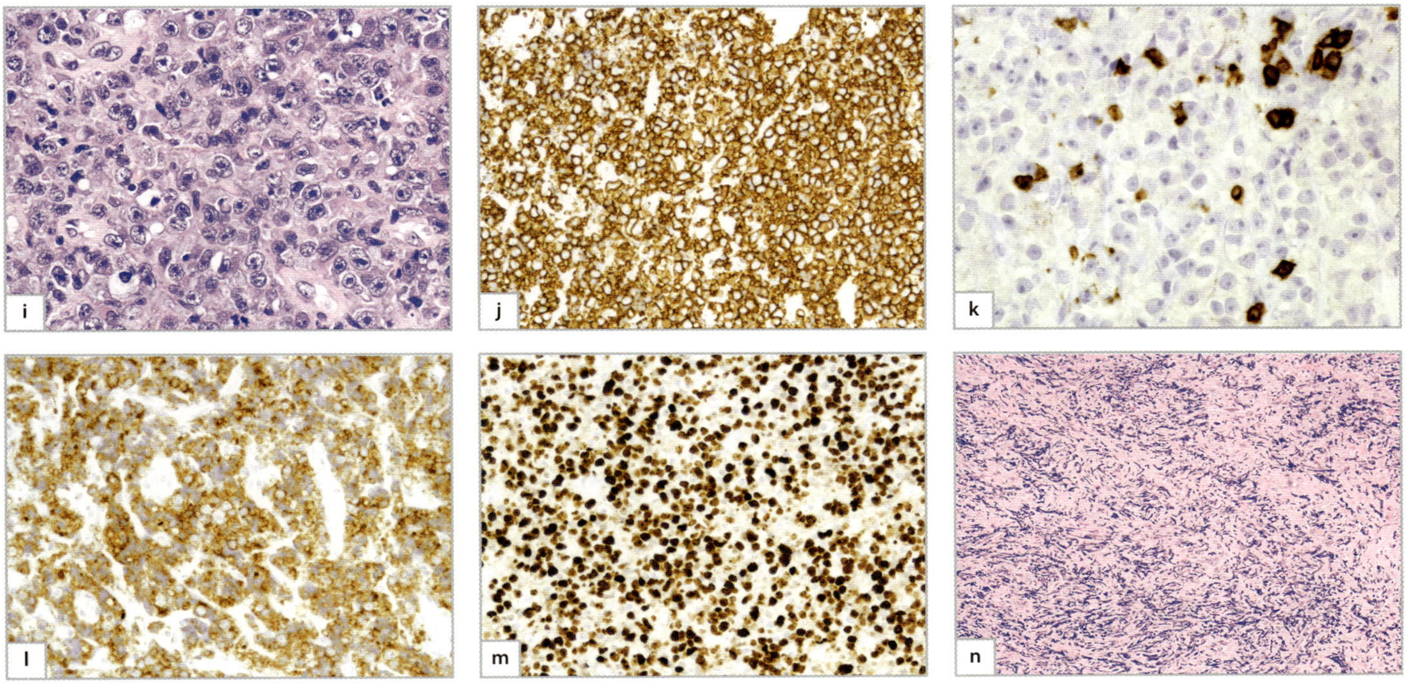

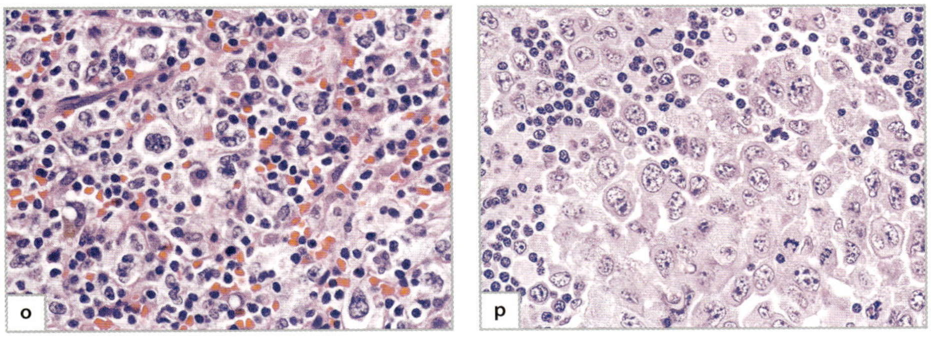

21.2i: AZF fixation, high magnification. Tumor cells are relatively large (for comparison, note the pale macrophage near the bottom left portion of the photo). Nuclei vary in size and contain moderately coarse chromatin. Single macronucleoli are common. Cell borders are indistinct, and the background is sclerotic. Individual cell necrosis is present. **21.2j**: Medium magnification, CD20 IHC stain. As expected the malignant B-cells diffusely and strongly express CD20 (brown chromogen). **21.2k**: Higher magnification, CD3 IHC stain. Tumor cells do not express CD3, a T-cell marker. However, a few T lymphocytes are intermingled among the malignant B-cells (brown chromogen). **21.2l**: Medium magnification, CD10 IHC stain. Diffuse large B-cell lymphomas may express a number of other markers. In this patient, the malignant cells also express CD10 (brown chromogen). **21.2m**: Medium magnification Ki-67 IHC stain. The patient's tumor has a high proliferation index with ~90% of malignant cells reactive for Ki-67 (brown chromogen). **21.2n**: Medium magnification, crush artifact. This second patient's biopsy is less than optimal due to crushing of malignant cells. Since malignant lymphoid cells are fragile, it is advisable to obtain the specimen in a manner that handles the tissue as gently as possible. **21.2o**: High magnification, second patient. This area of the biopsy is not crushed and reveals scattered multilobated neoplastic cells surrounded by reactive inflammatory cells including lymphocytes, histiocytes, and plasma cells. DLBCL of bone may assume a variety of morphologies including cleaved and non-cleaved nuclei, nuclei with prominent nucleoli, multilobated nuclei, scattered cells intermixed with reactive inflammatory cells as in this patient, and even a spindle cell appearance. **21.2p**: High magnification, third patient. This third comparison patient with DLBCL of bone discloses the large size of the cells compared with normal lymphocytes, and exhibits marked nuclear pleomorphism. The differential diagnosis of DLBCL of bone often includes other malignancies such as metastatic carcinoma, metastatic melanoma and another lymphoma. Ancillary testing is always advised to confirm the diagnosis.

tumor is preserved and consists of hyperlobated malignant lymphocytes intermixed with many reactive lymphocytes, plasma cells, and histiocytes (**Case fig. 21.2o**). When possible, the individual obtaining a biopsy of a potential lymphoma should perform the procedure in a manner minimalizing crushing. The morphology of these cells may cause them to be mistaken for Hodgkin lymphoma or a T-cell lymphoma. Both rarely present as primary lymphoma of bone, and both can be distinguished from the usual primary lymphoma of bone, DLBCL, by immunohistochemistry, flow cytometry, and, when necessary, genetic analysis. The malignant cells of a third patient with lymphoma of bone exhibit more nuclear pleomorphism than the patient presented (**Case fig. 21.2p**). Ancillary studies are required to establish the diagnosis of DLBCL.

Pathologic differential or, why isn't it one of the following?

Chronic osteomyelitis: Some primary bone lymphomas consist of relatively few tumor cells intermingled with reactive inflammatory cells including neutrophils, eosinophils, lymphocytes, and plasma cells. In such cases, osteomyelitis may enter the differential. However, most cases of primary bone lymphoma will feature cells with nuclear atypia. Mixed B and T cells will be seen in osteomyelitis.

Flow cytometry or gene rearrangement studies will fail to identify a clonal population.

Other lymphomas: The differential of DLBCL of bone may include other lymphomas and myeloma. T-cell lymphoma and Hodgkin lymphoma of bone are rare, and the latter is more likely to occur in the axial rather than appendicular skeleton. IHC and flow cytometry (and serum and urine protein electrophoresis in myeloma) enable a specific diagnosis. Burkitt lymphoma in African endemic form occurs preferentially in the maxilla or mandible, exhibits a starry sky pattern, is less pleomorphic cytologically, expresses CD10 (usually absent in DLBCL), and most harbor a t(8;14)(q24;q32).

Metastatic carcinoma: The discohesive malignant lymphoid cells and lack of gland or tubule formation could be consistent with a poorly differentiated metastatic carcinoma. Rarely, lymphoma of bone exhibits a signet ring cell morphology that can be mistaken for metastatic gastric adenocarcinoma. IHC will reveal expression of keratins in carcinoma and lack of lymphoid markers, while the obverse holds for lymphoma of bone.

Metastatic melanoma: Overlap can occur histologically, but melanoma expresses melanocytic markers in most cases. In the rare cases of metastatic melanoma lacking melanocytic marker expression, clinical history and/or lack of lymphoid marker expression should enable the diagnosis.

Metastatic or primary spindle cell sarcoma: DLBCL of bone may rarely assume a spindle cell morphology that could mimic sarcoma. Once more, IHC lymphoid marker expression enables the correct diagnosis of primary lymphoma of bone.

Oncology approach

Medical oncology

A staging work-up reveals metastatic disease to nodes and bones. The bone scan shows bilateral humeral lesions, the CT scan demonstrates extensive lymphadenopathies, and the bone marrow is involved with lymphoma.

Table 21.2 Summary pathology findings of Case 21.2

Diagnosis	Diffuse large B cell lymphoma presenting as a single lytic bone mass
Size	Large destructive lesion with extraosseous extension > 8 cm
Location	Humerus
Margin status	Not applicable: this is a curettage specimen of a hematopoietic malignancy
Histologic grade	'Aggressive' histology
Pathologic stage (Ann Arbor staging system)	Stage IVA (O+)(M+)(N+): bilateral humerus lesions, positive bone marrow and unilateral axillary adenopathy in a patient without B symptoms

The patient is enrolled in a clinical trial 'Phase III randomized study of R-CHOP (see Introduction) versus dose-adjusted EPOCH-R (etoposide, prednisone, vincristine, doxorubicin, and cyclophosphamide with rituximab) with molecular profiling in untreated de novo diffuse large B-cell lymphomas'. The patient completes 8 cycles of therapy on the dose-adjusted arm. A complete remission is documented by bone marrow biopsy and PET/CT scan six months after the onset of treatment.

This is a case of disseminated lymphoma that presents as a bone tumor. Twenty-five percent of patients who first present with a bone lymphoma have disseminated disease (Alencar, et al. 2010). In this case, the treatment follows the standard therapy for disseminated disease (Cabanillas 2010).

Radiation oncology

Initially chemotherapy is delivered followed by a course of palliative radiation therapy.

Patient outcome

Three years following treatment, the patient remains in remission. She will continue to have chest, abdomen and pelvis CT scans and selected laboratory studies and annually thereafter until five years from diagnosis.

REFERENCES

Alencar A, Pitcher D, Bryne G, et al. Primary bone lymphoma – the University of Miami experience. Leuk Lymhoma 2010;51:39–49.

Beal K, Alen L, Yahalom J. Primary bone lymphoma: treatment results and prognostic factors with long-term follow-up of 82 patients. Cancer 2006:106:2652–2656.

Cabanillas F. Front-line management of diffuse large B-cell lymphoma. Curr Opin Oncol 2010;22:642–5.

Cai L, Stauder MC, Zhang YJ, et al. Early-stage primary bone lymphoma: A retrospective, multicenter rare cancer network (RCN) study. Int J Radiat Oncol Biol Phys 2012;83(1):284–91.

Chesi M, Bergsagel L. Many multiple myelomas: making more of the molecular mayhem. Hematology 2011;344–353.

Dosoretz DR, Murphy GF, Raymond AK, et al. Radiation therapy for primary lymphoma of bone. Cancer 1983;51:44–6.

Fidias P, Spiro I, Sobczak ML, et al. Long-term results of combined modality therapy in primary bone lymphomas. Int J. Radiat Oncol Biol Phys 1999;45:1213–8.

Fletcher CDM, Krishnan Unni K, Mertens F (Eds). World Health Organization Classification of Tumours. Pathology and Genetics of Tumours of Soft Tissue and Bone. Lyon: IARC Press, 2002.

Folpe AL, Inwards CY, editors. Bone and Soft Tissue Pathology: a Volume in the Series Foundations in Diagnostic Pathology, series editor John R Goldblum. Philadelphia, USA: Saunders Elsevier, 2010.

Freeman C, Berg JW, Cutler SJ. Occurrence and prognosis of extranodal lymphomas. Cancer 1972;29:252–60.

Ghanem N, Lohrmann C, Engelhardt M, et al. Whole-body MRI in the detection of bone marrow infiltration in patients with plasma cell neoplasms in comparison to the radiological skeletal survey. Eur Radiol 2006;16(5):1005–14.

Hanrahan CJ, Christensen CR, Crim JR. Current Concepts in the Evaluation of Multiple Myeloma with MR Imaging and FDG PET/CT. Radiographics 2010;30(1):127–142.

Heyning FH, Hogendoorn PC, Kramer MH et al. Primary non-Hodgkin's lymphoma of bone: a clinicopathological investigation of 60 cases. Leukemia 1999;13:2094–2098.

Kilciksiz S, Karakoyun-Celik O, Agaoglu FY, et al. A review for solitary plasmacytoma of bone and extramedullary plasmacytoma. ScientificWorldJournal 2012;epub article ID 895765.

Kim SH, Smith SE, Mulligan ME. Hematopoietic tumors and metastases involving bone. Radiol Clin North Am 2011;29:1163–1183.

Kyle RA, Rajkumar SV. Criteria for diagnosis, staging, risk stratification and response assessment of multiple myeloma. Luekemia 2009;23:3–9.
Lal A, Bhurgri Y, Vaziri I, et al. Extranodal non-Hodgkin's lymphomas – a retrospective review of clinico-pathologic features and outcomes in comparison with nodal non-Hodgkin's lymphomas. Asian Pac J Cancer Pre 2008;9(3):453–8.
Li S, Siegal GP. Small cell tumors of bone. Adv Anatomic Pathol 2010;17:1–11.
Limb D, Dreghom C, Murphy JK, et al. Primary lymphoma of bone. Int Orthop 1994;18:180–3.
Lorsbach RB, Hsi ED, Dogan A, Fend F. Plasma cell myeloma and related neoplasms. American Journal Clin Pathol 2011;136:168–182.
Lorsbach RB. Update on the diagnosis and classification of the plasma cell neoplasms. Surg Pathol 2010;3:1061–1089.
Ludwig H, Durie BG, McCarthy P, et al. IMWG consensus on maintenance therapy in multiple myeloma. Blood 2012;119:3003–15.
Mahindra A, Laubach J, Raje N, et al. Latest advances and current challenges in the treatment of multiple myeloma. Nat Rev Clin Oncol 2012;9:135–43.
Matsui W, Borrello I, Mitsiades C. Autologous stem cell transplantation and multiple myeloma cancer stem cells. Biol Blood Marrow Transplant 2012;18:S27–32.
McGrory JE, Pritchard DK, Unni KK et al. Malignant lesions arising in chronic osteomyelitis. Clinical Orthop Relat Res 1999;181–189.
Mikhaeel NG. Overview: primary bone lymphoma. Clin Oncol 2012;24:366–370.
Miller TP, Dahlberg S, Cassady JR, et al. Chemotherapy alone compared with chemotherapy plus radiotherapy for localized intermediate- and high-grade non-Hodgkin's lymphoma. N Engl J Med 1998;339–21–6.
Modi ND, Lentzsch S. Bisphosphonates as antimyeloma drugs. Leukemia 2012;26:589–94.
Moreau P, Richardson PH, Cavo M, et al. Proteasome inhibitors in multiple myeloma: ten years later. Blood 2012;120(5):947–59.
Morgan GL, Walker BA, Davies FE. The genetic architecture of multiple myeloma. Nat Reviews Cancer 2012;12:335–348.
Mulligan ME, McRae GA, Murphey MD. Imaging features of primary lymphoma of bone. AJR 1999;173(6):169–7.
Munshi NC, Anderson KC, Bergsagel PL, et al. Consensus recommendations for risk stratification in multiple myeloma: report of the International Myeloma Workshop Consensus Panel 2. Blood 2011;117:4696–700.
Rajkumar S V. Multiple myeloma: 2011 update on diagnosis, risk-stratification, and management. Am J Hematol 2011;86:57–65.
Rajkumar SV, Gahrton G, Bergsagel PL. Approach to the treatment of multiple myeloma: a clash of philosophies. Blood 2011;118:3205–11.
Ramadan KM, Shenkier T, Sehn LH et al. A clinicopathological retrospective study of 131 patients with primary bone lymphoma: a population-based study of successively treated cohorts from the British Columbia Cancer Agency. Ann Oncol 2007;18:129–135.
Rathmell AJ, Gospodarowicz MK, Sutcliffe SB, et al. Localized lymphoma of bone: prognostic factors and treatment recommendations. The Princess Margaret Hospital Lymphoma Group. Br J Cancer 1992;66:603–6.
Scharschmidt TJ, Lindsey JD, Becker PS, et al. Multiple myeloma: diagnosis and orthopaedic implications. J Am Acad Orthop Surg 2011;19(7):410–419.
Sheppard D, Bredeson C, Allan D, et al. Systematic Review of Randomized Controlled Trials of Hematopoietic Stem Cell Mobilization Strategies for Autologous Transplantation for Hematologic Malignancies. Biol Blood Marrow Transplant 2012;18(8):1191–203.
Slovak, M. Multiple myeloma: current perspectives. Clin Lab Med 2011;31:699–724.
Warsame R, Gertz MA, Lacy MQ, et al. Trends and outcomes of modern staging of solitary plasmacytoma of bone. Am J Hematol 2012;87(7):647–51.
Zinzani PL, Carrillo G, Ascani S, et al. Primary bone lymphoma: experience with 52 patients. Haematologica 2003;88:280–5.

Chapter 22 Osteoclastic giant cell rich tumors of bone

OVERVIEW

Many bone tumors may contain multinucleated giant cells (MNGC) with features of osteoclasts. These include chondroblastoma, non-ossifying fibroma, benign fibrous histiocytoma, osteosarcoma, giant cell reparative granuloma, aneurysmal bone cyst, and brown tumor of hyperparathyroidism. Three tumors comprise the 2013 WHO osteoclastic giant cell rich tumors group: giant cell lesion of the small bones, giant cell tumor of bone (GCTB), and malignancy in GCTB. GCTB is distinctive because of its hallmark, even distribution of giant cells embedded among histiocytic mononuclear cells the nuclei of which morphologically match those of the giant cells. Although characteristic of this tumor, the MNGC represents a recruited, reactive cell rather than genetically altered, neoplastic cell.

Considered a benign tumor (except in exceptional sarcomatous transformation cases), GCTB nonetheless can 'metastasize' to the lungs, can destroy bone and extend into surrounding soft tissues and can recur. Fortunately, most patients do not develop metastases and most can be treated effectively, even those developing multiple local recurrences and/or lung implants.

CLASSIFICATION

Giant cell lesion of the small bones (GCLSB) is very rare and unrelated to giant cell tumor of bone. Giant cell tumor of bone is discussed in detail in this chapter, as it is relatively common, can cause significant morbidity and in rare cases may be fatal (**Table 22.1**). Interestingly, a pure soft tissue tumor morphologically identical to GCTB occurs rarely (giant cell tumor of low malignant potential). GCTB have been reported to undergo malignant change (less than 2% of cases) (Beebe-Dimmer et al. 2009, Errani et al. 2010). This is an exceptional occurrence as a de novo phenomenon (termed primary malignant giant cell tumor); most cases develop in incompletely resected tumors at least several years after radiation therapy. Primary malignant giant cell tumor of bone is diagnosed on pathology review which reveals unequivocal malignant features. Primary malignant giant cell tumor involves patients of the same age presenting with the same symptoms and involving the same bone locations as non-malignant giant cell tumor of bone (Domovitov et al. 2010). Understandably, because of the risk of sarcomatous transformation to secondary malignant giant cell tumor of bone (level of risk still to be determined: see Radiation Oncology section of this chapter), radiotherapy plays a limited role in GCTB and is used only as a last resort at body sites not amenable to surgery.

DEMOGRAPHICS

Although considered uncommon, GCTB represents about 5% of all primary bone tumors and 20% of all benign primary bone tumors (Fletcher et al. 2002). On average, a moderately sized orthopaedic oncology practice treats several patients annually. GCTB nearly always arises in a bone whose physis has closed, yet it seldom affects adults over the age of 55 years. Slightly more females develop the tumor than males, and since physes close sooner in females, younger patients tend to be female. Most patients come to medical attention in their 20s to 40s. However, when GCTB occurs in the hands and feet, which is uncommon, almost half of these patients are younger than 20 years of age (Yanagasawa et al. 2011, Gupta et al. 2008).

PATHOGENESIS

Despite decades of research and reviews of hundreds of patients, the cause of GCTB has not been determined. Questions that remain speculatively answered include why the tumor occurs almost exclusively in skeletally mature bones in the epiphysis or epiphysis equivalent, why certain unpredicted sites such as the distal radius and sacrum are relatively commonly involved, why females are more often affected than males, and why some tumors behave more aggressively than others by forming solitary or even miliary lung implants.

Some investigators suggest that GCTB begins as a reactive response to vascular insufficiency in the epiphysis commencing as profound hypoxia and acute hemorrhage. According to this theory, as osteoblast like cells become stimulated under these conditions, they release chemical promoters that recruit monocytes and induce osteoclast differentiation; these substances comprise M-CSF (monocyte colony stimulating factor), HIF-1α and HIF-2α (hypoxia inducible factor-1α and -2α). Multiple intertangled pathways then activate leading to pro-osteoclastic stimulation by osteoblasts and monocytes with mature osteoclasts themselves contributing. The result is a runaway process culminating in tumor formation, telomeric associations, and sometimes clonal genetic aberrations (Knowles et al. 2008, Ul Haque et al. 2008). This theory may explain why the vascularly delicate epiphysis is affected and why certain bones are more commonly involved than others.

Table 22.1 Table 22.1 WHO Classification of osteoclastic giant cell rich tumors of bone (2013)

Tumor	Behavior	Additional comments
Giant cell lesion of the small bones (GCLSB)	Benign	Rare to very rare Almost exclusive to hands and feet High non-aggressive local recurrence rate
Giant cell tumor of bone (GCTB)	Intermediate to malignant	Intermediate because of capacity for locally aggressive growth and rare implants in lungs Malignant in the exceptional cases of high grade malignant transformation in the absence of prior irradiation

At the genetic level, a high percentage of GCTB contain chromosomes whose ends have abnormally fused together without visible loss of material. These are called telomeric associations (tas), and they are a characteristic feature of this tumor seen on karyotyping (Zheng et al. 1999). If carefully looked for using especially detailed analyses, telomeric associations may be present in up to 100% of cases (Gorunova et al. 2009). Usually, tas occur in high grade tumors after loss of normal telomerase activity, but interestingly, there is no disruption of telomerase in GCTB (Forsyth RG et al. 2008). The tas may be clonal or non-clonal, and one tumor often contains both types. Certain chromosome sites are more commonly affected than others, and these include the following in order of frequency: 11p15>19q13>11p11>1q32=11q32 (Gorunova et al. 2009). Additional structural chromosomal changes can accrue in GCTB, and tas seem to predispose to such changes (which include a wide variety of alterations including translocations, deletions, duplications, inversions, and others).

Early evidence suggests that giant cell tumors of bone with complex clonal karyotypes have a higher risk for aggressive behavior (Moskovszky et al. 2009, Gorunova et al. 2009).

PATHOLOGY

GCTB contains three main cell types: the osteoclast-like giant cell, a mononuclear histiocytic cell, and a mononuclear round to spindle cell. The osteoclastic giant cells can contain greater than 100 nuclei; such large numbers are a helpful diagnostic feature when present. Characteristically, the giant cells are evenly dispersed among the mononuclear histiocytic cells, often blending in almost imperceptibly. Since the histiocytic mononuclear cells give rise to the osteoclastic giant cells, it is not surprising that the nuclei of both cell types are morphologically indistinguishable, a key feature in making the diagnosis. Only the round to spindle, non-histiocytic mononuclear cell is neoplastic and displays karyotypic abnormalities of telomeric associations and sometimes other chromosomal changes. The neoplastic cells are usually greatly outnumbered by the reactive mononuclear histiocytic cells and osteoclastic giant cells and may be difficult to find. Very rarely, a GCTB may contain only a few to no osteoclastic giant cells. In such cases, radiologic, clinical, and chromosomal findings must be strongly supportive in order the make the diagnosis (Folpe et al. 2010).

The most common skeletal sites for GCTB are the following, in order of frequency: distal femur, proximal tibia, pelvis, proximal humerus, sacrum and distal radius, although any bone can be affected, but the skull, scapula, and diaphyseal locations are only rarely involved. Knee bones are the site of origin in 40 to 50% of patients in several large recent series of 470, 349, and 219 individuals (Gupta et al. 2008, Errani et al. 2010, and Balke et al. 2008, respectively).

RADIOLOGY

Giant cell tumors (GCT) have aggressive clinical and radiographic features despite their non-malignant histology. GCT occurs in young adults; it is said that the open physis acts as a relative barrier to these lesions. With skeletal maturity, the physis heals and the GCT is able to grow into the epiphysis extending to the articular surface. GCT often has a characteristic radiographic feature that allows accurate diagnosis. They are typically lucent lesions without sclerotic borders that extend to the articular surface. They are commonly found around the knee - in the distal femur and proximal tibia. There is usually no visible matrix. Giant cell tumors exhibit a moderately aggressive appearance with a wide zone of transition. Sometimes they can show periosteal reaction and cortical breakthrough with a soft tissue mass.

The differential diagnosis for a lucent lesion of the epiphysis or subchondral region includes chondroblastoma and a degenerative subchondral cyst. Chondroblastoma typically has a sclerotic margin, occurs in a skeletally immature patient and is a relatively rare lesion. The subchondral degenerative cysts are usually easily identifiable by the associated osteoarthritic changes, and these cysts sometime have visible communication to the joint.

The workup for GCT often includes MRI to evaluate for soft tissue mass, and to confirm the presence of destructive features. The MR appearance is quite variable. The tumor is usually heterogeneous low signal on T1 and heterogeneously high signal on T2 or STIR with heterogeneous enhancement. Some tumors show cystic change. Giant cell tumors sometimes have significant hemosiderin deposition which appears as dark areas on all MR sequences.

SURGERY

Although GCTB are benign, they typically present with a substantial degree of bone destruction and treatment is associated with a high rate of local recurrence.

Curettage alone has resulted in a recurrence rate of >50%. Lower recurrence rates, in the order of 25%, have been achieved with 'extended curettage.' This technique involves margin extension following curettage by either mechanical (e.g. high-speed burr) or chemical/physical (phenol, liquid nitrogen, argon laser) means. Typically, extended curettage has been accompanied with placement of polymethylmethacrylate (PMMA or bone cement) which is thought to add further to the margin extension through the heat produced by the exothermic reaction of curing. Long term presence of PMMA in a subchondral location has not led to a substantial increase in significant degenerative change.

The polymerization of cement, liquid nitrogen and the argon beam are thought to extend the margins via thermal necrosis of cells for perhaps 1-2 mm (Lewis et al. 2007). The argon laser works in two ways: thermally and by discoloring the initial margin which is then removed with a burr. Liquid nitrogen is favored by a few centers for its thermal effect, although there is then an associated risk of fracture (Malawar et al. 1999). The high-speed burr is a purely mechanical means of extending the margin, and its use is very familiar to many orthopaedists. Phenol 5% is also widely used and extends the margin by producing local cellular death.

En bloc resection results in a much lower recurrence rate but at the expense of a procedure and associated reconstruction with much higher morbidity and potential dysfunction. En bloc resection should be reserved for multiply recurrent tumors, those associated with such a degree of bone destruction that reconstruction with existing bone plus PMMA is not possible, or potentially when the tumor occurs in expendable bones (rib, proximal fibula, iliac wing).

At our institution, we have witnessed an 88.5% local control rate with the use of extended curettage (high-speed burr and PMMA) over the past decade (six recurrences out of 52 patients).

Tumors involving the spine can present additional challenges, as margin extension can be dangerous when used in proximity to the spinal cord and/or nerve roots, and recurrences can present a surgical challenge. Wide margin resection is preferred, where it can be performed with acceptable morbidity and adequate reconstruction.

In the rare cases of pulmonary 'metastasis,' cure is usually effected with metastasectomy.

MEDICAL ONCOLOGY

Until recently, the treatment for giant cell tumor of bone was surgical only, and resection remains a mainstay of therapy in most patients (Balke et al. 2008). Many lesions can be successfully curetted, but sometimes the whole bone might need to be replaced (especially for vertebral lesions). Pulmonary lesions are usually optimally treated by excision.

Medical therapy is based on the biology of GCT. Osteoprotegerin is a receptor found on osteoclasts (Huang 2000). This receptor is specifically stimulated by the RANK ligand (RANKL), also known as CD254. RANKL is a member of the tumor necrosis factor cytokine family and is a surface-bound molecule found on osteoblasts (Buckley 2003). Trafficking between osteoblasts or mononuclear stromal cells (Haque et al. 2008, Wuelling et al. 2003) and osteoclasts is important for bone homeostasis and RANKL is important in bone metabolism (Collin-Osdoby et al. 2005). RANKL binds to osteoprotegerin to activate osteoclasts, which are the cells involved in bone resorption. The ligation causes differentiation and activation of the osteoclasts.

A new human IgG2 monoclonal antibody inhibitor of RANKL, denosumab, was recently approved by the FDA for prevention of osteoporosis in post-menopausal women. Fortuitously, this antibody is also very effective against GCT, because it blocks the very mechanism of osteoclast activation which is responsible for tumor development. A recent study showed that patients with GCT treated with denosumab had a rapid and profound correction of their symptoms. However, tumors do not resorb quickly, and physicians are left with tumors that seem to create a risk of fracture in patients that become quickly asymptomatic. More observation time is needed to understand the long term efficacy of denosumab.

In an open-label, single-group study, 37 patients with recurrent or unresectable GCT were enrolled and received subcutaneous denosumab 120 mg every 28 days, with loading doses on days 8 and 15 of month 1 (Thomas et al. 2010). The primary endpoint was tumor response, defined as elimination of at least 90% of giant cells or no radiological progression of the target lesion up to week 25. Thirty of 35 assessable patients had a tumor response by histology (100%) or by radiology (66%). The most common adverse events were pain in an extremity (n=7), back pain (n=4), and headache (n=4). The approved dose of denosumab is 120 mg every 4 weeks as a subcutaneous injection in the upper arm, upper thigh, or abdomen. However, the above study used a loading dose.

Calcium, magnesium, and vitamin D administration may be necessary to treat or prevent hypocalcemia that can occur with denosumab therapy. Calcium levels may need to be monitored. Patients with a creatinine clearance less than 30 mL/min or receiving dialysis are at greater risk of severe hypocalcemia. Two to 3 percent of patients receiving denosumab developed osteonecrosis of the jaw, which manifest as jaw pain, osteomyelitis, osteitis, bone erosion, tooth or periodontal infection, toothache, gingival ulceration, or gingival erosion. Persistent pain and slow healing after dental surgery might also be manifestations of this side effect.

In summary, denosumab therapy is recommended as front line treatment for inoperable or large GCT. Patients must be carefully followed, and surgery might be necessary for bone stabilization. Denosumab might replace surgery for all cases in the near future. Older medical treatments with lesser success are interferon, biphosphonate, and calcitonin. These agents have been supplanted by denosumab. Chemotherapy is not indicated.

RADIATION ONCOLOGY

Complete surgical resection is the treatment of choice for giant cell tumor of bone. Occasionally giant cell tumor of bone can originate in locations such as the axial skeleton (sacrum in particular) which would make complete surgical resection debilitating and place the patient at high risk for complications. Therefore, radiation therapy has been used in these circumstances. In general, high local control rates have been reported with the use of radiation therapy for giant cell tumor of bone.

Investigators from M.D. Anderson reported a series of thirteen patients with primary giant cell tumor of bone treated with radiation therapy who achieved an 83% local control rate at 5 years. On the other hand, recurrent giant cell tumor of bone treated with radiation therapy had only a 42% local control rate at 5 years. They concluded that perhaps radiation therapy should be delivered early because the success of radiation therapy is much lower for patients who have recurrent disease after failing initial therapy. They recommended a dose of 45 Gy for postoperative cases and up to 60 Gy for patients with large or recurrent disease (Caudell et al. 2003).

Another series of 20 patients treated with radiation therapy from a group at Massachusetts General Hospital reported an 85% local control rate at 10 years. This report also addressed the possibility of malignant transformation which is a major concern about the use of radiation therapy for giant cell tumor of bone. The authors pooled data from recent studies and found a less than 3% rate of malignant transformation after an average of 10 years of follow up. They also described cases of malignant transformation after surgery alone confirming (as has been previously discussed in the Pathology section of this chapter) that some cases of malignant transformation are not due to prior radiation therapy. Thus, a better estimate of the development of malignant transformation from radiation needs further study with more patients and longer follow up (Chakravarti et al. 1999).

CASES

Case 22.1 Giant cell tumor of bone

Clinical history and presentation

The patient is a 28 year old man who reports an eight month history of increasing left knee pain. Two weeks ago he was accidentally kicked in the knee by his daughter and has been on crutches since, unable to weight bear secondary to pain.

Surgical findings and comments

Physical examination reveals a firm soft tissue mass arising from the lateral aspect of the distal femur that is tender on palpation. Range of motion of the knee occurs from minus 25 degrees extension to 100 degrees of flexion.

Because imaging studies are consistent with giant cell tumor of bone, the patient is taken to surgery for curettage of the tumor, margin extension with a high speed burr and PMMA.

The patient does well initially after his procedure, but is lost to follow-up until he returns one year after his initial procedure with a three month history of recurrent and increasing knee pain.

Work-up now reveals recurrent tumor with extensive destruction of the distal femur and a large associated soft tissue mass. Due to the recurrent and destructive nature of the tumor, repeat curettage with retention of the femur does not appear reasonable or likely. Wide resection of the distal femur and reconstruction with a distal femoral replacement, rotating hinge total knee arthroplasty is performed.

Radiology findings

The plain radiographs show a lucent lesion of the distal femur extending to the articular surface. The lesion has destructive, lytic features with apparent cortical break through and soft tissue mass (**Case figs 22.1a** and **22.1b**). These findings together are essentially diagnostic of a GCT. The usual differential diagnosis for an epiphyseal lesion includes chondroblastoma and a degenerative subchondral cyst. Degenerative cyst can be excluded as there are no other findings of osteoarthritis, and degenerative cysts would usually have sclerotic margins. Likewise, chondroblastoma can be excluded because it is seen in younger patients and there is no sclerotic margin.

This particular GCT shows more expansion than typically seen, perhaps due to delay in presentation. The MR images confirm an aggressive lesion with soft tissue mass (**Case figs 22.1c** through **22.1m**). This particular GCT also shows fairly extensive cystic change and little hemosiderin. Given the degree of expansion, cystic change and soft tissue mass, this GCT has findings that are somewhat worrisome for an even more aggressive lesion such as telangiectatic osteosarcoma. However, no osteoid is seen, and the enhancement is only modestly intense. These findings would not entirely exclude a telangiectatic osteosarcoma and tissue diagnosis is warranted regardless. For comparison, please also see additional cases of giant cell tumor in **Case figs 22.1n** through 1s (second patient) and **Case figs 22.1t** through **22.1y** (third patient).

Pathology findings

Gross features

The initial curettage specimen consists of numerous gritty to hemorrhagic 1-5 mm fragments of tissue aggregating to 10.2 cm.

The resection comprises the left distal femur and attached soft tissues with additional shaved proximal femur, proximal tibia, and patella. Serial cut sections reveal six nodules in association with cement and/or bone ranging in size from 0.7 to 2.2 cm. In addition, a large 8.5 cm mass occupies the posterior soft tissues and abuts cortical bone. Upon sectioning, the nodules are soft to rubbery; the largest nodule contains numerous blood-filled cysts (**Case fig. 22.1z**). Tumor nodules closely approach surgical resection margins. Multiple sections are taken of the various nodules to include nearest margins.

Microscopic features

Low magnification: The curettage specimen contains abundant tumor that consists of two morphologies. The first comprises the classic appearance of giant cell tumor of bone: multinucleated, osteoclastic giant cells approximately evenly dispersed among round histiocytic cells (**Case figs 22.1aa** and **22.1bb**). The second pattern exhibits a spindle cell proliferation of uniform cells with only rare, small osteoclastic like giant cells. Extension of tumor into soft tissue is present.

Resection: The resection specimen is similar to the curettage specimen except for greater soft tissue penetration, early aneurysmal bone cyst change, and the presence of previously placed orthopaedic cement. At low magnification, the leading edge of tumor creates a shell of reactive new bone, a classic feature of GCTB as it invades soft tissues (**Case fig. 22.1cc**). Changes consistent with secondary aneurysmal bone cyst formation include blood-filled cystic spaces and strands of new bone, fibrosis and inflammation in the cyst septae (**Case fig. 22.1dd**).

High magnification: High magnification of the resection specimen reveals three appearances to the tumor: 1) classic areas with giant cells merging imperceptibly with surrounding monocytoid macrophage precursors (**Case fig. 22.1ee**), 2) a spindle cell area composed of uniform plump spindle cells without giant cells (**Case fig. 22.1ff**), and 3) early ABC change as described above. Some of the giant cells are very large and contain more than 50 nuclei, a feature often present in GCT of bone and rare in other tumors or lesions containing osteoclastic giant cells (**Case fig. 22.1gg**). Mitotic figures are numerous and average 10-12 per ten high magnification microscopic fields. There are no atypical mitoses.

Special studies: Cytogenetics reveals non-clonal telomeric associations. This is a common finding in giant cell tumor of bone and supports the histologic diagnosis. By immunohistochemistry, neoplastic mononuclear cells show nuclear expression of p63 (**Case fig. 22.1hh**) especially in the classic areas of the tumor. This is a sensitive but not specific marker of giant cell tumor of bone with ~90% negative predictive value, as it also labels nuclei of the histologic entities in the differential including chondroblastoma, aneurysmal bone cyst and non-ossifying fibroma (De la Roza, 2011).

Comparison microscopic images: To demonstrate a few of the other histologic appearances that can occur in giant cell tumors, several images from other patients are provided. A storiform (whirling or basketweave) proliferation of spindle cells is seen in **Case fig. 22.1ii**, an area of reactive bone formation in **Case fig. 22.1jj**, an area of fibroplasia and inflammation mimicking non-ossifying fibroma in **Case fig. 22.1kk**, and vascular invasion in **Case fig. 22.1ll**. These photos derive from three other patients with giant cell tumor of bone in which classic areas also were present. They illustrate the necessity for submitting multiple

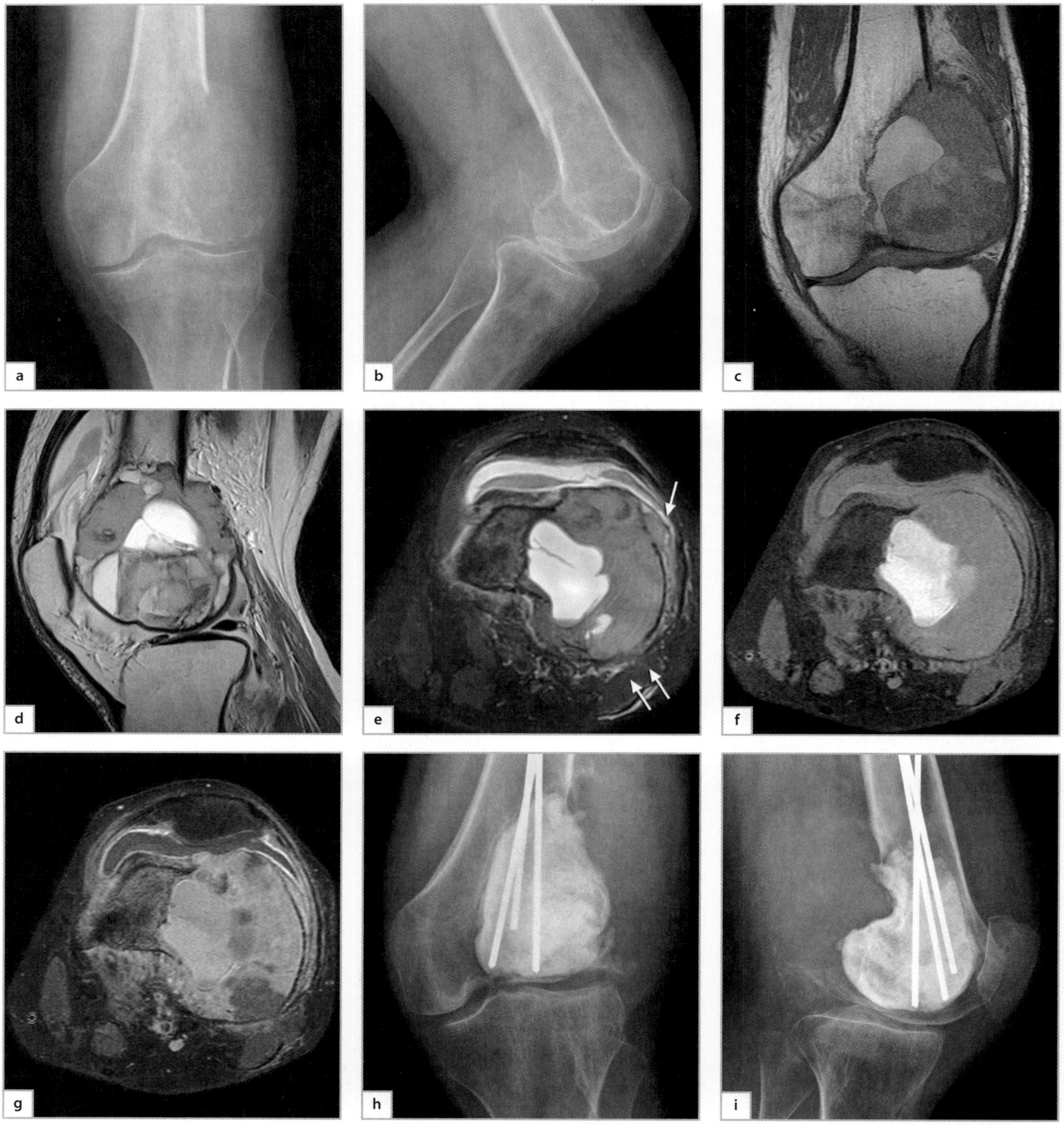

Case figures 22.1 Giant cell tumor. Radiology images. **22.1a** and **22.1b**: Anteroposterior and lateral radiographs show a lytic and expansile lesion of the distal femur. The lateral cortex may have breakthrough. The lesion extends to the articular surface without sclerotic margins evident. **22.1c**: Coronal T1. **22.1d**: Sagittal PD. **22.1e**: Axial STIR. **22.1f**: Axial T1 fat saturation. **22.1g**: Axial T1 fat saturation post-contrast. Preoperative MR images show a heterogeneous destructive lesion of the distal femur with cortical breakthrough as seen on 22-1e (arrows). This GCT shows numerous cystic spaces with fluid-fluid levels. There is heterogeneous enhancement. Note the extension to the articular surface. **22.1h** and **22.1i**: Anteroposterior and lateral radiographs show curettage and cement packing with pin fixation. There is a large lateral and posterior soft tissue mass with bone lysis extending into the medial femoral condyle. These findings indicate recurrent GCT.

Case figure 22.1: Continued from page 500

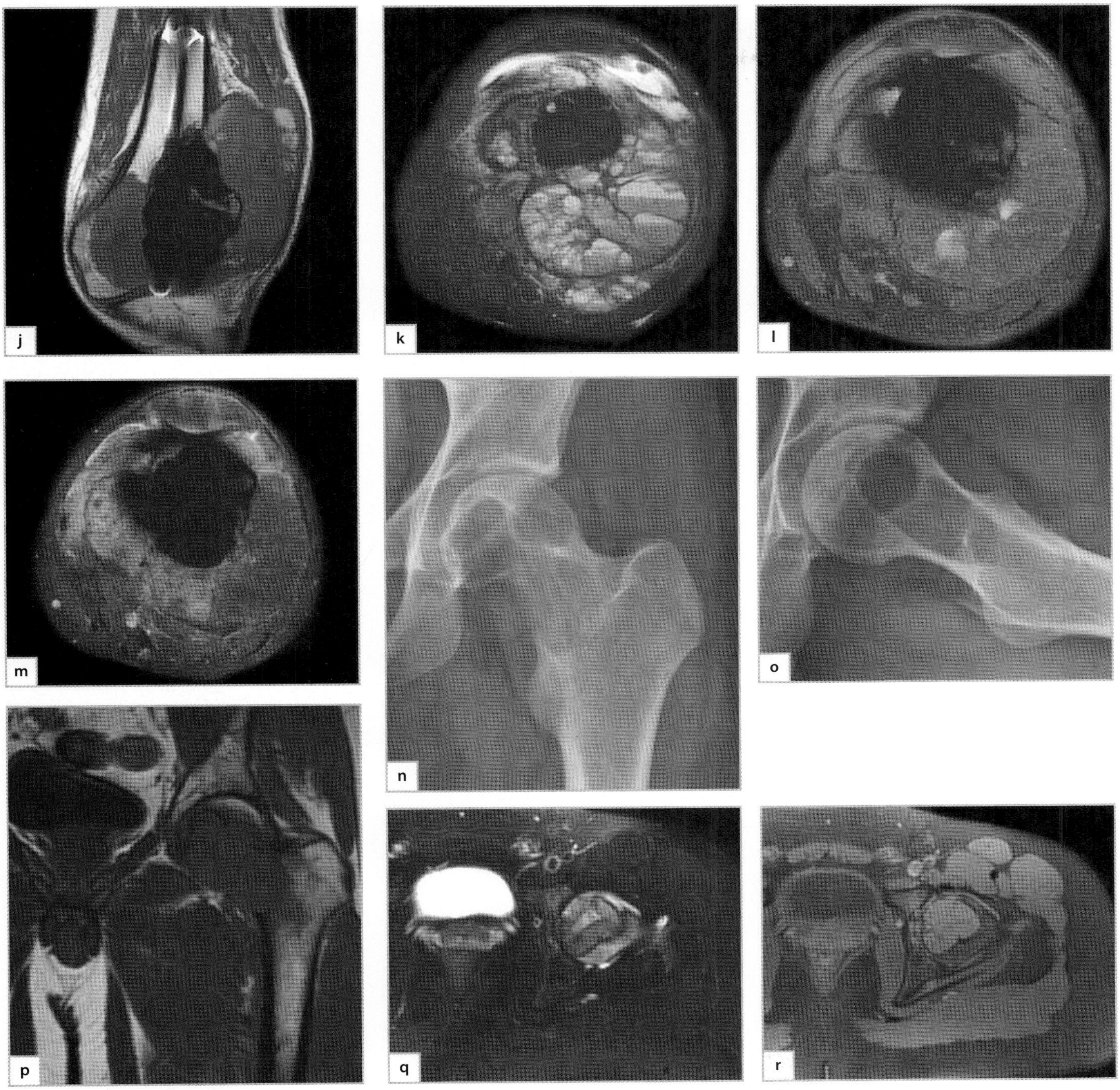

22.1j: Coronal T1. **22.1k**: Axial STIR. **22.1l**: Axial T1 fat saturation. **22.1m**: Axial T1 fat saturation post-contrast. MR images confirm the large soft tissue mass and extension of tumor into the medial femoral condyle. The axial STIR image shows the recurrence has strikingly similar gross appearance with numerous cystic spaces with fluid-fluid levels. *Case fig. 22.1n to Case fig. 22.1s are images of first additional patient with giant cell tumor.* **22.1n**: Anteroposterior and **22.1o**: Lateral views of the hip show a lucent lesion extending to the articular surface of the femoral head. There is no sclerotic border and no visible matrix. **22.1p**: Coronal T1, **22.1q**: Axial T2 fat saturation, **22.1r**: Axial T1 fat saturation.

Case figure 22.1: Continued from page 501

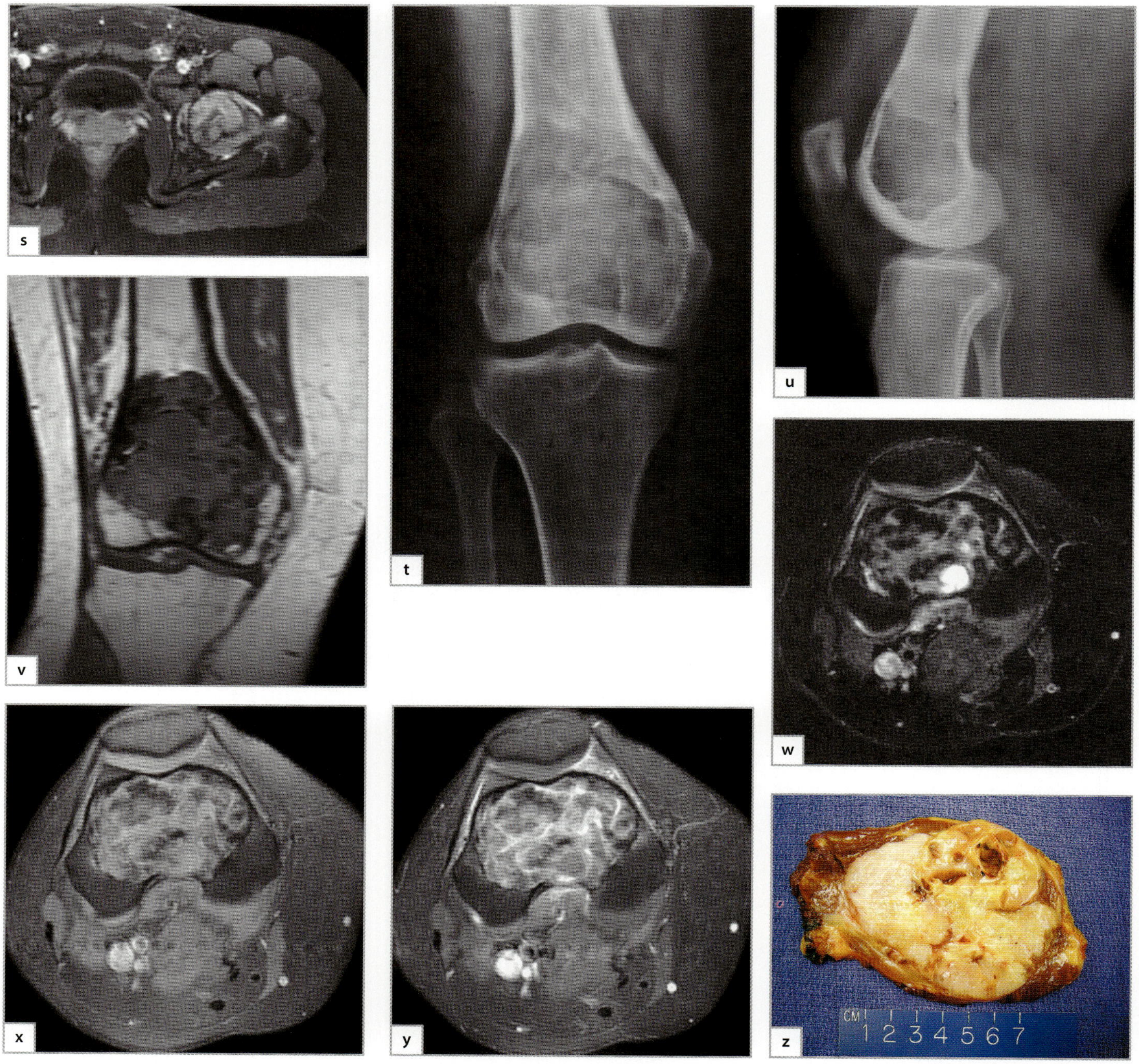

22.1s: Axial T1 fat saturation post-contrast MR images show a heterogeneous lesion of the proximal femur extending to the articular surface. There is moderate heterogeneous enhancement without soft tissue mass. *Case fig. 22.1t to Case fig. 22.1y are images of second additional patient with giant cell tumor.* **22.1t**: Anteroposterior. **22.1u**: Lateral views of the knee show a lucent lesion without matrix or sclerotic margin. The extension to the articular surface is best seen on the anteroposterior view. **22.1v**: Coronal T1. **22.1w**: Axial STIR. **22.1x**: Axial T1 fat saturation. **22.1y**: Axial T1 fat saturation post-contrast. The MR images show a heterogeneous signal lesion with moderate heterogeneous enhancement. This case of GCT is notable for the abundant areas of low signal on all sequences likely from extensive hemosiderin. **22.1z**: Gross photo of giant cell tumor of bone. The cut surface of the largest nodule exhibits pink to tan solid areas, cysts (early aneurysmal bone cyst change) and degenerative mottled yellow to gelatinous regions. These are non-specific findings that can be seen in a sarcoma. Notice the location is within soft tissue (skeletal muscle) and indicates a locally aggressive tumor that has broken through bone cortex.

Case figure 22.1: Continued from page 502

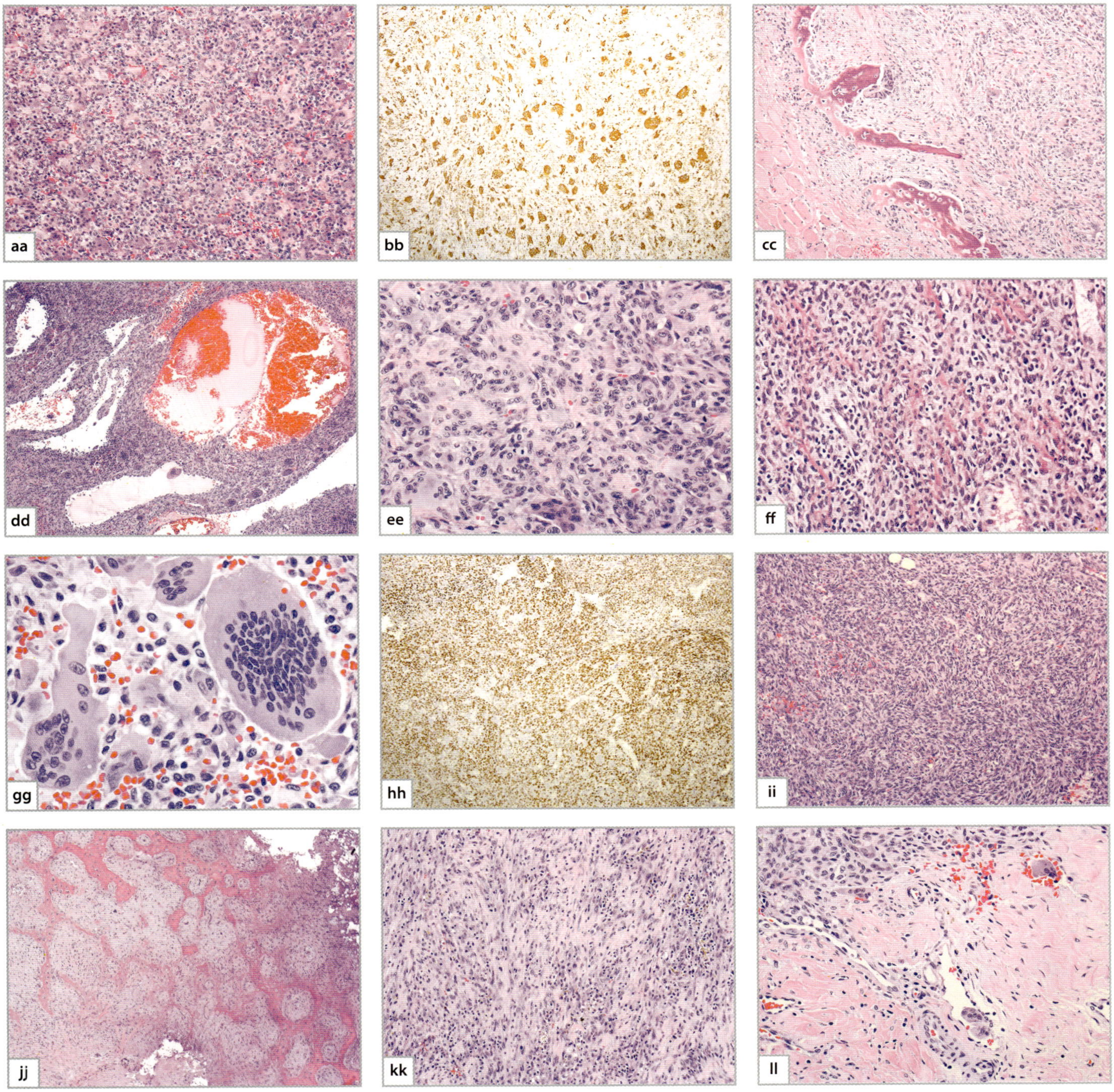

22.1aa Classic area of giant cell tumor at medium magnification. The giant cells are numerous and spaced evenly apart. Intermingled cells include histiocytes (precursors to the giant cells) and a few lymphocytes. **22.1bb**: CD68 immunostain of classic area at lower magnification. Both the giant cells and the mononuclear precursor histiocytes express CD68, a marker of macrophages and osteoclasts (and other cells). The stain highlights the even distribution of the osteoclastic giant cells, a key histologic feature of GCT. The mononuclear true tumor cells do not express CD68. **22.1cc**: Reactive cuff of new bone formation at the leading soft tissue edge of giant cell tumor of bone. The reactive new bone forms a discontinuous interface between normal soft tissue (in this case, skeletal muscle in the left side of the photo) from the tumor. Peripheral new bone formation occurs commonly with soft tissue expansion. **22.1dd**: Early ABC like change with blood filled cysts (not blood vessels) and focal streamer like deposition of collagen (visible as dark pink acellular bands). **22.1ee**: Nearly imperceptible blending of osteoclastic giant cells and background mononuclear macrophages. High magnification of a classic area of tumor demonstrating the identical nuclear features of the mononuclear cells and the osteoclastic giant cells. It is difficult to discern the cell borders of the giant cells so similar are the two cell types. One mitotic figure is present in a mononuclear cell (the giant cells do not undergo mitotic division). **22.1ff**: Spindle cell dominant area. This patient's resection consisted of approximately 50% ovoid spindle cell solid areas as seen at higher magnification in this photomicrograph. The cells are uniform with indistinct cell borders, and some are forming columns of collagen (eosinophilic acellular strands). This cell is the true neoplastic cell in GCT and exhibits the cytogenetic abnormalities including telomeric associations.

sections for microscopic review, as occasionally, the classic identifiable giant cell rich areas form only a minor component of the tumor.

Pathologic differential or, why isn't it one of the following?

In principle, the histologic differential diagnosis of giant cell tumor of bone is broad (**Case table 22.1b**). This is because giant cell tumor of bone can exhibit a number of features that can mimic other tumors, (see **Case table 22.1a**) and because other tumors can also contain osteoclastic giant cells.

In practice, in many cases, after consideration of the clinical presentation and radiologic features, by the time the pathologist reviews the biopsy, only a few tumors are realistic diagnostic contenders. For younger patients, the benign tumors in the differential include aneurysmal bone cyst (ABC, including the solid type), non-ossifying fibroma, and chondroblastoma, and the malignant entities in the differential consist of giant cell rich osteosarcoma and telangiectatic osteosarcoma. For older patients, the benign entities in the differential include ABC and fibrous histiocytoma, and the malignant tumors to consider include clear cell chondrosarcoma, giant cell rich osteosarcoma, and pleomorphic undifferentiated sarcoma with giant cells.

Aneurysmal bone cyst (classic and solid types): These lesions feature a mixture of reactive appearing cells from fibroblasts to histiocytes and siderophages which are mixed with linear streamers of fibrin and new bone with or without cystic, blood-filled spaces. The even distribution of osteoclastic giant cells blending well with background mononuclear histiocytoid cells and mononuclear neoplastic tumor cells is absent. Telomeric associations are not seen on cytogenetics; rather, abnormalities of chromosomes 17 or 16 (*USP6* fusion genes). Giant cell tumor is one of the main bone tumors that can show secondary ABC change. Therefore, it is important to thoroughly sample tumors with ABC features in order not to miss residual primary tumor such as GCT or chondroblastoma.

Non-ossifying fibroma and fibrous histiocytoma: These two tumors are histologically identical and contain a range of cell types in varying proportions such as spindle fibroblasts, xanthomatous histiocytes, and lymphocytes. The spindle cells are commonly arrayed in a storiform pattern sprinkled by inflammatory cells with massings of xanthomatous histiocytes. While giant cells are often present, they cluster around foci of hemorrhage and are neither evenly distributed nor similar in nuclear features to surrounding mononuclear cells.

Chondroblastoma: Chondroid matrix, epithelioid cells (round cells with distinct cell borders) with nuclear clefts, and 'chicken wire' calcifications (present in about 40% of cases) distinguish chondroblastoma from giant cell tumor of bone. Giant cells may be scattered but are small and dissimilar to the epithelioid tumor cells. Chondroid matrix is very rare in giant cell tumor of bone. Cytogenetically, telomeric associations are absent in chondroblastoma. Immunoreactivity is common in both giant cell tumor and chondroblastoma.

Clear cell chondrosarcoma: This rare epiphyseal to epiphyseal/metaphyseal tumor occurs in the same age group as giant cell tumor and, like GCT, in bones with a closed physis. Giant cells are present, but the mononuclear tumor cells are distinctly dissimilar to the osteoclastic giant cells being epithelioid (round cells with a low to moderate N/C ratio and distinct cell borders) with clear to granular eosinophilic cytoplasm and nuclei with prominent nucleoli. Tumor bone is often present interspersed among the epithelioid cells, and areas of conventional chondrosarcoma are noted in about 50% of cases (Folpe et al, 2010).

Giant cell rich osteosarcoma: Unlike GCT, the tumor cells are obviously malignant with hyperchromatic or vesicular nuclei of irregular shapes and sizes. Some of the giant cells may show malignant nuclear features, but osteoclastic giant cells similar to those of GCT are also present. The latter, however, do not usually reach the prodigious size of some osteoclastic giant cells in giant cell tumor of bone. Atypical mitotic figures can be seen; these are absent in giant cell tumor. In addition to the pleomorphic tumor cells, malignant osteoid (osteoid with embedded cytologically atypical osteoblasts) distinguishes giant cell rich osteosarcoma from giant cell tumor. GCT can form bone, but it is reactive only with histologic characteristics of woven bone.

Pleomorphic undifferentiated sarcoma with giant cells (PUS-GC): PUS-GC harbors cytologically malignant tumor cells that are spindled to polygonal with pleomorphic, hyperchromatic to vesicular nuclei. Osteoclast like giant cells are scattered throughout but are smaller than those noted in some giant cell tumors. Atypical mitotic figures are often present.

Oncology approach

Medical oncology

There is no indication for chemotherapy or use of denosumab, as the tumor has been entirely resected.

Radiation oncology

As long as complete surgical resection is accomplished, radiation therapy is not necessary. Fortunately, wide resection was performed on this patient for recurrent disease, and consequently, radiation therapy is not recommended.

Patient outcome

One year following his second procedure, the patient is doing well with no evidence of recurrence and has a fully functional knee with minimal pain.

22.1gg High magnification. Some of the giant cells in GCT are gargantuan, containing more than 50 or even 100 nuclei. Such behemoths are rarely seen in tumors or lesions other than GCT. **22.1hh**: Giant cell tumor with p63 expression. Many of the mononuclear cells express p63 in the nuclei (immunohistochemical stain; brown color is a positive reaction). This is typical of GCTB but is also found in other tumors in the histologic differential. **22.1ii**: Giant cell tumor with storiforming growth pattern. This is a relatively common architectural pattern in giant cell tumor of bone. Here the neoplastic cells are forming short interweaving bundles of spindle cells with sparse giant cells. **22.1jj**: Giant cell tumor with reactive bone formation. A lattice like network of new bone is present with a fibrotic background. This area is not diagnostic of GCT of bone. **22.1kk**: Giant cell tumor with area resembling non-ossifying fibroma. This area comprises fibroblasts mixed with chronic inflammatory cells, collagen and clusters of siderophages (macrophages containing hemosiderin pigment). This area is not diagnostic of GCT of bone. **22.1ll**: Giant cell tumor with vascular invasion. Just outside the leading edge of the tumor, two giant cells are partially plugging a thin-walled vessel. Finding vascular invasion does not alter the prognosis or predict pulmonary metastasis.

Case table 22.1a Variant features of giant cell tumor of bone

Feature	Frequency	Comment
Small giant cells (containing no more than 20 nuclei)	Common	Although very large giant cells containing 100 or more nuclei are characteristic of GCTB, they are not always present
Storiform pattern of spindle cells	Common	Mimics non-ossifying fibroma
Xanthogranulomatous inflammation	Common	Mimics non-ossifying fibroma
Hemosiderin deposition	Common	Hemosiderin deposition also commonly occurs in the other tumors in the histologic differential such as ABC, NOF, PVNS, and giant cell reparative granuloma
High mitotic rate	Common	A high mitotic rate (>10 mitoses/10 high magnification microscopic fields) does not predict more aggressive behavior
Reactive bone formation	Common	Often associated with pathologic fracture
Aneurysmal bone cyst change	Uncommon	Occurs in ~10% of cases Any older patient (greater than 20 years) with an epiphyseal 'aneurysmal bone cyst' requires thorough sampling of the lesion to exclude residual giant cell tumor
Hemangiopericytomatous vessels	Uncommon	Dilated thin-walled branching vessels vaguely shaped like staghorns
Extra-osseous extension	Uncommon	20-25% of patients. Recurrent tumor can be located in soft tissue
Vascular invasion	Uncommon	Does not affect prognosis
Sheets of spindle cell growth without osteoclastic giant cells	Uncommon	The true tumor cells in GCTB are mononuclear, round to plump to elongate spindle cells. In ~10% of tumors, they may form solid sheets of cells
Infarct like necrosis	Uncommon	Does *not* affect prognosis
Malignant transformation with marked pleomorphism, atypical mitoses	Rare	Most develop in the setting of prior radiation therapy but can occur de novo. In the latter instance, classic GCT areas are almost always present. The sarcoma is usually a high grade spindle cell tumor. It may, however, produce osteoid
Complete absence of giant cells	Rare	Must have corroborating clinical history, radiology and genetics to make the diagnosis of GCTB

Table 22.1b Differential diagnosis of bone tumors that contain giant cells

Lesion	Incidence	Patient age/sex	Location (in order of frequency)	Key microscopic features	Special laboratory studies
Giant cell tumor of bone (osteoclastoma)	Common	F slightly > M Peak 20s-40s Younger when in hands/feet	Closed epiphysis of distal femur, proximal tibia, distal radius, sacrum, vertebral bodies. Rarely in craniofacial bones, ribs, scapula. Can involve metaphysis.	Evenly spaced often large giant cells intermixed with round to polygonal mononuclear histiocytes of identical nuclear appearance. No atypical mitoses. Tumor spindle cells may be rare. Secondary changes common such as fibrosis, inflammation, reactive bone, xanthomatous reaction.	Telomeric associations (clonal or non-clonal) +/- other chromosomal changes
Non-ossifying fibroma (fibrous cortical defect, metaphyseal fibrous defect)	Common	F = M First two decades of life.	Metaphysis of distal femur, proximal tibia, or distal tibia; far less commonly other sites.	Looks identical to fibrous histiocytoma. Giant cells often cluster around areas of hemorrhage. Necrosis and normal mitoses can be seen.	None
Fibrous histiocytoma (fibroxanthoma, fibrous xanthoma, xanthofibroma, xanthogranuloma)	Very rare	F slightly > M Broad age range; most are adults	Epiphysis or diaphysis of long bones, most commonly femur, tibia. 25% occur in pelvic bones, especially ilium	Storiform pattern of spindle cells (fibroblasts) with small giant cells that often cluster. Foam cells few to abundant. Hemosiderin common.	None
Aneurysmal bone cyst, primary or secondary	Common	F = M First two decades of life most commonly but can occur at any age	Metaphysis of long bones, most commonly femur, tibia, humerus Vertebra posterior elements but any bone can be involved	Blood filled spaces with fibroblastic, reactive woven bone, inflammatory cells and giant cells 'blue bone' can be present but is not specific	Primary ABC often has rearrangements of chromosome 17 (most commonly) or 16 secondary ABC does not usually have chromosomal abnormalities
Brown tumor of hyperparathyroidism	Rare	F > M 30s to 60s most common.	Mandible, clavicle, ribs, pelvic bones most common.	Looks identical to giant cell reparative granuloma (solid ABC)	Serological evidence of hyperparathyroidism. May have MEN syndromes.

Case table 22.1b: Continued from page 505

Lesion	Incidence	Patient age/sex	Location (in order of frequency)	Key microscopic features	Special laboratory studies
Giant cell lesion of the small bones/ giant cell reparative granuloma (probably a solid variant of aneurysmal bone cyst, solid ABC)	Rare	F = M Peaks in first two decades	Maxilla/mandible and hands and feet. Rare elsewhere	Clusters of giant cells set in a moderately to highly cellular spindle cell (fibroblastic) background. Inflammation and reactive bone also present. GC clustering is usually around hemorrhage	May show same genetic findings as classic ABC. No consistent findings to date. One case with telomeric associations similar to GCTB
Giant cell rich osteosarcoma	Rare	M > F First two decades of life; second smaller peak in incidence in patients > 50 years	Distal femur, proximal tibia, proximal humerus; older patients also have higher numbers of cranial/facial, ribs and pelvis tumors	Pleomorphic tumor cells and tumor bone ('malignant osteoid') formation with scattered giant cells. Atypia is usually > > than in GCTB. Atypical mitoses +/-	Karyotype is usually aneuploid
Pleomorphic undifferentiated sarcoma with giant cells (when it arises in bone)	Very	Adults > 50 years	Distal femur, proximal tibia, pelvic bones	Storiform arrangement of spindle cells and pleomorphic tumor cells with interspersed giant cells in giant cell rich variant. Atypical mitoses. NO tumor osteoid	Karyotype is usually aneuploid May express myofibroblastic markers such as smooth muscle actin
Malignancy in giant cell tumor of bone	Very rare	F slightly > M Age is usually about 10 years later than average age for GCTB	Distal femur, proximal tibia; hands/feet and skull not affected	After radiation no residual benign GCT may remain. Tumor is spindled with marked pleomorphism. May have abrupt transition from benign to malignant GCT. Atypical mitoses +/-	No information on genetics
Chondroblastoma	Uncommon	M > F 10 to 25 years most common	Epiphysis or epiphysis/ metaphysis of distal femur, proximal femur, proximal tibial and proximal humerus Pelvic bones not uncommon. Uncommonly talus, calcaneus and patella	Epithelioid cells with pale clefted nuclei mixed with randomly distributed giant cells Pink to blue chondroid present. Rarely hyaline cartilage. Chicken wire calcifications in 50-75% of cases	No consistent specific genetic findings. Tumor cells usually express S-100 protein, often express keratins including keratin 19.
Clear cell chondrosarcoma	Very rare	M > F Adults in 20s to 50s most commonly but any age can be affected	Epiphysis or epiphysis/ metaphysis of proximal femur, proximal humerus, distal femur most common	Epithelioid clear and pink granular cells mixed with randomly dispersed giant cells and scarce to abundant osteoid formation. Conventional low grade chondrosarcoma may also be present. Mitoses usually rare	No consistent specific genetic findings. Clear and pink granular tumor cells contain abundant glycogen (PAS and PAS/D stains helpful). Tumor cells strongly express S-100 protein
Pigmented villonodular synovitis (diffuse type tenosynovial giant cell tumor) enters the differential with GCTB when it erodes bone	Uncommon	F = M Adults in 20s to 40s most common	Knee joint, shoulder joint, hip joints, ankle joints, temporal-mandibular joint	Mononuclear tumor cells (usually sparse) mixed with fibroblasts, randomly distributed GC, inflammatory cells, hemosiderin, and xanthomatous cells	Intracellular hemosiderin is often prominent. 50% of cases are aneuploid; may have trisomies of 5, 7 and abnormalities of 1p. Tumor cells may be desmin, clusterin, and podoplanin positive

Incidence note: 'Common to very common' indicates that a medium sized practice will treat at least several to dozens of patients with the lesion annually. 'Uncommon to rare' indicates the same practice size will treat one to two patients with the lesion every five years. 'Rare to very rare' indicates the same sized practice will see zero to one patient with the lesion every 20 years. GCTB: giant cell tumor of bone

Case table 22.1c Summary pathology findings of Case 22.1

Diagnosis	GCTB
Size	Multiple tumor nodules measuring up to 8.5 cm
Location	Closed epiphysis of distal femur
Margin status	Negative
Histologic grade	Not graded: benign
Pathologic stage (TNM Classification)	Not staged: benign

REFERENCES

Balke M, Schremper L, Gebert C, et al. Giant cell tumor of bone: treatment and outcome of 214 cases. J. Cancer Res. Clin Oncol 2008;134(9):969.

Beebe-Dimmer JL, Cetin K, Fryzek JP, et al. The epidemiology of malignant giant cell tumors of bone: an analysis of data from the Surveillance, Epidemiology, and End Results Program (1975-2004). Rare Tumors 2009;1:e52.

Buckley KA, Fraser WD. Receptor activator for nuclear factor kappaB ligand and osteoprotegerin: regulators of bone physiology and immune responses/ potential therapeutic agents and biochemical markers. Ann Clin Biochem 2003;39(Pt 6):551–6.

Caudell JJ, Ballo MT, Zagars GK, et al. Radiotherapy in the management of giant cell tumor of bone. Int J Radiat Oncol Biol Phys 2003;57(1):158–165.

Chakravarti A, Spiro IJ, Hug EB, et al. Megavoltage radiation therapy for axial and inoperable giant-cell tumor of bone. J Bone Joint Surg Am 1999;81:1566–1573.

Collin-Osdoby P. Regulation of vascular calcification by osteoclast regulatory factors RANKL and osteoprotegerin. Circ Res 2004;95(11):1046–57.

De la Roza. P63 expression in giant cell-containing lesions of bone and soft tissue. Arch Pathol Lab Med 2011;135:776–779.

Domovitov SV, Healey JH. Primary malignant giant-cell tumor of bone has high survival rate. Ann Surg Oncol 2010;17:694–701.

Durr HR, Maier M, Jansson V. Phenol as an adjuvant for local control in the treatment of giant cell tumor of the bone. Eur J Surg Oncol 1999;25(6):610–18.

Errani C, Ruggieri P, Nogales Asenzio MA, et al. Giant cell tumor of the extremity: a review of 349 cases from a single institution. Cancer Treatment Reviews 2010;36:1–7.

Folpe AL, Inwards CY (Eds). Bone and Soft Tissue Pathology. A volume in the series: Foundations in Diagnostic Pathology. Goldblum JR (series ed). Philadelphia: Elsevier Saunders, 2010.

Gorunova L, Vult von Steyern F, Storlazzi CT, et al. Cytogenetic analysis of 101 giant cell tumors of bone: nonrandom patterns of telomeric associations and other structural aberrations. Genes Chromosomes Cancer 2009;48:583–602.

Gupta R, Seethalakshmi V, Jambhekar NA, et al. Clinicopathologic profile of 470 giant cell tumors of bone from a cancer hospital in western India. Ann Diag Pathol 2008;12:239–248.

Haque AU, Moatasim A. Giant cell tumor of bone: a neoplasm or a reactive condition? Int J Clin Exp Pathol 2008;1(6):489–501.

Huang I, Xu J, Wood DJ, et al. Gene expression of osteoprotegerin ligand, osteoprotegerin, and receptor activator of NF-kB in giant cell tumor of bone. Amer J Pathol 2000;156(3):761–767.

Lewis VO, Wei A, Mendoza T. et al. Argon beam coagulation as an adjuvant for local control of giant cell tumor. Clin Orthop Rel Re 2007;454:192–97.

Malawar MM, Bickels J, Meller I, et al. Cryosurgery in the treatment of giant cell tumor. A long term follow-up study. Clin Orthop 1999;359:176–88.

Moskovszky L, Dezso K, Athanasou N, et al. Centrosome abnormalities in giant cell tumour of bone: possible association with chromosomal instability. Mod Pathol 2010;23:359–366.

Moskovszky L, Szuhai K, Krenacs T, et al. Genomic instability in giant cell tumor of bone. A study of 52 cases using DNA ploidy, relocalization FISH, and array-CGH analysis. Genes Chromosomes Cancer 2009;48:468–479.

Pietschmann MF, Dietz DA, Utzschneider S, et al. The influence of adjuvants on local recurrence rate in giant cell tumour of the bone. Acta Chir Belg 2010;110:584–89.

Takeuchi A, Tsuchiya H, Niu X, et al. The prognostic factors of recurrent GCT: a cooperative study by the Eastern Asian Musculoskeletal Oncology Group. J Orthop Sci 2011;16:196–202.

Thomas D, Henshaw R, Skubitz K, et al. Denosumab in patients with giant-cell tumour of bone: an open-label, phase 2 study. Lancet Oncol 2010;11(3):275–280.

Wuelling M, Delling G, Kaiser E. The origin of the neoplastic stromal cell in giant cell tumor of bone. Hum Pathol 2003;34:983–993.

Yanagisawa M, Okada K, Tajino T. A clinicopathologic study of giant cell tumor of small bones. Ups J Med Science 2011;116:265–268.

FURTHER READING

Campanacci M, Baldini N, Boriani S, et al. Giant cell tumor of bone. J Bone Joint Surg Am 1987;69:106–114.

Dorfman HD, Czerniak B. Bone Tumors. St Louis: Mosby, 1998.

O'Donnell RJ, Springfield DS, Motwani HK, et al. Recurrence of giant-cell tumors of the long bones after curettage and packing with cement. J Bone Joint Surg Am 1994;76:1827–1833.

Chapter 23 Notochordal lesions of bone

OVERVIEW

Notochordal tumorous lesions consist of benign notochordal cell tumor; and chordoma. Both are listed in **Table 23.1** which also includes chordoma variants. The more clinically significant tumor is chordoma.

Chordoma is a malignant tumor exhibiting notochordal cell differentiation. It arises in three sites in the axial skeleton and also exceptionally rarely in soft tissue or the lungs. It accounts for up to 4% of primary bone tumors and ranks as the most common primary malignant bone tumor of the spine (if one excludes myeloma). Recent gene expression profiling data suggest a close relationship with chondrosarcoma (Schwab et al. 2007). In fact, a variant of chordoma, chondroid chordoma, closely resembles chondrosarcoma. Fortunately, immunohistochemical panels enable an accurate diagnosis even in small needle core biopsies. Correct diagnosis is important due to new approaches to treatment of chordoma that would have little efficacy in its histologic mimics or would result in overtreatment.

Although the majority of tumors are histologically low grade, chordomas exhibit a high local recurrence rate and significant risk for distant metastases, especially over the long term. Dedifferentiated and poorly differentiated variants (which comprise a minority of chordomas) behave more aggressively. New experimental treatments targeting specific, abnormally activated cell pathways are beginning to boost long term survival rates.

CLASSIFICATION

Table 23.1 World Health Organization classification of notochordal lesions (2013)

Tumor	Behavior	Additional comments
Intraosseous benign notochordal cell tumor	Benign	Recently described benign lesion of vertebrae that is also radiologically non-aggressive Possibly slight risk for malignant transformation to chordoma
Chordoma including chondroid chordoma	Malignant	Most cases sporadic; a few are familial or rarely associated with tuberous sclerosis complex
Dedifferentiated chordoma	Malignant	Some cases associated with history of radiation therapy
Poorly differentiated chordoma	Malignant	Poor prognosis; pediatric age group

Benign: does not recur or recurs non-aggressively and does not metastasize. Intermediate: can recur locally agressively and/or rarely metastasizes (<5%). Malignant: can recur and commonly metastasizes.

DEMOGRAPHICS

Benign notochord tumors are more commonly found in adults with a mean age in the 7th decade. Males are more commonly affected than females (Yamaguchi et al. 2004). They occur in the same sites as chordoma, e.g. the skull base (clivus), spine and sacrum. Vestiges of notochord (also known as notochord remnants) are found in intervertebral discs as small lesions, in vertebral bodies or base of skull: these are all histologically distinct from the intraosseous benign notochordal tumor and usually smaller (Wang et al. 2008).

For chordoma, Surveillance, Epidemiology and End Result (SEER) data were evaluated from 13 registries during a 15 year period (U.S.A., 1994-2008). This section will focus on three malignant histologic types (with the ICDO-3 code presented parenthetically): chordoma, NOS (9370/3), chondroid chordoma (9371/3), and dedifferentiated chordoma (9372/3). All tumors presented here arise in the bone.

The average annual incidence rate is 0.6 per million for chordoma, NOS. Males have a higher incidence rate (0.8 per million) than females (0.5 per million). Chondroid chordoma tumors are very rare – the average annual incidence rate is 0.0 per million. There is no statistically significant difference between males and females. No cases of dedifferentiated chordoma of the bone are documented for the selected registries and time period.

The number of cases reported in 13 SEER registries is shown in **Figure 23.1**.

The mean ages for the selected notochordal tumors are 54.1 years for chordoma, NOS and 44.6 years for chondroid chordoma. The age distribution of these tumors is shown in **Figure 23.2**.

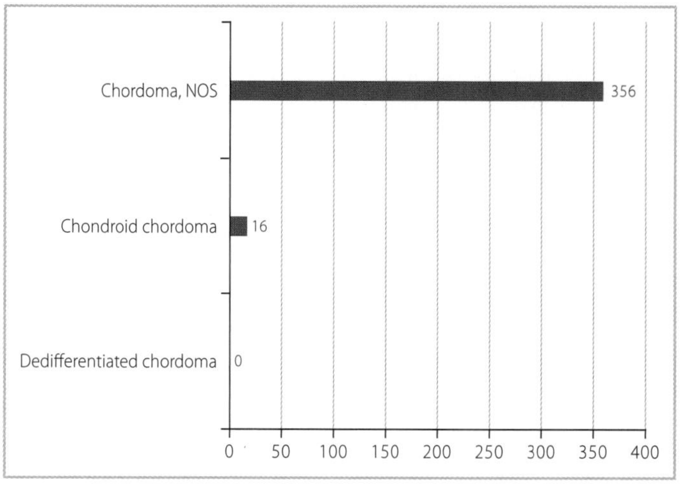

Figure 23.1 Frequency of notochordal tumors of the bone in 13 SEER registries between the years 1994 and 2008.

PATHOGENESIS/ETIOLOGY

Notochord vestiges or remnants represent persistent, residual notochordal elements. Autopsy studies suggest that notochordal cells normally undergo involution, and nearly all disappear entirely by the end of childhood. Ecchordosis physaliphora is another term given to these vestiges which may be located at the base of the skull, the spine or in the sacrum. At the skull base, lesion size may reach 3.5 cm (Zeinab et al. 2010). Some notochord cell remnants are located in the intervertebral disks, specifically the nucleus pulposus which normally is acellular by late childhood and represents the normal, post-embryonic outcome of the human embryonic notochord.

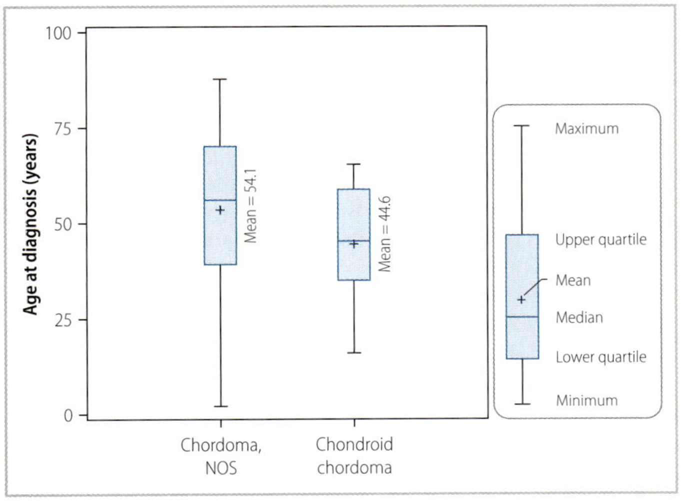

Figure 23.2 Age distribution of notochordal tumors of the bone among cases in 13 SEER registries during the time period 1994.

The etiology of benign notochordal cell tumor (BNCT) is unknown. They may increase in number with advancing age, and thus origin from notochordal remnants, which primarily disappear by age 4 years, is improbable (Yamaguchi et al. 2004). The skeletal distribution of BNCT is identical to that of chordoma suggesting a relationship between the two entities. However, only scant evidence by way of a few case reports hints that benign notochordal cell tumor may serve as a precursor to chordoma. As most benign notochordal cell tumors are asymptomatic, do not transform to chordoma over long periods of time, and those that are treated surgically remain without recurrence long after resection, the precursor supposition is tenuous but may hold for rare cases (Yamaguchi et al. 2002). However, scant but tantalizing genetic data (assessed in three cases of BNCT) noted a loss of MTAP and CDKN2A protein expression in two and three cases respectively which compared to loss of expression in 40 and 70% of chordomas, respectively (Sommer et al. 2010). These findings indicate BNCT shares at least a few molecular alterations with chordoma.

Since virtually all chordomas histologically resemble notochordal elements and share with normal notochordal cells expression of brachyury, a protein found in few other cells (whether normal or abnormal), it is conjectured that chordomas arise from a notochordal differentiating cell. The heterogeneous genetic nature of chordoma appears to invalidate any simple, stepwise progression explaining the transition from vestigial notochordal cell to malignant tumor. The usual accrual of gene alterations with advancing age can be invoked, as most patients are older, and only 5% are children/adolescents. **Table 23.2** lists some of the genetic findings reported to date for chordoma.

By contrast with BNCT, genetic information for chordoma is copious despite its relative rarity. Multiple chromosomal and specific gene abnormalities have been described, some of which have led to promising, targeted therapies (see Medical Oncology section of this chapter). A few chordomas occur in a familial setting. Affected family members of different kindreds show chromosome 7q33, 6q27

Table 23.2 Genetics of notochordal lesions of bone

Tumor or lesion	Chromosomal abnormality	Genes involved	Percentage of lesions with abnormality
Notochord remnants (vestigial notochord)	Not enough data; most likely no abnormalities	Not enough data	No data; most likely no abnormalities
Benign notochordal cell tumor (intraosseous giant notochordal tumor, giant vertebral notochordal rest)	Not enough data	Loss of expression of MTAP protein (this is also reported in some chordomas). Loss of expression of CDKN2A protein (also reported in some chordomas)	Not enough data
Chordoma including chondroid chordoma	May be diploid or hypodiploid (33-44 chromosomes). Common losses: areas of 1p, 3p, 3q, 4, 9p, 10, and 13, 17q. Common gains: areas of 1q, 5q, 7q, 7p, 7, 19, 20 Rare patients with tuberous sclerosis complex develop chordoma	Some familial cases and many sporadic cases have duplications of 6q27 or polysomy 6 (brachyury gene); other familial and sporadic cases have LOH at 1p36 and 7q33. O-E PDGFR and KIT receptors, EGFR, c-MET and STAT3. Activation of P13K-AKT, IGF1R and RAS-MAPK pathways. Tuberous sclerosis genes TSC1 (9q34) or TSC2 (16p.13.3) mutations in TSC patients with chordoma	A few familial cases and some sporadic cases show 6q27 or 1p36 alterations (possibly ~70% for 1p36 in sporadic cases). Fifty percent of sporadic chordomas may have 6q27 alterations. Unknown percentage of tumors with 7q33 alterations Unknown percentage of tumors with specific overexpressed genes and/or activated pathways, but likely the majority show varying combinations of these specific gene and pathway abnormalities
Dedifferentiated chordoma	May have complex aneuploidy in dedifferentiated area	Unknown	Majority of cases may show complex aneuploidy in dedifferentiated region
Poorly differentiated chordoma	Complex polyploidy (but only rare cases analyzed)	SMARCB1/INI1 (22q11.23) gene deletion	Majority may have SMARCB1/INI1 deletions (n = 4 cases studied)

Amp: amplification. O-E: over-expressed. LOH: loss of heterozygosity.
See References for papers and texts pertaining to this table. This static list of genetic abnormalities must be viewed in the context of continuing discovery and refinement of genetic findings.

(brachyury gene site), or 1p36 alterations (Dewaele et al. 2011, Larizza et al. 2005). Additionally, patients with tuberous sclerosis complex are at increased risk for development of chordoma implicating a role for the mutated genes TSC1 or TSC2 in some cases (Larizza et al. 2005). Interestingly, all affected TSC patients develop chordoma before the age of 16 years, while only 5% of chordomas overall occur in the pediatric age group (McMaster et al. 2011).

Sporadic chordomas share with familial cases alterations at chromosomes 7q33, 1p36, and 6q27. However, chordomas are genetically heterogeneous tumors, and no chromosomal gains or deletions are found recurrently in 100% of tumors. What is apparent from recent intensive study of these tumors is the important causal or at least growth contributory role of receptor tyrosine kinases such as EGFR, PDGFB, and others, most of which interact via the PI3K-AKT or RAS-MAPK pathways (Dewaele et al. 2011, Shalaby et al. 2011, Scheipl et al. 2012, Yang et al. 2009, Dobashi et al. 2009, Presneau et al. 2011).

PATHOLOGY

Table 23.3 briefly describes the incidence and histologic features of notochordal lesions. As shown in **Figure 23.3**, chordoma NOS tumors are found in the skull, face and associated joints, as well as the pelvic bones, sacrum, coccyx and associated joints, and vertebral column. Almost all of the chondroid chordoma tumors are seen in the skull, face and associated joints.

Histologic grading

Benign notochordal tumors and notochord remnants do not display cytologic atypia.

Chordomas are not formally graded, and in fact, there is no universally accepted formal system of grading of bone tumors as exists for soft tissue tumors (the FNCLCC and NCI systems).

However, classic chordoma and chondroid chordoma generally show mild to at most moderate nuclear atypia comprising nuclear hyperchromasia, nuclei with smudgy chromatin, and irregularly shaped nuclei. Mitotic activity is most commonly absent but if present seldom exceeds 3/10 hpf. 'Cellular chordoma' differs from usual chordoma in lack of a myxoid or myxochondroid matrix. The degree of cytologic atypia is similar to that seen in conventional chordoma.

Dedifferentiated chordomas consist of tumors with regions showing classic features combined with a high grade sarcoma. The high grade component most commonly comprises a spindle cell pleomorphic sarcoma NOS, but osteosarcoma, rhabdomyosarcoma, and chondrosarcoma have also been reported. Extensive sampling may be required to find the chordoma component.

Poorly differentiated chordoma may resemble epithelioid sarcoma or rhabdoid tumor and contains small round cells with either uniform oval or irregularly shaped nuclei. In either case, nuclei are enlarged and vesicular with prominent nucleoli. Mitotic figures and necrotic areas are often present (Hoch et al. 2006).

Behavior

Benign notochordal tumors are usually asymptomatic. However, symptomatic tumors most commonly present with back pain (chronic or acute); coccydynia, limitation of movement, numbness at various sites, and back, buttock or shoulder stiffness occur less frequently (Amer et al. 2010). A very small number may transform to chordoma.

Table 23.3 Notochordal lesions grouped by behavior

Tumor or lesion	Incidence	Age and sex distribution	Body site (in order of frequency)	Histopathology description including IHC: Medium magnification	Histopathology description including IHC: High magnification
Benign: does not recur and does not metastasize					
Notochord remnant (vestigial notochord) including ecchordosis physaliphora	Very rare	More common in children; may rarely persist into adulthood	Base of skull, extraosseous (ecchordosis physaliphora), intervertebral discs (nucleus pulposus), vertebral bodies	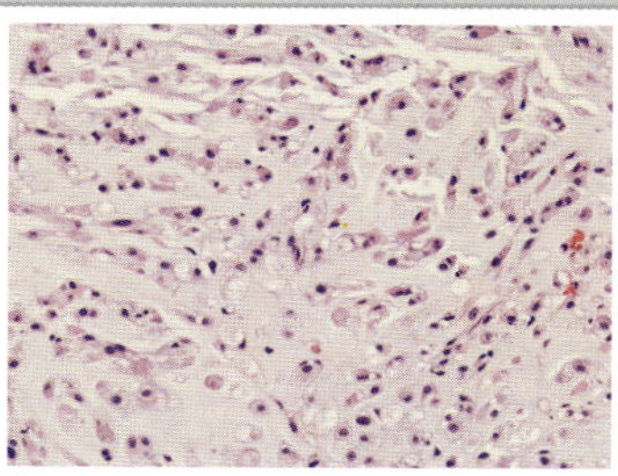	
Clusters or strands of eosinophilic, round notochordal cells without cytologic atypia or mitotic activity (small pyknotic nuclei). Myxoid matrix. No lobular or infiltrative growth. Chordoma does not occur in intervertebral disk. IHC: Lesional cells + for keratins including keratin 18.					
Intraosseous benign notochordal cell tumor (intraosseous giant notochordal tumor, giant vertebral notochordal rest)	Common* (incidence in autopsy series; not resected and so rare in practice)	All ages but adults most commonly Usually incidentally detected	Skull base (clivus) sacrum and vertebral bodies (cervical, lumbar) = similar to chordoma	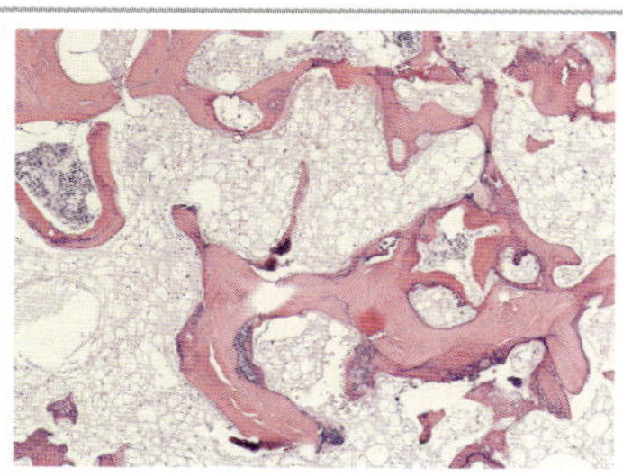	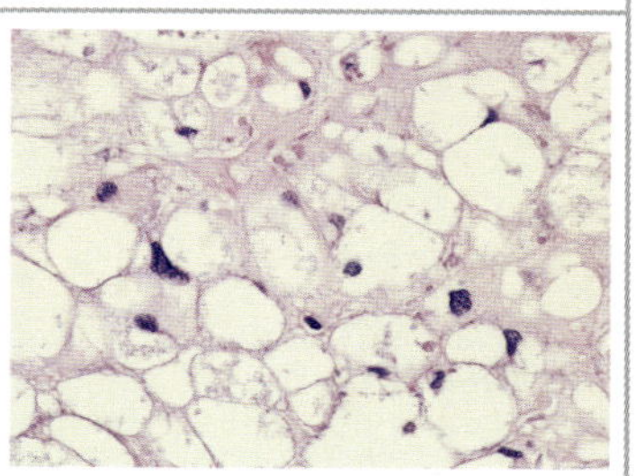
Sheets rather than lobules of large vacuolated cells resembling vacuolated fat cells and large eosinophilic cells. Native bone (often sclerotic), fatty marrow and hematopoietic marrow often entrapped in the tumor. Eosinophilic colloid like pools may be present and intracytoplasmic eosinophilic globules. Minimal nuclear atypia. No mitoses or necrosis. No myxoid matrix.					

Table 23.3: Continued from page 510

Tumor or lesion	Incidence	Age and sex distribution	Body site (in order of frequency)	Histopathology description including IHC	
				Medium magnification	High magnification
Malignant: can recur and can metastasize					
Chordoma including chondroid chordoma	Rare	Adults, usually middle aged; ~5% occur in children. M > F by ~2:1	Skull base, mobile spine (vertebral bodies cervical and lumbar), sacrum Children more commonly have skull base tumors. However, the rare children with chordoma and tuberous sclerosis more typically have sacral tumors Chondroid chordoma is usually located at the skull base	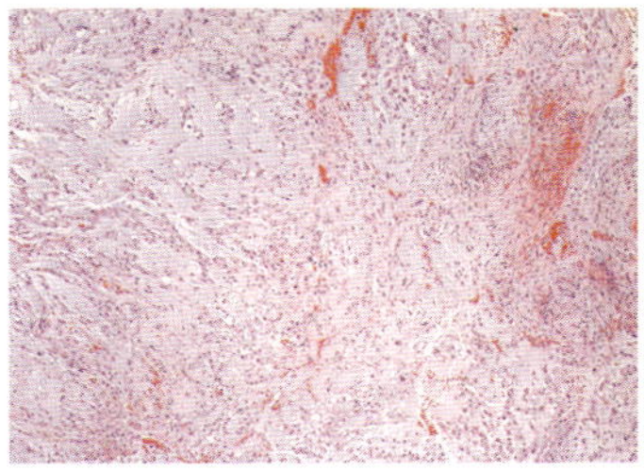	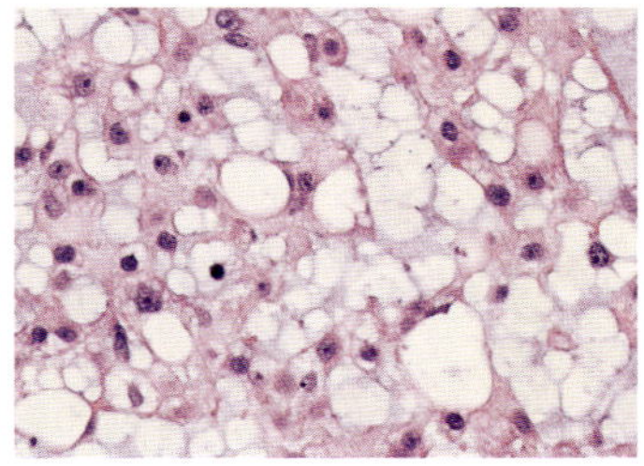
Classic chordoma: Lobulated infiltrative tumor destructive of bone trabeculae. Tumor cells are clear to eosinophilic mildly to moderately atypical with mutivacuolation, round to multilobulated nuclei often with prominent nucleolus. Rarely, spindled cells may ber present. Prominent myxoid or chondromyxoid stroma. Mitotic figures, necrosis and hemorrhage may be present. *'Cellular chordoma'*: classic chordoma that lacks myxoid or chondromyxoid stroma. *Chondroid chordoma:* areas of classic chordoma present in addition to hyaline-like cartilage. IHC: Brachyury (>90%), keratin (100%), EMA (100%), S-100 protein (~60-85%).					
Dedifferentiated chordoma	Very rare	Adults, usually middle aged or older M > F		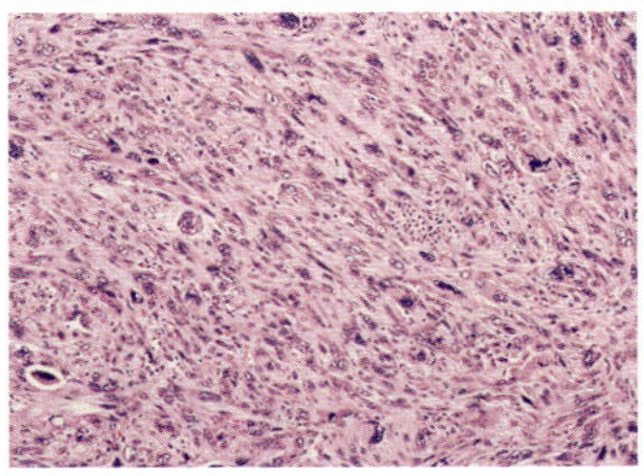	
Classic chordoma plus high grade sarcoma, usually pleomorphic spindle cell NOS. IHC: classic chordoma areas stain like chordoma; dedifferentiated areas may be negative for brachyury, keratins, EMA, S-100 protein.					
Poorly differentiated chordoma	Very rare	Children, usually under 5 years M = F		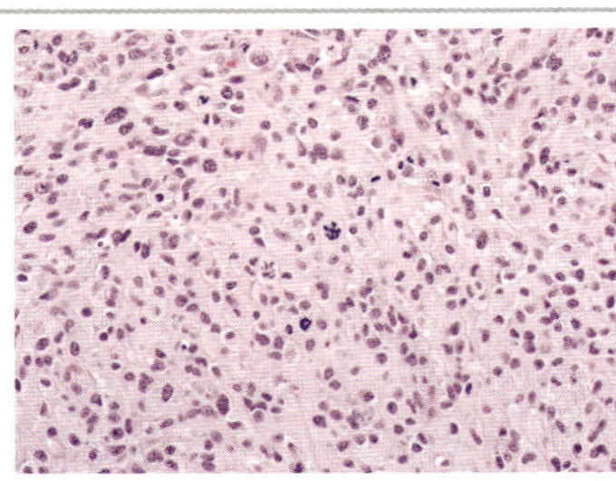	
Sheets of epithelioid, eosinophilic or clear tumor cells without physaliferous cells. Nuclei oval to irregular. Increased tendency for mitotic activity, necrosis and nuclear atypia compared to classic chordoma or cellular chordoma. IHC: Reactive for keratins and EMA. Limited data for brachyury but reported positive in few cases studied (nuclear expression). Possibly majority show loss of INI1 (SMARCB1) expression.					
M: male. F: female. IHC: immunohistochemistry Incidence note: 'Common to very common' indicates that a medium sized practice will treat at least several to dozens of patients with the lesion annually, 'Uncommon to rare' indicates the same practice size will treat one to two patients with the lesion every five years, 'Rare to very rare' indicates the same sized practice will see zero to one patient with the lesion every 20 years.					

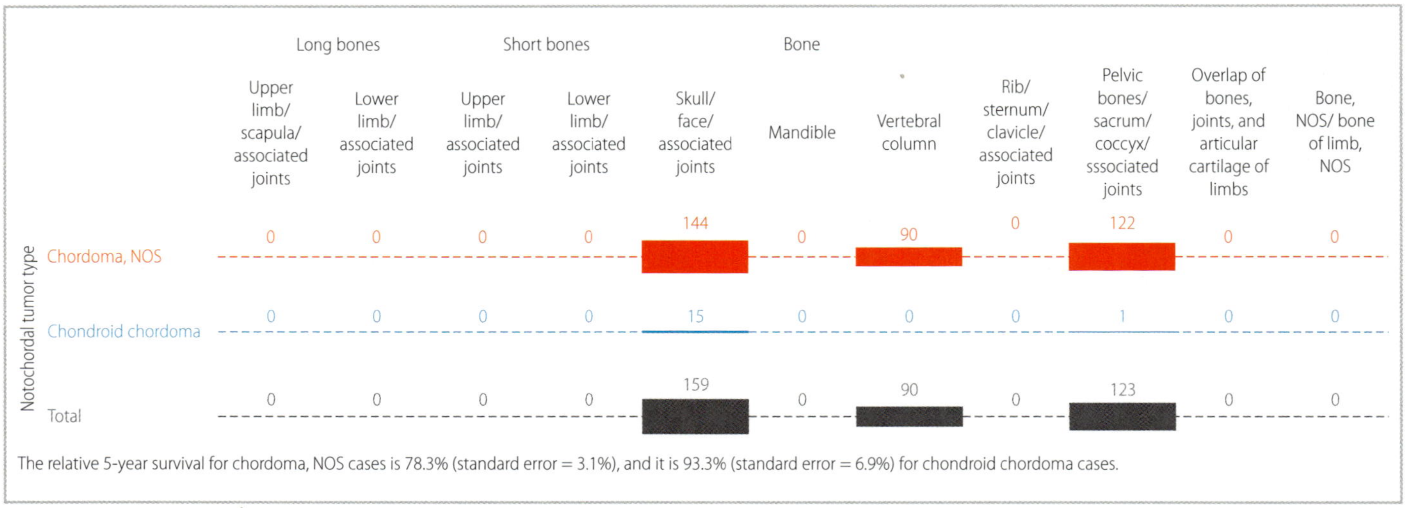

Figure 23.3 Notochordal tumors of the bone by site for cases in 13 SEER registries diagnosed between 1994 and 2008.

The natural history of classic or chondroid chordoma is repeated local recurrence and eventual death due to metastasis or uncontrolled local growth. A recent review of 89 chordoma patients with skull based tumors treated with surgery +/- proton beam radiotherapy reported a 10 year survival rate of 74% for de novo cases and 48% for recurrent cases. Ten year, recurrence-free survival rate for de novo chordoma dropped from 74% to 40% when patients showed residual tumor on post-operative MRI (Almefty et al. 2007). Other adverse prognostic factors determined in various studies include upper cervical spine location and involvement of contiguous vertebral levels (Zhou et al. 2010, n = 37), loss of heterozygosity of 1p36 (Longoni et al. 2008, n = 16 skull based tumors), overexpression of phosphorylated Stat3 (Yang et al. 2009, n = 70), elevated proliferation rate as assessed by Ki67 percentage, deletion at 9p21 (both Horbinski et al. 2010, n = 28 skull based tumors), presence of phosphorylated IGF1R (Sommer et al. 2010, n = 30) and large tumor size (Lee et al. 2012, n = 409), among others.

Dedifferentiated and poorly differentiated chordomas behave aggressively (Hoch et al. 2006, Ridenour et al. 2010).

Additional laboratory testing

Immunohistochemistry

The differential diagnosis of notochordal tumors includes metastatic carcinoma (especially renal cell carcinoma), chordoid meningioma, chondrosarcoma, extraskeletal myxoid chondrosarcoma, epithelioid sarcoma, and extra-renal rhabdoid tumor, among others. All notochordal tumors express brachyury, and thus far, only hemangioblastoma has been reported to express this protein (Tirabosco et al. 2008). Thus, it is exceptionally discriminatory for a commercial antibody in diagnosing notochordal cell tumors. Brachyury is also demonstrable in 100% of chondroid chordomas (Jambhekar et al. 2010). Chordomas also express keratins (including keratin 19) and EMA, and S-100 protein is also frequently expressed, although reactivity is often patchy; staining is usually both nuclear and cytoplasmic. Particularly useful negative reactivity is recorded for GFAP (helpful when differential includes strongly positive chordoid glioma), and D2-40 (helpful when differential includes commonly positive enchondroma, low grade chondrosarcoma and intraosseous myxoid chondrosarcoma) (Sangoi et al. 2009).

Routine cytogenetics

Routine cytogenetic analysis is not of great use in chordoma diagnosis, although the finding of an abnormal karyotype might corroborate the diagnosis when the differential diagnosis includes notochordal remnant.

Molecular genetics

As treatment strategies become more targeted, it will be essential to evaluate a patient's chordoma for specific pathway abnormalities, akin to the assessment of Her2/neu gene amplification in breast carcinoma. This requirement for molecular analysis may apply in only a few years (**Table 23.4**).

RADIOLOGY

The notochord gives rise to the neural plate and spinal column. The notochord normally regresses completely, however it can leave remnants that create a spectrum of benign tumors and a single malignant tumor, the chordoma. The spectrum of benign notochord remnant entities has confusing terminology. A notochord remnant within the intervertebral disk is benign and is known as a vestige or rest. An extra-osseous, extra-vertebral notochord remnant can also occur, most commonly adjacent to the occiput and is known as ecchondrosis physaliphora spheno-occipitalis. They are seen in 0.38% of autopsies (Wyatt et al. 1971). An asymptomatic, intra-vertebral, <1cm benign notochord remnant that is not visible with imaging is called ecchordosis physaliphora vertebralis. The final benign notochord remnant is the controversial entity of a symptomatic, larger lesion that can be seen with imaging. This had originally been given several names including: giant notochordal rest, giant notochordal hamartoma of intraosseous origin and benign chordoma. Ultimately, the term benign notochordal cell tumor (BNCT) has come into favor to encompass the full spectrum of all benign notochord remnant lesions (Amer 2010). There are reported cases of BNCT coexisting or being associated with chordoma (Deshpande et al. 2007, Yamaguchi et al. 2002). There is controversy whether a large symptomatic BNCT can incidentally co-exists with chordoma or is in fact a precursor of chordoma.

Chordoma is a rare malignant tumor derived from notochord remnants. Chordomas can occur anywhere along the neuraxis with

57% occurring in the sacro-coccygeal region, in which case patients may present with intra-abdominal complaints and a mass growing anteriorly in the lower abdomen, and 27% in the spheno-occipital region, particularly affecting the clivus, and the remaining 16% occur in the vertebrae. The imaging appearance is a lytic, destructive lesion often having a large soft tissue mass component. The appearance per se is non-specific; however, the location along the midline of the neuraxis may be the best clue to the diagnosis. On MRI, the notochord lesions show T1 low or isointense signal and T2 high signal. Chordoma usually has intense enhancement and shows destructive, aggressive features absent in the spectrum of BNCT. The differential for chordoma includes chondrosarcoma. Both can show relatively indolent course despite their ultimate malignant behavior. Calcifications can be present in both; chondroid matrix may be identifiable in a chondrosarcoma. Metastases of chordomas are seen in up to 45% of patients with spread to the skin and bone being most common. Metastasis to lung and lymph nodes can also occur (Chambers et al. 1979).

SURGERY

Wide surgical resection is the principal treatment modality for these tumors. The length of recurrence-free survival is directly proportional to the adequacy of the surgical margins. Tumors distal to S2 can generally be resected with satisfactory margins, low complexity, good functional result, and low risk of local recurrence. The reality, however, is that these indolent tumors are typically quite large when they present and mostly involve the upper sacrum or, less frequently, the vertebral bodies or clivus. Wide resection of large tumors involving the upper sacrum and spine can represent the most challenging of operations. Even in the best of hands, obtaining satisfactory margins is extremely difficult, the surgery exceedingly complex, complications common, and significant and disabling neurologic compromise the rule rather than the exception. If a total sacrectomy is necessary, the spino-pelvic junction must be reconstructed which adds an additional complex procedure, also associated with a high complication rate in its own right.

MEDICAL ONCOLOGY

Chordoma classically presents as a slow growing lytic, cervical lesion in 35% which might cause brain stem compression, or anterior sacral (50%), in which case patients may present with intra-abdominal complaints and a mass growing anteriorly in the lower abdomen. The clinical differential diagnosis includes a giant cell tumor of the bone (in younger patients or cervical cancer (in women). The prognosis is relatively good with a 10-year disease-free survival of 46% (Fuchs, et al. 2005). Despite radical surgical resection, these tumors have a tendency to recur locally. Rarely, chordoma is genetically transmitted through a duplication of the brachyury gene (Yang, et al. 2009).

There are no drugs currently approved to treat chordoma. This tumor is usually resistant to chemotherapy. Thus participation in a clinical trial is highly recommended.

Aggressive chemotherapy should be reserved for dedifferentiated cases (Fleming, et al. 1993). A prospective study of 9-nitrocampthotecin induced one partial response in a series of 15 chordoma patients and a median progression-free survival of 47% and 33% at 3 and 6 months, respectively (Chugh, et al. 2005). Single case experiences of responses to vinca alkaloids and alkylating agents have been reported (Al-Rahawan, et al. 2011, Razis, et al. 1974).

The burgeoning understanding of molecular pathways has led to a biological approach to therapy. For example, a case report of response

Table 23.4 Cell pathways and targetable genes in chordoma

Pathway activation	N	Gene involved and alteration	References
mTOR signaling	10/10	Phosphorylation of Ribosomal protein s6	Han, et al. 2009
	58/59	Phosphorylation of EIF4EBP1	Han, et al. 2009
		Deletion of PTEN gene	Han, et al. 2009
		Deletion of CDKN2A (p16)	Hallor, et al. 2008
		Deletion of CDKN2B (p15)	Hallor, et al. 2008
	41/49	Phosphorylation of AKT	Presneau, et al. 2009
	47/49	Phosphorylation of TSC2	Lee-Jones, et al. 2004
	21/21	Overexpression of PDGFR-b	Tamborini, et al. 2006
	14/21	Overexpression of EGFR	Shalaby, et al. 2011
	7/21	Overexpression of CD117	Tamborini, et al. 2006
	62%	Overexpression of CSPG4	Schwab, et al. 2009

EIF4EBP1: Eukaryotic translation initiation factor 4E-binding protein. PTEN: Phosphatase and tensin homolog. CDKN2: Cyclin dependent kinase 2. AKT: Protein Kinase B. TSC: Tuberous sclerosis complex. PDGFR-b: (Platelet-derived growth factor receptor-β). EGFR: Epidermal growth factor receptor). CD117: c-Kit. CSPG4: Chondroitin sulfate proteoglycan 4 (or molecular weight melanoma associated antigen.

to thalidomide, an antiangiogenetic agent, was recently published (Chay, et al. 2011). Because of the PDGF expression of chordoma, imatinib, a PDGFR inhibitor was tested (Casali, et al. 2004,Ferraresi, et al. 2010) In the first case report series, five of 6 patients had a partial response to imatinib at a dose of 400 mg twice a day. A phase II trial of imatinib mesylate at 800 mg daily dose was then performed in 56 patients with unresectable or metastatic chordomas. The clinical benefit rate (complete response plus partial response plus stable disease ≥ 6 months) was 73% and 38% were free of progression at 1 year (Stacchiotti, et al. 2012). There was also a subjective improvement of pain in 64% of 39 symptomatic patients. We successfully treated one patient with recurrent chordoma in the low anterior abdominal wall with imatinib. This patient had chronic renal disease with a glomerular filtration rate below 25 ml/min related to sequelae of surgical therapy for the chordoma. A renal dose of 100 mg per day was given, and the patient remains in remission at 2 years. In this case, response to imatinib was slow but continuous over many months (unpublished data). Other molecularly target agents (cetuximab, gefitinib) have been reported in single cases of chordomas (Hof et al. 2006).The addition of sirolimus to imatinib is active as a salvage therapy in patients whose tumors progressed on imatinib alone (Stacchiotti et al. 2009). Chordoma is difficult to manage medically when the tumor has grown beyond a surgical or radiotherapy approach. Imatinib might be useful if the tumor overexpresses PDGFR. A multidisciplinary approach is favored.

RADIATION ONCOLOGY

Following surgical resection of chordoma with widely negative margins, observation is recommended. However, obtaining such widely negative margins is usually difficult in this disease and therefore surgery followed by post-operative radiation is preferred and is associated with higher rates of disease-free survival. However, clival-based tumors are largely inoperable, and therefore definitive RT is recommended. Sacral chordomas are typically more amenable to surgery.

Reviews of the literature demonstrate that higher radiation doses (> 60 Gy) yield better outcomes than doses < 60 Gy. Traditionally, photon beam therapy has been used for treatment, given its wider availability. Advances in treatment delivery, such as Intensity modulated radiotherapy (IMRT), has allowed for increased coverage of the tumor volume and sparing of critical structures. Due to the rarity of these tumors, no large series are available describing patients who have been uniformly treated with IMRT. Single institution retrospective series contain a wide heterogeneity of patient treatments, making it difficult to compare outcomes. Debus et al (2000) reported on 45 patients with chordoma or chondrosarcoma who received post-operative photon RT, with a median dose of 66.6 Gy. The 5 year local control rate was 50%, and survival was 82%.

With its more favorable dose-depth characteristics, charged-particle therapy such as proton beam therapy allows for escalation of radiation dose to the tumor while improving the level of sparing of radiation dose to the surrounding critical structures, such as brainstem, optic nerves, and optic chiasm. In cases of clival chordomas, the use of proton therapy can be very advantageous, and therefore there is a growing clinical experience using this particular type of radiation in this disease. When comparing outcomes of protons vs. photons, better results have been achieved with proton therapy. A recent report included 40 patients who underwent surgery and proton therapy (Yasuda et al. 2012). The mean dose was 68.9 Cobalt-gray equivalents (CGE). The 5-year progression free survival was 70%, while the overall survival was 83%. Terahara et al. (1999) reported on a series of 132 patients with skull base chordoma treated with a combination of photon and proton radiation. Prescribed doses ranged from 66.6 CGE to 79.2 CGE. The 5-year actuarial local control rate was 59%.

CASES

Case 23.1 Benign notochordal cell tumor

Clinical history and presentation

The patient is a 68-year-old man who presents with an incidental finding of an L5 destructive lesion discovered during workup of unexplained penile pain. He denies any low back pain or neurologic symptoms. Physical examination is unremarkable.

Surgical findings and comments

Needle biopsy is consistent with chordoma. En bloc spondylectomy is performed with satisfactory wide margins. An instrumented arthrodesis with autograft is performed for reconstruction.

Radiology findings

Our case, **Case figs 23.1a** through **23.1h**, involves a 68 year old man. The plain radiograph and bone scan show very subtle findings that might go unnoticed. It is cross sectional imaging which reveals the lesion best with CT showing an irregular sclerotic lesion with a tiny area of cortical breakthrough. The MR best demonstrates the lesion showing that its true extent involves the entire L5 vertebral body with a small soft tissue mass adjacent to the left L5 nerve root. This soft tissue mass has identical appearance to a herniated disc. However, the remainder of the disc shows only minimal disease and the presence of the vertebral body lesion with cortical destruction leads to the correct diagnosis of an underlying tumor. The differential for this large solitary lesion of the vertebrae includes malignancies such as myeloma or a metastasis, and tissue diagnosis is needed. In general, a midline tumor of the spine, especially involving the clivus or sacrum, suggests chordoma.

Pathology findings

Gross features

The needle core biopsy consists of a 0.3 cm in aggregate of wispy soft tissue fragments.

The resected vertebra measures 6.5 × 5 × 5 cm, and cross sections show spongy medullary bone with a slightly mottled hemorrhagic appearance. A well-defined lesion is not identified. The specimen is abundantly sampled for microscopic exam.

Microscopic features

Needle core biopsy: The needle core biopsy contains disrupted tumor fragments that consist of variably sized, vacuolated cells with a very low N/C ratio and no significant atypia (**Case fig. 23.1i**). Immunohistochemistry staining reveals diffuse keratin and patchy S-100 protein expression (also repeated on the resection specimen). A diagnosis of chordoma is rendered. The patient is referred to the University Hospital for further treatment.

Resection low magnification: The tumor envelops but does not destroy trabecular bone. It replaces most of the marrow, but islands of normal marrow elements remain (**Case fig. 23.1j**). The trabecular bone is reactively sclerotic with variable amounts of appositional new bone.

Resection high magnification: At medium magnification, the tumor looks a bit like ischemic marrow fat with enlarged, vacuolated cells resembling adipocytes (**Case fig. 23.1k**). Importantly, there is no myxoid matrix as would be seen in chordoma. Instead, intracytoplasmic eosinophilic material is scattered throughout the tumor as small globules or pools (**Case fig. 23.1l**). Tumor nuclei vary slightly in size and shape with generally inconspicuous nucleoli (**Case fig. 23.1m**). Most of the cells are univacuolated, but a few physaliphorous cells (bubbly cells with multiple clear vacuoles) are present. There is no necrosis or mitotic activity.

Special studies: The tumor cells are diffusely strongly reactive for keratins AE1/AE3 (**Case fig. 23.1n**). Scattered cells also express S-100 protein (**Case fig. 23.1o**).

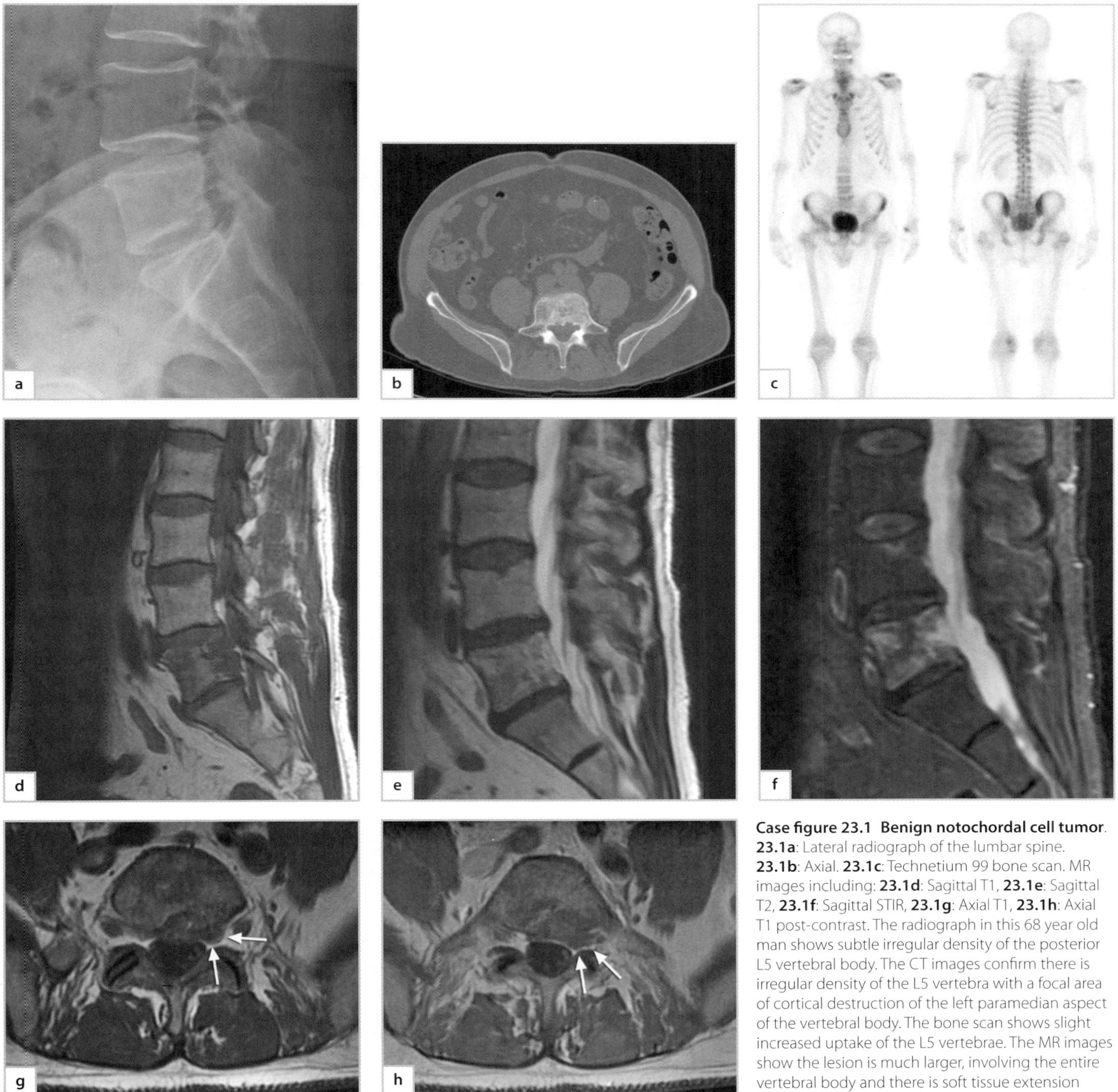

Case figure 23.1 Benign notochordal cell tumor. **23.1a**: Lateral radiograph of the lumbar spine. **23.1b**: Axial. **23.1c**: Technetium 99 bone scan. MR images including: **23.1d**: Sagittal T1, **23.1e**: Sagittal T2, **23.1f**: Sagittal STIR, **23.1g**: Axial T1, **23.1h**: Axial T1 post-contrast. The radiograph in this 68 year old man shows subtle irregular density of the posterior L5 vertebral body. The CT images confirm there is irregular density of the L5 vertebra with a focal area of cortical destruction of the left paramedian aspect of the vertebral body. The bone scan shows slight increased uptake of the L5 vertebrae. The MR images show the lesion is much larger, involving the entire vertebral body and there is soft tissue extension along the left paramedian aspect adjacent to the left exiting L5 nerve root, white arrows in Case fig. 23.1g and 23.1h. The mass has non-specific T1 low signal with T2 heterogeneous signal and STIR sequence high signal. The lesion has no appreciable enhancement.

Case figure 23.1: Continued from page 515

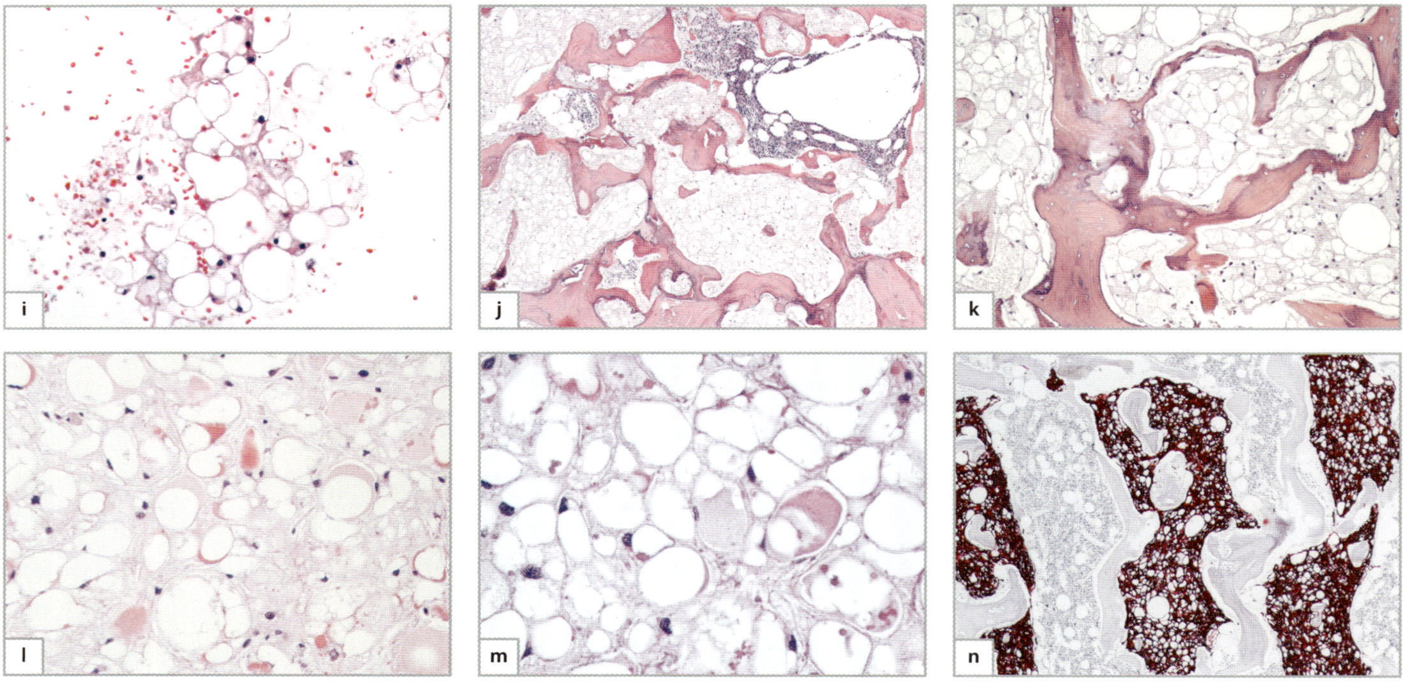

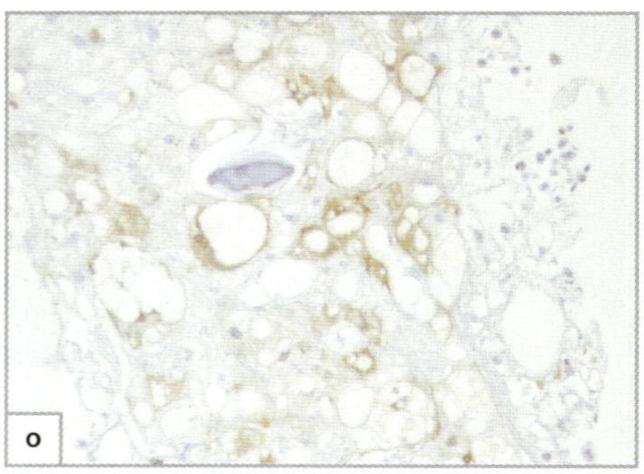

23.1i: Needle core biopsy. The small fragments comprise clusters of clear and eosinophilic cells with a low nuclear to cytoplasmic ratio. Some cells are bubbly (with multiple vacuoles) consistent with physaliphorous cells. **23.1j**: Resection at low magnification. Unlike chordoma, BNCT grows as sheets of cells between bone trabeculae. It surrounds but does not destroy trabecular bone. Islands of normal marrow are also present. **23.1k**: Resection at medium magnification. The trabecular bone is thickened by appositional new bone, a reactive response to the tumor. In this field, the tumor has completely replaced normal bone marrow. At a quick glance, it resembles fat. **23.1l**: Resection at higher magnification. Distinctive from chordoma, BNCT produces intracytoplasmic eosinophilic globules and pools rather than a gray myxoid or chondromyxoid matrix. **23.1m**: Resection at highest magnification. Tumor nuclei are only mildly variable in size and shape, and nucleoli are generally inconspicuous. **23.1n**: Resection with mixed keratin antibody IHC stain. Tumor cells strongly and diffusely express keratins (AE1/AE3 keratin mixture with red chromagen). Notice the preserved marrow elements sandwiched between sheets of tumor. **23.1o**: Resection with S-100 protein antibody IHC stain. Reactivity for S-100 protein is scattered, a common pattern in notochordal cell lesions.

Pathologic differential or, why isn't it one of the following?

Chordoma: Chordoma is usually radiologically an aggressive lesion, unlike this patient's lesion. Microscopically, it can erode cortex and destroys rather than surrounds trabecular bone. In most cases, at low magnification, it demonstrates lobulation with fibrous trabeculae, a feature absent in benign notochordal cell tumor (BNCT). Except for the cellular variant in which matrix is scant, a myxoid or myxochondroid stroma is prominent in chordoma and lacking in BNCT. Chordomas may exhibit necrosis (35% of sacral cases). The nuclei of a chordoma may show prominent nucleoli, and scattered cells can display hyperchromatic, large or multilobulated nuclei; such cells are absent in BNCT. Immunohistochemically, the cells of both tumors would express the same set of antigens, so IHC is not diagnostically helpful. Cytogenetics may be useful but not typically necessary because of major differences in histologic features. However, small needle core biopsy samples can be challenging as was the case with this patient first evaluated at an outlying hospital, and consideration could be given to obtaining additional material for karyotyping in cases where the radiologic features are not classic for either lesion.

Metastatic carcinoma such as renal cell carcinoma: The clear cell variant of renal cell carcinoma contains keratin positive vacuolated tumor cells arranged in sheets. Trabecular bone could be preserved but often is destroyed. The carcinoma cells are considerably smaller than the cells in BNCT and would display at least some nuclear atypia consisting of prominent nucleoli and possibly mitotic activity. RCC can express S-100 protein, keratins and EMA like BNCT. It is negative for brachyury. Additionally, clear cell RCC also expresses RCC antigen and CD10 both of which would be absent in BNCT.

Metastatic liposarcoma: Well differentiated liposarcoma consists of sheets of vacuolated fat cells and lipoblasts that could mimic BNCT. However, it often destroys rather than preserves trabecular bone. Eosinophilic pools and globules are absent. Liposarcomas express S-100 protein like BNCT but not brachyury or keratins. Unlike BNCT, most cases will reveal abnormal nuclear expression of MDM2 and CDK4.

Oncology approach

Medical oncology

This is a benign tumor with no role for medical oncology.

Radiation oncology

Benign notochordal cell tumor is not treated with radiation.

Patient outcome

Twenty months postoperatively the patient has no symptoms, normal neurologic function, and no evidence of recurrence.

Case table 23.1 Summary pathology findings of Case 23.1

Diagnosis	BNCT
Size	6.5 × 5 × 5 cm
Location	Entire body of lumbar vertebra (L5)
Margin status	Negative
Histologic grade (FNCLCC grading system)	Tumor is benign and therefore not graded
Pathologic stage (AJCC TNM classification)	Tumor is benign and therefore not graded

FNCLCC: Fédération Nationale des Centres de Lutte Contre le Cancer (French Federation of Cancer Centers). AJCC: American Joint Committee on Cancer

Case 23.2 Chordoma

Clinical history and presentation

The patient is a 76-year-old man who presents with a six month history of right leg weakness. He denies any pain, numbness, or bowel/bladder symptoms.

Physical examination reveals no obvious abnormalities of the spine or sacrum. He has 1/5 strength L5 and S1 distribution right lower extremity. He has slightly diminished sensation in the L5 and S1 dermatomes right lower extremity.

Needle biopsy is consistent with chordoma.

Surgical findings and comments

Due to the patient's advanced age and the morbidity which would be associated with wide resection of the tumor, the patient and surgeon elect to proceed with laminectomy and tumor debulking followed by radiation therapy.

Radiology findings

This 76 year old man (**Case figs 23.2a** through **23.2e**), is a classic case of chordoma with a bulky, destructive mass of the midline sacrum. The image characteristics themselves are not specific, but this is clearly an aggressive tumor that requires tissue diagnosis. The differential would include chondrosarcoma, but no cartilage matrix is found on CT. This is not a BNCT given the large size and the aggressive features seen. In general, it is the location of a destructive tumor involving the midline sacrum or clivus that suggests the diagnosis of chordoma.

Pathology findings

Gross features

The tumor is evaluated by frozen section at the time of resection, and a diagnosis of 'chordoma' is rendered. The subsequently excised tumor consists of a 5 × 3 × 2.5 cm aggregate of mixed bone spicules and gelatinous to dusky red hemorrhagic soft tissue. A portion is banked for possible research, and multiple cassettes are sent to Histology for routine processing.

Microscopic features

Low magnification: Less disrupted parts of the tumor show a well-defined lobular architecture with fibrous trabeculae (**Case fig. 23.2f**). This fibrous septation is classic for chordoma.

High magnification: Medium magnification reveals cords, strands and webs of neoplastic cells suspended in an abundant gray, myxoid matrix (**Case fig. 23.2g**). Tumor cells comprise two basic types: a population with eosinophilic, slightly granular cytoplasm, and a second intermixed set of cells with single to multiple vacuoles imparting in some a bubbly appearance (physaliphorous cells) (**Case fig. 23.2h**). In general, the nuclear to cytoplasmic ratio is low. Nearly all the tumor cells contain round nuclei with fine chromatin and many feature single round nucleoli. A few cells are multinucleated but marked nuclear pleomorphism or hyperchromasia is absent (**Case fig. 23.2i**). Approximately 10% of the tumor is necrotic. Mitotic figures are not identified.

Special studies: Tumor nuclei diffusely express brachyury. Of additional IHC stains performed, tumor cells are also strongly and diffusely reactive for keratin 19 (**Case fig. 23.2j**) with membranous reactivity for EMA, and scattered cells reactive for S-100 protein. There is no expression of CEA, smooth muscle actin, HMB-45, or D2-40.

Pathologic differential or, why isn't it one of the following?

Poorly differentiated chordoma: Poorly differentiated chordoma occurs in the pediatric age group with most tumors located in the clivus. It comprises sheets of eosinophilic or clear cells without myxoid matrix. Most cases display nuclear atypia and mitotic activity. At least some cases lack nuclear INI1 expression by IHC (Mobley et al. 2010), which is preserved in conventional chordoma.

Metastatic carcinoma: Tumors with vacuolated cells such as renal cell carcinoma or adrenal cell carcinoma enter the differential with chordoma. Immunohistochemistry aids in the differential, as some metastatic tumors express relatively specific markers lacking in chordoma (including RCC antigen, ER/PR, CDX2, TTF-1, PSA, inhibin, and Melan A). No carcinomas are known to express brachyury which starkly contrasts with nearly 100% of chordomas.

Primary sacral chondrosarcoma: Intraosseous chondrosarcoma can exhibit a myxoid matrix and cords and nests of cells similar to

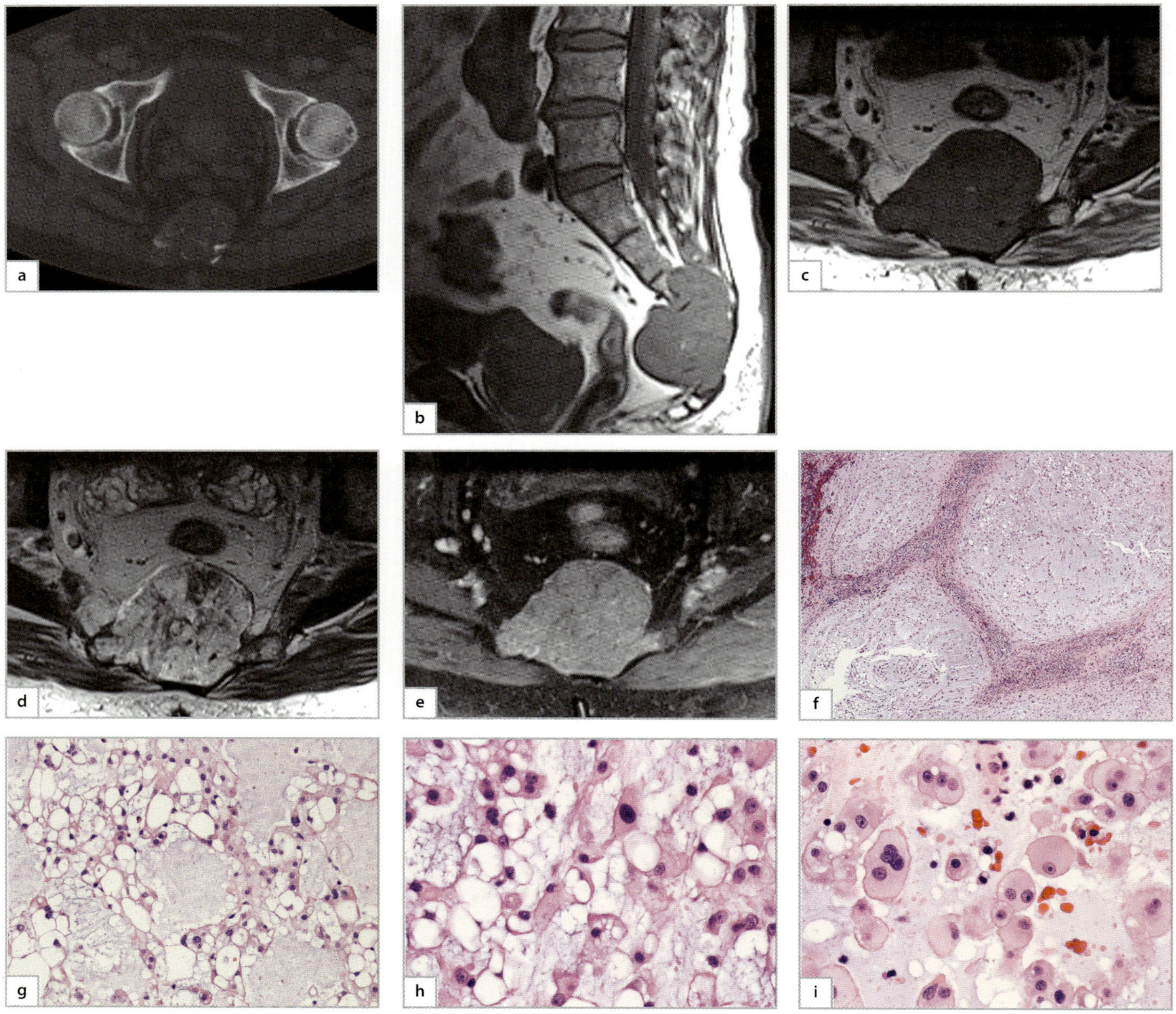

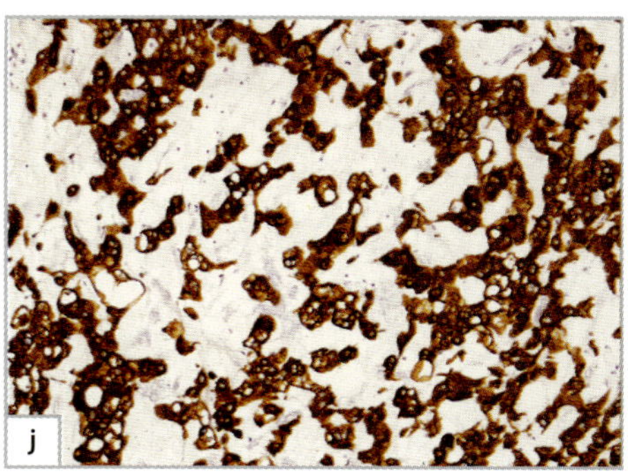

Case figure 23.2 Chordoma. 23.2a: Is a post contrast axial CT image. MR images including: **23.2b**: Sagittal T1, **23.2c**: Axial T1, **23.2d**: Axial T2 and **23.2e**: Axial T1 fat saturated post-contrast. The MR images in this 76 year old man show a 4.6 × 7.4 × 6.5 cm mass destroying the sacrum. The mass shows non-specific T1 low signal and T2 heterogeneous high signal with intense diffuse enhancement. The CT images show scattered coarse calcifications without specific matrix pattern. **23.2f**: Low magnification. Chordoma displays distinct lobulation (when not too fragmented from the surgical procedure). Tumor cells and matrix are separated by fibrous bands. This is a characteristic feature of chordoma not seen in benign notochordal cell tumor. **23.2g**: Medium magnification. Tumor cells form a web or strands and cords of cohesive cells floating in abundant myxoid matrix. **23.2h**: High magnification. Three cell types occur in classic or conventional chordoma: the famous physaliphorous cell (a bubbly, clear multivacuolated tumor cell), an eosinophilic granular cell and a clear, univacuolated cell. The nuclear to cytoplasmic ratio is low, and the cell types freely intermingle. Nuclei exhibit mild variability in size, and some cells contain single nucleoli. **23.2i**: High magnification. In this field, the cells are more discohesive. Multinucleation is present. Foci of increased nuclear atypia (including multinucleation, pleomorphism, and hyperchromasia) can occur in conventional chordoma but with retention of a low N/C ratio. **23.2j**: Keratin 19 IHC stain, brown chromagen. Most chordomas strongly and diffusely express keratin 19, a helpful diagnostic marker in the differential with chondrosarcoma and certain carcinomas.

chordoma. Spindle cells and delicate intercellular connections rather than broad, back to back appositions (as is typical of chordoma) are more common in chondrosarcoma. Hyaline cartilage can occur in chondrosarcoma, but only in skull based chordomas (if it is the dominant matrix component, the tumor is designated 'chondroid chordoma'). IHC is again very helpful in small biopsies or skull based tumors because chordomas express brachyury (absent in chondrosarcoma) and keratins including keratin 19 and EMA (rare in chondrosarcoma) (Oakley et al. 2008).

Case table 23.2 Summary pathology findings of Case 23.2

Diagnosis	Chordoma
Size	At least 5 cm but less than 8 cm
Location	Sacrum with extension into soft tissue
Margin status	Positive
Histologic grade (FNCLCC grading system)	Low grade
Pathologic stage (AJCC TNM classification)	IA (T1/N0/M0)

FNCLCC: Fédération Nationale des Centres de Lutte Contre le Cancer (French Federation of Cancer Centers). AJCC: American Joint Committee on Cancer

Oncology approach

Medical oncology

This patient was not referred to Medical Oncology. However, if the patient becomes more symptomatic, the recommendation would be either participation in a clinical trial or imatinib therapy, which targets PDGFR, a receptor usually expressed on the cell surface of chordoma. Imatinib induces a clinical benefit rate > 50%, with symptomatic improvement, but few true partial responses (Stacchiotti, et al. 2012). Immunohistochemistry could be performed to demonstrate the PDGFR expression, but it is not yet a clinically approved test. The dose of imatinib is 400 mg twice a day (Casali, et al. 2004). In the absence of response, pharmacokinetics of imatinib could be performed to establish the specific metabolic pattern of the treated patient (Gurney, et al. 2007).

Future studies should evaluate the use of PDGFR inhibitors as neoadjuvant treatment for chordoma. Current clinical trials include tumor banking, radiotherapy protocols, and studies of PDGFR inhibitors. Chemotherapy is usually inactive. The Chordoma Foundation is a good source of information.

Radiation oncology

As the patient undergoes tumor debulking only, radiation therapy is necessary in the case to optimize local control of his disease. With gross disease remaining, a minimum radiation dose of 66 Gy is required. A post-operative MRI for treatment planning is also necessary to accurately delineate the target volume, which consists of the gross disease seen on MRI and an additional margin. Using photon beam radiation, intensity modulated radiation therapy (IMRT) would be needed to allow for dose escalation while minimizing dose to the surrounding normal structures, such as small bowel, rectum, bladder, and femoral heads. The use of charged particles such as protons has been shown in multiple single institutional series to yield superior local control outcome compared to historical series of patients treated with traditional photon beams, although the extent of surgical resection remains a confounding variable (Yasuda et al 2012). Doses of 70-80 cobalt-gray equivalents (CGE) can be delivered with proton beam treatment.

Patient outcome

Eighteen months postoperatively, the patient is noted to have a persistent foot drop right lower extremity and persistent numbness in the L5/S1 distribution. He denies back pain. He has normal bowel and bladder function. Imaging reveals slowly progressive recurrent disease.

REFERENCES

Al-Rahawan MM, Siebert JD, Mitchell CS, et al. Durable complete response to chemotherapy in an infant with a clival chordoma. Pediatr Blood Cancer 2012;59(2):323–5

Amer HZ, Hameed M. Intraosseous benign notochordal cell tumor. Arch Pathol Lab Med 2010;134(2):283–8.

Casali PG, Messina A, Stacchiotti S, et al. Imatinib mesylate in chordoma. Cancer 2004;101:2086–97.

Chambers PW, Schwinn CP. Chordoma. A clinicopathologic study of metastasis. Am J Clin Pathol 197;72(5):765–776.

Chay WY, Teo M, Sittampalam K, et al. Effective use of thalidomide in the treatment of recurrent metastatic chordoma. J Clin Oncol 2011;29:e477–80.

Chungh R, Dunn R, Zalupski MM, et al. Phase II study of 9-nitro-camptothecin in patients with advanced chordoma or soft tissue sarcoma. J Clin Oncol 2005;23:3597–604.

Debus J, Schulz-Ertner D, Schad L, et al. Stereotactic fractionated radiotherapy for chordomas and chondrosarcomas of the skull base. Int J Radiat Oncol Biol Phys 2000;47(3):591–6.

Deshpande V, Nielsen GP, Rosenthal DI, et al. Intraosseous benign notochord cell tumors (BNCT): further evidence supporting a relationship to chordoma. Am J Surg Pathol 2007;31(10):1573–7.

Dewaele B, Maggiani F, Floris G, et al. Frequent activation of EGFR in advanced chordomas. Clin Sarcoma Res 2011;1(1):4.

Dobashi Y, Suzuki S, Sato E, et al. EGFR-dependent and independent activation of Akt/mTOR cascade in bone and soft tissue tumors. Mod Pathol 2009;22(10):1328–1340.

Eriksson B, Gunterberg B, Kindblom LG. Chordoma. A clinicopathologic and prognostic study of a Swedish national series. Acta Orthop Scand 1981;52(1):49–58.

Ferraresi V, Nuzzo C, Zoccali C, et al. Chordoma: Clinical characteristics, management and prognosis of a case series of 25 patients. BMC Cancer 2010;10:22.

Fleming GF, Heimann PS, Stephens JK, et al. Dedifferentiated chordoma. Response to aggressive chemotherapy in two cases. Cancer 1993;72:714–8.

Franz DN, Weiss BD. Molecular therapies for tuberous sclerosis and neurofibromatosis. Curr Neurol Neurosci Rep 2012;12(3):294–301.

Fuchs B, Dickey ID, Yaszemski MJ, et al. Operative management of sacral chordoma. J Bone Joint Surg Am 2005;87:2211–6.

Gil Z, Fliss DM, Voxkoboinik N, et al. Cytogenetic analysis of three variants of clival chordoma. Cancer Genet Cytogenet 2004;154(2):124–30.

Gurney H, Wong M, Balleine RL, et al. Imatibin disposition and ABCB1 (MDR1, P-glycoprotein) genotype. Clin Pharmacol Ther 2007:82:33–40.

Hallor KH, Staaf J, Jonsson G, et al. Frequent deletion of the CDKN2A locus in chordoma: Analysis of chromosomal imbalances using array comparative genomic hybridization. Br J Cancer 2008;98:434–42.

Han S, Polizzano C, Nielsen GP, et al. Aberrant hyperactivation of akt and Mammalian target of rapamycin complex 1 signaling in sporadic chordomas. Clin Cancer Res 2009;15:1940–6.

Hoch BL, Nielsen GP, Liebsch NJ, et al. Base of skull chordomas in children and adolescents. A clinicopathologic study of 73 cases. Am J Surg Pathol 2006;30(7):811–8.

Hof H, Welzel T, Debus J. Effectiveness of cetuximab/gefitinib in the therapy of a sacral chordoma. Onkologie 2006;29:572–4.
Horbinski C, Oakley GJ, Cieply K, et al. The prognostic value of Ki-67, p53, epidermal growth factor receptor, 1p36, 9p21, 10q23, and 17p13 in skull base chordomas. Arch Pathol Lab Med 2010:134(8):1170–6.
Lee J, Bhatia NN, Hoany BH, et al. Analysis of prognostic factors for patients with chordoma with use of the California Cancer Registry. J Bone Joint Surg Am 2012;94(4):356–63.
Lee-Jones L, Aligianis I, Davies PA, et al. Sacrococcygeal chordomas in patients with tuberous sclerosis complex show somatic loss of TSC1 or TSC2. Genes Chromosomes Cancer 2004;41:80–5.
Longoni M, Orzan F, Stroppi M, et al. Evaluation of 1p36 markers and clinical outcome in a skull base chordoma study. Neuro Oncol 2008;10(1):52–60.
McMaster ML, Goldstein AM, Bromley CM, et al. Chordoma: incidence and survival patterns in the United States, 1973-1995. Cancer Causes Control 2001;12:1–11.
McMaster ML, Goldstein AM, Parry DM. Clinical features distinguish childhood chordomas associated with tuberous sclerosis complex (TSC) from chordoma in the general paediatric population. J Med Genet 2011;48(7):444–9.
Mobley BC, McKenney JK, Bangs CD, et al. Loss of SMARCB1/INI1 expression in poorly differentiated chordomas. Acta Neuropathol 2010;120(6):745–753.
Paolo Dei Tos A. Unveiling the molecular pathogenesis of chordoma: a new paradigm for molecular targeting of rare cancers. J Pathol 2011;223(5): 565–566.
Presneau N, Shalaby A, Idowu B, et al. Potential therapeutic targets for chordoma: P13K/AKT/TSC1/TSC2/mTOR pathway. Br J Cancer 2009;100:1406–14.
Presneau N, Shalaby A, Ye H, et al. Role of the transcription factor T (brachyury) in the pathogenesis of sporadic chordoma: a genetic and functional-based study. J Pathol 2011;223(3):327–35.
Razis DV, Tsatsaronis A, Kyriazides I, et al. Chordoma of the cervical spins treated with vincristine sulfate. J Med 1974;5:274–7.
Ridenour RV 3rd, Ahrens WA, Folpe AL, et al. Clinical and histopathologic features of chordomas in children and young adults. Pediatr Dev Pathol 2010;13(1):9–17.
Scheipl S, Froehlich EV, Leithner A, et al. Does insulin-like growth factor 1 receptor (IGF-1R) targeting provide new treatment options for chordomas? A retrospective clinical and immunohistochemical study. Histopathol 2012;60(6):999–1003.
Schwab JH, Boland PJ, Agaram NP, et al. Chordoma and chondrosarcoma gene profile: implications for immunotherapy. Cancer Immunol Immunother 2009;58(3):339–49.
Shalaby A, Presneau N, Ye H, et al. The role of epidermal growth factor receptor in chordoma pathogenesis: a potential therapeutic target. J Pathol 2011;223:336–46.
Stacchiotti S, Longhi A, Ferraresi V, et al. Phase II study of imatinib in advanced chordoma. J Clin Oncol 2012;30:914–20.
Stacchiotti S, Marrari A, Tamborini E, et al. Response to imatinib plus sirolimus in advanced chordoma. Ann Oncol 2009;20:1886–94.
Tamborini E, Miselli F, Negri T, et al. Molecular and biochemical analyses of platelet-derived growth factor receptor (PDGFR) B, PDGFRA, and KIT receptors in chordomas. Clin Cancer Res 2006;12:6920–8.
Terahara A, Niemierko A, Goitein M, et al. Analysis of the relationship between tumor dose inhomogeneity and local control in patients with skull base chordoma. Int J Radiat Oncol Biol Phys 1999;45(2):351–8.
Walcott BP, Nahed BV, Mohyeldin A, et al. Chordoma: current concepts, management, and future directions. Lancet Oncol 2012;13(2):e69–76.
Wang WL, Abramson JH, Ganguly A, et al. The surgical pathology of notochordal remnants in adult intervertebral disks. A report of 3 cases. Am J Surg Pathol 2008;32(8):1123–9.
Wyatt R, Schochet S Jr, McCormick WF. Ecchordosis physaliphora: an electron microscopic study. J Neurosurg 1971;34(5):672–677.
Yamaguchi T, Suzuki S, Ishiiwa H, et al. Benign Notochordal Cell Tumors. A comparative histological study of benign notochordal cell tumors, classic chordomas, and notochordal vestiges of fetal intervertebral discs. Am J Surg Pathol 2001;28(6):756–61.
Yamaguchi T, Yamato M, Saotome K. First histologically confirmed case of a classic chordoma arising in a precursor benign notochordal lesion: differential diagnosis of benign and malignant notochordal lesions. Skeletal Radiol 2002;31(7):413–8.
Yang C, Schwab R, Schoenfeld AJ, et al. A novel target for treatment of chordoma: signal transducers and activators of transcription 3. Mol Cancer Ther 2009;8(9):2597–605.
Yang XR, Ng D, Alcorta DA, et al. T (brachyury) gene duplication confers major susceptibility to familial chordoma. Nat Genet 2009;41:1176–8.
Yasuda M, Bresson D, Chibbaro S, et al. Chordomas of the skull base and cervical spine: clinical outcomes associated with a multimodal surgical resection combined with proton-beam radiation in 40 patients. Neurosurg Rev 2012;35(2):171–83.

FURTHER READING

Sciubba DM, Cheng JJ, Petteys RJ, et al. Chordoma of the sacrum and vertebral bodies. J Am Acad Orthop Surg 2009;17:708–717.
Dorfman HD, Czerniak B. Bone Tumors. St Louis: Mosby, 1998.
Folpe AL, Inwards CY (eds). Bone and Soft Tissue Pathology. A volume in the series: Foundations in Diagnostic Pathology. Goldblum JR (series ed). Philadelphia: Elsevier Saunders, 2010.
Fletcher CDM, Bridge JA, Hogendoorn P, Mertens F (eds). WHO Classification of Tumours of Soft Tissue and Bone, 4th ed. Lyon: IARC Press, 2013.

Chapter 24 Vascular tumors of bone

OVERVIEW

Hemangioma of bone is a common lesion that is seldom biopsied. The other vascular tumors of bone are very rare. Treatment of malignant, intraosseous vascular tumors demands a team approach. As with other sarcomas, targeted gene therapy will most likely soon compose an essential aspect of treatment.

CLASSIFICATION

Table 24.1 provides the 2013 World Health Organization (WHO) classification of vascular tumors of bone. **Table 24.2** offers a second proposed classification of bone vascular tumors (Verbeke et al. 2011). The current classification of vascular tumors of bone follow the same classification scheme created for those occurring in soft tissue (Fletcher et al. 2013, O'Connell et al. 2001, Errani et al. 2011). Tissue location (bone vs soft tissue vs skin) should not alter the characteristic, classifiable features of a tumor. Of course, there are exceptions to this general rule even in well-established soft tissue tumors. For example, schwannoma, solitary fibrous tumor, and perineurioma look microscopically different when they occur in soft tissue versus the GIT, around the orbit or in a nerve, respectively. Nonetheless, despite superficial differences, these tumors still are identified as schwannoma, solitary fibrous tumor, and perineurioma. Intraosseous location should not prevent a specific diagnosis. For example, if a tumor in the bone fulfills all the histologic criteria of composite hemangioendothelioma, it should be labeled specifically as such and not just termed 'hemangioendothelioma of bone'.

DEMOGRAPHICS

Benign vascular lesions of bone

Hemangiomas occur across a broad age range without a strong gender proclivity. Most patients present in young adulthood. While the lesions are very common (found in 10% of the spines of adults in one autopsy series), they are usually asymptomatic and are not biopsied or resected. The lesions may be multifocal. Epithelioid hemangioma is notable for occasional cortical destruction with soft tissue extension, a ~10% risk for local recurrence, and a 3% risk for regional lymph node involvement. Angiomatosis of the skeleton usually presents in childhood or adolescence, and males are more frequently affected.

Malignant vascular tumors of bone

Primary malignant vascular tumors of bone are very rare. Surveillance, Epidemiology, and End Results (SEER) registry data were evaluated from 13 registries during a 15 year period (1994-2008). This section focuses on 5 malignant histologic types (with the ICDO-3 code presented parenthetically): hemangiosarcoma (angiosarcoma) (9120), malignant hemangioendothelioma (9130), malignant epithelioid

Table 24.1 WHO Classification of vascular tumors of bone (2013)

Tumor	Behavior	Additional comments
Hemangioma	Benign	Extremely common but seldom symptomatic
Epithelioid hemangioma	Intermediate (locally aggressive)	Can be confused histologically with EHE
Epithelioid hemangioendothelioma (EHE)	Malignant	May be solitary or associated with multiorgan disease such as with concurrent involvement of liver, lung or soft tissue
Angiosarcoma	Malignant	Rare
Benign: does not recur and does not metastasize. Intermediate: can recur but does not metastasize. Malignant: can recur and can metastasize. RMS: rhabdomyoscarcoma		

Table 24.2 One proposed classification of vascular tumors of bone (Verbeke et al. 2011)

Tumor or lesion	Behavior	Comments
Hemangioma Cavernous, capillary	Benign	Some or all may represent hamartomas rather than clonal neoplasms
Angiomatosis Non-aggressive regional Non-aggressive disseminated (cystic) Aggressive or massive osteolysis or Gorham Stout's Disease (GSD)	Benign	Soft tissue or spleen involved in 60-70% GSD results in destruction of one or more bones in a regional distribution. Half of cases are associated with trauma
Epithelioid hemangioma	Intermediate	Considered benign in WHO vascular soft tissue tumors classification although behavior is is in some cases intermediate: can recur and rarely spreads to regional lymph nodes; does not metastasize or dedifferentiate
Epithelioid hemangioendothelioma	Malignant	Same histologic features as in soft tissue
Angiosarcoma Primary Irradiation-induced Bone infarction associated	Malignant	Ranges from low to high grade. One third are multifocal in the skeleton Comprise <1% of primary malignant bone tumors

hemangioendothelioma (9133), Kaposi sarcoma (9140), lymphangiosarcoma (9170). All tumors presented in these figures originated in the bone.

The average annual incidence rate is 0.1 per million for hemangiosarcoma, and 0 per million for malignant hemangioendothelioma, malignant epithelioid hemangioendothelioma, and Kaposi sarcoma. There is no statistically significant difference between males and females. No cases of lymphangiosarcoma of the bone are documented for the selected registries and time period.

The number of cases reported in 13 SEER registries is shown in **Figure 24.1**.

The mean ages for the selected vascular tumors of the bone are very similar (hemangiosarcoma (angiosarcoma) = 58.0 years, malignant epithelioid hemangioendothelioma = 56.7 years, malignant hemangioendothelioma = 60.2 years). Patients with Kaposi sarcoma are typically much younger at diagnosis. **Figure 24.2** depicts the age distribution of vascular tumors of the bone.

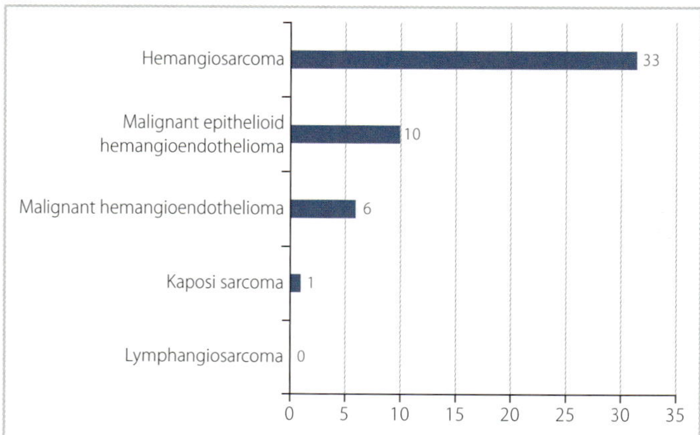

Figure 24.1 Frequency of vascular tumors of the bone in 13 SEER registries between the years 1994 and 2008. (Hemangiosarcoma is synonymous with angiosarcoma.)

PATHOGENESIS/ETIOLOGY

Benign vascular lesions of bone

Some hemangiomas may represent hamartomas or vascular malformations. A few syndromes are associated with malformations or hemangiomas (Blue rubber bleb nevus syndrome, Klippel-Trenaunay syndrome, Proteus syndrome, venous malformations with TIE2 gene mutation, Parkers-Weber syndrome, von Hippel-Lindau syndrome, Osler-Weber-Rendu disease, and others). Epithelioid hemangioma, with its distinctive histology and sometimes aggressive local growth with rare spread to regional lymph nodes, is distinctive, but no specific genetic alterations have yet been identified. It does not bear the t(1;3)(p36;q25) of epithelioid hemangioendothelioma.

Malignant vascular lesions of bone

Risk factors for development of intra-osseous angiosarcoma may include those implicated in soft tissue examples. However, the vanishingly few number of skeletal angiosarcomas make it difficult to confirm these risks. It is established that a few cases are related to prior irradiation or bone infarction (Verbeke et al. 2011). As with other mesenchymal tumors, a mixture of environmental, genetic and epigenetic events is likely to be causative. At least for angiosarcoma of soft tissue, characteristic altered cell pathways are being identified (see Chapter 10 for a list of some of the implicated genes).

The list of sarcomas harboring specific gene translocations continues to grow and now includes epithelioid hemangioendothelioma. Many cases demonstrate a t(1;3)(p36;q25) translocation which fuses the *WWTR1* gene (a transcriptional coactivator highly expressed in endothelial cells) with *CAMTA1* (a DNA binding transcriptional regulator)(Tanas et al. 2011).

PATHOLOGY

Table 24.3 lists the key pathologic features of vascular tumors of bone including incidence and demographics. Conceivably, any soft tissue vascular tumor could also occur in the skeleton, and skimming PubMed one can find a smattering of case reports of primary skeletal

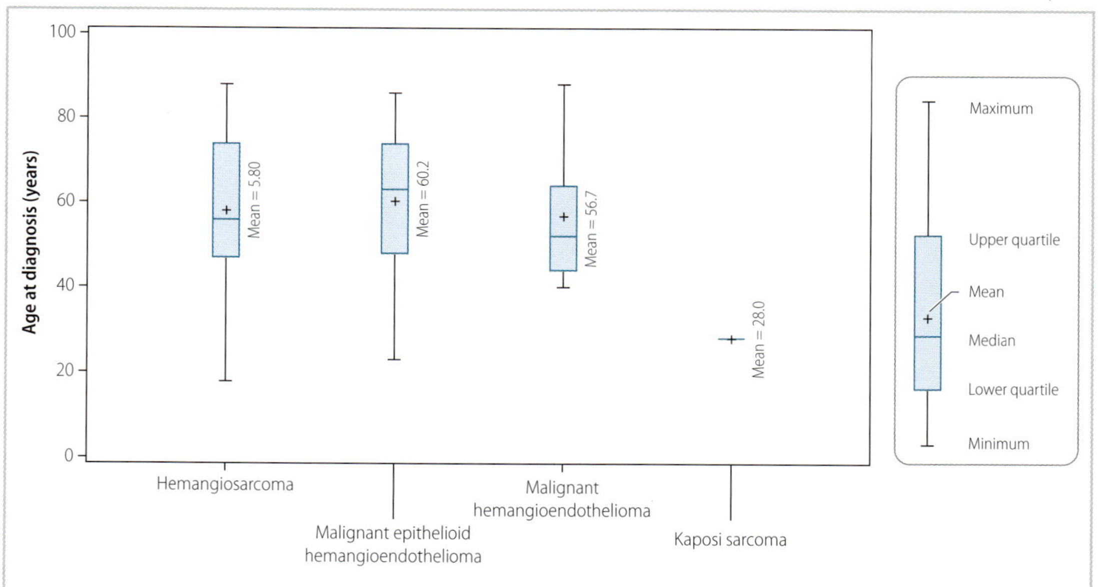

Figure 24.2 Age distribution of vascular tumors of the bone among cases in 13 SEER registries during the time period 1994-2008 (n=50).

Table 24.3 Vascular tumors of bone grouped by behavior

Tumor	Incidence	Age and sex distribution	Bone site (in order of occurrence)	Histopathology description including IHC	
				Medium magnification	High magnification
Benign: does not recur or recurs non-aggressively and does not metastasize					
Hemangioma	Common	All ages but young to middle aged adults most commonly. F slightly > M	Vertebrae and skull >> long bones > others	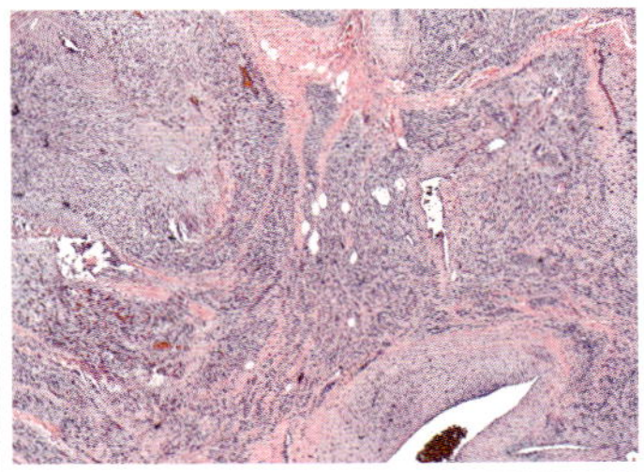	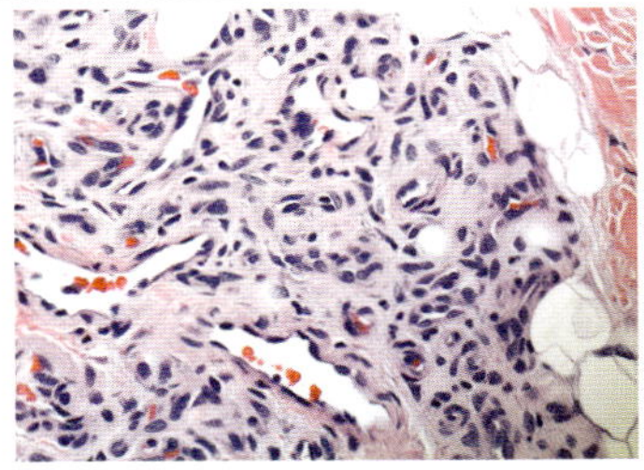
Variants include lobular capillary hemangioma, cavernous hemangioma, and sclerotic hemangioma. All consist of well-formed, mature vessels but of differing calibers. Look identical to soft tissue counterparts. Positive for vascular markers including CD31, CD34, ERG (C-terminus directed), and FLI-1.					
Intermediate: can recur locally aggressively and/or rarely metastasizes (<5%)					
Epithelioid hemangioma	Rare	All ages but young adults (20s-30s) most commonly. M slightly > F	Long bones ~20% multifocal	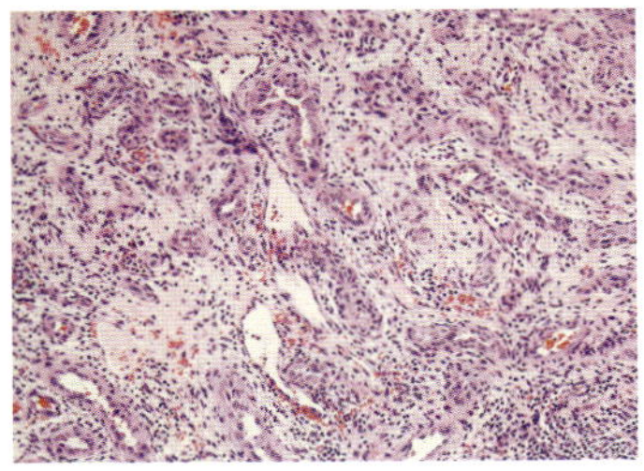	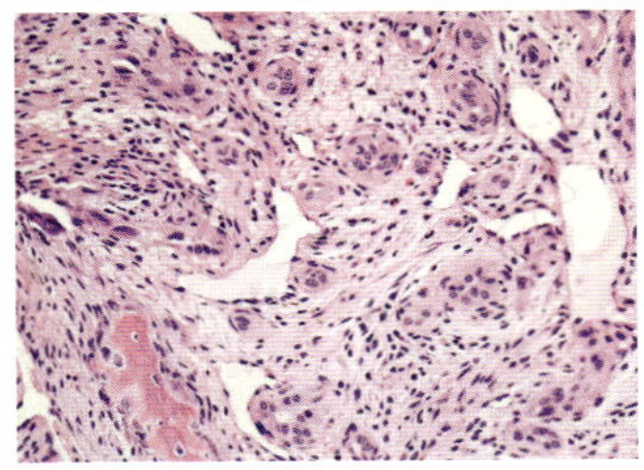
Capillary or venular sized vessels lined by plump epithelioid endothelial cells. May have zonal pattern with less epithelioid vessels at periphery then epithelioid vessels then central solid or solid appearing areas. Less commonly inflamed than soft tissue counterpart. Often mitotically active but without atypical division figures. Some cases may have spindle cells. Positive for CD31, CD34, ERG (C-terminus directed), and FLI-1. Keratins and EMA also often positive.					
Malignant: can recur locally aggressively and commonly metastasizes					
Epithelioid hemangioendothelioma (EHE)	Rare	All ages but teenagers and young adults most commonly. M > F	Long bones ~60% multifocal including visceral involvement	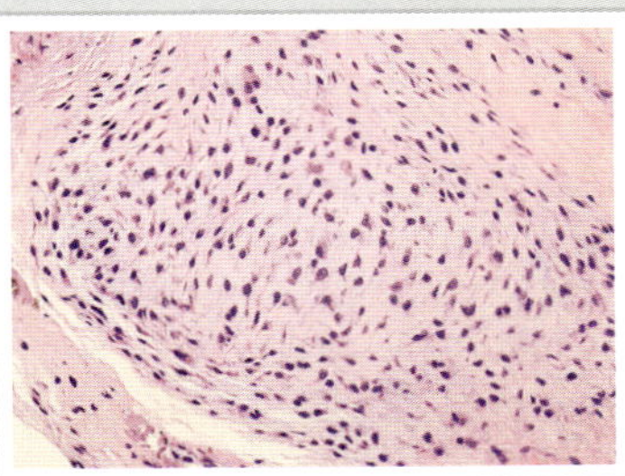	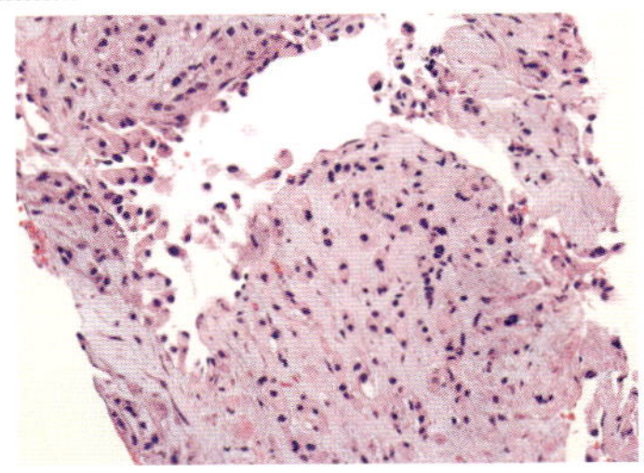
Cords, nests, and single cells embedded in a myxochondroid or hyaline matrix. Few if any primitive vessels. Tumor cells are epithelioid (rounded with distinct cell borders and medium N/C ratio). Classic type has little mitotic activity or pleomorphism. 'Malignant' or 'high grade' EHE is more anaplastic with more mitotic activity. Positive for CD31, FLI-1 and ERG (C-terminus directed) in almost all cases; often positive for CD34, simple keratins, and smooth muscle actin.					
Angiosarcoma	Very rare	All ages most common in middle age and elderly (50s through 70s) M >> F	Long bones, vertebrae ~33% multifocal	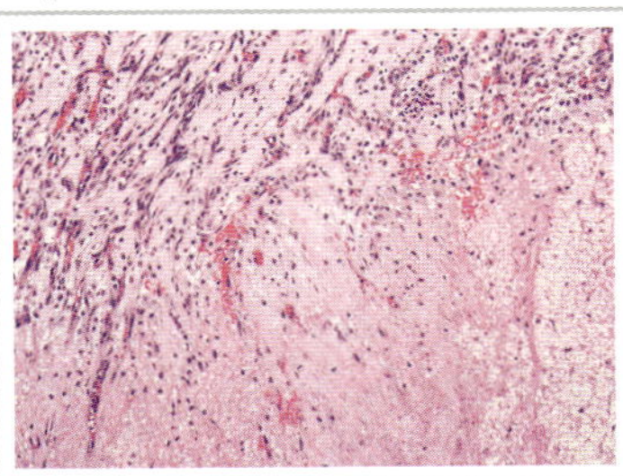	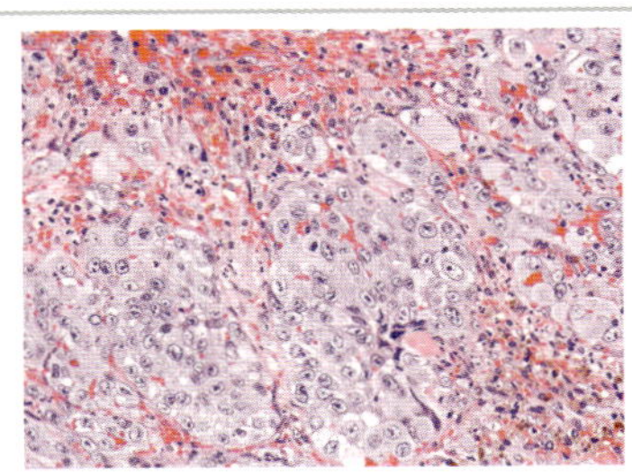
Three grades as in soft tissue counterpart. Epithelioid variant may dominate over spindle cell morphology in most cases. Lower grades show obvious vessel formation with minimal atypia but permeative, destructive growth. High grade tumors may have only focal to no primitive vessel formation other than intracytoplasmic lumena. Nuclear pleomorphism and mitotic activity increase with grade. All grades often associated with acute hemorrhage. Positive for CD31(>90%), FLI-1 (>80%), CD34 (40-100%, especially in better differentiated tumors), ERG (C-terminus directed), and sometimes simple keratins (25-75%). May also be positive for D2-40 and SMA (in pericytic differentiated tumor cells; usually confined to lower grade tumors).					
Incidence note: 'Common to very common' indicates that a medium sized practice will treat at least several to dozens of patients with the lesion annually. 'Uncommon to rare' indicates the same practice size will treat one to two patients with the lesion every five years. 'Rare to very rare' indicates the same sized practice will see zero to one patient with the lesion every 20 years.					

spindle cell hemangioma, papillary intralymphatic angioendothelioma, retiform hemangioendothelioma and kaposiform hemangioendothelioma (McCarthy et al. 1999, Ma et al. 2011, Zhang et al. 2012). For histologic descriptions of these tumors, please refer to Chapter 10, Vascular Tumors of Soft Tissue.

Figure 24.3 depicts the distribution of malignant vascular tumors of bone in the skeleton (n= 50, SEER data 1994-2008). Based on a relatively large series of cases, most angiosarcomas are intermediate to high grade, approximately 57% feature well-formed, identifiable blood vessels but ~80% also feature solid areas, 98% contain cells with intracytoplasmic vacuoles (early vessel lumina), and a large majority are associated with a lymphocytic infiltrate (Verbeke et al. 2011).

Histologic grading

Benign vascular lesions of bone

Benign lesions are not histologically graded. However, these lesions can be cellular and mitotically active, and such features do not by themselves denote malignancy. Epithelioid hemangioma (EH) is notorious for being confused with epithelioid hemangioendothelioma (EHE) as both feature round, pink, epithelioid endothelial cells often with nucleoli, mitotic activity, and sometimes solid growth and small foci of necrosis. Despite their names, both may also contain spindle tumor cells. However, EH produces recognizable small vessels and lacks the myxochondroid or hyaline matrix of EHE. It grows in a contained, lobular manner rather than in the permeative pattern of EHE.

Malignant vascular lesions of bone

The classic version of epithelioid hemangioendothelioma exhibits mild nuclear atypia, a low mitotic rate, and little solid growth (generally the cells are disposed singly, in cords, or nests). A high grade version 'high grade EHE' or 'malignant EHE' consists of more pleomorphic cells with hyperchromatic, variably sized nuclei, increased necrosis, often solid growth, and a higher mitotic rate. Some experts favor placing 'malignant EHE' into the angiosarcoma category.

Angiosarcoma (AS) ranges from well differentiated tumors with extensive, mature vessel formation and minimal atypia but with telltale permeative growth to high grade sarcomas with marked nuclear pleomorphism and little to any vessel formation. Some high grade AS may contain lower grade regions. Angiosarcoma is formally graded by the FNCLCC system.

Behavior

Benign vascular lesions of bone

Hemangiomas and angiomatoses are benign. Exceptionally, an angiosarcoma can develop from a benign precursor; this is case reportable. Epithelioid hemangioma, as previously mentioned, can recur, can aggressively penetrate cortex and extend into periskeletal soft tissue, and can rarely spread to regional lymph nodes. It has no risk for distant metastasis.

Malignant vascular lesions of bone

Limited data are available for behavior of primary malignant vascular tumors of bone. Intra-osseous epithelioid hemangioendothelioma may behave similarly to its soft tissue counterpart with a 20-30% risk for metastasis and 20% disease specific mortality. However, cases of EHE with aggressive radiologic features may be more likely to metastasize and cause death (Deyrup et al. 2007).

The histologic grade of intra-osseous angiosarcoma may exert a small effect on behavior. One group reported that tumors with prominent nucleoli, a mitotic rate >3/10hpf and <5 eosinophils/10hpf behave aggressively with a worse outcome (Verbeke et al. 2011). In general, angiosarcoma primary to bone exhibits a poor outcome with a five year survival rate of ~33% (Verbeke et al. 2011).

Additional laboratory testing

Immunohistochemistry: Benign and malignant vascular tumors express CD31, CD34, FLI-1, and ERG (C-terminus specific) in the majority of cases. Some high grade angiosarcomas and a few EHE lack CD34 expression. Other proteins that may be expressed include D2-40 (podoplanin), smooth muscle actin in tumor cells differentiating towards pericytes, and simple keratins such as keratins 8 and 18 with some tumors also reactive for antibody to keratin 7. New antibodies are regularly developed, because none of the highly sensitive vascular markers (CD31, CD34, and FLI-1) are uniquely specific for blood

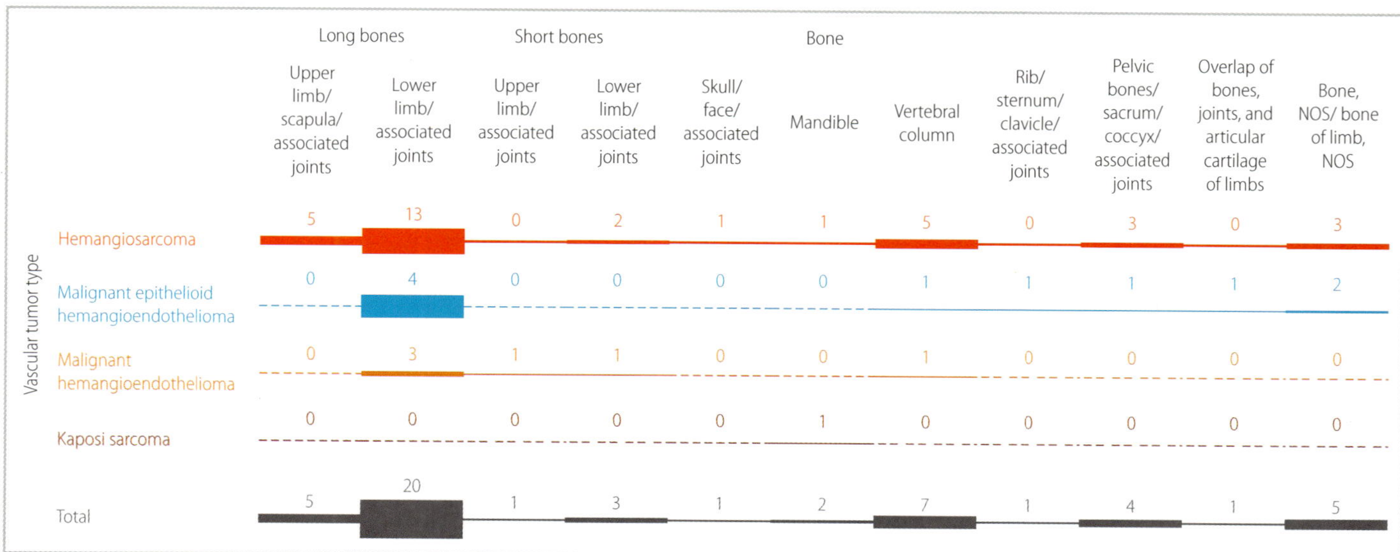

Figure 24.3 Vascular tumors of the bone by site for cases in 13 SEER registries diagnosed between 1994 and 2008.

vessels. As always, use of immunohistochemistry must be informed and discerning, coupling the histologic and IHC features to clinical and radiologic findings.

***Routine cytogenetics*:** Most angiosarcomas display a complex aneuploid karyotype. This can support a diagnosis of malignancy but is otherwise non-specific. Epithelioid hemangioendothelioma cases often contain a t(1;3)(p36;q25) which can be detected by standard karyotyping and FISH.

Molecular genetics: Thus far, the role of molecular genetics in vascular tumors is limited. PCR for the gene fusion of t(1;3) can be performed, if necessary. As altered cell pathways are mapped for the malignant tumors, molecular genetic methods may be employed to detect the alterations and guide targeted gene therapy. This approach is in its early stages.

RADIOLOGY

Hemangiomas of bones are very common lesions, often seen in the marrow space of the axial skeleton. There are several subtypes including the capillary, cavernous, venous, and mixed which are named for the type of vessels comprising the lesion.

The most common hemangiomas of the skeleton are the cavernous and capillary. Both have a flattened endothelial lining. The cavernous hemangiomas have dilated vascular spaces as opposed to capillaries. The cavernous hemangiomas commonly occur in the skull. These can occasionally become quite large and disfiguring. The capillary hemangioma is the most common overall and is frequently seen in the vertebral body. These are essentially incidental findings commonly seen on routine spine MR imaging. Hemangiomas can rarely cause symptoms by extra-osseous extension into the neuroforamina or spinal canal. The capillary hemangiomas typically have T1 high signal and are variably high signal on T2 images. Not all hemangiomas have T1 high signal, but when they do, the diagnosis is virtually pathognomonic for a benign lesion, such as a capillary hemangioma or lipoma. Hemangiomas of the spine usually are spherical lesions with somewhat lobulated, irregular margins. One can often see stippled low signal foci on transverse slices representing thick trabeculae. The thick trabeculae may give a corduroy appearance on longitudinal slices.

The radiologist is often confronted with marrow lesions, especially in the axial skeleton. Metastasis and multiple myeloma are common marrow malignancy and these are almost uniformly T1 low signal thus distinguishing them from hemangiomas. Marrow malignancies will look similar to hemangiomas on T2 and STIR imaging where they both show variable high signal. Hence, the T1 images are of crucial importance to the radiologist, as the distinction between benign and malignant cannot be made without them. There are only a few settings when malignancy can potentially have T1 high signal such as hemorrhage and a melanin producing melanoma (Premkumar et al. 1996). However, these are typically heterogeneously T1 high signal and not the uniform T1 high signal of a hemangioma. Unless there is known melanoma metastases, the radiologist can usually confidently diagnose a T1 high signal lesion as benign, representing a hemangioma or an intra-osseous lipoma, and no further workup is required (McMenamin et al. 2007).

SURGERY

Hemangioma

The vast majority of hemangiomas of bone are asymptomatic. Rarely, tumors of the spine may cause pain and even neurologic deficit and treatment may be indicated in these cases. Radiation therapy or embolization can often provide symptomatic relief without surgery, which can be associated with extensive hemorrhage. Vertebroplasty has been associated with good pain relief when pathologic fracture occurs, although long term results may be disappointing. If surgery is indicated, such as in cases with symptoms refractory to more conservative treatment or neurologic compromise, pre-operative transarterial embolization followed by surgical resection of the involved bone decreases associated blood loss and demonstrates good long term results with low recurrence.

Angiosarcoma

Wide resection is the surgical treatment of choice for this malignancy.

MEDICAL ONCOLOGY

Hemangioma

Some unresectable hemangiomas might respond to interferon α (Appelbaum 1990, Takahashi, et al. 2005).

Angiosarcoma

The medical oncologist will mainly treat metastatic epithelioid hemangioendothelioma or high grade angiosarcoma. These types of tumor can affect any portion of the skeleton. One third of cases occur in the axial skeleton, one third in long tubular bones, and on third in the small bones of the hands and feet. High grade angiosarcoma of the bone can present as multiple lesions in a single bone, two or more adjacent bones, or perhaps all the bones of one limb. When localized, the course remains indolent with a good prognosis. The second presentation is that of single or multiple rapidly progressive lesions that metastasize to other bones or to the lungs. This form is highly lethal. Tumor might arise in association with a bone infarct or Paget's disease.

Because these lesions can be multifocal, they pose a diagnostic challenge between a non-secretory plasma cell myeloma and a metastatic carcinoma. A high degree of suspicion is necessary. Once the diagnosis is established, the medical oncology treatment is similar to the one of soft tissue or visceral angiosarcoma (see Chapter 10). However, even in case of metastatic disease, a local treatment to stabilize the bone might be necessary and referral to the interventional radiologist for embolization or the orthopedic oncology surgeon might be appropriate.

RADIATION ONCOLOGY

While benign vascular tumors of bone are common, they are rarely of clinical significance. In those rare cases where severe local symptoms exist, surgical resection is the most common treatment. When these are so large that surgical resection is not possible or in locations where surgery is not feasible, radiation therapy may be utilized. This appears to be most commonly in the head or spine. Radiation therapy is also utilized as a postoperative treatment for concern of margins or residual disease in larger resected lesions. Because of the rarity, the medical literature is confined to case reports and reviews. Consequently, strong or generalized recommendations are difficult. Radiation usually results in partial response or stability by radiological imaging. Typically, these responses are durable.

Malignant vascular tumors of bone (angiosarcoma) are quite rare. Typically radiation therapy may be recommended after surgical resection in localized disease. This is in an effort to achieve cure as well as local control. Local control can often be a serious clinical issue. Most of the treatment approaches are extrapolated from angiosarcoma of soft tissues. Typically these are aggressive cancers, both locally and systemically, and difficult to control, with poor outcomes.

CASES

Case 24.1 Cavernous hemangioma of bone

Clinical history and presentation

The patient is an eight year old girl who presents with a three month history of left hip, thigh, and knee pain with an intermittent limp. Symptoms increase with activity and decrease with rest.

Physical examination reveals no masses. She has mild tenderness on palpation over the left greater trochanter and mild pain in the left groin with internal rotation of the left hip.

Surgery is scheduled. Two days prior to surgery she sustains a fall and suffers a pathologic fracture through her femoral lesion.

Surgical findings and comments

Findings at surgery include a thinned and expanded cortical shell containing a multi-loculated cystic lesion. Curettage is performed along with allograft packing of the defect and internal fixation of the pathologic fracture.

Radiology findings

This is a predominantly cystic lesion with mild expansion of the proximal femur in an eight year old girl (**Case figs 24.1a** through **24.1e**). Fortunately, no aggressive feature such as cortical breakthrough or periosteal reaction is seen. There is minimal enhancement of the margins and the trabeculae without nodularity or focal mass. The differential might include a unicameral bone cyst or cavernous hemangioma.

For comparison, a second case of a vertebral hemangioma is also presented (**Case figs 24.1f** through **24.1h**).

Pathology findings

Gross features

The curettings comprise bony fragments mixed with blood clot aggregating to 3 × 2.3 × 0.9 cm. A small portion is submitted fresh

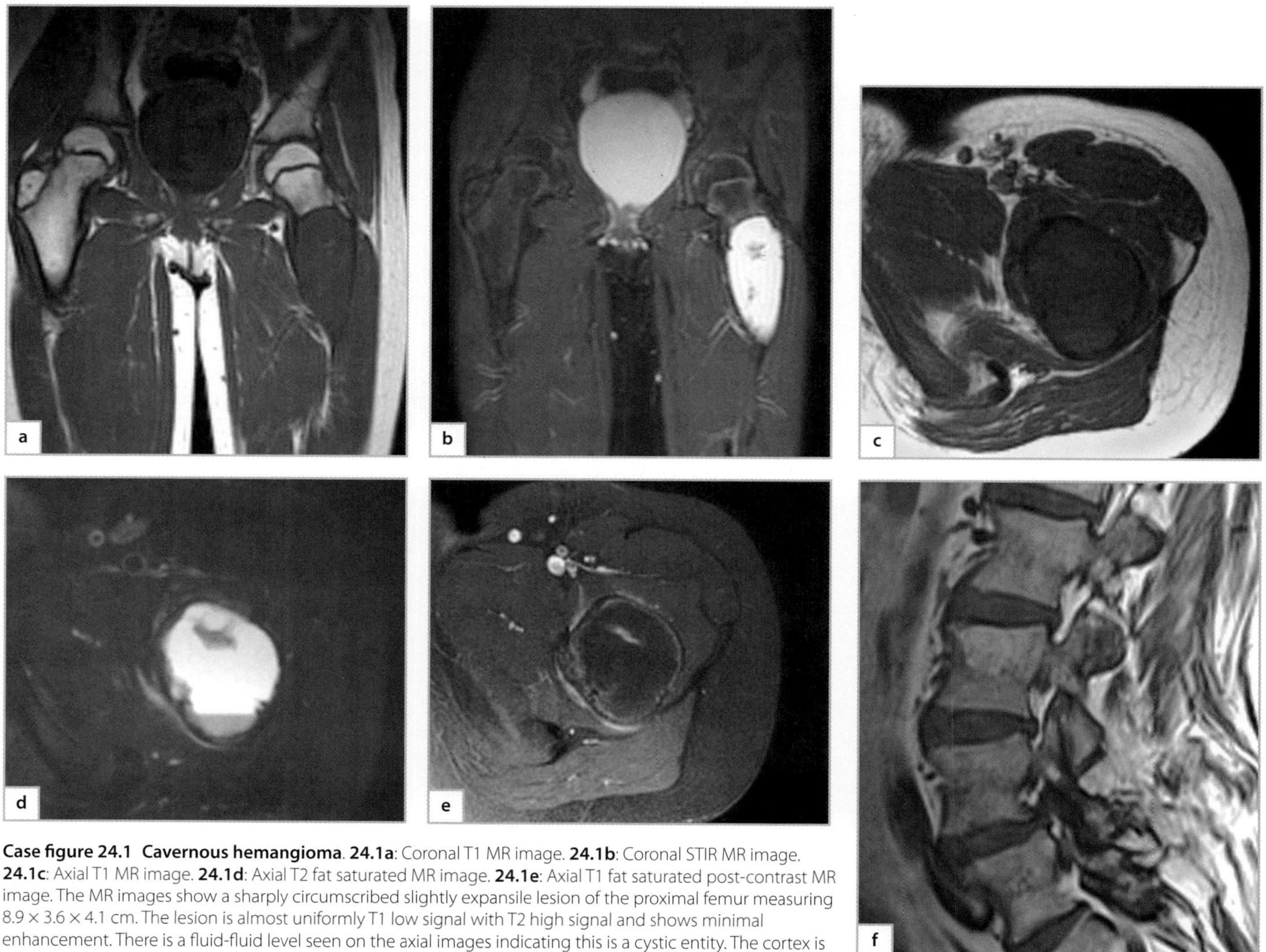

Case figure 24.1 Cavernous hemangioma. **24.1a**: Coronal T1 MR image. **24.1b**: Coronal STIR MR image. **24.1c**: Axial T1 MR image. **24.1d**: Axial T2 fat saturated MR image. **24.1e**: Axial T1 fat saturated post-contrast MR image. The MR images show a sharply circumscribed slightly expansile lesion of the proximal femur measuring 8.9 × 3.6 × 4.1 cm. The lesion is almost uniformly T1 low signal with T2 high signal and shows minimal enhancement. There is a fluid-fluid level seen on the axial images indicating this is a cystic entity. The cortex is preserved despite the mild expansion. No nodular component or soft tissue mass seen. *Additional case, Case fig. 24.1f through Case fig. 24.1h, of a vertebral body capillary hemangioma.* **24.1f**: Sagittal T1 MR image.

Case figure 24.1: Continued from page 526

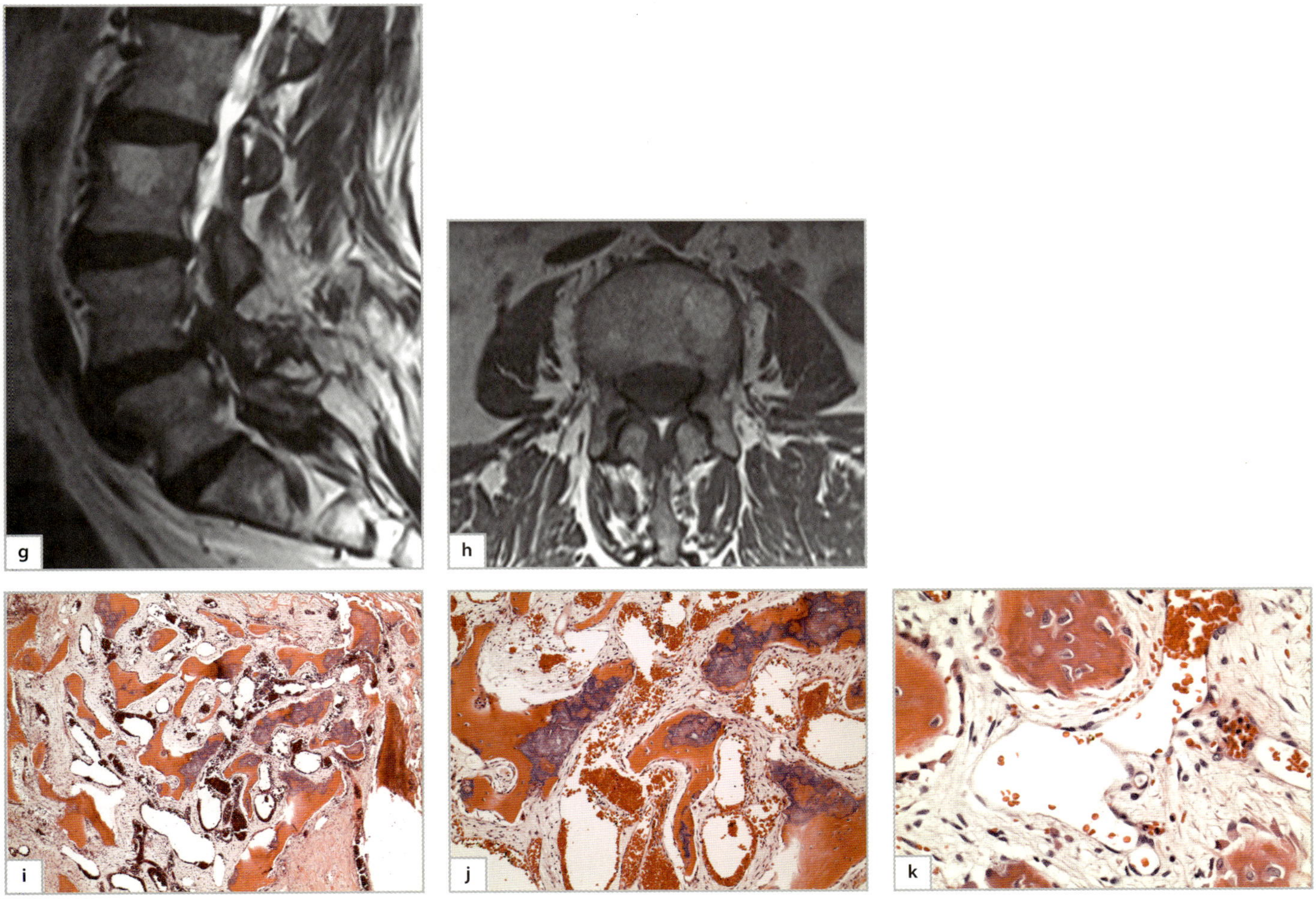

24.1g: Sagittal T2 MR image. **24.1h**: Axial T1 MR image. The MR images show a nearly uniform T1 and T2 high signal lesion of the L3 vertebral body. There is subtle stippled appearance likely from prominent trabeculae. There is no extra-osseous extension or encroachment of the foramina and spinal canal. **24.1i**: Low magnification. The lesion comprises thin-walled vessels embedded in a hypocellular spindle cell stroma. Thin layered, streams of reactive bone skirt the upper right corner of the photomicrograph consistent with the patient's history of recent fracture. **24.1j**: Medium magnification. Multiple thin-walled vascular channels of varying caliber intercolate between bone spicules. The bone trabeculae are thickened and irregular in shape, a common finding in hemangioma. Normal marrow fat and hematopoietic elements are absent. **24.1k**: High magnification. The abnormal vessels are lined by uniform, non-atypical endothelial cells without a discernable muscularis or adventitia. Such thin-walled vessels are characteristic of cavernous hemangioma.

to Cytogenetics. The remainder is processed for histology after decalcification.

Microscopic features

Low magnification: The lesion consists of numerous blood vessels embedded in a hypocellular, spindle cell stroma (**Case fig. 24.1i**). The dilated, thin-walled vessels of varying caliber intertwine among oddly shaped, sclerotic, trabecular bone spicules (**Case fig. 24.2j**).

High magnification: High magnification confirms that the dilated spaces are vessels. They are lined by well-formed endothelial cells and contain red blood cells (**Case fig. 24.2k**). Nuclear atypia is absent.

Special studies: Cytogenetics reveals a normal karyotype of 46,XX.

Pathologic differential or, why isn't it one of the following?

Vascular malformation: This may be a semantic argument only, as some hemangiomas of bone most likely represent vascular malformations or hamartomas. This especially pertains to cavernous hemangiomas which are composed of ectatic veins and do not differ histologically from known congenital vascular lesions of similar vessel caliber. Whether called a hemangioma, hamartoma, or malformation, there is no treatment difference when these lesions occur in the bone.

Lymphangioma: Another probable malformation but in this instance of lymphatic channels. Lymphangiomas usually exhibit extremely thin walls in many areas composed only of lining endothelium. Lymphoid aggregates may be prominent. A few vessels may exhibit a thin muscularis that is most commonly interrupted or incomplete. Lymphangiomas express D2-40 and may also react with antibodies to CD31 and CD34. Cavernous hemangiomas do not usually express D2-40. Veins generally have a more continuous smooth muscle layer (tunica media) and tunica adventitia, a band of collagen and elastic fibers. Numerous intraluminal red blood cells are helpful in distinguishing small, ectatic veins from lymphatic channels.

Oncology approach

Medical oncology

This is a benign lesion with no role for medical oncology.

Radiation oncology

In this case of a young child, a recurrence would not be life-threatening and surgical salvage is unlikely to be associated with significant morbidity or mortality. Radiation is associated with decreased bone growth, potential hip arthropathy, and possible future malignancy. Consequently, radiation therapy is not recommended.

Case table 24.1 Summary pathology findings of Case 24.1

Diagnosis	Hemangioma of bone, cavernous subtype
Size	7 × 4 × 4 cm
Location	Femur
Margin status	Positive
Histologic grade (FNCLCC grading system)	This is a benign tumor and therefore not graded
Pathologic stage (AJCC TNM classification)	This is a benign tumor and therefore not staged

FNCLCC: Fédération Nationale des Centres de Lutte Contre le Cancer (French Federation of Cancer Centers). AJCC: American Joint Committee on Cancer

Patient outcome

Nine months postoperatively, the patient is noted to have recurrence of the tumor. She is returned to the operating room for repeat curettage, allograft packing, and internal fixation.

Five years postoperatively, the patient has normal limb lengths and no evidence of recurrent tumor.

Case 24.2 Angiosarcoma of bone

Clinical history and presentation

This is an 84 year old woman who six years ago underwent a right total knee arthroplasty. She did very well postoperatively for about five years. About six months prior to presentation she developed pain in her right ankle which was treated conservatively. Since then, she has had progressively worsening pain in her right ankle as well as the right knee, in the area of the proximal tibia.

Physical examination of the right lower extremity reveals significant point tenderness to palpation about the distal tibia as well proximal tibia. She also has an area of point tenderness about mid fibula shaft. There is no palpable soft tissue mass.

Surgical findings and comments

Because of the need for diagnostic tissue and the concern for the possibility of a pathologic fracture through the proximal tibia lesion, the patient is taken to surgery where curettage of the proximal tibial lesion is performed. The defect is reconstructed with polymethylmethacrylate and pins to prevent pathologic fracture.

Radiology findings

Unfortunately, due to a fire at a storage facility, the plain films and other imaging studies were destroyed. However, the patient did present with multiple lytic lesions of the right tibia.

Malignant vascular tumors of bone include a range of tumors spanning from hemangioendothelioma at the low grade end, up through angiosarcoma at the high grade end of the spectrum. There is also the entity of epithelioid hemangioendothelioma. Together, these are relatively uncommon tumors amongst sarcomas and unfortunately, we do not have imaging of this case to present. These tumors all have a broad spectrum of distribution in the skeleton but mainly involve the femur, tibia and humerus. They also have broad range of age at presentation but tend to occur in adulthood. These vascular tumors of bone share a similar radiographic appearance with multiple lytic lesions (Wenger et al. 2000).

Angiosarcoma may be multicentric throughout the skeleton, whereas epithelioid hemangioendothelioma may be multicentric within one extremity or one region of the skeleton. Angiosarcoma will also show permeative destruction of bone with a soft tissue mass. The differential for multiple lytic lesions in an adult include metastatic disease, multiple myeloma and multicentric lymphoma. In pediatric patients, the differential would also include Langerhans cell histiocytosis and brown tumor, while metastatic disease and myeloma are unusual. It is difficult to distinguish amongst these without tissue diagnosis. Given the multicentric nature, skeletal survey is needed to assess disease burden and determine the easiest lesion for biopsy. This can be performed with radiographs or with bone scan. MRI is helpful to determine extent of soft tissue and marrow disease.

Pathology findings

Gross features

The curettage comprises small bits of bone and purple to red soft tissue aggregating to 2.8 cm maximally. A small portion is sent fresh to Cytogenetics, and touch preps are also made. The remainder is processed for histology.

Microscopic features

Low magnification: Low magnification reveals fragmented bone trabeculae mixed with blood clot and densely cellular areas.

High magnification: The densely cellular areas comprise sheets of large cells that are round to polygonal. There is no evidence of gland

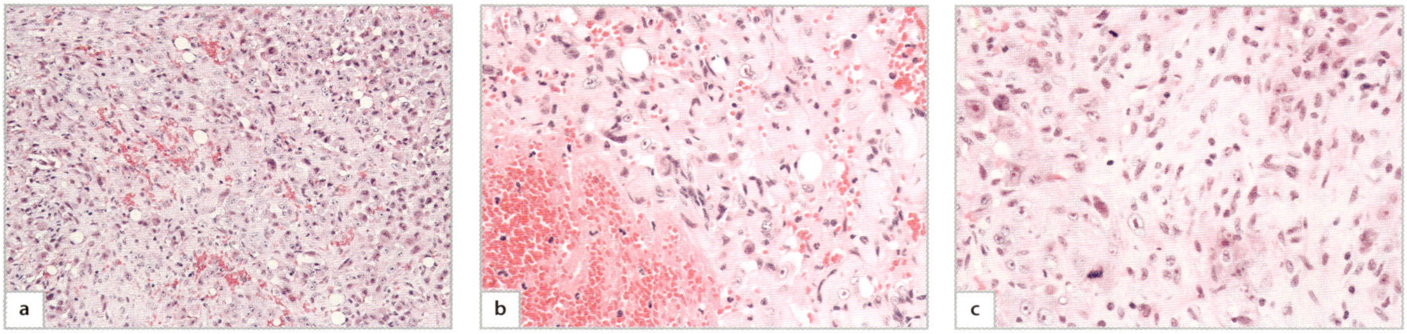

Case figure 24.2 Angiosarcoma of bone. **24.2a** Medium magnification. The tumor forms sheets of pleomorphic round to polygonal cells with foci of hemorrhage. Glands and tubules are absent. The round clear spaces comprise residual bone marrow fat cells. **24.2b**: High magnification. In this field, some tumor cells exhibit intracytoplasmic clear spaces. These are consistent with early attempts at vessel formation. **24.2c**: High magnification. The tumor is highly proliferative (three mitotic figures are present in this field). Tumor nuclei are pleomorphic with a range of size and shapes. Often, high grade angiosarcomas feature vesicular (cleared or pale) nuclei with prominent nucleoli as is the case here. Nucleoli may even by misshapen (most noticeable in Case fig. 24.2b).

or tubule formation (**Case fig. 24.2a**). Slit-like vascular channels lined by atypical cells are also absent. Hemorrhage is intermixed with tumor cells (**Case fig. 24.2b**). The cells contain abundant eosinophilic cytoplasm and variably shaped vesicular (pale) nuclei with prominent nucleoli. A few nucleoli are abnormally shaped. These nuclear features are high grade. Mitotic activity is brisk and estimated at greater than 25 mitoses/10 high magnification microscopic fields (**Case fig. 24.2c**). Small foci of necrosis are present.

Special studies: Because the tumor cells are epithelioid and because the patient is elderly with multiple lesions, a number of tumors must be excluded from the differential including metastatic tumors. Thus, several antibodies are used. Tumor cells are strongly positive for CD31 in a membranous pattern of reactivity. Rare tumor cells are reactive for CD34. Tumor cells diffusely express simple keratins (CAM5.2) without reactivity for keratins 7 or 20. Tumor cells are negative for S-100 protein, MelanA-103, CD45, and CD79a.

The patient's karyotype is aneuploid: 45-47,X,-X,add(1)(q21),add(3)(p21),add(7)(p22),-9,-9,add(10)(p13),+11,-16,-17,add(19)(q13.1),-21,-22,+4-7mar[cp11]/46,XX[9]. This is consistent with a high grade sarcoma such as angiosarcoma. There are only a few reports describing the karyotypes of angiosarcomas. However, this patient's karyotype does not contain any of the changes found with increased frequency in soft tissue angiosarcoma (Guillou et al. 2010).

Pathologic differential or, why isn't it one of the following?

Cellular hemangioma: Hemangioma can certainly involve multiple bones or locations within one bone. It is most common in the vertebral column and skull. The marked nuclear atypia and necrosis of this specimen would not be seen in hemangioma. Many hemangiomas are mitotically active, but usually the number is less than 5/10 high magnification microscopic fields.

Epithelioid hemangioendothelioma (EHE): The degree of atypia exceeds that of classic EHE, although not the 'malignant' or 'high grade' variant (which some experts suggest should just be termed angiosarcoma). The characteristic myxochondroid or hyaline matrix of EHE is absent. Some angiosarcomas contain tumor vessels lined by hobnailed malignant endothelial cells. Such vessels are absent to very sparse in EHE. Unfortunately, this patient's tumor consists only of sheets of tumor cells. Intracytoplasmic lumen formation is common to both EHE and angiosarcoma. Both EHE and angiosarcoma express CD31, CD34, ERG (C-terminus directed), FLI-1 and simple keratins, so immunohistochemistry is not diagnostically useful. Many EHE of soft tissue show a t(1;3) WWTR1/CAMTA1 rearrangement. Presumably, a similar large proportion of bone EHE would also contain this translocation which is absent in angiosarcoma.

Metastatic carcinoma: There is no evidence of gland or tubule formation. However, these may not develop in high grade carcinomas or may not be sampled in a small curettage specimen. Cytoplasmic vacuoles can be present in both angiosarcoma (early vessel lumen formation) or carcinoma (may have contained lipid or glycogen or may be a degenerative change). Most carcinomas have more extensive epithelial marker expression than just CAM5.2, and very few are CD31 reactive (especially in a membranous pattern of reactivity). The patient has no history of carcinoma, and a workup reveals no other tumors elsewhere.

Metastatic melanoma: Melanoma can commonly exhibit an epithelioid cytomorphology. Cytoplasmic vacuolation can be seen. The discohesion and lack of tubule or gland formation in this specimen would also be seen in melanoma. However, there is no expression of markers used to identify melanoma, and rarely does melanoma express CD31.

High grade lymphoma: This is an unusual morphology for lymphoma: epithelioid. However, rare high grade lymphomas may show this appearance. There is no reactivity for lymphoma markers, and keratin expression would also be very unusual for lymphoma.

Case table 24.2 Summary pathology findings of Case 24.2

Diagnosis	Angiosarcoma of bone
Size	Three discontinuous (skip) lesions, 2.5, 3 and 4.5 cm
Location	Tibia, right: proximal, mid-shaft, and distal lesions
Margin status	Biopsy only
Histologic grade (FNCLCC grading system)	High grade (Grade 3)
Pathologic stage (AJCC TNM classification)	III = T3/N0/M0

FNCLCC: Fédération Nationale des Centres de Lutte Contre le Cancer (French Federation of Cancer Centers). AJCC: American Joint Committee on Cancer

Osteosarcoma: The rare epithelioid variant of osteosarcoma easily could match the patient's histopathology. However, tumor bone or malignant osteoid is absent and required for a diagnosis of osteosarcoma. CD31 would not be expected to be expressed in osteosarcoma. Epithelioid OS can express simple keratins, however. The complex karyotype in this patient could also be similar to one found in osteosarcoma.

Oncology approach

Medical oncology

Because this lesion is a high grade angiosarcoma of the bone, chance for long term survival is limited with local treatment only. Most angiosarcomas recur within 1 year of diagnosis, usually with lung, bone, and liver metastases. Thus the clinical question in this case is whether adjuvant chemotherapy with an antiangiogenic agent is appropriate (See Chapter on vascular tumors for chemotherapy discussion). The decision should be made individually, depending on the patient presentation and current state of health. In this case, the lesion remained localized for at least 6 months, which might bear a better prognosis. The local surgical treatment was definitively appropriate. The need for systemic therapy is not established. Specifically, this patient was lost to follow-up and a discussion of adjuvant treatment did not take place.

Radiation oncology

If the patient had a localized angiosarcoma, post-operative radiation therapy would be recommended. However, this patient has multiple lytic lesions. If the patient had evidence of distant metastases, I would recommend radiation for palliative purposes only. This of course would be contingent on her having a good performance status.

Patient outcome

The patient failed to return for follow-up postoperatively. Unfortunately, the patient is likely to do poorly given her T3 disease and high grade features (including macronucleoli and mitotic rate >3 mitoses/10 hpf) (Verbeke et al. 2011).

REFERENCES

Appelbaum FR. Introduction and overview of interferon alfa in myeloproliferative and hemangiomatous diseases. Semin Hematol 1990;27:1–5.

Deyrup AT, Montag AG. Epithelioid and epithelial neoplasms of bone. Arch Pathol Lab Med 2007;131:205–216.

Evans HL, Raymond AK, Ayala AG. Vascular tumors of bone: a study of 17 cases other than ordinary hemangioma, with an evaluation of the relationship of hemangioendothelioma of bone to epithelioid hemangioma, epithelioid hemangioendothelioma, and high-grade angiosarcoma. Hum Pathol 2003;34:680–689.

Ma J, Shi Q-L, Jiang S-J, et al. Primary kaposiform hemangioendothelioma of a long bone: two cases in unusual locations with long-term follow-up. Pathol Int 2011;61:382–386.

McCarthy EF, Lietman S, Argani P, et al. Endovascular papillary angioendothelioma (Dabska tumor) of bone. Skeletal Radiol 1999;28:100–103.

McMenamin DS, Stuckey SL, Potgieter GJ. T1 hyperintense vertebral column melanoma metastases. Am J Neuroradiol 2007;28:1817–1818.

O'Connell JX, Nielsen GP, Rosenberg AE. Epithelioid vascular tumors of bone: a review and proposal of a classification scheme. Adv Anat Pathol 2001;8:74–82.

Premkumar A, Marincola F, Taubenberger J, et al. Metastatic melanoma: correlation of MRI characteristics and histopathology. J Magn Reson Imaging 1996;6(1):190–194.

Takahashi A, Ogawa C, Kanazawa T, et al. Remission induced by interferon alfa in a patient with massive osteolysis and extension of lymph-hemangiomatosis: a severe case of Gorham-Stout syndrome. J Pediatr Surg 2005;40:E47–50.

Verbeke SLJ, Bertoni F, Bacchini P, et al. Distinct histological features characterize primary angiosarcoma of bone. Histopathol 2011;58:254–264.

Verbeke SLK, Bovée JVM. Primary vascular tumors of bone: a spectrum of entities? Int J Exp Pathol 2011;4:541–551.

Wenger DE, Wold LE. Malignant vascular lesions of bone: radiologic and pathologic features. Skeletal Radiol 2000;29:619–631.

Zhang HZ, Jiang ZM, Zhou J, et al. [Primary intermediate hemangioendothelioma of bone: a study of five cases.] Zhonghua Bing Li Xue Za Zhi 2012;41:39–43.

FURTHER READING

Dorfman HD, Czerniak B. Bone Tumors. St Louis: Mosby, 1998.

Folpe AL, Inwards CY (eds). Bone and Soft Tissue Pathology. A volume in the series: Foundations in Diagnostic Pathology. Goldblum JR (series ed). Philadelphia: Elsevier Saunders, 2010.

Acosta FL, Sanai N, Chi JH, et al. Comprehensive management of symptomatic and aggressive vertebral hemangiomas. Neurosurg Clin N Am 2008;19(1):17–29.

Fox MW, Onofrio BM. The natural history and management of symptomatic and asymptomatic vertebral hemangiomas. J Neurosurg 1993;78(1):36–45.

Fletcher CDM, Krishnan Unni K, Mertens F (Eds). World Health Organization Classification of Tumours. Pathology and Genetics of Tumours of Soft Tissue and Bone. Lyon: IARC Press, 2013.

Chapter 25 Uncommon primary bone tumors

OVERVIEW

This chapter is more an amalgam of disparate entities than a rational grouping based on tumor relatedness. The list primarily includes tumors that normally occur with much greater frequency in the soft tissues but which can rarely arise in the bone. These comprise myogenic, myofibroblastic, neural and lipogenic tumors, among others.

Two other tumors are also featured: phosphaturic mesenchymal tumor, a rare neoplasm that affects with equal frequency bone and soft tissue and which has recently been well characterized. The final tumor is adamantinoma, another unusual tumor with a marked propensity for the tibia but which histologically resembles ameloblastoma of the gnathic bones (the old name for which was adamantinoma).

Virtually any primary soft tissue sarcoma has also been reported to occur as a primary intraosseous tumor. For most sarcomas, bone origin is unusual to extraordinary. However, when faced with a histologically unusual, malignant bone tumor that does not appear to be osteosarcoma, chondrosarcoma or Ewing sarcoma (basically any of the more expected primary bone sarcomas), it is worth considering exotics when mundane possibilities are carefully excluded. A favored site of metastasis for soft tissue sarcomas is the bone; therefore, when dealing with a sarcoma that otherwise typically arises in soft tissue, it is imperative to exclude distant spread from a soft tissue-situated sarcoma before diagnosing it as a rare primary intraosseous example.

Specific sarcoma diagnoses can be achieved even when these tumors develop de novo in bone. However, because diagnosis of some tumors relies heavily on immunohistochemistry, it is important to optimize antigenicity in bone abiding tumors. This entails sectioning tumors fresh and, whenever possible, collecting a sample that will not require decalcification, because the acidic process of softening the tumor for Histology also can alter or destroy antigens and thus change the protein expression profile of a tumor. This can cause confusing results. If decalcification cannot be avoided for all the blocks of tumor, fixation should also occur simultaneously. Paying strict attention to positive internal normal tissue controls is essential to confirm preservation of antigenicity in decalcified sections.

CLASSIFICATION

The classification of the tumors that primarily occur as soft tissue neoplasms is covered in other chapters. For example, the classification of myogenic tumors is detailed in Chapter 8.

DEMOGRAPHICS

Most of the tumors in this chapter are rare when they arise in bone even though the same tumor may be relatively common in a primary soft tissue site, or rare even when bone is a common origin (as with phosphaturic mesenchymal tumor) or rare when bone is the only origin (adamantinoma of long bones). In fact, the title of the chapter overstates the incidence of these tumors. However, it is important to be aware of them, as appropriate treatment depends on accurate diagnosis.

Table 25.2 lists rare primary bone sarcomas registered with the Surveillance Epidemiology and End Results (SEER) program from 1994 through 2008. Some tumors are not specifically diagnosed being labeled only descriptively such as 'spindle cell sarcoma' or 'sarcoma'. The age ranges of affected patients are broad but match the range of ages when these tumors arise in soft tissues. For example, rhabdomyosarcomas occur most commonly in children whether developing in bone or soft tissue.

The SEER database was also examined for adamantinoma of the long bones (ICDO-3 = 9261). The average annual incidence rate is 0.1 per million, and the ages of diagnosis for these tumors range from 4 to 75 years, with a mean of 31.5 years, as shown in **Figure 25.1**. Of the 33

Table 25.1 World Health Organization (WHO) classification of uncommon primary bone tumors (2013)

Tumor	Behavior	Additional comments
Myogenic tumors		
Smooth muscle tumors	Benign	Please see Chapter 8 for classification of smooth muscle tumors
	Malignant	
Myofibroblastic tumors	Benign	Please see Chapter 6 for classification of myofibroblastic tumors
	Malignant	
Lipogenic tumors	Benign	Please see Chapter 5 for classification of lipogenic tumors
	Malignant	
Neural tumors	Benign	Please see Chapter 13 for classification of neural tumors
	Malignant	
Phosphaturic mesenchymal tumor – mixed connective tissue type	Benign	Relatively few cases studied. Thus far, malignant cases seem to be histologically distinguishable from benign cases
	Malignant	
Adamantinoma	Low grade malignant	Differentiated variant has very low risk for malignant behavior

Benign: does not recur and does not metastasize. Intermediate: can recur but does not metastasize. Malignant: can recur and can metastasize.

Table 25.2 Selected uncommon primary bone tumors from 13 SEER registries, 1994–2008

Histology group	ICD-O-3 code	Histologic type	Total number	Male to female ratio	Age at diagnosis (years)		
					Mean	Median	Range
Sarcomas categorized descriptively only (no specific diagnosis) and sarcoma, NOS	8800	Sarcoma, NOS	78	35:43	61.7	66.5	4-104
	8801	Spindle cell sarcoma	37	21:16	54.4	51.0	16-95
	8804	Epithelioid sarcoma	10	4:1	36.8	35.5	13-75
	8805	Undifferentiated sarcoma	11	8:3	37.2	43.0	2-77
Fibromatous and myofibroblastic neoplasms	8810	Fibrosarcoma, NOS	30	4:11	47.5	45.0	0-92
	8811	Low grade fibromyxoid sarcoma	4	3:1	55.5	63.5	29-66
	8815	Solitary fibrous tumor, malignant	2	0:1	60.5	60.5	53-68
	8830	'Malignant fibrous histiocytoma' – currently most cases are considered high grade pleomorphic undifferentiated sarcoma	82	43:39	58.2	60.0	15-95
Lipomatous neoplasms	8851	Liposarcoma, well differentiated	2	0:1	57.0	57.0	46-68
	8852	Myxoid liposarcoma	3	1:2	67.3	83.0	32-87
Myomatous neoplasms	8890	Leiomyosarcoma, NOS	27	8:19	50.9	51.0	8-96
	8900	Rhabdomyosarcoma	2	1:1	24.0	24.0	5-43
	8910	Embryonal rhabdomyosarcoma, NOS	6	5:1	8.2	4.0	0-34
	8920	Alveolar rhabdomyosarcoma	3	2:1	10.7	11.0	7-14
Synovial sarcoma	9040	Synovial sarcoma, NOS	5	3:2	37.6	43.0	14-55
	9041	Synovial sarcoma, spindle cell	4	1:0	49.8	51.0	38-59
	9043	Synovial sarcoma, biphasic	4	3:1	35.3	36.0	22-47
Nerve sheath tumors	9540	Malignant peripheral nerve sheath tumor	7	3:4	58.6	52.0	35-92

SEER data were evaluated from 13 registries during a 15 year period (1994-2008). Six histology groups and 18 histologic types were selected for review, all of which occur in the bone as a primary site. As seen in Table 25.2, gender differences and ages at diagnosis for these tumors vary widely by sub-type.

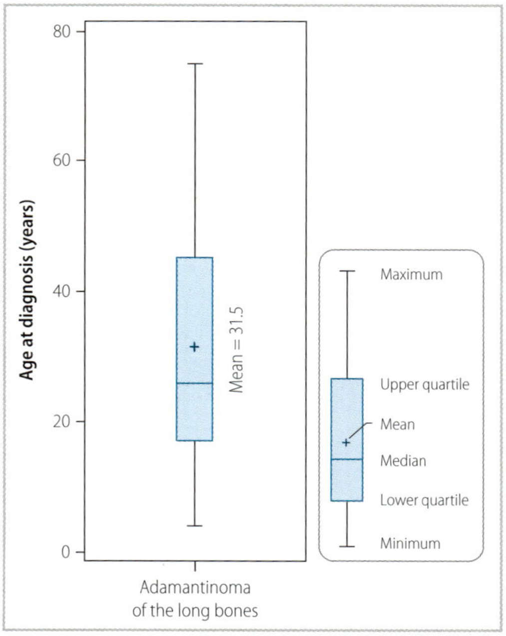

Figure 25.1 Age distribution of adamantinomas of the long bone among cases in 13 SEER registries during the time period 1994-2008 (n=33).

cases diagnosed in this time period (1994-2008) 19 cases were male (57.6%) and 14 cases were female (42.2%). These numbers illustrate the rarity of this tumor.

PATHOGENESIS/ETIOLOGY

Presumably, many of the same factors leading to the development of sarcomas in soft tissue apply to those arising in the bone. The pathogenesis often involves genetic or epigenetic abnormal events that may occur in the setting of increasing age and certain exposures. For example, radiation can induce intraosseous sarcoma development, and the radiation may be iatrogenic. Sarcomas arising in radiated fields may include undifferentiated high grade pleomorphic sarcoma (old name pleomorphic-storiform malignant fibrous histiocytoma) and specific soft tissue type sarcomas such as leiomyosarcoma.

A unique predisposing factor to the development of primary bone sarcoma consists of long-in-place orthopaedic hardware. Given the huge number of metal implants placed annually, the phenomenon, though real, is noticeably rare. The most common tumor reported is osteosarcoma, but undifferentiated high grade pleomorphic sarcoma is a close second (Keel et al. 2001) and specific tumors including malignant peripheral nerve sheath tumor have been reported. See the

Case presentations section of this chapter for a case of leiomyosarcoma associated with a metal implant.

PATHOLOGY

Please refer to the specific chapters on muscle (Chapter 8), myofibroblastic (Chapter 6), neural (Chapter 13) and lipogenic (Chapter 5) tumors for tables providing representative images and descriptions of those tumors.

Adamantinoma and phosphaturic mesenchymal tumor-mixed connective tissue variant are detailed in **Table 25.4** and **Table 25.5**.

Histologic grading

Smooth muscle tumors

Refer to Chapter 8 for histologic descriptions and grading of myogenic tumors. Primary osseous leiomyoma is case reportable and in fact, less than 10 cases are to be found in the recent medical literature. Primary osseous leiomyosarcoma is marginally more common with approximately 107 cases reported to date (Adelani et al. 2009). Most are histologically high grade with conventional morphology of long sweeping fascicles of spindled cells with scattered markedly pleomorphic tumor cells and moderate nuclear pleomorphism in the spindled nuclei. However, other histologic variants may also occur de novo in bone including pleomorphic LMS, areas of epithelioid LMS, and LMS with large numbers of osteoclast-like giant cells (Antonescu et al. 1997, Rekhi et al. 2011).

Myofibroblastic tumors

Refer to Chapter 6 for histologic descriptions and grading of myofibroblastic tumors. As of 2010, there are nine cases of low grade myofibroblastic sarcoma reported in the English medical literature. Most occur in the femur or iliac bone. Histologically, the tumors are identical to their soft tissue counterparts consisting of short fascicles and cartwheels of spindled cells with pale eosinophilic cytoplasm and elongate tapered nuclei. Unlike LMS of bone, the tumors show more fibrosis or collagen deposition, and those reported to date are negative for desmin expression and reactive for SMA (Arora et al. 2010). Distinguishing between LMS and myofibroblastic sarcoma can be challenging, and some authors suggest that ultrastructural examination may sometimes be necessary to do so. Few clinical pathology laboratories retain this ability to perform electron microscopic analysis, and the diagnosis rests on morphology and immunohistochemistry which unfortunately are not always perfect discriminators in this diagnostic setting.

Lipogenic tumors

Refer to Chapter 5 for histologic descriptions and grading of lipogenic tumors. Intraosseous lipomas are more common than primary intraosseous liposarcoma. As of 2004, there were ~175 cases of primary bone lipoma reported in the medical literature. The tumors match the histology of soft tissue lipoma but also often contain fat necrosis with fibrosis and calcifications (Campbell et al. 2003, Radl et al. 2004).

Table 25.3 Genetics of uncommon primary bone tumors (see Chapters 5, 6, 8, and 13 for details of genetics of adipose tumors, myofibroblastic tumors, smooth muscle tumors, and neural tumors, respectively)

Tumor	Chromosomal abnormality	Genes involved	Percentage of tumors with abnormality
Phosphaturic mesenchymal tumor-MCT	Limited information thus far: three cases (including the case in this chapter) show variable gains and losses of whole or partial chromosomes and/or translocations	FGF-23 gene (12p13) is expressed	90% of TIO positive patients show expression of *FGF-23* by rtPCR and 75% of cases not associated with TIO
Adamantinoma	No consistent single specific finding. One or more extra copies of chromosomes 7,8,12,19, 21 most commonly often with additional translocations, inversions and marker chromosomes	Unknown	Majority have extra chromosome copies, especially of 19. Cytogenetic findings are the same for classic and differentiated adamantinoma
TIO = Tumor-induced osteomalacia See References for papers pertaining to this table. This static list of genetic abnormalities must be viewed in the context of continuing discovery and refinement of genetic findings.			

Table 25.4 Predominantly pediatric uncommon bone tumors grouped by behavior

Tumor	Incidence	Age and sex distribution	Body site (in order of occurrence)	Histopathology description including IHC	
				Medium magnification	High magnification
Benign: does not recur and does not metastasize					
Adamantinoma, differentiated variant	Rare to extremely rare	Most patients < 20 years M = F	Tibia diaphysis >>> fibula>>rarely other bones Tibia and fibula may be synchronously involved	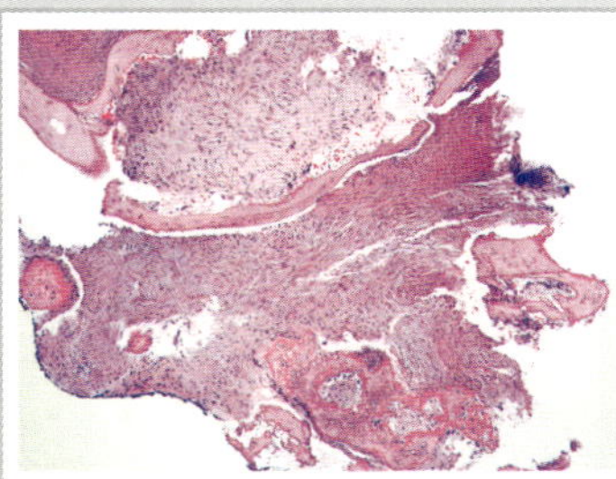	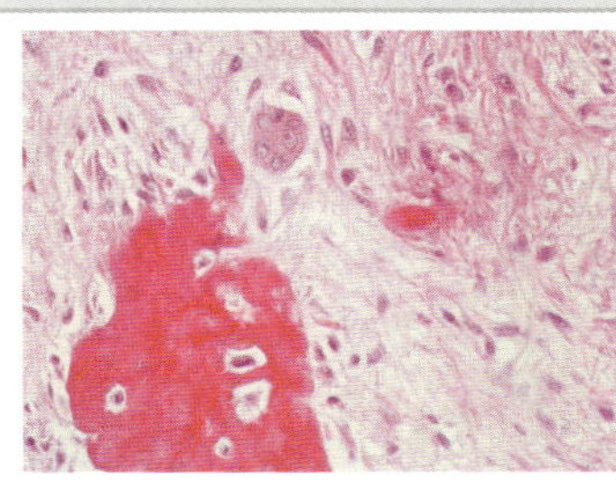
Most exhibit a zonal pattern of peripheral fused trabecular bone with more central area of irregularly shaped bone trabeculae prominently rimmed by osteoblasts set in a fibrous stroma. Subtle strands and clusters of epithelial cells are present on H&E stains mostly centrally. IHC for keratin (keratins AE1/AE3, 14 and 19 especially with minimal expression of 8 and 18) highlights the sparse epithelial component. Rare tumors can recur and may transform to classic adamantinoma.					
Incidence note: Rare to extremely rare: a medium sized practice will see zero to one patient with the lesion every 20 years.					

Table 25.5 Predominantly adult uncommon bone tumors grouped by behavior

Tumor	Incidence	Age and sex distribution	Body site (in order of occurrence)	Histopathology description including IHC: Medium magnification	Histopathology description including IHC: High magnification
Malignant: can recur and can metastasize					
Adamantinoma classic variant	Rare to extremely rare	Most patients > 20 years M = F	Tibia diaphysis >>> fibula>>rarely other bones (ulna, humerus, femur, tarsals, etc) Tibia and fibula may be synchronously involved in 10-15% of cases	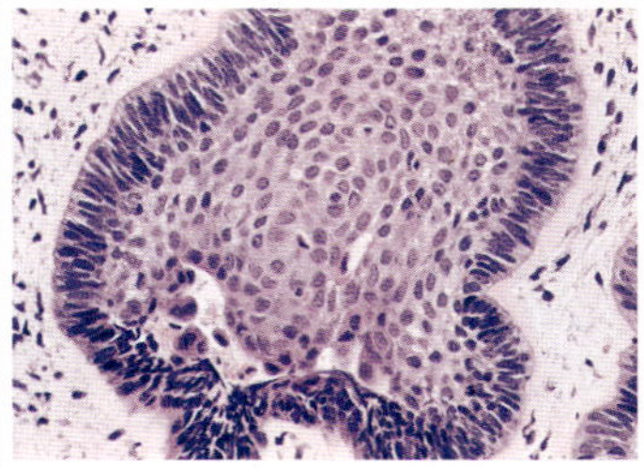	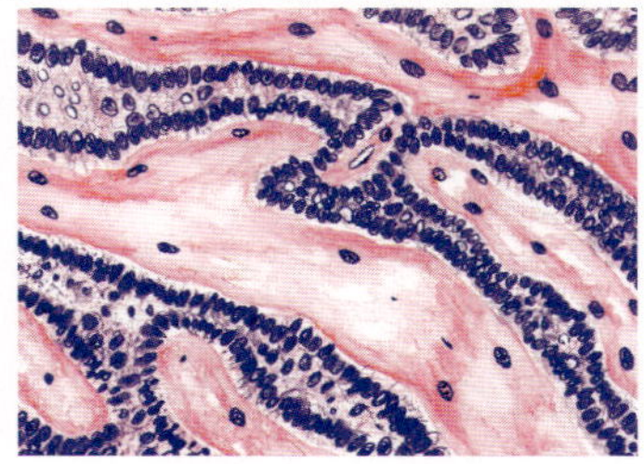
				All tumors have a fibroosseous stroma similar to differentiated adamantinoma. However, unlike in differentiated adamantinoma, the epithelial component is prominent. The epithelial patterns listed below are often found mixed in one tumor. All epithelial areas and some spindle cells are positive for keratins, EMA, p63, and D2-40. Basaloid epithelial pattern: nests of cells with ovoid nuclei and peripheral palisading like BCC of skin; nest centers are often cystic (medical illustration at top right).	
				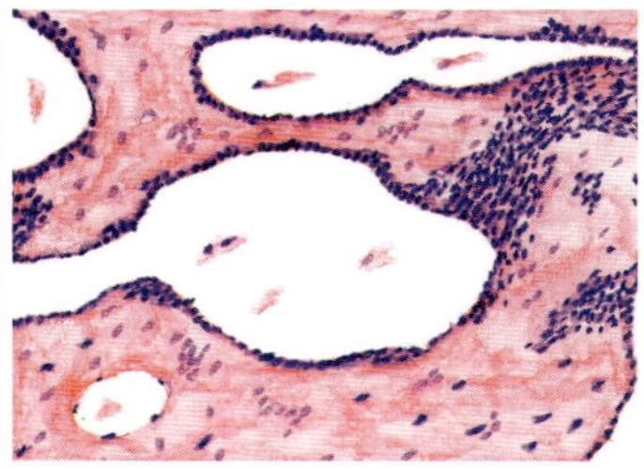	
				Pseudovascular or tubular epithelial pattern: round or cylindrical spaces lined by flat or cuboidal cells simulate glands or vessels.	
				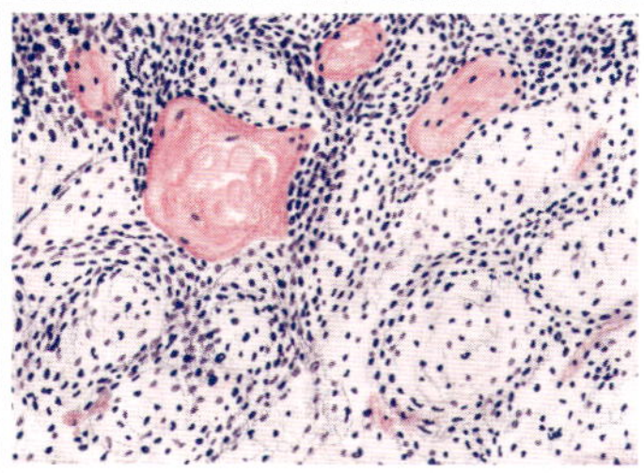	
				Squamoid epithelial pattern: nests of cells some of which exhibit keratinization including eosinophilic, glassy cytoplasm and pyknotic nuclei.	
				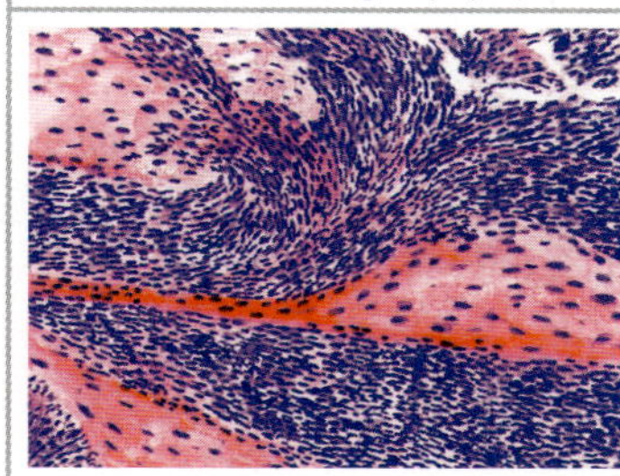	
				Spindled epithelial pattern: Tight streams and whorls of elongate spindle cells that are strongly epithelial marker positive. These nests usually are well defined and stand out from the osteofibrous stromal background.	

Table 25.5: Continued from page 534

Tumor	Incidence	Age and sex distribution	Body site (in order of occurrence)	Histopathology description including IHC	
				Medium magnification	High magnification
Intermediate: can recur but does not metastasize					
Phosphaturic mesenchymal tumor	Rare to extremely rare	Median age ~50 years but broad range of 9-80 years. M = F	50% located in bone: any site in axial or appendicular skeleton; small lesions can produce rickets 50% located in soft tissue: most commonly extremities including hands and feet	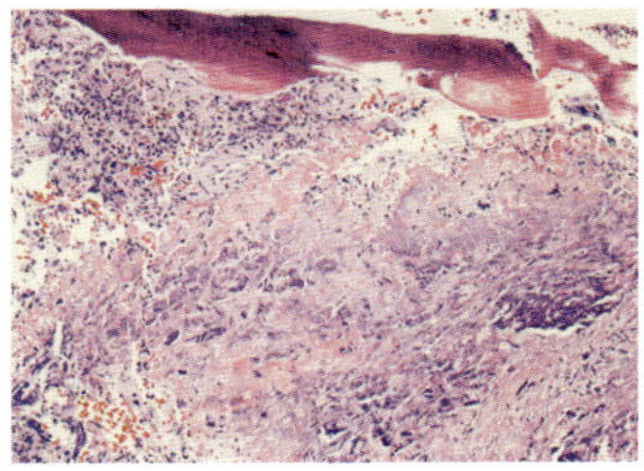	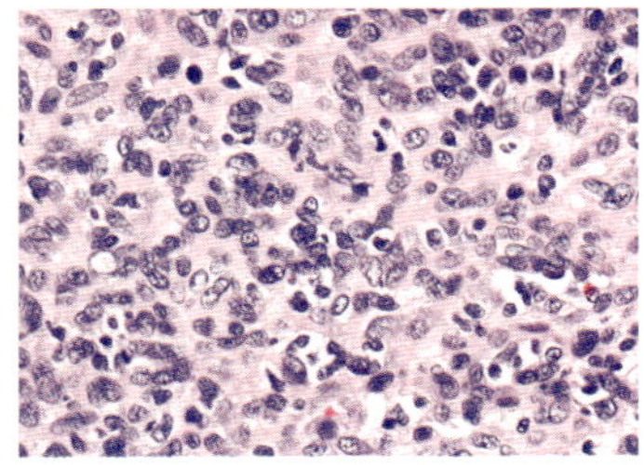
Irregularly heterogeneous tumor composed of flocculent 'grungy' or blotchy calcifications, mixed with bland spindle cells or ovoid cells, osteochondroid matrix, and hemorrhage. Myxoid stroma, microcysts and adipose tissue may also be present. Rare tumors are histologically malignant with increased celluarity, cellular pleomorphism and mitotic activity.These can metastasize. Most tumors express FGF-23. Focal staining for SMA and EMA also reported.					
Incidence note. Rare to extremely rare: a medium sized orthopaedic oncology practice will see zero to one patient with the lesion every 20 years.					

Neural tumors

Refer to Chapter 13 for histologic descriptions and grading of neural tumors. Primary benign intraosseous neural tumors include schwannoma and neurofibroma (and there is one case report of intraosseous perineurioma). Malignant peripheral nerve sheath tumor primary to the bone has also been reported. Benign and malignant types are quite rare as primary bone tumors with only scattered case reports in the literature. The histologic features are identical to their soft tissue counterparts.

Adamantinoma

Both the differentiated and classic variants of adamantinoma are histologically low grade tumors. However, in extremely rare instances, classic adamantinoma dedifferentiates to a high grade sarcoma. These tumors usually are recognized because areas of classic adamantinoma are retained. The high grade areas comprise large epithelioid or epithelioid and spindle cells with a high mitotic rate. Malignant chondroid and osteoid may be present. In three of four reported cases, the high grade areas as well as low grade areas expressed keratins (Izquierdo et al. 2010, Hazelbag et al. 2003).

Phosphaturic mesenchymal tumor-mixed connective tissue variant

Most of these tumors are morphologically low grade. However, a subset exhibit increased cellularity coupled with increased mitotic figures (>5/10 hpf) and cellular atypia.

Behavior

Smooth muscle tumors

Intraosseous leiomyoma may cause pathologic fracture but otherwise is benign. Primary leiomyosarcoma of bone demonstrates a five year overall survival similar to conventional intramedullary osteosarcoma (59%) with lower grade, lower stage patients faring better (Adelani et al. 2009).

Myofibroblastic tumors

Six of eight reported patients with myofibroblastic sarcoma of bone have had long term survival with no evidence of disease at 2-16 years post-surgery (Arora et al. 2010). Thus, the tumor appears to have an excellent prognosis. However, long-term follow-up is warranted, as soft tissue myofibroblastic tumors can recur and metastasize decades after initial presentation.

Lipogenic tumors

Intraosseous lipoma is most often asymptomatic but can cause pain and pathologic fracture. Too few intraosseous liposarcomas have been reported to reliably predict behavior.

Neural tumors

Intraosseous schwannoma and neurofibroma can cause pain, weakness (when located in the spine) or pathologic fracture. Primary bone origin is rare but reported most frequently in the mandible, spine including sacrum, and tibia. Primary malignant peripheral nerve sheath tumor is also vanishingly rare, and the most common site is mandible, also. Too few cases have been reported to reliably predict behavior.

Adamantinoma

After wide local excision, the local recurrence rate for classic adamantinoma is ~20%, the mortality rate is ~13%, and >25% may metastasize, most commonly to the lungs with lymph node involvement also possible (Deyrup et al. 2007, Szendroi et al. 2008). Recurrences and metastases of classic adamantinoma may be found many years after initial surgery, so long term follow-up is required. Metastases may consist of spindle cell or epithelial elements (Deyrup et al. 2007). Factors which may be associated with a more aggressive course in patients with classic adamantinoma include: male sex, age less than 20 years, short duration of symptoms, pain, lack of squamous component, and local recurrence (Camp et al. 2008, Jain et al. 2008).

The less common differentiated adamantinoma (osteofibrous dysplasia-like adamantinoma) exhibits a more indolent behavior akin to osteofibrous dysplasia, and very few progress to metastasis (Folpe et al. 2010). Metastatic potential is acquired when the tumor recurs as classic adamantinoma. In the absence of an extensive or deforming lesion, treatment of these patients may reasonably be conservative with careful, close, radiologic follow-up (Gleason et al. 2008)

The extremely rare dedifferentiated adamantinoma behaves like a high grade sarcoma (Izquierdo et al. 2010).

Phosphaturic mesenchymal tumor-mixed connective tissue variant

Most tumors behave in a benign fashion, and excision results in dramatic improvement of osteomalacia. A few histologically benign tumors may locally recur, sometimes many years after initial treatment. Rare, histologically malignant cases often locally recur and may metastasize and cause death (Folpe et al. 2004). As with many sarcomas, the lungs are the favored metastatic site.

Additional laboratory testing

Immunohistochemistry

Smooth muscle tumors: In general, 90% of smooth muscle tumors are reactive for smooth muscle actin or muscle specific actin and 70-80% are also reactive for desmin. Calponin is also reactive in many cases. Caldesmon is a more specific marker of smooth muscle differentiated cells and is expressed in approximately 70% of tumors overall.

Myofibroblastic tumors: Myofibroblastic tumors overlap smooth muscle differentiated tumors in immunoexpression. At least 90% express SMA or MSA, but only a small percentage express desmin (~5-10%). Caldesmon is infrequently expressed in myofibroblastic tumors (~5%) and if present is usually focal or weak.

Lipogenic tumors: S-100 protein is expressed in more differentiated lipogenic tumors. It may be focal or absent in high grade liposarcomas. CDK and MDM2 are usually expressed in the nuclei of well-differentiated liposarcomas.

Neural tumors: Schwannomas are diffusely reactive for S-100 protein, while neurofibromas also demonstrate extensive positivity within a tumor. Expression is nuclear as well as cytoplasmic. MPNST characteristically exhibits only focal reactivity for S-100 protein and may be reactive for neurofilaments and/or GFAP. Cytogenetic or molecular testing may be required to differentiate MPNST from synovial sarcoma, however, as the latter may also express all the antigens seen in MPNST.

Adamantinoma: Both classic and differentiated adamantinoma must show reactivity for keratins in the epithelial component. The positive keratins include 4,19 and AE1/AE3, among others with diminished expression for keratins 8 and 18. Some of the spindle stromal cells will also react for these epithelial markers indicating a close relationship of the spindle cell stroma to the epithelial component (transitional fibro-epithelial cells with features of fibroblasts and epithelial cells are also identified on ultrastructural examination) (Gleason et al. 2008). Other antibodies that are often reactive in the epithelium and some stromal spindle cells include p63, EMA, and D2-40 (Kashima et al. 2011, Dickson et al. 2011). Osteofibrous dysplasia also contains rare dispersed spindle stromal cells that react for epithelial markers consistent with a close relationship between OFD and adamantinoma.

Phosphaturic mesenchymal tumor-mixed connective tissue variant (PMT-MCT): Fibroblast growth factor-23 (FGF-23) is expressed in the majority of PMT-MCT. It is fairly specific for this tumor, although it may also be seen in rare other tumors such as aneurysmal bone cyst and chondromyxoid fibroma. As of early 2012, a commercial antibody was not yet available for FGF-23. Otherwise, there is minimal antigen expression in PMT-MCT; a few cases show focal SMA or EMA expression. D2-40 is expressed in lining cells of intratumoral lymphatic channels in ~90% of cases (Williams et al. 2007). Dentin matrix-protein 1 can also be detected in the matrix and in a paranuclear position in the cells of PMT-MCT (Toyosawa et al. 2004). DMP-1 normally helps regulate matrix mineralization in teeth, bone, and hypertrophic cartilage. Its overexpression in PMT-MCT may contribute to the development of oncogenic osteomalacia (also known as tumor induced osteomalacia).

Routine cytogenetics

Smooth muscle tumors: Refer to Chapter 8 for information on the cytogenetic findings of myogenic tumors.

Myofibroblastic tumors: Refer to Chapter 6 for information on the cytogenetic findings of myofibroblastic tumors.

Lipogenic tumors: Refer to Chapter 5 for information on the cytogenetic findings of lipogenic tumors.

Neural tumors: Refer to Chapter 13 for information on the cytogenetic findings of neural tumors.

Adamantinoma: Karyotyping may be of value in distinguishing differentiated adamantinoma from osteofibrous dysplasia. Thus far, osteofibrous dysplasia (OFD) shares with differentiated adamantinoma the finding of extra chromosome copies of 7,8,12, and 21 but not extra copies of chromosome 19 which is lacking in OFD. Osteofibrous dysplasia usually does not have additional changes seen in most adamantinomas such as translocations, inversions, and marker chromosomes.

Phosphaturic mesenchymal tumor-mixed connective tissue variant (PMT-MCT): The karyotype may be complex and is distinctly different from the karyotypes of some of the tumors in the differential including chondromyxoid fibroma (rearrangements of 6p23-25, 6q12-15, and 6q23-27) (Romeo et al. 2010), giant cell tumor of bone (telomeric fusions), and primary aneurysmal bone cyst (translocations of 16q22 and/or 17p13). However, only three PMT-MCT karyotypes have been reported to date, so information is limited.

Molecular genetics

Smooth muscle tumors: Refer to Chapter 8 for histologic descriptions and grading of myogenic tumors.

Myofibroblastic tumors: Refer to Chapter 8 for histologic descriptions and grading of myogenic tumors.

Lipogenic tumors: Refer to Chapter 8 for histologic descriptions and grading of myogenic tumors.

Neural tumors: Refer to Chapter 8 for histologic descriptions and grading of myogenic tumors.

Adamantinoma: There are no specific molecular genetic tests for adamantinoma.

Phosphaturic mesenchymal tumor-mixed connective tissue variant (PMT-MCT): FGF-23 expression may be detected by rtPCR when immunohistochemistry is negative. It can thus be of diagnostic aid.

RADIOLOGY

There are several unusual primary bone tumors that we have categorized in this chapter. The leiomyosarcoma of bone and myofibroblastic sarcoma of bone are rare tumors. Leiomyosarcoma of bone has non-specific imaging features of a complex, aggressive tumor originating in and destroying bone. Leiomyosarcoma of bone has a predilection for the long bones (64%) predominantly around the knee with an average age of presentation of 44 years, (Antonescu et al. 1997). Myofibroblastic sarcoma of bone is a very rare tumor with scant published literature describing its appearance.

The phosphaturic mesenchymal tumor is also rare, but presents as a cause of unexplained osteomalacia, or in our case, rickets. The removal of the tumor is curative of rickets. Hence, the radiologist and clinical care team must be vigilant for the opportunity to find this unusual tumor. Fibroblast growth factor 23 (FGF23) has been identified as one of the circulating phosphatonins, and is elevated in phosphatemic diseases. This hormone appears to maintain serum phosphate and counter regulates the effects of vitamin D. High levels of FGF23 are found in hypophosphatemic rickets, fibrous dysplasia and tumor induced osteomalacia (Beck-Nielsen et al. 2010). Furthermore, high serum levels of FGF23 appear to distinguish between patients having tumor induced osteomalacia or X-linked hypophosphatemic rickets from other causes of hypophosphatemic diseases such as vitamin D deficiency, Fanconi's syndrome and Cushing's syndrome (Endo et al. 2008). Some have advocated whole body MR imaging with STIR sequences to diagnose this tumor when clinically suspected. In our case the lesion was visible by MR, however, a PET-CT happened to have been performed initially. Ideally, a non-radiation based imaging would be performed to minimize exposure, especially in the pediatric population.

Next, this chapter includes adamantinoma, a rare low-grade malignant tumor with aggressive appearance. Typically, adamantinoma occurs in the tibia or less commonly in the fibula and usually has mixed lytic and sclerotic appearance. Adamantinoma occurs in the diaphysis 91% of the time with extension to the metaphysis in 9%. There is periosteal reaction in only 32% and sclerotic margins in 41% with anterior bowing in 5% (Bloerm et al. 1991). The radiographic appearance shows lytic destruction of the cortex, sometimes with multifocal involvement that can create the classic 'soap bubble' appearance. Metastasis can also occur with a propensity for spread to the lung. Recurrence can occur up to 20 years after surgery, (Szendroi et al. 2009), emphasizing the importance of long term followup. There are rare cases of dedifferentiation into sarcomatoid tumors. (Izquierdo et al. 2010)

There has been a long standing challenge and controversy surrounding the differentiation of adamantinoma from osteofibrous dysplasia (OFD). Part of the difficulty stems from the clinical overlap in these entities. Both have a strong predilection for occurring in the tibia in young individuals. Radiographically, they both have lucent and sclerotic areas with an overall aggressive appearance. Both can progress and may require resection and are fraught with risk of recurrence. However, adamantinoma is a malignancy and thus can metastasize whereas OFD is benign. In a series of 68 patients showed the ability to correctly identify adamantinoma in 95% of cases and fibrous dysplasia (osteofibrous dysplasia) in 87% of cases using a combination of radiographic features and patient age (Bloerm et al. 1991). The features proving most useful in identifying fibrous dysplasia were younger age, presence of ground glass density and anterior bowing, absence of multilayered periosteal reaction and absence of moth-eaten destruction. In their series, all patients with fibrous dysplasia were younger than 38 years old with a peak age range of 11-15 years, while adamantinoma has a peak incidence of 11-30 years. In a series of 12 patients with adamantinoma the average age was 30 years (Desai et al. 2006).

Tibial osteofibrous dysplasia-like adamantinoma may recur with the histology of classic adamantinoma (Hatori et al. 2006). These entities are not only confusing for their overlapping clinical and imaging presentation, but they can show histologic overlap with progression over time from OFD-like adamantinoma to classic adamantinoma.

The last case is an intraosseous lipoma which is a benign lesion of bone often encountered incidentally on imaging studies. Milgram has described three stages of development for intraosseous lipoma. These begin with stage 1 which is a homogeneous fat lesion, evolving to stage 2 lesions which have variable calcification or ossification centrally and finally stage 3 which have further cystic change and bone formation, (Milgram et al. 1988). The imaging appearance of stage 1 lesions is usually diagnostic (Murphey et al. 2004). Radiographs will show a lucent lesion with sclerotic margins during stage 1 and a variable central calcification and trabeculation as stage 2/3 evolution occurs. CT or MR imaging will show fat density or fat signal tissue comprising the lesion. There may be slight bulging of the cortex especially in smaller bones with less space to accommodate the lesion. There should be no periosteal reaction or edema and the lesion is usually homogeneous. A classic case of intraosseous lipomas occurs in the anterior third of the calcaneus with variable central calcification (see Case fig. 25.5). These lipomas can also occur in the long bones, especially the intertrochanteric portion of the femur. This location is more troubling for diagnosis as the radiologist must be confident the lesion is not fibrous dysplasia or a liposclerosing myxofibrous tumor. Cross sectional imaging and follow up are probably warranted for a fatty lesion of the intertrochanteric region if the lesion shows any heterogeneity or complexity as there is a 10% malignant transformation rate with LSMF tumor (Kransdorf et al. 1999).

SURGERY

Leiomyosarcoma of bone

These tumors should be resected with wide margins. Adjuvant therapy should be strongly considered in addition to surgery.

Myofibroblastic sarcoma of bone

These tumors should be resected with negative margins. Adjuvant therapy has not been shown to be of significant benefit.

Lipogenic tumors of bone

Intraosseous lipomas are benign and rarely require intervention. If the structural integrity of the bone is felt to be compromised, simple curettage and bone grafting can be performed. Recurrence is unlikely.

Neural tumors of bone

Neurofibroma: These tumors rarely present in an intraosseous location in the absence of neurofibromatosis. In the rare instance when they do, simple curettage is generally curative.

With neurofibromatosis, an association with congenital pseudarthrosis of the tibia has been reported. The treatment of this condition is complex and beyond the scope of this text. Soft tissue neurofibromas can erode into the cortex and even intramedullary canal of long bones. Excision of the soft tissue tumor will halt, and generally reverse, the bony changes although bone grafting, and rarely even prophylactic internal fixation will be required.

Schwannoma: These tumors can rarely occur within bone. When bone is involved, changes are generally secondary from an adjacent schwannoma or from a tumor involving a nerve passing through foramina. Rare cases of intraosseous involvement are usually successfully treated with curettage.

Malignant neuroepithelioma, malignant schwannoma, and malignant peripheral nerve sheath tumor: As with most primary malignant bone tumors, these are best treated with wide resection, often in conjunction with adjuvant radiation therapy.

Metastatic neuroblastoma: Patients with this condition are treated with systemic chemotherapy aimed at control of the primary and systemic disease. Bony lesions are treated in a manner typical of metastatic tumors, where treatment is typically aimed at palliation and avoidance of pathologic fracture rather than as a primary curative modality.

Adamantinoma

Wide resection is indicated for this tumor and surgery alone results in a high cure rate.

Phosphaturic mesenchymal tumor

Complete excision results in cure in a large majority of cases. This includes resolution of oncogenic osteomalacia.

MEDICAL ONCOLOGY

Most patients are cured with surgical eradication. Because these tumors are so rare, there are no series defining the optimal medical therapy. Thus if a patient is a candidate for a clinical trial, this would be the recommended option. Any high grade rare tumor of the bone should be treated following the principles outlined for the same tumors originating from soft tissue. Benign or low malignant potential tumors are not candidate for chemotherapy treatments.

Paraneoplastic manifestation with calcium or phosphate imbalance, usually respond to treatment that eradicate the disease. Hypercalcemia should be treated with biphosphonate, either pamidronate at 60 to 90 mg intravenously or Zoledronic acid 4 mg intravenously, with dose adjustments depending on the kidney function.

RADIATION ONCOLOGY

Since uncommon primary bone tumors are rare disease entities, there are not many reports on the use of radiation therapy for the treatment of these tumors. In fact, only case reports and small retrospective reviews exist on the use of radiation therapy for some uncommon primary bone tumors. Due to the lack of evidence for the effectiveness of radiation therapy, treatment decisions should be individualized based on the specifics of each case. Treatment decisions may also be based on the more abundant existing evidence for the use of radiation therapy for these tumors when they originate from soft tissue. In general, most reports advocate wide surgical resection as the treatment of choice in which case radiation therapy has no proven benefit. Adamantinoma is the only uncommon primary bone tumor which originates exclusively in bone. Radiation therapy has never been shown to be effective for adamantinoma except for palliation in a patient who is not a surgical candidate presenting with medically refractory hypercalcemia (Lyons et al. 1999).

CASES

Case 25.1 Leiomyosarcoma of bone

Clinical history and presentation

The patient is a 51 year old man who was involved in a motorcycle accident 28 years prior to presentation, during which he sustained bilateral femur fractures treated with bilateral intramedullary rodding. He was subsequently well until six months prior to presentation when he sustained a mild twisting injury of the left leg. Work up at that time was felt to be consistent with osteomyelitis of the left femur, and he was treated with a course of antibiotics. Despite the antibiotics, he has failed to improve and presents with progressively increasing left thigh pain and swelling.

Physical examination reveals pronounced fusiform swelling of the left thigh with a palpable but ill-defined deep seated, firm soft tissue mass.

Surgical findings and comments

Open biopsy is performed. Staging work-up reveals no evidence of metastatic disease.

Wide resection of the entire femur with reconstruction is performed six months after initiation of chemotherapy with neoadjuvant docetaxel and gemcitabine. Satisfactory margins are obtained.

Radiology findings

Our patient's lesion (**Case figs 25.1a** through **25.1e**) shows a typical highly aggressive appearing sarcoma that appears to originate from the femur in this 51 year old man. The mass appears to stream out of the bone, invading and displacing the thigh musculature. There are central areas without enhancement which may well represent necrosis in such a large tumor. Presumably, the tumor's growth has exceeded the available blood supply resulting in necrosis. The axial T1 image (**Case fig. 25.1c**) shows the frank destruction of cortex in this highly aggressive tumor.

The one year follow-up CT exam shows pleural, pericardial and lung parenchymal metastatic disease.

Pathology findings

Gross features

The open biopsy consists of aggregates of gritty, white to tan bony and soft tissue.

The resection comprises a femur with associated skeletal muscle and scant skin. After fixation and decalcification, the femur is serially sectioned parallel to the longitudinal axis. Sections reveal a

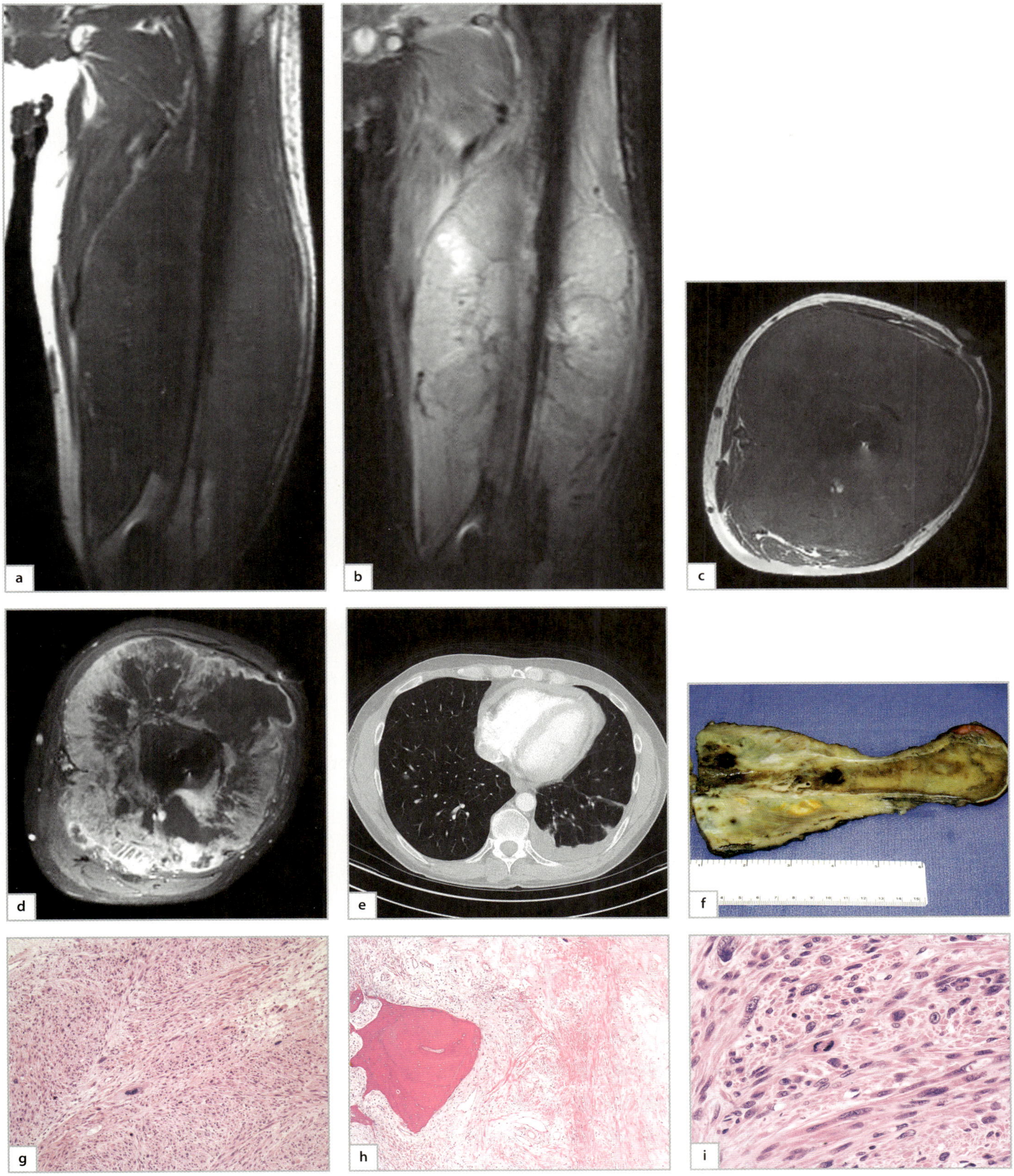
a
b
c
d
e
f
g
h
i

Case figure 25.1: Continued from page 539

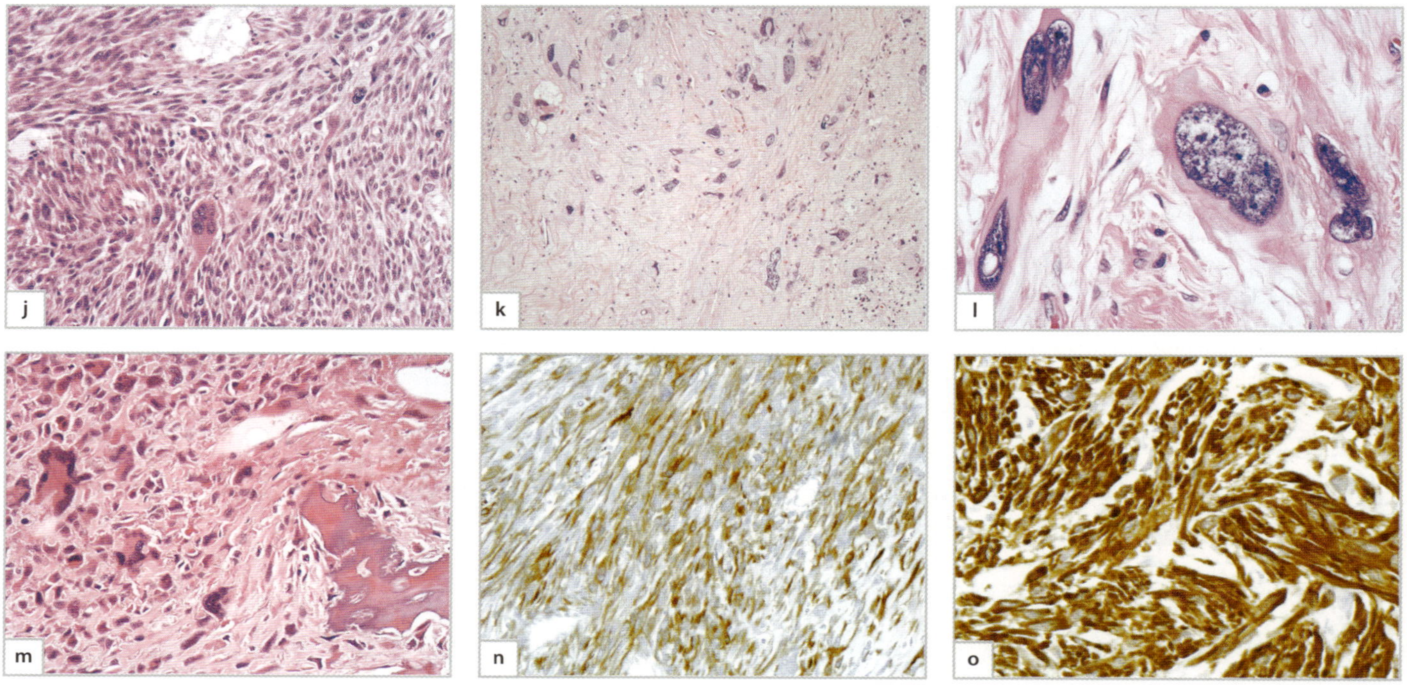

Case figure 25.1 Leiomyosarcoma of bone. **25.1a**: Coronal T1, **25.1b**: Coronal STIR, **25.1c**: Axial T1, **25.1d**: Axial T1 fat saturation post-contrast MR images in this 51 year old man show a very large mass (21 × 13.1 × 14.1 cm) of the left femur, destroying it and expanding aggressively into the soft tissues. The mass has heterogeneous enhancement with extensive non-enhancing areas likely from necrosis. **25.1e**: Axial CT post contrast image obtained 1 year after the initial MR exam shows lung metastasis with two right lower lobe lobulated nodules, pericardial effusion and left pleural effusion. **25.1f**: Gross photo of cross section of resected femur. The tumor is large, replace most of the medullary cavity, and focally extends into skeletal muscle. Hemorrhage and necrosis are apparent. **25.1g**: Biopsy at low magnification. The tumor is hypercellular and consists of spindle cells arranged in intersecting fascicles. Scattered cells are larger with greater nuclear pleomorphism, and cellular eosinophilia is striking. This is a classic appearance of leiomyosarcoma. **25.1h**: Resection at low magnification. The tumor surrounds scant residual medullary bone trabeculae. Post-neoadjuvant chemotherapy, the tumor is variably fibrotic as seen in this field, while other changes include hemorrhage, necrosis, and giant cell or 'monstrocellular' change. **25.1i**: Biopsy at high magnification. Features typical of LMS are present: streaming spindled eosinophilic cells with blunt ended nuclei, scattered paranuclear vacuoles, and cytoplasmic condensation suggestive of contraction bands. A pleomorphic giant cell is scattered among the moderately atypical spindle cells. This smatter pattern of more pleomorphic cells is also a typical though not specific feature of classic LMS histology. **25.1j**: Resection at high magnification. The typical alternating right angled fascicular architecture of classic LMS is also present in some of the resection specimen. **25.1k**: Medium magnification. Scattered among the more typical fascicular areas of tumor are groups of giant, highly atypical cells with extreme variation in nuclear and nucleolar size and shape. These are 'monstrocellular' cells and may be a result of neoadjuvant chemotherapy. **25.1l**: Resection at high magnification. The extremely pleomorphic tumor cells (also termed 'monstrocellular cells') exhibit no degenerative changes (smudgy chromatin, breaks in nuclear rim, dual colored cytoplasm, cytoplasmic vacuoles) which can accompany chemotherapy effect. These cells may be a part of the native tumor (consistent with pleomorphic LMS) or they may be the result of endomitosis induced by the neoadjuvant regimen. **25.1m**: Resection medium magnification. This heterogeneous tumor also features epithelioid cells (rounded tumor cells with discrete cell borders). **25.1n**: Smooth muscle actin IHC stain. Tumor cells in the biopsy express smooth muscle actin with weak to moderate intensity (chromogen is DAB). **25.1o**: Calponin IHC stain. Reactivity for calponin is diffuse and strong (calponin is another marker expressed in myoid tumors and a few other tumor types)(chromogen is DAB).

predominantly intra-osseous, white to tan, 15 × 9 × 8 cm mass that involves the majority of the medullary cavity, breaks through cortex, and extends into adjacent skeletal muscle (**Case fig. 25.1f**). Sixty eight blocks are submitted that entirely encompass one longitudinal section of femur, tumor, and adjacent soft tissues.

A separate specimen submitted for frozen section consultation includes a previously placed metal rod and closely adherent, necrotic tumor.

Microscopic features

Low magnification: The open biopsy discloses a fascicular, spindle cell neoplasm with scattered pleomorphic giant cells (**Case fig. 25.1g**). Even at low magnification, the tumor cells are strikingly eosinophilic. Some of the specimen is necrotic in keeping with the radiologic impression.

Resection: Sections of resected tumor are more heterogeneous than observed in the biopsy. This is presumably due to much broader sampling in the resection allowing other inherent elements to be captured, and also due to the morphology altering effects of neoadjuvant chemotherapy. Trabecular bone is entrapped by tumor, and the number of normal bone spicules is greatly reduced (**Case fig. 25.1h**).

***High magnification**, Open biopsy:* The streaming spindle tumor cells exhibit moderate nuclear atypia with scattered, markedly atypical giant cells. Most of the tumor nuclei demonstrate a blunt ended or cigar shape characteristic of smooth muscle differentiation. A rare paranuclear vacuole is also evident; this is another feature of smooth muscle differentiation (but can also be seen in gastrointestinal stromal tumors and rarely in myofibroblastic tumors). The cytoplasm is clumped and condensed in some cells with peripheral clearing mimicking the contraction bands of normal smooth muscle. Mitotic figures are easily found (**Case fig. 25.1i**).

Resection: Areas of hemorrhage, fibrosis, 'monstrocellular' giant cell clusters, and epithelioid cells are interspersed with more typical LMS fascicular regions identical to the biopsy (**Case figs 25.1j, 25.1k, 25.1l, 25.1m**). The very large, multinucleated tumor giant cells (monstrocellular cells) may be a result of chemotherapy effect.

Special studies: The biopsy specimen is stained with a limited panel of antibodies, and tumor cells show moderately intense reactivity for smooth muscle actin (SMA; **Case fig. 25.1n**) with no reactivity for desmin. The resection specimen also reveals similar reactivity for SMA and desmin. In addition, there is multifocal weak staining for caldesmon and strong reactivity for calponin (**Case fig. 25.1o**). This pattern of reactivity supports a diagnosis of a myogenic tumor; more specifically a smooth muscle differentiated tumor.

PATHOLOGY PEARL

Since antigenicity may be lost or weakened by decalcification methods, whenever possible, it is helpful to process a portion of an intraosseous tumor without decalcification. This is possible in cases where some of the intraosseous lesion is grossly soft and not gritty. Simultaneously, a portion of fresh tumor can be submitted for cytogenetic analysis and frozen for tissue banking.

Pathologic differential or, why isn't it one of the following?

Osteosarcoma: Although osteosarcoma can grow as fascicles of spindle cells, malignant osteoid must also be identified to enable a diagnosis of osteosarcoma. Copious sampling of this patient's tumor shows no malignant osteoid (also known as tumor osteoid). Moreover, the morphology of this patient's neoplastic cells is nearly emblematic of LMS: eosinophilic spindle cells with cigar shaped or blunt ended nuclei, scattered paranuclear vacuoles and contraction bands. Osteosarcoma cells may express smooth muscle actin, but the reactivity in this patient's tumor is diffuse and also includes reactivity for muscle specific actin, calponin, and focally caldesmon. This extended panel of muscle marker reactivity would be very unusual in an osteosarcoma. SATB2 is expressed in osteosarcoma and thus far has not been described in leiomyosarcoma (Conner et al. 2013)

Myofibroblastic sarcoma: Myofibroblastic sarcoma is a myoid tumor and will express some muscle markers including smooth muscle actin, muscle specific actin (also known as HHF-35 actin), and less commonly desmin. It does not usually express caldesmon as this patient's tumor does. High grade myofibroblastic sarcoma is not well-defined in the pathology literature, but it should feature areas that resemble the low grade version; namely, pale spindle cells with elongate tapered nuclei and lack of contraction bands and paranuclear vacuoles. No such regions are present in this patient's tumor.

Case table 25.1 Summary pathology findings of Case 25.1

Diagnosis	Primary intraosseous leiomyosarcoma
Size	15 × 9 × 8 cm
Location	85% intraosseous in the medullary cavity with 15% soft tissue component
Margin status	Negative (> 1.0 cm)
Histologic grade (FNCLCC grading system)	High grade
Pathologic stage (AJCC TNM classification)	IIB = T2 (>8 cm) and high grade without nodal or distant metastases

Metastatic sarcoma: Leiomyosarcoma can certainly metastasize to the bones. The origin can include the uterus and deep soft tissue. For this patient, there is no evidence of a mass elsewhere. Also, the tumor is intimately associated with metal hardware that had been placed in the femur nearly 30 years previously. A recognized risk factor for intraosseous soft tissue sarcoma is longstanding metal hardware insertion. Occurrence of primary intraosseous LMS has been described in this setting.

Oncology approach

Medical oncology

Neoadjuvant chemotherapy is initiated with seven cycles of docetaxel and gemcitabine, and minor response is noted. Three months after wide resection, the combination of doxorubicin and ifosfamide is administered because of a new finding of metastases to several thoracic vertebral bodies. Nine months postoperatively, the patient is noted to have pulmonary metastases on routine imaging. Multiple chemotherapy regimens are tried over the next few months including a Phase I protocol, re-induction with doxorubicin (discontinued due to profound toxicity), and sorafenib.

Radiation oncology

The patient underwent wide resection of the primary tumor in the left femur with satisfactory margins. Therefore, he was not referred for radiation therapy initially. After the patient develops metastatic disease, he receives a palliative course of radiation therapy to the spine and right hip.

Patient outcome

Widespread bone and lung metastatic disease continues to progress despite multiple therapeutic attempts at control. The patient, on maximum pain medication and restricted to a powered wheelchair, chooses hospice care. He succumbs to metastatic disease 21 months after surgical resection. This aggressive course is consistent with sarcoma developing in the setting of longstanding metal hardware placement.

Case 25.2 Myofibroblastic sarcoma (myofibrosarcoma) of bone

Clinical history and presentation

The patient is a 56 year old man who presents with a one year history of right knee pain which began spontaneously and has been slowly progressive. He denies a history of antecedent trauma.

Physical examination reveals no soft tissue masses, swelling or joint effusion. He has mild tenderness on deep palpation of the right distal femur. He has full and painless range of motion of the knee.

Surgical findings and comments

Open biopsy is performed, revealing the diagnosis of myofibroblastic sarcoma of bone. Staging workup is negative for metastatic disease. Wide resection of the distal femur with reconstruction is performed.

Radiology findings

This case illustrates the challenges faced by the radiologist. **Case figs 25.2a** through **25.2e** show a lucent lesion extending to the articular surface without a sclerotic margin in this 56 year old man. These are typical radiographic findings for a giant cell tumor (GCT). Indeed, GCT can be quite aggressive and may show soft tissue breakthrough in advanced cases. At age 56, however, this patient is older than typically seen for GCT. Tissue diagnosis proved to be the very rare entity of myofibroblastic sarcoma of bone.

Pathology findings

Gross features

Biopsy: The biopsy comprises approximately 1.5 cm in aggregate of finely gritty, white tissue fragments mixed with blood clot. The specimen is entirely submitted for microscopic review.

Resection: The resection consists of distal femur transected through the mid-shaft with associated skeletal muscle and an ellipse of previously incised skin. Shaved tibial plateau comprises the second specimen. Proximal marrow margin is sent separately for frozen section. Serial sectioning of the fresh specimen using a commercial grade band saw reveals an 11 × 8.5 × 5 cm, intramedullary, tan to white, expansile tumor with distinct sharp margins. The tumor is predominantly located in the epiphysis and metaphysis without obvious bone or cartilage formation (**Case fig. 25.2f**). Likewise, necrosis and hemorrhage are grossly absent.

Microscopic features

The histologic features of the biopsy match those of the resection specimen. Therefore, only photomicrographs of the resection are presented.

Low magnification: The tumor is predominantly composed of one unusual pattern: fascicles of spindle cells interrupted by bands of hyalinized collagen. The collagen bands encircle ectatic blood vessels and stream through the tumor like a branching river delta flowing around islands (**Case fig. 25.2g**).

High magnification: Nearly all the medium sized vessels are wrapped by hyalinized collagen. These collagen bands impart a river delta like appearance coursing and anastomosing between cellular tumor areas (**Case fig. 25.2h**). A minority of the tumor comprises pure fascicular growth of spindle cells (**Case figs 25.2i** and **25.2j**) a rounded, more cellular appearance (**Case fig. 25.2k**) or a myxoid/microcystic appearance (**Case fig. 25.2l**). There is very focal cortical breakthrough, and necrosis is present in 5% of sections, possibly secondary to effects of biopsy.

Most tumor cells are spindled with pale eosinophilic cytoplasm and indistinct cell borders. Paranuclear vacuoles and contraction bands suggestive of smooth muscle differentiation are absent. Most tumor nuclei are spindled with tapered ends and fine chromatin. A few tumor cells are polygonal or stellate in hypercellular and myxoid regions, respectively (**Case figs 25.2k** and **Case fig. 25.2j**). Marked pleomorphism, individual cell apoptosis, prominent nucleoli, and atypical mitoses are absent. Mitoses range up to 3 per 10 high magnification fields. Lymphovascular invasion is not identified. All margins are negative for tumor by at least 1.0 cm.

Special studies: Consistent with myofibroblastic differentiation, tumor cells are diffusely strongly reactive for smooth muscle actin (SMA) and muscle specific actin (MSA). The staining is accentuated in a parallel subplasmalemmal manner for SMA, and MSA reactivity shows mixed subplasmalemmal accentuation and globular staining (**Case figs 25.2m** and **25.2n**, respectively). Tumor cells are negative for expression of desmin, caldesmon, EMA, S-100 protein and ALK-1 (anaplastic lymphoma kinase).

The karyotype is hypodiploid with numerous structural and numerical abnormalities noted in 14 cells including marker chromosomes and whole chromosome losses: 40,XY,-1,-2,der(3)t(3;11)(q11.2;q12),der(9)t(1;9)(q12;p13),-11,-14,add(14)(q32),-15,add(16)(p11.2),-18,-19,del(20)(q13.1),-20,-21,-22,+r,+3mar[14]/46,XY[6].

A t(7;16)(p13;p11) or t(11;16)(p13;p11) characteristic of low grade fibromyxoid sarcoma is absent. Interestingly, there is an addition of 16p11.2. A mixture of partial chromosome gains and losses has been reported in a recent comparative genomic hybridization study of myofibroblastic sarcoma (Meng et al. 2009).

Pathologic differential or, why isn't it one of the following?

Leiomyosarcoma: The streaming fascicles of this patient's tumor are also characteristic of many LMS. However, the neoplastic cells in this patient's tumor do not exhibit nuclear or cytoplasmic features suggestive of smooth muscle differentiation (see Presentation case 25.1). The reactivity for SMA and MSA is also usually strong and diffuse in LMS. However, in this patient, there is no reactivity for desmin or caldesmon both of which are often positive in leiomyosarcoma. The SMA subplasmalemmal accentuated expression is more typical of myofibroblasts than smooth muscle differentiated cells. The karyotype is not specific and therefore not helpful in distinguishing the two tumors. The tumor was not stained with antibody to fibronectin, which has recently been reported to be helpful in distinguishing myofibroblastic tumors (strongly positive) from smooth muscle tumors (negative) (Guo-zhao et al. 2007).

Low grade fibromyxoid sarcoma (LGFMS): LGFMS shows mixed fibrotic and myxoid areas with arcades of blood vessels and sometimes large collagen rosettes. This architecture is absent. At least 40% up to 90% of LGFMS are reactive for EMA; EMA is negative in this patient's tumor. Finally, characteristic translocations of LGFMS are not found in the patient's tumor karyotype. The tumor was not stained with antibody to MUC4 which is reported to be a sensitive and relatively specific marker for LGFMS (Doyle et al. 2010).

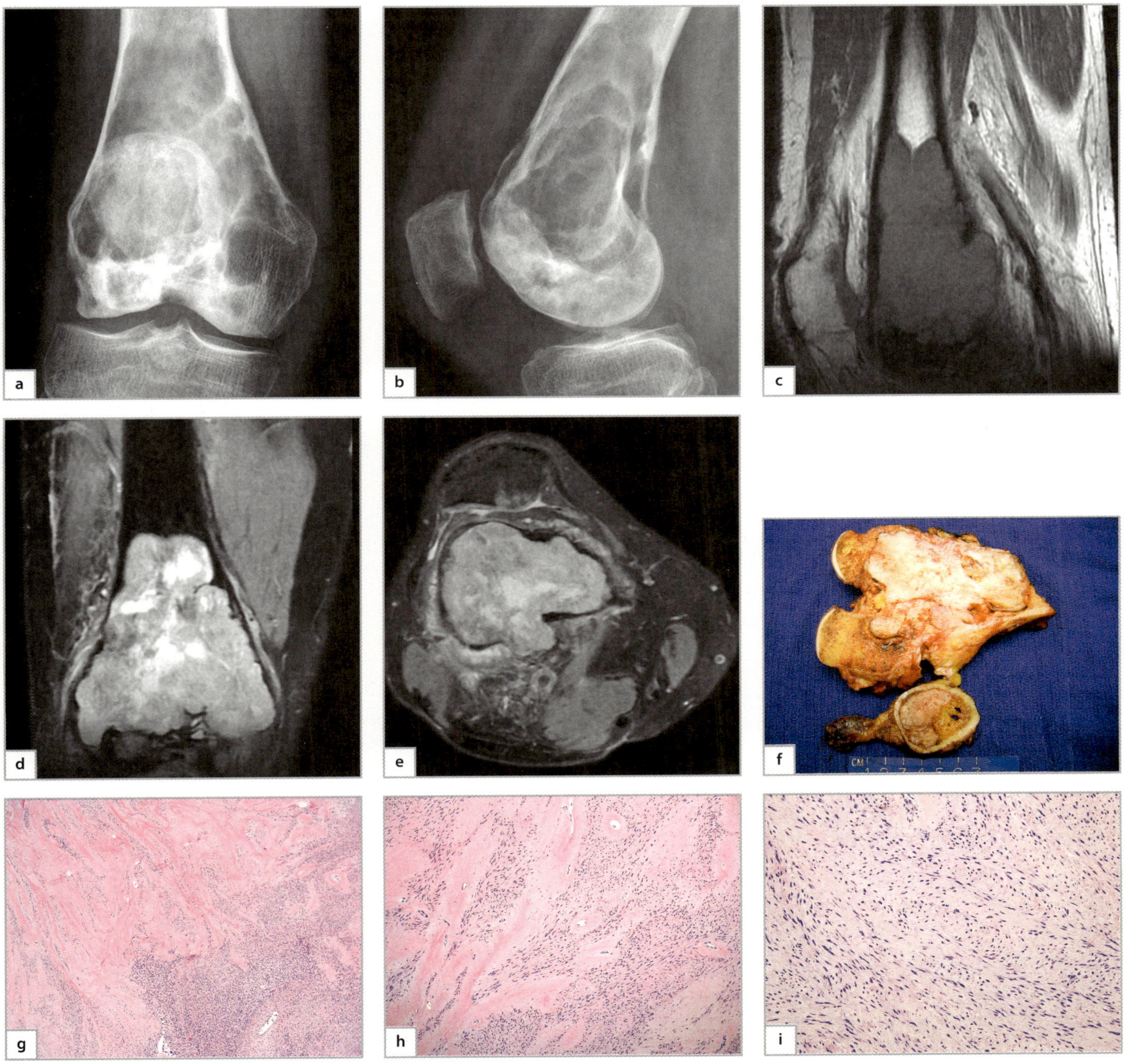

Case figure 25.2 Myofibroblastic sarcoma of bone. **25.1a**: Anteroposterior and **25.1b**: Lateral radiographs of the knee. **25.1c**: Sagittal T1 MR image. **25.1d**: Coronal PD fat saturated MR image. **25.1e**: Axial PD fat saturated MR image. The radiographs show a lucent lesion without sclerotic margin of the distal femur which extends to the articular surface of this 56 year old male. There is no visible matrix. There is marked posterior cortical thinning, possibly with breakthrough. The MR images show an 8.3 × 6.9 × 9.8 cm homogeneously T1 low signal lesion with high signal on the fluid sensitive sequences. The mass has posterior soft tissue breakthrough. **25.2f**: Cross section of resection, gross photo. The tumor is intramedullary, multinodular and located in the distal femoral metaphysis and epiphysis. There is no gross evidence of cortical breakthrough although the cortex is markedly eroded in areas. **25.2g**: Low magnification. Most of the tumor consists of long bands of collagen separating hypercellular areas. **25.2h**: Medium magnification. Reminiscent of branches in a river delta, bands of hyalinized collagen stream through the tumor. The collagen bands appear for the most part to enwrap and follow the course of medium sized blood vessels. **25.2i**: Some areas are devoid of collagen bands and exhibit the fascicles of spindled cells typical of many myofibroblastic tumors.

Case figure 25.2: Continued from page 543

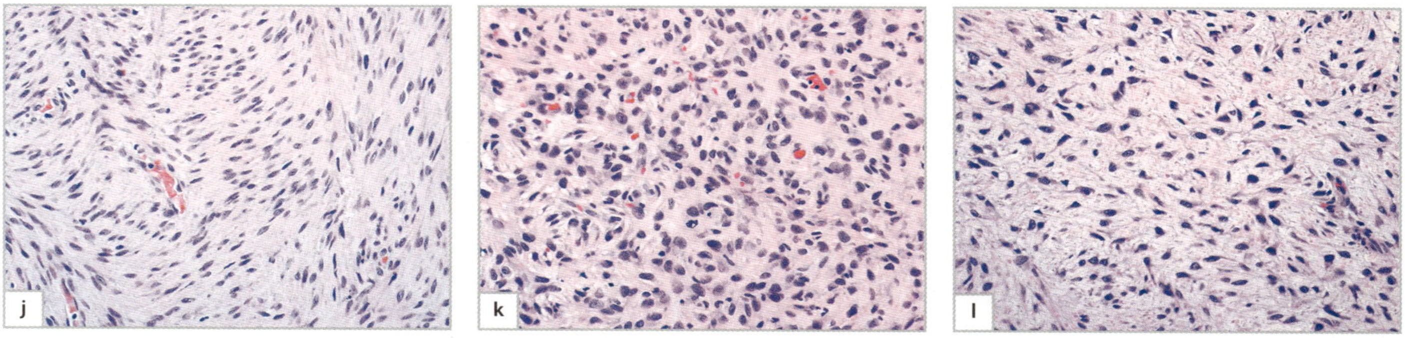

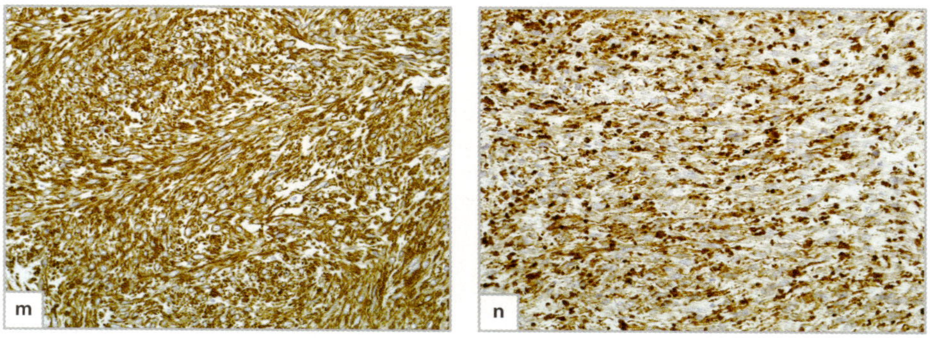

25.2j: High magnification. The great majority of tumor cells are spindled with pale eosinophilic cytoplasm and indistinct cell borders. Most of the tumor nuclei are elongate, tapered, fairly uniform and contain fine, evenly distributed chromatin. There is minimal nuclear pleomorphism in this field. **25.2k**: High magnification. Scattered throughout the tumor are small hypercellular foci composed of polygonal cells. Nuclear atypia is still mild to moderate, and mitotic figures are present. **25.2l**: High magnification. A myxoid area (a minor component of this tumor) reveals stellate, uniform tumor cells suspended in matrix. **25.2m**: Smooth muscle actin IHC stain. Tumor cells are diffusely positive and show subplasmalemmal accentuated expression commonly seen in myofibroblastic cells (DAB is chromogen). **25.2n**: Muscle specific actin, IHC stain. Muscle specific actin is also diffusely strongly expressed in a mixed peculiar globular and accentuated subplasmalemmal pattern (DAB is chromogen).

Osteosarcoma: This tumor was thoroughly sampled and showed no evidence of tumor osteoid, a necessary requirement for the diagnosis of osteosarcoma. Moreover, the strong diffuse staining for SMA and MSA would be highly unusual for osteosarcoma. SATB2 IHC staining was not performed but would be predicted to be negative in the patient's tumor and positive in osteosarcoma.

Metastatic sarcoma: Although it is possible that soft tissue or visceral myofibrosarcoma could metastasize to the bone, there is no evidence of a primary tumor elsewhere on staging workup.

Oncology approach

Medical oncology

Because the tumor is entirely resected, and there is no evidence of metastasis, chemotherapy is not advocated. Moreover, myofibrosarcoma of soft tissues and viscera generally is chemoresistant also arguing for a conservative approach.

Radiation oncology

The patient is not referred for radiation therapy as wide resection is performed. As the risk of recurrence after wide resection is thought to be low, there is no evidence proving effectiveness of adjuvant radiation therapy for myofibroblastic sarcoma of bone.

Case table 25.2 Summary pathology findings of Case 25.2

Diagnosis	Myofibroblastic sarcoma primary of bone, low to intermediate grade
Size	11 × 8.5 × 5 cm
Location	Metaphysis and epiphysis of distal femur with very focal soft tissue extension
Margin status	Negative (all margins >1 cm from tumor)
Histologic grade (FNCLCC grading system)	High grade (2 points moderate nuclear atypia, 1 point mitotic rate, 1 point focal necrosis) = high grade because FNCLCC Grade 2 tumors are now lumped with Grade 3 tumors as high grade)
Pathologic stage (AJCC TNM classification)	IIB = T2 (>8 cm) and high grade without nodal or distant metastases

Patient outcome

The patient remains active, functional, and free of disease two years after resection. However, he will be closely followed with periodic imaging because of the unpredictable nature of myofibroblastic sarcoma which can metastasize and cause death in a minority of cases, sometimes many years after initial presentation.

Case 25.3 Phosphaturic mesenchymal tumor-mixed connective tissue variant of bone

Clinical history and presentation

This is a 15 year old teenage boy, diagnosed one year previously with hypophosphatemic rickets, who now presents with a new fragility fracture of the femur and poor clinical response to his treatment of rickets.

Work-up has revealed a suspicious neoplasm of the left proximal fibula.

Surgical findings and comments

Curettage of the tumor is performed.

Radiology findings

The radiographs (**Case figs 25.3a** through **25.3g**) show a classic example of rickets with the broad physes with frayed margins in this 14 year old boy. The PET-CT scan performed two years later at age 16 show a puzzling small lesion of the fibula with marked increase FDG uptake. MR imaging follow up shows a non-specific expansile heterogeneous mass with enhancement. The axial MR images show an intact cortical rind successfully containing the mass indicating it is slow growing, allowing time for the cortex to remodel. Fortunately for the child, this tumor is discovered and its removal cures the rickets.

Oncogenic osteomalacia (tumor-induced osteomalacia) patients have hypophosphatemia, hyperphosphaturia and low 1,25-dihydroxycholecalciferol levels with resulting diffuse osteomalacia. This paraneoplastic syndrome is rare but has been reported with various benign mesenchymal tumors including myopericytoma (Brunschweiler et al. 2009), hemangiopericytoma (Ghosh et al. 2009). However, oncogenic osteomalacia has also been reported with sarcomas including fibrosarcoma (Nitzan et al. 1989) and a so called malignant fibrous histiocytoma (Rico et al. 1986).

Pathology findings

Gross features

The curetted tumor comprises fragmented hemorrhagic pink to tan soft and slightly gritty tissue aggregating to 2.5 cm maximally. A small portion is submitted to Cytogenetics for karyotyping.

Microscopic features

Low magnification: The tumor is heterogeneous incorporating cellular and fibrotic regions spotted by osteoid. The nodules of osteoid variably meld with osteochondroid and cluttered calcifications (**Case fig. 25.3h**). Focally, ectatic, blood filled sinuses impart a look of aneurysmal bone cyst (**Case fig. 25.3i**).

High magnification: Matching the mixed mesenchymal patterns present, the tumor also features a variety of blood vessels and lymphatic channels. Some are thick walled with secondary hyalinization (**Case fig. 25.3j**), some are thin-walled, dilated, and angulated (hemangiopericytoma like) and some are capillary-sized. Some phosphaturic mesenchymal tumor-mixed connective tissue (PMT-MCT) also contains adipose tissue, hemorrhage, myxoid areas, non-atypical spindle cells, and osteoclast-like giant cells. This patient's tumor contains only rare osteoclast-like giant cells, myxoid areas are absent, and hemorrhage is difficult to assess in this curettage specimen. The main components of this patient's tumor are represented in **Case fig. 25.3k**: streaming ovoid cells, flocculent 'grungy' calcifications and osteochondroid matrix, and blobby or toothpaste like collagen. A key feature of PMT-MCT seen in all cases is the 'grungy' blotchy or mottled, ragged calcifications that is usually fairly abundant in a particular tumor (**Case fig. 25.3l**). The most cellular areas of the patient's tumor comprise vaguely streaming, plump spindle cells with indistinct cell borders and ovoid nuclei with fine chromatin and inconspicuous nucleoli (**Case fig. 25.3m**). There is no significant cytologic atypia, no necrosis, pleomorphism is absent, and mitoses number up to 2 per 10 high magnification fields.

Special studies: The patient's radiologic evidence of osteomalacia matches laboratory values showing hypophosphatemia, hyperphosphaturia, mildly elevated serum alkaline phosphatase and low serum calcium.

By immunohistochemistry, approximately 1% of tumor cells express smooth muscle actin and up to 5% express epithelial membrane antigen (EMA). Antibody to CD34 highlights the pervasive, mixed thin and thick vessels but is non-reactive in tumor cells. Nearly all PMT-MCT express fibroblast growth factor 23 (FGF-23) by immunohistochemistry (Folpe et al. 2004, Bahrami et al. 2009), especially those causing oncogenic osteomalacia as this patient's tumor does. However, given the classic appearance with exquisitely correlating clinical, radiologic, and serological findings, it was not considered necessary to test the tumor with this non-commercially available antibody.

The karyotype of the tumor is hypodiploid with extensive structural and numerical abnormalities in three of 19 cells: 39~41,X,-Y,add(4)(q12),-5,-7,add(8)(p21),-9,-13,add(13)(q34),add(14)(q32),-15,add(16)(p13.3),-19,+1~2mar[cp3]/46,XY[16].

Two other PMT-MCT karyotypes have been reported and both were abnormal; one with a t(X;3;14)(q13;p25;q21)[15]/46XY[5] and the other with five clones: 46,XY,add(2)(q31),add(4)(q31.1)[2]/92,slx2[3]/46,sl,der(2)t(2;4)(q14.2;p14),der(4)t(2;4)(q14.2;p14),add(4)(q31.1)[10]/46,sdl,add(13)(q34)[4]/92,sdl2x2[1] (Graham et al. 2011).

This patient's karyotype shows plasticity in chromosome number similar to the second reported patient's, and shares an addition of 13q34.

Pathologic differential or, why isn't it one of the following?

Giant cell tumor of bone (GCTB): At least some portion of giant cell tumor of bone comprises evenly dispersed osteoclast-like giant cells, often containing increased numbers of nuclei (>40) that mingle with mononuclear cells harboring identical nuclear features. There are no such areas in this patient's tumor. The 'grungy' or mottled calcifications are not a feature of giant cell tumor of bone. Although reactive new bone can be found in GCTB, composites of new bone nodules, osteochondroid, and ragged calcifications typical of PMT-MCT are lacking in giant cell tumor of bone.

Aneurysmal bone cyst (ABC): Some areas of this patient's tumor bear a likeness to ABC because of blood filled sinuses with intervening fibrous and cellular areas including new bone formation. However, ABC does not contain the mottled ragged calcifications consistently present in PMT-MCT. Instead, it often contains honeycomb basophilic calcifications forming in loose fibrous tissue. Some examples of PMT-MCT also feature myxoid areas and adipose tissue; two other elements absent in ABC. The solid type of ABC may be particularly difficult

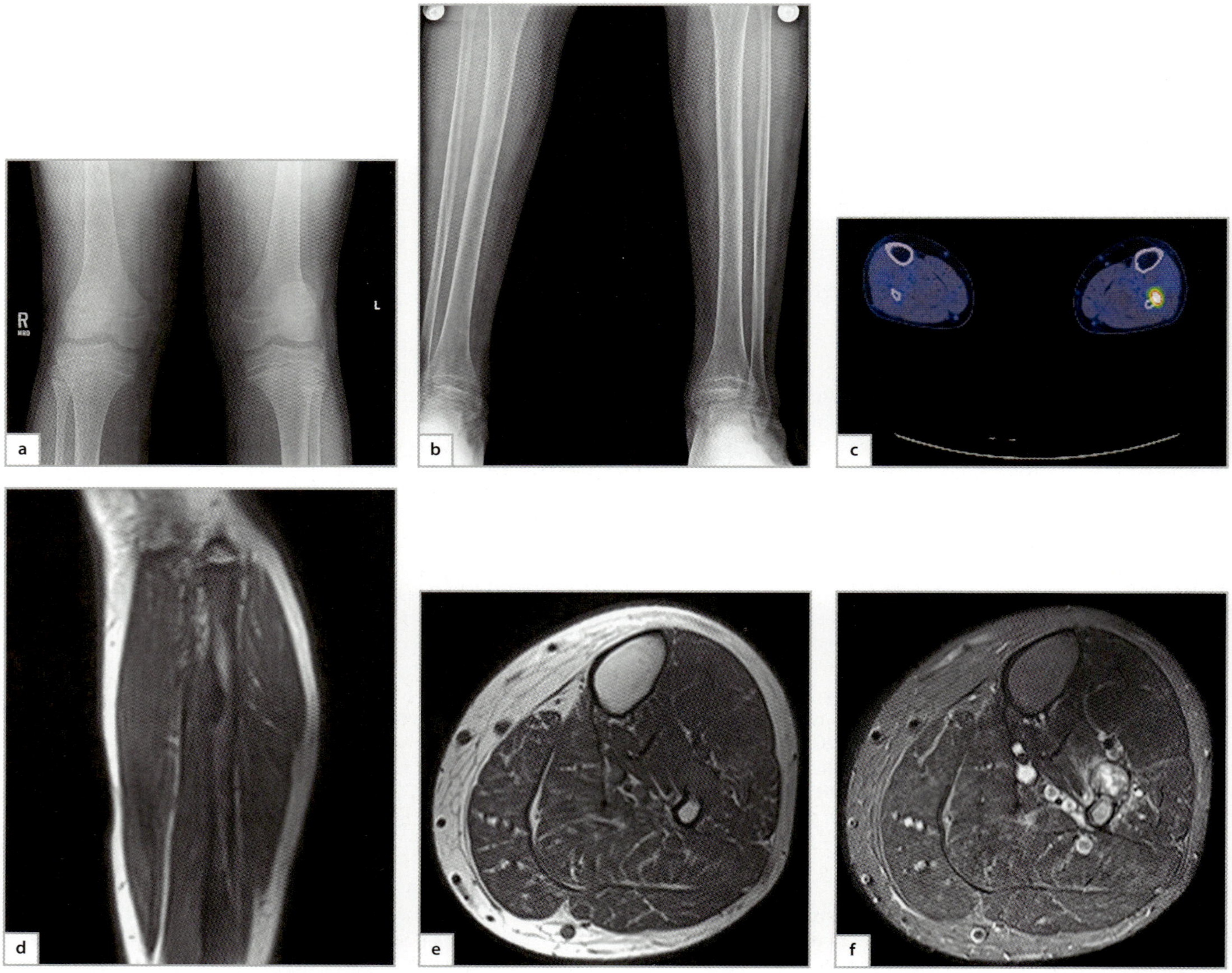

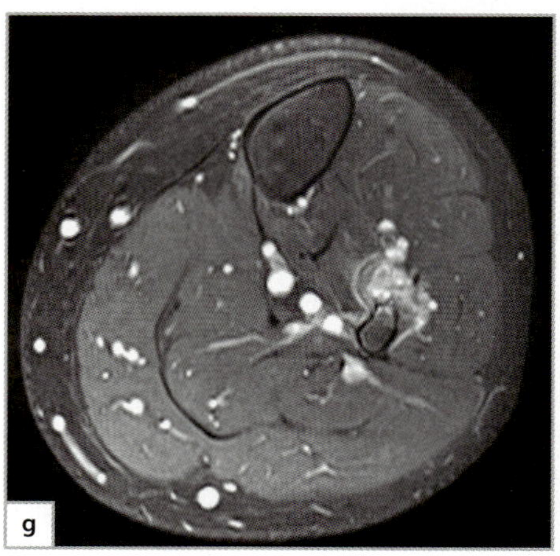

Case figure 25.3 Phosphaturic mesenchymal tumor. **25.3a**: Anteroposterior radiographs of the knees in this 14 year old boy. **25.3b**: Anteroposterior radiographs of the tibia and fibula 19 months later. The radiographs show diffusely widened, frayed appearing physes typical of rickets. Note there is no proximal fibular tumor visible on either radiograph. One month later at age 16. **25.3c**: PET-CT fusion image shows a small focus of marked increased FDG uptake in the proximal fibular diaphysis. MR imaging with: **25.3d**: Sagittal T1, **25.3e**: Axial T1, **25.3f**: Axial STIR, and **25.3g**: Axial T1 fat saturation post-contrast images show a small, 1.7 × 1.3 × 3.8 cm expansile heterogeneous mass of the fibula, correlating with the PET-CT images. The mass measures 1.7 × 1.3 × 3.8cm and has non-specific T1 isointensity with STIR heterogeneous high signal and intense heterogeneous enhancement.

Case figure 25.3: Continued from page 546

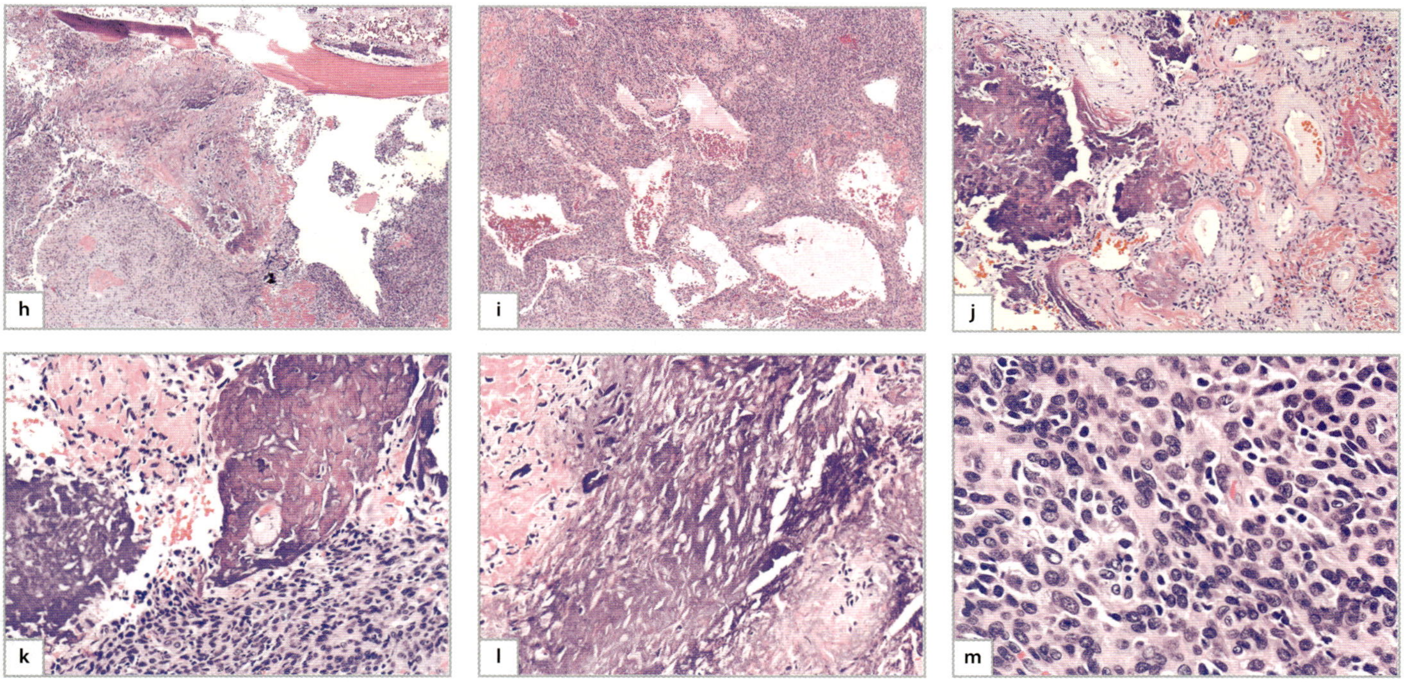

25.3h: Low magnification. The tumor is expansile and destroys trabecular bone (residual spicule is seen in top portion of photo). At scanning (low) magnification, the tumor shows a messy, disorganized jumble of cellular areas merging with fibrotic regions with interspersed osteoid and osteochondroid nodules and clustered calcifications. **25.3i**: Low magnification. Other areas resemble aneurysmal bone cyst with dilated sinuses filled with blood and fibrotic to cellular stroma. **25.3j**: Medium magnification. The tumor features numerous vessels of various caliber and lymphatic channels. In this field, thick walled vessels with partial hyalinization are prominent. **25.3k**: Higher magnification. This patient's PMT-MCT contains four distinct types of tissue: 1) flocculent, 'grungy' blotchy or mottled calcifications (left), 2) dense, sometimes hyaline collagen (upper left), 3) ragged, mottled osteochondroid that also include small nodules of osteoid (upper right; plain osteoid not present in this photomicrograph), and 4) streaming or tumbling plump spindle to glomoid (resembling glomus cells) cellular areas. **25.3l**: Higher magnification. A key component nearly reaching the status of sine qua non is the flocculent, 'grungy' mottled or blotchy calcifications that unevenly speckle the tumor. **25.3m**: High magnification. This patient's tumor is relatively cellularbut without other the features associated with malignant behavior in PMT-MCT: pleomorphic nuclei and elevated mitotic rate. Tumor cells are uniform with ovoid nuclei and indistinct cell borders. Chromatin is fine, and nucleoli are absent.

to distinguish from PMT-MCT. In such cases, antibody staining for FGF-23 may be helpful, although rare cases of ABC are positive for this antibody (Bahrami et al. 2009). Finally, cytogenetically, 70% or more of primary ABC contain a *USP6* fusion gene.

Chondroblastoma (CB): Chondroblastoma does not contain woven bone, although the chondroid material is often a pink hue. 'Chicken-wire' calcifications are also present in about 50% of cases; these are absent in PMT-MCT. The tumor cells of chondroblastoma are round, often grow in a pavement like manner, and commonly feature nuclei with longitudinal grooves. Such cells are not seen in PMT-MCT. Often the tumor cells of chondroblastoma are reactive for S-100 protein, and most cases also express keratins 8 and 18. DOG-1 is also expressed in chondroblastoma. PMT-MCT exhibits a very limited immunohistochemical staining profile that includes FGF-23 and occasionally focal smooth muscle actin expression.

Osteosarcoma: Cytologic atypia and osteoid formed by cytologically malignant cells would be present in an osteosarcoma of the degree of cellularity present in this patient's tumor; this tumor is devoid of both. FGF-23 expression has not been described in osteosarcoma and would be positive in >90% of PMT-MCT cases. Both tumors may cause oncogenic osteomalacia. SATB2 is expressed in osteosarcoma in PMT-MCT has not been reported.

Malignant phosphaturic mesenchymal tumor-mixed connective tissue variant (malignant PMT-MCT): These compose a minority of all PMT-MCT. Defining features consist of high cellularity, marked nuclear pleomorphism, and mitotic rate >5/10 high magnification fields (>5/10 hpf) (Folpe et al. 2004). Sarcomatous areas may comingle with typical PMT-MCT. While this patient's tumor is focally moderately cellular, there is no nuclear atypia, and the mitotic rate is at most 2/10 hpf.

Case table 25.3 Summary pathology findings of Case 25.3

Diagnosis	PMT-MCT variant
Size	3 cm
Location	Fibula, left proximal
Margin status	Positive (lesion is curetted)
Histologic grade (FNCLCC grading system)	Presumed low grade because of no atypia, few mitotic figures, and lack of necrosis.
Pathologic stage (AJCC TNM classification)	IA = T1 (G1 or G2,<or=8 cm), N0, M0

Oncology approach

Medical oncology

The patient presents typically with profound hypophosphatemia, hyperphosphaturia, and reduced or inappropriately normal 1.25-dihydroxyvitamin D level. Elevated serum alkaline phosphatase with normal serum calcium and parathyroid hormone levels are seen. This particular patient's tumor is not histologically malignant. Rare PMT-MCT examples metastasize, but such cases demonstrate increased mitotic activity and cytologic atypia. Morphologically, this patient's tumor falls into the range of benign PMT. Therefore, chemotherapy is not indicated.

Radiation oncology

The patient is being followed for tumor progression after curettage only. At the time of progression, wide resection may be performed. Therefore, there is no role for radiation therapy.

Patient outcome

The patient is doing well with improvement of his hypophosphatemic rickets and normalization of serum chemistries. However, he is at risk for tumor recurrence which would require wide resection to achieve negative margins.

Case 25.4 Adamantinoma (differentiated subtype)

Clinical history and presentation

The patient is a six year old girl who complains of pain in her right leg which is especially noticeable after running.

Surgical findings and comments

Biopsy is performed after radiology reveals an anterior cortical lesion of the right tibia. Following diagnosis of differentiated adamantinoma, wide resection of the right mid-shaft of the tibia is performed with contralateral vascularized fibula reconstruction.

Radiology findings

This patient, **Case figs 25.4a** through **25.4d**, only had MR imaging available. The MR appearance per se is non-specific in this 6 year old girl showing T1 low signal and high signal on T2 or STIR sequences. Had gadolinium contrast been given, there probably would have been heterogeneous enhancement. The lesion is multiloculated and causes expansion of the cortex. There is cortical destruction, perhaps best shown with the axial T1 image. There is also mild adjacent marrow and soft tissue edema indicating a more aggressive lesion. No pathologic fracture is found, although this often is the presenting feature of adamantinoma and osteofibrous dysplasia (OFD). Despite the non-specific appearance of the lesion, the location and young age of the patient is strongly suggestive of adamantinoma. The differential for a complex, aggressive lesion of the mid tibia includes adamantinoma, OFD and neurofibromatosis. Imaging alone cannot reliably distinguish these, although as discussed above, features favoring OFD include: young age, presence of ground glass, absence of periosteal reaction and absence of moth eaten appearance. At a minimum, close imaging surveillance should be performed; often tissue diagnosis is required to avoid delaying definitive management of adamantinoma.

Three other radiographic cases of adamantinoma and one case of OFD are also presented for comparison. **Case figs 25.4e** and **25.4f** is of a 15 year old teenaged boy with a classic 'soap-bubble' appearance of the lesion. The location is also typical with the lesion centered in the diaphysis having cortical expansion and destruction. Note there is no ground glass portion which would favor OFD.

Case figs 25.4g and **25.4h** is of a 57 year old woman with advanced adamantinoma. Note the extensive disease involving the entire diaphysis with extensive area of bone destruction. This is much more aggressive appearing than an OFD or neurofibromatosis. There is also a pathologic fracture of the proximal metaphysis with a large lytic area worrisome for possible sarcomatous dedifferentiation. Interestingly, the only periosteal reaction is associated with the healing pathologic fracture. This becomes a pertinent negative finding to distinguish from other potential extensive aggressive lesion of the tibia such as chronic osteomyelitis or end stage Paget disease. Both of these entities would have extensive periosteal reaction at various stages of formation and maturity. Also, there is only mild anterior bowing of the tibia. Typically, when OFD, neurofibromatosis or Paget disease involves an entire weight-bearing bone, there is more severe bowing.

Case figs 25.4i through **25.4j** is of a 61 year old woman with a fibular adamantinoma. The fibula is the second most common location for adamantinoma after the tibia. Note the dominant portion of the lesion has a bland uniform density that might reasonably be called 'ground-glass' density and thus might erroneously lead the interpreter to think this is a OFD case (of course, the patient age is far too old for this condition). However, there are worrisome features of wide zone of transition and cortical near breakthrough that compel the radiologist to refer this case for tissue diagnosis. Nevertheless, the case underscores the difficulty in diagnosing adamantinoma, in particular, distinguishing it from OFD.

Case figs 25.4k through **25.4l** is of a 21 year old man with tibial OFD. There is an expansile proximal tibial diaphyseal lesion with areas possible ground glass density. One might consider performing a CT to definitively exclude cortical breakthrough and to better assess for ground glass matrix. Note the absence of periosteal reaction or moth-eaten destruction. There is only modest anterior bowing evident. These feature help guide the radiologist to the diagnosis of OFD. The lateral view shows a developing stress fracture through the proximal aspect of the lesion. As these cases illustrate, there can be much overlap in the appearance of OFD and adamantinoma and distinguishing between them can be difficult.

Pathology findings

Gross features

The biopsy and curettage specimens contain fragments of hemorrhagic red to tan gritty material.

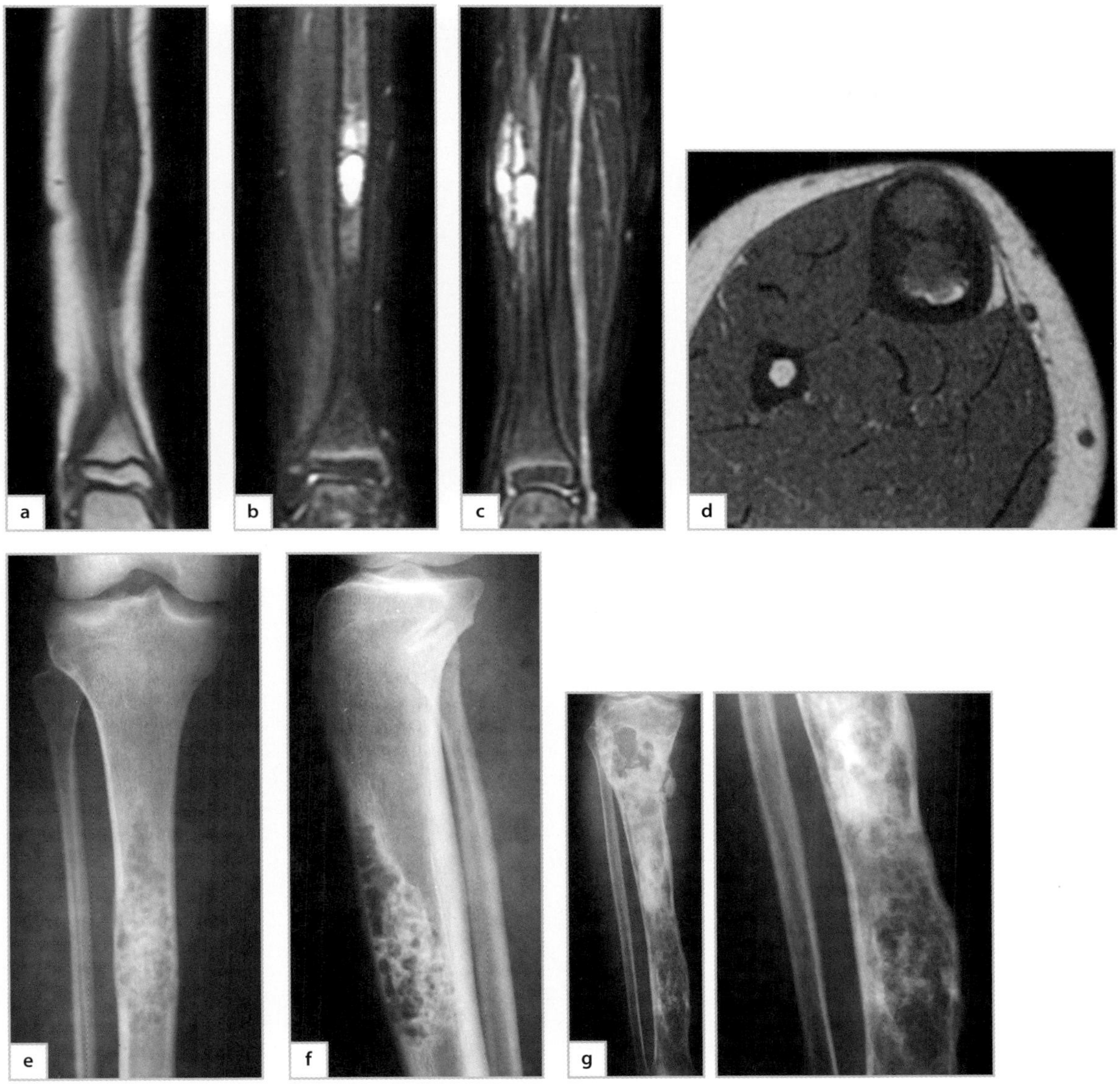

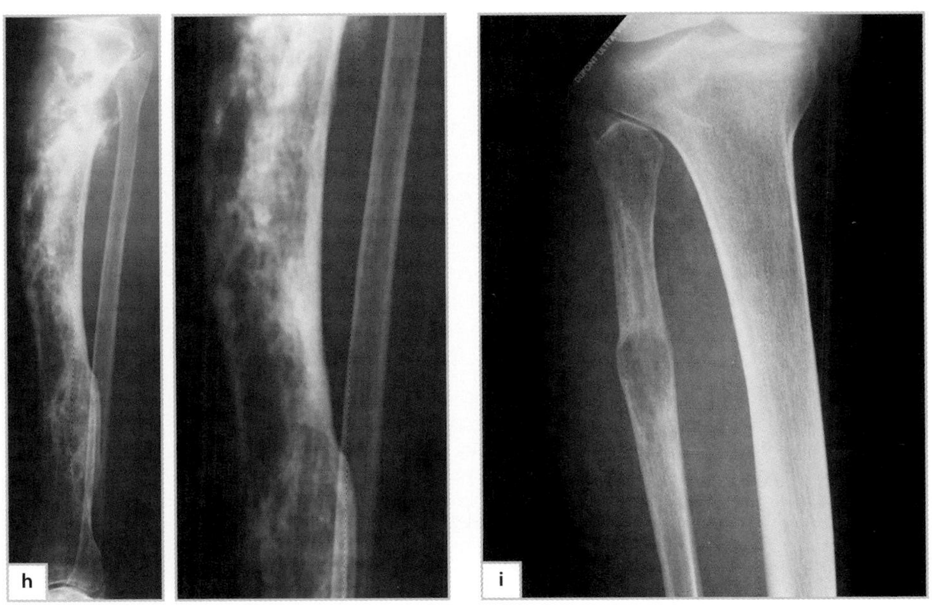

Case figure 25.4 Adamantinoma. **25.4a**: Coronal T1 MR image. **25.4b**: Coronal STIR MR image. **25.4c**: Sagittal T2 fat saturated MR image. **25.4d**: Axial T1 MR image. The MR images in this 6 year old girl show a complex expansile lesion centered in the proximal cortex of the mid tibial diaphysis. There is no appreciable bowing and no soft tissue component. The lesion is T1 low signal and high signal on T2 and STIR images. The MR image characteristics are non-specific, however the location in this skeletal immature individual is worrisome for adamantinoma with a differential including osteofibrous dysplasia and neurofibromatosis. Case figs *25.4e to 25.4f are an additional case of adamantinoma*. **25.4e**: Anteroposterior radiograph of the tibia and fibula. **25.4f**: Lateral radiograph in a 15 year old male. There is a lucent and sclerotic muliloculated expansile cortical lesion of the anterior tibial diaphysis. The lesion has the classic 'soap-bubble' appearance. Note the absence of any periosteal reaction, which is only seen in 32% of adamantinomas. Case figs *25.4g to 25.4h are an additional case of adamantinoma*. **25.4g**: Anteroposterior radiograph of the tibia and fibula with detailed image of the mid diaphysis.

Case figure 25.4: Continued from page 549

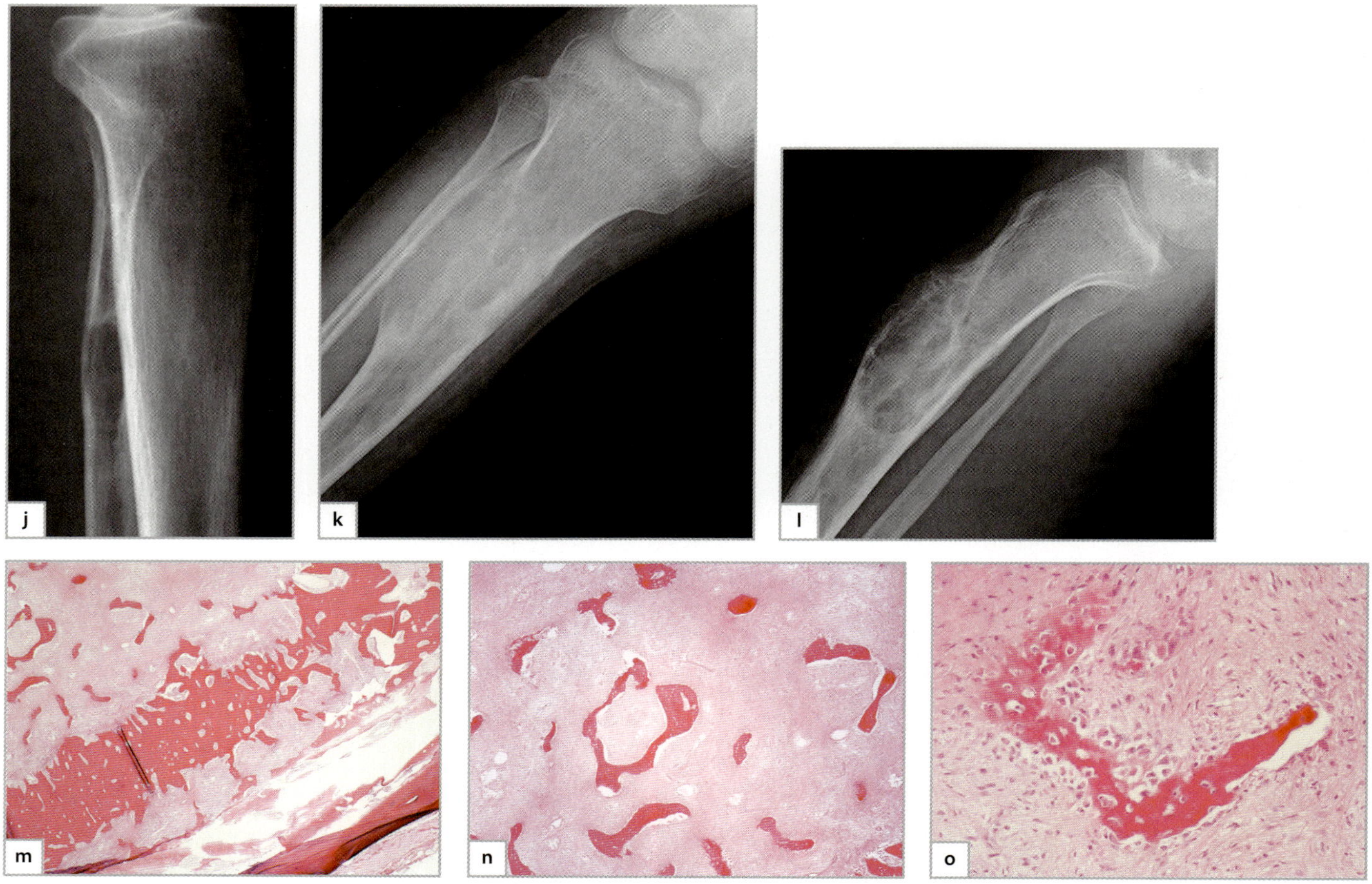

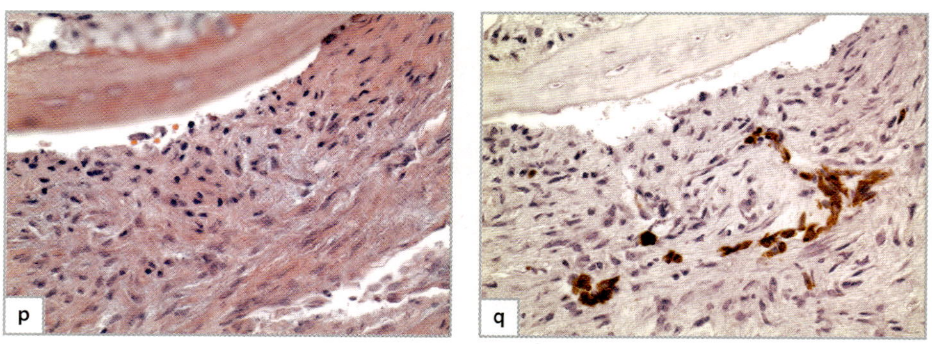

25.4h Lateral radiograph with detailed image of the mid diaphysis in this 57 year old female. There is an extensive lytic destructive lesion involving the entire tibial diaphysis. There is a pathologic fracture of the proximal metaphysis. Note the only periosteal reaction in this extensive aggressive lesion is associated with the healing pathologic fracture. There is only mild anterior bowing. Case figs *25.4i to25.4j are an additional case of adamantinoma.* **25.4i**: Anteroposterior and **25.4j**: Lateral radiograph of the proximal leg in this 61 year old woman. There is a predominantly lucent lesion with ground glass like appearance seen in the proximal fibular diaphysis. There is no periosteal reaction, soft tissue mass or fracture. The lesion shows a worrisome wide zone of transition of its proximal and distal margins. Also, there is focal cortical thinning with near cortical breakthrough along the lateral margin. The lesion is more aggressive than typically seen with fibrous dysplasia and referral for tissue diagnosis is probably warranted. Case figs *25.4k and 25.4l are an additional case of osteofibrous dysplasia.* **25.4k**: Anteroposterior, **25.4l**: Lateral radiographs in this 21 year old man show an expansile lucent and sclerotic lesion of the proximal tibia. There is mild anterior bowing with a developing pathologic fracture seen proximally. The lesion expands the cortex but no soft tissue mass or cortical breakthrough is seen. There are areas with a suggestion of ground glass density appearance; this is difficult to appreciate with the overall heterogeneity of the lesion. Importantly, there is no periosteal reaction and no moth-eaten destruction evident. **25.4m**: Differentiated subtype, low magnification. The tumor shows a zonal pattern common to osteofibrous dysplasia and both variants of adamantinoma with peripheral condensation of woven bone in areas converting to lamellar bone and a center that is more typical tumor. **25.4n**: Differentiated subtype, low magnification: The central region of this patient's tumor comprises dispersed ossicles of woven bone embedded in a fibrous stroma. Epithelial components are not identified at this magnification. **25.4o**: Differentiated subtype, high magnification. The woven bone in the center of OFD and adamantinoma tends to be rimmed by prominent osteoblasts in contrast to the trabeculae of fibrous dysplasia which generally have no to only a rare rimming osteoblast. **25.4p**: Differentiated subtype, high magnification. The epithelial cells in this case are very subtle and consist of strips of slightly more cohesive cells dispersed in the central portion of the tumor. **25.4q**: Differentiated subtype, keratin IHC, high magnification. Immunohistochemistry highlights the epithelial cells. The exact cut-point between OFD and differentiated adamantinoma is controversial; some experts require recognition of epithelium on H&E to confer a diagnosis of adamantinoma while others require only clusters of keratin positive cells to reach the diagnosis.

Microscopic features

Low magnification: The tumor is zonal with peripheral fusion of woven bone trabeculae with centrally more typical tumor (**Case fig. 25.4m**). The tumor's center consists of oddly shaped, woven bone spicules strewn about in a fibrous stroma (**Case fig. 25.4n**).

High magnification: A closer view of the one of the bone trabeculae discloses many rimming osteoblasts disposed along the edges of the bone. This is characteristic of adamantinoma (and also OFD) and rare in the much more prevalent fibro-osseous lesion, fibrous dysplasia (**Case fig. 25.4o**). The epithelial cells in the differentiated variant of adamantinoma can be extremely subtle requiring painstaking examination of the stroma. They are found more frequently in the central than peripheral region (**Case fig. 25.4p**).

Special studies: The spare and subtle epithelial clusters and strands are much more apparent on immunohistochemistry staining, as they show strong keratin expression (broad spectrum keratin antibody, **Case fig. 25.4q**).

Pathologic differential or, why isn't it one of the following?

Osteofibrous dysplasia (OFD): OFD and differentiated adamantinoma exhibit slim histologic differences that are not definitionally firmly defined. However, this patient's tumor meets the stricter criteria espoused by some experts: clusters or strands of sparse epithelial cells must be observed on standard, hematoxylin and eosin staining. That is the case here. A more expansive view of differentiated adamantinoma includes cases where the epithelium is identified only on keratin immunohistochemical staining. Here is the murky area, because OFD also features keratin positive cells strewn throughout the fibrous stroma. These cells are spindled, however, or if epithelial in shape, are dispersed as single cells without clustering. In this patient's tumor, small clusters and strands of epithelium are identifiable on H&E (just barely), and many more clusters of rounded cells are appreciated on keratin IHC.

Fibrous dysplasia (FD): Fibrous dysplasia replicates the osteofibrous pattern of OFD and differentiated adamantinoma down to the level of oddly shaped spicules of woven (and uncommonly lamellar) bone jumbled in a fibrous stroma. However, many of the trabeculae in OFD and adamantinoma are rimmed by osteoblasts; these are absent in FD which instead features spicules bare of osteoblasts. In addition, there are no keratin positive cells in the stroma of FD.

Adamantinoma, classic type: The classic adamantinoma contains abundant epithelial elements with or without OFD-like areas. The epithelium can appear basaloid, squamoid, tubular (pseudovascular) and spindled, and one tumor commonly demonstrates more than one pattern. The appearance mimics ameloblastoma (previously called adamantinoma). The differential diagnosis for classic adamantinoma is not in reality differentiated adamantinoma but other tumors including monophasic and biphasic synovial sarcoma, vascular tumors, and metastatic carcinoma.

Oncology approach

Medical oncology

Lung metastases, although extremely rare, have been described decades after the diagnosis of the primary tumor. The role of chemotherapy is limited to the rare cases that do metastasize. Tumor regression has been observed with a combination of etoposide and platinum (Lokich et al. 1994) or drug combinations usually used for Ewing sarcoma. Additionally, paraneoplastic hypercalcemia might require treatment with a bisphosphonate or the newer denosumab, a Rank ligand inhibitor.

Radiation oncology

There is no proven role for the use of radiation therapy for adamantinoma except for palliation of hypercalcemia in patients who are not surgical candidates. This patient underwent wide resection, and no further treatment was recommended.

Patient outcome

Eight years after surgery, the patient is doing well with no evidence of recurrence.

Case table 25.4 Summary pathology findings of Case 25.4

Diagnosis	Adamantinoma, differentiated (osteofibrous dysplasia-like adamantinoma)
Size	7 × 1.8 × 2.0 cm
Location	Tibia, right, cortex
Margin status	Negative
Histologic grade	Low grade
Pathologic stage (AJCC TNM classification)	IA = T1 (G1 or G2,<or=8 cm), N0, M0

Case 25.5 Lipoma of bone

Clinical history and presentation

The patient is a 44 year old man who feels pain in his heel. He has recently avoided jumping on it because the pain intensifies. However, he continues a high activity level including running triathlons. The patient has a known history of a cystic lesion in the calcaneus for at least 10 years when he first noticed some the heel pain. He is coming for further treatment because of increasing discomfort with exercise.

On physical exam, the patient has slight tenderness on palpation of the plantar, medial heel. There is no swelling, the tendons are intact, and he is non-tender around his calcaneus.

X-rays reveal no change in the size of the lesion since it was imaged more than 10 years previously. The patient desires resolution of the problem and is agreeable to a recovery regimen involving non-weight bearing for six weeks followed by a walking cast.

Surgical findings and comments

The lesion is easily curetted. It is packed with iliac crest bone graft.

Radiology findings

This patient (**Case fig. 25.5a**) is a 44 year old man with a lucent lesion with a central calcified nidus. Although, the lesion is well circumscribed, the typically sclerotic margin is not seen with these projections. A lucent area in the anterior third of the calcaneus has a classic differential of intraosseous lipoma, pseudo-lesion and cyst. These are all benign entities with the pseudo-lesion simply resulting from the relative decreased density seen between the major zones of trabeculation in the calcaneus. If further imaging is clinically warranted, MR or CT can diagnose the presence of fat tissue and can confirm the nonaggressive appearing margins.

We present two additional cases (**Case figs 25.5b** through **25.5c**) of intraosseous lipoma of the calcaneus. The location and size is quite consistent in the calcaneus, the central calcification is variable. The intraosseous lesion in the 13 year old boy, **Case fig. 25.5b**, correlates with a Milgram stage 1 whereas the lesion in the 55 year old man, **Case fig. 25.5c** is probably a late Milgram stage 2 or 3.

Pathology findings

Gross features

The curettage consists of hemorrhagic fragments of soft and gritty tissue aggregating to 3 cm maximally.

Microscopic features

Low magnification: The lesion consists of mature adipose tissue with secondary degenerative and ischemic changes including fibrosis and dystrophic calcifications (**Case fig.25.5d** and **25.5e**).

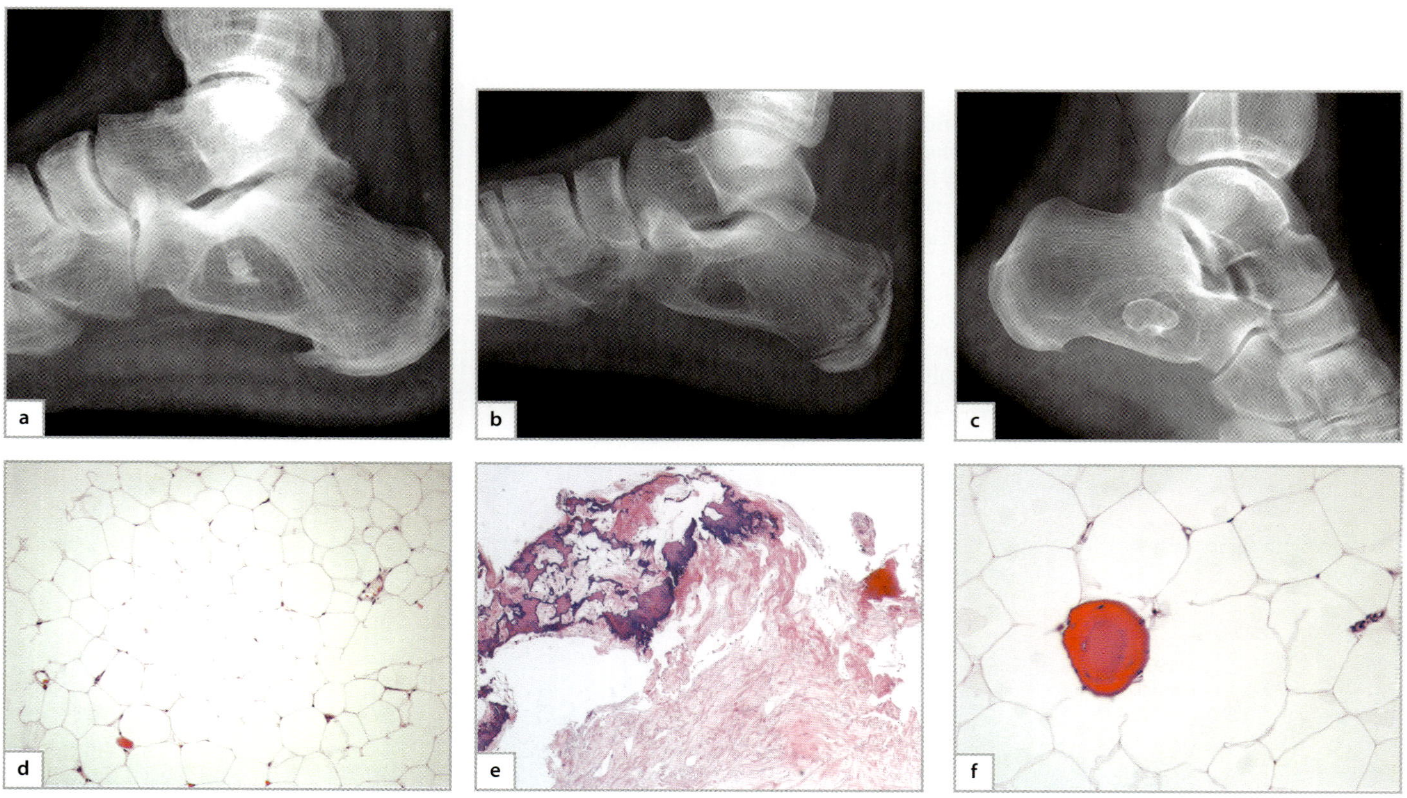

Case figure 25.5 Intraosseous lipoma. **25.5a**: Lateral radiograph of the heel in a 61 year old male shows a lucent somewhat triangular lesion of the anterior third of the calcaneus. There is a dense irregular calcification centrally. The lesion margin shows a narrow zone of transition although an actual sclerotic margin is not visible with this view. There is no cortical bulging. *Case figs 25.5b to 25.5c show an additional case of intraosseous lipoma.* **25.5b**: Lateral radiographs of the heel in a 13 year old male, and **25.5c**: Lateral radiograph in a 55 year old male. Both cases show a lucent lesion with sclerotic margin in the anterior third of the calcaneus. There is subtle inferior cortical bulging seen in figure 25.5c. Note there is no cortical destruction or periosteal reaction. Central calcification is variable. **25.5d**: Low magnification. The tumor is histologically identical to lipoma of soft tissue comprising mature, evenly sized adipocytes. **25.5e**: Low magnification. Centrally, the tumor has undergone necrosis with ensuing fibrosis and dystrophic calcifications. **25.5f**: High magnification. Most of the bone trabeculae are effaced by the lipoma but in this field a residual spicule is surrounded by histologically bland neoplastic adipocytes.

High magnification: The tumor is histologically identical to lipoma of soft tissue (**Case fig. 25.5f**).

Special studies: There is no need for special stains or cytogenetics because of the classic appearance of the tumor.

Pathologic differential or, why isn't it one of the following?

Bone infarct: A bone infarct will retain the bone trabeculae and more commonly shows a ring of peripheral calcifications, while intraosseous lipoma shows the converse: loss of most or all of the bone spicules and central rather then peripheral calcification.

Liposarcoma, metastatic or primary to bone: Primary intraosseous liposarcoma is extraordinarily rare. Metastatic liposarcoma can exhibit the range of features seen in the soft tissue types. In contrast to lipoma, atypical cells will be present including malignant lipoblasts.

Oncology approach

Medical oncology

This is a benign tumor with no role for chemotherapy.

Case table 25.5 Summary pathology findings of Case 25.5

Diagnosis	Intraosseous lipoma
Size	~ 3 cm
Location	calcaneus
Margin status	Positive but expected as preferred treatment is a curettage
Histologic grade (FNCLCC grading system)	Not graded as the lesion is benign
Pathologic stage (AJCC TNM classification)	Not staged as the lesion is benign

Radiation oncology

This patient requires only curettage as this is a benign tumor. There is no role for radiation therapy.

Patient outcome

The patient is doing well and has returned to his vigorous running routine.

REFERENCES

Adelani MA, Schultenover SJ, Holt GE, et al. Primary leiomyosarcoma of extragnathic bone: clinicopathologic features and reevaluation of prognosis. Arch Pathol Lab Med 2009;133:1448–1456.

Antonescu CR, Erlandson RA, Huvos AG. Primary leiomyosarcoma of bone: a clinicopathologic, immunohistochemical, and ultrastructural study of 33 patients and a literature review. Am J Surg Pathol 1997;21(11):1281–94.

Arora R, Gupta R, Sharma A, et al. A rare case of low-grade myofibroblastic sarcoma of the femur in a 38 year old woman: a case report. J Med Case Reports 2010:4:121.

Bahrami A, Weiss SW, Montgomery E, et al. RT-PCR analysis for FGF23 using paraffin sections in the diagnosis of phosphaturic mesenchymal tumors with and without known tumor induced osteomalacia. Am J Surg Pathol 2009;33:1348–1354.

Beck-Nielsen SS, Pedersen SM, Kassem M, et al. Fibroblast growth factor 23 – a phosphate regulating hormone. Ugeskr Laeger 2010;172(20):1521–1527.

Bloerm JL, vander Heul RO, Schuttevaer HM, et al. Fibrous dysplasia vs adamantinoma of the tibia: differentiation based on discriminant analysis of clinical and plain film findings. AJR 1991;156(5):1017–23.

Brunschweiler B, Guedj N, Lenoir T, et al. Oncogenous osteomalacia and myopericytoma of the thoracic spine: a case report. Spine (Phila Pa 1976)2009;34(23):E857–860.

Campbell RSD, Grainger AJ, Mangham DC, et al. Intraosseous lipoma: report of 35 new cases and review of the literature. Skeletal Radiology 2003:32:209–222.

Conner JR, Hornick JL. SATB2 is a novel marker of osteoblastic differentiation in bone and soft tissue tumors. Mod Pathol 2013;26(Supp 2):11a.

Desai SS, Jambhekar N, Agarwal M, et al. Adamantinoma of Tibia: a study of 12 cases. J Surg Oncol 2006;93(5):429–33.

Deyrup AT, Montag AG. Epithelioid and epithelial neoplasms of bone. Arch Pathol Lab Med 2007;131:205–216.

Dickson BC, Gortzak Y, Bell RS, et al. p63 expression in adamantinoma. Virchows Arch 2011;459:109–113.

Endo I, Fukumoto S, Ozono K, et al. Clinical usefulness of measurement of fibroblast growth factor 23 (FGF23) in hypophosphatemic patients: proposal for diagnostic criteria using FGF 23 measurement. Bone 2008;42(6):1235–1239.

Fisher C. Myofibrosarcoma. Virchows Arch 2004;445:214–233.

Folpe AL, Fanburg-Smith JC, Billings SD, et al. Most osteomalacia-associated mesenchymal tumors are a single histopathologic entity: An analysis of 32 cases and a comprehensive review of the literature. Am J Surg Path 2004;28:1–30.

Ghosh S, Sinha R, Bandyopadhyay R, et al. Oncogenous ostoemalacia. J Cancer Res Ther 2009;5(3):210–212.

Gleason BC, Liegl-Atzwanger B, Kozakewich HP, et al. Osteofibrous dysplasia and adamantinoma in children and adolescents: a clinicopathologic reappraisal. Am J Surg Pathol 2008;32:363–376.

Hatori M, Watanabe M, Hosaka M, et al. A classic adamantinoma arising from osteofibrous dysplasia-like adamantinoma in the lower leg: a case report and review of the literature. Tohoku J Exp Med 2006;209(1) 53–9.

Hazelbag HM, Laforga JB, Roels HJL, et al. Dedifferentiated adamantinoma with revertant mesenchymal phenotype. Am J Surg Pathol 2003;27:1530–1537.

Izquierdo FM, Ramos LR, Sanchez-Herraez S, et al. Dedifferentiated classic adamantinoma of the tibia: a report of a case with eventual complete revertant mesenchymal phenotype. Am J Surg Pathol 2010;34(9):1388–92.

Jain D, Jain VK, Vasishta RK, et al. Adamantinoma: a clinicopathologic review and update. Diag Pathol 2008;3:8.

Kashima TG, Dongre A, Flanagan AM, et al. Podoplanin expression in adamantinoma of long bones and osteofibrous dysplasia. Virchows Arch 2011;459:41–46.

Keel SB, Jaffe KA, Neilsen GP, et al. Orthopaedic implant-related sarcoma: a study of twelve cases. Mod Pathol 2001;14:969–977.

Kransdorf MJ, Murphey MD, Sweet DE. Liposclerosing myxofibrous tumor: a radiologic-pathologic-distinct fibro-osseous lesion of bone with a marked predilection for the intertrochanteric region of the femur. Radiology 1999;212(3):693–8.

Lokich J. Metastatic adamantinoma of bone to lung. A case report of the natural history and the use of chemotherapy and radiation therapy. Am J Clin Oncol 1994;17(2):157–9.

Lyons JA, Budd GT, Crownover RL. Hypercalcemia caused by metastatic adamantinoma: response to radiotherapy. Sarcoma 1999;3(1):33–5.

Meng G-Z, Zhang H-Y, Zhang Z, et al. Myofibroblastic sarcoma vs nodular fasciitis: a comparative study of chromosomal imbalances. Am J Clin Pathol 2009;131:701–709.

Milgram JW. Intraosseous lipomas. A clinicopathologic study of 66 cases. Clin Orthop Relat Res 1988;(231):277–302.

Most MJ, Sim FH, Inwards CY. Osteofibrous dysplasia and adamantinoma. J Am Acad Orthop Surg 2010;18:358–366.

Murphey MD, Carroll JF, Flemming DJ, et al. From the archives of the AFIP: benign musculoskeletal lipomatous lesions. Radiographics 2004;24(5):1433–66.

Nitzan DW, Horowitz AT, Darmon D, et al. Oncogenous osteomalacia: a case study. Bone Miner 1989;6(2):191–197.

Qiu X, Montgomery E, Sun B. Inflammatory myofibroblastic tumor and low-grade myofibrblastic sarcoma: a comparative study of clinicopathologic features and further observations on the immunohistochemical profile of myofibroblasts. Hum Pathol 2008;39:846–856.

Radl R, Leithner A, Machacek F, et al. Intraosseous lipoma: retrospective analysis of 29 patients. Int Orthopaedics 2004:28:374–378.

Rekhi B, Kaur A, Puri A, et al. Primary leiomyosarcoma of bone- a clinicopathologic study of 8 uncommon cases with immunohistochemical anlaysis and clinical outcomes. Ann Diag Pathol 2011;15:147–156.

Rico H, Fenandez-Miranda E, Sanz J, et al. Oncogenous osteomalacia: a new case secondary to a malignant tumor. Bone 1986;7(5):325–329.

Szendroi M, Antal I, Arato G. Adamantinoma of long bones: a long-term follow-up study of 11 cases. Pathol Oncol Res 2009;15(2):209–16.

Toyosawa S, Tomita Y, Kishino M, et al. Expression of dentin matrix protein 1 in tumors causing oncogenic osteomalacia. Mod Pathol 2004;17:573–578.

Williams K, Flanagan A, Folpe A, et al. Lymphatic vessels are present in phosphaturic mesenchymal tumors. Virchows Arch 2007;451:871–875.

FURTHER READING

Fletcher CDM, Bridge JA, Hogendoorn P, Mertens F (eds). World Health Organization Classification of Tumours of Soft Tissue and Bone, 4th Ed. Lyon: IARC Press, 2013.

Nielsen P, Rosenberg A, Deshpande V, et al (eds). Diagnostic Pathology Bone. Salt Lake City: AMIRSYS, 2012.

Chapter 26 Bone tumors of undefined nature

OVERVIEW

A few of the tumor in the World Health Organization (WHO) category are associated with specific genetic changes. Osteofibrous dysplasia is included by the WHO in this group, but it is discussed with adamantinoma in Chapter 25, as the two tumors are closely related (in fact, some cases of osteofibrous dysplasia may be 'differentiated' adamantinomas).

CLASSIFICATION

Table 26.1 lists the bone tumors of undefined nature according to the 2013 WHO classification.

DEMOGRAPHICS

Aneurysmal bone cyst

Primary aneurysmal bone cyst (ABC) most commonly is diagnosed in the first two decades of life and may be slightly more common in females. Secondary ABC occurs in the age range of the underlying primary tumor; for example, young to middle aged adults in cases of secondary ABC arising in the setting of giant cell tumor of bone.

Unicameral (simple) bone cyst

Boys outnumber girls by ~3:1, and most patients are under the age of 20 years.

Fibrous dysplasia

The monostotic form occurs over a broad age range and affects both genders equally. The polyostotic form usually presents in early childhood and may be more common in females. For both types, the first symptoms occur before age 15 in 80% of cases (Michou et al. 2011).

Langerhans cell histiocytosis

Langerhans cell histiocytosis (LCH) has a variety of presentations and occurs from infancy to old age. However, most patients are children to young adults. Males outnumber females by 2:1. Male infants are more likely to develop multisystem LCH (Type I LCH: Letterer-Siwe disease) or self-healing LCH (Hashimoto-Pritzker syndrome, respectively), young children more often present with unisystem multifocal LCH (Type II LCH: Hand-Schüller Christian syndrome), and adults more often present with localized LCH (Type III LCH: eosinophilic granuloma, Histiocytosis X) (Jones 2010, Walia et al. 2004).

Erdheim-Chester disease

Although children to the elderly may be affected, most patients are middle-aged. Males and females are equally affected.

Rosai-Dorfman disease

Young adults are most commonly affected, but all ages have been reported. Females outnumber males.

Chest wall hamartoma

This is almost exclusively a mass discovered in the neonatal period. Very rare cases in older children and a young adult have been reported. Males outnumber females by 2:1 (Serrano-Egea et al. 2001). Fewer than 70 cases have been reported in the literature.

Table 26.1 Bone tumors of undefined neoplastic nature (WHO 2013)

Lesion	Behavior	Additional comments
Aneurysmal bone cyst (ABC)	Intermediate, locally aggressive	Rare transformation to sarcoma or metastatic behavior in the absence of transformation may occur Primary ABC (~70%): true neoplasm with specific genetic translocations Secondary ABC (~30%): ABC-like changes that arise in the setting of another primary bone tumor
Simple bone cyst (unicameral bone cyst)	Benign	Prior to newer treatment methods, local recurrence occurred in up to 20% of cases
Fibrous dysplasia	Benign	Rarely, fibrous dysplasia may undergo malignant transformation Monostotic is 6-8 fold more common than polyostotic form Two syndromes associated with polyostotic form: McCune-Albright syndrome and Mazabraud syndrome
Langerhans cell histiocytosis	Intermediate, locally aggressive	Monostotic form much more common then polyostotic form Relatively rare bone disorder
Erdheim-Chester disease	Intermediate, Locally aggressive	Infiltrative disease of lipid laden histiocytes that also affects extraskeletal sites in ~60% of cases Rare disease that may be related to LCH
Rosai-Dorfman disease (sinus histiocytosis with massive lymphadenopathy)	Benign	Rare A disease of histiocytes Occurs in the setting of visceral disease with only rare isolated primary bone disease
Chest wall hamartoma	Benign	Very rare; almost all occur in infants to young children Mix of ABC-like cysts and mature hyaline cartilage some with endochondral ossification with additional fibroblastic and chondroblastic components The tumor is usually more intrathoracic than extrathoracic in location arising from the undersurface of the ribs

Benign: does not recur and does not metastasize. Intermediate: can recur but does not metastasize or only rarely metastasizes (<5%). Malignant: can recur and commonly metastasizes.

BEHAVIOR

Aneurysmal bone cyst

Primary ABC is an expansile, locally destructive lesion that may cause significant morbidity. Primary ABC exhibits a recurrence rate of 19% to 30.5% when curettage is combined with cryosurgery or phenol application (de Silva et al. 2003). Almost all cases occur within two years, but occasional patients recur 10 or more years after initial treatment. Rare cases of ABC transform to sarcoma including osteosarcoma, undifferentiated pleomorphic sarcoma, and chondrosarcoma. One case report of a lethal metastasizing ABC in the absence of sarcomatous transformation was large (27 cm), and the patient was treated with possibly sarcomagenic bevacizumab (van de Luijtgaarden et al. 2009). A few primary ABC may spontaneously regress (de Silva et al. 2003).

Predictors of behavior have not been reproducible across study populations. The presence or absence of *USP6* translocations and the specific translocation partner do not predict behavior. Two studies found certain histologic features correlated with recurrence, but the methods used differed, and no confirmatory studies have followed (de Silva et al. 2003, Docquier et al. 2010).

Unicameral (simple) bone cyst

Although benign, unicameral (simple) bone cyst (UBC) may recur in up to 20% of cases and is associated with pathologic fracture in up to 66% of cases. A few cases spontaneously regress.

Fibrous dysplasia

Pain, pathologic fracture and disfigurement are the most common morbidities of monostotic fibrous dysplasia (FD), although in most cases it is discovered incidentally. The natural history usually is of an asymptomatic lesion that may remain stable over time or may grow with bone growth and then subsequently stabilize after skeletal maturation. However rarely, osteomalacia and sarcomatous transformation may occur in both monostotic and polyostotic FD. The sarcomas may or may not be associated with prior irradiation and include osteosarcoma, fibrosarcoma, chondrosarcoma and undifferentiated pleomorphic sarcoma.

McCune-Albright syndrome is a rare subtype of polyostotic FD associated with irregularly edged café au lait ('coast of Maine') spots, hyperfunctioning endocrinopathies and occasionally other organ or metabolic abnormalities (Fletcher et al. 2002). Mazabraud syndrome combines intramuscular myxomas and polystotic FD and is also rare. The majority of polyostotic FD are not associated with syndromes. The disease may progress with new lesions in affected segments of the body (usually one side) until skeletal maturity is attained.

Langerhans cell histiocytosis

LCH exhibits a broad range of behavior from spontaneous regression to cure to apparent cure but with relapse (reactivation rate of 30-40%) to aggressive multisystem involvement with a mortality rate of approximately 20% (Minkov et al. 2011). Outcome depends on the types and number of organs involved. Spleen and liver involvement are considered 'risk' organs indicating that patients with LCH at these sites have a greater complication rate. CNS involvement is also considered a risk site because of neurodegenerative consequences including diabetes insipidus (Donadieu et al. 2012). LCH is divided into practical clinical categories of 'single system LCH': one organ or one system is involved which may include risk sites, and 'multisystem LCH' consists of two or more systems involved that may include risk organs. Disease activity is assessed using a semi-quantitative scoring system.

Erdheim-Chester disease

Similar to LCH, E-CD is a rare histiocytosis, and the two may be related. It involves multiple body sites but mainly the skeleton, lungs, skin, retro-orbital soft tissue, CNS, blood vessels, kidney, heart and retroperitoneum (Arnaud et al. 2012). Morbidity and mortality directly relate to the number and extent of organ/tissue involvement. Almost all E-CD patients (>97%) have skeletal lesions (De Filippo et al. 2009). Some patients may only have asymptomatic bone lesions. CNS involvement is an independent predictor of death (Haroche et al. 2012). Up to 16% of E-CD patients also have concordant LCH (most commonly) or Rosai-Dorfman disease (Haroche et al. 2012). The disease is a chronic disorder that may wax and wane, but no formal disease activity score has been established as for LCH. Prior to interferon α therapy, the mean survival was 19.2 months; after IFN α treatments began, the five year survival has improved to 68% (Arnaud et al. 2011).

Rosai-Dorfman disease

This is another histocytic disease that only rarely involves bone. It is indolent, and most patients with bone lesions are adequately treated by curettage (Nielsen et al. 2013). Patients with bone lesions most often present with pain. More than 70% of patients experience spontaneous resolution of symptoms, but a few will relapse or develop multiple bony and/or additional extranodal lesions. A review of 15 patients (12 with follow-up; mean of ~50 months) with primary R-DD of the bone reported that 5 developed extra-osseous lesions, two developed additional bone lesions, and five remained free of disease after treatment (Demicco et al. 2010). Additional lesions became apparent within two years of initial diagnosis.

Chest wall hamartoma

Chest wall hamartoma (CWH) is a benign lesion that is cured by surgical resection. Rare cases may spontaneously regress (Fletcher et al. 2002).

PATHOGENESIS/ETIOLOGY

Aneurysmal bone cyst

Primary ABC is a monoclonal neoplasm with a characteristic recurrent genetic finding of *USP6* gene rearrangements. Secondary ABC may be a degenerative rather than neoplastic lesion, as it lacks balanced translocations of *USP6* (Sciot et al. 2000). Only a subpopulation of spindle cells in primary ABC exhibit *USP6* alterations; the other cells in ABC including monocytes, osteoclasts, osteoblasts and some fibroblasts/myofibroblasts lack genetic abnormalities and are interpreted as normal cells recruited to the tumor.

The most common genetic abnormality in primary ABC is a translocation of *USP6*, (also known as *TRE2* or *TRE17* and located on chromosome 17p13) with the promoter region of *CDH11* (on chromosome 16q22) (Panoutsakopoulos et al. 1999, Oliveira et al. 2004). Translocations of the *USP6* gene occur in 60% of primary ABC cases including the solid variant. Five fusion partners have been identified, and all swap in a highly active promoter region upstream to the functional portion of *USP6* resulting in its transcriptional upregulation. Overexpression of the USP6 gene inhibits osteoblastic maturation and induces matrix metalloproteinase production and thus may account for bone loss and destruction in ABC (Lau et al. 2010, Ye et al. 2010). The multinucleated giant cells of ABC are true osteoclasts which form by a RANKL dependent mechanism and which also contribute to bone resorption/destruction (Taylor et al. 2012).

Activation of *USP6* does not have an effect on tumor cell proliferation, based on initial experiments (Lau et al. 2010), so it does not account for all findings in ABC. However, the ubiquitin-specific proteases to which USP6 belongs play a role in multiple processes such as DNA-damage response, inflammation and tumor formation (Ye et al. 2010).

Unicameral (simple) bone cyst

The cause of UBC is not known but it is speculated to be a developmental or reactive defect and not a true neoplasm. Cytogenetic abnormalities have been reported in a few cases by karyotyping without consistent findings (Greenspan et al. 2007). Simple bone cysts have been uncommonly associated with other lesions such as fibrous dysplasia (Martini et al. 2010). Analogous to secondary ABC, these may represent 'secondary' UBC.

Fibrous dysplasia

FD is a post-zygotic, genetically driven, abnormal fibro-osseous proliferation of the skeleton. Both the monostotic and polyostotic forms are caused by activating missense mutations of the *GNAS1* gene located on chromosome 20q13. It is a signal transducing membrane protein, a G-protein: guanine nucleotide-finding protein, α-stimulating activity polypeptide 1. Gene expression takes the form of multiple splice variants and is regulated by imprinting (Riminucci et al. 2010). The relevant gene product in FD consists of an abnormal 'a' subunit of stimulatory G protein that causes increased cyclic AMP activity, a potent phosphorylator of serine/threonine kinases and indirect activator of the protein kinase C pathway (Fletcher et al. 2002). It may be considered a stem cell disease in which the lesional cells are progenitor cells capable of differentiating into woven bone spicules and cartilage and inducing osteoclastogenesis by release of various cytokines such as IL6 (Riminucci et al. 2010).

Fibrous dysplasia is also sometimes associated with phosphate-wasting syndrome due to increased number of lesional cells producing FGF-23 (Dorfman et al. 2010).

While the cause of FD is genetic, FD is not a monoclonal neoplasm but rather a somatic mosaic abnormality with intermixed normal and mutated stem/progenitor cells. The proportion of the genetically abnormal stem cells varies from patient to patient, affects other tissues than bone marrow such as in McCune-Albright and Mazabraud syndromes and may decrease with time in a single patient leading to reversion to normal of the affected site.

The phenotype may depend on the point in embryogenesis or postnatal period when the GNAS mutation occurs with early events being more severe (such as the polyostotic form) (Michou et al. 2011).

Additional genetic abnormalities that may be found in FD include structural alterations of chromosomes 3,8,10,12 and 15 (Dorfman 2010).

Langerhans cell histiocytosis

Whether LCH is a neoplastic process, a reactive lesion or an aberrant immune response is still being debated, but accumulating data support a neoplastic designation, specifically a myeloid neoplasm. The non-pulmonary forms and some pulmonary LCH are monoclonal consistent with but not definitive for neoplasia (Willman et al. 1994, Yousem et al. 2001).

One theory proposes that the lesional cells of LCH represent aberrant immature Langerhans cells, possibly neoplastic, that recklessly release a rampant cytokine storm (Egeler et al. 2010, Filipovich et al. 2010).

Recent revelations indicate the origin of the lesional LCH cell is a myeloid-monocyte progenitor residing in the bone marrow. The majority of LCH cases harbor activating, somatic BRAF V600E mutations, especially those in patients younger than 10 years (76% vs 44% for <10y vs 10y or older) (Badalian-Very et al. 2012). However, BRAF V600E mutations do not unquestionably signify a neoplasm, because polyclonal proliferations such as melanocytic nevi commonly contain those (Badalian-Very et al. 2012). It is probable that additional genetic and possibly epigenetic alterations will be discovered in LCH that will stratify with LCH type and behavior and suggest specific therapy targets.

Erdheim-Chester disease, chondromesenchymal hamartoma

Interestingly, BRAF V600E mutations have also been detected in cases of Erdheim-Chester disease, a non-Langerhans cell histiocytosis. A recent examination of 24 cases found the mutation in 13 patients (54%) (Haroche et al. 2012). Like LCH, many of the disease manifestations are likely due to tissue damage ensuing from exuberant cytokine release by the lesional cells and recruited inflammatory cells, 'a systemic immune T-h-1 oriented perturbation' (Haroche et al. 2012, Blombery et al. 2012). It is possible that the pathogenesis and pathology of LCH and E-CD are similar (Haroche et al. 2012). Several cases (n=11) of combined E-CD and LCH has also been recently reported hinting at one abnormal progenitor cell subsequently diverging into two phenotypes possibly due to a shifting cytokine milieu (Pineles et al. 2011, Marchal et al. 2011).

Rosai-Dorfman disease

The etiology of R-DD is unknown. As the lesion most commonly develops in lymph nodes and involves histiocytes, an infectious and/or deranged autoimmune response have been hypothesized but remain unproven. The most common presentation is bilateral cervical adenopathy. A subset of patients may have increased IgG4 plasma cells and this group may be related to IgG4 disease (Zhang et al. 2013).

Chest wall hamartoma

CWH is considered an extremely rare developmental abnormality leading to hamartomatous overgrowth of chest wall cartilaginous and fibrous tissue often with secondary aneurysmal bone cyst changes.

PATHOLOGY

Table 26.2 provides a brief description of the incidence, body site locations and pathologic features of these bone tumors of undefined neoplastic nature.

Additional laboratory testing

Immunohistochemistry

Immunohistochemistry is not routinely used to make the diagnosis of ABC, UBC, fibrous dysplasia, or chest wall hamartoma. However, lack of CDK4 and MDM2 reactivity helps exclude low grade osteosarcoma and lack of keratin or p63 reactivity helps exclude osteofibrous dysplasia when those entities figure into the differential of fibrous dysplasia such as in a small needle core biopsy specimen.

IHC is nearly mandatory in the identification of the lesional cells of LCH which are reactive for S-100 protein, langerin (CD207) and CD1a. Of these three antibodies, CD1a is the most specific. E-CD is characterized by lack of reactivity for S-100 protein in 80% of cases, lack of reactivity for CD1a and expression of CD68 by IHC (Haroche et al. 2012).

Table 26.2 Bone tumors of undefined neoplastic nature

Tumor or lesion	Incidence	Age and sex distribution	Body site (in order of frequency)	Histopathology description including IHC Medium magnification	 High magnification
Benign: does not recur or recurs non-aggressively and does not metastasize					
Unicameral bone cyst (UBC) also termed simple bone cyst	Common	First two decades of life most commonly but may affect middle aged and elderly. M > F by 3:1.	Humerus, femur >> other sites In older patients (>20years) pelvis, or calcaneus have an increased rate of involvement Spares epiphysis	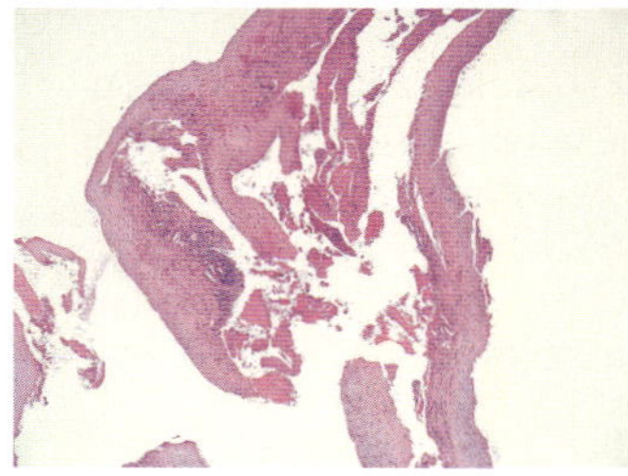	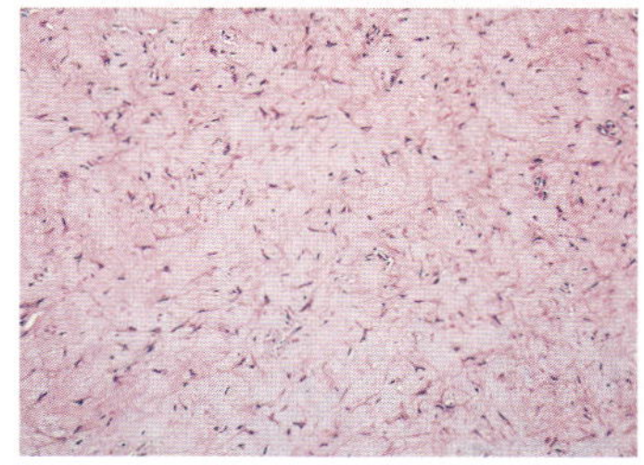
Usually unilocular cyst filled with serous to sanguinous fluid with thin, membranous wall. Wall is fibrotic to mildly cellular. Secondary changes due to micro-injury or fracture are common including woven bone, granulation tissue, hemosiderin, calcifications, and inflammation. Cementum like ossicles may also be present (10% of cases).					
Fibrous dysplasia (FD)	Common	Children to middle age but most common in children to age 15y. M = F	Bone always affected including in syndromes. Monostotic: jaws, base of skull, ribs, proximal femur, tibia, pelvis and arm but any bone may be affected Polyostotic: Same sites as above but pelvis and humerus more commonly involved. Almost always spares the epiphysis or articular surface Almost always intramedullary but rare cases are apposed to outer cortex: 'fibrous dysplasia protuberans' Other organs involved in syndromic cases	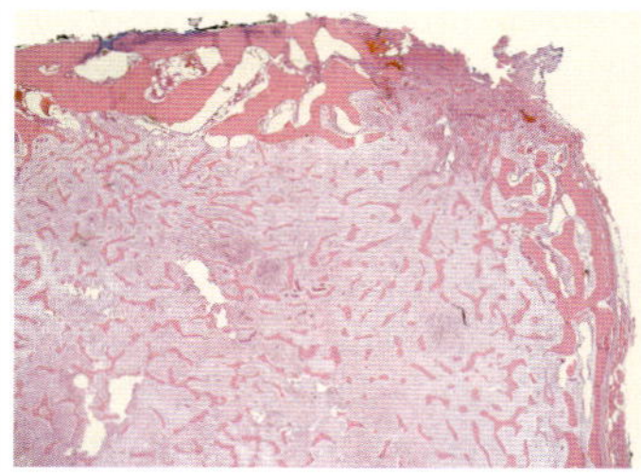	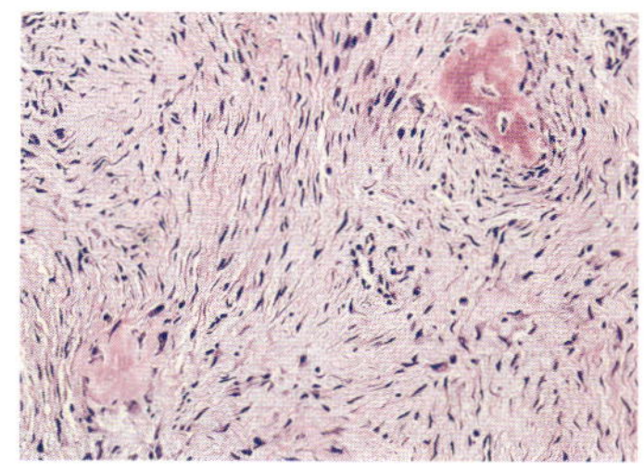
Variably cellular, plump to slender spindle cell proliferation with embedded, oddly shaped woven bone spicules. Spicules are not rimmed by osteoblasts (or these are focal and inconspicuous). Usually intramedullary but rarely may be exophytic. At periphery, extends between host bone trabeculae and may incite shell of reactive woven bone rimmed by osteoblasts. Cartilage may also be present and may be prominent. Secondary changes d/t trauma may be present, most commonly in rib lesions. Cystic change consistent with secondary ABC or simple cyst may be present. Rare cases of malignant transformation to sarcoma.					
Rosai-Dorfman disease	Very rare in bone, Rare otherwise	Young adults most commonly but all ages affected F slightly > M	Most commonly affects cervical lymph nodes then sinonasal extranodal tissues; bone affected in 8% of cases usually with extranodal sites also involved Any bone can be affected; some studies suggest most common is calvarial bones	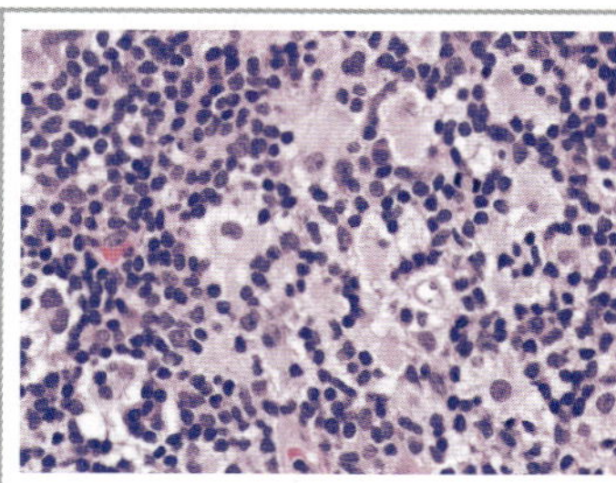	
Invasive infiltrate of large histiocytes that have eosinophilic cytoplasm with at least some showing emperipolesis (engulfment of lymphocytes, plasma cells and/or neutrophils). Lesional cells grow around bone trabeculae and into Haversian canals. Background contains mixed inflammatory cells sometimes prominent neutrophils and granuloma-like aggregates of non-lesional histiocytes. Lesional cells are S-100, CD68, CD163 positive. Negative for CD1a and langerin.					
Chest wall hamartoma, chondromesenchymal hamartoma	Very rare	Neonatal period (birth to 1 year) with exceptional cases in childhood to early adulthood.	Chest wall mass that is predominantly intrathoracic Arises from posterior or lateral aspect of one or more ribs Rare cases are multifocal or bilateral	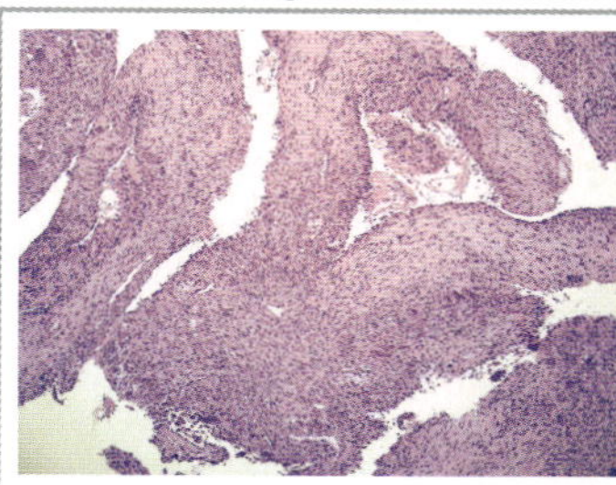	
Heterogeneous appearance histologically with mature cartilage often showing endochondral ossification, fibrous solid areas, chondroblastoma like areas and secondary ABC changes; most prominent is the cartilage component. IHC: Not performed.					

Table 26.2: Continued from page 558

Tumor or lesion	Incidence	Age and sex distribution	Body site (in order of frequency)	Histopathology description including IHC Medium magnification	 High magnification
Intermediate: can recur locally aggressively and/or rarely metastasizes (<5%)					
Aneurysmal bone cyst (ABC)	Common	Most common in first two decades of life but extends into middle age. F = M	Metaphysis of long bones, posterior arch and spinous processes of vertebra, but almost any bone may be affected Multifocal disease is rare but when present, affects spine most commonly Secondary ABCs occur when and where primary tumors arise	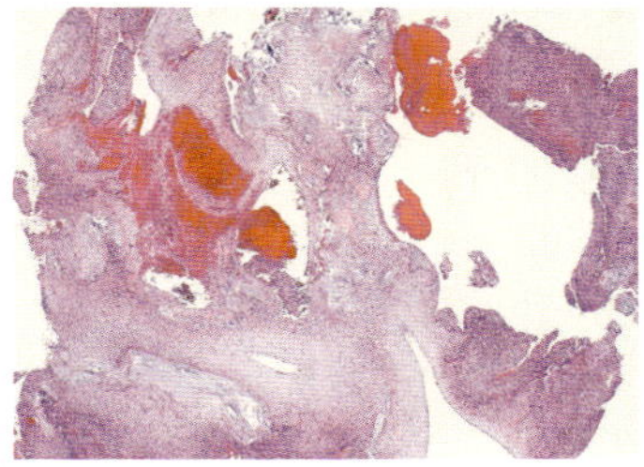	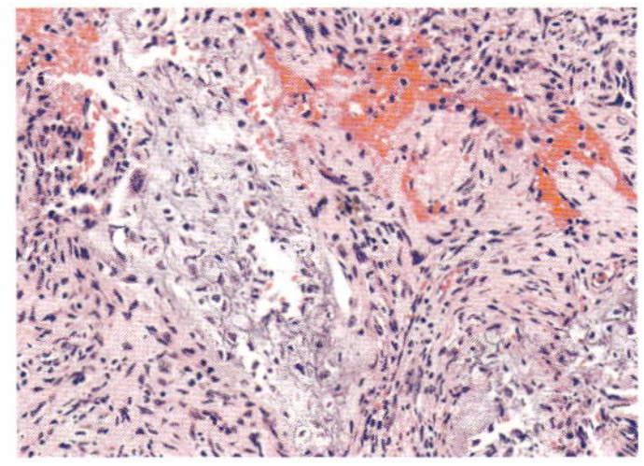
Classic variant: Multiple blood filled cystic cavities with cellular fibrous septa containing fibroblasts, osteoclasts, sinuous bands of pink osteoid, +/- blue calcified osteochondroid, +/- hemosiderin and +/- chronic inflammation. Solid variant: Same constituents as classic variant but without cysts. Rare cases of malignant transformation to sarcoma.					
Langerhans cell histiocytosis (LCH)	Rare	Children more commonly than adults. M > F by ~2:1 Multisystem disease much more common in infants and young children.	Bone most common followed by skin and lymph nodes Spleen, liver, other sites involved in multisystem disease Bone sites: Calvarium, femur, pelvis, ribs, mandible, other bones but rarely hands/feet Single bone site disease > multi-bone disease by > 5:1	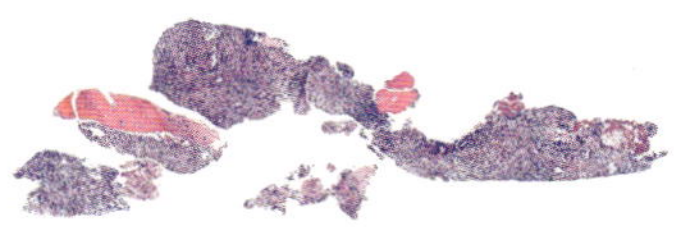	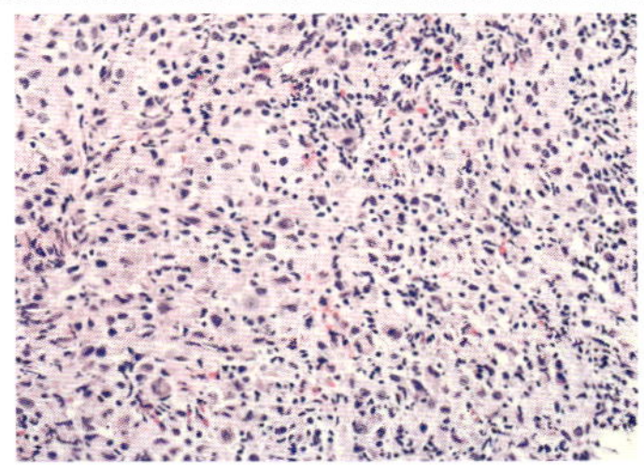
Sheets of moderately sized histiocytes with pale eosinophilic cytoplasm and indented or grooved oval to reniform nuclei. Often associated with multinucleated osteoclastic giant cells and infiltrates of eosinophils, lymphocytes, small, non-clonal histiocytes, and neutrophils. IHC: most are positive for S-100 protein, Langerin (CD207), and CD1a in varying proportions. CD68 and fascin positive. Negative for lysozyme.					
Erdheim-Chester disease (E-CD)	Very fare	Middle aged patients predominantly but children to elderly may be affected. M > F	Bone most common site (>97%): long bones of legs, long bones of arms; bilateral and symmetric changes in metaphyses and diaphyses are characteristic Does not usually affect axial skeleton and mandible Other sites affected in up to 66% of cases include a long list such as cardiovascular, endocrine organs, skin, renal, lung, kidney, retro-orbital soft tissues and CNS	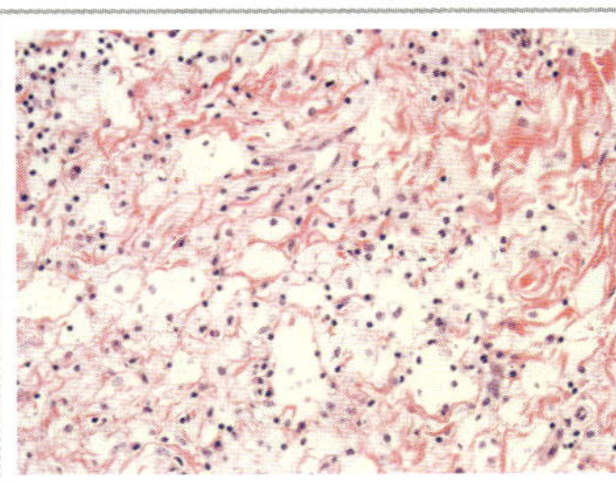	
Diffuse infiltrate of foamy (xanthomatous) histiocytes with fibrosis and secondary inflammatory cells including lymphocytes, plasma cells and Touton giant cells. Host bone is sclerotic with intense woven bone reaction resembling Pagetoid bone. IHC: Only 20% positive for S-100 protein. Negative for Langeran and CD1a. Positive for CD68.					
M: male. F: female. IHC: immunohistochemistry Incidence note: 'Common to very common' indicates that a medium, sized practice will treat at least several to dozens of patients with the lesion yearly; 'Uncommon to rare' indicates the same practice size will treat one to two patients with the lesion every five years; and 'Rare to extremely rare' indicates the same size practice will see zero to one patient with the lesion every 20 years.					

Routine cytogenetics and molecular genetics

Genetic analysis is not routine in the pathology work-up of ABC, UBC, FD, or chest wall hamartoma. However, for LCH and E-CD, BRAF V600E mutation analysis may be performed, the test is readily available in larger clinical laboratories, and potentially it may help direct therapy, although mutation status has not yet been established as a treatment guide.

RADIOLOGY OF BENIGN MIMICKERS

Aneurysmal bone cyst

ABC is a benign vascular lesion which may coexist with a number of other bone lesions. Giant cell tumor is the most common secondary lesion accounting for approximately 25% of cases. Other underlying lesions include chondroblastoma, fibrous dysplasia, osteoblastoma, chondromyxoid fibroma and nonossifying fibroma (Kransdorf et al. 1995). In approximately one third of cases, a preexisting lesion can by pathologically identified. When it occurs secondarily, ABC may be secondary process caused by a vascular abnormality of the primary lesion such as venous obstruction or arteriovenous malformation. ABC usually occurs before 20 years of age, and typically is an eccentric lesion in the metaphysis of a long bone. It will cause variable expansion and thinning of the cortex. ABC can have periosteal reaction in 25% of cases (Freeby et al. 1995). Flocculent calcifications similar to chondroid matrix can be seen in about 15% of cases. Approximately 25% of ABCs can also occur in the spine where it usually involves the posterior elements (Kransdorf et al. 1995). There should never be a soft tissue mass or cortical breakthrough or else telangiectatic osteosarcoma is a diagnostic possibility. MR imaging is invaluable for determining if there is soft tissue mass. CT scan is invaluable for assessing cortical integrity.

Given the differential may include the highly malignant telangiectatic osteosarcoma (TOS), the radiologist should not hesitate to utilize both CT and MRI for evaluation. Cross sectional imaging will typically show an ABC to have multiple cystic spaces with fluid-fluid levels containing blood degradation products. The MR signal characteristics are thus highly variable dependent on the age of blood products. There is usually thin, smooth enhancement of the margins of the cysts. There should be no mass or nodular component, or TOS is a possibility. It is difficult to exclude TOS in the setting of pathologic fracture of an ABC due to the traumatically altered cortex and the soft tissue hemorrhage and hematoma.

Unicameral bone cyst

UBC, also called simple bone cyst, is an idiopathic benign cyst of bone commonly presenting before the age of 20. These tend to occur centrally in the metaphysis of long bones and most commonly affect the humerus and femur. They often present after pathologic fracture. Radiographs will show a central, lucent lesion with minimal expansion and no matrix or periosteal reaction. The lesion may have minimal septation or multiloculation but as the name implies, these should be single chamber cysts. Pathologic fracture may result in the classic fallen fragment sign where a portion of fractured cortex displaces within the cystic space. This sign only proves the lesion has a cystic portion and hence could represent an UBC or fibrous dysplasia or an aggressive lesion of bone. MR imaging of a UBC will show a well circumscribed lesion with signal consistent with water; T1 low signal and T2 high signal. There may be thin, smooth enhancing margins without nodularity or mass.

The differential for a lucent lesion of the metaphysis in a young patient might include aneurysmal bone cyst, cavernous hemangioma and osteomyelitis. Signs of systemic illness should be present with osteomyelitis, and infection can cross the physis. Aneurysmal bone cyst may have much more expansion of bone and can have periosteal reaction. ABC and cavernous hemangiomas will have multiple fluid-fluid levels with complex MR signal with multiloculated morphology.

Fibrous dysplasia

FD is a benign disease of bone which can be monostotic or polyostotic. FD has a highly variable appearance ranging from a simple ground glass density lesion to an aggressive appearing lesion with expansion, periosteal reaction, wide zone of transition and mixed density. The radiologist may not be able to diagnose FD when the lesion has this heterogeneous or aggressive appearance. Fortunately, the typical lesion has ground glass density with somewhat irregular sclerotic margins and minimal expansion or distortion of the cortex and the diagnosis can be made with sufficient confidence to support conservative management.

On MR imaging, FD has a highly variable appearance depending on the amount of bone, fibrous tissue, cartilage and cystic component present. Enhancement is variable. Radiographs are usually the most specific imaging modality for diagnosing FD. However, CT may be helpful to confirm matrix type and CT is best for assessing extent of craniofacial disease. Leontiasis ossea or lion facies describes the deformity of the face and orbits when there is extensive craniofacial disease. This is not specific to FD and can also be seen with Paget disease and leprosy. Typically, FD involves and expands the outer table of the skull distinguishing it from Paget disease which predominantly involves the inner table. Bone scan is probably best for skeletal survey for initial assessment of monostotic versus polyostotic disease.

There are benign and malignant complications of FD. The abnormal bone will deform under load and weight bearing bones such as the femur will develop the shepherd crook deformity (see Figure 26.3e in the Case Presentation section of this chapter). The abnormal bone is also more prone to pathologic fracture. There are rare instances of malignant degeneration into sarcoma with osteosarcoma being most frequent, followed by fibrosarcoma and chondrosarcoma. Malignant degeneration is more likely to occur in polyostotic disease (Campanacci et al. 1979). Polyostotic disease is unilateral in 90% of cases.

There are several syndromes associated with fibrous dysplasia. McCune Albright is the association of polyostotic fibrous dysplasia, café-au-lait lesions of the skin and endocrinopathies. This occurs almost exclusively in girls with the endocrine abnormality usually being precocious puberty. Mazabraud syndrome is the association of polyostotic fibrous dysplasia and benign soft tissue myxomas.

Langerhans cell histiocytosis

LCH is an idiopathic disease of Langerhans cell overgrowth resulting in a broad spectrum of clinical disease. Previous nomenclature described three clinical entities including; eosinophilic granuloma (EG) with isolated skeletal disease and the best prognosis. Hand-Schüller-Christian disease involved the triad of bone lesions, exophthalmos and diabetes insipidus due to involvement of the pituitary stalk. Letterer-Siwe disease was the most fulminant version of disease presenting at the youngest age and involved multiple organs and the skeleton.

So called EG accounts for up to 60% of cases of LCH and may be monostotic or polyostotic. Skeletal disease usually involves the skull, spine, pelvis, ribs and mandible. Long bone disease typically involves the diaphysis but can occur in the metaphysis with the physis acting as a barrier to spread. Patients may present with bone pain, fever and can have a palpable tender mass. Bone lesions are lucent, sharply circumscribed with a punched out appearance. Lesions can sometimes have an aggressive appearance with permeative or moth-eaten destruction of bone and irregular periosteal reaction and soft tissue mass. In the skull, the lesions will affect both the inner and outer table resulting in a beveled edge appearance. Occasionally, there will be a dense central calcification called a button sequestrum. In the spine, an LCH lesion may have develop pathologic fracture and collapse of the vertebra causing a vertebra plana appearance. Interestingly, healing of the lesion may lead to recovery of vertebral body height (David et al. 1989). In the mandible, the lucent destructive lesion may give the appearance of floating teeth.

Erdheim-Chester disease

ECD is a rare non-Langerhans cell histiocytosis characterized by inflammatory infiltration of bone and other organs. Prognosis is poor with less than 50% survival at 3 years. The disease predominantly affects the long bones symmetrically, particularly of the lower extremity. Patients present with bone pain and can also have diabetes insipidus, exophthalmos, renal failure, pulmonary fibrosis, and heart failure. Radiographs typically show sclerosis of long bone diaphysis in 76% of cases. Osteolytic lesions can be seen in the skull and ribs in 14% (Veyssier-Belot et al. 1996). The cortex becomes thickened with narrowing of the medullary cavity and loss of the corticomedullary junction. The epiphyses are spared as can be seen with progressive diaphyseal dysplasia (Camurati-Engelmann disease) which is an inherited hyperostosis of long bones. There can be bone infarcts and periostitis (Ihde et al. 2011).

Rosai-Dorfman disease

This very rare disease of histocytes can affect any bone without preference. This includes all appendicular and axial bones, the gnathic bones and calvarium. Similarly, any part of a long bone may be affected (epiphysis, metaphysis, or diaphysis). The lesion is typically lytic with clearly defined margins that are occasionally sclerotic. Size is usually between 0.5-5 cm, and a soft tissue component may be present. MRI shows low signal intensity on T1 imaging and high signal on T2 with or without surrounding edema (Gupta et al. 2008). The radiologic features encompass a broad differential from infections to metastasis to myeloma, sarcoidosis, Langerhans cell histiocytosis, and lymphoma. Whole body MRI scan or radioisotope scans will identify multiple lesions

Chest wall hamartoma

Hamartoma of the chest wall is a rare benign lesion of infancy and childhood. These often present as a deforming chest wall mass found at birth, but can be found incidentally on chest radiography later in life. The mass always arises from a rib and involves the posterior rib in 79% of cases (Groom et al. 2002). Sixty four percent of cases show calcification with most having cartilaginous matrix evident. Also, hemorrhagic cavities with fluid-fluid levels are seen in 64% of cases with CT imaging and 80% of cases with T2 MR imaging, indicating secondary aneurysmal bone cyst formation. On MRI, the lesions are mostly T1 intermediate signal with some areas showing T1 high signal likely related to hemorrhage. The tumors show mild to moderate enhancement and are heterogeneous on T2 images.

SURGERY OF BENIGN MIMICKERS

Aneurysmal bone cyst

Although spontaneous regression of these tumors has been reported, most represent aggressive lesions that grow fairly rapidly and can cause substantial bone destruction. Curettage and bone grafting is the preferred method of treatment for these tumors. Recurrence rates as high as 30% have been reported. The use of mechanical (burr) or chemical adjuvants (phenol, cryotherapy, polymethylmethacrylate) may reduce the rate of recurrence. Wide resection may be indicated with multiple recurrences particularly in expendable bones. More significant reconstructive procedures may be necessary if the tumor has caused substantial bone loss.

Pre-operative embolization may be employed in an effort to reduce surgical blood loss which may be significant, particularly with axial lesions. Several studies support the role of sclerotherapy in the treatment of these tumors as an alternative to surgery.

SURGERY GRAY AREA

Although recurrence rates for these tumors can be relatively high with standard treatment, it should be remembered that eradication is generally accomplished with persistence. Since these tumors have negligible malignant potential, more aggressive procedures performed in an attempt to lower the recurrence rate at the cost of higher potential complications or compromised function should be considered cautiously.

Unicameral bone cyst

Because most UBCs will resolve after skeletal maturity, specific treatment is not always required. Asymptomatic cysts discovered incidentally which do not particularly appear to weaken the bone and remain stable over time can be observed, particularly if they occur in non-weight bearing bones. Traditional treatment has involved corticosteroid injection into the cyst or curettage and bone grafting (particularly for larger cysts). Recurrence rates vary from 15% to 88% after an average of three injections. Following curettage and grafting, recurrence rates have been reported as high as 45%. Multiple different agents have been introduced by injection or as an adjuvant to surgery with little overall change in the recurrence rates.

Most unicameral bone cysts present after pathologic fracture. Generally, the fractures are non-displaced and heal readily. Performing surgery early on these cases would require curettage of the cyst along with internal fixation of the fracture. As the added surgery required for fracture fixation is often unnecessary and increases the extent of the procedure and risk of complications, most surgeons advocate conservative management of the fracture followed by treatment of the cyst after the fracture has healed. An exception would perhaps be a high-stress area such as the subtrochanteric femur where early fixation of the fracture is likely indicated. Historically, the belief was that many cysts underwent involution following a fracture, but longer term follow-up has shown that this in fact rarely occurs.

Fibrous dysplasia

This dysplastic condition is extremely difficult to eradicate, particularly in the immature patient and/or in the presence of polyostotic disease. Asymptomatic lesions can be observed. Symptomatic lesions, and those associated with pathologic fracture or deformity prove more challenging. Curettage and bone grafting is rarely curative, as the bone graft is replaced by the same type of immature woven bone. Cortical bone graft is more resistant to degradation and may increase the time to recurrence. Intravenous bisphosphonates have proven successful in at least short term management of symptoms, however longer outcome term is unknown, and this treatment can be associated with other complications such as osteonecrosis of the jaw and stress fractures of the femur.

SURGERY GRAY AREA

Because of the difficulty eradicating this disease, current treatment often involves prophylactic fixation of the bone with intramedullary hardware without any specific attempt to treat the disease itself. This technique can be quite successful in controlling symptoms, preventing pathologic fracture, and minimizing associated deformity.

Langerhans cell histiocytosis

Multi-focal or disseminated forms of histiocytosis are generally treated systemically; surgery rarely plays a role. In the more common form of isolated bony lesions, eosinophilic granuloma, surgery may play a role. Despite the typically aggressive radiographic features, these lesions tend to behave in a relatively benign fashion and respond well to limited intervention. Even cases with substantial vertebral collapse rarely have associated neurologic findings. These lesions can be paucicellular so adequate tissue sampling during biopsy is required. Once the diagnosis is secured, many lesions will heal spontaneously and the bone will reconstitute even in cases of vertebra plana. Lesions often will respond to percutaneous corticosteroid injection. If operative intervention is chosen as the preferred treatment modality, simple curettage with or without bone graft generally results in resolution of the lesion.

Rosai-Dorfman disease

Most patients are treated conservatively with observation alone. However, if symptoms persist, or there are additional complications from the site of involvement, curettage can be performed.

MEDICAL ONCOLOGY

Aneurysmal bone cyst

Although this disease is usually not traditionally treated by Medical Oncology, the overexpression of RANK ligand might make the use of denosumab potentially attractive (Lange, 2013).

Langerhans cell histiocytosis

Histiocytic diseases in children and adults include three major classes of disorders, LCH, E-CD (primarily found in adults) and juvenile xanthogranuloma (diagnosed in children and adults). LCH is a dendritic cell disorder and the latter two, macrophage disorders. Other disorders of the macrophage/monocytoid lineages include benign disorders such as R-DD and hemophagocytic lymphohistiocytosis or malignant disorders including malignant histiocytosis of various histiocyte lineages (formerly called histiocytic sarcoma) and the monocytic or myelomonocytic leukemias. A good resource is the Histiocytosis Association and the Histiocytosis Society LCH includes a variety of syndromes; histiocytosis X, eosinophilic granuloma, Abt-Letterer-Siwe disease, Hand-Schüller-Christian disease, or diffuse reticuloendotheliosis. Gene expression profile revealed that the same myeloid dendritic precursor is responsible for these entities. The clinical spectrum includes acute disseminated disease (Letterer-Siwe disease), intermediate acuity (Hand-Schüller-Christian disease which presents with the triad of diabetes insipidus, proptosis, and lytic bone lesions) and indolent lesions (eosinophilic granulomas). A congenital variant is self-healing (Hashimoto-Pritzker disease).

The nomenclature used for LCH indicates the disease extent. LCH may involve a single organ (single-system LCH), either unifocally or multifocally, or multiple organs (multisystem LCH), which may be limited to a few organs or could be disseminated.

PEARL

Langerhans cells of the epidermis are different by morphology, phenotype, and gene expression from the clonal proliferation of the immunophenotypically and functionally immature cells seen in LCH (Allen et al. 2010).

Medical Oncology focuses on adult LCH. The disease incidence is rare, with 1 to 2 cases per million, and occurs in the fourth decade with a slight male preponderance (Arico et al. 2003).

In the German registry, 62% of patients have single-organ involvement and 38% multisystem involvement, with lung involvement in 34%, followed by bone and skin (Gotz et al. 2004). Any organ could be involved. Pulmonary LCH is seen in young adult smokers. Diabetes insipidus is a common manifestation of the disease (Garcia Gallo et al. 2010) and is treated symptomatically with desmopressin acetate (DDAVP). Symptoms in order of decreasing frequency include dyspnea, polydipsia and polyuria, bone pain, weight loss, fever, ataxia, and memory problems. Patients present with skin rash, scalp nodules, lymphadenopathies,soft tissue swelling near bone lesions, gingival hypertrophy, and hepatosplenomegaly.

The diagnosis is established by biopsy.

Treatment of adult Langerhans cell histiocytosis

Treatment varies with the clinical presentation. The lack of clinical trials limits evidence-based recommendations for adult patients. Treatment follows the guidelines established in pediatrics.

Localized treatments are reserved for single-system disease. An isolated bone lesion can be treated surgically or by radiotherapy (Cantu et al. 2012). However, mutilating surgery should be avoided and patients referred for chemotherapy. The bisphosphonate, pamidronate, has been administered to control severe bone pain in patients with multiple osteolytic lesions (Farran et al. 2001, Morimoto et al. 2011). Pulmonary involvement requires smoking cessation because of the probable causative effect in pulmonary LCH, since most adults have gradual progression of disease with continued smoking. Smoking avoidance might prevent the need for long term immunosuppression with drugs such as azathioprine or chemotherapy. Lung transplant may be necessary for adults with extensive pulmonary destruction from LCH (Suri et al. 2012). Skin involvement has been treated with various agents and techniques including topical tacrolimus, imiquimod, psoralen with long-wave ultraviolet radiation (PUVA), and oral isotretinoin (Park et al. 2012).

Chemotherapy is administered to patients with multisystem LCH or recurrent disease. Etoposide and vinblastine, with or without steroids, has been the mainstay of chemotherapy until recently (Gadneret al. 2008, Minkov et al. 2000). Newer therapies include cladribine (2-CdA) (Saven et al. 1999, Weitzman, et al. 2009) and the combination of MACOP-B (methotrexate, doxorubicin, cyclophosphamide, vincristine, prednisone and bleomycin), a lymphoma regimen (Derenzini et al. 2010).

Biological therapies have included imatinib mesylate which has been effective in a few cases (Caponetti et al. 2012, Montella et al. 2004). Thalidomide and lenalidomide have also been used in a few cases. The BRAF mutation V600E was demonstrated in about 40% of LCH. Thus drug targeting this mutation, such as vemurafenib, could be helpful for the treatment of LCH (Badalian-Very, et al. 2012, Sahm, et al. 2012). Other potential treatments include monoclonal antibody targeting with indium-labeled anti-CD1a, alemtuzumab, low-dose oral cyclophosphamide, and all-*trans* retinoic acid.

For refractory or fulminant disease, allogenous bone marrow transplantation should be considered.

Erdheim-Chester disease

This very rare disease is not currently curable. There are no well-established treatment regimens. Some minor success has been achieved in individual patients using steroids, interferon, or various chemotherapeutic agents.

Rosai-Dorfman disease

Patients requiring treatment comprise individuals with recurrent or relapsing symptoms or those who have neurologic symptoms from lesional extension into the spinal canal. Many patients respond to steroids. A few will require chemotherapy such as methotrexate, vinblastine, 6-MP, thalidomide or Gleevec.

RADIATION ONCOLOGY OF UNDEFINED NEOPLASTIC NATURE

Most bone tumors of undefined neoplastic nature are benign. Radiation therapy is not indicated for these benign entities. Included in the benign group of bone tumors of undefined neoplastic nature are the ABC, simple bone cyst, FD, osteofibrous dysplasia, and chest wall hamartoma.

Radiation therapy has been used to treat the other types of bone tumors of undefined neoplastic nature. First, LCH is generally curable with surgery alone. If surgery is not possible, then radiation therapy may be used with good success. Usually, between 6 to 10 Gray is sufficient to achieve an 80-90% local control rate. LCH may induce diabetes insipidus. Radiation therapy delivered within 1 week of diagnosis of this condition is recommended for optimal results. A dose of 15 Gray is usually prescribed in these circumstances.

Radiation therapy has been used in patients with R-DD as adjunctive treatment. Doses range from 20-30 Gy.

Finally, palliative radiation therapy has been used for E-CD. A dose between 10 to 20 Gray can induce excellent short term palliation. Unfortunately, the duration of palliation is usually short lived. This may be due to the repopulation of the treated area with abnormal histiocytes and recurrence of symptoms (Miller et al. 2006).

Table 26.3 Clinical trials for LCH

Trial	Drugs	Outcome	Reference
European cooperative clinical trial	Vinblastine, etoposide, and prednisone for 6 weeks, followed by mercaptopurine, vinblastine, and prednisone for 1 year with addition of etoposide for soft tissue lesions and methotrexate for organ dysfunction	Disease-free survival rate, 77% at 6 years	Gadner, et al. 1994
LCH-I trial	Etoposide or vinblastine for 24 weeks	Equivalent responses at week 6 with similar effects on survival and disease recurrence	Gadner, et al. 2001
LCH-II trial	Vinblastine, oral prednisone, and mercaptopurine with or without etoposide for 24 weeks	Etoposide has marginal benefit	Gadner, et al. 2003
LCH-III trial	Vinblastine and prednisone with or without methotrexate for 6 to 12 months	Methotrexate has marginal benefit	Minkov 2011

CASES

Case 26.1 Aneurysmal bone cyst

Clinical history and presentation

The patient is a 5 year old girl who sustained an injury to the right leg 3 months previously during a minor fall. Pain resolved after one week and she is currently asymptomatic.

Physical examination of the right leg is unremarkable. Imaging studies reveal a lesion in the right tibia suspicious for ABC.

Surgical findings and comments

Curettage and allografting of the tibial lesion are performed.

Radiology findings

Our case, **Case figs 26.1a** through **Case fig. 26.1d**, shows a multi-loculated mass of the proximal tibial metaphysis of this 5 year old girl. The dominant feature of the lesion is the multiple fluid - fluid levels with mild expansion but no cortical breakthrough. The differential for this includes telangiectatic osteosarcoma which should have cortical breakthrough and a soft tissue mass but may not show calcifying osteoid. Please also see Case presentation 17.4 (Chapter 17) of telangiectatic OS for comparison. Cross sectional imaging is invaluable to assess for cortical integrity and the presence of soft tissue mass. The distinction is critical, and the radiologist should not hesitate to employ both CT for cortical assessment and MRI for soft tissue assessment in this clinical setting. Unfortunately, these lesions can present with pathologic fracture which can greatly complicate imaging assessment, as an ABC will then have soft tissue hematoma that can masquerade as a soft tissue tumor of TOS. Tissue diagnosis may then be required.

The additional case of ABC, **Case figs 28.1e** through **Case fig. 26.1n**, show a markedly expansile lesion with fluid-fluid levels but no cortical breakthrough and no soft tissue mass. The radiographs do not definitively prove the intact cortex. The MR exam excludes a soft tissue mass, but the anterior portion of the lesion has marked cortical thinning with possible cortical breakthrough. The CT scan was crucial in this case to show cortical integrity and thus exclude telangiectatic OS.

Pathology findings

Gross features

The specimen consists of a 2 cm aggregate of tan to red fibroconnective tissue with intermixed bone splinters. A small amount is sent to Cytogenetics, and the remainder is submitted in two cassettes.

Microscopic features

Low magnification: The lesion is mixed solid and cystic with free-floating strips of cyst walls and areas of acute hemorrhage (**Case fig. 26.1o**).

High magnification: The fibrous septa separating cystic spaces range in cellularity and collapse together when cyst contents are expelled after curettage (**Case fig. 26.1p**). Cellular septa feature two types of osteoid: ribbons of pink osteoid and chunks of pale basophilic 'blue bone' (**Case fig. 26.1q**). A more solid area forming 15% of the entire lesion consists of crowded, round to spindled cells with loose clusters of relatively small osteoclastic giant cells (**Case fig. 26.1r**). This field resembles giant cell reparative granuloma. Basophilic bone exhibits a mottled ragged appearance and is composed of partly calcified osteo chondroid (**Case fig. 26.1s**). The blue bone is not specific to ABC and can be found in osteoblastoma, Nora's lesion (bizarre parosteal osteochondromatous proliferation), and phosphaturic mesenchymal tumor, among others. Tumor cells show mild nuclear shape variability, but chromatin is fine (**Case fig. 26.1t**).

Special studies: The karyotype is 46,XX[20]. Many primary ABC demonstrate translocation of the *USP6* gene (17p13) with active promoters of several other genes, the most common of which is *CDH11* resulting in a t(16;17)(q22;p13)(van de Luijtgaarden et al. 2009). Other partners are located at 1p34, 3q21, 9q22, and 17q21 (Geiersbach et al. 2011). Secondary ABCs lack *USP6* rearrangements (Oliveira et al. 2004).

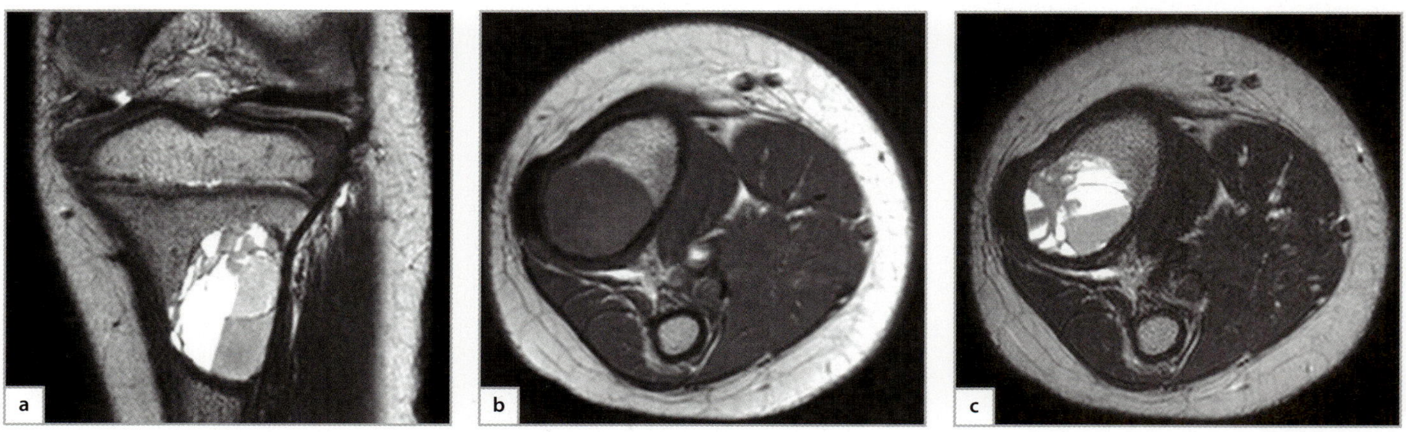

Case figure 26.1 Aneurysmal bone cyst. MR images including; **26.1a**: Coronal T2, **26.1b**: Axial T1, **26.1c**: Axial T2.

Case figure 26.1: Continued from page 564

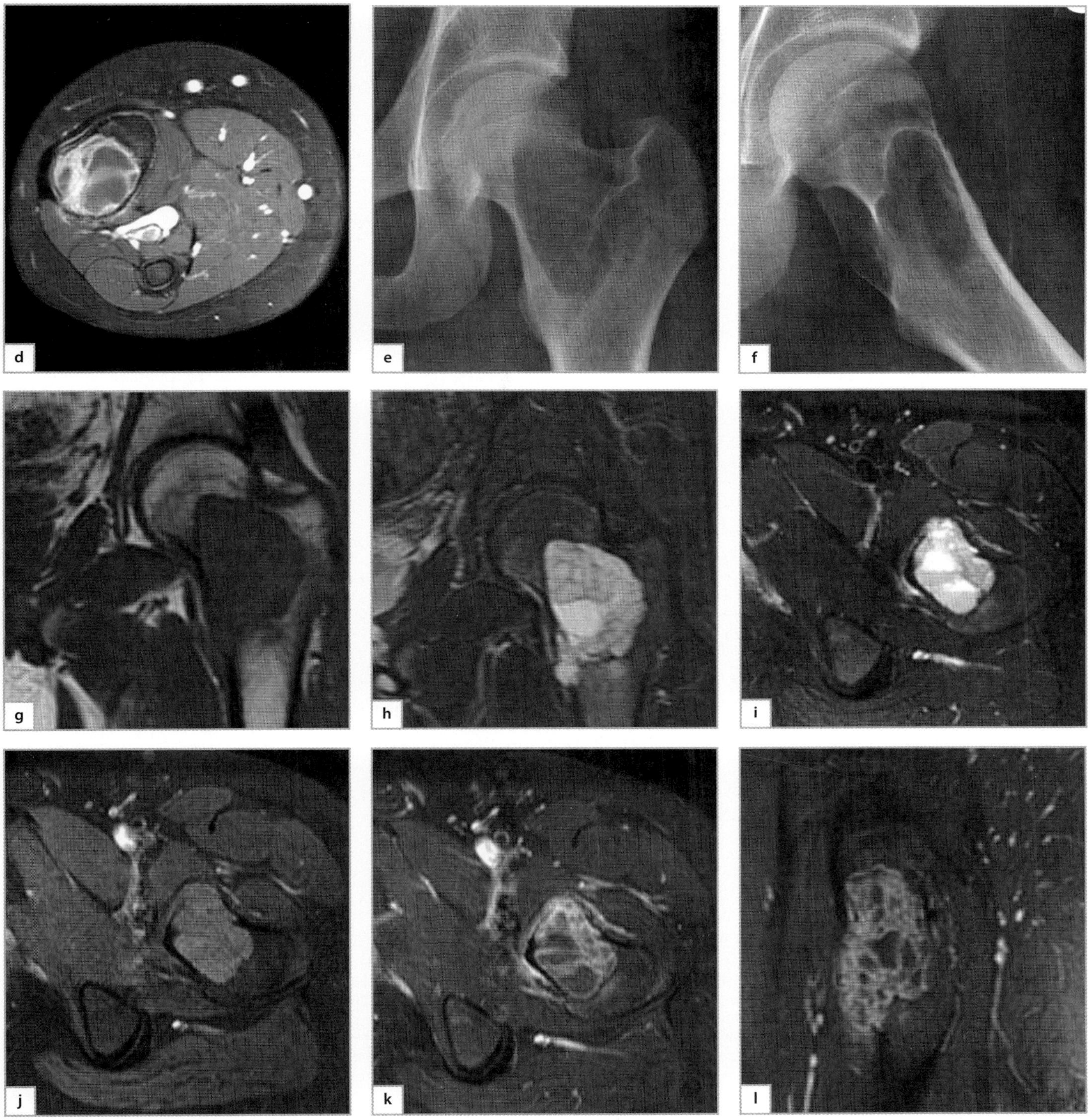

26.1d Axial T1 fat saturated post-contrast are presented of the proximal tibia in this 5 year old female. There is a mutiloculated 3.1 × 2 × 2 cm mass with fluid – fluid levels. There is mild expansion of the overlying cortex with mild cortical thinning but no soft tissue mass or full thickness breakthrough. The lesion is predominantly T1 iso-intense to muscle with variable T2 signal depending on the hemorrhage and protein content of the fluid. The lesion shows intense thin rim enhancement without nodularity or solid component. *Additional case of ABC in a 19 year old man with a femoral neck lesion.* **26.1e**: Anteroposterior, **26.1f**: Frog lateral radiographs show a lucent lesion of the femoral neck without matrix or sclerotic margin. The lesion causes anterior expansion as seen on lateral view with a subtle shell of calcification. It is not definitively clear from the radiograph if the expanded cortex is intact.

Case figure 26.1: Continued from page 565

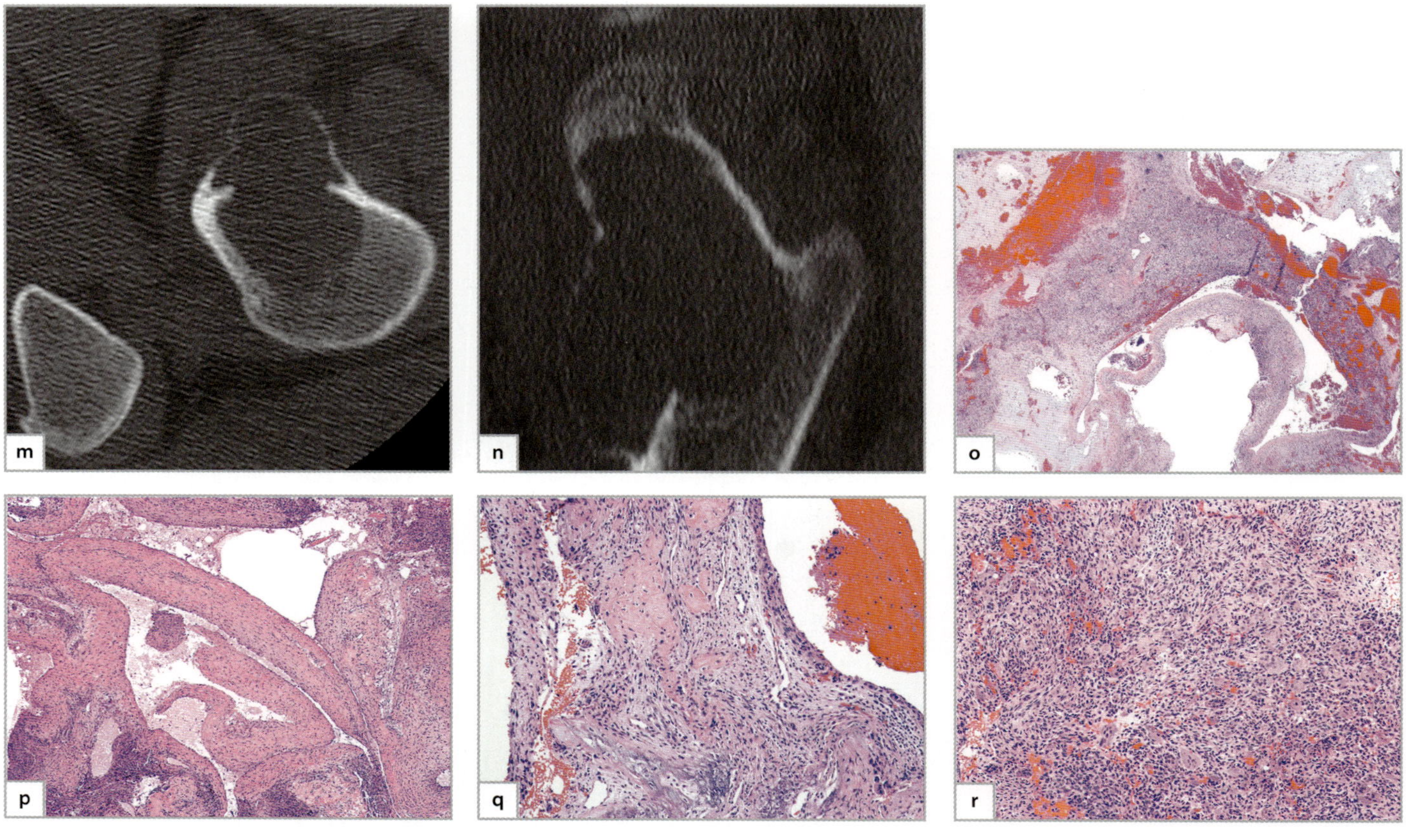

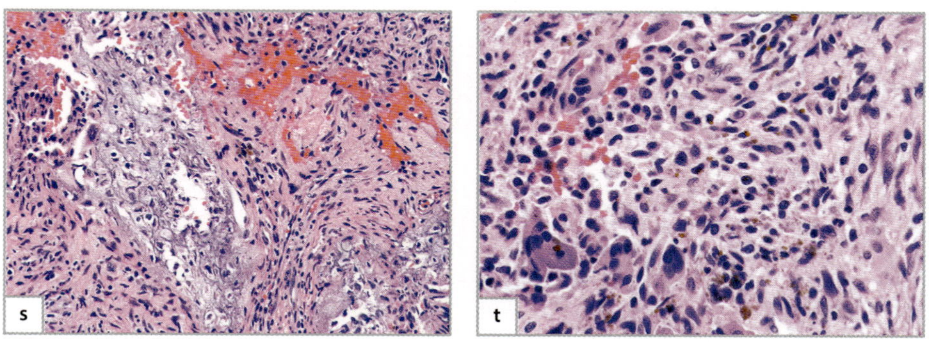

MR images include: **26.1g** Coronal T1, **26.1h**: Coronal STIR, **26.1i**: Axial STIR, **26.1j**: Axial T1 fat saturated, **26.1k**: Axial T1 fat saturated post-contrast, **26.1l**: Sagittal T1 fat saturated post-contrast. The MR images show an expansile lesion with T1 low signal and STIR high signal and multiple fluid-fluid levels. There is rim enhancement without nodularity or definite soft tissue mass. The axial STIR image, **26.1i**: Shows marked anterior cortical thinning with possible breakthrough. However, the CT exam, **26.1m**: axial image and, **26.1n**: Coronal reformation image show that despite marked expansion and thinning, the anterior cortex remains intact. No soft tissue mass is found. **26.1o**: Aneurysmal bone cyst (ABC), low magnification. The lesion is multiloculated with cystic spaces and variably cellular fibrous septa. Acute hemorrhage is present. **26.1p**: Medium magnification. The fibrotic septa collapse against each other. **26.1q**: Medium magnification. A band of pink osteoid curls up the middle of this septum. At the lower left is 'blue bone'. **26.1r**: Medium magnification. A more solid area consists of round to spindled cells with small foci of acute hemorrhage and somewhat clustered, relatively small osteoclastic giant cells. Solid areas of ABC are often histologically identical to giant cell reparative granuloma and Brown tumor of hyperparathyroidism. **26.1s**: High magnification. Mottled, partly calcified, basophilic osteo chondroid ('blue bone') is present arising in a fibrotic, spindle cell matrix. Blue bone is common in ABC but not specific. **26.1t**: High magnification. The tumor cells vary mildly in nuclear size, but worrisome features such as macronucleoli and coarse chromatin are absent. Fibroblasts, osteoblasts, histiocytes and osteoclastic giant cells compose the majority of the tumor. Hemosiderin as well as fresh hemorrhage may also be present as in this field.

Pathologic differential or, why isn't it one of the following?

Giant cell tumor of bone (GCT) with secondary ABC changes: The characteristic features of GCT of bone must be present comprising an even distribution of large, multinucleated osteoclastic giant cells with a mononuclear stromal cell component that matches the giant cells in nuclear characteristics. GCT of bone occurs in skeletally mature bones and is epiphyseal, while many ABC occur in the metaphysis of skeletally immature bones or the posterior element of the vertebral body. Genetically, ABC exhibits USP6 gene rearrangements (~60% of primary ABC), while GCT of bone commonly demonstrates telomeric associations.

Chondroblastoma of bone with secondary ABC changes: Chondroblastoma must be present and is composed of sheets of round to polygonal cells with grooved or clefted nuclei with interspersed nodules of blue to pink chondroid and scattered osteoclastic giant cells. Osteoid is absent. The chondroblastoma cells are often reactive for S-100 protein and smooth muscle actin and may express DOG-1, a protein of unknown function expressed in gastrointestinal stromal tumors. Chondroblastoma and ABC occur in an overlapping age group of predominantly children to young adults. Chondroblastoma is generally epiphyseal rather than metaphyseal in location. *USP6* gene alterations are absent in chondroblastoma.

Phosphaturic mesenchymal tumor, mixed connective tissue type: Although highly vascular, phosphaturic mesenchymal tumor (PMT) lacks the blood filled cystic spaces of ABC. It contains usually bland spindled to stellate fibroblasts mixed with myxochondroid matrix with mottled calcifications, and numerous osteoclastic giant cells. 'Blue bone' may be present. PMT more commonly affects middle-aged adults and is typically associated with osteomalacia with phosphaturia, hyperphosphatemia and low or normal serum levels of vitamin D. Most cases demonstrate expression of fibroblast growth factor-23 (FGF23) by RT-PCR or IHC (Graham et al. 2012). Interestingly, approximately 40% of ABC also expresses FGF23 by RT-PCR (Graham et al. 2012). Chondromyxoid fibromas and fibrous dysplasia may also overexpress FGF23 by RT-PCR (Kobayashi et al. 2006). ABC is not associated with osteomalacia, and patients have normal serum and urine phosphate levels. *USP6* gene translocations have not been found in PMT.

Telangiectatic osteosarcoma: Telangiectatic osteosarcoma (TOS) and ABC may appear radiologically similar, and both occur in children in the metaphysis of long bones most commonly. TOS exhibits nuclear atypia, a high mitotic rate and may contain atypical mitotic figures. Genetically, TOS exhibits a complex aneuploid karyotype and lacks *USP6* translocations, while primary ABC is diploid, and most reveal *USP6* translocations.

Case table 26.1a Variant pathology features of ABC

Feature	Frequency	Comment
Primary ABC: Blood filled cystic spaces separated by fibrous septa	Common	This is the classic appearance of ABC. Fibrous septa range in cellularity but may be highly cellular Lesional cells comprise fibroblasts, mononuclear histiocytes, osteoclasts, and osteoblasts lining reactive woven bone Chronic inflammation is also present in varying amounts
'Solid ABC': Solid growth only without cysts	Uncommon	~10% of primary ABC This may be equivalent to giant cell reparative granuloma. Cellular components are as above
Pink bands or ribbons of osteoid running along the long axis of fibrous septa	Common	This is a characteristic feature of ABC
'Blue Bone' = mottled, calcified basophilic osteoid and bone found in fibrous septa	Uncommon	Seen in approximately 25% of ABC Not specific for ABC but relatively restricted to a few tumors including osteoblastoma, phosphaturic mesenchymal tumor, and bizarre parosteal osteochondromatous proliferation of the hands and feet
Chondromyxoid foci	Uncommon	May become focally calcified and merges with appearance of 'blue bone'
Cortical breakthrough with eggshell rim of reactive periosteal new bone	Common	Attests to the aggressive local growth of ABC
Cortical breakthrough with ABC abutting normal soft tissue	Uncommon	Lacks a permeative pattern
Necrosis	Rare	Usually associated with pathologic fracture
Mitotic activity	Common	Atypical mitoses are absent
Hemosiderin	Common	May be extracellular or within macrophages (siderophages) May be surrounded by a ring of osteoclastic giant cells
FGF23 Expression by RT-PCR	Common	Found in 40% of primary ABC in one study (Graham et al. 2012). FGF23 is also expressed in most phosphaturic mesenchymal tumors, some chondromyxoid fibromas and a few fibrous dysplasias
USP6 gene rearrangements in primary ABC	Common	Found in majority of primary ABC. Common partners are: 16q22, 1p34, 3q21, 9q22, and 17q21
Diploid karyotype	Common	Typical of primary ABC
Secondary ABC: ABC-like changes that arise in the background of another bone tumor	Common	Tumors associated with secondary ABC include giant cell tumor of bone, osteoblastoma, fibrous dysplasia, chondroblastoma, and osteosarcoma, among others
Soft tissue location of primary ABC	Rare	Has histologic features of solid ABC May mimic myositis ossificans USP6 translocations are present
Malignant transformation to osteosarcoma	Rare	Must exclude primary osteosarcoma with secondary ABC formation
Metastatic behavior in absence of radiation or sarcomatous transformation	Very rare (1 case report)	Tumor was diploid by karyotype, metastasized to lungs and showed USP6 gene translocation The patient had a 27 cm pelvic ABC with multiple surgical interventions and bevacizumab therapy (van de Luijtgaarden et al. 2009)

Case table 26.1b Summary pathology findings of Case 26.1

Diagnosis	Aneurysmal bone cyst
Size	3.1 × 2 × 2 cm
Location	Proximal tibial metaphysis
Margin status	Positive (curettage specimen)
Histologic grade	Not graded: benign lesion
Pathologic stage	Not staged: benign lesion

Oncology approach

Medical oncology

Medical oncology is not indicated for aneurysmal bone cyst.

Radiation oncology

Radiation therapy is not indicated for aneurysmal bone cyst.

Patient outcome

Three years postoperatively the patient has no symptoms, normal function, and no radiographic evidence of recurrence.

Case 26.2 Unicameral bone cyst

Clinical history and presentation

The patient is a 12 year old boy who presents with a three month history of left hip pain. Symptoms began while playing sports but he denies a specific history of injury. Pain is increased with activity and relieved with rest. He denies pain at rest or at night.

Physical examination reveals full range of motion of the left hip with mild pain at extremes.

Surgical findings and comments

Curettage and allografting of the femoral lesion are performed.

Radiology findings

Our case, **Case figs 26.2a** and **26.2b** show a lucent lesion of the proximal femoral metaphysis of a 12 year old boy. The lesion is non-aggressive as evidenced by the uniform sclerotic margins without periosteal reaction or expansion. UBCs can sometimes have scallops or partial bone septa that can give the lesion a multiloculated appearance. The differential might include a cavernous hemangioma of bone and fibrous dysplasia. Cross sectional imaging may help distinguish between these. MRI might show multiple fluid levels and true multi-loculations in a cavernous hemangioma. CT would typically show ground glass matrix in fibrous dysplasia. A UBC will have a thin featureless margin with no solid components. The classic radiographic finding of a UBC is the fallen fragment sign which can occur after pathologic fracture. We present two additional cases with fallen fragments, **Case figs 26.2c** and **26.2d**. The fallen fragment simply indicates there is a cystic space in the bone lesion where a cortical fragment might settle dependently. The presence of a cyst is not necessarily specific for a UBC, and the radiologist must be careful that the cyst represents the entirety of the lesion before diagnosing UBC.

Pathology findings

Gross features

The specimen consists of 3 cm in aggregate, fibromembranous connective tissue fragments mixed with trabecular bone fragments. A small portion is submitted fresh for karyotyping, and the remainder is submitted in two casettes for routine histology.

Microscopic features

Low magnification: The lesion consists primarily of collapsed, hypocellular strips of fibrous tissue. A more solid region is also hypocellular but relatively vascular and consistent with early reparative fibroplasia (**Case fig. 26.2e**).

High magnification: Some areas feature fibrosis, reactive woven bone, and cholesterol clefts from fat necrosis (**Case fig. 26.2f**) consistent with tissue injury after microtrauma. A small amount of hypocellular myxoid fibrous tissue is also present featuring spindled fibroblasts without nuclear atypia (**Case fig. 26.2g**).

Special studies: The karyotype is 46,XY.

Pathologic differential or, why isn't it one of the following?

Aneurysmal bone cyst: UBC may be multiloculated like ABC and may contain blood especially in cases of pathologic fracture. Radiologic features can help distinguish the two lesions. Pathologic fracture can result in increased cellularity in a UBC with fibroblasts, osteoclasts, hemosiderin, fibrin deposits, cholesterol clefts, inflammation and reactive bone. This increased cellularity can mimic ABC. However, long strands of pink osteoid in fibrous septa and 'blue bone' are absent in UBC. ABC demonstrates *USP6* translocations absent in UBC.

Fibrous dysplasia: FD can have a cystic component that can resemble UBC or ABC. However, classic areas are characterized by cellular fibrotic stroma with embedded woven bone spicules of varying size and shape devoid of osteoblastic rimming. These areas are generally more cellular than UBC. The solid areas in UBC are usually composed of reactive tissue such as granulation tissue or fibrosis.

Intraosseous ganglion: Intraosseous ganglion (IOG) occurs in middle aged and older patients in contrast to UBC which largely affects children. IOG is usually subchondral and contains abundant mucoid material. The wall is similar to UBC in being thin, hypocellular and fibrous. A few more solid areas consist of myxoid degeneration of fibrous tissue.

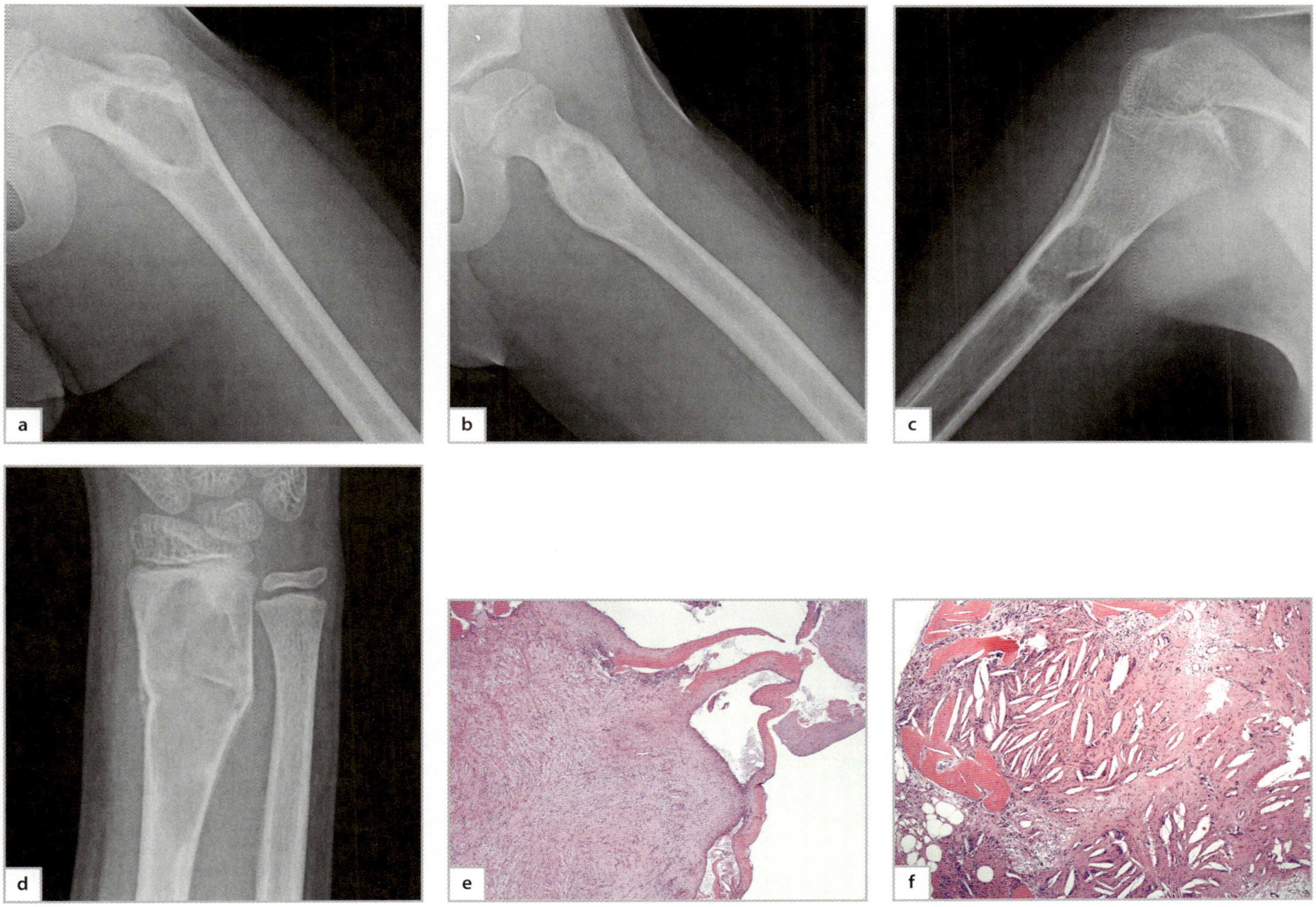

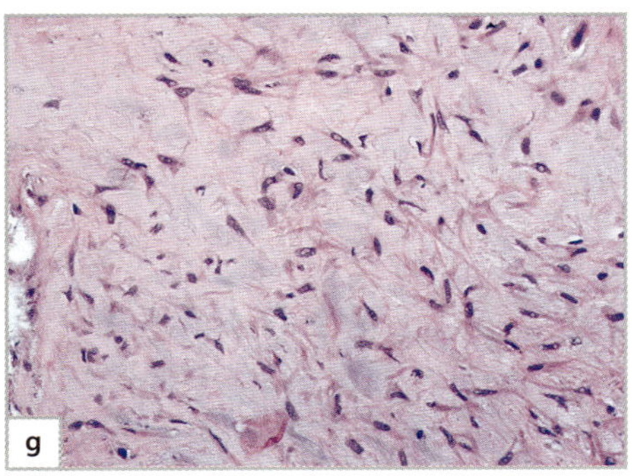

Case figure 26.2 Unicameral bone cyst 26.2a: Anteroposterior, **26.2b**: Frog leg lateral views of the left hip are presented in this 10 year old boy. There is a 2.1 × 4.2 × 3.1 cm lucent lesion of the proximal femoral metaphysis. There is a smooth sclerotic margin of uniform thickness. There are no aggressive features such as periosteal reaction, erosion or soft tissue mass. No matrix or fracture is apparent. Two additional cases of Bone Cysts. **26.2c**: Is an anteroposterior radiograph of the proximal humerus in an 11 year old boy. There is a non-displaced fracture with a fallen fragment of cortex projecting adjacent to the medial cortex. The second additional case, **26.2d**: Is an anteroposterior radiograph in a 9 year old boy showing a distal radial metaphyseal fracture with a fragment of cortex that has fallen into a rotated position oriented transversely. **26.2e**: Low magnification. The lesion consists of strips of hypocellular fibrous tissue focally attached to more solid areas that are also hypocellular and fibrous. **26.2f**: Medium magnification. A few areas exhibit fat necrosis with cholesterol cleft formation, fibrosis and reactive woven bone consistent with microtrauma. **26.2g**: High magnification. Wispy, myxoid hypocellular fibrous tissue is focally present. The elongate fibroblasts have hypochromatic, non-atypical nuclei.

Table 26.2a Variant pathology features of UBC

Feature	Frequency	Comment
Cystic cavity with or without septations filled with serous or sanguinous fluid	Common	The lesion does not expand the bone unlike most ABC
Cyst wall and septa are usually hypocellular	Common	Septa are not as common as in ABC and cyst lining is grossly usually thin, often membranous
Reactive woven bone	Common	Typical pink osteoid with rimming osteoblasts and osteocytes
Findings consistent with microfracture or pathologic fracture	Common	Cholesterol clefts, hemosiderin, granulation tissue, hemorrhage, osteoclasts, fibrin, fibrosis and calcifications can be present
Cementum like bodies	Uncommon	Calcified fibrin nodules that resemble cementum
'Solidified' UBC	Rare	Consists of hypocellular fibrous and myxofibrous tissue without a prominent cyst cavity. Controversial entity

Case table 26.2b Summary pathology findings of case 26.2

Diagnosis	UBC also termed simple bone cyst
Size	2.1 × 4.2 × 3.1 cm
Location	Proximal femoral metaphysis
Margin status	Positive (curettage specimen)
Histologic grade	Not graded: benign lesion
Pathologic stage	Not graded: benign lesion

Oncology approach

Medical oncology

Medical oncology is not indicated for UBC.

Radiation oncology

Radiation therapy is not indicated for UBC.

Patient outcome

Sixteen months postoperatively the patient has no symptoms, normal function, and no radiographic evidence of recurrence.

Case 26.3 Fibrous dysplasia

Clinical history and presentation

The patient is an 18 year old woman with a known history of FD of the right proximal femur initially diagnosed and treated nine years previously with curettage, bone grafting, and internal fixation. She has been well until two months ago when she developed insidious onset recurrent hip pain which has been progressive.

Physical examination reveals a scar over the lateral aspect of the right proximal thigh. She has full range of motion of the right hip but experiences groin pain with extreme internal rotation.

Radiographs reveal progressive tumor.

Surgical findings and comments

Repeat surgery is performed with replacement of the internal fixation device, curettage of the tumor and bone grafting with a combination of crushed cancellous and cortical strut allograft.

Radiology findings

Our case, **Case figs 26.3a** through **26.3d**, show a ground glass density lesion of the proximal femur in an 18 year old woman. The lesion shows a sclerotic margin without aggressive features. The presence of ground glass matrix indicates fibrous matrix and strongly suggests fibrous dysplasia. FD can have a markedly variable appearance with cystic change, expansion and mixed density. FD can be polyostotic, in which case 90% are unilateral. Bone scan or radiographic survey of the skeleton may be warranted to diagnose the extent of involvement. FD can lead to deformities, especially in weight bearing bones, and early intervention may prevent morbidity.

We present three additional cases of fibrous dysplasia in **Case figs 26.3e** through **26.3j**. These demonstrate the heterogeneous appearance of FD. Note the differing degree of lesion expansion, deformity and mixed density. The presence of ground glass matrix is highly variable in FD.

Pathology findings

Gross features

The specimen comprises 5.5 × 5 × 2 cm in aggregate of tan-brown to golden yellow soft tissue fragments with interspersed bone spicules. The specimen is submitted in 6 cassettes with two requiring light decalcification.

Microscopic features

Low magnification: The tumor is located in the medullary portion of the bone and expands outward with a minimally invasive border around pre-existing bone trabeculae (**Case fig. 26.3k**).

High magnification: The new bone formed by the lesional cells has been likened to Chinese characters or alphabet soup. They are abnormally shaped with highly variable branches and curves (**Case fig. 26.3l**). The bone spicules are always composed of woven (immature) bone (**Case fig. 26.3m**). Polarization can confirm the woven nature of the bone, and the increased number of osteocytes is another clue to its immaturity. The stroma is focally hypercellular (**Case fig. 26.3n**). Storiforming areas of stroma can resemble non-ossifying fibroma or desmoplastic fibroma (**Case fig. 26.3o**). High magnification of a spicule reveals a lack of rimming osteoblasts and comb-like extensions of collagen from bone edge into stroma like Sharpey's fibers (**Case fig. 26.3p**). The lesional spindled cells are not cytologically atypical. Necrosis is absent.

Special studies: Special studies are not performed, because the patient has a history of biopsy diagnosed fibrous dysplasia at the same site, the radiology is consistent with FD, and the current histopathology is classic.

Pathologic differential or, why isn't it one of the following?

Low grade osteosarcoma: Low grade central osteosarcoma can appear similar histologically to fibrous dysplasia. Lamellar bone may even be found in well-differentiated osteosarcoma, a stage of maturation not achieved in FD. Subtle cytologic atypia is present in the spindle tumor cells of low grade osteosarcoma that is lacking in fibrous dysplasia. This is manifested as increased nuclear size and coarse chromatin. Additionally, most low grade osteosarcomas express MDM2 and/or CDK4 by IHC (Dujardin et al. 2011), and FD does not.

Osteofibrous dysplasia: This lesion is rare compared with fibrous dysplasia and is closely related to adamantinoma of long bones. It is nearly always diagnosed in young childhood and only

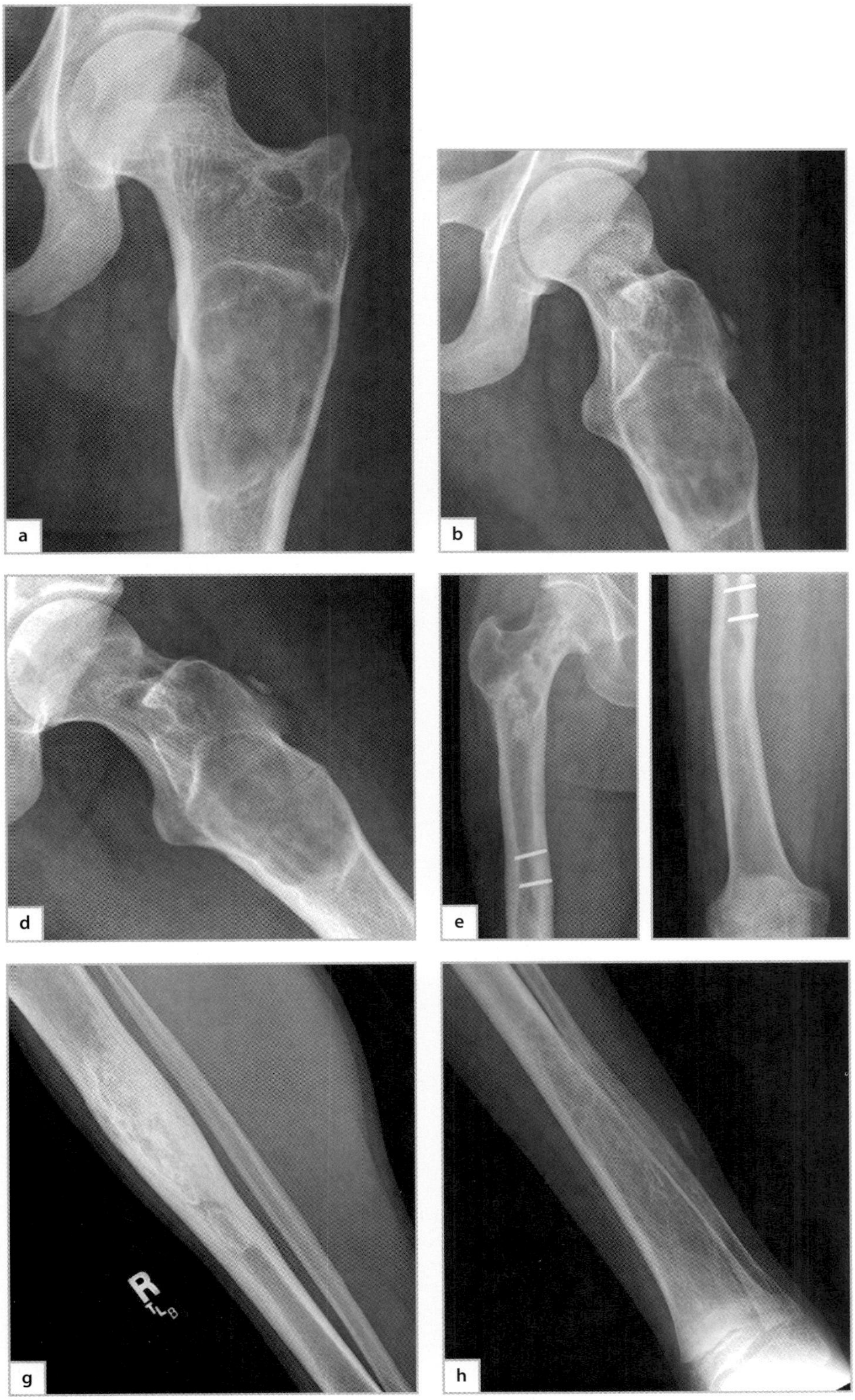

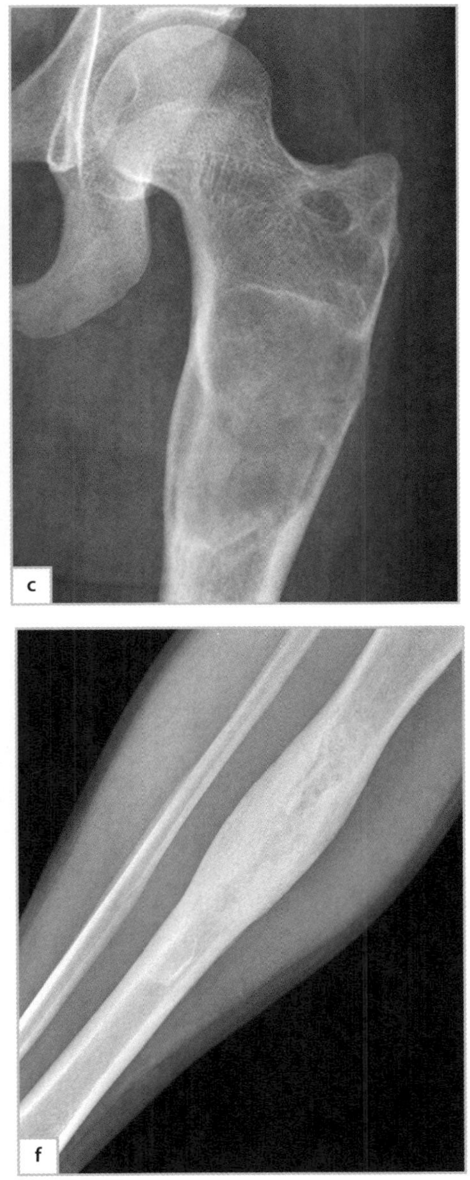

Case figure 26.3 Fibrous dysplasia.
26.3a Anteroposterior, **26.3b**: Frog lateral views of the left hip in this 20 year old woman show a lucent lesion with ground glass density. The margin is sclerotic with mildly irregular thickness. There are also some areas showing mild expansion of the cortex with minimal thinning. There are no aggressive features such as periosteal reaction, soft tissue mass or erosion destruction. The follow-up radiographs. **26.3c**: Anteroposterior, **26.3d**: Frog lateral view were obtained 14 weeks later show a non-displaced pathologic fracture. *Three additional cases of fibrous dysplasia.* **26.3e**: Anteroposter or views of the right femur in a 50 year old male with polyostotic disease showing a mild bowing deformity convex laterally called a shepherd crook deformity. The lesion shows mixed density with retained screw fragments from previous fixation hardware. **26.3f**: Anteroposterior, **26.3g**: Lateral views of the right tibia showing an expansile lesion with mixed density. The second case is also a patient with polyostotic fibrous dysplasia involving a 9 year old boy. **26.3h**: Anteroposterior.

Case figure 26.3: Continued from page 571

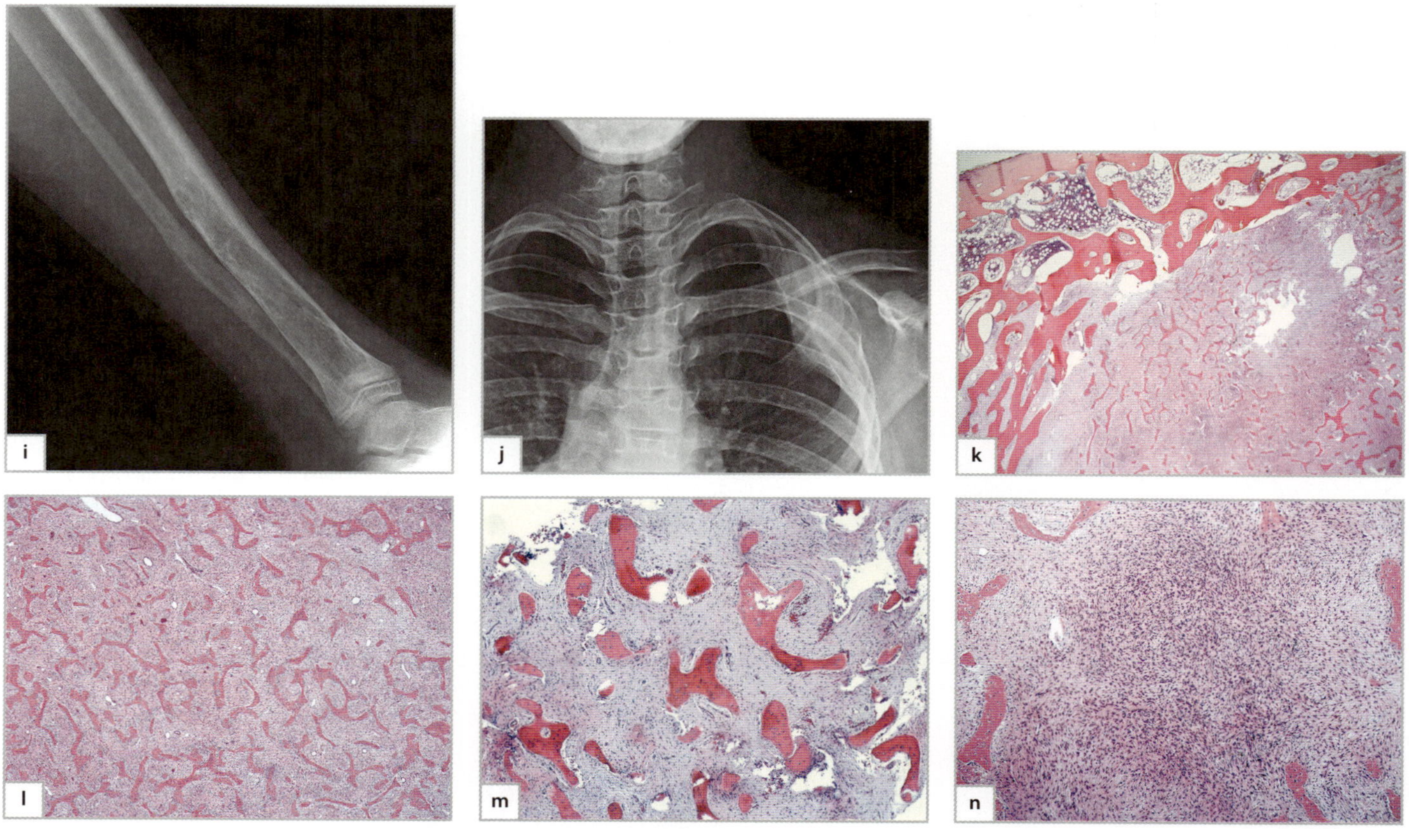

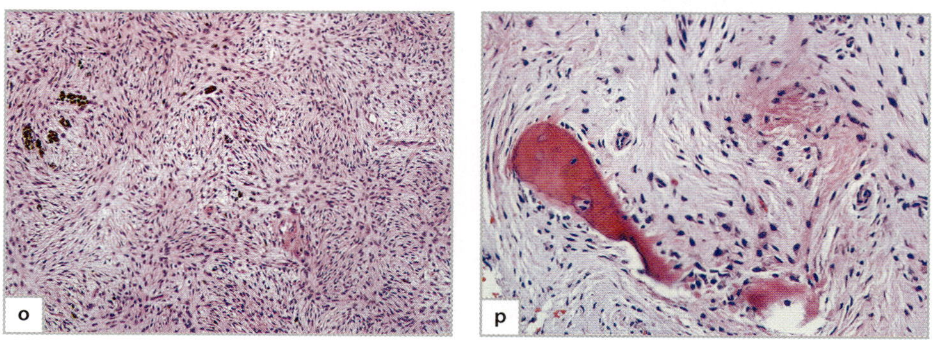

26.3i: Lateral views of the tibia and fibula show mixed density mildly sclerotic lesions of the distal metaphyses. The third case of fibrous dysplasia affects a 13 year old girl. **26.3j**: Anteroposterior view of the left ribs show an expansile ground glass density lesion of the 3rd rib without associated lung disease. **26.3k**: Low magnification of presented case. The tumor expands outward from its central medullary base. It exhibits a minimally invasive border with adjacent slightly thickened host trabecular bone. At the leading edge of the lesion, normal bone marrow is being replaced. Notice, in this case, the small size of the FD spicules compared to the patient's native trabecular bone. **26.3l**: Medium magnification. The woven bone formed in fibrous dysplasia is famous for fanciful shapes, curves and branches and in the past has been compared with Chinese characters (they are more like shorthand script) and alphabet soup. In this case, the proportion of bone to fibrous stroma is consistent. **26.3m**: Medium magnification. The bone in FD is always woven (immature). Woven bone contains more osteocytes than mature lamellar bone, and its mat-like collagen deposition is easily appreciated on polarization. **26.3n**: Medium magnification. The stroma in this field is cellular. The new bone formed by the tumor may be sparse or irregularly distributed and can cause diagnostic difficulty on a small needle core biopsy. **26.3o**: Higher magnification. Here the stroma is prominently storiforming. Such areas on a small biopsy could be mistaken for non-ossifying fibroma or desmoplastic fibroma. Notice the hemosiderin deposition which is fairly common in FD, especially lesions in the ribs. **26.3p**: High magnification. Few if any osteoblasts rim the woven bone present in FD. Instead, the spicules seem to arise out of the fibrous stroma de novo. This spicule shows a thin outer layer of unmineralized new bone and short anchoring collagen bands similar to Sharpey's fibers of normal cortical bone.

rarely occurs at sites other than the cortex of the tibia and fibula. In contrast to FD, the spicules of osteofibrous dysplasia (OFD) are prominently rimmed by osteoblasts. The spindle cell stroma is histologically similar between the two entities by H&E staining. However, OFD often reveals scattered individual fibroblasts that express keratin or podoplanin (Kashima et al. 2011) both of which are absent in FD.

Desmoplastic fibroma: The leading edge of desmoplastic fibroma may be mistaken for FD, because the tumor can entrap spicules of host bone that lack rimming osteoblasts. However, the strangely shaped trabeculae of FD are absent. FD with sparse woven bone may also resemble DF, but adequate sampling distinguishes the two entities. DF lacks *GNAS1* gene mutations. DF is very rare compared to FD.

Case table 26.3a Variant pathology features of FD

Feature	Frequency	Comment
Variably cellular plump to slender spindle cell proliferation with embedded, strangely shaped and small, rounded woven bone spicules devoid of rimming osteoblasts	Common	This is the classic appearance of fibrous dysplasia. The woven bone ranges from early intramembranous like ossification foci to distinct, oddly shaped (alphabet soup especially C, S, Y shapes) spicules. Calcification in the woven bone spicule may be centrally prominent wrapped by a thin layer of unmineralized osteoid. A few contracted, rimming osteoblasts may be present focally in lesional woven bone
Peripheral superficial infiltration between normal bone trabeculae	Common	This occurs at the leading edge of the FD lesion. Bone marrow is replaced first before normal host bone trabeculae are re-absorbed. Reactive host bone may be present at this interface and will feature variably prominent rimming osteoblasts
Storiforming stroma	Common	The woven bone may be irregularly distributed in the stroma with large areas lacking bone spicules
Hypocellular dense fibrous stroma	Common	Often mixed with the other stroma types
Myxoid stroma	Common	Often mixed with the other stroma types
Nodules of hyaline cartilage	Common	If abundant, the lesion may be termed: 'fibrocartilaginous dysplasia'. Often the nodules undergo endochondral ossification at their edges
Nonspecific cystic degeneration	Common	May resemble UBC
Secondary ABC changes	Uncommon	Histologically indistinguishable from primary ABC
Cementum like bodies	Uncommon	Concentric, lamellated bodies that looks similar to cementum ossicles. If abundant, the lesion has been termed: 'cementomatous variant of fibrous dysplasia'
Short collagen fibers joining the woven bone to the stroma like normal Sharpey's fibers	Common	Not specific for fibrous dysplasia but a typical feature. Also known as 'combed bone'
Secondary changes presumably due to microtrauma or pathologic fracture	Common	These include aggregates of osteoclastic giant cells around foci of hemorrhage or hemosiderin, sheets of xanthoma cells, granulation tissue, and host reactive woven bone with rimming osteoblasts
Mutation of GNAS1 gene (at 20q13) (Guanine nucleotide-finding protein, α-stimulating activity polypeptide 1 gene)	Common	Present in monostotic and polyostotic cases. Mutation occurs in embryogenesis: polyostotic. Mutation occurs postnatally: monostotic. Results in mosaicism for this gene
Monostotic form	Common	Outnumbers polyostotic form by 8-10:1
Polyostotic form	Uncommon	Associated with syndromes in 3% of cases: McCune-Albright (precocious puberty, other endocrinopathies and FD). Café au lait ('coast of Maine') skin lesions may also be present. Mazabraud (deep myxomas and FD)
Exophytic FD	Rare	Also called 'FD protuberans'. The lesion grows on the surface of the bone instead of within the medullary cavity. Can radiologically mimic other tumors such as osteochondroma or parosteal osteosarcoma
Malignant transformation to sarcoma	Rare	Estimated to occur in <0.5% of cases. Occurs in absence or presence of prior irradiation. Sarcomas include osteosarcoma, spindle cell sarcoma NOS, undifferentiated pleomorphic high grade sarcoma, and rarely chondrosarcoma

Table 26.3b Summary pathology findings of Case 26.3

Diagnosis	FD
Size	10.4 × 5.5 × 4 cm
Location	Right proximal femur
Margin status	Positive (lesion is curetted)
Histologic grade	Not graded: benign lesion
Pathologic stage	Not staged: benign lesion

Oncology approach

Medical oncology

Medical oncology is not indicated for fibrous dysplasia.

Radiation oncology

Radiation therapy is not indicated for FD.

Patient outcome

Three years postoperatively, the patient is asymptomatic with normal function and no evidence of significant disease progression.

Case 26.4 Langerhans cell histiocytosis

Clinical history and presentation

The patient is a newborn male infant with an extensive maculopapular skin rash and a large right thigh mass. He is described as a 'blueberry muffin' baby.

Physical examination confirms an extensive maculopapular skin rash and a large right thigh mass.

Surgical findings and comments

Punch biopsies of the skin rash and an incisional biopsy of the deep thigh mass are performed.

Radiology findings

Our case, **Case figures 26.4a** through **26.4g** shows a large thigh soft tissue mass in a 1 day old boy. The plain radiographs show ill-defined calcifications in the mass. There is no lytic lesion or periosteal reaction or bone deformity. The mass shows minimal edema signal without necrosis or enhancement suggesting an indolent lesion. The differential for a congenital soft tissue mass in an extremity would include hematoma, vascular malformation and rhabdomyosarcoma. Hematoma would be associated with fracture or birth trauma. The absence of enhancement militates against the other aggressive tumors.

Pathology findings

Gross features

The right thigh mass incisional biopsy comprises multiple portions of pink to purple-red soft tissue aggregating to 2 × 1 × 0.3 cm. After 10 touch prep slides are made, the specimen is submitted in two cassettes for routine processing. The thigh mass is biopsied three days after punch biopsies of skin lesions are diagnosed as LCH.

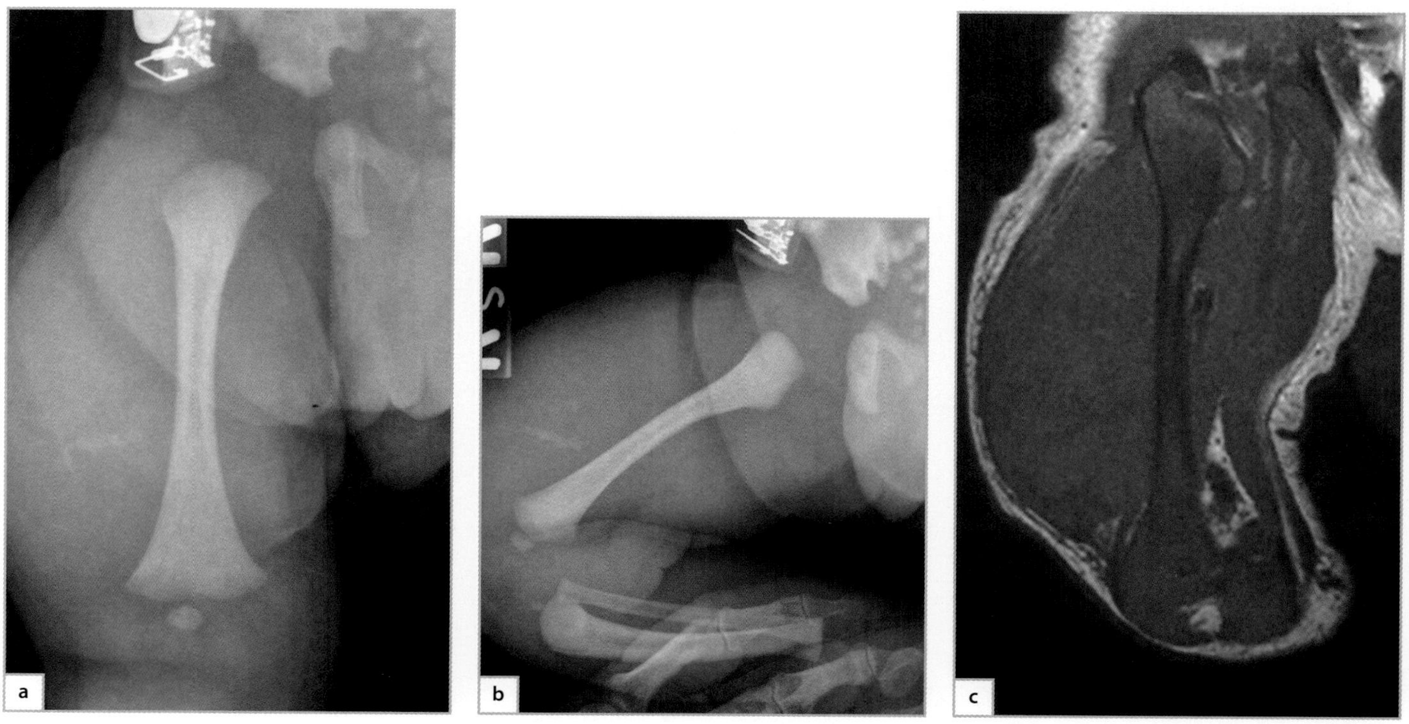

Case figure 26.4 Langerhans cell histiocytosis. **26.4a**: Anteroposterior, **26.4b**: Lateral view of the right thigh in this 1 day old boy show a soft tissue mass with a few irregular calcifications. MR images include; **26.4c**: Coronal T1.

Case figure 26.4: Continued from page 574

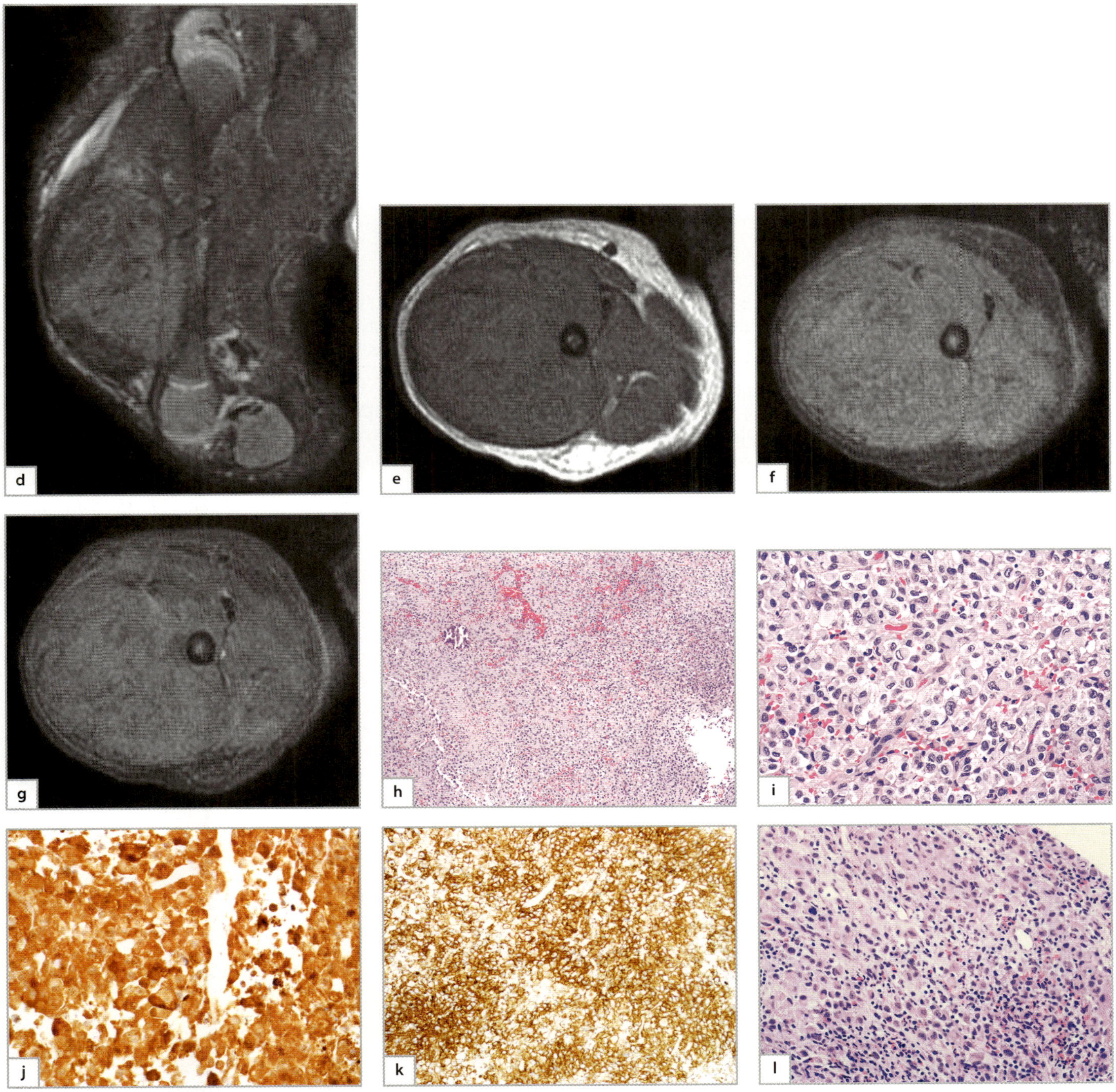

26.4d: Coronal STIR, **26.4e**: Axial T1, **26.4f**: Axial T1 fat saturated, **26.4g**: Axial T1 fat saturated post-contrast. The MR images show a heterogeneous measuring 6.1 $\times$ 3.7 $\times$ 2.8cm with T1 and STIR low signal. There is no appreciable edema or enhancement and the adjacent femur appears normal. **26.4h**: Low magnification. The soft tissue thigh mass features sheets of mononuclear cells with interspersed calcifications and acute hemorrhage. Small foci of necrosis are also present. **26.4i**: High magnification. Tumor cells are moderately sized, round with pale, slightly frothy cytoplasm and eccentrically located round to reniform nuclei. Scattered nuclear grooves are present. Mitoses are few overall, and none are observed in this field. Marked nuclear atypia is absent. **26.4j**: High magnification S-100 IHC stain. Tumor cells are strongly and diffusely positive for S-100 protein (brown chromogen). **26.4k**: Medium magnification, CD1a IHC stain. Tumor cells diffusely strongly express CD1a. From the near universal reactivity, it is clear that very few non-neoplastic cells are present. **26.4l**: *Comparison patient, medium magnification*. This osseous lesion shows less well preserved nuclear features secondary to decalcification. Eosinophils, neutrophils and lymphocytes infiltrate among the tumor cells, a common finding in LCH.

Microscopic features

Low magnification: The incisional biopsy comprises sheets of mononuclear cells with interspersed acute hemorrhage, focal necrosis and calcifications (**Case fig. 26.4h**).

High magnification: The lesional cells are moderate in size with pale amphophilic cytoplasm and eccentrically located nuclei (**Case fig. 26.4i**). The tumor nuclei are hypochromatic, oval to reniform, and scattered nuclear grooves are notable. Mitotic activity is sparse (<1 mitosis/10 hpf). A few histiocytes are present, but multinucleated osteoclastic giant cells and eosinophils are not found. Marked cytologic atypia is absent.

Special studies: Tumor cells strongly and diffusely express S-100 protein and CD1a by IHC (**Case figs 26.4j** and **26.4k**). The previously obtained punch biopsies were also analyzed by IHC with similar staining results for S-100 protein and CD1a.

Additional patient for comparison: A 7 year old with single site LCH in the skull shows the appearance of the cells after decalcification. Notice the typical infiltrates of eosinophils, lymphocytes and neutrophils (**Case fig. 26.4l**).

Pathologic differential or, why isn't it one of the following?

Sarcomatous LCH: This high grade version of LCH shows marked nuclear atypia and a high mitotic rate and is more common in adults over the age of 40 years.

Xanthogranuloma (juvenile type) (JXG): JXG may present at birth as multiple skin and subcutaneous nodules and so could be a pre-biopsy consideration. Microscopically, it consists of foamy, lipid laden histiocytes (xanthoma cells) with or without scattered Touton type giant cells, plasma cells and eosinophils. In some cases, nuclear atypia is present. Mitotic activity may be very high. The cells may react for S-100 protein. They also express HHF-35, HAM56, CD68 and factor XIIIa. In contrast, in LCH, the histiocytic cells exhibit clefted or grooved nuclei, osteoclastic giant cells are often found but generally not Touton type giant cells, and LCH cells express not only S-100 protein but also CD1a and langerin (CD207) by IHC.

Case table 26.4 Summary pathology findings of Case 26.4

Diagnosis	LCH
Size	Diffuse dermal lesions and one soft tissue lesion in thigh
Location	Thigh soft tissue
Margin status	Positive (not relevant as this is a diffuse hematopoietic disease)
Histologic grade	Classic LCH (not high grade sarcomatous LCH)
Pathologic stage	There is no specific staging system for LCH Treatment is based on whether the patient has 'single-system' or 'multisystem' LCH and whether the involved sites are 'low risk' or 'high risk'

Oncology approach

Medical oncology

After confirmatory diagnosis of LCH, the patient is treated with systemic vinblastin and prednisone for a period of one year. Treatment commences after consultation with a national medical oncologist expert in LCH.

Radiation oncology

This is a baby with LCH of the right thigh who undergoes biopsy followed by chemotherapy for one year. The patient will be reevaluated after the chemotherapy for further treatment.

Patient outcome

Six months post-treatment, the patient is in complete remission by physical exam, skeletal survey and MRI of the thigh. He is meeting all developmental milestones. He will be carefully followed in case of relapse.

REFERENCES

Allen CE, Li L, Peters TL, et al. Cell-specific gene expression in Langerhans cell histiocytosis lesions reveal a distinct profile compared with epidermal Langerhans cells. J Immunol 2010;184:4557–67.

Arico M, Girschikofsky M, Genereau T, et al. Langerhans cell histiocytosis in adults. Report from the International Registry of Histiocyte Society. Eur J Cancer 2003;39:2341–8.

Arnaud L, Hervier B, Neel A, et al. CNS involvement and treatment with interferon-α are independent prognostic factors in Erdheim-Chester disease: a multicenter survival analysis of 53 patients. Blood 2011;117:2778–2782.

Badalian-Very G, Vergilio JA, Degar BA, et al. Recent advances in the understanding of Langerhans cell histiocytosis. Br J Haematol 2012;156:163–72.

Blombery P, Wong SQ, Lade S, et al. Erdheim-Chester disease harboring the BRAF V600E mutation. J Clinical Oncology 2012;30:1–2.

Campanacci M, Bertoni F, Capanna R. Malignant degeneration in fibrous dysplasia (presentation of 6 cases and review of the literature). Ital J Orthop Traumatol 1979;5(3):373–81.

Cantu MA, Lupo PJ, Bilgi M, et al. Optimal therapy for adults with Langerhans cell histiocytosis bone lesions. PLoS One 2012;7:e43257.

Caponetti GC, Miranda RB, Althof PA, et al. Immunohistochemical and molecular cytogenetic evaluation of potential targets for tyrosine kinase inhibitors in Langerhans cell histiocytosis. Hum Pathol 2012;43(12):2223–8.

David R, Oria R, Kumar R, et al. Radiologic features of eosinophilic granuloma of bone. Am J Roentgenol 1989;153(5):1021–26.

De Filippo, Ingegnoli A, Carloni A et al. Erdheim-Chester disease: clinical and radiologic findings. Radiol Med 2009;114:1319–1329.

Derenzini E, Fina MP, Stefoni V, et al. MACOP-B regimen in the treatment of adult Langerhans cell histiocytosis: experience on seven patients. Ann Oncol 2010;21:1173–8.

De Silva MVC, Raby N, Reid R. Fibromyxoid areas and immature osteoid are associated with recurrence of primary aneurysmal bone cysts. Histopathol 2003;43:180–188.

Docquier P-L, Delloye C, Galant C. Histology can be predictive of the clinical course of a primary aneurysmal bone cyst. Arch Orthop Trauma Surg 2010;130:481–487.

Donadieu J, Chalard F, Jeziorski E. Medical management of Langerhans cell histiocytosis from diagnosis to treatment. Expert Opin Pharmacother 2012;13:1309–1322.

Dorfman HD. New knowledge of fibro-osseous lesions of bone. Int J Surg Pathol 2010;18:62S–65S.

Dujardin F, Bui Nguyen Binh M, Bouvier C, et al. MDM2 and CDK4 immunohistochemistry is a valuable tool in the differential diagnosis of low-grade osteosarcomas and other fibro-osseous lesions of the bone. Mod Pathol 2011;24:624–637.

Egeler RM, van Halteren AGS, Hogendoom PCW, et al. Langerhans cell histiocytosis: fascinating dynamics of the dendritic cell-macrophage lineage. Immuno Rev 2010:234:213–232.
Farran RP, Zaretski E, Egeler RM. Treatment of Langerhans cell histiocytosis with pamidronate. J Pediatr Hematol Oncol 2001:23:54–6.
Filipovich A, McClain K, Grom A. Histiocytic disorders: recent insights into pathophysiology and practical guidelines. Biol Blood Marrow Transplant 2010;16:S82–S89.
Freeby JA, Reinus WR, Wilson AJ. Quantitative analysis of the plain radiographic appearance of aneurysmal bone cysts. Invest Radiol 1995;30(7):433–9.
Gadner H, Grois N, Arico M, et al. A randomized trial of treatment for multisystem Landerhans' cell histiocytosis. J Pediatr 2001;138:728–34.
Gadner H, Grois N, Potschger U, et al. Improved outcome in multisystem Langerhans cell histiocytosis is associated with therapy intensification. Blood 2008;111:2556–62.
Gadner H, Heitger A, Grois N, et al. Treatment strategy for disseminated Langerhans cell histiocytosis. DAL HX-83 Study Group. Med Pediatr Oncol 1994;23:72–80.
Garcia Gallo MS, Martinez MP, Abalovich MS, et al. Endocrine manifestations of Langerhans cell histiocytosis diagnosed in adults. Pituitary 2010;13:298–303.
Geiersbach K, Rector LS, Sederberg M, et al. Unknown partner for USP6 and unusual SS18 rearrangement detected by fluorescence in situ hybridization in a solid aneurysmal bone cyst. Cancer Genetics 2011;204:195–202.
Gotz G, Fichter J. Langerhans'-cell histiocytosis in 58 adults. Eur J Med Res 2004;9:510–4.
Graham R, Krishnamurthy S, Oliveira A, et al. Frequent expression of fibroblast growth factor-23 (FGF23) mRNA in aneurysmal bone cysts and chondromyxoid fibromas. J Clin Pathol 2012;65:907–909.
Graham RP, Hodge JC, Folpe AL, et al. A cytogenetic analysis of 2 cases of phosphaturic mesenchymal tumor of mixed connective tissue type. Hum Pathol 2012;43:1334–1338.
Greenspan A, Jundt G, Remagen W. Differential Diagnosis in Orthopaedic Oncology, 2nd ed. Philadelphia: Lippincott, Williams and Wilkins, 2007.
Groom KR, Murphey MD, Howard LM, et al. Mesenchymal Hamartoma of the Chest Wall: Radiologic Manifestations with Emphasis on Cross-sectional Imaging and Histopathologic Comparison. Radiology 2002;222(1):205–11.
Haroche J, Arnaud L, Amoura Z. Erdheim-Chester disease. Rheumatology 2012;24:53–59.
Haroche J, Charlotte F, Arnaud L, et al. High prevalence of BRAF V600E mutations in Erdheim-Chester disease but not other non-Langerhans cell histiocytoses. Blood 2012;120:2700–2703.
Ihde LL, Forrester DM, Gottsegen CJ, et al. Sclerosing Bone Dysplasias: Review and Differentiation from Other Causes of Osteosclerosis. Radiographics 2011;31(7):1865–82.
Jones D. Histiocytic and dendritic cell neoplasms. Surg Pathol Clin 2010;3:1165–1183.
Kashima TG, Dongre A, Flanagan AM, et al. Podoplanin expression in adamantinoma of long bones and osteofibrous dysplasia. Virchows Arch 2011;459:41–46.
Kobayashi K, Imanishi Y, Koshiyama H, et al. Expression of FGF23 is correlated with serum phosphate level in isolated fibrous dysplasia. Life Sci 2006;78:2295–2301.
Kransdorf MJ, Sweet DE. Aneurysmal bone cyst: concept, controversy, clinical presentation, and imaging. AJR 1995;164(3):573–80.
Lange T, Stehling C, Fröhlich B, et al. Denosumab: a potential new and innovative treatment option for aneurysmal bone cysts. Eur Spine J Mar 1. 2013;22(6):1417-1422
Lau AW, Pringle LM, Quick L, et al. TRE17/Ubiquitin-specific protease 6 (USP6) oncogene translocated in aneurysmal bone cyst blocks osteoblastic maturation via an autocrine mechanism involving bone morphogenetic protein dysregulation. J Biol Chem 2010;285:37111–37120.
Marchal A, Cuny JF, Montagne K, et al. Associated Langerhans cell histiocytosis and Erdheim-Chester disease. Ann Dermatol Venereol 2011;138:743–747.
Michou L, Brown JP. Genetics of bone diseases: Paget's disease, fibrous dysplasia, osteopetrosis and osteogenesis imperfecta. Joint Bone Spine 2011;78:252–258.
Miller RC, Villa S, Kamer S, et al. Palliative treatment of Erdheim-Chester disease with radiotherapy: a Rare Cancer Network study. Radiother Oncol 2006;80(3):323–6.
Minkov M, Grois N, Heitger A, et al. Treatment of multisystem Langerhans cell histiocytosis. Results of the DAL-HX 83 and DAL-HX 90 studies. DAL-HX Study Group. Klin Padiatr 2000;212:139–44.
Minkov M. Multisystem Langerhans cell histiocytosis in children: current treatment and future directions. Paediatr Drugs 2011;13:75–86.
Montella L, Insabato L, Palmieri G. Imatinib mesylate for cerebral Langerhans'-cell histiocytosis. N Engl J Med 2004;351:1034–5.
Morimoto A, Shioda Y, Imamura T, et al. Nationwide survey of bisphosphate therapy for children with reactivated Langerhans cell histiocytosis in Japan. Pediatr Bloo d Cancer 2011;56:110–5.
Oliveira AM, Perez-Atayde AR, Inwards CY, et al. USP6 and CDH11 oncogenes identify the neoplastic cell in primary aneurysmal bone cysts and are absent in so-called secondary aneurysmal bone cysts. Am J Pathol 2004;165:1773–1780.
Panoutsakopoulos G, Pandis N, Kyriazoglou I, et al. Recurrent t(16;17)(q22;p13) in aneurysmal bone cysts. Genes Chromosomes Cancer 1999;26:265–266.
Park L, Schiltz C, Korman N. Langerhans cell histiocytosis. J Cutan Med Surg 2012;16:45–9.
Pineles SL, Liu GT, Acebes X, et al. Presence of Erdheim-Chester disease and Langerhans cell histiocytosis in the same patient: a report of two cases. J Neuro-Opthalmol 2011;31:217–223.
Riminucci M, Robey PG, Saggio I, et al. Skeletal progenitors and the GNAS gene: fibrous dysplasia of bone read through stem cells. J Mol Endocrinol 2010;45:355–364.
Rosenberg AE, Nielsen GP, Fletcher JA, et al. Tumours of undefined neoplastic nature. In: Fletcher CDM, Krishnan Unni K, Mertens F (Eds). World Health Organization Classification of Tumours. Pathology and Genetics of Tumours of Soft Tissue and Bone. Lyon: IARC Press, 2002.
Sahm F, Capper D, Preusser M, et al. BRAFV600E mutant protein is expressed in cells of variable maturation in Langerhans cell histiocytosis. Blood 2012;120:e28–34.
Saven A, Burian C. Cladribine activity in adult Langerhans-cell histiocytosis. Blood 1999;93:4125–30.
Sciot R, Dorfman H, Brys P, et al. Cytogenetic-morphologic correlations in aneurysmal bone cyst, giant cell tumor of bone, and combined lesions. A report from the CHAMP Study Group. Mod Pathol 2000;13:1206–1210.
Serrano-Egea A, Santos-Briz A, Garcia-Munoz H, et al. Chest wall hamartoma report of two cases with secondary aneurysmal bone cysts. Pathol Res Practice 2001;197:835–839.
Sukov WR, Franco MF, Erickson-Johnson M, et al. Frequency of USP6 rearrangements in myositis ossificans, brown tumor and cherubism: molecular cytogenetic evidence that a subset of 'myositis ossificans-like lesions' are the early phases in the formation of soft-tissue aneurysmal bone cyst. Skeletal Radiol 2008;37:321–327.
Suri HS, Yi ES, Nowakowski GS, et al. Pulmonary Langerhans cell histiocytosis. Orphanet J Rare Dis 2012;7:16.
Taylor RMI, Kashima T, Hemingway FKE, et al. CD14- mononuclear stromal cells support (CD14+) monocyte-osteoclast differentiation in aneurysmal bone cyst. Lab Investi 2012;92:600–605.
Van de Luijtgaarden ACM, Veth RPH, Slootweg PJ, et al. Metastatic potential of an aneurysmal bone cyst. Virchows Arch 2009;455:455–459.
Veyssier-Belot C, Cacoub P, Caparros-Lefebvre D, et al. Erdheim-Chester disease. Clinical and radiologic characteristics of 59 cases. Medicine 1996;75(3):157–69.
Walia M, Paul P, Mishra S, et al. Congenital Langerhans Cell Histiocytosis: the self-healing variety. J Ped Hematol Oncol 2004;26:398–402.
Weitzman S, Braier J, Donadieu J, et al. 2'-Chlorodeoxyadenosine (2-CdA) as salvage therapy for Langerhans cell histiocytosis (LCH) results of the LCH-S-98 protocol of the Histiocyte Society. Pediatr Blood Cancer 2009;53:1271–6.
Willman CL, Busque L, Briffith BB, et al. Langerhans'-cell histiocytosis (histiocytosis X) – a clonal proliferative disease. New Eng J Med 1994;331:154–160.
Ye Y, Pringel LM, Lau AW, et al. TRE17/USP6 oncogene translocated in aneurysmal bone cyst induces matrix metalloproteinase production via activation of NF-kB. Oncogene 2010;29:3619–3629.
Yousem SA, Colby TV, Chen YY, et al. Pulmonary Langerhans' cell histiocytosis: molecular analysis of clonality. Am J Surg Pathol 2001;25:630–636.

Chapter 27 Benign mimics of bone and soft tissue tumors

OVERVIEW

This collation of benign mimics of bone and soft tissue tumors is not all-inclusive. Experienced, ensuingly wary clinicians and radiologists could likely add other lesions. However, this chapter is designed to draw attention to lesions that can occasionally dupe a clinician or radiologist into favoring a diagnosis of sarcoma. The chapter excludes pseudosarcomas (the different types of fasciitis, myositis ossificans, or reactive periosteal lesions) that, even at the level of pathology review, can resemble a sarcoma. Instead, the focus is on various inflammatory or infectious conditions, post-traumatic lesions, and a rare, enigmatic entity, massive localized lymphedema.

The majority of individual examples of the lesions presented in this chapter are diagnosable after careful clinical history is obtained, physical exam is performed, imaging studies are reviewed, and relevant laboratory studies are obtained. However, a subset may not be clearly deducible as non-neoplastic until a biopsy is evaluated in Pathology. A rush to judgment may unduly increase patient anxiety, delay appropriate therapy, or result in the wrong treatment.

Obversely, rare sarcomas may present clinically and radiologically as hematomas or abscesses. Case reports describe epithelioid sarcoma, synovial sarcoma, and pleomorphic undifferentiated high grade sarcoma being mistaken originally for a non-neoplastic benign lesion (Niimi et al. 2006, Liarmakopoulos et al. 2011, Dion et al. 2001, Agarwal et al. 2010). The authors of this text have treated two patients with inguinal masses that were initially considered a chronically expanding hematoma (angiomatoid fibrous histiocytoma on biopsy) and draining abscess (superinfected high grade myxofibrosarcoma on biopsy). Obtaining a biopsy is a prudent response to a patient presenting with an ambiguous soft tissue lesion. Though more complicated to perform, a bone biopsy usually also resolves the question of whether an intraosseous lesion is neoplastic.

CLASSIFICATION

Table 27.1 lists the entities discussed in this chapter.

DEMOGRAPHICS, ETIOLOGY, AND PATHOLOGY

Osteomyelitis

Osteomyelitis (OM) occurs in children and adults. Hematogenous spread is more common in the pediatric age group but can occur in adults particularly those who are immunocompromised. Infections in IV drug abusers may not be accompanied by fever or chills instead manifesting only as localized pain, and thus the diagnosis can be initially missed. In addition, microbiology cultures may be negative, and radiology imaging may suggest malignancy.

Up to 20% of diabetic patients with foot ulcers develop osteomyelitis (Game 2009). These cases of osteomyelitis are seldom misdiagnosed as sarcoma but may be under-diagnosed, as most arise from bacterial spread of contiguous soft tissue infection. Contiguous spread from an entry wound is the most common source of bone infection for adults. The most common organisms causing pediatric osteomyelitis are *Staphylococcus aureus* (*SA*), *Streptococcus pyogenes* (*SP*) and *Haemophilus influenzae*. In adults, *SA* and *SP* remain common pathogens, with *Staphylococcus epidermidis*, gram-negative

Table 27.1 Benign mimics of bone and soft tissue tumors

Lesion	When it can mimic a neoplasm	Consequent clinical and radiologic differential
Osteomyelitis	Minimal serologic or clinical findings of inflammation multifocal disease	Metastatic carcinoma, metastatic melanoma, multiple myeloma, lymphoma
Seroma/hematoma	The seroma or hematoma is large and spontaneous The seroma or hematoma is 'ancient': it presents years after the initial trauma	High grade sarcoma is a strong consideration given the size and imaging characteristics Bursal cyst or inflammatory process Myositis ossificans (when the seroma/hematoma is calcified) Infectious cyst
Granulomatous inflammation at a surgical scar site of a prior sarcoma resection	Any new nodules at the site of a prior sarcoma resection should raise a healthy suspicion for recurrent tumor	Recurrent sarcoma Suture granulomas Hypertrophic scar Infection
Bursitis	This rarely raises the possibility of a mesenchymal tumor, but long persisting, large lesions are most likely to be less straightforward	Benign soft tissue tumor such as schwannoma, neurofibroma or myxoma Rarely, low grade sarcomas such as low grade myxofibrosarcoma
Massive localized lymphedema	When no cause such as malformation or infection can be found	Atypical lipomatous tumor
Localized soft tissue infection (abscess or mycetoma)	When the patient lacks laboratory or clinical findings of infection Ulcers or draining fistulas are absent In the case of mycetoma, when the lesion only becomes clinically apparent years after the initial traumatic introduction of the causative organism	Benign soft tissue tumor Malignant soft tissue tumor Metastatic tumor, especially if the lesion is painful

rods, *Pseudomonas* species, and mixed bacteria able to successfully infect the bone of immunocompromised or IV drug abusing patients (Bullough 2010). However, numerous case reports attest to the ability of exotic organisms to cause OM.

Organisms such as *Candida* species that seldom caused OM in the past are gaining new footholds due to increased numbers of immunosuppressed patients, more invasive surgeries, implementation of broad-spectrum antibiotics, and placement of central venous catheters (Slenker et al. 2012). If OM is a clinical suspicion on biopsy of a bone lesion, rapid delivery of fresh specimen directly from the operating room to the microbiology laboratory may be vital in determining the pathogen.

Histologically, acute OM is characterized by necrotic trabecular bone spicules surrounded by marrow infiltrates of neutrophils and eosinophils. Normal marrow hematopoiesis is absent and fat necrosis of marrow adipose is common. Reactive woven bone may be prominent and may use non-viable bone trabeculae as a base. Chronic OM may continue to exhibit acute inflammation, but marrow fibrosis and plasma cell infiltrates predominate. Necrotic trabecular bone and reactive immature bone are present in both acute and chronic OM. Some organisms elicit a granulomatous inflammatory response; these include fungi and mycobacteria.

Non-infectious OM is a diagnosis of exclusion. The two forms of this peculiar disease are termed chronic recurrent multifocal OM (CRMO) and SAPHO syndrome (synovitis, acne, pustulosis, hyperostosis, and osteitis). Patients with CRMO may also develop a skin lesion (pustulosis palmoplantaris) and the two diseases overlap to some extent in symptoms and findings. CRMO occurs preferentially in children but also affects young adults, while classic SAPHO occurs in adults. The clinical findings in children may mimic OM or a small round blue cell tumor such as Ewing sarcoma or lymphoma. In adults, the main differential is multifocal metastatic carcinoma or multifocal primary bone lymphoma. CRMO and SAPHO may represent an infectious OM, but no organism has been isolated to date. Both are currently considered an inter-related auto-inflammatory disease (Gikas et al. 2009, Hashkes et al. 2012). A recent German review estimated an annual incidence of 0.4/100,000 with a mean age of 11.4 years and female predominance (Jansson et al. 2011). Approximately 10% of patients with spine involvement suffered one or more vertebral fractures. Patients may have a protracted disease course with painful flare-ups despite aggressive therapy, and additional complications include leg length discrepancy, bony overgrowth, and generalized growth failure (Catalano-Pons et al. 2008). Nonphysical complications include impaired education and inability to work. Treatment consists not of antibiotics but anti-inflammatory agents including NSAIDs, and corticosteroids.

CRMO and SAPHO are typically histologically indistinguishable from bacterial OM. Early lesions resemble acute OM with acute inflammation, dead bone and appositional reactive new bone, while late lesions commonly contain markedly sclerotic bone trabeculae, diffuse marrow fibrosis, and sparse chronic inflammation (Reith et al. 1996). It can be unifocal, but in one study, the largest number of discrete lesions in one individual was eighteen, and some of the more commonly affected bones include the clavicle, femur, tibia, ribs, tarsals, and carpals, but any bone may become involved (Tlougan et al. 2009, Gikas et al. 2009, Cimolai 2011). Disease in the sternum, clavicle or mandible in a child or young adult is particularly suggestive of CRMO. Symptoms may persist in 25-59% of patients with chronic pain or bone deformities being the most common sequelae (Wipff et al. 2011).

Seroma/hematoma

Although a patient of any age may incur a seroma or hematoma, generally it is adults rather than children with the lesion who are more commonly assessed as having a probable sarcoma. Patients with 'ancient hematoma' are those individuals who present months to many years (up to 6 decades) after trauma with deep-seated, expanding hematomas that clinically and radiologically mimic aggressive sarcoma (Mentzel et al. 1997, Negoro et al. 2012). These lesions have also been termed calcific myonecrosis, chronic expanding hematoma, or post-traumatic cyst of soft tissue.

Abruptly forming, spontaneous hematomas may also mimic a soft tissue neoplasm. These are also rare lesions compared to the vast majority of hematomas that are related to a specific injury or predisposing condition (such as hemophilia) and that eventually resolve.

Granulomatous inflammation consistent with deep granuloma annulare

Deep granuloma annulare (DGA) is a necrobiotic granulomatous process of unknown etiology that most commonly occurs in young children (Pesce et al. 2010). It is also known as pseudorheumatoid nodule. The subcutaneous nodules may be mistaken for epithelioid sarcoma or, as inferable from its alternate name, rheumatoid nodules. The unusual cases occurring in adults are prone to pre-operative misdiagnosis. Pathogenetic mechanisms proffered comprise altered immune response to trauma or altered immune response to prior infection of various types (McDermott et al. 1998, Pesce et al. 2010, Stefanaki et al. 2007). It may represent a Th-1 delayed-type hypersensitivity reaction that induces matrix destruction (Stefanaki et al. 2007).

Biopsy of DGA reveals scattered palisading granulomas containing central degenerating collagen. Inflammation is histiocytic, but multinucleated giant cells are absent to rare. Alcian blue stains may reveal mucinous degenerative material in the granulomas. A perivascular and perigranulomatous lymphocytic response is typical.

Most granulomas arising in a surgical resection site are of the foreign body type reacting to suture material. These are often nonpalpable but if clinically apparent are usually small and located close to the scar. Fine needle aspiration biopsy can be performed to confirm the diagnosis. Multinucleated giant cells are numerous, suture material is identified, and necrobiotic collagen is absent.

Bursitis

Bursitis, inflammation of the synovial lined, fluid filled, cushioning sacs around joints, usually occurs in adults after repetitive use of the joint. Other causes include rheumatoid arthritis, infection and gout. Bursitis does not typically suggest a diagnosis of mesenchymal tumor, but large chronic lesions without a history of over-use may raise the possibility of a neoplasm.

Histologically, non-infectious bursitis demonstrates fibrosis, sparse chronic inflammation, fibrin deposition with or without loose bodies, and neovascularization. Dystrophic calcifications and hemosiderin may also be present. The synovial lining may be abraded, hyperplastic or both. Infectious bursitis will feature acute inflammation and tissue necrosis. Organisms may be identified on special stains.

Massive localized lymphedema

This is a rare, pseudoneoplastic lesion that occurs due to excess, pendulous fat compressing draining lymphatic channels. Most patients live with the lesion for years, or it may become apparent after sudden weight loss (Farshid et al. 1998, Manduch et al. 2009). Nearly all patients are morbidly obese adults. A recent review of 22 patients noted a mean weight of 186 kg (411 pounds) and a mean age of 42 years with a range of 25-70 years (Manduch et al. 2009). Most cases involve the lower extremity especially the thigh (Farshid et al. 1998). A few patients may have had prior lymphadenectomy of the affected limb or hypothyroidism in addition to obesity (Wu et al. 2000, Wang et al. 2010, Manduch et al. 2009).

Clinically, the mass is often interpreted as pendulous pannus. However, when it affects an entire limb, infectious causes of massive lymphedema may also be considered, and secondary cellulitis may certainly develop. In most cases, the radiologic and clinical features are more consistent with a non-neoplastic process than a tumor. This is because the lesion is long-standing, obviously extensively involves the superficial tissues with skin thickening ('cobblestoning' or warty changes) or edema ('peau d'orange' effect), and because the patient is almost invariably morbidly obese.

However, in some instances, the clinician and the pathologist may entertain the possibility of atypical lipomatous tumor (ALT). Histologically, massive localized lymphedema (MLL) shows a remarkable degree of homogeneity from case to case. Suprafascial changes include dermal fibrosis, epidermal thickening in chronically rubbed areas, and perivascular lymphocytic inflammation with prominent capillary aggregates. The subcutaneous fat features normal sized fat cells with edematous interlobular septa, numerous vessels, many of which are dilated, and often clusters of capillaries located between dermis and fat. Fat necrosis, myxoid change and chronic inflammation may also be focally present. The deep fat is abundant, with normal fat cell morphology, and has thick, variably edematous fibrous trabeculations noticeable grossly and microscopically. Some septal stromal cells may be multinucleated, but the nuclear hyperchromasia noted in the atypical stromal cells of ALT are absent. Lipoblasts are also absent as are adipocytes with greater than 10 fold size variation as commonly prevails in ALT.

Cutaneous angiosarcoma may complicate MLL. This is not surprising; given the risk chronic lymphedema poses in other settings (Stewart-Treves syndrome, for example). The angiosarcomas occurring in MLL are high grade with mixed spindled, epithelioid and vasoformative areas (Shon et al. 2011). Of four patients recently reported with follow-up, one patient died of disease, one died of therapy-related complications, and two were alive without disease (mean tumor size 15.0 cm with range of 6 -28.5cm) (Shon et al. 2011).

Soft tissue abscess and mycetoma

Soft tissue abscesses may be confused with sarcoma if there are no recognized antecedent associations such as prior surgery, nearby OM, bacteremia, endocarditis, trauma, diabetes, corticosteroid therapy, other immunosuppressive condition, or myxedema. Abscess with myonecrosis is usually due to trauma (most common in children) as well as the above factors. However, it can also occur in the absence of a known precipitating source of infection (Brook 2008). Deep neck abscesses are commonly associated with dental infections and upper airway infections (Wang et al. 2010).

Methicillin-resistant *Staphylococcus aureus* (MRSA) is a common cause of subcutaneous abscess in the US. In some studies, it comprises the majority of infections, including those that are community acquired (Nalmas et al. 2009, Rossini et al. 2011). However, the relative proportion of methicillin resistant SA in clinical isolates of *staphylococcus aureus* in clinical isolates is much lower in countries such as France (14.5%) and the Netherlands (3.1%)(Watkins et al. 2012). Other important pathogens causing soft tissue abscesses include group A β-hemolytic streptococci and indigenous aerobic and anaerobic local microflora including *Staphylococcus lugdunensis* and actinomycetes (Brook 2007, Klotchko et al. 2011).

Histologically, abscesses consist of varying amounts of pus (neutrophils, viable and necrotic mixed with fibrin) and necrotic tissue usually walled off by a fibrotic, hypervascular pseudocapsule. Bacteria may be identified on routine H&E stains but visualization is optimized with tissue gram or silver stains. In many cases, no organisms are found.

Mycetoma refers to discrete nodular infections in subcutaneous and deep soft tissues caused by true fungi (eumycetes) or actinomycetes (*Actinomycosis* and *Nocardia* species). Patients may present with a chronic, relatively painless nodule that has been present for years, usually on the extremities (lower > upper). Although most mycetomas form fistulas, some do not, and these are especially subject to being mistaken for a soft tissue tumor. Mycetomas are more common in parts of the world between latitudes 15^0 south and 30^0 north (tropical and subtropical areas), but immigrants may present with the lesion in other geographic locales (Lichon et al. 2006). Males are more commonly affected than females with a ratio of 3-5:1, and most patients present between ages 20 and 40 years (Lichon et al. 2006). *Madurella mycetomatis* is the most common fungal cause, and eumycetes outnumber actinomycetes as the involved pathogen. However, geography determines the most likely organism with actinomycetes being more common causes in Central America and Mexico, and *Pseudallescheria boydii* responsible for the majority of U.S. cases (Lichon et al. 2006).

Histologically, mycetoma is characterized by granulomatous inflammation with superimposed foci of acute inflammation, fibrosis, and lymphoplasmacytic inflammation. The granulomas contain 'grains' (also known as 'granules' or 'sclerotia') which consists of large tight mats of the fungus or actinomycete. These grains may be shed through a draining ulcer, and their color may enable differentiation of the organism into eumycete or actinomycete. However, ancillary laboratory studies are required for speciation.

RADIOLOGY

Chronic osteomyelitis

The imaging of bone infection, OM, is a frequent and challenging imaging problem for the radiologist. OM has a highly variable appearance on all imaging modalities depending on the chronicity, microbiology, and clinical setting. Furthermore, the imaging findings have significant overlap with other diseases. The radiologist must carefully interpret the constellation of soft tissue and bone findings with the clinical setting to reach the correct diagnosis.

The bone findings on radiography include focal osteopenia, cortical erosion, and bone destruction with irregular periosteal reaction. These findings are not specific and only indicate an aggressive process. If there is history of penetrating trauma, open fracture or overlying loss of skin integrity, then the diagnosis of OM can be made. Unfortunately, the history of a soft tissue wound is often omitted and the wound itself may not be visible on imaging or the wound may have already healed. The history of overlying skin violation is crucial for correct interpretation. If radiographic findings are uncertain, cross sectional imaging may be helpful. CT scan allows definitive evaluation for cortical erosion but does not show marrow edema well. Generally, MRI is more useful than CT because it has exquisite sensitivity for both marrow and soft tissue edema. Indeed, a normal MR exam excludes inflammation and thus rules out OM. On the other hand, the presence of edema has little specificity because any injury, inflammation, healing, infection or neoplastic process can cause edema.

The cornerstone of the diagnosis of OM is the combination of bone destruction with adjacent soft tissue violation. Intravenous contrast is not needed for the diagnosis of OM but IV contrast is usually given to help visualize soft tissue abscess, bone sequestrum, and assess bone viability.

Acute OM (AOM) presents with several common clinical scenarios. AOM in pediatrics may occur spontaneously with seeding of the distal metaphysis of one or more long bones. Radiographs may show a lucent focus indicating a Brodie's abscess that can eventually track to the surface of the bone and then may develop a draining wound. Pediatric patients can also present with AOM from penetrating trauma in which case history is crucial to guide diagnosis.

In adults, AOM can occur due to seeding from a wound, penetrating trauma, post-surgical complication or from an open fracture. History is equally important for correct diagnosis. Occasionally, AOM can develop from spread of an infected joint or even hematogenous seeding.

The burgeoning epidemic of diabetes and obesity has increased the incidence of AOM and chronic osteomyelitis (COM) of the foot due to the plethora of deep soft tissue ulcers with direct seeding of bone. These cases are challenging for the radiologist, as these patients often have neuropathy and altered walking mechanics which will commonly cause marrow edema of multiple bones, typically throughout the mid-foot. This edema indicates stress response and could progress to stress fracture or may represent the early stages of neuropathic joint disease (Charcot foot). No imaging modality can definitively exclude osteomyelitis in the setting of neuropathic changes. Some advocate bone scan with an additional tag white cell scan however, in our experience, these cases remain a diagnostic dilemma.

COM has a much more complex appearance due to the superimposition of ongoing bone destruction with concomitant healing response. The patient may have had numerous episodes of acute infection with multiple courses of antibiotics and multiple surgical debridements. COM usually shows mixed lytic, destructive features with sclerotic areas of healing and maturing periosteal reaction. Deformities may develop due to the chronically weakened bone. Osteomyelitis can develop a lucent abscess space called an involucrum. Occasionally a sequestrum, or fragment of necrotic bone will develop within the involucrum. The sequestrum serves as a nidus for persistent infection and often requires surgical resection. The radiologist must be cautious as a sequestrum is not specific for COM. A radiographic sequestrum simply represents a calcified focus within a lucent area of bone and can be seen in a broad spectrum of entities such as osteomyelitis, intraosseous lipoma, osteoid osteoma, eosinophilic granuloma, radiation necrosis and some malignancies (Jennin et al. 2011).

The most common infectious microbe causing osteomyelitis is *Staphylococcus aureus*. Tuberculosis and fungal infections will have a more indolent appearance with relative preservation of bone density. Madura foot represents diffuse soft tissue and bone fungal infection of the foot seen in the tropics. Fungal infection, especially in an immune compromised patient may require amputation to treat. Sickle cell disease predisposes for bone infarct and infection which can cause dactylitis. In sickle cell patients, *S. aureus* remains the most common bacteria, with salmonellae being the second most common infectious agent. Discitis is usually a secondary process due to spread of infection from the adjacent vertebral body that is presumably seeded hematogenously. Biopsy of the disc often results in no growth on microbial culture. The clinical care team often must treat discitis empirically.

Hematoma and seroma

Hematomas have a heterogeneous complex appearance depending on the age of hemorrhage products and whether there are recurring hemorrhages. Radiography may show a soft tissue density mass. Ultrasound will show a complex echogenic mass likely with septations and fluid areas. The ultrasound appearance is least specific amongst the cross sectional imaging tests but is a convenient method of imaging guidance should needle aspiration be needed. CT scan typically shows a complex mass without internal enhancement. CT scan may demonstrate adjacent injury or vascular lesion to account for the presence of the hematoma. On MRI, the hematoma will typically appear as a complex mass with variable T1 and T2 signal. In particular, there are areas of high T1 signal is due to met-hemoglobin or the presence of proteinaceous material. There may be irregular rim enhancement of a hematoma. Gradient echo sequences will show hemosiderin as markedly low signal. Compared to a spin echo T2 image, the hemosiderin will bloom and appear larger on gradient echo sequences due to susceptibility artifact.

A seroma is the evolving fluid collection resulting from previous hematoma. These will typically have fluid-fluid levels due to blood breakdown products. There is commonly T1 high signal fluid present due to protein or met-hemoglobin. Seromas may remain stable for some time, but usually slowly resolve over several weeks to months. The fluid collection may show collapsing configuration of the walls as the volume decreases. In the setting of post-operative follow up for sarcoma surgery, the radiologist must be vigilant for enhancing nodular or mass like areas that might indicate tumor residual or recurrence. The MR findings can then direct subsequent biopsy as needed. If a seroma develops thick, irregular walls with adjacent edema, abscess formation from secondary infection may have developed.

Granuloma annulare

Granuloma annulare (GA) is an idiopathic inflammatory process characterized by dermal papules and annular plaques. Imaging rarely plays a role in the diagnosis of GA. There are several forms of GA, the most common is the localized form which will have violaceous skin lesions. The subcutaneous form predominates in children and has firm asymptomatic nodules.

Bursitis

A bursa is a synovial lined collection of fluid, usually near a joint that serves to cushion and dissipate friction between adjacent mobile structures. These develop in utero and are consistently present anatomic structures. On the other hand, an adventitial bursa can develop de novo in any location related to repetitive friction or trauma. For instance, an adventitial bursa can develop over the medial malleolus in ice skaters (Brown et al. 2005). An adventitial bursa is lined by synovial-like tall columnar cells and not actual synovial cells. Bursitis indicates inflammation or infection of the bursa and is usually exquisitely painful.

Bursitis can develop from systemic illness such as crystal arthropathy or from synovial disease such as rheumatoid arthritis. Alternatively, repetitive injury or overuse may lead to bursal inflammation. This is common with the subacromion-subdeltoid bursa of the shoulder and the olecranon bursa of the elbow. Often physical exam and the clinical setting are diagnostic. If imaging is warranted, MR is most helpful to evaluate the bursa and to exclude ancillary pathology such as a rotator cuff tear in a patient with shoulder pain. On MR imaging, acute bursitis will show fluid distention of the bursa with intense enhancement of the wall and adjacent soft tissue edema. More commonly, bursitis is chronic and the fluid may show debris and synechiae from prior acute inflammatory episodes. The lining of the bursa may become thickened over time.

Massive lymphedema

Patients with massive lymphedema present with marked enlargement of a limb or a large mass of a limb invariably occurring in adult patients with morbid obesity. The patients may have had preceding disturbance of the lymphatics, such as lymphadenectomy, trauma or radiation. Stewart-Treves syndrome is the association of long standing lymphedema with subsequent development of angiosarcoma. Despite the striking clinical presentation, the diagnosis may not always be clear and imaging may be employed to evaluate for underlying abscess or sarcoma.

Soft tissue abscess

Soft tissue abscess refers to a localized infectious process that has formed a collection of liquid pus. Abscesses are common and occur throughout the body. Abscesses of the soft tissues and extremities are often associated with penetrating trauma, ulcerated wounds, foreign bodies and drug abuse. On occasion, a soft tissue abscess can develop from infection that began in bone, lymph node or joints. Soft tissue abscess are usually of bacterial etiology. For skin and soft tissue infections, *Staphylococcus aureus* were the most common aerobic bacteria identified regardless of IV drug abusers status. Amongst IV drug abusers patients, oral flora was isolated in 67% of cases (Summanen et al. 1995). Fungal infection and mycobacterial vectors are less common but imply compromised host immunity.

Imaging is commonly utilized for the diagnosis of intra-abdominal and soft tissue abscesses. Ultrasound can be useful for imaging guidance and percutaneous drainage of an abscess and can identify superficial foreign bodies. However, the inability of ultrasound to visualize deeper structures, particularly in patients with large body habitus or intervening bowel gas and bone, limits its overall diagnostic utility. CT with IV contrast or MRI with IV contrast can provide excellent overall visualization of abscess and more importantly, they have adequate sensitivity to also exclude the presence of an abscess. CT can also show bone erosion and periosteal reaction. CT may show foreign bodies well if they have significant density difference from soft tissue. Plastic is usually less dense (appears lucent) than soft tissue whereas metal, mineral structures (calculi, dirt and stones) and most glass are higher density than soft tissue. MR offers the best imaging ability to exclude osteomyelitis because of its high sensitivity for marrow edema. MR has modest utility for foreign body detection, with most foreign bodies having signal void or susceptibility artifact. In general, CT is the preferred modality for abscess evaluation because of its overall soft tissue, bowel and skeletal visualization. CT scan is also clinically more robust for imaging ill patients who cannot tolerate a long MR exam that may require multiple breath holds. Abscess will have similar appearance on CT and MR with a focalized fluid collection that has a thick, irregular enhancing wall. There is typically adjacent soft tissue edema and enhancement of soft tissues indicating inflammation. It is important to remember that the appearance of abscess is similar to both hematoma and sarcoma especially when there is central non-enhancing matrix or necrosis. The clinical setting is crucial to distinguish between these.

> **GRAY AREA**
>
> It is important to remember that the appearance of abscess is similar to both hematoma and sarcoma especially when there is central non-enhancing matrix or necrosis. The clinical setting is crucial to distinguish between these.

SURGERY

Osteomyelitis

Treatment of OM is a textbook discussion in itself. In general, surgical treatment is aimed at the evacuation of any related abscess and debridement of related avascular bone and soft tissue to maximize the ability of antibiotics to eradicate any residual infection. Multiple operations may be necessary for successful treatment. Potential success of combined surgical and antibiotic treatment is related to the virulence of the organism, susceptibility to antibiotics, and systemic and local conditions of the host (largely related to systemic immunocompetency and vascularity of the involved local tissues). Local tissue vascularity may be substantially compromised due to underlying vascular disease, diabetes mellitus, scar tissue from prior surgery, and prior radiation. Compromised vascularity at the local level impairs delivery of systemic antibiotics thereby decreasing the likelihood of successful eradication of the infection. In refractory cases, particularly in the immunocompromised host, amputation is occasionally necessary for eradication of infection.

> **GRAY AREA**
>
> Placement of antibiotic impregnated bone cement into the bony void created by debridement of infected tissue may increase treatment success.

> **GRAY AREA**
>
> Infections involving foreign material, such as the metal and polyethylene of joint implants, are particularly difficult to eradicate. Often, successful treatment of infection in the presence of foreign material requires removal of the hardware, placement of an antibiotic 'spacer,' and reimplantation following resolution of the infection.

> **GRAY AREA**
>
> If a disabling amputative procedure is necessary to eradicate the infection, patients and their treating doctors may elect for chronic antibiotic suppression. This does not eradicate the infection, runs the risk of sepsis in the immunocompromised host, and often is associated with chronic drainage. Nevertheless, in some patients with complex and refractory infection faced with a debilitating amputation, suppression is a worthwhile alternative.

Seroma and hematoma

Seroma formation is common after many surgical procedures. A seroma generally resolves spontaneously. In large resection operations, such as those associated with removal of a tumor, where a 'dead space' is left behind, part of the seroma may persist indefinitely. This is particularly true if the local area has been irradiated, either prior to or following surgery. Evacuation of a seroma is rarely successful in preventing recurrence unless the dead space is filled, such as with a muscle flap. Rarely, a seroma may become secondarily infected and form an abscess.

A hematoma generally develops following trauma which causes bleeding within the involved tissue. Occasionally, a hematoma may form spontaneously or following minimal trauma, as a result of coagulopathy or due to the presence of an underlying neoplastic process. Rarely, a hematoma may form in a completely spontaneous setting. In most cases, the hematoma will resolve spontaneously.

In those cases involving coagulopathy or neoplasm, treatment should be directed to the underlying process. A hematoma that is persistent or significantly symptomatic may require evacuation and hemostasis if the bleeding remains persistently active.

GRAY AREA

Tumors, particularly sarcomas, can occasionally present as a soft tissue hematoma. The clinician should be wary of a patient presenting with a spontaneous hematoma with no or minimal trauma, who does not have an underlying predisposition to bleeding (bleeding dyscrasia or anti-coagulant medication). Formal biopsy should be performed if an index of suspicion exists and open biopsy is generally preferred as a malignancy may represent a rather small component of the overall mass.

Granuloma annulare

This is generally a self-limited disease; therefore surgery does not generally have a role in treatment. However, a small biopsy is often required to make the diagnosis.

Localized disease generally resolves spontaneously in one to two years. Disseminated disease can prove more difficult to treat, but local therapy with steroids (topical or injected) or liquid nitrogen and/or systemic medical or ultraviolet treatment is used.

Bursitis

Bursitis is generally a self-limited inflammatory disease that responds to rest and anti-inflammatory agents. Rarely, a surgical bursectomy is performed in refractory cases. Recurrence following bursectomy is relatively common unless the underlying cause is addressed.

Massive lymphedema

Chronic primary lymphedema is a frustrating malady for which there is no good treatment. Generally, this condition can be controlled conservatively with compression stockings and manual lymph drainage therapy. Surgery is occasionally indicated in refractory cases and may consist of lymphatic-venous bypass procedures, debulking, and even amputation in cases of uncontrolled massive lymphedema.

Abscess

Drainage of any abscess is indicated to facilitate cure of infection. This can be accomplished by percutaneous drain placement or open evacuation of the abscess along with debridement.

MEDICAL TREATMENT

Because these are not tumors neither medical oncology nor radiotherapy interventions are necessary. Consultations with infectious disease and rheumatology specialists are warranted.

CASES

Case 27.1 Chronic osteomyelitis (chronic recurrent multifocal osteomyelitis)

Clinical history and presentation

The patient is a 22 year old man with a history of heavy alcohol and methamphetamine use who presents with an eight month history of pain which initially began in the left hip but has recently become more localized to the left knee. He also describes new onset of pain in the right knee.

Left hip symptoms began insidiously and have been progressive. Pain occurs with activity but also at rest. He receives no relief of pain with anti-inflammatory medication. He denies fevers or chills. He denies rashes.

Physical examination reveals full range of motion of the involved hip and knees, but pain with motion. The patient has no adenopathy.

CT images reveal lytic destruction of the left ilium and acetabulum with mild changes in the femoral head and neck. A bone scan reveals increased uptake in the left ilium, acetabulum and femoral neck, distal right femur and proximal left tibia. A white blood cell count is mildly elevated, and serum alkaline phosphatase is 2x normal range. The remainder of the patient's CBC and serum chemistries are within normal range.

Surgical findings and comments

Open biopsy is performed of the left ilium lesion with findings of softened bone but no soft tissue purulence or other abnormality.

Pathologic analysis is consistent with chronic OM. Cultures are negative.

Because no abscess or devitalized bone is present, no further surgery is indicated.

Radiology findings

We present an interesting case, **Case figs 27.1a** through **27.1i** of a 22 year old man show multifocal areas of intense uptake on bone scan and even more areas of severe edema as seen with MRI. The radiographs only have subtle heterogeneous areas of low density. The radiographic findings would be easy to overlook without relevant history. The left hip does not have an effusion as seen by MR (the lateral right knee file showed no effusion, not included). Commonly, when acute OM abuts a joint, there will be an associated effusion and the presence of joint sepsis must be ruled out. There is no abscess demonstrated on MR exam, however typically IV contrast would be given to evaluate for sequestrum or abscess.

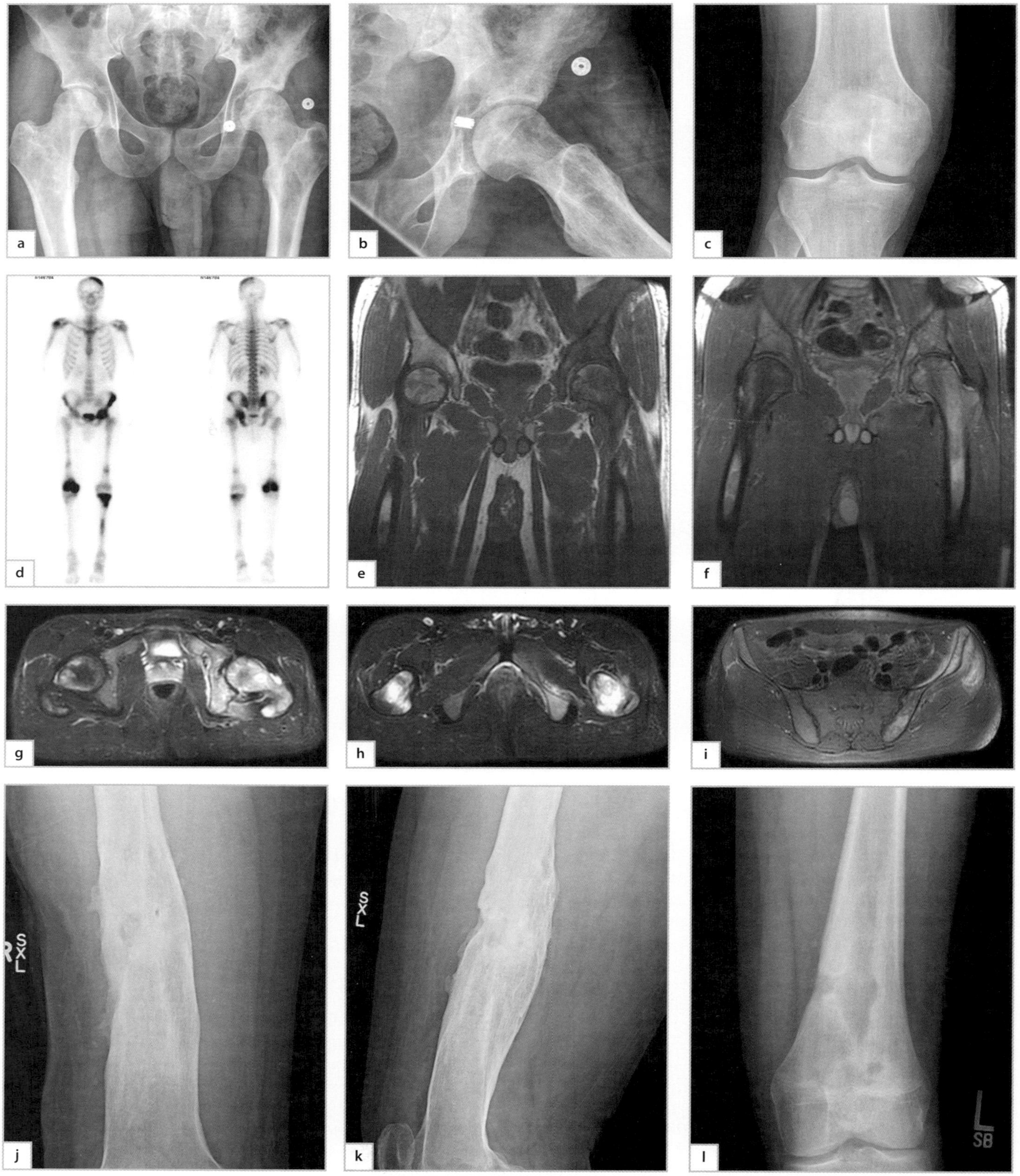

Case figure 27.1 Chronic osteomyelitis. Chronic recurrent multifocal osteomyelitis. Radiographs of a 22 year old male including **27.1a**: Anteroposterior view of the pelvis, **27.1b**: Frog lateral view of the left hip, **27.1c**: Anteroposterior view of the right knee. There is mild mottled decreased density throughout much of the left hemi pelvis and the proximal left femur. The proximal right femur shows slight increased density. The right knee radiographs appear normal. There is no knee effusion (lateral view not included) and no periosteal reaction or sequestrum seen.

Case figure 27.1: Continued from page 584

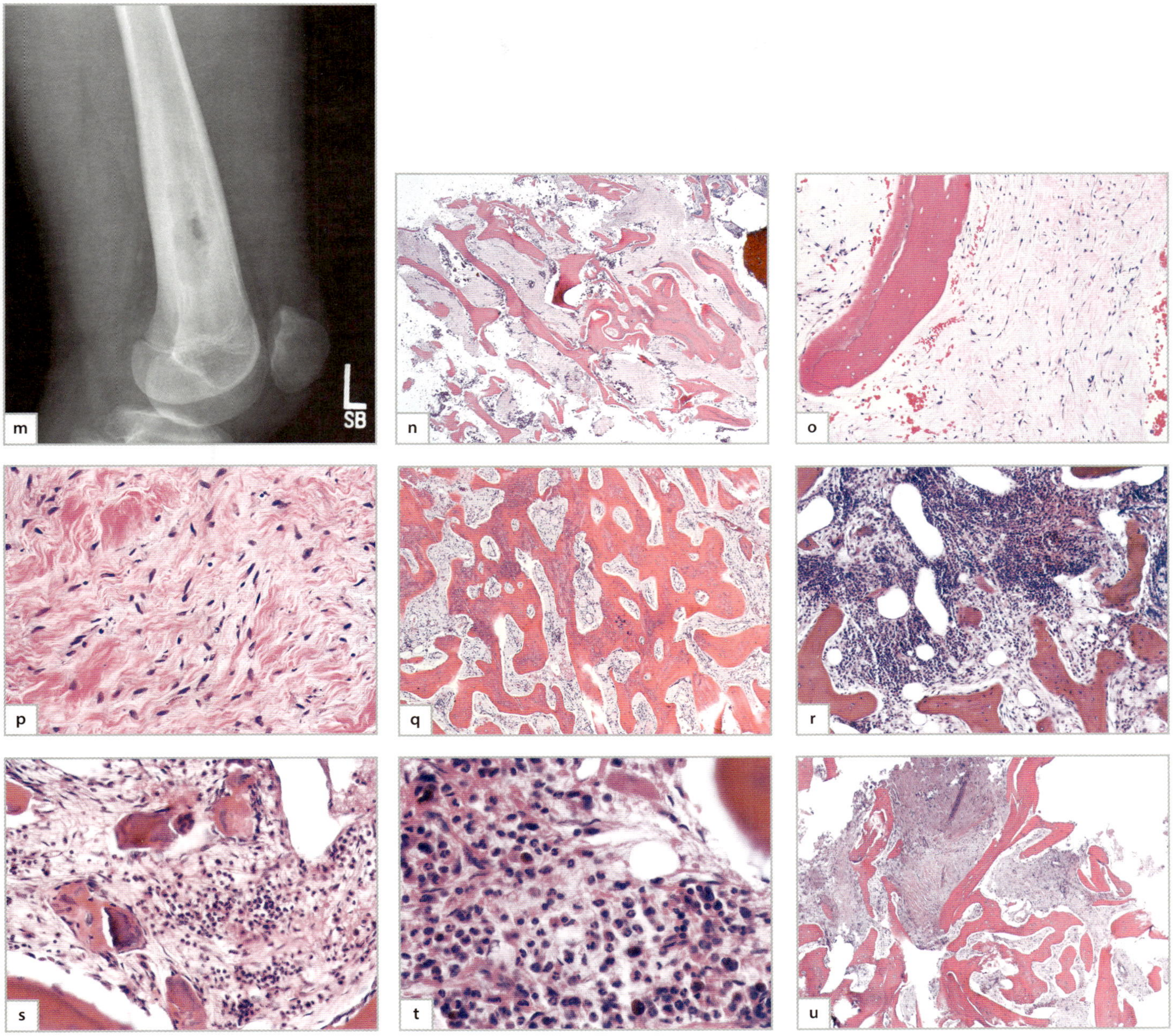

27.1d: Nuclear medicine bone scan. shows multiple areas of intense uptake with much greater disease than seen with radiography. Note the discordant appearance between bone scan and the radiographs with marked increased uptake of the distal right femur that appears normal on radiographs. MR images including; **27.1e**: coronal T1, **27.1f**: Coronal PD fat saturated images show extensive T1 low signal and corresponding PD fat saturated high signal involving the proximal left femur, the left acetabulum and the right femoral diaphysis. **27.1g**: Axial STIR through the femoral heads, **27.1h**: Axial STIR at the level of the intertrochanteric femoral neck again show the intense edema of the both femurs. **27.1i**: Axial PD fat saturated of the mid pelvis shows high signal edema of the left iliac bone with adjacent edema of the left iliacus and gluteal muscle. Note the absence of left hip effusion. Note also the discordant appearance of the intertrochanteric femurs between the MR STIR images (Case fig. 27.1h) which show intense marrow edema and the bone scan (Case fig. 27.1d) which shows near normalcy. We present two additional cases of chronic OM. **27.1j**: Anteroposterior, **27.1k**: Lateral views of the distal femur show extensive chronic periosteal reaction with remodeling. There is a central lucent defect of the femur, likely an involucrum. There is a lateral soft tissue wound defect. **27.1l**: Anteroposterior, **27.1m**: Lateral view of the distal femur in a 14 year old boy. There is a serpentine lucent tract of the medullary space extending to the lateral surface indicating a Brodie's abscess. Note the extensive periosteal reaction. **27.1n**: Low magnification. The biopsy reveals irregularly remodeled trabecular bone set in a fibrotic stroma. Normal marrow is obliterated by the fibrosis. **27.1o**: Chronic recurrent multifocal osteomyelitis (CRMO), medium magnification. Characteristic of OM, new reactive bone is laid down on dead bone. The surrounding marrow is hypocellular and fibrotic. **27.1p**: Chronic recurrent multiocal osteomyelitis (CRMO), High magnification. The affected marrow is no longer recognizable and consists of scattered spindled fibroblasts producing abundant wiry collagen. In some areas (not seen in this field) clusters of neutrophils and plasma cells indicate ongoing inflammation. **27.1q**: Chronic recurrent multifocal osteomyelitis (CRMO), low magnification. Lattices of reactive new bone are also present with a vascularized non-fibrotic but still abnormal stroma. **27.1r**: Comparison patient no.2, acute OM, lower magnification. In contrast to the bone marrow of the presented patient, this patient's marrow is highly cellular because of aggregates of acute inflammatory cells. **27.1s**: Comparison patient no. 2, acute OM, medium magnification. In this field, acute inflammatory cells congregate in slightly fibrotic marrow next two fragments of necrotic bone. New bone is partly engulfing the devitalized bone. **27.1t**: Comparison patient no. 2, acute OM, high magnification. Consistent with an acute process, the inflammatory cells consist predominantly of neutrophils with scattered eosinophils.

Case figure 27.1: Continued from page 585

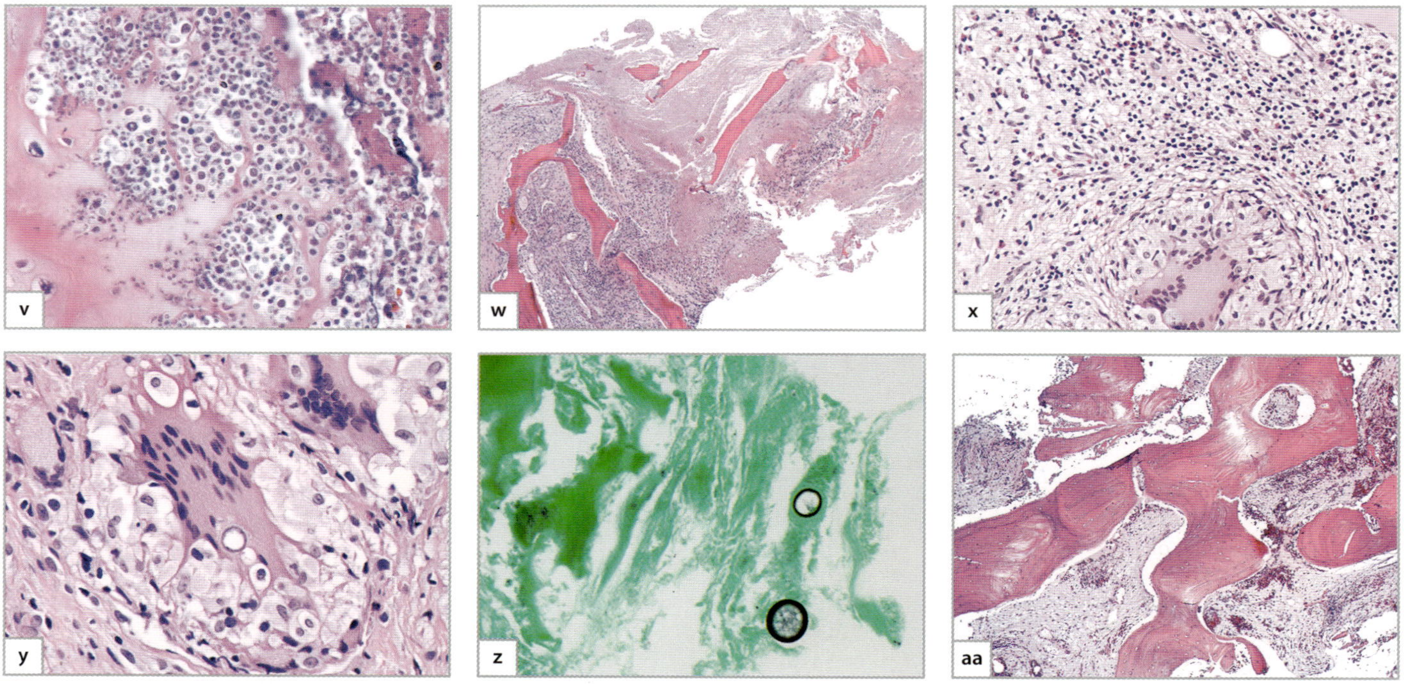

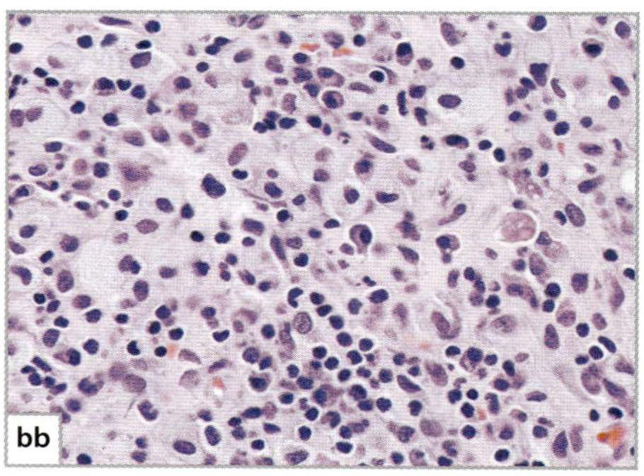

27.1u Comparison patient no. 2, acute OM, low magnification. Although most of the process comprises acutely inflamed marrow and dead bone fragments, areas also show marrow fibrosis similar to the patient with CRMO. CRMO may be indistinguishable from infectious OM, because both can exhibit acute inflammation, chronic inflammation, necrotic bone, and marrow fibrosis, even simultaneously. **27.1v**: Comparison patient no. 2, acute OM, high magnification. The cause of this patient's OM is revealed to be Candida fungal infection. Here the yeast forms and a few hyphae are invading hyaline cartilage. The species was identified on Microbiology cultures. **27.1w**: Comparison patient no. 3, OM, low magnification of bone biopsy. This patient's biopsy is uncommonly dramatic with large swathes of necrosis and corroded, necrotic bone. **27.1x**: Comparison patient no. 3, OM, medium magnification. At medium magnification, the marrow contains scattered small granulomas and a mixed inflammatory infiltrate of lymphocytes, histiocytes, and eosinophils. In the center of the granuloma sits a large, multinucleated giant cell. **27.1y**: Comparison patient no. 3, OM, high magnification. The central giant cell has ingested a relatively large round fungal structure, an empty spherule. **27.1z**: Comparison patient no. 3, OM, GMS stain. A silver stain highlights the spherules of Coccidiomycosis (black round structures). **27.1aa**: Comparison patient no. 4 Chronic OM, low magnification. This patient with chronic osteomyelitis shows thickened bone trabeculae and fibrotic marrow with sprinkles of inflammatory cells. **27.1bb**: Comparison patient no. 4 chronic OM, high magnification. The inflammation consists of plasma cells and lymphocytes with a scattered histiocyte (one of which contains hemosiderin or hematoidin pigment). This degree of chronic inflammation is typical in many biopsies of chronic OM.

We present two additional cases of chronic OM. **Case fig. 27.1j** anteroposterior and **Case fig. 27.1k** lateral radiographs of the distal femur in a 55 year old man with longstanding history of recurrent chronic OM. He had surgery 40 years prior and presented with a draining abscess. The lucent focus in the mid femoral diaphysis likely represents a bone abscess or involucrum. The adjacent lateral soft tissue defect is likely an ulcer with the draining wound. Note the mature periosteal reaction medially and the overall normal bone density indicating longstanding healing response. **Case fig. 27.1l** anteroposterior and **Case fig. 27.1m** are lateral radiographs in a 14 year old boy with a Brodie's abscess of the distal femur. There is a clear lucent track extending to the medial surface of the femoral metaphysis allowing pus to drain from the bone. There is diffuse mature appearing periosteal reaction of the metadiaphysis.

Pathology findings

Gross features

The specimen comprises multiple fragments of bony and hemorrhagic soft tissue aggregating to 3.5 cm maximally. A portion is submitted fresh for flow cytometry analysis. The remainder is submitted for Histology after mild decalcification.

Microscopic features

Low magnification: The biopsy shows abnormally shaped bone trabeculae embedded in dense, fibrotic marrow (**Case fig. 27.1n**). Normal marrow is absent. Even at low magnification, the bone appears irregularly remodeled.

High magnification: Very little inflammation is present but characteristic dead bone acts as a scaffold for reactive new bone

(**Case fig. 27.1o**). The marrow is replaced by dense fibrous tissue (**Case fig. 27.1p**). In a few areas (not sampled here) clusters of neutrophils and plasma cells are noted. Normal hematopoiesis is absent. Reactive new bone is also present associated with a vascularized marrow (**Case fig. 27.1q**).

Special studies: Flow cytometry is negative for a monotypic B-cell or abnormal T-cell population. Microbiology cultures on a portion of bone sent directly from the operating room do not grow organisms.

Additional comparison patients: Because the patient presented is quite unusual, the pathology of three other patients is also provided. Patient no. 2 is an elderly man post-sternotomy for coronary artery bypass surgery. He develops OM at the sternotomy wound site. This patient presents with a florid acute and chronic OM. At medium magnification, the marrow is filled with acute inflammatory cells (**Case fig. 27.1r**). Higher magnification reveals small fragments of necrotic bone serving as scaffolding for new bone formation (**Case fig. 27.1s**). High magnification reveals the inflammatory infiltrate to be composed of neutrophils and eosinophils (**Case fig. 27.1t**). However, other areas of the process appear similar to the main patient presented, with marrow fibrosis and irregular reactive new bone formation (**Case figure 27.1u**). The OM in this patient extends to the articular cartilage, which is invaded by yeast forms and incipient hyphae of culture proven Candida species (**Case fig. 27.1v**). Of note, the clavicle is a relatively common site for Candidal OM (Slenker et al. 2012).

Patient no. 3 is a 43 year old, immunocompetent man from Southwest New Mexico with femoral OM. Biopsy reveals widespread marrow and bone necrosis (**Case fig. 27.1w**). The viable marrow contains small granulomas surrounded by a mix of lymphocytes, eosinophils, and histiocytes (**Case fig. 27.1x**). Careful searching reveals large empty round fungal structures in dead tissue and in multinucleated giant cells (**Case fig. 27.1y**). A GMS (Gomori methenamine silver) stain highlights the spherules which are consistent with Coccidiomycosis (**Case fig. 27.1z**).

Patient no. 4 is a young adult with a long history of intermittent bone pain and fevers. The humerus biopsy reveals thickened trabecular bone and a mixed fibrotic and inflamed, abnormal marrow (**Case fig. 27.1aa**). High magnification of a more cellular area of the fibrotic marrow discloses increased plasma cells intermixed with lymphocytes consistent with chronic OM (**Case fig. 27.1bb**).

Pathologic differential or, why isn't it one of the following?

Infectious osteomyelitis: No organism is isolated. The patient has a history of substance abuse, but denies IV drug use, so the widespread, multifocal nature of the disease is unusual. He does not respond to antibiotics (two trials) and develops new lesions. He does respond to a tentative trial of steroids. All these findings are consistent with a diagnosis of exclusion: the auto-inflammatory disease, chronic recurrent multifocal OM.

Lymphoma: Multifocal bone lesions in a young adult should raise the diagnostic possibility of lymphoma which can form multiple lytic or lytic/blastic bone lesions. However, the patient does not have adenopathy, had only mildly abnormal CBC findings, and the biopsy shows no evidence of lymphoma histologically or by flow cytometric cell surface marker analysis.

Low grade osteosarcoma: Low grade osteosarcoma will not usually form multiple lesions. This patient's marrow is replaced by fibrotic tissue consistent with a mesenchymal tumor, but cytologic atypia is absent and would be present in low grade osteosarcoma. Most low grade OS express CDK4 and MDM2 in the neoplastic spindle cells; these antigens are absent in CRMO.

Oncology approach

This is not a neoplasm, and therefore chemotherapy and radiation are not indicated.

Patient outcome

The patient does not respond to two courses of antibiotics. He experiences continued pain. Repeat imaging reveals new lesions including in the skull. The Infectious Disease team is consulted. After careful review of his history, they render a diagnosis of CRMO. The patient responds well to a trial course of steroids.

Case table 27.1 Summary pathology findings of Case 27.1

Diagnosis	CRMO
Size and location	Disease is multifocal involving left pelvis and proximal femur, right distal femur and proximal tibia
Microbiology cultures and stains	Multiple blood and bone marrow cultures are negative for bacteria, viruses, and fungi. Special stains are negative for organisms.

Case 27.2 Hematoma of soft tissue

Clinical history and presentation

The patient is an 82 year old man who presents with a six week history of a right calf mass. The mass was noted spontaneously and has been persistent. He denies a history of trauma. He relates no symptoms referable to the mass. It has not changed in size.

Physical examination demonstrates a large mass associated with the right medial gastrocnemius. The limits of the mass are poorly defined.

Surgical findings and comments

Open biopsy of the soft tissue mass is performed.

Although pathologic analysis of the biopsy specimen reveals only hematoma, suspicion remains for an underlying malignancy given the persistent nature of the hematoma and lack of identifiable precipitating cause or risk factors (bleeding disorder). Therefore, the patient and surgeon elect for a myectomy of the medial gastrocnemius.

Radiology findings

Our case, **Case figs 27.2a** through **27.2c,** show a heterogeneous mass of the calf with non-enhancing areas of T1 high signal consistent with areas of hemorrhage products or protein. The lacy peripheral enhancement is unusual and likely represents contrast slowly oozing into the liquid spaces of the seroma. The margins are low signal likely from hemosiderin. Had gradient echo sequences been performed on MR, there would be blooming with apparent thickening of the wall due to susceptibility artifact caused by the iron in the hemosiderin. With time, the seroma should decrease in size and may develop collapsed appearing margins.

The imaging appearance is not specific for hematoma or seroma, as a hemorrhagic tumor could have similar appearance. Follow up either with imaging or clinical exam is warranted to assure complete resolution thus excluding an underlying malignancy. Abscess should have appropriate clinical setting and would have enhancing walls with adjacent edema and inflammation of the soft tissues.

Pathology findings

Gross features

The biopsy consists of multiple fragments of hemorrhagic tissue aggregating to 3.5 cm. The specimen is entirely submitted in five cassettes.

The resection comprises a 16 × 10 × 7.5 ovoid mass that appears encapsulated and is variably fluctuant and firm to palpation. After inking the margins, it is serially sectioned and reveals a soft, hemorrhagic to pale yellow laminated interior with central cystic cavity formation (**Case fig. 27.2d**). No tan or white tumor mass is identified. Sixteen cassettes are submitted for Histology, and the edge of the lesion is collected fresh for Cytogenetics.

Microscopic features

Low magnification: The biopsy consists of acellular fibrin and blood clot (**Case fig. 27.2e**). The resected mass consists almost entirely of organizing hematoma encased by a shell of mildly inflamed fibrous tissue containing cholesterol clefts consistent with blood breakdown (**Case fig. 27.2f**).

High magnification: The hematoma consists primarily of non-viable cell ghosts (degenerated inflammatory and red blood cells) embedded in fibrin (**Case fig. 27.2g**). The enmeshing fibrin is more easily appreciated in **Case fig. 27.2h**. Acute inflammation in association with fresh hemorrhage forms a minor component of the mass (**Case fig. 27.2i**).

Special studies: Multiple abnormal clones are identified after long term culturing and derive from a single flask: 46,XY,t(3;10)(q12;q22)[3], 46,XY,t(15;16)(q22;p13.3)[3], 46,X-Y[4], and 46,XY[13]. One non-clonal aberration of +8 is also found. Because there is no histologic evidence of a neoplasm, these abnormalities (albeit three are clonal) are considered to be an artifact of long-term culture.

Additional comparison patients: Two additional patients are briefly presented to illustrate the range of pathologic features of seromas and hematomas. Patient no. 2 has a combined seroma hematoma with fibrin bands separating serum and blood in the cystic cavity (**Case fig. 27.2j**). Hypervascular granulation tissue walls off the seroma/hematoma (**Case fig. 27.2k**).

Patient no. 3 exhibits an unusual myxochondroid change in the seroma. This could represent residual bursal tissue blends imperceptibly with fibrin deposits and mats of ghost cells (**Case fig. 27.2l**). At high magnification the gray blue matrix is studded with fibroblasts

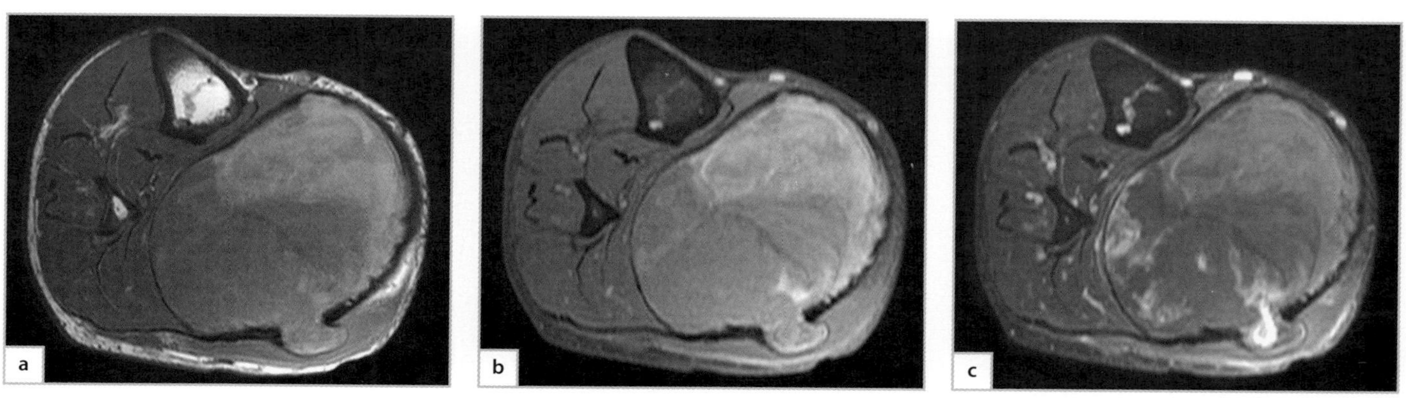

Case figure 27.2 Seroma/hematoma. MR images including; **27.2a**: Axial T1. **27.2b**: Axial T1 fat saturated, **27.2c**: Axial T1 fat saturated post-contrast are presented of this 82 year old man. There is a 9 × 6.9 × 10.9 cm heterogeneous mass in the posterior compartment of the calf. The mass shows areas of T1 high signal that do not enhance and do not show fat saturation indicating proteinaceous material or hemorrhage products (met-hemoglobin). The wall of the mass is well defined and very low signal with minimal irregularity. Although there is no T2 or gradient echo imaging to show blooming, the wall probably has hemosiderin accounting for the low signal. The mass has lacy peripheral enhancement without nodularity likely representing contrast slowly leaking into the fluid spaces of this seroma.

Case figure 27.2: Continued from page 588

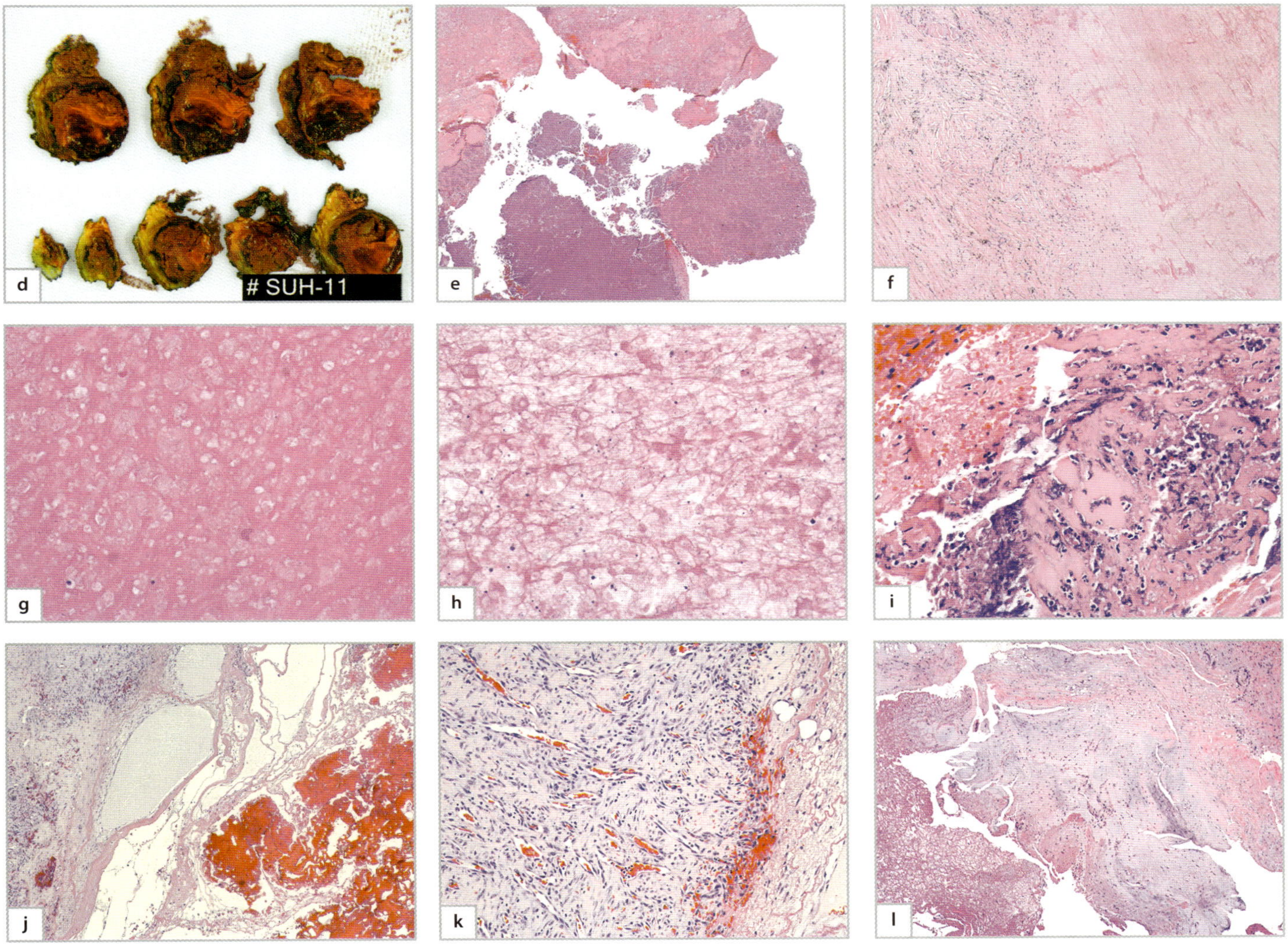

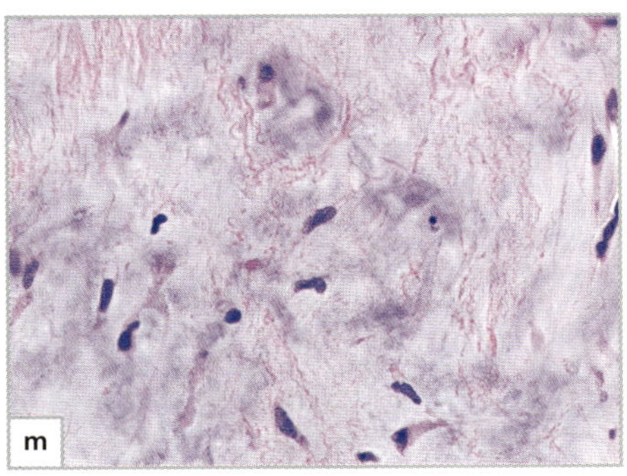

27.2d: Serial sections of 'tumor'. By gross inspection, this large mass is either an organizing hematoma or a completely infracted tumor with secondary hemorrhage. Lamination is present consistent with hematoma, and firm, tan or white areas suggestive of tumor are absent. Surrounding adipose tissue and muscle are grossly edematous and atrophic respectively. **27.2e**: Biopsy low magnification. The biopsy reveals acellular fibrin and blood clot. **27.2f**: Resection at low magnification. The organizing hematoma is surrounded by a rind of fibrous tissue that contains cholesterol clefts and scattered histiocytes and lymphocytes. **27.2g**: High magnification. Much of the resected lesion consists of cell ghosts embedded in fibrin. These necrotic cells are consistent with inflammatory cells and red blood cells. **27.2h**: High magnification. The fibrin meshwork is readily apparent in this field. A few degenerated nuclear bits form small balls strewn among ghost cells. **27.2i**: High magnification. In a few areas, acute inflammation and fresh hemorrhage are present. **27.2j**: Comparison patient no. 2, low magnification. This patient has an organizing seroma with hemorrhage. Mutiple fibrin bands cross a cystic cavity filled with serum and blood. The wall is fibrotic and hypervascular. **27.2k**: Comparison patient no. 2, high magnification. The wall of this patient's seroma/hematoma consists of hypervascular granulation tissue (cyst contents are partly seen on the right). **27.2l**: Comparison patient no. 3, edium magnification. An unusual myxochondroid change accompanies the fibrin and ghost cells in this patient's seroma. **27.2m**: Comparison patient no. 3, high magnification. The myxochondroid appearing area contains scattered fibroblasts responsible for the blue-gray myxoid matrix.

(**Case fig. 27.2m**). This myxoid character to the fibroblastic response is unusual but does not signify a neoplasm.

Pathologic differential or, why isn't it one of the following?

Sarcoma: Extensive sampling and careful gross examination of the biopsy and resection fail to reveal any evidence of a neoplasm. Although the cytogenetics reveals clonal populations, these are all derived from one flask in long term culture conditions and are considered spurious. The patient is followed carefully, and he shows no evidence of residual or metastatic tumor. Spontaneous hematomas may be quite large and are thus worrisome for malignancy. This patient's presentation is unusual but not exceptional. It is possible that the patient sustained an injury many years prior to developing the lesion, presenting with an 'ancient hematoma' (Mentzel et al. 1997). However, most patients present within six months of the inciting trauma (Negoro et al. 2012).

Infection: The patient had no signs or symptoms of infection. The few inflammatory cells present in the lesion were enmeshed in fibrin without abscess formation. Greater than 99% of the lesion consisted only of fibrin, blood clot, and amorphous debris.

Case table 27.2 Summary pathology findings of Case 27.2

Diagnosis	Spontaneous hematoma mimicking a soft tissue sarcoma
Size	15 × 9 × 7 cm
Location	Lower leg, intramuscular

Oncology approach

This is not a neoplasm, and therefore chemotherapy and radiation are not indicated.

Patient outcome

One year following surgery, the patient is asymptomatic, has normal function, and has had no signs of malignancy either on physical exam or repeat MRI. He has resumed an active lifestyle including golfing.

Case 27.3 Granulomatous inflammation suggestive of granuloma annulare at site of prior sarcoma resection mimicking recurrent sarcoma

Clinical history and presentation

The patient is a 23 year old man with a history of embryonal rhabdomyosarcoma involving the right paratesticular and spermatic cord region initially treated six years previously with chemotherapy (cyclophosphamide, actinomycin-D, and vincristine) and surgery (right orchiectomy and exploratory laparotomy with pelvic node dissection).

The patient is being followed at regular intervals and with reassuring results until he noticed a mass one month prior to presentation in the right lower quadrant soft tissue above the inguinal ligament.

Physical examination reveals a firm solid soft tissue mass in the right lower quadrant of the abdomen. It is fixed to underlying deep tissue and non-tender.

Surgical findings and comments

At surgery, a 4-cm firm fixed mass is excised. No surrounding tissue is grossly concerning. The mass is cephalad to the inguinal ligament and caudad to the iliac crest approximately 10 cm from the umbilicus. Marginal excision is performed.

Pathologic analysis reveals sarcoma inconsistent with rhabdomyosarcoma. Margins are positive. The patient is returned to surgery for wide resection, following which pathologic analysis reveals residual tumor with a very close deep margin.

Postoperatively, the patient develops a wound infection which resolves with local care and antibiotics.

After satisfactory resolution of the infection and wound healing, the patient is returned for surgery three months later for wide resection of the residual tumor bed.

Radiology findings

Our case, **Case figs 27.3a** through **27.3d**, is complicated in that this 23 year old patient develops a second primary sarcoma many years after his initial paratesticular embryonal rhabdosarcoma was treated. The second sarcoma is discovered on routine surveillance imaging, **Case fig. 27.3b**, with a new nodule in the right inguinal region developing in a region of stable postoperative scaring. The patient then develops a post-operative seroma, a relatively common non-alarming occurrence. However, just 5 months post-operatively, the seroma has resolved and there is another new solid nodule in the right inguinal region. Quite reasonably, this is thought to represent an early recurrence of the second primary sarcoma. But fortunately for the patient, it proves to be non-infectious granulomatous inflammation.

Pathology findings

Gross features:

The third resection specimen consists of an ellipse of skin and underlying tan soft tissue 4.5 × 3 × 1.6 cm. After careful inking of the margins, serial sections reveal central defect in the soft tissue without a discrete tumor mass. A sample around the defect is submitted for Cytogenetics, and the remainder is submitted in 10 cassettes.

Microscopic features

Low magnification: Low magnification reveals multiple nodules studding the dermis (**Case fig. 27.3e**). Most of the nodules have a pink center similar to surrounding collagen.

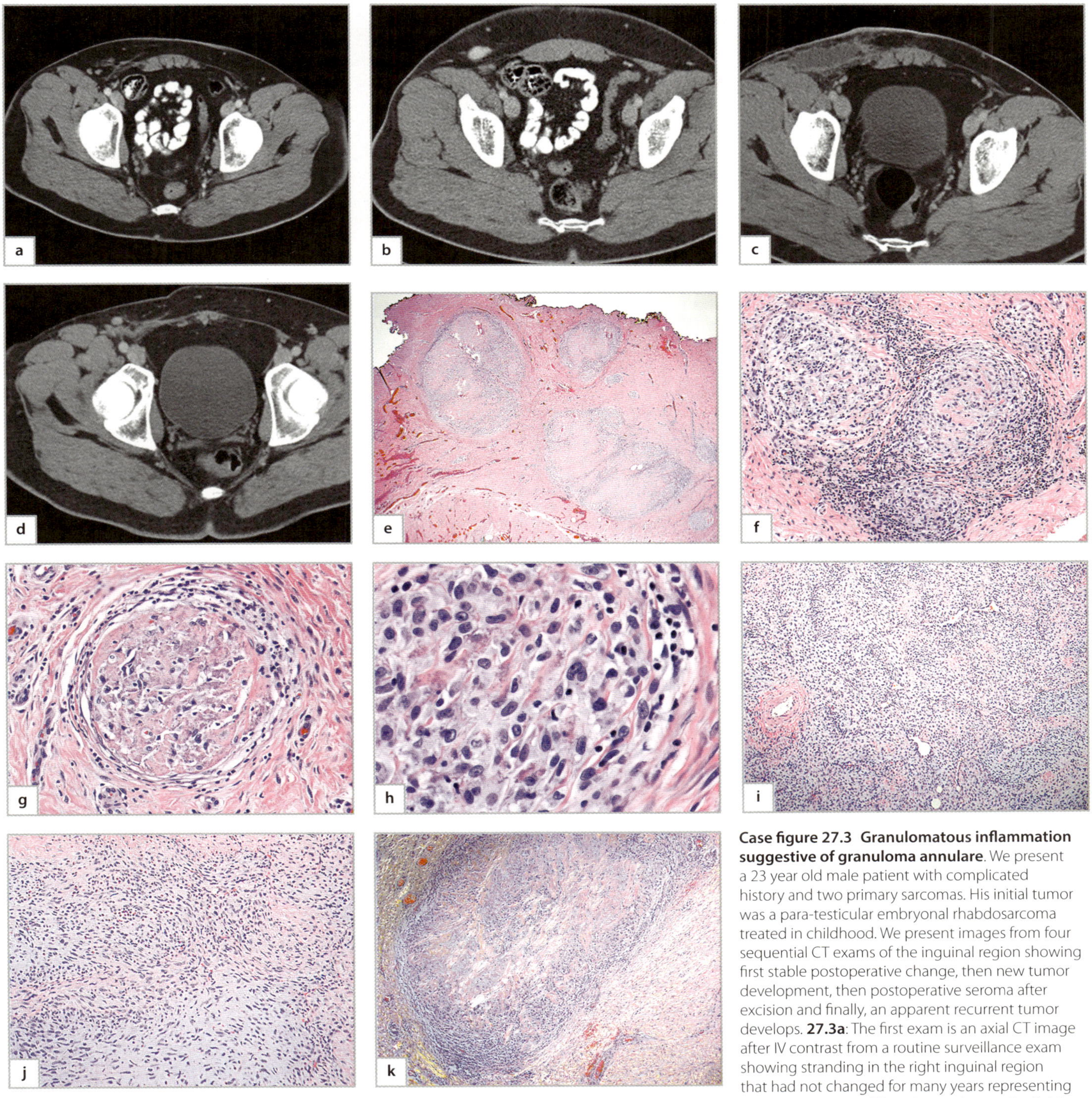

Case figure 27.3 Granulomatous inflammation suggestive of granuloma annulare. We present a 23 year old male patient with complicated history and two primary sarcomas. His initial tumor was a para-testicular embryonal rhabdosarcoma treated in childhood. We present images from four sequential CT exams of the inguinal region showing first stable postoperative change, then new tumor development, then postoperative seroma after excision and finally, an apparent recurrent tumor develops. **27.3a**: The first exam is an axial CT image after IV contrast from a routine surveillance exam showing stranding in the right inguinal region that had not changed for many years representing post-operative scar. There is no adenopathy, fluid collection or mass. **27.3b**: This image is a post-IV contrast CT image obtained one year later showing a hyperdense mass measuring 21 × 13 × 24 mm had developed in the right inguinal region subcutaneous tissues. Biopsy was performed at an outside institution and this proved to be a new primary sarcoma. **27.3c**: This image is a post-IV contrast CT image obtained 3 months later showing a fluid collection in the right groin with partially collapsed appearing margins indicating a resolving seroma. There is no adenopathy or solid tumor identified. **27.3d**: This image is the final post-IV contrast CT image obtained 2 months later showing a small new solid mass measuring 7 × 8 × 12 mm in the right groin. This was thought to represent an early recurrence of the second sarcoma. **27.3e**: Low magnification. The dermis is studded with well-defined nodules. These nodules are located in normal and fibrotic dermis, indicating they extend beyond the area of prior surgery. **27.3f**: Medium magnification. Some of the smaller nodules are cellular, surrounded by chronic inflammatory cells and contain relatively little acellular pink material. **27.3g**: Medium magnification. Degenerating acellular eosinophilic material consistent with necrobiotic collagen compose the center of most of the nodules. **27.3h**: High magnification. Epithelioid histiocytes form the nodules. Multinucleated giant cells are absent. **27.3i**: Low magnification. The patient's preceding intermediate grade sarcoma forms moderately cellular swirls in the dermis centering around ectatic blood vessels. This is the tumor seen in the prior two biopsies. **27.3j**: High magnification. The sarcoma is myxoid, spindled and elicits an eosinophil-laden inflammatory response. Granulomas are absent in the two biopsies that contain sarcoma. **27.3k**: Polarization of an H&E slide confirms that the eosinophilic material in the granulomas is collagen as it polarizes exactly as adjacent dermal collagen.

High magnification: A few of the smaller nodules are cellular with a cuff of chronic inflammatory cells and contain only scant pink material (**Case fig. 27.3f**). However, most are predominantly filled with acellular eosinophilic material consistent with degenerated collagen (**Case fig. 27.3g**). The main cell type located in and/or at the edges of the nodules is the epithelioid histiocyte (**Case fig. 27.3h**). Multinucleated histiocytes are conspicuously absent.

The granulomas bear no resemblance to the sarcoma that had been resected in the same site. The sarcoma consists of relatively hypocellular swirls of cells centered around dilated blood vessels (**Case fig. 27.3i**). The lesional cells are spindled, float in a pale myxoid matrix, and incite an eosinophil rich inflammatory response (**Case fig. 27.3j**). There are no granulomas present at this stage in the patient's course.

Returning to the granulomas, polarization confirms the collagenous material within the nodules which polarizes exactly as surrounding dermal collagen (**Case fig. 27.3k**).

Special studies: Special stains including AFB (for mycobacteria), GMS (for fungi and bacteria), Tissue Gram (for most bacteria) and PAS/D (for fungi) are all negative for organisms.

The karyotype is 46,XY [18] with two non-clonal abnormalities of t(X;19)(p11.4;p13.3)[1] and der(17)t(1;17)(q24;p13)[1].

Pathologic differential or, why isn't it one of the following?

Foreign body granulomas: Granulomatous inflammation responding to suture or keratin is common at the site of prior surgery. However, such granulomas often feature multinucleated histiocytes (which are absent in these nodules) and suture material. The material present in these granulomas is collagen undergoing dissolution. By definition, these are necrobiotic granulomas. Necrobiotic granulomas occurring at the site of prior vaccination or trauma have been termed deep granuloma annulare (DGA) (McDermott et al. 1998, Pesce et al. 2010). However, DGA is also associated with a number of other conditions such as various infections and autoimmune or immunosuppressed states (Stefanaki et al, 2007).

Case table 27.3 Summary pathology findings of Case 27.3

Diagnosis	Necrobiotic granulomatous inflammation suggestive of granuloma annulare
Size	Multiple nodules involving approximately 2 cm of dermis
Location	Dermis including scarred dermis at prior sarcoma resection site

Infectious granulomas: After two resections, the patient developed a wound infection. He was treated successfully, and five months later was noted to have this nodule at the surgical scar. There is no evidence the granulomas are infectious, as no organisms are identified. Furthermore, the nature of the granulomas is necrobiotic with central dissolving masses of collagen. It is possible these granulomas are related to the prior infection and represent an aberrant immune response (Pesce et al. 2010).

Oncology approach

This final resection consists of non-neoplastic granulomatous inflammation and therefore chemotherapy and radiation are not indicated.

Patient outcome

Two years postoperatively, the patient has no evidence of tumor. There is no detectable granulomatous inflammation.

Case 27.4 Bursitis

Clinical history and presentation

The patient is a 77 year old woman who presents with a two year history of right knee pain associated with degenerative arthritis. She relates an associated mass which has also been present for two years. Fluid has been drained repeatedly from the mass but it remains persistent.

Physical examination reveals a large (10x15x5 cm) mass overlying the anteromedial aspect of the left leg just below the knee. It is fluctuant and compressible. It is non-tender.

Surgical findings and comments

Surgical excision is elected to rule out neoplasm. At surgery, the mass is noted to consist of an encapsulated cystic structure. The cyst lining is excised.

Radiology findings

We present three cases (**Case figs 27.4a** through **27.4g**) of bursitis unrelated to the pathology case. Commonly, the clinical setting allows diagnosis as there is focal soft tissue swelling with exquisite pain and point tenderness. Only if there is clinical concern for other pathology is imaging undertaken. MR is often utilized because it can best diagnose or exclude associated or confounding pathology. In particular, the adjacent tendon and its bone attachment are important sites to assess for associated injury.

Pathology findings

Gross features

The specimen consists of greater than 10 fragments of gray soft tissue mixed with mucoid material aggregating to 8.5 × 6.5 × 2.5 cm. Cross sections reveal edematous and mucinous surfaces. Representative sections are submitted in ten cassettes.

Microscopic features

Low magnification: The specimen comprises a mix of fibrous and adipose tissue. The fibrous tissue fragments contain multiple partially compressed spaces filled with fibrin (**Case fig. 27.4h**). A synovial lining is absent, but the spaces are circumscribed by bands of dense connective tissue.

High magnification: Medium magnification of the fibrotic wall of a cyst shows increased vascularity appearing as blooms of small

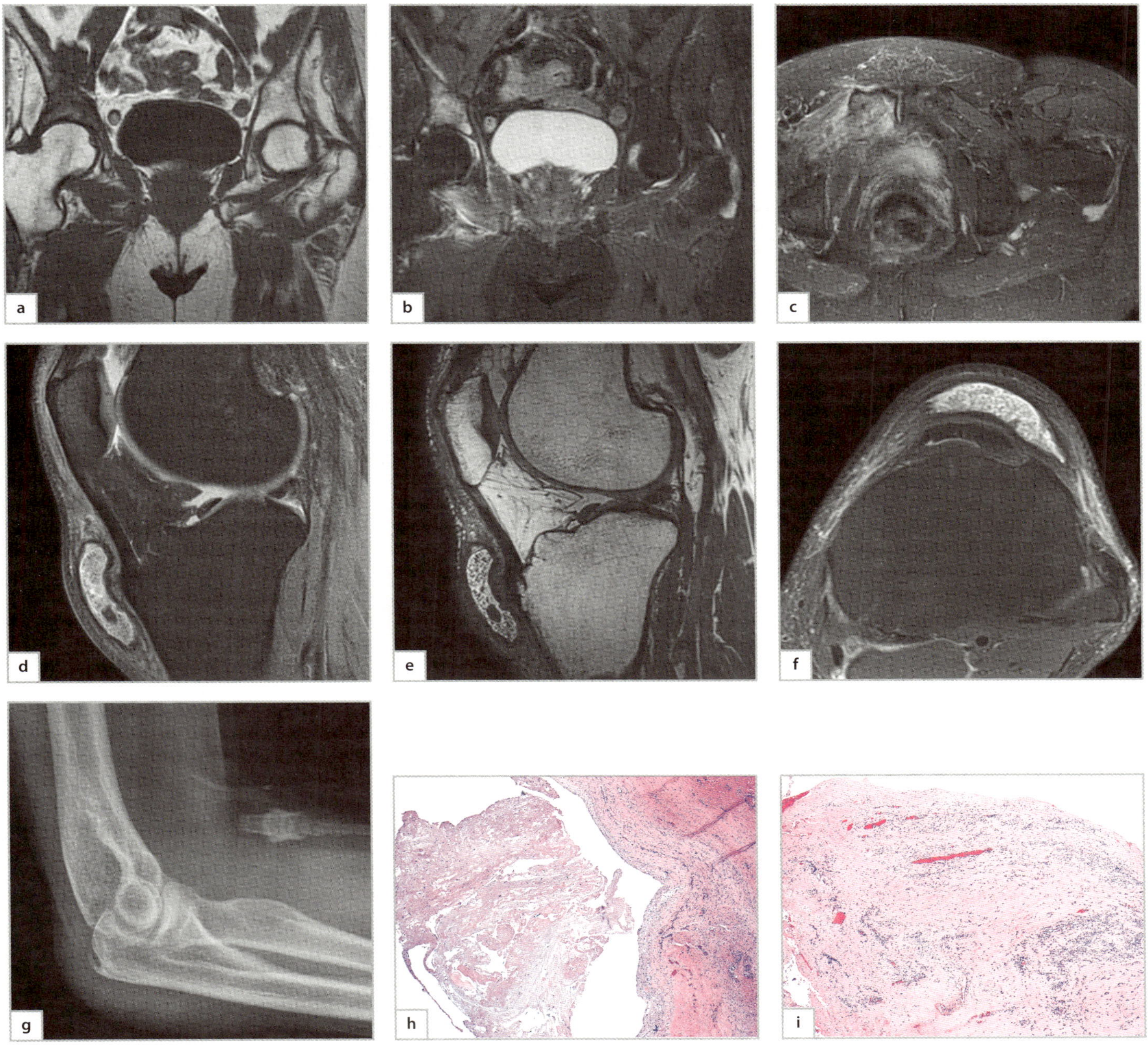

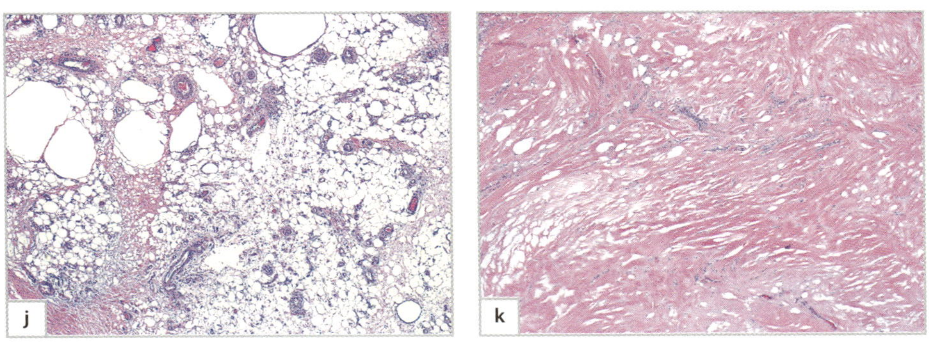

Case figure 27.4 Bursitis. We do not have imaging associated with the pathology case. However, we present three unrelated cases of bursitis involving the greater trochanter bursa, the infrapatellar bursa and the olecranon bursa. **27.4a**: Coronal T1, **27.4b**: Coronal STIR, **27.4c**: Axial STIR MR images of an 80 year old woman show moderate fluid in the left greater trochanteric bursa. This causes distention of the bursa posteriorly and there is adjacent soft tissue edema indicating active inflammation. There are also fractures of the right pubic bone and right supra-acetabular iliac bone. Note, the greater trochanter and gluteal tendon insertions are normal. **27.4d**: Sagittal PD fat saturated, **27.4e**: Sagittal T2 3D space, **27.4f**: Axial PD fat saturated MR images of a 48 year old man with infra-patellar bursitis. The fluid is heterogeneous, having numerous 'rice bodies' as can be seen with rheumatoid arthritis. This appearance may be related to chronic inflammation with the accumulation of debris. The bursal walls are thickened and low signal indicating there is probably scaring from chronic disease. Note, the patellar tendon and tibial tubercle are normal.

vessels with sparse perivascular chronic inflammation (**Fig. 27.4i**). The adjacent adipose tissue exhibits fat necrosis and regeneration (**Case fig. 27.4j**) or hyalinization (**Case fig. 27.4k**).

Special studies: None are performed.

Pathologic differential or, why isn't it one of the following?

Realistically, there is no histologic differential for this lesion which shows classic features of bursitis including septal fibrosis, fibrin deposits, inflammation, and neovascularization. In this case, diagnostic consideration of a neoplasm occurred at the clinical and radiologic phases of the patient's care. The typical pathology findings of bursitis resolves this concern.

Case table 27.4 Summary pathology findings of Case 27.4

Diagnosis	Chronic bursitis
Size	15 × 10 × 5 cm
Location	Bursal tissue of knee
Margin status	Not relevant

Oncology approach

This is not a neoplasm, and therefore chemotherapy and radiation are not indicated.

Patient outcome

Three months postoperatively, the cyst is noted to have recurred. She is scheduled for total knee arthroplasty in the hope that this procedure will treat her underlying arthritis and the associated cyst.

Case 27.5 Massive lymphedema

Clinical history and presentation

The patient is a 32 year old man with a history of massive chronic swelling of the left leg over the previous three years. Prior to onset of swelling, he was an active individual without disability, including a tour of four years of duty in the military.

Physical examination of the right lower extremity reveals massive swelling below the groin. Clinical pre-operative photos are shown in **Case figs 27.5a** and **27.5b**.

The patient has exhausted all conservative measures and is substantially disabled by his condition with inability to ambulate and chronic pain. He was extensively evaluated at another national specialist institution to attempt to find an infectious cause, and none were identified. The patient requests an amputation. His family and spouse are present during the initial treatment discussion and subsequent consultations, and all are aware of the significant risk of surgery (10-15% mortality rate). He decides to proceed with amputation.

Surgical findings and comments

Left hip disarticulation is performed with primary wound closure. Because of numerous, dilated torturous vessels, bleeding is significant (~6 liters). After amputation, thick, copious lymphatic tissue is debulked and two drains and a wound-vac are placed. Postoperatively, he develops a wound dehiscence and infection which resolves with negative pressure wound care and antibiotics.

Radiology findings

Imaging is not performed.

Pathology findings

Gross features

The massively enlarged leg weighs 165 kg (363 lbs). Redundant folds of skin and fat drape over the inferior anterior leg. In these pendulous areas, the skin is corrugated and markedly hyperkeratotic consistent with reaction to chronic contact rubbing. Ulcers are not identified. Sectioning through the leg confirms that the enlargement is due to excess mature adipose tissue (**Case fig. 27.5c**). No discrete tumors are found. Multiple sections are submitted for histology review. Samples are also collected fresh for cytogenetics and tissue banking.

Microscopic features

Low magnification: Many sections of the patient's deep adipose tissue are histologically normal (**Case fig. 27.5d**). However, approximately 20% exhibit increased variability in fat cell size and increased fibrous trabeculations (**Case fig. 27.5e**).

High magnification: Myxoid change and sparse chronic inflammation are present in some of the sampled adipose tissue (**Case fig. 27.5f**). Some of the small vessels show edema and mild reactive nuclear changes (enlargement). Some vessel nuclei are pyknotic consistent with necrosis (**Case fig. 27.5g**). The lower leg with areas of grossly apparent hyperkeratosis correlates with microscopic areas of marked hyperkeratosis, dermal fibrosis, and perivascular inflammation of dermal capillaries (**Case fig. 27.5h**). The most abnormal dermal sections exhibit diffuse fibrosis and foci of lymphoplasmacytic inflammation near clusters of capillaries and venules (**Case fig. 27.5i**).

The final case of bursitis, **27.4g** Lateral view of the elbow in a 69 year old woman show posterior soft tissue swelling without erosion or calcification. The findings are classic for olecranon bursitis. **27.4h**: Low magnification. Some of the specimen consists of partially compressed spaces filled with fibrin. The walls enclosing the spaces comprise dense connective tissue with adherent fibrin and scant inflammation. A synovial lining is not observed. **27.4i**: Medium magnification. The inflamed bursal walls are thickened and exhibit neovascularization and mild chronic inflammation. Smaller new vessels cluster around congested larger vessels. **27.4j**: Medium magnification. Interestingly, the adjacent cushioning adipose tissue is also abnormal, displaying fat necrosis and regeneration. **27.4k**: Medium magnification. Some of the adipose tissue has undergone hyalinization.

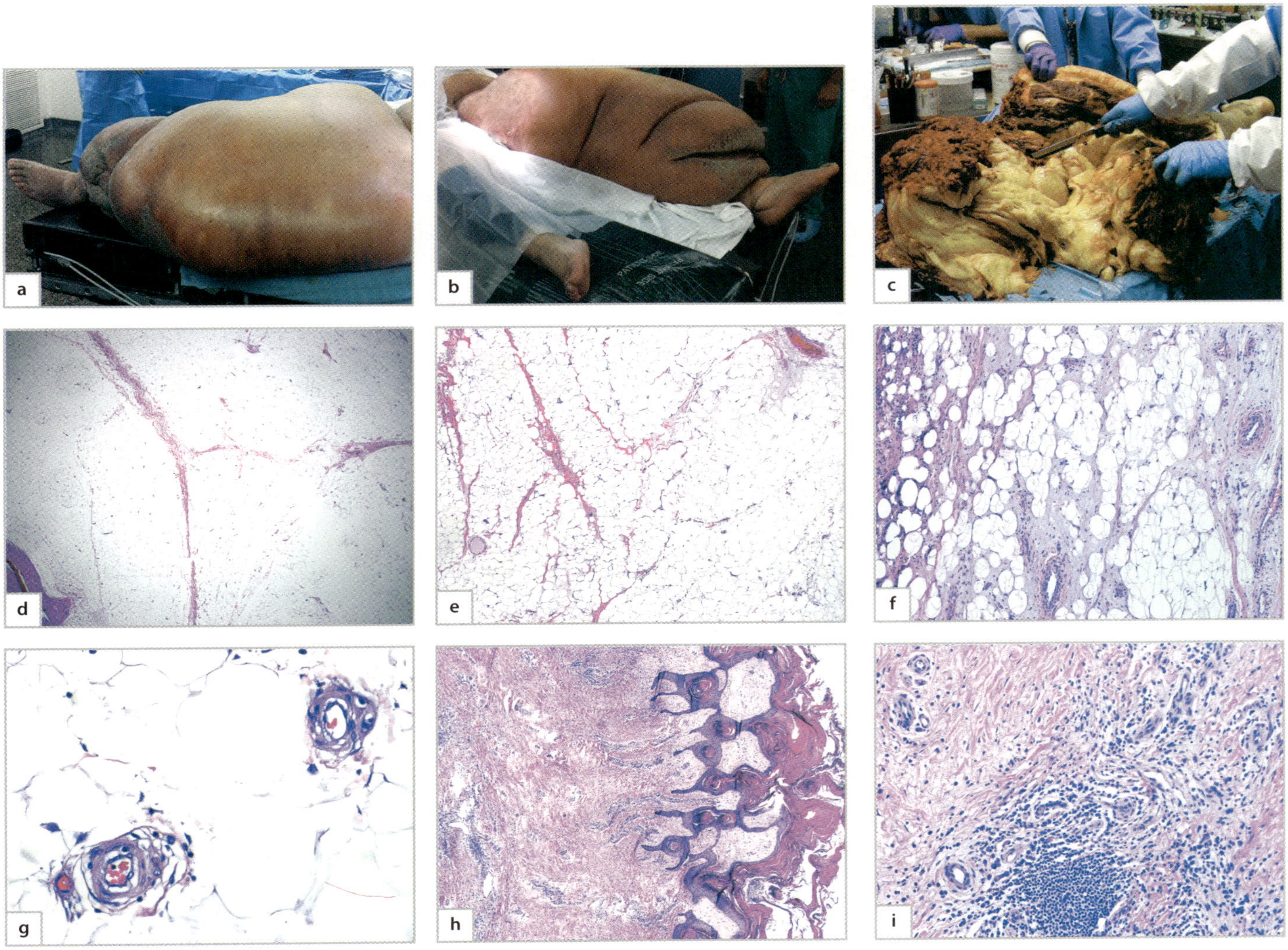

Case figure 27.5 Massive lymphedema 27.5a: The patient's leg with the anterior surface shifted laterally on the operating table. Note the relatively normal sized foot and the callous like thickening of the inferior skin **27.5b**: The patient is otherwise moderately obese. The affected leg lacks ulcers or hyperemic areas. **27.5c**: Cross section of leg. Sectioning through the leg reveals an extreme amount of mature appearing yellow adipose tissue. There are no discrete tumor masses, and fat necrosis is also absent. Vessels are patent without atherosclerotic changes. The subcutaneous fat is only mildly thickened (observed to the right of the purple-gloved hand); it is the deep inter-muscular fat that has massively expanded. **27.5d**: Low magnification. Most of the deep adipose tissue is histologically normal. **27.5e**: Low magnification. Twenty percent of the sections reveal subtle changes of increased variability in fat cell size, more fibrous septae, and mild edema. **27.5f**: Medium magnification. Myxoid change is present focally along with sparse chronic inflammation. Atypical stromal cells and lipoblasts are absent. **27.5g**: High magnfication. Some of the small vessels in the deep fat appear damaged with edema or cytoplasmic vacuolation, nuclear pyknosis, mild reactive nuclear enlargement. **27.5h**: Medium magnification. The thickened skin noted grossly corresponds microscopically to marked papillomatous hyperkeratosis, dermal fibrosis, and perivascular dermal chronic inflammation. **27.5i**: High magnification. The dermis beneath the hyperkeratotic epidermis reveals lymphoplasmacytic inflammation in association with increased numbers of small blood vessels. Cytologic atypia is absent.

Special studies: The patient's karyotype is 46,XY[19] with one nonclonal aberration of del(7)(q10). The normal karyotype is expected for lymphedema.

Pathologic differential or, why isn't it one of the following?

Atypical lipomatous tumor, lipoma-like variant: Atypical lipomatous tumor (ALT) forms a distinct mass rather than diffusely involving a limb. It contains atypical stromal cells, marked variation in adipocyte size, and lipoblasts may also be present. Many of the neoplastic adipocytes express p16, CDK4 and/or MDM2 by IHC. CDK4 and MDM2 gene amplification are usually present.

Case table 27.5 Summary pathology findings of Case 27.5

Diagnosis	Massive lymphedema
Size	Entire leg (165 kg)
Location	Left leg

Lymphedema lacks CDK4 and MDM2 IHC overexpression or gene amplification.

Lymphedema due to an infectious organism: The patient was carefully examined for evidence of infection such as filariasis. However, no organisms were found.

Oncology approach

This is not a neoplasm, and therefore chemotherapy and radiation are not indicated.

Patient outcome

Six months postoperatively, the patient is ambulatory with crutches, regularly undergoing physical therapy and awaiting a prosthesis. He is quite happy with his outcome.

Case 27.6 Mycetoma

Clinical history and presentation

A 70 year old male presents with a decade long history of a right medial elbow mass. The mass initially occurred following a trauma but has been persistent and has continued to slowly enlarge over the years. He relates mild tenderness associated with the mass.

Physical examination reveals a 3×7 cm, firm deep soft tissue mass over the medial aspect of the elbow. It is fixed to underlying deep structures. It is minimally tender. There are no neurologic deficits. The skin over the mass is focally discolored which the patient states represented a 'pimple' which 'popped' the week prior.

The clinical impression is inflammatory granulomatous type tissue persistent after trauma. However, histopathology is required for definitive diagnosis.

Surgical findings and comments

The mass is excised, with finding of largely solid material containing an admixture of purulence.

Radiology findings

Imaging is not performed.

Pathology findings

Gross features

The specimen comprises an 8 × 7 × 3 cm portion of focally hyperemic yellow lobulated adipose tissue. After the margins are inked, it is cross sectioned and reveals four cysts up to 2.5 cm in diameter containing viscous, somewhat mucinous, yellow-brown material. The cysts are surrounded by variable amounts of dense, fibrous, tan tissue. Multiple sections are submitted for histology review.

Microscopic features

Low magnification: Multiple inflammatory nodules are dispersed in dense fibrous tissue which also shows more diffuse inflammation (**Case fig. 27.6a**).

High magnification: High magnification of a crescent shaped structure in the nodule of inflammation reveals a mat of non-pigmented fungal hyphae encased by serum-like glassy eosinophilic debris (**Case fig. 27.6b**). Neutrophils and histiocytes surround this granule (also known as a grain). The lesion displays a range of inflammatory responses including abscess like areas (**Case fig. 27.6c**), xanthomatous inflammation (**Case fig. 27.6d**), and chronic plasmacytic inflammation (**Case fig. 27.6e**). Some fields contain acute inflammation, chronic inflammation, and multinucleated giant cells (**Case fig. 27.6f**).

Special studies: Because there was no indication that the specimen might represent an infectious process, no tissue is taken fresh for microbiology cultures. A silver stain (GMS) performed on the formalin-fixed, paraffin embedded tissue highlights the fungal hyphae which are thicker than 1 micron in diameter and relatively non-septate (**Case fig. 27.6g**).

Additional comparison patients: Because mycetoma is far less common than soft tissue abscess, two patients with bacterial abscesses are also presented for histologic comparison. Patient no. 2 has a subcutaneous bacterial abscess that has produced a pseudocapsule (**Case fig. 27.6h**). Abscess contents comprise viable and necrotic neutrophils mixed with fibrin (**Case fig. 27.6i**).

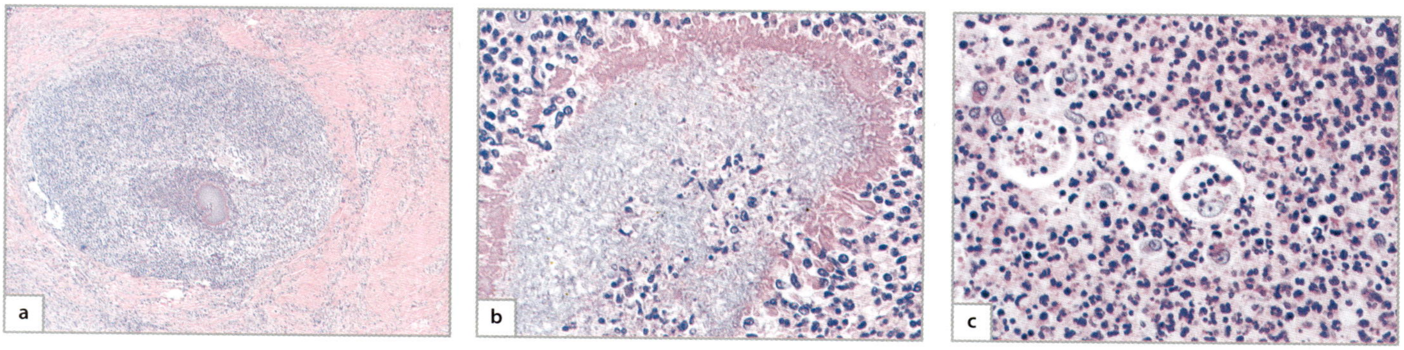

Case figure 27.6 Soft tissue mycetoma 27.6a: Low magnification. Multiple nodules are dispersed in fibrotic tissue that itself is variably inflamed. Even at low magnification, a crescent shaped structure rimmed by red material is apparent in the inflammatory nodule. **27.6b**: High magnification. A typical granule or grain (mat of fungal hyphae) encased by eosinophilic glassy material and surrounded by neutrophils and histiocytes. **27.6c**: High magnification. A single mycetoma may simultaneously demonstrate different types of inflammatory response, and this patient's lesion is no exception. In this field, abscess like findings include abundant neutrophils with tingible body macrophages stuffed with phagocytosed dead neutrophils.

Case figure 27.6: Continued from page 596

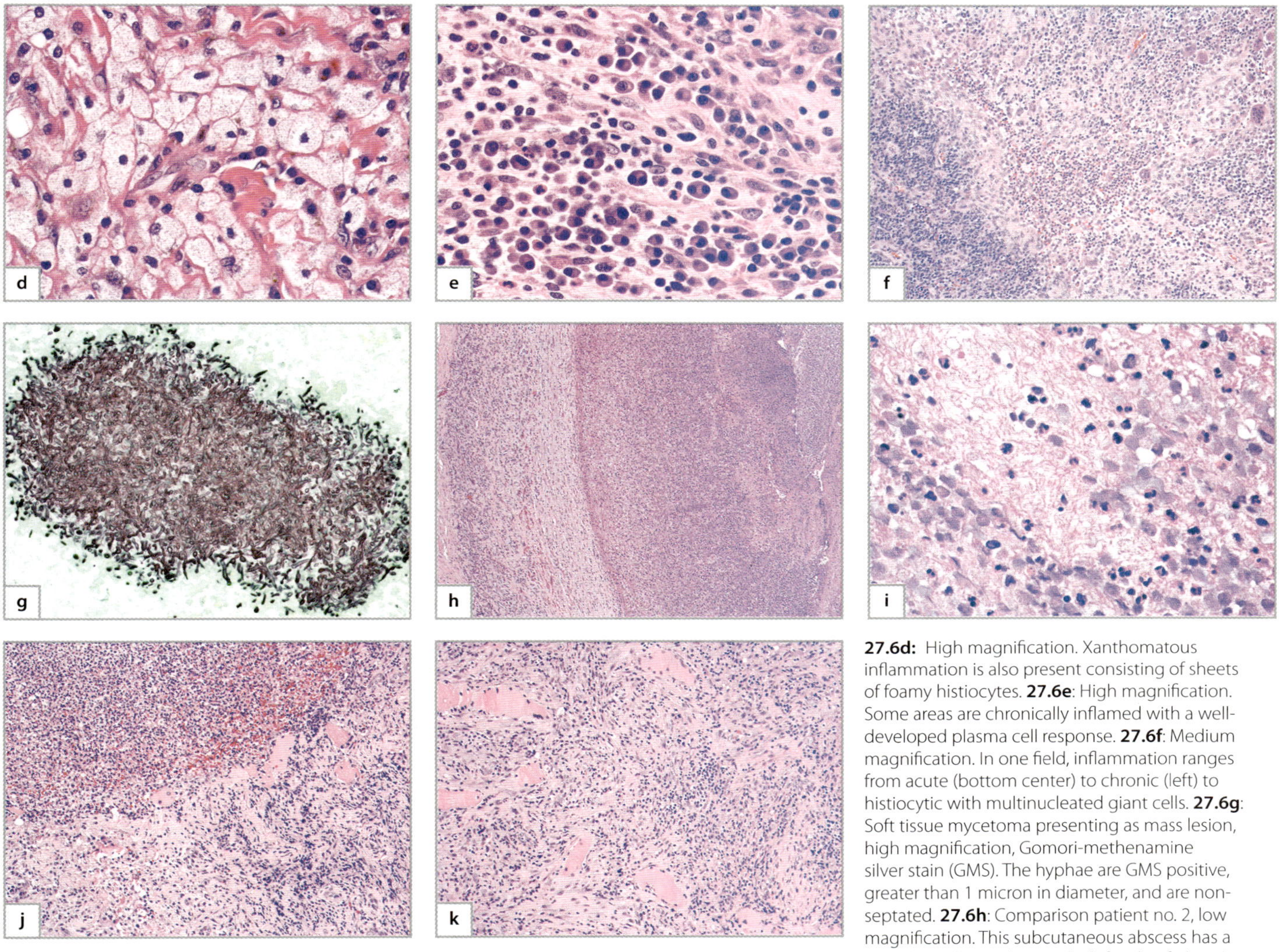

27.6d: High magnification. Xanthomatous inflammation is also present consisting of sheets of foamy histiocytes. **27.6e**: High magnification. Some areas are chronically inflamed with a well-developed plasma cell response. **27.6f**: Medium magnification. In one field, inflammation ranges from acute (bottom center) to chronic (left) to histiocytic with multinucleated giant cells. **27.6g**: Soft tissue mycetoma presenting as mass lesion, high magnification, Gomori-methenamine silver stain (GMS). The hyphae are GMS positive, greater than 1 micron in diameter, and are non-septated. **27.6h**: Comparison patient no. 2, low magnification. This subcutaneous abscess has a vascularized pseudocapsule (left side of photo). **27.6i**: Comparison patient no. 2, high magnification. The abscess contents consist of viable and necrotic neutrophils mixed with fibrin. **27.6j**: Deep soft tissue abscess, patient no. 3, low magnification. This deep abscess does not have a pseudocapsule. **27.6k**: Deep soft tissue abscess, comparison patient no. 4, medium magnification. The tissue immediately surrounding the abscess is also markedly abnormal with myonecrosis, fibrosis and chronic inflammation.

Patient no. 3 has a deep muscular abscess that is not walled off from surrounding tissue and comprises a center of acute inflammatory cells and hemorrhage and an edge of necrotic myofibers mingled with chronic inflammatory cells (**Case fig. 27.6j**). The tissue surrounding the purulent center is also quite abnormal with myonecrosis, fibrosis and chronic inflammation (**Case fig. 27.6k**).

Pathologic differential or, why isn't it one of the following?

The microscopic finding of fungal granules or grains is characteristic of mycetoma, so at the histology level, there is no diagnostic differential. This is another case where consideration of mesenchymal tumor only occurs clinically and at imaging. Ultrasound-guided, fine needle aspiration biopsy may enable a pre-operative diagnosis of mycetoma.

Speciation of the causative organism may be accomplished in some cases by microbiology cultures and biochemical testing (requires 2 weeks), serologic analysis of specific antibodies, or PCR amplification of a ribosomal gene complex (Lichon et al. 2006). It is important to distinguish *Actinomyces* and *Nocardia* causes of mycetoma from true fungal mycetoma, as medical therapy differs.

A rough idea of the species involved may be attempted by examining the size, color, and texture of the granules formed by the organisms. *Actinomyces* and *Nocardia* species do not produce

Case table 27.6 Summary pathology findings of Case 27.6

Diagnosis	Mycetoma caused by true fungal species
Size	Granulomatous, acute and chronic inflammation involving an 8 × 7 × 3 cm area
Location	Subcutaneous tissue of right elbow

black granules, but both true fungi (eumycetes) and the actinomycetes can produce white granules. Yellow granules are found only in actinomycetes (Ahmed et al. 2004). In this case, granules were not described by the prosector. The granules identified on microscopy are consistent with a filamentous fungus rather than *Actinomyces* or *Nocardia*.

Oncology approach

This is not a neoplasm, and therefore chemotherapy and radiation are not indicated.

Patient outcome

Three years following excision and treatment with anti-fungal agents, the patient has had no recurrence.

REFERENCES

Agarwal N, Kauer N, Panwar P, et al. Synovial sarcoma of the thigh mimicking chronic hematoma: a rare manifestation. J BUON 2010;15:192.

Ahmed AOA, van Leeuwen W, Fahal A, et al. Mycetoma caused by Madurella mycetomatis: a neglected infectious burdern. Lancet Infect Dis 2004;4:566–574.

Becker C, Assouad J, Riquet M, Hidden G. Postmastectomy lymphedema: long-term results following microsurgical lymph node transplantation. Ann Surg 2006;243(3):313–5.

Brook I. Microbiology and management of soft tissue and muscle infections. Int J Surgery 2008;6:328–338.

Brook I. The role of anaerobic bacteria in cutaneous and soft tissue abscesses and infected cysts. Anaerobe 2007;13:171–177.

Brown RR, Rosenberg ZS, Schweitzer ME, et al. MRI of medial malleolar bursa. Am J Roentgenol 2005;184(3):979–83.

Bullough P. Orthopaedic Pathology, 5th ed. Maryland Heights: Mosby, 2010.

Catalano-Pons C, Comte A, Wipff J, et al. Clinical outcome in children with chronic recurrent multifocal osteomyelitis. Rheumatology 2008;47: 1397–1399.

Cebesoy O, Tutar E, Arpacioglu O. Spontaneous giant expanding thigh hematoma mimicking soft tissue neoplasm. Joint Bone Spine 2008;75:64–66.

Cimolai N. Chronic recurrent multifocal osteomyelitis: is infectious causation a moot point? J Infection Public Health 2011;4(4):157–168.

Dion E, Forest M, Brasseur JL, et al. Epithelioid sarcoma mimicking abscess: a review of the MRI appearance. Skeletal Radiol 2001;30:173–7.

Farshid G, Weiss SW. Massive localized lymphedema in the morbidly obese: a histologically distinct reactive lesion simulating liposarcoma. Am J Surg Pathol 1998;22:1277–1283.

Ferguson PJ, Sanu M. Current understanding of the pathogenesis and management of chronic recurrent multifocal osteomyelitis. Curr Rheumatol Rep 2012;14:130–141.

Game F. Management of osteomyelitis of the foot in diabetes mellitus. Nat Rev Endocrinol 2009;6:43–47.

Gikas P, Islam L, Aston W, et al. Nonbacterial osteitis: a clinical, histopathological, and imaging study with a proposal for protocol-based management of patients with this diagnosis. J Orthop Sci 2009;14:505–516.

Hashkes PJ, Toker O. Autoinflammatory syndromes. Pediatr Clin North Am 2012;59:447–70.

Jansson AF, Grote V, ESPED Study Group. Nonbacterial osteitis in children: data of a German Incidence Surveillance Study. Acta Paediatrica 2011;100:1150–7.

Jennin F, Bousson V, Parlier C, et al. Bony sequestrum: a radiologic review. Skeletal Radiol 2011;40(8):963–75.

Kothari NA Pelchovitz DJ, Meyer JS. Imaging of musculoskeletal infections. Radiol Clin North Am 2001;39:653–71.

Klotchko A, Wallace MR, Licitra C, et al. Staphylococcus lugdunensis: an emerging pathogen. South Med J 2011;104:509–514.

Liarmakopoulos E, Lampropoulos P, Marinis A, et al. Soft tissue paraspinal inflammatory malignant fibrous histiocytoma presenting as a lumbar abscess. Case Rep Oncol 2011;4:343–349.

Lichon V, Khachemoune A. Mycetoma: a review. Am J Clin Dermatol 2006;7:315–321.

Manduch M, Oliveira AM, Nascimento AG, et al. Massive localized lymphedema: a clinicopathologic study of 22 cases and review of the literature. J Clin Pathol 2009;62:808–811.

McDermott MB, Lind AC, Marley EF, et al. Deep granuloma annulare (pseudorheumatoid nodule) in children: clinicopathologic study of 35 cases. Pediatr Dev Pathol 1998;1:300–308.

Mentzel T, Goodlad JR, Smith MA, et al. Ancient hematoma: a unifying concept for a post-traumatic lesion mimicking an aggressive soft tissue neoplasm. Mod Pathol 1997;10:334–10.

Nalmas S, Bishburg E, Shah M, et al. Skin and soft tissue abscess: 1 year's experience. J Cutan Med Surg 2009;13:257–261.

Negoro K, Uchida K, Yayama T, et al. Chronic expanding hematoma of the thigh. Joint Bone Spine 2012;79:192–194.

Niimi R, Matsumine A, Kusuzaki K, et al. Soft-tissue sarcoma mimicking large haematoma: a report of two cases and review of the literature. J Ortho Surgery 2006;14(1):90–5.

Pesce V, Notarnicola A, Moretti B. Diagnostic dilemma of a subcutaneous nodule following trauma in a child: immunohistochemical examination put the final diagnosis of deep granuloma annulare. Musculoskelet Surg 2010;94:49–51.

Reith JD, Bauer TW, Schils JP. Osseous manifestations of SAPHO (Synovitis, Acne, Pustulosis, Hyperostosis, Osteitis) Syndrome. Am J Surg Pathol 1996;20(11):1368–77.

Rossini CJ, Moriarty KP, Tashjian DB, et al. Geographic distribution of community-acquired methicillin-resistant Staphylococcus aureus soft tissue infections. J Pediatr Surg 2011;46:1089–1092.

Shon W, Ida CM, Boland-Froemming JM, et al. Cutaneous angiosarcoma arising in massive localized lymphedema of the morbidly obese: a report of five cases and review of the literature. J Cutan Pathol 2011;38:560–564.

Slenker AK, Keith SW, Horn DL. Two hundred and eleven cases of Candida osteomyelitis: 17 case reports and a review of the literature. Diag Micro Inf Dis 2012;73:89–93.

Stefanaki K, Tsivitanidou-Kakourou, Stefanaki C, et al. Histological and immunohistochemical study of granuloma annulare and subcutaneous granuloma annulare in children. J Cutan Pathol 2007;34:392–396.

Summanen PH, Talan DA, Strong C, et al. Bacteriology of skin and soft-tissue infections: comparison of infections in intravenous drug users and individuals with no history of intravenous drug use. Clin Infect Dis 1995;20 Suppl 2:S279–82

Tlougan BE, Podjasek JO, O'Haver J, et al. Chronic recurrent multifocal osteomyelitis (CRMO) and synovitis, acne, pustulosis, hyperostosis, and osteitis (SAPHO) syndrome with associated neutrophilic dermatoses: a report of seven cases and review of the literature. Pediatr Dermatol 2009;26:497–505.

Wang LF, Tai CF, Kuo WR, et al. Predisposing factors of complicated deep neck nfections: 12-year experience at a single institution. J Otolaryngol Head Neck Surg 2010;39:335–41.

Wang NS, Walters RF, Warren SJ. Massive localized lymphedema: a soft tissue process that may present to dermatologists. Am J Dermatopathol 2010;32:380–383.

Watkins RR, David MZ, Salata RA. Current concepts on the virulence mechanisms of methicillin-resistant Staphylococcus aureus. J Med Micro 2012;61:1179–1193.

Wipff J, Adamsbaum C, Kahan A, et al. Chronic recurrent multifocal osteomyelitis. Joint Bone Spine 2011;78:555–560.

Wu D, Gibbs J, Corral D, et al. Massive localized lymphedema: additional locations and association with hypothyroidism. Hum Pathol 2000;31:1162–1168.

Index

Note: Page numbers in *italics* refer to figures.